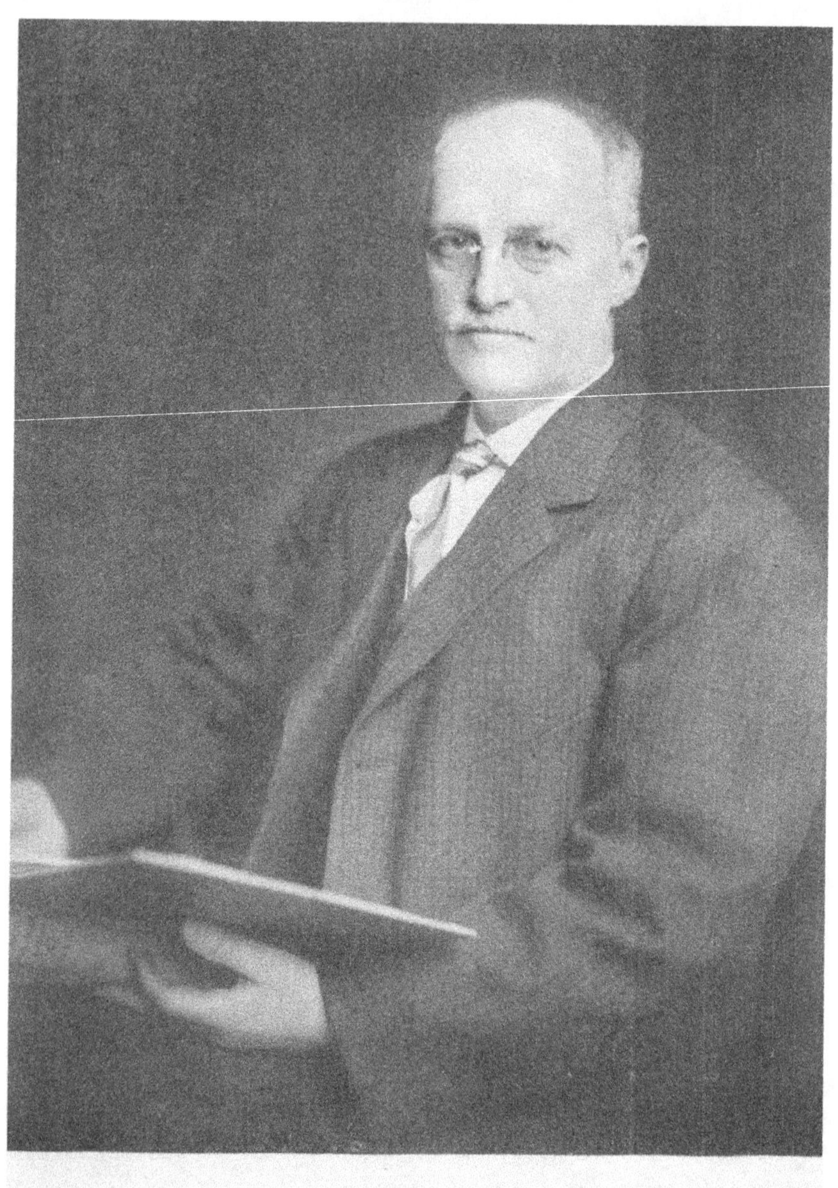

T. J. Ritter M.D.

May 12th 1910

MOTHERS' REMEDIES

Over One Thousand

Tried and Tested Remedies from Mothers of the United States and Canada.

Also

Symptoms, Causes, Prevention, Diet, Nursing, Treatments, Etc., of Every Known Disease.

Poisons, Accidents, Medicinal Herbs and Special Departments on Women, Children and Infants,

by

DR. T. J. RITTER

Formerly connected with Medical Faculty of University of Michigan at Ann Arbor, Mich.

REVISED

with

INTRODUCTION

by

DR. W. E. ZIEGENFUSS

ISBN: 978-1-84902-280-4

TABLE OF CONTENTS

LIST OF ILLUSTRATIONS

PREFACE.

Medicine is not an exact science, and it is reasonable to presume that even Time, with all its qualifying influences, will fail in its effects on this one branch of science. As the millions of faces seem each to present some differentiating feature, so each human system seems to require special study of its individual temperament.

So physicians find it necessary to have more than one remedy for a given ill; they still find truth in the old adage, "What is one man's meat is another's poison." But Mother finds a variety of remedies necessary for another reason. Her medicine-chest is usually lacking the full quota of drugs required to meet the many emergencies, and she must turn to the "remedy at hand."

Necessity has again proved its influence and with the years thousands of simple home concoctions have found their way to the relief of the daily demands on Mother's ingenuity. These mothers' remedies have become a valuable asset to the raising of a family, and have become a recognized essential in a Mother's general equipment for home-making.

For fifteen years the Publisher has handled so-called home medical works; during that time he has had occasion to examine practically all the home medical works published. He has been impressed with the utter uselessness of many, perhaps most, of these books because the simple home remedies were lacking.

A few years ago he conceived the idea of gathering together the "Mothers' Remedies" of the world. This one feature of this book he claims as distinctly his own. Letters were sent by him to Mothers in every state and territory of the United States, and to Canada and other countries, asking for tried and tested "Mothers' Remedies." The appeal was met with prompt replies, and between one thousand and two thousand valuable remedies were collected in this way.

Through courtesy to these Mothers who helped to make this book possible, the book was named "MOTHERS' REMEDIES."

Dr. T. J. Ritter, of Ann Arbor, Michigan, a graduate of the regular School of Medicine at the University of Michigan, at Ann Arbor, and later one of the medical staff of the University, consented to furnish the necessary material to complete the Medical Department. Dr. Ritter, in over thirty years of actual practice, has met with all the exigencies of both city and country practice which have brought to him the ripe experience of what would be called a "physician's life-time." His success has been, in part, due to his honesty, kindliness and conscientiousness, as well as to his thorough training and natural adaptability to the profession.

Besides writing the Causes, Symptoms, Preventives, Nursing, Diet, Physicians' Treatment, etc., he has examined each and every one of the

Mothers' Remedies and added, when possible, the *reason why that remedy is valuable.* In short, he supplied in his remarks following each Mother's Remedy the Medical virtue or active principle of the ingredients. This lifts each Mother's Remedy into the realm of science,--in fact, to the level of a Doctor's Prescription.

In writing his part, Dr. Ritter consulted, personally or through their works, considerably over one hundred of the acknowledged Medical Specialists of the world. Thus he has brought to you the latest discoveries of modern science,--the Medical knowledge of the world's great specialists.

Dr. Ritter, therefore, wishes to acknowledge his indebtedness to the following: On the subject of Theory and Practice, to Dr. Wm. Osler, Oxford University, England; Dr. James M. Andres, Ph. D., Medico-Chirurgical College, Philadelphia, Pa.; Dr. Hughes Dayton, Vanderbilt Clinic-College of Physicians and Surgeons; Dr. Hobart A. Hare, Jefferson Medical College, Philadelphia, Pa.; Dr. Temple S. Hoyne, Hahnemann Medical College, Chicago, Ill.; Dr. A. E. Small, Hahnemann Medical College, Chicago, Ill.; Dr. C. G. Raue, Hahnemann Medical College, Philadelphia, Pa.; Dr. John King, Eclectic Medical Institute, Cincinnati, Ohio. On the subject of Materia Medica to Dr. John Shoemaker, Medico-Chirurgical College, Philadelphia, Pa.; Dr. Hobart A. Hare; Drs. Hemple and Arndt, Homeopathic, and others. On the subject of Obstetrics, to Dr. W. P. Manton, Detroit Medical College, and others. On the subject of Surgery, to the American Text Book on Surgery, edited by Drs. Keen and White, of Philadelphia, and many contributors. On the subject of Nervous Diseases, to Dr. Joseph D. Nagel and others. On the subject of the Eye, to Dr. Arthur N. Alling, of Yale University. On the subject of the Ear, to Dr. Albert H. Buck, College of Physicians and Surgeons, New York City; Dr. O. A. Griffin, University of Michigan and others. On the Nose and Throat, to Dr. James B. Ball, London, England. On the Skin, to Dr. James N. Hyde, Rush Medical College, Chicago, Ill.; Dr. Alfred Schalek, Rush Medical College, Chicago, Ill. On the Rectum and Anus, to Dr. Samuel G. Gant, Ph. D., Post-graduate College, New York City. On the Diseases of Children, to Dr. L. Emmett Holt, College of Physicians and Surgeons, New York City; Dr. Koplik, New York City; Dr. Charles Douglas, Detroit College of Medicine; Dr. Henry E. Tuley, University of Kentucky; Dr. Tooker, Chicago. On the subject of Nursing, to Isabel Hampton Robb, and on Dietetics, to Dr. Julius Friedenwald, College Physicians and Surgeons, Baltimore, Md. On the Baby to Drs. Holt, Douglas, Tooker, Koplik and Coolidge. On Insanity, to Dr. Selden Talcott, formerly superintendent of the Middleton State Hospital for the Insane, New York State. Besides the above a great many other physicians and their works might be mentioned, and to all appreciation is gratefully acknowledged.

Mrs. Elizabeth Johnstone, who writes the department on "Manners and Social Customs," is the only daughter of the late Francis Gardiner, one of the early settlers of Washtenaw County, Michigan. She was educated at the State Normal School, now the Normal College at Ypsilanti, and taught for several years after graduation. In 1880 she married the late Robert Ferguson Johnstone, editor of the Michigan Farmer, and after his death became editor of the Household Department of that paper. In 1895, the Farmer having passed into other ownership, she became a member of the Editorial Staff of the Detroit Free Press, where,--continuing to write under the pseudonym of "Beatrix" she has become widely known through the vast circulation of that paper.

Years of experience have enabled her to write on topics of interest to women with comprehension of their needs, and to answer social inquiries with exactness.

Miss Edna Gertrude Thompson, who supplies the chapter on Domestic Science, is a graduate of the Northern State Normal of Michigan. She was for a time a teacher in the Public Schools of Michigan and New York State. Miss Thompson later graduated from and is now the director of the Domestic Science Department of the Thomas Normal Training School of Detroit, Michigan.

Miss Thompson has won an enviable reputation in Domestic Science work. She has avoided all of the quackery, self-exploitation and money schemes, which have proved a temptation to many in the work, and which have tended to brand the science as an advertising scheme, and confined herself to study, teaching and the legitimate development of the science. Her work in the Normal and in giving lectures on Domestic Science brings her in touch with large numbers of intelligent and practical women who realize that housekeeping and cookery must be reduced to a science. Luxuries of fifty years ago are necessities today. The increase in the cost of living without a corresponding advance in wages has made it imperative that method and system he installed in the home.

Domestic Science is still in the embryo, but let us hope it will, in a measure at least, prove a panacea for modern domestic ills and receive the encouragement and speedy endorsement that it deserves.

PHYSICIAN'S INTRODUCTION

"Of the things which man can do or make here below, by far the most momentous, wonderful, and worthy, are the things we call Books."

--CARLYLE.

"A good book may be among the best of friends. It is the most patient and cheerful of companions. It does not turn its back upon us in times of adversity or distress. It always receives us with the same kindness."

--S. SMILES.

Of making books there seems no end. Some are good, some bad, and many just an encumbrance upon the book-shelves, neither of much use nor particularly harmful. Some books are to be read for cheer and amusement; some for reproof and correction; others to be studied for useful information and profit.

The Ideal Book.--There is a wide felt need for a worthy book of sound hygienic and medical facts for the non-medical people. The **Ideal Book** for this mission should be compact in form, but large enough to give the salient facts, and give these in understandable language; it must not be "loaded" with obsolete and useless junk of odds and ends which have long ceased to be even interesting; it must carry with it the stamp of genuine reliability; it should treat all the ordinary and most common forms of ailments and accidents; it must be safe in its teachings; it needs to be free from objectionable language and illustrations, so that all of any family may study and use it with profit; it must frequently warn of dangers ahead and urge the summoning of professional skill promptly, for there are many cases requiring the services of experienced physicians and surgeons in their treatment; it should advise remedies readily obtainable, as well as those for which long journeys to a drug store are required; and finally the book should be reasonable in price that those who most need it can afford to own it.

Need of Brevity.--The facts of hygiene and therapeutic measures are widely scattered through medical literature, and extend over hundreds of years of time. Many volumes have been written on diseases of the eye, the heart, liver, and stomach, brain and other organs, to understand which requires special technical education. It would be the height of folly to present these discussions to the laity in their original form, hence the necessity for condensation and presentation of the needful facts in the language of the people in whose interests the book is printed. In a book of fiction there may be need for useless verbiage for the sake of "making pages," but facts of vital importance and usefulness in our daily welfare need to be well boiled down and put into shape for ready reference. This has been done in "Mothers' Remedies" and I think it quite fulfills the ideal I have outlined above.

The title is rather odd upon first seeing it, but the most plausible when you become acquainted with its import. It surely becomes the best friend of the whole family. "It does not turn its back upon us in times of adversity," but cheerfully answers a thousand and one questions of vital importance to the household. In the hour of distress, when illness or accident befalls the dear ones, you may turn again and again to its pages without meeting disappointment.

Its Value.--There are many books on household medicines, but in my opinion this is the most useful of them all, a very present help in time of need. You can go to it for helpful information without failing to find it. Is there serious illness in the house? It will tell you about it concisely and plainly, describing its symptoms, nature and course, and advise you to consult the family physician if of a serious nature before it is too late. In the chapters on accidents, emergencies and poisons, it tells you what to do at once while awaiting the doctor's arrival. He will be much pleased to see that you have made the proper effort to treat the case. Prompt treatment makes for prompt recovery.

The real value of any book, or what is sometimes called its intrinsic value, or utility, consists in what it avails to gratify some desire or want of our nature. It depends, then, wholly upon its qualities in relation to our desires. That which contributes in ever so small degree to the wellbeing of humanity is of greater value than silver or gold. This book contains hundreds of prescriptions, anyone of which will repay the small cost in money that it requires to possess it. In fact, the financial investment is so small when compared with the benefit derived from its pages that this feature need not be considered.

Examples.--In the stillness and loneliness of the night, away from medical help, there comes the hoarse barking cough of the child, perhaps, and a case of croup is upon the responsibility of the parents. The struggles and terror of the little patient throws the household into consternation, and all is excitement in a moment. If the mother ever knew what to do in such a case she is likely not able to recall the exact remedy at this time, the doctor is miles away, and **the case is urgent.**

A reference to the medical index of "Mothers' Remedies" under croup shows that on pages 27, 28 and 29, is a full description of the attack, and there are fifteen (15) home remedies given, many of which can be found in the house, and the spasm may be stopped by the use of one of them.

This is only one example of the use of this book. There are innumerable times when cases come up in the home, or accidents befall a dear one and a ready remedy is required; the book most likely contains it, and is willing to tell you if you consult it carefully.

Tuberculosis.--The article on tuberculosis is full of valuable rules on diet and hygiene for every person, whether he has the disease or not. A knowledge of the dangers and mode of spreading the disease is the best safeguard against having it. Where one person in every seven (7) dies of consumption it becomes imperative that full knowledge of the disease and its prevention should become widespread.

Accidents and Poisons.--Another department that illustrates the value of the book is that on Accidents and Poisons, where quick action is needed to prevent great suffering and danger and the salvation of life itself. One cannot always get the doctor in time. A quick reference to this part of the book will give the proper course of action to follow. The indicated mother's remedy or the physician's treatment as given here applied in the "nick of time" will save many a life in cases of burns, or accidental poisoning, or hemorrhage. I have been called in such cases where a simple drink of warm mustard water promptly used would have saved a life in carbolic acid poisoning. It is in the emergencies where a ready knowledge of the ways and means necessary to conserve life is most valuable; and it is in just such emergencies that one is most apt to forget what is best to do that a copy of Mothers' Remedies becomes a priceless boon of helpfulness.

All About Baby.--The Woman's Department, and the chapter on "All About Baby," alone contain priceless information for the guidance of the women of the home. It is like having a good doctor right in the house who is ready and able to answer more than 500 questions of vital interest about Baby. The book is thoroughly reliable, free from exaggerated statements and written in the plainest language possible so as to make it useful to every member of the home. The Herb Department gives a brief description of the more common and most useful plants and roots, with the time for gathering them, and the dose and therapeutic indication for their use. The botanical illustrations are correct and worthy of careful study.

THE INDEX.--Mothers' Remedies is unique in arrangement, and full of detail, but so well indexed that any portion of it, or any disease and remedy, can be readily found, and when found you will have a choice of home remedies ready at hand. This is one of the features of the book that distinguishes Mothers' Remedies from the usual home medical books heretofore sold.

This feature of the book cannot be too strongly impressed. Its value becomes apparent as soon as one consults its pages. Long chapters of descriptive reading filled with high sounding, technical terms may look very learned because the average reader does not understand it fully. But it is what one can obtain from a book that is usable that makes it valuable. In **Mothers' Remedies** this idea has been excellently carried out.

The Home Remedies.--If there was any question regarding the success of the book in this homelike arrangement, the utilization of the home remedies, in addition to the strictly medical and drug-store ingredients; it was promptly dispelled when the book was printed and presented to the people interested. It has proved to be the most wonderful seller on the market--the most usable and useful book ever offered the non-medical reader; because never before has a medical book contained the hundreds of simple home remedies from mothers. Because a physician tells you why the remedies are useful--the reason why the things used are efficacious.

Medical Terms.--Frequently one comes across technical terms in the secular papers which, unless understood, obscure the sense of the reading. There is a dictionary of medical terms as a separate department which adds much to the usefulness of the work; the spelling, -pronunciation and definition being concisely given in English.

Other Departments.--There are other departments, such as chapters on Manners and Social Customs, by an expert. Nursery Hints, Candy Making, Domestic Science, and Miscellaneous departments which interest every member of any average family in health as well as in sickness. The Candy Department provides many an evening's enjoyment for the young people.

In addition, the book gives under each disease the physician's remedies, the symptoms, causes, preventives wherever important, the diet, nursing, necessity for operations, and much other needful information for the sick-room. A complete chapter on Nursing and a detailed account of the Baby and its care is perhaps the most useful portion of the book to the mothers who desire to learn all about the baby. Many home medical books are of doubtful value by reason of exaggerated statements or vague and unusable directions regarding treatments. **Mothers' Remedies** stands squarely upon the foundation of utility and practical every-day usefulness. No matter how many other home medical books one may have, this is also needful because there's none other on the market like it. One of the missions of **Mothers' Remedies** in the home is the prevention of disease through its sound sanitary teachings. It was written exclusively for home use, and its instructions can be followed by anyone who can understand plain English, and the home remedies are extensively explained and recommended so that in emergencies one can always find something of value to use while awaiting the surgeon's arrival. It is a well-spring of usefulness in any home, and it gives me genuine pleasure to call attention to it in these few lines, and to bespeak for it the continued enthusiastic reception with which it has met heretofore.

(Signed) WM. ELLWOOD ZIEGENFUSS, M.D.

Detroit, July 2, 1914.

The National Narcotic law makes it practically impossible for the laity to have prescriptions filled which contain opiates or cocaine.

We therefore have substituted other remedies quite as good whenever this was possible and still retain the efficiency of the prescription.

DR. W. E. ZIEGENFUSS.

August, 1918.

MEDICAL DEPARTMENT

MOTHERS' DIAGNOSIS STRIKING, CHARACTERISTIC SYMPTOMS

of Many Diseases for Quick Reference and Comparison

WHEN IN DOUBT BEFORE CALLING THE DOCTOR.

APPENDICITIS.--Loss of appetite. There may be nausea and vomiting; there is usually a sudden onset of pain, often sharp and severe in the whole or part of the abdomen. Later the pain settles in the right groin. Patient lies on his back with his right knee drawn up. The muscles become rigid on the right side and later a lump appears in the right groin (iliac fossa).

ANEMIA.--This disease is a diminution of the total quantity of the blood of its red cells, or red corpuscles or of their Haemoglobin, the coloring matter of the red corpuscles. Some difficulty of breathing. Palpitation on least exertion, tendency to faint, headache, tired, irritable, poor or changeable appetite, digestive disturbances, constipation, cold hands and feet, difficult and painful menstruation (dysmenorrhea), irregular menstruation, leucorrhea. And when the skin is pale, yellowish green tinge, with perhaps flushed cheeks, it might properly be called chlorosis or "green sickness."

ADDISON'S DISEASE.--Great weakness, stomach and bowel disorders, weak heart and dark coloring (pigmentation) of the skin.

BRIGHT'S DISEASE.--Albumin and casts in the urine. The onset is usually gradual. There is paleness and puffiness of the eyelids, ankles or hands in the morning. Later increased dropsy of face and the extremities, pasty yellow complexion, dyspepsia, constipation and heart symptoms.

BRONCHITIS, ACUTE. (Cold on the Chest.)--There is a feeling of tightness under the breastbone, with a dry hard cough and headache. This cough may make the chest feel raw and sore, especially in front.

CHOLERA MORBUS.--The onset is usually sudden with nausea, vomiting, and cramp-like bowel pains; vomits at first the stomach contents. Purging follows; vomiting and purging with severe cramps in abdomen and legs.

CROUP.--Child wakes up suddenly, perhaps at midnight, with a harsh barking cough, with difficulty of breathing, and it looks as if it could not get another breath. Then there is an easy spell and soon the spasm recurs.

CANCER OF THE STOMACH.--There is anemia and a gradual loss of weight. A peculiar color of the skin (cachexia), irregular vomiting, some bleeding of "coffee-ground" color. Progressive loss of weight. Dragging or burning in the region of the stomach.

CHICKEN POX.--Slight fever, chilly feelings. In twenty-four hours the eruption appears upon the body, face and forehead often only a few separate red pimples which soon become rounded vesicles; however, there may be few or many.

DIABETES.--The onset is gradual, glucose (sugar) is persistently in the urine. Great quantity of urine passed; six to forty pints in twenty-four hours. Thirst is great. Large quantities of water is taken. Loss of strength and weight, mouth is dry, tongue is red and glazed, skin is dry and wrinkled.

DIPHTHERIA.--This disease begins gradually, as a rule, with chilly feelings, pain in the back and limbs, pulse is faster, with a general redness of the throat before the formation of the membrane; with such symptoms there are great weakness, paleness, and a bad smelling breath. Soon a spot or spots may be seen on the tonsils, uvula or soft palate, but in a day or two a dirty white patch is seen on the tonsils and this may spread, and with it there is increased weakness, pallor, loss of appetite and fever. When the membrane is taken off of the tonsils there is left a raw surface, and the membrane rapidly reforms.

DYSENTERY.--The onset may be marked by diarrhea, followed by a severe, cramp-like bowel pain, with frequent small stools containing blood and mucus and accompanied by much straining (tenesmus).

DYSPEPSIA, ACUTE. (Acute Gastritis, Acute Indigestion).---Distress in the stomach, headache, thirst, nausea, vomiting, tongue heavily coated, foul breath, distaste for food, tender stomach.

ERYSIPELAS.--The onset is sudden, high fever, and a local redness with a sharply defined margin between it and a healthy skin. It frequently appears upon the nose and spreads over one cheek or both. It may show only a smooth raised skin, or there may be vesicles.

EARACHE.--This is very common in children. It comes frequently as an extension through the eustachian canal of a cold. The ache is only an evidence of congestion or inflammation in the ear. The child bursts out crying violently and nothing seems to make it stop. It may cry for some time then stop. When it is very young it is restless, and wants to move constantly, and refuses to be comforted by the soothing embraces of its mother. It is quiet only a few moments at a time and again renews its cries and restlessness. The cries are moaning and seem like hopeless cries. A child or infant that cries that way and will not be quieted, should be suspected of having earache, and hot applications of dry or wet heat should be applied to the ear. If such symptoms are neglected, in a few days you are likely to have a discharge running from the external canal (meatus) and perhaps permanent injury may be done to the drum membrane by ulceration. Warm water poured in the ear frequently relieves common earache.

GALL STONES.--Sudden agonizing pain in the right upper abdomen in the region of the liver, with vomiting, prostration, tenderness in that region. Pain generally comes at intervals in paroxysms. There may be pains in the stomach during the weeks when the attack is absent and the patient may think the stomach is the seat of the trouble.

IRITIS.--Pain is severe and worse at night, the iris looks cloudy, muddy, the pupil is small. There is congestion around the iris (ciliary congestion).

KIDNEY STONES.--Pain goes from the kidneys down through the ureter into the bladder and into the scrotum. There may be sand in the urine that makes it look like blood.

LA GRIPPE--The onset is usually sudden, with a chill, and all of the symptoms of an active fever, headache, bone-ache, a general ache all over. A feeling of extreme weakness; feels miserable and sick.

LOCK-JAW (Tetanus).--History of a wound. The muscles of the jaw may be stiff and set. When there are spasms the muscles remain stiff and hard for some time.

MALARIAL FEVER.--Chill, fever, and sweat, or one stage may be absent. There may be only a slight chilly feeling with fever almost all day and then remission.

MUMPS.--The swelling is in front and below and behind the ear. Hard to eat and the swallowing of vinegar is almost impossible.

MEASLES.--Comes on gradually. There is a feeling of tiredness and languor, headache followed shortly by sneezing, cold symptoms, running at the eyes, dry throat, cough, much like an ordinary cold in the head, but with a persistent, hard racking cough. The eruption appears first in the sides of the mouth, in the inner surface of the cheeks, lips, gums and soft palate, in size from that of a pin-head to that of a split pea. It appears then about the eyes and then on the face, chest and extremities. It is first in red spots and then gets blotchy. This is usually three to six days after the appearance of the cold (catarrh) symptoms.

MEASLES (German).--Chilliness, slight fever, pain in the back and legs, coryza. The eruption appears on the first or second day, on the face, then on the chest and in twenty-four hours over the whole body. The glands under the jaw enlarge.

OPHTHALMIA NEONATORUM. (Inflammation of Eyes at Birth).--A severe conjunctivitis in the newly-born baby, swelling and redness usually of both eyes, occurring on the second or third day after birth; very soon there is a discharge and shortly it becomes creamy pus which runs from the eyes when the lids are parted.

PLEURISY.--The onset may be sudden or gradual. Sudden with a chill, fever, a severe sharp pain, stitch in the side, made worse by respiration, coughing or moving. The cough is dry. The pain is near the breast and sometimes it extends to the back.

PNEUMONIA.--It begins with a chill, fever, pain in the lungs, expectoration with cough, and the material spit up may be mixed with blood (rusty sputa). Then also rapid rise of temperature, "grunting" breathing, the nostrils dilate, and the cheeks are flushed.

RHEUMATIC FEVER OR INFLAMMATORY RHEUMATISM.--A number of joints become involved. It spreads from one joint to another, very painful joints; profuse sweating.

SMALLPOX.--The onset is sudden and ushered in by a chill, nausea and vomiting, headache, and severe pains in the back and legs, without grip symptoms. There is a rapid rise of temperature. Usually on the fourth day after the onset small red pimples appear on the forehead, along the line of the hair and on the wrists. The temperature falls with the appearance of the eruption.

SPOTTED FEVER.--Marked loss of appetite, chill, projectile vomiting, severe headache, pain and stiffness of the back and neck. Later head is drawn back, often the back is rigid. The muscles of the neck and back are very tender.

SCARLET FEVER. (Scarlatina).--Comes on suddenly with loss of appetite, headache, sick stomach, perhaps vomiting, high fever, sore throat, vomiting may persist. The tongue is coated, edges are red; later it is red and rough; the so-called strawberry tongue. Usually within twenty-four hours an eruption appears, first upon the neck and chest which spreads rapidly over the face and the rest of the body. The eruption consists of red pimply elevations about the size of a pin-head, very close together, so that the body seems to be covered with a scarlet flush. If you look closely you can see these little pimply elevations.

TUBERCULOSIS OF THE LUNGS.--Irregular temperatures, respiration is more frequent than normal, pulse is rapid, cough, expectoration, night sweats, perhaps, and general failure of strength.

TONSILITIS. (Smooth and Follicular).--Commences with a

chill, rapid rise of temperature, general aching in the back, and legs especially. The tonsils are large and red and spots may appear on them in a few hours. There may be no spots but a smooth; red, swollen tonsil, sometimes swollen to an enormous size. The spot and membrane, if any exists, are easily rubbed off and when this is done a glistening surface is seen, but not raw, as in diphtheria.

TYPHOID FEVER--There is a feeling of illness for a week or two and the patient is not able to work much, does not sleep well, dreams, has a dull headache, back of the neck may be stiff, nosebleed sometimes, with a feeling as if there was some fever, increasing feeling of weakness, and sick feeling. Finally the fever, etc., becomes more prominent with constipation and diarrhea.

ULCER OF THE CORNEA.--Light hurts the eyes very much, tears run freely and there is a feeling of something in the eye. The eyeball shows a rim of pink congestion about the cornea. The ulcer can be seen.

ULCER OF THE STOMACH.--Pain, local tenderness, bleeding. Distress after eating and vomiting of a very acid fluid. Pain in the region of the stomach and usually sharp pain in the back is the most constant symptom. It is increased by food at once and relieved by vomiting. The tenderness upon pressure is usually marked and is localized.

WHOOPING-COUGH.--Begins with symptoms of a cold in the eyes, nose, and the chest. The cough gradually becomes worse, usually in from seven to ten days; it comes in paroxysms (spells) and then the whoop.

RESPIRATORY DISEASES
Including CROUP, COLDS, SORE-THROAT, HOARSENESS, BRONCHITIS, ASTHMA, HAY-FEVER, PLEURISY, ADENOIDS, PNEUMONIA, ETC.
With Definition, Cause, Symptoms, Preventives, Mothers' Remedies, Physicians' Treatment; also Diet, Nursing and Sanitary Care; all for Home Use and Reference.

THE ANATOMY OF THE NOSE.--The nose is divided by a middle partition (septum) into two cavities (nasal chambers or fossae) each being a wedge-shaped cavity, distinct by itself and extending from the nostril or anterior nares in front to the posterior openings behind and from the base of the skull to the hard palate below. Where the posterior opening or nares ends is called the nose-pharynx, The pharynx joins there with the cavities and hence called nose-pharynx. The partition (septum) is thin, one-tenth to one-eighth of an inch in thickness and is composed in front of cartilage (gristle) and behind of bone. In its normal state this partition (septum) should be perfectly straight, thin and in the middle line, The cartilaginous (gristle) portion is seldom found in this condition as, owing to its prominent location and frequent exposure to injury, blows and falling on the nose, the partition (septum) is often bent or turned to one side or the other so far in some cases as to close the nostril. The posterior part is composed of bone, and being well protected, is seldom found out of position or displaced, even when the cartilaginous portion is often badly deformed, The floor of the nose is formed by the upper jaw bone (maxillary) and the palate bone. The outer wall of the nose or nose cavity is the most complicated, for it presents three prominences, the turbinated bones, which extend from before backwards and partially divide the nose cavity into incomplete spaces called meatus passages. The turbinated bones are three in number, the inferior, middle and superior. They vary in size and shape, and owing to the relations they hear to the surrounding parts, and to the influence they exert on the general condition of the nose and throat, are of great importance. The inferior or lower turbinate bone is the largest and in a way is the only independent bone. The middle and superior are small. They are all concave in shape and extend from before backwards, and beneath the concave surface of each one of the corresponding passages or openings (meatus) is formed. The inferior or lower (meatus) opening or passage is that part of the nasal (nose) passage which lies beneath the inferior turbinate bone and extends from the nostrils in front to the passage behind the nose (postnasal) (posterior nares) toward the pharynx. The middle opening (meatus) lies above the inferior turbinate bone and below the middle turbinate bone. The superior opening (meatus) is situated above the middle turbinate bone.

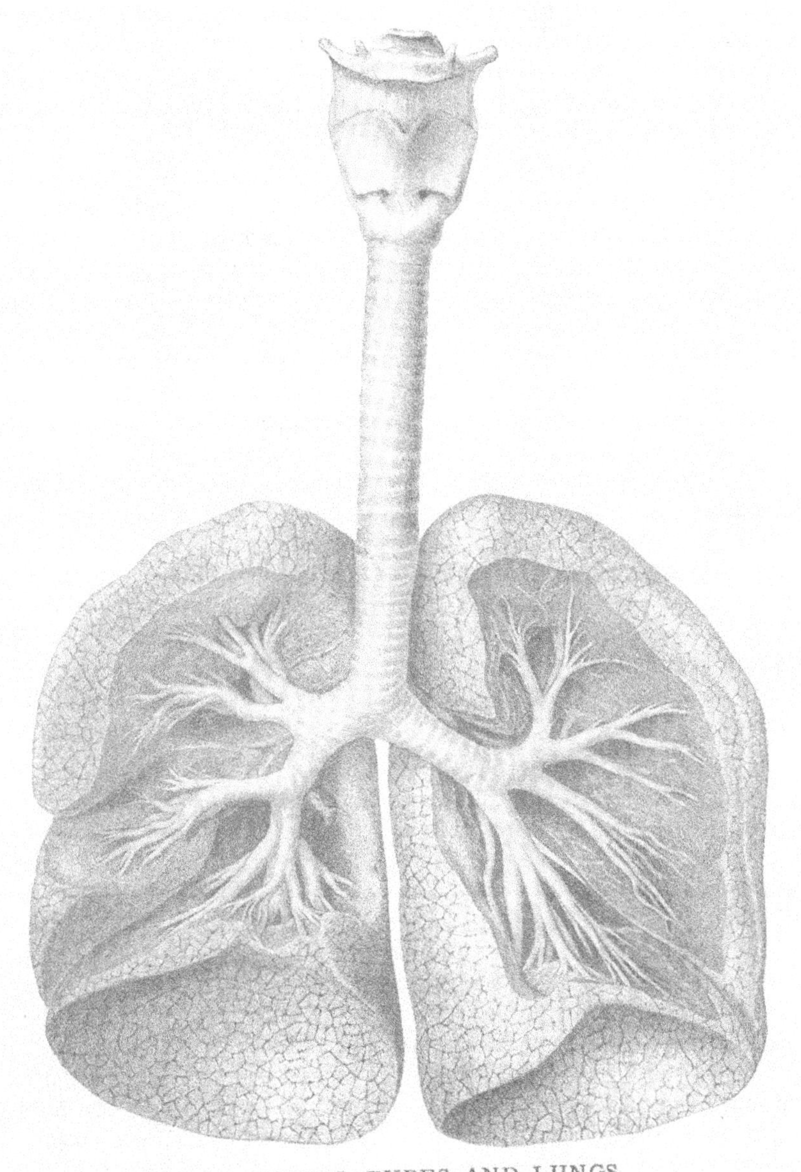

BRONCHIAL TUBES AND LUNGS.

Bronchial Tubes and Lungs

The mucous membrane lining the nasal passages is similar to other mucous membranes. It is here called the Schneiderian membrane after the name of a German anatomist named Schneider. It is continuous through the ducts with the mucous membrane of all the various accessory cavities of the nose. It is quite thin, in the upper part over the superior turbinate bone and partition (septum) while it is quite thick over the lower turbinate bone, the floor of the nose cavity and the lower part of the partition. It is well supplied with blood vessels, veins, and glands for producing the necessary secretion.

The nose is an organ of breathing (respiration) and it warms and moistens the air we breathe and arrests particles of dust in the air before they enter the lungs. If the air we breathe is of an uneven temperature, or of marked degree of dryness, or if it is saturated with impurities, it always acts as a source of irritation to the mucous membrane of the upper respiratory tract, like the larynx. By the time the air reaches the pharynx, through the nose, it has become almost as warm as the blood, and also is well saturated with moisture. The mucous membrane that lines the nose cavity and especially that part over the lower turbinate bone, secretes from sixteen to twenty ounces of fluid daily. This fluid cleanses and lubricates the nose and moistens the air we breathe. Conditions may arise which interfere with this natural secretion. This may be due to the fact that some of the glands have shrunk or wasted (atrophied) and the secretion has become thick. This collects in the nose, decomposes and forms scabs and crusts in the nostrils. In this condition there will be dropping of mucus into the throat. This condition is usually only a collection of secretions from the nose,--which are too thick to flow away,--collect in the space behind the nose, and when some have accumulated, drop into the pharynx.

In order to be in good health it is necessary to breathe through the nose, and to do this there must be nothing in the nose or upper part of the pharynx to interfere with the free circulation of the air through these cavities. The cavities of the nose may be partly closed by polpi (tumors) on the upper and middle turbinate bone, a spur on the (septum) partition, deviation of the partition or enlarged turbinate bones, or adenoids in the upper part of the pharynx. These troubles almost close up the nose sometimes and the person is compelled to breathe through his mouth. He not only looks foolish, talks thick, but is laying up for himself future trouble. By correcting the trouble in the nose and removing the adenoids in the upper part of the pharynx the patient can breathe through the nasal passages. If you take a tube you can pass it straight back through the lower channel (meatus) into the pharynx. It will touch the upper back wall of the pharynx. If the tube has a downward bend you can see it behind the soft palate and by attaching a string to that end you can draw it back out through the nostrils. In that way we plug the posterior openings (nares). The upper part of the pharynx reaches higher up behind than a line drawn horizontally above the tip of the nose to the pharynx. It reaches forward above the soft palate on its front surface. Its front surface is almost directly on a vertical line with tonsil, above the soft palate. On its upper part and on the side near the nose cavity is the opening of the eustachian tube.

The name naso-pharynx means the junction of the nose and pharynx. Sometimes the upper posterior wall of the pharynx, called the vault of the pharynx, especially the part behind each eustachian tube, is filled almost full with adenoids. These are overgrowths or thickenings of the glandular tissue in the upper posterior wall of the pharynx (vault of the pharynx).

ADENOIDS. (Pharyngeal Tonsil, Lursehkas Tonsil, Adenoid Vegetation, Post-nasal Growth.)--Adenoids are overgrowths or thickenings of the glandular tissue in the vault (top) of the pharynx. They are on the upper posterior wall of the pharynx, often filling the whole space, especially the part behind the ear-tube--eustachian tube.

They are a soft pliable mass, well supplied with blood vessels, especially in children. Some are firmer and these are the kind seen in adults. The color varies from pale pink to dark red. The structure is similar to enlarged tonsils.

Symptoms.--Children breathe chiefly or wholly through the mouth. They are apt to breathe noisily, especially when they eat and drink. They sleep with their mouth open, breathe hard and snore. They have attacks of slight suffocation sometimes, especially seen in young children. There may be difficulty in nursing in infants; they sleep poorly, toss about in bed, moan, talk, and night terrors are common.

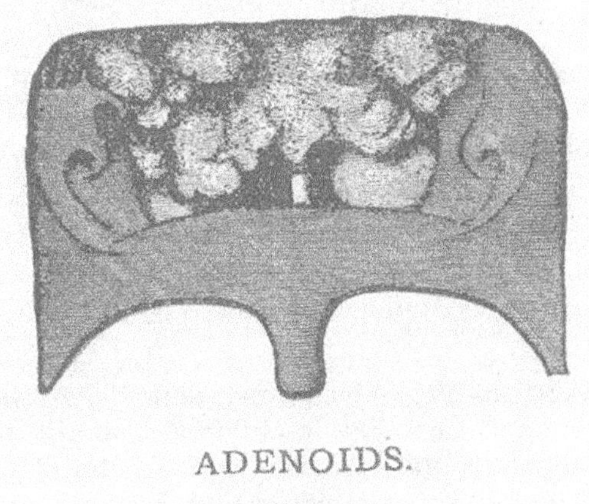

Adenoids

They may also sweat very much during sleep. A constant hacking or barking cough is a common symptom and this cough is often troublesome for some hours before going to bed. Troubles with the larynx and pharynx are common and spasmodic laryngitis appears to be often dependent upon adenoids. Bronchial asthma and sneezing in paroxysms are sometimes connected with them. The chest becomes deformed. The prolonged mouth-breathing imparts to adenoid patients a characteristic look in the face. The lower jaw is dropped and the lips are kept constantly apart. In many cases the upper lip is short, showing some part of the upper teeth. The dropping of the jaw draws upon the soft parts and tends to obliterate the natural folds of the face about the nose, lips, and cheeks. The face has an elongated appearance and the expression is vacant, listless, or even stupid. The nose is narrow and pinched, from long continued inaction of the wings of the nose (alae nasi). The root of the nose may be flat and broad. When the disease sets in during early childhood, the palate may become high arched. If the disease continues beyond second teething, the arch of the palate becomes higher and the top of the arch more pointed. The upper jaw elongates and this often causes the front teeth to project far beyond the corresponding teeth in the lower jaw. The high arched palate is often observed to be associated with a deflected partition (septum) in the nose.

The speech is affected in a characteristic way; it acquires a dead character. There is inability to pronounce the nasal consonant sounds; *m, n,* and *ng* and the *l, r,* and *th* sounds are changed. Some backwardness in learning to articulate is often noticed.

Deafness is frequently present, varying in degree, transient and persistent. Attacks of earache are common and also running of the ears. The ear troubles often arise from the extension of catarrh from the nose-pharynx through the eustachian tubes to the middle ear. Sometimes the adenoids block the entrance to the tubes. The ventilation of the middle ear may be impeded. Dr. Ball, of London, England, says: "Ear troubles in children are undoubtedly, in the vast majority of cases, dependent upon the presence of adenoid vegetation" (growths).

Children with adenoids are very liable to colds in the head, which aggravate all the symptoms, and in the slighter forms of the disease the symptoms may hardly be noticeable, except when the child is suffering from a cold.

Chronic catarrh is often caused by adenoids. A chronic pus discharge often develops, especially in children. There is often a half-pus discharge trickling over the posterior wall of the pharynx from the nose-pharynx. And yet some children with adenoids never have any discharge from the nose. There may be more or less dribbling of saliva from the mouth, especially in young children, and this is usually worse during sleep. Headache is not uncommon when these growths persist into adult life: they continue to give rise to most of the symptoms just described, although these symptoms may be less marked because of the relatively larger size of the nose-pharynx. The older patients seek relief, usually, from nasal catarrh symptoms. They complain of a dry throat on waking and they hawk and cough, In order to clear the sticky secretion from the throat. The adenoids have often undergone a considerable amount of shrinking, but they frequently give rise to a troublesome inflammation of the nose and pharynx. Rounded or irregular red elevations will often be seen on the posterior wall of the pharynx, outgrowths of adenoid tissue in this region. Similar elevations are sometimes seen on the posterior pillars of the fauces. The tonsils are often enlarged. A good deal of thick discharge will sometimes be seen in the posterior wall of the pharynx proceeding from the nose-pharynx.

Although adenoids, like the normal tonsil, usually tend to diminish and disappear with the approach of youth, they constitute during childhood a constant source of danger and trouble and not infrequently inflict permanent mischief. Also children afflicted with adenoids are less able to cope with diphtheria, scarlet fever, measles, whooping-cough, etc.

Deafness, mouth-breathing habit, and imperfect resonance of the voice, as well as the characteristic expression of the face, will often remain as permanent effects of the impairment of function due to these growths in childhood, even though they have more or less completely disappeared. The collapsed state of the wings of the nose, and wasted condition of their muscles, resulting from long disease, often contributes to the perpetuation of the mouth-breathing habit. On the other hand the rapid improvement, after a timely removal of the growths, is usually very striking.

Treatment.--The only thing to do is to remove them soon, no matter how young the patient may be. An anesthetic is usually given to children. The operation does not take long and the patient soon recovers from its effects. The result of an operation, especially in young children, is usually very satisfactory. Breathing through the nose is re-established, the face expression is changed for the better. The symptoms as before described disappear to a great extent.

COLDS. (Coryza. Acute Nasal Catarrh. Acute Rhinitis).--This is an inflammation of the mucous membrane lining the nose.

Causes.--Exposure to cold or wet when the body is overheated; sudden or extreme changes in the atmosphere; inhaling irritating fumes or dust.

Symptoms.--A chilly feeling, limbs ache, tendency to sneeze, severe headache above the nose, eyes are dry, stopped-up feeling in the nostrils. Then there is a thin watery discharge, usually of an irritating character, very thin at first, but it soon becomes thicker; sometimes the ears ring (tinnitus). The nose and lining is red and swollen.

MOTHERS' REMEDIES.--1. Colds. Borax for Cold Settled in Throat. "For a cold in the throat, dissolve a piece of borax, the size of a pea, in the mouth and don't talk. It will work like a charm." This is an old and well tried remedy and is very good for colds or sore throat. It acts by contracting the tissues and in that way there is less congestion in the parts.

2. Colds, Valuable Caution and Treatment for.--Mrs. Maxwell, of Cleveland, writes in the Cleveland Press as follows: "If you intend to treat the cold yourself, take it up at the outset. Don't wait for it to develop. To break it up, nothing is better than the full hot bath at bed time, or the foot bath with mustard, followed by a hot drink. It is old-fashioned, but scientific, for nine colds out of ten are due to clogged pores. Benjamin Franklin said a hundred years ago that all colds come from impure air, lack of exercise, and over-eating, and nobody has ever bettered his conclusion. Even contagious colds will not be taken if the bodily resistance is kept at par. More fresh air, less grip. Avoid people who have colds, and keep out of badly ventilated rooms. Stuffy street cars are responsible for half the hard colds, not because people get chilled, but because the air is foul. And when you have a cold keep away from the baby. If the baby takes a cold, let it have medical attention at once. Don't experiment upon it with remedies intended for grown-ups."

3. Colds, Molasses-Vinegar Syrup for.--"One-half cup of molasses, butter the size of a hickory nut, one tablespoon vinegar, boil together. Dose: One teaspoonful or less as the case requires. Take often until relieved." This is an old remedy and a good one.

4. Colds, Quinine and Ginger for.--"Give plenty of quinine and drink hot water with ginger in it." Quinine, as we all know, is an old remedy for colds and therefore we all know how it acts. The ginger warms up the system and produces sweating. Care should be taken when using this remedy not to take cold, as the pores are all opened by the quinine.

5. Colds, Boneset for.--"Boneset tea steeped and drank cold cures a cold." Boneset simply acts by causing a better circulation in the system and in that way sweating is produced and we all know that a good sweat will usually cure a cold if taken in time.

6. Severe Cold or Threatened Consumption.--"One pint of molasses; one pint of vinegar; three tablespoonfuls of white pine tar; let this boil not quite half down; remove from the stove and let stand until next day; then take and skim tar off from the top, throwing tar away. Jar up and take as often as necessary. Spoonful every half to two hours."

7. Colds, Rock Candy Syrup for.--"Ten cents worth of rock candy; one pint of whisky; one pint of water; fifteen cents worth of glycerine; mix all together; this will syrup itself." Take one teaspoonful as often as necessary. This is excellent.

8. Colds, Skunk's Oil for.--"Skunk's oil has cured colds quickly by rubbing on chest and throat." The oil penetrates quickly and relieves the congestion. This remedy can always be relied upon.

9. Colds, Lemons and Mustard for.--"A hot lemonade taken on going to bed and put the feet in a hot mustard bath; taken in time will break up a cold." The idea of the foot bath is to equalize the circulation, as so many of our colds begin in the head and by drawing the blood from the head the congested parts of the head are relieved.

10. Colds and Cough, Hops or Catnip Poultice for.--"Hops or catnip put in little bags and steamed until hot, then placed on lungs and throat." This is a very good remedy, as the hot bags act as a poultice and draw the congestion from the diseased parts. It produces not only local, but general perspiration.

11. Colds, Honey for.--"Eat honey. I have tried this many times and it is very good." The honey is very soothing, but if a little hoarhound or lemon is added it would make it much more effective. This is a good remedy for children, as they most all like honey.

12. Colds, to Break Up at the Outset.--"To break up a cold soak the feet in hot water and drink all the cold water you can." This has been known to cure many severe colds if taken at the beginning.

13. Cold in the Chest, Mutton Tallow and Red Pepper for.--"If cold is in the chest, render enough mutton tallow for one cupful and add one teaspoonful of red pepper and rub on chest and apply a flannel to keep out the cold. This is an old-time remedy and a good one."

14. Colds, Lard and Turpentine for.--"Melt a half cupful of lard and add one and one-half teaspoonfuls of turpentine, rub on chest and apply flannel cloth."

15. Cold, Milk and Cayenne as a Preventive.--"Drink a glass of milk with a pinch of cayenne in it. This will warm the stomach and prevent headache."

PHYSICIANS' TREATMENT for Colds.--Preventive. Avoid the known causes of the trouble. A daily cold bath, if well borne, is held to be an effectual prevention against taking cold. Have the adenoids removed if your physician so recommends it. If seen early it can frequently be aborted. Bathe the feet in hot mustard water, a small handful of mustard to a pail half full of hot water. At the same time, drink hot teas, like hoarhound, ginger, lemonade, etc. Then put the patient to bed and place hot water fruit jars around him. This treatment will produce a good sweat. After the sweating has continued for some time and the patient feels uncomfortable because of the sweat, bathe him with a towel dipped in warm water, and dry the parts as you go along. Of course, all of this is done under cover. After you have bathed and dried the patient, put on a clean and well-aired night shirt and clean sheets, also well aired. This simple treatment will abort most colds. The patient should keep in bed for at least twelve hours after such a sweating. Plenty of cold water and lemonade can be given, especially after the patient has become cooler. Plenty of water is good for any cold; hot outside and cool for the inside. The bowels should be opened with salts. A Dover's powder (ten grains) will produce sweating, but why use it when sweating can be produced by the means first mentioned.

1. Camphor and Vaseline Mixed, or Camphor and Cream, rubbed in the nose is good to stop the cold and soreness.

2. A few drops (two or three) of camphor taken internally every three hours will abort some colds, especially if the nose is all the time pouring out drops of water.

3. Aconite in small doses, one-tenth of a drop, every two hours is a splendid remedy at the beginning. My experience has shown me that aconite does better work in these small doses. Put one drop in ten teaspoonfuls of water and give one teaspoonful at a dose.

4. The following is good for a thick discharge: in oil spray.

Menthol	6 grains
Chloroform	5 drops
Camphor	5 grains
Liquid Alboline	2 ounces

Mix and make into a solution. Use in an atomizer, every two hours.

To cleanse the nostrils wash out each nostril gently with a solution made of one teaspoonful of listerine, or glyco-thymoline, or borolyptol, or one-quarter teaspoonful of common salt in a half glass of warm water.

You can use a vaporizer and this solution:

Menthol	5 grains
Camphor	5 grains
Compound tincture benzoin	1 dram
Liquid Alboline	1 ounce

Mix and make solution and use frequently in a nebulizer.

Never snuff a solution into the nose, and do not blow the nose hard after using. Some of the solution or nasal discharge may be forced into the eustachian tube.

5. Lard or camphorated oil rubbed on the nose and throat twice a day is good.

6. To Restore the Loss of the Voice.--

Oil of wintergreen	2 drams
Lanolin or vaseline	1 ounce

Mix and rub on the throat at night and put on flannel until morning. This will relieve the loss of voice very promptly.

7. Put a quart of boiling water in a pitcher; add from two to four drams of the compound tincture of benzoin and inhale the hot vapor. Wrap both head and pitcher in a towel. This is very good for sore throat also.

8. Herb Teas for.--Ginger tea, catnip, hoarhound, pennyroyal, etc.; hot, are all good to produce sweating and thus relieve cold.

9. From Dr. Ball, a London, England, Specialist.--

Menthol	30 grains
Eucalyptol	30 drops
Carbolic acid	2 drams
Rectified spirits of wine	1 dram

Mix thoroughly; a teaspoonful to be put into a pint (or less) of hot water and the steam to be inhaled through the nose for four or five minutes. This is *useful* in acute colds, especially in the later stages, and in chronic catarrh, etc.

10. When the stage is rather marked or prolonged spray or syringe out the nose with tepid solution once or twice a day using the following:

Bicarbonate of soda	3 to 5 grains
Borax	3 to 5 grains
Tepid water	1 ounce

Use a spray, douche, or gargle in chronic catarrh and chronic pharyngitis. When you wish to use a large quantity, mix an equal quantity each of soda and borax and put a couple teaspoonfuls to each pint of warm water and use.

CATARRH. (Chronic Inflammation of the Nose, Chronic Rhinitis). Causes.--Frequent attacks of colds, irritating gases and dust, adenoids, enlarged tonsils, spurs on the septum (partition bone) or foreign bodies in the nose, like corn, beans, stone, etc.

Symptoms and Course.--There are alterations of the secretions: the amount varies in the same case at different times. Sometimes it is thin and watery, or thick, sticky mucus or this may alternate with more watery discharges. It may be mucus and pus or entirely pus. Frequently the secretions discharge into the throat and cause efforts to clear it by hawking and spitting. The secretion sometimes dries and forms crusts in the fore part of the turbinated bones and partition. Patients frequently pick the nose for this crust and ulceration may result at that point from its doing. Bleeding often occurs from picking the scales from the ulcers, and perforation of the partition may take place from extension of the ulceration. There is a feeling of stuffiness. There is some obstruction to breathing. If there is much thickness of the structures, nasal obstruction is a persistent symptom. Changed voice, mouth-breathing, etc., are noticed. A sensation of pain or weight across the bridge of the nose is sometimes complained of and this symptom is especially found associated with enlargement of the middle turbinated body on one or both sides, etc.

MOTHERS' REMEDIES. 1. Catarrh, Successful remedy for.--- "Dissolve in one-half ounce olive oil as much camphor gum as it will take up. Moisten a little finger with the oil, rub into the nostrils and snuff well up into the head." The olive oil is very soothing to the diseased parts and the camphor contracts the swollen mucous membranes, thereby relieving the catarrh. This is an excellent remedy.

2. Catarrh, Cleansing Antiseptic Remedy for.--"Snuff about one teaspoonful of salt in cup of warm water every morning in nostrils. I have found this remedy simple but fine for catarrh and also having sleeping room well ventilated summer and winter will help in curing disease." This remedy will be found very effective in catarrh because it loosens up the secretions and cleanses the nose of the foul secretions and also has an antiseptic action. This can be used twice daily. Snuffing should be done very gently so as not to draw the water too far back.

3. Catarrh, Witch-Hazel for.--"Pond's extract applied with nose spray." Pond's extract is simply witch-hazel water and everyone knows that witch-hazel water is healing and soothing to the membranes of the nose. This may be used regularly twice a day.

4. Catarrh, Cure for.--

Menthol	10 grains
Camphor Gum	10 grains
Chloroform	10 drops
Fluid Alboline	8 ounces

Mix. Apply in the nasal cavities with alboline atomizer.

5. Catarrh of head, Mullein Leaves. Treatment, etc., for.-- "Smoke dried mullein leaves and blow the smoke through the nose, and in addition to this, put a heaping tablespoonful of powdered borax in a quart of soft water; syringe this up in the nose, and in addition to both of the above, frequently inhale a mixture of two drams of spirits of ammonia, half a dram tincture of iodine and fifteen drops of carbolic acid; smoke the mullein, syringe the borax water and inhale the last mixture all as frequently as convenient and it frequently will cure if kept up faithfully."

6. Catarrh, Milk and Salt Wash for.--"Mix together one teaspoonful common salt, a teacupful milk, and half pint of warm water. Inject this into the nostrils three times a day. You may use the same quantity of borax in place of the salt, if you choose to do so."

PHYSICIANS' TREATMENT for Catarrh.--If the patient is run down, give tonics, plenty of fresh air and sunshine in the sleeping room, change of climate to a dry, unchangeable climate is sometimes necessary.

Local.--Attend to any disturbing cause, such as adenoids, spurs on the partition, turbinate bone, etc. It is first necessary to render the parts clean, through the use of some mild antiseptic solution, such as glycothymoline, listerine, borolyptol, salt, etc. Salt should not be used stronger than one-quarter teaspoonful in a glass half full of water. The others can be used in one to two teaspoonfuls, to same amount of warm water. The solution should always be mild and warm. To use any solution pour it gently through the nose, tilting the head backward, with the mouth open; then as the solution flows through the head should be put forward and downward. The solution flows out of the mouth, and also out of the other nostril. A nasal douche cup made purposely should be used if possible.

1. Spray for.--After cleansing the nostrils with the solution the following soothing mild spray will be found of great benefit.

Menthol	5 grains
Camphor	5 grains
Liquid Alboline	2 ounces

Mix and make a solution. Use in an atomizer or nebulizer.

2. Powders for.--Antiseptic powders are also very useful in some cases, such as, compound stearate of zinc and boric acid, or compound stearate of zinc and alum or compound stearate of zinc and menthol.

One or two drams is enough to buy at once as it is very light; always use it in a powder in the following way:

First take a long breath and while holding the breath, puff some of the powder into each nostril; then gently puff the breath out through each nostril. Do not snuff powder up the nose or use the powder--blower while breathing. If this is done, some will get into the pharynx and larynx and cause annoying coughing.

3. Solution for.--

Bicarbonate of soda	1/2 ounce
Borax	1/2 ounce
Salt	1/2 ounce
White sugar	1 ounce

Mix all. Half a teaspoonful to be dissolved in one-half tumbler of warm water; used with spray producer or a syringe.

4. Spray, for.--

Bicarbonate of soda	1-1/2 drams
Listerine	6 drams
Water	1 ounce

Use as a spray.

OZENA.--(Foul odor from nose, not breath, due to catarrh of the nose). The membrane is dry and shrunken. It is a very offensive odor, thus called "ozena."

Causes.--It is usually seen in people who are very much debilitated, in young factory girls, and sometimes in healthy boys. Retained secretions in the nose, usually cause the odor. These decompose and ferment. The nose is large and roomy, the nostrils are filled with scabby secretions; hard masses are formed which sometimes fill the nostril.

PHYSICIANS' TREATMENT.--The first few weeks, cleansing the nose with peroxide of hydrogen will stop the odor. First, remove the scabs with forceps and then wash and cleanse the nose with the peroxide solution. It can be used from one-quarter strength to full strength, but warm. This will leave the nose in a foamy, soapy condition and this can be cleansed with a mild solution of glyco-thymoline or salt water.

HOME TREATMENT.--This is very important. The patient should use a douche three or four times a day. In the solution glyco-thymoline or borolyptol one or two teaspoonfuls to one-half cup of warm water, and follow by a nebulizer or atomizer in which the following solution can be used:

1.	Lysol	10 drops
	Oil of Pine	15 drops
	Liquid Alboline	2 ounces

Mix and make a solution, spray into the nose after douching.

2. The following ointment can be used if there is no atomizer or nebulizer at hand:

Iodol	5 grains
Boric Acid	10 grains
Cold cream	2 ounces

Mix and make into an ointment, and rub a little into each nostril before retiring.

3. Dr. Ferguson of New York uses the following: A new antiseptic enzymol. This is used as follows.--Use one part of enzymol, three parts of warm water. Rub and cleanse the nose thoroughly with the solution, saturate a piece of absorbent cotton with this solution, place it in the nostril and leave it there fifteen to twenty minutes.

HAY FEVER. (Rose Cold, June Cold or Hay Asthma).--This inflammation of the nose occurs in August and September. It is really a nervous affection of the nose membrane.

Causes.--A predisposition: A peculiar sensitive area in the mucous membrane of the nose. An exciting cause circulating in the air, the dust or pollen of certain plants, such as rag-weed, hay and barley; the odor of certain flowers, such as roses and golden rod; dust of some drugs as ipecac and benzoic acid; the odor of some animals. It usually comes about the same date each year, growing worse each year and, in time, affects the bronchial tubes.

Symptoms.--The earliest symptoms are, usually, an itching sensation in the roof of the mouth and the palate, or itching and burning at the inner corner of the eyes. Irritation within the nose is also experienced and very soon spells of sneezing set in. The nose soon feels stuffy and obstructed, and there is a clear water discharge from the nose, which is especially copious after sneezing. The eyes look red and watery and the eyeballs pain and there is also pain in the forehead above the nose. It may take several days to develop these symptoms. They are usually worse in the morning. After some days these symptoms become more persistent and severe. The nostrils are completely closed, and the patient must breathe through the mouth, and the spells of sneezing are very violent. The conjunctiva becomes congested and red, a profuse watery discharge runs from the eyes and the lids are swollen. In severe cases the face looks red and swollen. The mucous membrane of the mouth, pharynx and tonsils is more or less reddened and irritated, smell and taste are impaired and sometimes the patient is slightly deaf. The patient feels tired, weak, and it is hard to study or do manual labor. Slight feelings of chillness are common.

MOTHERS' REMEDIES. 1. Hay fever, Quick Relief from.--"For hay fever and other slight forms of diseases which produce sneezing, there is no remedy more quickly effective, and often curative, than a vapor of heated salt and alcohol. Heat it very hot and breathe the vapor for ten minutes at a time, four or five times a day."

2. Hay fever, Remedy Worth Trying for.--"A mixture composed of ten grains of sulphate of zinc, half teaspoonful of borax, and about four ounces of rose water. This is very good to inject into the nostrils if there is much irritation of eyes and nostrils."

3. Hay fever, Our Canadian Remedy for.--"Inhale smoke from ground coffee (sprinkle over coals). This relieved a case for me of five years standing."

4. Hay Fever, Medicine That Helps.--"Use phenol sodique as directed on the bottles. This was recommended to me by Mrs. Levi Weller, who said her husband had found more relief from this remedy than any other he had tried."

PHYSICIANS' TREATMENT for Hay Fever.--1. The following gives relief from the distressing symptoms. (But first the nose should he examined, for often there is local trouble there.). Then give suprarenal extract tablets, each five grains. Take one every four or five hours.

2. Pill Blennostasin.--Each pill contains five grains. Take one every four hours.

3. The following solution gives temporary relief:--

Dionin	10 grains
Adrenalin (1 to 1000)	5 drams
Water	2 ounces

Mix solution and spray into the nose every two hours.

4. After using the above spray which will shrink the mucous membrane apply the following oil spray:--

Thymol	5 grains
Menthol	5 grains
Camphor	5 grains
Liquid Alboline	1 ounce

Mix and make a solution and spray into the nose three or four times a day.

5. In some cases a drying powder does well, such as compound stearate of zinc and alum one dram; puff it into the nose with a powder-blower every hour.

6. Dr. Ball of London, England, gives the following.--A spray of a four per cent of cocaine, or direct application of cotton-wool soaked in a stronger solution will be found to afford immediate relief. But the after effect is likely to be bad. Hence menthol is a better application.

7. Another from Dr. Ball.--A one to five per cent solution of menthol in liquid paraffin may be painted or sprayed on the mucous membrane, or a little cotton-wool soaked in an oily solution may be inserted in the nostrils. We must confess our weakness as physicians, when we treat this disease. There are local measures, such as give relief for the time being, but they must be carefully used. Diseases of the nose, tumors or "spurs" frequently cause in the first place; bad tonsils, and adenoids are likely to aggravate the trouble. A change of climate is the only real help. Tone the general health. If the patient is very nervous fifteen grains of bromide of sodium three or four time a day gives relief. People subjected to hay fever should be treated between the attacks to make them strong and to remove any local nose trouble and just before the time of year arrives for the attack it is well to take five grains three times a day of the suprarenal tablets or blennostasin the same way, and also spray the nose twice daily with a mild adrenalin solution as the following:-

Adrenalin (1 to 1000)	1 dram
Water	2 ounces

Change of climate is frequently quite beneficial. Some are relieved in the dry mountain air, while others are more benefited by the seashore or an ocean trip.

TUMOR OF THE NOSE. (Nasal Polypus).--This tumor consists of a soft jelly-like whitish growth, usually found in the upper front part of the nostril. It may extend to the bottom (floor) of the nose, is quite soft and moveable, being easy to push aside with a probe. The air passing through the nostril will move it backward and forward. There may be one or several and they may completely fill the nostril. They sometimes grow from the back end of the middle turbinate bone, and gradually extend backward filling up the back part of the nostril and even extending into the space behind the nose and, if large, they may be seen below the soft palate.

PHYSICIANS' TREATMENT.--The only thing to do is to remove them. This is usually done by a wire placed around the polypus and by the thumb-screw in the instrument, tighten the wire until it has cut through the base.

DEVIATION OF THE SEPTUM (Partition).--Deviation is the bending or curving of the partition (septum) to one side or the other, leaving one nostril very large and roomy and closing the other nostril wholly or partly.

Causes.--Blows, falls, etc., high-arch palate. It is seldom seen under seven years of age.

PHYSICIANS' TREATMENT.--The treatment is to replace if possible, the part in the proper position. This requires an operation.

NOSEBLEED. Mothers' Remedies.--1. Nosebleed; remedy sent us by a Public School Teacher.--"Make a compress of paper soaked in cold water; put it under the upper lip and have the patient press the lip with the fingers. Remarks.--Tried with success in many cases by a school teacher." By putting under the lip and pressing on it, you press on an artery and stop bleeding. Be careful to use nothing but white paper, as ink or colors would come out when wet.

2. Nosebleed, Alum as a cure for.--"Apply cold water to face and back of neck; snuff powdered alum." The powdered alum contracts the blood vessels, thereby shutting off the supply of blood. The cold water applied to the back of the neck affects the nervous system in such a manner that the blood vessels are contracted and so the blood supply is diminished.

3. Nosebleed; Remedy that succeeded in a severe case.--"Put pieces of ice in cloth. Lay a piece each side of the nose and on the back of the neck. Remarks.--My neighbor's daughter had nosebleed which refused to stop until they were much frightened but this treatment soon stopped it, after which she rested quietly for a time,"

4. Nosebleed, Simple Remedy for.--"Place the finger on the side of the nose tight for ten or fifteen minutes. My mother has stopped her nose from bleeding when other remedies failed." This shuts off the circulation and helps to form a clot.

5. Nosebleed, Another Home Remedy for.--"Hold the head back as far as possible, press up the end of the nose with the end of the finger." Best to lie on the side so blood will not run down the throat and choke the patient.

6. Nosebleed, Puff-Ball for.--"Find an old brown puff-ball from the ground, pick out the soft inside part and put it in nose and let remain for some time."

7. Nosebleed, Vinegar and Water for.--"Wet a cloth in very cold water or strong cold water and vinegar and apply to back of neck, renewing as it gets warm. Have seen this tried and know it to be good."

PHYSICIANS' TREATMENT for Nosebleed.--Place the patient on his side half lying, head and shoulders raised and apply a cold compress to the forehead, nose, and to the back of the neck. Press the end of the nose firmly against the partition between the nostrils, for some minutes. This presses directly upon the bleeding point, as a rule. Also, when lying in this position, the blood does not flow into the throat so readily. Raise the arms above the head, apply cold to the spine or to the scrotum of men and breasts of women. Mustard foot baths are good, injection of cold water, or the injection of hot water, 120 F., into the nostril will often help: Cold water, Or salt water, can be gently snuffed. Alum solution on a cloth put in the nostril often helps. A piece of bacon cut to bits and placed in the nostril often stops it. Vinegar injected into the nostril is good, or you can use a cloth saturated with vinegar and placed in the nostril. White oak bark tea, strong, is effective; juice of lemon applied same way or injected is helpful.

How to plug the nostrils; (front or anterior nares).--Do this with narrow strips of sterilized gauze, by placing the first piece as far back as possible, then with a narrow pair of forceps pushing in a little at a time until the nostril is filled. The gauze should be only one-half inch wide. If the bleeding still continues the posterior opening (nares) should be plugged. This can be known by seeing the blood flowing down the throat (pharynx).

How this is done? Pass a soft rubber catheter, along the floor (bottom) of the nose until its end is seen passing down behind the soft palate into the throat. Grasp this with a pair of forceps and pull it forward into the mouth. Tie a stout string to the end of the catheter (about 1-1/2 feet long) and tie the other end of the string around the center of a plug of lint or gauze, 1-1/2 inches long and three-quarters of an inch wide. Then pull the catheter back through the nostril, very gently. This will pull the plug into the posterior opening of the nose, and plug it. . Hold this same end firmly and with a pair of forceps fill the anterior nostril with strips (1/2 inch wide) of gauze, pushing them back to the posterior plug. The end of the string in the mouth may be fastened to a tooth or to the side of the cheek (if long enough) with a piece of adhesive plaster. The plug should not be left in position more than forty-eight hours, and it should be thoroughly softened with oil or Vaseline before it is removed. Remove the anterior part first, gently and carefully and then with cocaine (if necessary) and more oil, the posterior plug is softened and removed by pulling the end of the string which is in the mouth gently and slowly.

SORE THROAT (Acute Pharyngitis--Acute Pharyngeal Catarrh--Inflammation of the Pharynx--Simple Angina).--This is a common complaint especially among some adults. A predisposition to it is often due to chronic pharyngitis, chronic enlargement of the tonsils and adenoids of the wall of the pharynx as well as chronic nasal obstruction. Rheumatic persons are especially subject to it and acute articular rheumatism is often observed to be preceded by an attack of pharyngitis. Tonsillitis is said to have the same influence also.

Symptoms.--The throat is dry and feels stiff. There may be tenderness at the angle of the jaw and outside of the neck. Pains some to swallow. In a day or two there is a mucous secretion, making the patient inclined to clear the throat by hawking or coughing. The throat looks red and in the early stage this is more noticeable on the anterior pillars of the fauces, the soft palate and uvula. On the back wall you see bright red spots, the inflamed lymph follicles. It usually gets well in two to seven days. It may become chronic after repeated acute attacks.

Chronic.--This is very common in persons who smoke or drink to excess, also people who use their voice in public speaking as preachers do, or in calling loudly as hucksters, railroad brakemen, stationmen, etc.

Prevention of chronic kind.--Ascertain the cause and remove it. Too hot food or too much spiced food cause the chronic kind. Rest the voice. Remove any existing catarrh.

Prevention of acute kind.--Avoid undue exposure to cold and wet, wear warm comfortable flannel underwear. Bath the neck and chest daily with cold water. This is good cold preventive. The wearing of handkerchiefs, mufflers, around the neck is injurious unless you are driving. Accustom your neck to the cold from the beginning in the fall and winter months. Wearing a full beard is said to be a good preventive.

MOTHERS' REMEDIES.--1. Sore throat, Used for Years Successfully.--"Salt pork dipped in hot water then covered thick with black pepper. Heat in the oven and lay or bind on the throat or lungs. This has been a favorite remedy with us for years." Sew the pork to a piece of cotton cloth and bind over the sore parts after you have sprinkled the pork with salt and pepper. Leave this on as long as the patient can endure it. When the pork is removed, rub the affected parts with cold cream or Vaseline and put a clean muslin cloth on to keep person from taking cold.

2. Sore throat, Splendid Liniment for.--

"Olive oil	1/2 pint
Ammonia	1/2 pint
Turpentine	1/2 pint
One egg.	

Shake till it forms emulsion. This can be used as a blister."

This is a very effective remedy, but you must watch the throat very carefully as this will blister quickly. After removing the liniment, grease the parts with oil or cold cream.

3. Sore throat, Simple Gargle for.--

"Soda	1 teaspoonful
Salt	1 teaspoonful
Borax	1 teaspoonful

Dissolve in pint of warm water; use as a gargle frequently."

This is a very good gargle. It contracts the parts and acts as an antiseptic and thoroughly cleanses the parts.

4. Sore throat, Home Made salve for.-

"Beeswax	1 ounce
Rosin	1 ounce
Camphor gum	1 ounce

Lard about the size of an egg."

Mix the above ingredients together and apply to the outside of the throat. This causes the skin to become red thus drawing the inflammation out of the throat and relieving the trouble.

5. Sore Throat, Cold Packs, Sure Cure for.--"Put cold packs on the throat. Remarks: Was in Washington once and my little girl had a very sore throat. I put cold packs on the throat the first half of the night and the next day she was out seeing the sights as well as ever." Gargle with very hot water and a little soda. This makes it very effective.

6. Sore Throat, Ointment for.--

Oil Turpentine	1/2 ounce
Oil of Hemlock	1/2 ounce
Oil of Peppermint	1/2 ounce
Oil of Encaliptus	1/2 ounce

Mix with one cup warm lard, apply warm to the throat."

7. Sore Throat, Remedy from a mother in Johnson City, Tenn.--"Fat meat stewed in vinegar and bound to the neck. Kind friends:--After waiting so long I will help you what I can, and where is the mother that won't want the book? I am truly glad you have such an interest in the welfare of suffering humanity. I hope this book will soon be out on its good mission. Kind friends, I think it a wonderful kindness to the rich as well as the poor to have a friend in time of need. I think a good honest book of home remedies tried by our good mothers and grandmothers will be accepted and looked to by all mothers, for we all think mother knows best. I certainly want this book completed and in my home."

8. Sore Throat, Gargle and Local Application for.--

"Common salt	2 tablespoonfuls
Strained honey	2 tablespoonfuls
Vinegar	3 tablespoonfuls
Camphor	1/2 teaspoonful"

Use as a gargle. External applications, wring a cloth out of salt and cold water and keep it quite wet, bind tightly about the neck and cover with a dry cloth. It is best to use this at night."

9. Mild Sore Throat, Vinegar Gargle for.--"Gargle with vinegar and hot water. This will help to sooth the irritation and in a mild sore throat is a sure cure."

10. Sore Throat, Alum and Vinegar for.--"One glass of warm water; one tablespoonful of vinegar; one teaspoonful of sugar; one-half teaspoonful of alum; dissolve well and gargle throat several times daily."

11. Sore Throat, Kerosene for.--"Dip a flannel cloth in coal oil, (kerosene) and bind on the throat. I have tried this; in fact it is what I always use. It is almost sure to cure."

12. Sore Throat and Cough, Remedy always at hand.--"Equal parts of alcohol and glycerin make a good gargle, or use three tablespoonfuls of vinegar and one of salt to a tumbler of water. Or simply hot water and salt when nothing else is to be had. The hot water alone is very good."

13. Tickling in Throat, Simple Remedy for.--"Take bread crumbs and swallow them."

PHYSICIANS' TREATMENT for Sore Throat.--1. Inhalation of steam either with or without medicine is good. (See treatment of tonsillitis-Inhaling steam) I treated a man once who had a terrific pharyngitis, All the parts were so terribly swollen, that he was unable to swallow or talk. I induced him to inhale steam from a teakettle. He was able to put his mouth over the spout of the kettle and he was relived in a few minutes. I think it saved his life. I put no medicine in the water for that case. Very few persons can inhale the steam directly from the kettle. Other method is given under tonsillitis. A dose of salts at first is good. Remain in the house for a few days.

2. Sulphur and Cream for.--Mix some sulphur with cream and put some of it on the sore membrane.

3. Good Old Mother's Remedy.--"Steep a medium sized red pepper in one-half pint of water, strain and add one-fourth pint of good vinegar and a heaping teaspoonful each of salt and powdered alum and gargle with it as often as needed. This is a very good remedy.

1. Physicians' Local Treatment.--A wet compress on the neck is useful at the onset. Sucking ice or gargling with ice or cold water, or applying an ice bag to the throat will be found useful.

Later on, warm gargles and steam inhalation are more grateful. If there is great pain in swallowing, cocaine painted on the throat or sucking a cocaine lozenge before taking food will be found very useful.

2. When the attack is mild medicine may not be needed. When there is fever and the throat is real sore, you can use one drop doses of tincture of aconite every hour. This will frequently check it.

3. I like the following at the beginning. Give tincture of aconite and mercury biniodide, called the pink tablet, alternately. Put ten drops of the aconite in one-half glass of water and give from one-half to two teaspoonfuls everyone or two hours, alternating with one or two tablets of one-hundred grain tablet of mercury biniodide. After the first twenty-four hours stop the acoite and give the mercury biniodide every three hours.

4. For Chronic Catarrh remaining after, lozenges containing rhatany or tannin are useful.

5. Other gargles.--

Menthol	3 to 5 grains
Camphor	2 to 4 grains
Liquid paraffin	1 ounce

For irritable and catarrhal conditions of nasal membrane use a spray.

8. Snuff.-

Hydrochloride of Cocaine	1 grains
Menthol	1 grain
Sugar of Milk	2 drams

Mix very thoroughly.

When using the Menthol preparation do not use the preparation very hot.

HOARSENESS. Inflammation of the Larynx. (Acute Laryngitis) Causes.--Due to taking cold or over using the voice; hot liquids, poisons. It may occur in influenza and measles; from irritating gases; some are subject to it.

Symptoms.--Tickling in the larynx; cold air irritates, and breathing may cause some pain; dry cough; the voice may be altered. At first it may be only husky. In children breathing may be very difficult, after a day or two there may be a light expectoration and finally there may be a loose cough and a slight fever. The trouble is in the region of "Adam's Apple." There is little or no danger in these attacks if proper care is taken. The attack generally lasts two to four days.

MOTHERS' REMEDIES. Hoarseness, Borax for.--"For hoarseness dissolve a piece of borax the size of a pea in the mouth and don't talk. It will work like a charm." The borax does away with the inflammation of the inflamed parts and gives relief very quickly.

2. Hoarseness, Egg and Lemon for.--"Beaten white of one egg, juice of one lemon, with sugar enough to thicken, then add one teaspoonful olive oil." Take one teaspoonful every hour until relieved.

3. Hoarseness, Horseradish for.--"Horseradish root; eat plenty of it. This has been tried and proved successful."

4. Hoarseness, Successful Remedy for Adults.--"Take two ounces of fresh scraped horseradish root, infuse in a close vessel in one-half pint of cold water for two or three hours; then add four ounces of acid tincture of lobelia and one-half pound of honey. Boil altogether for one-half hour, strain and take a teaspoonful four times a day. This is a very good remedy, especially for adults."

5. Hoarseness, Lemon and Sugar for Children.--"Take the juice of one lemon and saturate with sugar, take a teaspoonful several times a day. It is sure to give relief. This is very pleasant to give to children, as they most all like it."

PHYSICIANS' TREATMENT for Hoarseness.--1. Rest of the voice and if the case is severe keep in bed in a room with an even temperature and the air saturated with moisture from a steaming teakettle, etc.

2. An ice bag on the throat or cold water cloths to the front of the throat often give relief.

3. Tincture of Aconite.--This is given in the beginning when there is fever. The dose depends upon the age, and the amount of fever. You can give it to a child by putting one drop of aconite in twelve teaspoonfuls of water and then give one teaspoonful every one to three hours according to the case. For an adult you can put ten drops of aconite in ten teaspoonfuls of water and give one teaspoonful every hour or two.

4. Citrate of Potash is given every four to five hours in adults.

5. Full dose of five grains of Dover's powders at night for the irritating cough.

6. For a cough, for a child one year old you can give one-half teaspoonful, every two hours, of the following:--

Syrup of Dover's powder	1 fluid dram
Tincture of Aconite	10 drops
Simple syrup	Enough to make two ounces

Shake before using.

TICKLING IN THROAT. Mothers' Remedies. Mullein Leaf Smoke Beneficial for.--"Smoke dried mullein leaves, just a few puffs are needed, and should be drawn into the throat. Myron H. Grinnel of Albion, Mich., says his grandmother always gathers mullein leaves for this purpose and finds them an excellent remedy. Too much would cause dizziness." Mullein leaves are good for inflamed membranes like the ear and throat. If a person does not wish to gather the leaves themselves they may buy them at a drug store.

2. Tickling in Throat, Good Northern Canada Remedy for.---"Chew some of the bark of slippery elm and gargle the throat with saliva. This stops tickling in a few minutes." **3. Tickling in Throat, Tested Gargle for.**--"Gargle from four to six times daily with following:--

Strong Sage Tea	1 pint
Salt	2 tablespoonfuls
Cayenne Pepper	2 tablespoonfuls
Vinegar	2 tablespoonfuls
Honey	2 tablespoonfuls

Mix thoroughly and bottle for use."

The above ingredients are all excellent for sore throat and it is an old tried remedy and can easily be obtained. If it is too strong dilute with warm water to the desired strength.

SWELLING OF THE GLOTTIS. (Oedematous Laryngitis. Oedma of the Glottis).--Swelling or oedma of the glottis or more correctly of the structure which forms the glottis, is a very serious affection. It may follow acute laryngitis or may be met with in chronic diseases of the larynx and from other diseases. It is dangerous.

Symptoms.--Difficulty of breathing which increases in intensity so that the condition becomes very serious in a short time. There is whistling breathing, the voice is husky and disappears.

Acute Laryngitis.--Inhalations and sprays.

Menthol	10 grains
Oil of pine	1 dram
Tincture of benzion	1 dram
Liquid alboline	2 ounces

Make a solution. Use one teaspoonful in a pint of boiling water; inhale with a cone placed over the dish or put a shawl over the head and dish and inhale the steam. Or this one to inhale same way:

Tincture of benzoin	1 dram
Oil of tar	1 drain
Liquid alboline	2 ounces

Make a solution and use one teaspoonful to a pint of boiling water as above.

It may be necessary in order to save life, to have a physician make an opening by incision into the windpipe for the admission of air into the lungs. This process is called Tracheotomy.

Diet in Laryngitis.--Hard and dry toasts should be avoided, for they give pain on being swallowed, same reason applies to highly seasoned foods. Milk, custards, eggs, scraped beef may be taken. Difficulty in swallowing may be overcome by allowing the patient to lie flat on the bed, etc., with his face over the edge. Food can be sucked through the tube from a vessel placed below; or the patient can lean forward while eating.

"CHILD CROWING" (Spasm of the Glottis.)--This is usually peculiar to children.

Cause.--It is purely a nervous affection and it occurs between six months and three years, and is most commonly seen in children with rickets.

Symptoms.--It may come in the night or day; or when the child awakes. The breathing is arrested, the child struggles for breath, the face is flushed, and then with a sudden relaxation of the spasm, the air is drawn into the lungs with a high pitched crowing sound. Convulsions may occur. Death rarely occurs. There may be many attacks during the day.

PHYSICIANS' TREATMENT of Child Crowing. Preventive.--The gums should be carefully examined and if they are swollen and hot they should be lanced. The bowels should be carefully regulated, and as these children are usually of a delicate nature and afflicted with rickets, nourishing food and the treatment in diet and medicine should be given for rickets. Cod liver oil is a good general remedy. (See rickets).

Cold Sponging.--In severe cases, the child should be placed in a warm bath tub and the back and chest thoroughly sponged for a minute or two with cold water. This plan may be used even when a child is in a paroxysm, though the attack is severe and the child looks blue, it is much better than to dash cold water in the face. Sometimes the attack can be stopped by introducing the finger far back into the throat.

CROUP, Spasmodic.--This disease gives the parents a terrible shock if they have never seen any attacks of the kind. The symptoms which attend the attack are out of all proportion to the real danger. It is generally the result of exposure to cold or to the cold wind. Irritating, undigested food, often causes it.

Symptoms.--Usually the child goes to bed perfectly well, or has a slight cold and wakes up an hour or two later, coughing and gasping for breath, due to a spasm in the wind pipe. The cough is shrill, more like a bark; the cough is repeated at intervals and soon the patient breathes quickly and laboriously. It must sit up for it can breathe easier sitting. The voice is oftentimes nearly or quite lost, or at least only a hoarse whisper; the face is bluish or perspiring. The spasm lasts for a variable period, but rarely exceeds one-half hour, sometimes only a few minutes. The croupy cough and oppressed breathing may last longer than this, but these too subside after a time, after which the child drops to sleep and usually rests quietly for the rest of the night. There is a tendency to recurrence on succeeding night unless obviated by treatment.

Treatment. Preventive.--Guard against such children's exposure to cold winds and dampness, dress them warmly. The living and sleeping rooms should not be too warm. Do not give them food hard to digest at any time, especially before bedtime. Foods hard to digest frequently cause the attack.

MOTHERS' REMEDIES. Croup, Cold Application for.--"Apply to throat a flannel wrung out of cold water, lay a dry cloth over it." This is an excellent remedy for a mother to try in case of an emergency when no other medicine can be obtained. This very often will relieve a child until other remedies can be secured and has been known to save many children's lives: The cold water helps to draw the blood away from the larynx and air passages and also dilates the tubes and gives relief. Take great care not to wet the child, as this will cause it to take more cold and may prove fatal.

2. Croup, Sure Cure for.--"Give child anything that will make it vomit, soak feet in hot water, apply onion drafts to bottom of feet, roast onions and put on the chest, keep warm. My mother has cured me at least one hundred times with the above remedy. She generally gave me pig's foot oil, or oil from the feet of a chicken, sometimes melted lard. Croup has to be attended to at once or it is fatal with the child." This is a very good remedy.

3. Croup, Immediate Relief from Steaming.--"Put a small shawl over the child's head to retain steam, then put a small chunk of unslaked lime in a bowl of water under shawl. The steam affords immediate relief, usually, if child inhales it." This is very good; shawl should cover the child's head and bowl in which lime is dissolved.

4. Croup, for Baby or Older Child.--"Take a teaspoonful alum, pulverize it and sprinkle it on the whites of two fresh eggs in a cup or glass, let it stand for a few minutes, until the combination has turned to water, or water is produced; then give one-half teaspoonful to a child six months old or less and increase the dose to one teaspoonful for older children, and repeat the dose in fifteen or thirty minutes as the case may require. Remarks: From personal experience in my own and neighbors' families, I have never known a case where it did not bring relief and cure. The dose must produce vomiting."

5. Croup, Remedy that Never Fails.--"Two tablespoonfuls of liquor or brandy and one-quarter teaspoonful of glycerin, one teaspoonful of sugar, one tablespoonful of water; stir up well and give one teaspoonful every hour or oftener if necessary. Then at same time take a flannel and soak well in cold water, wring it gently and put around neck with a heavy, dry flannel over the damp one. If damp flannel becomes hot take it off, dampen it in more cold water and apply again, and so on until relieved. Do not allow the patient to get chilled. Better results are obtained if patient will go to bed. Remarks: I have used this in my family, and have always found it to be the best croup cure I have ever seen, and it will be found to give immediate relief. The external application is extremely good."

6. Croup, Coal Oil (kerosene) and Sugar for.--"Coal oil and sugar; put a few drops on a teaspoonful of sugar." The coal oil produces vomiting, relieving the trouble. If the first dose does not have this effect upon the child, repeat it.

7. Croup, Pork and Onion Poultice for.--"Put pork and onions on the throat. Drink plenty of hot water." Bind the pork and onions on the throat, acting as a poultice. The virtue of this can be increased by cooking the onions and pork together. Onion syrup may be given internally to produce vomiting, even in very small babies.

8. Croup, Bloodroot for.--"One teaspoonful powdered bloodroot mixed with molasses or sugar. Have taken this myself and it relieved at once. If one dose does not seem enough it may be repeated." This is a very effective remedy, but is very weakening. Care should be taken not to repeat dose any oftener than absolutely necessary.

9. Croup, Time Honored Remedy for.--"Pulverized alum and sugar or honey or molasses; mix together and give half teaspoonful doses or less. For infants use only in emergency cases." This is one of the good old-fashioned remedies that nearly every mother has used. It acts simply by producing vomiting and causing the air tubes to relax. Repeat in five to twenty minutes until it causes vomiting.

10. Croup, Ipecac for.--"One-third teaspoonful of powdered ipecac dissolved in one teaspoonful of water, one tablespoonful of sugar; pour on one teacupful of boiling water and let boil down to a half cup, Dose: One teaspoonful for adults; children in proportion every two hours; or, if needed to vomit children give again in ten or fifteen minutes." If you cannot secure the powdered ipecac, the syrup can be bought at any drug store, and is already prepared, Dose: Ten to fifteen drops as the case may need.

11. Croup, Vaseline for.--"Vaseline rubbed on the chest, cover with a hot flannel, and take 1/4 teaspoonful of Vaseline internally occasionally." Dissolve Vaseline and repeat dose if necessary to produce vomiting.

12. Croup, Ice Application for.--"Ice applied to the throat is almost instant relief." It is best to break the ice up fine and sprinkle salt on same, putting it in a cheese cloth bag, binding on the throat with a flannel, and change as soon as it shows signs of wetting.

13. Croup, Salt for.--"Parched salt put on the throat hot." The parched salt acts the same as mustard plaster, by producing a redness on the throat. Salt is something that we can always have on hand and by using this remedy we are always prepared for an emergency in case of croup.

14. Croup, Castor Oil Breaks up.--"Castor oil, given before bedtime, is good. Dose.--From one-half to one teaspoonful. I have taken this when I was small." Castor oil is good when the bowels are constipated or the stomach is full.

15. Croup, Coal Oil, Turpentine and Snuff, a Canadian Remedy for.--"A little coal oil and a few drops of turpentine soaked up by snuff, and used as plaster. Makes the child sneeze after a few minutes. The poultice loosens the phlegm and the sneezing throws it off."

PHYSICIANS' TREATMENT for Croup.--Active. 1. Dr. Douglas says wring cloths out of cold water and apply very freely to the throat, and recommends the following syrup:

Syrup of Ipecac	3 fluid drams
Hive Syrup	4 fluid drams
Water	1-1/2 ounces

Mix, and give one teaspoonful every half hour until the child vomits, then repeat the dose every two hours as needed.

2. Place the child in a hot bath, wrap hot or cold cloths about the throat and put one teaspoonful of common soda in a glass of water and give one teaspoonful every fifteen minutes until relieved.

3. Dr. Holt of New York, says.--The room should be very warm, hot cloths or poultices should be applied over the throat (Adam's apple and below) and either a croup kettle or ordinary teakettle kept boiling in the room. This is more efficacious if the child is placed in a tent made by a raised umbrella or some like method with a sheet thrown over it, and the steam introduced beneath the tent. If the symptoms' are urgent ten drops of the syrup of ipecac should be given every fifteen minutes until free vomiting occurs.

Whenever the symptoms reach a point where the breathing becomes difficult, a doctor should be summoned without delay. It might be some other disease.

4. Home Treatment.--One-half teaspoonful of alum mixed with molasses or honey will produce vomiting and help. This is very good when the croup is due to indigestion. At the same time, fry onions in lard and put them on the neck in front, or hot wet cloths may do. The alum can be given once or twice if necessary, half an hour apart, about in one-fourth or one-half the first dose.

5. Goose grease, or lard dissolved, and enough given to produce vomiting will do good. This idea is not only to cause vomiting but to cause a sick feeling after and at that time, which will cause the spasms to relax. A very good thing to do in addition is to put the child's feet in hot water, while local applications are put on the throat. These things tend to relax the muscles and this relieves the spasm.

6. Steam is Very Useful. It relaxes the spasm by local contact and by producing general sweating. Cover the child's head and a pitcher with a shawl and inhale the steam from the boiling water in pitcher. You can put in the pitcher one teaspoonful of oil of tar or one to two teaspoonfuls of tincture of benzoin. This can be kept up for some time.

COLD IN THE CHEST. (Acute Bronchitis. Inflammation of Bronchial Tubes).--This is an acute inflammation of the larger and medium sized bronchial tubes.

Causes.--Youth and old age are more predisposed to it. Lack of fresh air and exercise, dusty work, poor general health, dampness and changeable weather in winter and early spring. It may be secondary to cold, pharyngitis, measles, typhoid fever, malaria, asthma, and heart disease.

Symptoms.--There is a feeling of oppression with chilliness and pain in the back, a dry, tight feeling beneath the breastbone with a dry harsh cough. This may cause headache and pain, and a raw feeling in the chest, chiefly in front. There may be a temperature of one hundred or one hundred three or less. After a few days there is a thick, sticky secretion; it is profuse. The other symptoms, except the cough, subside. This generally stops in ten days in a favorable case, or it may become chronic. In infants or old people it may extend to the smaller tubes causing broncho-pneumonia. There is more danger in infants than in older people.

MOTHERS' REMEDIES. Bronchitis, Camphor and Lard for.--1. "Grease a cloth well with lard to which has been added some camphor gum, then sprinkle on some dry baking soda and lay it on the chest. The camphor and lard should be made into a salve, then put on the soda. The lard and camphor gum penetrates the affected parts, relieving the inflammation and tightness in the chest. It is well in children to put a layer of cotton cloth over the chest keeping them warm and getting better results from the remedy.

2. Bronchitis, Grandmother's Remedy for.--

"Hoarhound	5 cents worth
Hops	5 cents worth
Wild cherry bark	5 cents worth
Licorice root	5 cents worth

Boil and simmer altogether in two quarts of water long enough to get the strength out of the ingredients, strain, add three cups sugar, then add enough good whisky to keep from souring, say a half pint." This combination is not only good for bronchitis, but for the cough left from the effects of bronchitis. The hoarhound, wild cherry bark and licorice root have a very soothing effect on the bronchial tubes, and the hops quiets the nervous system. This is also good for a common cough.

3. Bronchitis, Antiphlogistine Plaster for.--"Antiphlogistine is fine for bronchitis, where there is any inflammation, pleurisy, any kind of a scratch, especially rusty nails; pneumonia, Set can in water long enough to heat, but not hot, spread on with case knife as thick as a silver dollar, spread cotton batting over it, keep on twenty-four hours, before changing. This is a very useful remedy to keep on hand." Antiphlogistine is very good to apply to the body wherever inflammation is present, as it withdraws the blood from the organ or part of the body that is affected. It does this by drawing the blood into the external circulation. It has the same effect upon the diseased parts as the old-fashioned mustard, but does not blister. In using the mustard plaster you are in fear of blistering, and then having the outward blister and inward inflammation to contend with. The antiphlogistine can be purchased at drug stores. Set the can in warm water until it is warm, then spread on a piece of cotton cloth and apply to the affected parts, where it may remain for twenty-four hours, then repeat if necessary. Should always be put on warm, but not *hot.* It usually drops off when dry and no longer effective.

4. Bronchial, or any Severe Cough. One of the best Home Remedies.--

"Hoarhound (herb form)	1 ounce
Irish moss	1 ounce
Flax Seed (the seed not pulverized)	1 ounce
Boneset	1 ounce
Licorice Root (cut up fine)	1 ounce

Place the above in some suitable pan or dish for such purpose in a gallon of cold water, and put it on the back of the stove, so that it will simmer slowly until reduced to one-half gallon, which may require one day or more, then strain and place in a bottle, or bottles. Dose.--One wineglassful three times a day. Add a little sugar if desired." This is a very fine cough remedy, as the hoarhound loosens the cough, the flax seed soothes the membrane, and the boneset by its general action on the system produces sweating. The Irish moss is a sort of food for the whole system and helps to build a person up.

5. Bronchitis, Camphorated Oil and Steaming for.--"Bathe the chest and throat up around the head with camphorated oil; drink water and steam the throat and mouth over hot water. Have tried this recipe and found it effectual. Have a bronchial cough now and am treating it myself." The camphorated oil seems to have a very soothing effect upon the chest, in fact it acts about the same as camphor and lard, only is more pleasant to use, and can be bought already prepared. Drinking plenty of water cleanses the system by acting upon the stomach, bowels and kidneys, carrying off the impurities. The breathing of steam is very soothing and healing to the throat and air passages.

6. Bronchitis, General Relief for.--"Dose of castor oil every night; one teaspoonful for child. Grease well with camphorated oil or any good oil." The castor oil is very good for carrying off the phlegm from the stomach and bowels that children always swallow instead of coughing up like an older person. It is well in addition to the above remedy to give a little licorice or onion syrup to relieve the bronchial cough.

7. Bronchitis, Lard Poultice for.--"Take a piece of cotton batting large enough to cover chest and fit up close to the neck; wring out of melted lard as hot as the patient can stand it, and apply. Change as often as it gets cold. Also give dose of castor oil."

8. Bronchitis, Mustard Plaster for.--"Mustard plasters are very good." This acts as a counter-irritant, as it draws the blood to the surface and relieves the inflamed bronchial tubes.

9. Bronchitis, Well-Known Remedy for.--

"Cod Liver Oil	2 ounces
Ginger Syrup	2 ounces
Mucilage of Gum Arabic	2 ounces
Oil of Cloves	6 drops

Dose :-Teaspoonful before meals and at bedtime."

This is a very good remedy, as the cod liver oil by its general action tones up the whole system. The ginger tones and stimulates the stomach and takes away the sickening effect of the cod liver oil.

10. Bronchitis Remedy and General Tonic.--"Take small doses of glycerin and one teaspoonful three times a day of codfish oil." This remedy, though simple, is very effective. The glycerin and codfish oil are both soothing to the affected parts, and the codfish oil is a very good tonic to tone up the general system.

1. PHYSICIANS' TREATMENT for Bronchitis. Sweating Remedy for.--Take a hot bath and then go to bed, and take hot drinks after. See that the bowels are open. Nourishment is especially important in infants and old age. You can sweat them as directed under la grippe. Drink hot drinks, such as hoarhound, ginger, flaxseed, hot lemonade or slippery elm. These will produce sweating and will give much relief. An onion poultice applied over the breastbone where the pain and tightness are, will do good.

2. Steaming Remedy.--Inhaling steam from plain boiling water is good, or you can add one to two teaspoonfuls of compound tincture of benzoin or turpentine. The steaming will be more effective if you make a tent, by fastening four sticks to the cradle or bed and cover with a sheet, introducing the steam underneath this at the foot of the bed, etc. A rubber tube can be fastened to the kettle. In this same way you can produce, if you wish, sweating by putting the end of the tube under the clothes elevated a little above the patient. Be careful not to scald the patient.

3. Steaming With Pitcher.--If the soreness of the bronchial tubes is not relieved by this means, inhalations of steam arising from boiling water may be practiced, either through a cone, one end of which covers the top of a pitcher, and the other end of which covers the mouth and nose of the patient, or by covering the head and pitcher with a towel. The usefulness of this method may be much increased by the addition of from two teaspoonfuls to one tablespoonful of compound tincture of benzoin to each pint of water in a pitcher. This latter method can also be used in tonsillitis, pharyngitis and quinsy.

4. Rub the chest with a camphor liniment and give the following:

Tincture of Aconite	10 drops
Sweet Spirits of Nitre	2 drams
Distilled water to make	4 ounces

Mix--One-half teaspoonful to a child, or dessert spoonful to an adult in water every hour.

5. For Adults.--Compound licorice mixture one to two drams every three to four hours; or five grains of Dover's powders every three to four hours.

Diet in Bronchitis (similar to Laryngitis).--Drinks are useful in the dryer forms, such as hot flaxseed tea sweetened and flavored with lemon juice. It should be taken in large quantities. Hot milk and lemonade are also useful.

CHRONIC BRONCHITIS. Causes.--People over middle age are more liable to it. It comes chiefly in winter, in changeable, cold and damp climates. It may follow repeated acute attacks.

Symptoms.--These are variable and are present chiefly in winter and damp weather. The cough is worse at night, and in the morning, expectoration is usually great. There may be slight fever at times. Often the patients are entirely free from the trouble during the summer.

PHYSICIANS' TREATMENT for Chronic Bronchitis. Preventive.--Warm equable climate, such as southern California, Florida, or the south of France, especially in the colder months; warm clothing, avoid exposure and fatigue.

1. First you can take three grains of ammonium chloride three to four times a day.

2.	Ammonium Chloride	2 drams
	Fluid Extract of Licorice	2 drams
	Distilled water brought to	3 ounces

Mix and take one teaspoonful every three hours.

3. If the cough is troublesome the following is good:

Ammonium Chloride	2 drams
Hive Syrup	4 drams
Fluid Extract Licorice	1 ounce
Paregoric	6 drams
Distilled water enough to make	2 ounces

Mix. Teaspoonful every three to four hours.

COUGHS. Causes.--There are many causes; inflammation of the larynx, bronchial tubes, lungs, also stomach and liver; and a nervous cough is present in our day. Remove the cause when possible. There are many good cough medicines now put up, and they can be bought at any drug-store. Cough lozenges of all kinds are plenty, and a sure cure is claimed by each.

MOTHERS' REMEDIES. Dry Cough and Tickling.--l. "Raspberry Tincture. Take one-half pound of honey, one cup water; let these boil; take off scum; pour boiling hot upon one-half ounce lobelia herb and one-half ounce cloves; mix well, then strain and add one gill of raspberry vinegar. Take from one teaspoonful to a dessertspoonful four times a day. Pleasant to take,"

2. Cough, Honey and Vinegar for.--"Honey and vinegar." This is an old and tried remedy and a good one. The vinegar cuts the phlegm in the throat and bronchial tubes, and the honey is very soothing.

3. Cough of Long Standing, Excellent Syrup for.--

"Carbonate Ammonia	40 grains
Syrup Senega	6 drams
Paregoric	4 drams
Syrup Wild Cherry	6 drams
Syrup Tolu	4 ounces"

This is a very good syrup, and is especially good for chronic cough or chronic bronchitis. Dose.--One teaspoonful every three hours.

4. Cough, Reliable Mixture in Severe Cases.--

"Oil of Anise	1/2 ounce
Syrup of Balsam of Tolu	1/2 ounce
Black Stick Licorice	1/2 ounce
Best Rye Whisky	1 pint

Shake well before using. Dose:--One teaspoonful at intervals of one hour or oftener; if cough is very bad."

5. Cough, Mullein Leaf Tea for--"Mullein leaves steeped with loaf sugar cures a cough." Take four ounces of mullein leaves and boil for ten minutes in water: then add the loaf sugar. This is very soothing to the sore parts and also helps to loosen up the secretion so it can be raised easily.

6. Cough, Lemon Juice and Sugar for.--"Lemon juice and sugar is a good remedy for coughs." It is surprising to see how quickly the lemon juice will cut the phlegm in throat, and sugar is always good for cold.

7. Cough, Standard Remedy for.--

"Hoarhound	Five cents worth
Hops	Five cents worth
Wild cherry bark	Five cents worth
Licorice root	Five cents worth

Boil or simmer altogether in two quarts of water long enough to get the strength out of the ingredients; strain, add three cups sugar. Add enough good whiskey to keep from souring, say one-half pint. This will cure a stubborn cough."

8. Cough, Ipecac Syrup for.--"One-third teaspoonful of ipecac dissolved in one teaspoonful of water; one tablespoonful of sugar; pour on one teacupful of boiling water and let it boil down to half cup. Dose.--One teaspoonful for adults, and children in proportion, every two hours, or, if needed to vomit children give again in ten or fifteen minutes."

9. Cough Remedy for Adults (not for children).--

"Laudanum	Three cents worth
Anise	Three cents worth
Essence of Peppermint	Three cents worth
Licorice (liquid)	Three cents worth
Brown Sugar	1 cup
Molasses	1 cup
Boiling water	2 cups

Let this come to a little more than a boil. Take a teaspoonful of it as often as necessary." This is for adults. Do not use for children.

10. Coughs, Very Simple Remedy for.--"Take one-half tablespoonful hogs' lard or salt pork grease, heat it hot, fill spoon with coal oil and swallow while hot. Have used this, will stop and cure the worst cough." Not to be given to children.

11. Coughs, Glycerin, Brandy and Paregoric with Lemon, Good for.--"Glycerin, one ounce; brandy, one ounce; paregoric, one ounce; lemon juice, one ounce. Mix well; one teaspoonful every hour." This makes a very effective cough syrup. The glycerin and brandy cut the phlegm, and the paregoric is soothing and quieting. The lemon juice is healing to the membranes of the throat.

PHYSICIANS'TREATMENT. For Coughs.--

1.	Flaxseed (unground)	3 teaspoonfuls
	Extract of Licorice	30 grains
	Boiling water	10 ounces

Allow the mixture to stand one to four hours in a warm place. Then add a little lemon juice and sugar and place one to two teaspoonfuls of gum arabic in the pitcher containing the mixture." A little paregoric (ten drops to the dose for adults) can be taken with it if the cough is very bad. Dose.--Drink freely every two to three hours.

2. A good combination is the following:

Chloride of Ammonia	2 drams
Fluid Extract of Licorice	2 drams
Distilled water	20 ounces

Mix. Teaspoonful every two hours or longer.

3.	Ammonium Carbonate	1/2 dram
	Syrup Senega	4 drams
	Wine of Ipecac	3 drams
	Syrup Totu	1 ounce
	Spirits of Chloroform	3 drams
	Syrup of Wild Cherry enough to make	4 ounces

Mix. Take one to two teaspoonfuls every hour or two until better.

4.	Ammonia Chloride	2 drams
	Hive Syrup	5 drams
	Paregoric	6 drams
	Syrup of Wild Cherry	4 ounces

Mix. Teaspoonful every three hours until cough is better.

5. Many other combinations could be given. Hoarhound tea. Sugar enough to sweeten makes a good cough remedy.

6. Onion syrup is good for children. The bowels should always be kept open.

BRONCHIAL ASTHMA. (Spasmodic Asthma.) Causes.--It occurs in all ages, but usually begins in the young, particularly males. It often follows whooping-cough. It may come from diseases of the mouth such as adenoids, polypi. Exciting causes are change of climate and residence, dust, smoke, odors, errors in diet, emotion, and cold.

Symptoms.--The onset is often sudden, often during the night. Difficulty of breathing is intense. The patient cannot lie down, but often sits at an open window, resting the elbows on a table. The face is pale and the expression is anxious. There is a feeling of great oppression in the chest and often dread of suffocation. Respiration (breathing) though labored, is not unusually frequent, as expiration (out breathing) is much prolonged. In severe or prolonged attacks there are blueness, sweating, coldness of the extremities, with small and frequent pulse and great drowsiness. The attack lasts a few minutes to many hours, and may pass off suddenly, perhaps to recur soon, or on several successive nights, with slight cough and difficulty in breathing in the intervals. The cough is nearly dry at first and the sputum is very tenacious.

MOTHERS' REMEDIES. 1. Asthma, Raspberry Tincture for Adults.--"Take a half pound of honey, one cup water; let these boil, take off the scum; pour boiling hot upon one-half ounce lobelia herb and one-half ounce cloves; mix well, then strain and add one gill of raspberry vinegar. Take from one teaspoonful to a dessertspoonful four times a day. Pleasant to take." The above remedy is very effective, as the honey has a soothing effect upon the inflamed parts, and the lobelia causes the bronchial tubes to dilate, relieving the patient. The raspberry tincture makes it more pleasant to take. In severe cases it will be necessary to give enough of the above remedy to cause vomiting which relieves the phlegm.

2. Asthma, Simple but Effective Remedy for.--"Take pieces of ordinary blotting paper and saturate it with a strong solution of saltpetre, then dry the paper. When a paroxysm is felt ignite a piece of the paper and inhale the smoke. This remedy is very good and acts quickly, doing away almost entirely with the distressing symptoms and shortens the paroxysm."

3. Asthma, Lobelia Tea for.--"There is no medicine that is half so effective as lobelia in removing the tough, hard ropy phlegm from the asthmatic persons." This remedy is very good, but care should be taken not to give it to consumptives, because it is too weakening. To obtain the best results, enough of the remedy should be given to produce relaxation of the bronchial tubes. Dose.--For adults should be from fifteen to sixty drops according to the strength of the patient. This will cause a little sickness of the stomach and vomiting, thus relaxing the muscles and relieving the asthma.

PHYSICIANS' TREATMENT for Asthma.--1. Inhale chloroform, or break a pearl of amyl nitrite in a handkerchief and inhale the fumes; or smoke saltpetre paper; or cigarettes containing stramonium (thornapple). Sometimes hot coffee fumes are good.

To Prevent Recurrence.--Take five to twenty grains of iodide of potash three times a day. Do not eat much at night. Do not eat foods that cause gas or that are hard to digest. A change of climate is often good. Hot foot baths and hot drinks are helpful. Tincture of lobelia can be given in severe cases, fifteen drops repeated every half hour until the patient feels sick at the stomach.

2. Vapo-Cresolene burned in a room is very good. This can be bought in twenty-five cent bottles in any drug store, with directions around the bottle.

3. Tartar Emetic in one-hundredth grain, two given every half hour until there is a little sickening is a very good remedy. These can be bought at a drug store or from a homeopathic doctor or pharmacist.

BLEEDING FROM THE WIND-PIPE AND LUNGS. (Haemoptysis).--This is a spitting of blood. It may come from the small bronchial tubes and less frequently from the blood vessels in the lung cavities or their walls.

Symptoms.--In incipient consumption of the lungs, bleeding develops suddenly as a rule, a warm salty taste, lasting but a few moments, generally preceded by the spitting up of blood. The blood is coughed up and the bleeding may last only a few minutes or it may continue for days, the sputum being apt to remain blood-stained for a longer time. The immediate effect of the bleeding is to alarm the patient and family, no matter how slight it may be, inducing heart palpitation and other nervous symptoms. A small bleeding is not attended with any bad result, but large ones give rise to the symptoms of shock (sometimes immediate death) combined with anemia following the loss of blood. When the bleeding is large, blood by the mouthful may be ejected with each cough, and in these instances of such profuse bleeding is shown by dizziness, faintness, cold extremities, excessive pallor, sweating and rapid, small feeble pulse. This is followed, if the attack does not prove speedily fatal, by restlessness, and later by mild delirium and some fever. In few cases does the patient have a single bleeding; more frequently there are several at shorter or longer intervals. Large or small bleedings may precede by weeks, months, or even years any rational symptoms of consumption.

Quantity.--This varies greatly. There may be less than an ounce or it might amount to a pint or more before the bleeding stops. In advanced cases, in which large cavities have formed, large blood vessels may be eaten through and this followed by copious and alarming bleeding.

MOTHERS' REMEDIES.--1. Bleeding from the Lungs. Salt Water for.--"Give the patient half a teaspoonful of common salt every hour or two until hemorrhage abates."

2. Bleeding from the Lungs. Herb Tea for.--"Two ounces each of bistory root, tormentil root, oak bark, and comfrey root, boil in three quarts of water down to one pint, strain and add one tablespoonful of ground ginger. Give a wine glass full every half hour until relieved.

Place the feet in hot mustard water, keep the bowels open with a little senna and ginger tea and if necessary give a vapor bath,"

3. Bleeding from the Lungs, Effective Remedy for.--

"Powdered Sugar	3 ounces
Powdered Rosin	3 ounces

Mix. Dose one teaspoonful three times a day."

4. Bleeding from the Lungs, Tannin and Sugar for.-

"Tannin	30 grains
Powdered Sugar	1 dram

Mix. Make ten powders and give one every ten minutes until relieved."

Either one of the above remedies is excellent for this trouble, as the tannin and rosin contract the arteries and acts as an astringent.

PHYSICIANS' TREATMENT for Bleeding of the Wind-pipe and Lungs.--In many cases the bleeding is slight and no more need be done than to keep the patient quiet and absolute rest. If the bleeding is free, the patient should be placed in bed, not allowed to speak above a whisper nor to change his position.

1. First Thing to Do.--Eating ice, and using ice drinks are useful measures. The drinking of a little salt water at a time with one tablespoonful of salt in a glassful of water is good. In most cases more can be done by assuring the patient he will not die and keeping him quiet and at rest. Medicines should be given to satisfy the patient and family. The most cases stop of themselves.

2. If Caused by Coughing.--If cough causes the bleeding one-half grain of opium should be given to control it, hypodermically, or even morphine one-eighth grain.

3. Alum for.--Alum solution six grains to three ounces of water in fine spray is good. This goes right to the wind-pipe and contracts the vessels; use a vaporizer.

4. White Oak Bark Tea can be used as a spray in a vaporizer. If these produce coughing, they should be discontinued.

5. Hot Water and Salt for.--A teaspoonful of salt in a pint of hot water is good also, used as a spray, or to inhale. But the patient must lie down.

6. Other Easily Obtained Remedies.--Ergot in dose of one-half to one teaspoonful is very good; this contracts the vessels. Bromide of potash in a dose of five to fifteen grains; or chloral hydrate in dose of five to seven grains, if there is not heart trouble. If there is, chloral hydrate cannot be used. These quiet the nervous system and do much good. Strong hop tea will do the same thing if taken freely. Witch-hazel water thirty drops at a dose is good.

Cautions.--Quiet the patient; keep quiet yourself. If the bleeding is bad the extremities should be bandaged, beginning at the toes and fingers.

Thirst.--Give small quantities at a time of ice-water.

Diet.--Peptonized or plain milk, liquid beef peptonoids, fresh beef juice, bouillon, should be given in small quantities, two or three ounces every two or three hours. If there is a tendency to constipation give rectal enemata. Return to the regular diet as soon as possible. Alcohol in any form is best avoided. If given as a stimulant it should be given in small quantities.

BRONCHO-PNEUMONIA. (Acute Inflammation of the Smaller Tubes and Lungs).--

Causes.--Most common under two years and in old people. Taking cold, whooping cough and measles.

Symptoms.--A primary case begins suddenly with a convulsion or chill, vomiting and rapid rise of temperature. Breathing is frequent and brain symptoms are marked.

Secondary Cases.--After an ordinary case of whooping-cough, measles, bronchitis, etc., there is more fever. The pulse is more frequent, and also the respiration, difficulty in breathing and severe and often painful cough. Temperature rises to 102 to 104; respirations are very fast, up to 60 to 80; the breathing (inspiration) is hard, labored, while the wings of the nose dilate; expiration may be grunting. Face looks anxious and bluish. This color may increase, other symptoms decreasing as suffocation deepens, rattling in chest and death from heart weakness.

Prevention.--Avoid exposure to sudden changes of temperature. For the attack, jacket of oil silk or flannel to prevent sudden exposure, keep the temperature warmed up to 68 to 70 degrees night and day; the air must be fresh and pure and changed regularly.

Children should be given ample room and not hampered by extra clothing, as they like change of position, to get relief. The hot bath must be used often to redden the skin and relieve the pressure on the lungs, till they can be given relief. If you wish to use a poultice the following is a nice way to make it. Take a piece of muslin or linen, or cheese-cloth, wide enough when doubled to reach from the lower margin of the ribs to well up under the arm pits, and long enough to go a little more than around the chest, open the double fold and spread the hot mass of poultice on one-half of the cloth and fold the other over it. It should be applied as hot as it can be comfortably borne and covered with oil silk or paraffin paper, so as to the longer retain the heat and moisture. The poultice should be renewed as often as it gets cold, and a fresh poultice should be all ready to put on when the old one is taken off. Place the end of the poultice uppermost, so that the contents will not fall out.

MOTHERS' REMEDIES. 1. Pneumonia, Herb Tea and Poultice for.--"Congestion of the lungs. One ounce of each of the following, slippery elm bark, crushed thyme, coltsfoot flowers, hyssop or marshmallow. Simmer in two quarts of water down to three pints; strain and add one teaspoonful of cayenne. Dose:--Wineglassful every half hour. Apply hot bran poultices or chamomile scalded in vinegar, changing often until the violence of the symptoms abate. If the bowels are confined, give an injection of half pint of hot water in which one-half teaspoonful each of gum myrrh, turkey rhubarb and ginger powder have been well mixed. If possible give vapor bath. Apply hot stones or bottles to the feet."

2. Pneumonia, Home Remedy for.--"This can easily be relieved by the use of cayenne and vapor bath. This promotes the circulation in every part of the body, diminishing the pressure upon the lungs. These baths produce a regular circulation throughout the whole body, thus relieving the pressure upon the lungs by decreasing the amount of blood in the lungs. These baths should be taken but once a day, as they are weakening."

3. Pneumonia, Hot Vinegar Applications for.--Congestion of Lungs.--"Over the lungs lay cloths wet in clear hot vinegar. They should be five or six inches square and several thicknesses. Over the cloths lay a hot plate or hot water bottle; change as often as necessary to keep them hot. This treatment will soon give relief, after which rub as much oil into the lungs as possible."

PHYSICIANS' TREATMENT for Pneumonia.--A doctor must be called. For high fever, one to one and a half drops of aconite, for adults every hour; for children, about one-twelfth to one-eighth of a drop. For cough, chloride of ammonium, one to two grain doses. For pain, hot applications.

Diet.--Milk, broth and egg albumen and plenty of water to drink. (See laryngitis for diet.)

ACUTE PLEURISY (Inflammation of the Pleura).--The pleura covers the wall of the chest cavity and infolds or surrounds the lungs. Pleurisy means the inflammation of this pleura or covering.

Causes.--Exposure to cold, etc. Onset may be gradual or sudden, with chills fever and sharp stitches in the side near the arm pit or breast. The patient lies on the affected side during the attack, the pain is made worse by breathing, coughing or motion. The cough is dry and painful, with difficult breathing. The temperature 102 to 103. Sometimes there is fluid accumulated in the cavity. In about seven to ten days the fever and other symptoms disappear. The fluid is absorbed quickly if it is scanty, often very slowly if abundant. This fluid is contained in the cavity of the pleura. The pleura covers the lungs. Its outer layer is attached to the ribs and costal cartilages in front and ribs behind, goes around the foot of the lungs underneath, then turns around under the side of the lungs and comes in front, making a sac. The two layers in health touch each other, but are separated when there is fluid in the cavity. The inner layer covers the lungs and drops into the grooves of the lungs. You can thus readily understand how easy it is for the pleura to be attacked. Also when the lung is inflamed we have what we call pleura-pneumonia. Pleurisy is a very painful disease. It hurts to move, breathe, or cough. The patient holds his chest when he coughs. The fluid that forms is poured out from the inflamed membrane, sometimes it is so great in quantity it must be drawn off,--tapped; we then call this hydrothorax,--water in the chest.

Diet and Nursing--The patient should be kept quiet and in the easiest position.

Milk diet is the best to use. There should not be much liquid diet, except milk. The milk may be diluted with lime water if necessary. Malted milk, Mellin's food, imperial granum, can be used when the milk cannot be taken.

PHYSICIANS' TREATMENT for Pleurisy.--1. Home Remedy.--The patient must go to bed and remain there. It is a good thing to get the patient in a sweat. For this purpose you can use the corn sweat described under treatment of la grippe. This will ease the patient and may shorten the attack.

I have great faith in this remedy in most inflammatory diseases. I had a patient sick with pleurisy; she did not get along fast enough to suit me, her color was a yellow-green. I advised the corn sweat and she improved fast from that time. Her night dress was green in color after the sweat. I have saved pneumonia cases in the same way. Of course, some cases may be too weak to stand it.

2. Other Home Remedies.--Another way to produce sweating is by placing fruit cans filled with hot water about the patient. This will stop the chilly cold feeling and also will relieve the pain. If you have a rubber water bottle, put hot water in that and place it near the sorest spot. It may hurt the patient by its weight; if so, use less water, at the same time you can give hot drinks freely. Almost any kind will do. If the stomach feels bad, ginger or peppermint is best. Hoarhound tea is especially good for chest trouble.

3. Fomentations.--Of hops or wormwood or smartweed, or catnip applied frequently and hot to the affected side often bring relief. They must always be hot, and you must be careful not to get the night robes or covers wet.

4. Camphorated Oil for.--Rub the side with camphorated oil and cover over with a cotton jacket. This is good unless it makes the patient too warm.

5. Adhesive Plaster Zinc Oxide.--Use a roll two or two and one-half inches wide. Commence at the backbone and cross directly over the ribs to the further side of the breastbone. The first strip should be at the lower part of the chest. In putting on the succeeding strips make them lap one-half inch over the next lower. Bandage almost up to the arm-pit. It may take eight strips for an adult. After you have the strips on, place a piece at each end, part on the flesh and part on the plasters, to keep them from giving any. The patient should have his arms over his head when you are putting on the strips. This strapping will hold that side of the chest quieter. The breathing will be less full and consequently less motion and pain.

6. Tincture of aconite in doses of one-tenth to one drop can be given everyone to three hours at the beginning, if there is much fever, dry hot skin, and full bounding pulse. Dover's powder can be given at night.

7. A hypodermic of morphine is frequently given when the pain is intense.

ABSCESS OF THE LUNGS. Causes.--Lobular pneumonia from abscesses in pyemia, from septic pleurisy, etc.

Symptoms.--Fever, pain, difficult breathing, cough, and expectoration containing or consisting of pus of offensive odor, etc.

PHYSICIANS' TREATMENT of Abscess of the Lungs.--Incision and drainage. You must depend entirely upon your physician.

EMPHYSEMA.--A condition in which there is air or gas in tissues that normally have none, or an excess of air in tissues that normally contain a certain quantity of it. A condition of the lungs characterized by a permanent dilation of the air cells of the lung with dwindling of the air cell walls and the blood vessels, resulting in a loss of the normal elasticity of the lung tissue.

Causes.--Heredity; it occurs in glass blowers, in musicians using wind instruments. It occurs also after whooping-cough, asthma, etc.

HYDROTHORAX.--This is an exudation (liquid) in the pleural cavity.

Causes.--Comes from disease causing dropsy, kidney disease, lung trouble, pleurisy, etc.

PHYSICIANS' TREATMENT.--Treat disease that causes it. An operation to remove the fluid may be necessary. A trusted physician must advise you.

NIGHT SWEATS.--These are common in "consumption" and

constitute one of the most distressing features of the disease. They usually occur when the fever drops in the early morning hours, or at any time of the day when the patient is sleeping. They may come on early in the disease, but are more persistent and frequent after cavities have formed in the lungs; some of the patients escape it altogether.

MOTHERS' REMEDIES.-l. Night Sweats, Salt Bath for.-- "Bathe the body in salt water every other day. Just before retiring take a cup of sage tea, and eat nourishing food," The salt acts as an astringent as it slightly closes up the pores, and the sage establishes a better circulation and at the same time helps the sweating. This is a very simple and effective remedy.

2. Night Sweats, Cold Sage for.--"Drink cold sage tea, before retiring." This cold sage tea is only to be used when the patient has a fever and needs a cold drink. In case of this kind it would be effective.

PHYSICIAN'S TREATMENT for Night Sweats.--l. Atropine in doses of 1-120 to 1-60 grain is good to stop the sweating. It must be used carefully, three doses in twenty-four hours are enough.

2. Tonics to keep up the appetite like gentian, nux vomica or quinine may be given. The patient should wear flannel night-dresses, as the cotton night-shirt, when soaked with perspiration, has a cold, clammy feeling. Bathe the patient in the morning with tepid water and afterwards rub gently with alcohol diluted one-half with water. Night sweating occurs in rickets but mainly around the head. They also occur when one is run down, but they are not so debilitating and constant. In such cases, building up treatment is needed. Proper diet, bathing, outdoor life, bitter tonics, etc.

ANIMAL PARASITES, DISEASES CAUSED BY.

ROUND WORM.--(Ascariasis Lumbricoides).--The round worm resembles the angle worm in form; is the most common human parasite and is found chiefly in children. The female is seven to twelve inches long, the male four to eight inches. It is pointed at both ends. The parasite occupies the upper part of the small bowel and there is usually only one or two present, but sometimes they occur in enormous numbers. They migrate in a peculiar manner. They may pass into the stomach, whence they may be thrown out by vomiting, or they may crawl up the gullet, and enter the pharynx and cause serious trouble. They may go up the eustachian tube and appear at the external meatus (opening of ear). The serious migration is into the bile-duct. There is a specimen in the Wister-Horner Museum of the University of Pennsylvania in which not only the common bile-duct, but also the main branches throughout the liver, are enormously distended, and packed with numerous round worms. The bowel may be blocked or in rare instances an ulcer may be perforated; even the healthy bowel may be perforated.

Symptoms.--Picking of the nose, grinding of the teeth, a whitish paleness around the mouth, restless sleep; sometimes convulsions, or presence of worms in the stool. Bad health, cross, peevish, irritable and dumpy, when the child is naturally the opposite.

MOTHERS' REMEDIES.--l. Round or Pin Worms, Sage Tea for.--"Sage tea is a fine remedy for children troubled with worms, taken before breakfast or on going to bed." Sage tea may help; I have known other mothers to have faith in it. Its virtue may consist in being a laxative and an antiseptic which in themselves would add to the general health of the child.

2. Round and Pin Worms, Tansy remedy for.--"Tansy leaves may be crushed and put in whisky or dried and crushed with sugar. This is the best vermifuge I ever used." A tea made of tansy leaves must be used carefully as it is strong and never given to pregnant women.

3. Round and Pin Worms, Peach Leaf Tea for.--"Half an ounce of dried peach leaves may be infused in a pint of boiling water and a tablespoonful given for a dose three times a day." They are laxative and exert a sedative influence over the nervous system. They have been frequently used for worms with reported success. An infusion is highly recommended in irritability of the bladder, in sick stomach and in whooping cough.

PHYSICIANS' TREATMENT.--l. Dr. Osler, of Oxford, England, recommends as follows: Santonin in doses of two or three grains for an adult; one or two a day for three or four days, followed by salts or calomel; one-half to one grain for children in the same way. This seems to me to be unnecessarily large.

2. Dr. Ritter's Santonin Remedy.--

I always give it thus:

Santonin	1/10 grain
Calomel	1/10 grain

Give four a day for two days, then miss two days, then give again for two days and stop. Salts can be given after this. I then follow this treatment by giving one drop doses of tincture of cina (Homeopathic preparation) four times a day for one or two weeks. Before giving any of these remedies it is well to move the bowels freely and also after the medicine has been stopped.

3. Dr. Douglass of Detroit, Michigan, recommends the following for a child five to ten years old:

Santonin	12 grains
Calomel	3 grains

Divide into six powders, and give one night and morning while fasting.

4. The following is from Professor Stille:

Spigelia	1/2 ounce
Senna	2 drams
Fennel seed	2 drams
Manna	1 ounce
Boiling water	1 pint

Mix and make into an infusion (tea). Dose for a child, one or two teaspoonfuls. For an adult, one or two wineglassfuls.

THREAD WORM OR PIN WORM.--(Oxyuris Vermicularis.)--This common worm occupies the rectum and colon. They produce great irritation and itching, particularly at night, symptoms which become intensely aggravated by the nightly migration (traveling) of the parasite. They sometimes in their travels enter the vagina. Occasionally abscesses are formed around the bowel (rectum) containing numbers of worms. The patient becomes extremely restless and irritable, for the sleep is very often disturbed, and there may be loss of appetite and also anemia. These worms are most common in children, but they can occur in all ages. The worms can easily be seen in the feces. The infection takes place through the drinking of water and possibly through salads, such as lettuce and cresses, and various other means. A person who is the subject of worms passes ova (eggs) in large numbers in the feces, and the possibility of reinfection must be guarded against very scrupulously.

MOTHERS' REMEDIES.--1. Pin worms, Aloes treatment for.--"Pin worms or seat worms are usually found in children and sometime cause a great deal of annoyance to the child. They are usually very restless at night and pull at the rectum both day and night. This condition may be relieved by an injection, of powdered aloes,--five grains; hot water one-half pint." This is sufficient for two injections and should be used at about blood heat.

2. Pin worms, Pink Root for.--"Take one ounce pink root, and one pint of water. Make a decoction of this by boiling the above to half a pint. Give a teaspoonful three times a day for two days, following this up by a good dose of castor oil or cream of tartar to thoroughly cleanse the system."

3. Pin worms, Quassia chips for.--"I knew of a child who had not slept three hours a night for several months, and several doctors had been called and none of them seemed to get down to the real trouble. Finally the mother tried an injection made by steeping quassia chips for two or three hours slowly, then straining it and injecting about one pint (luke warm) once a day. This gave the child immediate relief and improvement could be seen within a week."

4. Pin worms, Lime-water injection for.--"A very simple remedy is an injection of a teacupful of lime water once a day, preferably in the morning, as the worms are usually lodged in the rectum and this injection will bring them away, giving the child relief at once."

5. Worms-Stomach, Salt Remedy for.--"Encourage the child to eat as much salt as possible and give an injection of salt and water, about one teaspoonful of salt to two quarts of water, once a day."

PHYSICIANS' TREATMENT.--1. Santonin in small doses and mild purgatives like rhubarb. Santonin in doses of one-tenth of a grain can be given for two days, three or four times a day, preceded by spiced syrup of rhubarb, one dram dose, and also followed by the rhubarb. In children the cold injections of strong salt and water is effective. They should be repeated for ten days. The hips should be well elevated so that the injection can be retained for some time.

2.	Quassia chips	1 ounce
	Common salt	1/2 ounce
	Water	1 pint

Soak over night and inject slowly all the bowels will hold. Repeat once each week till all are removed.

3. Dr. Tooker of Chicago, Illinois, recommends the following:--Give an injection of an infusion of fresh garlic for two or three nights in succession, using, to make the infusion, a small bunch of garlic in a pint of water, steeped down to one-quarter pint.

4. Dr. Tooker gives another method which is often successful.

Anoint the anus for several nights in succession with sweet oil, using the little finger to insert the oil as far into the rectum as the fingers will reach.

5. Another Remedy. Inject cod-liver oil (pure) into the bowel or make into an emulsion with the yolk of an egg and then inject.

6. Spearmint Remedy.--Make an infusion of the common spearmint and inject some in the bowel every night for one week. Some can be taken internally at the same time.

Oil of Wormseed	1/2 ounce
Oil of Turpentine	1-1/2 dram
Castor Oil	2 ounces
Fluid extract of Pink Root	3 drams
Hydrastin	10 grains
Syrup of Peppermint	4 drams

One teaspoonful three times a day one hour before meals to a child ten years old. If it physics to much give less often. Good for both kinds of worms.

8. Tincture of Cina; to accompany any injection.--I give the Tincture of Cina (Homeopathic preparation) in from one-quarter to two or three drop doses, three or four times a day, always after I have given the other worm remedies. It can be given for weeks without producing bad effects. The dose can be made less for weakly children; or greater in grown people. It is good to give in small doses in pin worms when injections are used. It seems to prevent their formation. It is also a good remedy for the worms puppies are troubled with. I have saved the lives of a good many little fellows with this remedy.

TAPE WORM, PORK.-(Taenia Solium). It is six to twelve feet long, but it is not a common form in this country. The head is small, round, not so large as the head of a pin and provided with four sucking ducts and a double row of hooklets. By these hooklets and disks, the parasite attaches itself to the mucous membrane of the small intestine in man. Below the head is a constricted neck, which is followed by a large number of segments, increasing in size from the neck onward. Each segment contains the generative organs of both sexes. The parasite (worm) becomes fully grown in three to three and one-half months. Segments then continually break off and are discharged at stool. Each ovum (egg) contains a single embryo, armed with six hooklets and contained in a thick shell. When swallowed by a pig or man these shells are digested and the embryos migrate (travel) to various parts of the body, where they change to Cysticerci or "Measles." Each contains a scolex or tape-worm. When meat, improperly cooked and containing "measles," is eaten, the cyst is dissolved in the human stomach and the free scolex or head attaches itself to the intestinal mucous membrane and grows into a tapeworm.

TAPE WORM, BEEF.--(Taenia Saginata). This is a larger and longer parasite than the Pork Tape Worm. It is the common form found in this country. It may grow fifteen to twenty feet or more and possesses a large head in comparison with the Taenia Solium. It is square shaped and has four large sucking disks, but no hooklets. The ripe segments are larger and they are passed as in the Taemia Solium, and are eaten by cattle, in the flesh or organs of which the eggs develop into the Cysticerci.

Symptoms.--These worms (parasites) are found at all ages. They are not uncommon in children, and may be found in nursing children. They may cause excessive appetite, nausea, vomiting, diarrhea, or abdominal pain or sometimes anemia. The knowledge of the presence of this worm may cause great nervousness or depression. The presence of the segment in the stools proves their presence in the bowels.

Treatment, preventive.--This is most important. Careful attention should be given to three points: *First,* all tapeworm segments should be burned. They should never be thrown into the water-closet or outside; *secondly,* special inspection of all meat; and, *thirdly,* cooking the meat sufficiently to kill the parasites.

MOTHERS' REMEDIES.--1. Tape Worms, Pumpkin Seed Tea for.--"One pint pumpkin seeds skinned and steeped. Add water enough to make three tumblers. Take one tumbler every half hour, then a good dose of castor oil. The worm will come with oil. My mother helped prepare the seeds and saw the tapeworm which came from a woman as a result of this dose."

2. Tape Worms, Another good Remedy for.--

"Powdered Kamala	3 drams
Syrup simple	3 ounces

Two doses of this mixture hardly ever fails to bring the worm. Give oil and turpentine two hours after the last dose." Of the oil and turpentine an average dose would be a half ounce of castor oil and fifteen drops of turpentine.

3. Tape Worm, Ontario Mother's Remedy for.--"Don't eat until very hungry (extremely so), then eat one-half pint of pumpkin seeds. This is good and will remove the worm every time." This remedy is different from the above in that you eat the seeds instead of making a tea.

4. Tape Worm, Successful Remedy for Children or Adult.--

"Turpentine	15 drops
Castor Oil	1 teaspoonful
Milk	1 teacupful

Mix and for adult take at one dose. If not successful repeat the next day. For child under ten years, one-half the quantity."

PHYSICIANS' TREATMENT.--Preparing the Patient; Giving the Remedy, and Receiving the Worm.--Whenever a round or tape worm is to be attacked, the patient must be starved for at least twelve to twenty-four hours, in order that no food in the intestinal (bowel) tract may protect the worm from the action of the drug. During this time a little milk can be given, and after a night of fasting, before breakfast, the worm medicine (anthelmintic) must be swallowed. In addition, nearly all the drugs must be followed by purges in order to dislodge the intruder while he is paralyzed and has lost his hold; and in many it is well to have a basin of salt and water ready so that when a passage occurs a rectal injection may be given to wash out the segments of the worm which remain in the rectum. I am giving many remedies and the different ways of administering them. Not every one can be cured with the same remedy. One will act better in some people than in others. So I give a variety and they are all good.

1. For two days prior to the administration of the remedies the patient should take a very light, diet and have the bowels moved by a saline (salts) cathartic. As a rule the male fern acts promptly and well. The etheral extract of male fern in two dram doses may be given; fast, and follow in the course of a couple of hours by a brisk purgative; that is, calomel followed by salts.

Fasting means this: Light diet for a day or two and a cathartic at night, no supper except a glass of milk before the worm medicine is given. Then at bed-time take two to three grains of calomel with ten grains of bicarbonate of sodium; rochelle salts, one-half to one ounce, upon awakening. As soon as the bowels have moved give oleorisin of aspidium, one dram in capsules. A saline cathartic should be given one-half to one hour later. Never give castor oil or any oil after this remedy, When calomel is given it should be given about one hour after taking the worm medicine and followed in one or one and one-half hours by a half to one ounce of salts.

2. Pelletierine Remedy for.--This comes in bottles of the proper dose. It is dear, but effective. It must be taken lying down, and followed by some cathartic or a dose of epsom salts in two hours after taking.

3. Infusion and Emulsion for.--An infusion of

Pomegranate root	1/2 ounce
Pumpkin seeds	1 ounce
Powdered ergot	1 dram
Boiling water	10 ounces

To an emulsion of the male fern (a dram of the ethereal extract) made with acacia powders, two drops of croton oil are added. The patient should have had a low diet on the previous day and have taken a dose of salts in the evening.

The emulsion and infusion are mixed and taken at nine in the morning. If the bowels do not move in two hours, salts should be taken.

4. An Old Remedy.--Chew freely of slippery elm bark. This, it is stated, is very effective and as it is cheap and will not injure, it is worth a thorough trial. I am often surprised at the value of the seemingly simple remedies.

TRICHINIASIS (Trichinosis).--The disease is caused by the trichina spiratis, a parasite introduced into the body by eating imperfectly cooked flesh of infected hogs. The "embryos" pass from the bowel and reach the voluntary muscles, where they finally become "encapsulated larvae,"--muscle trichinae. It is in the migration of these embryos that the group of symptoms known as trichiniasis is produced. When the flesh containing the trichinae is eaten by man or by any animal in which the development can take place, the capsules are digested and the trichinae are set free. They pass into the small intestine and about the third day attain their full growth and become sexually mature. The young produced by each female trichina have been estimated at several hundred. The time from the eating of the flesh containing the muscle trichinae to the development of the brood of embryos in the intestines (bowels) is from seven to nine days. The female worm penetrates the intestinal wall and the embryos are probably discharged into the lymph spaces, thence into the venous system, and by the blood stream to the muscles, which constitutes their seat of election. After a preliminary migration in the inter-muscular connective tissue, they penetrate the primitive muscle-fibres and in about two weeks develop into the full grown muscle form. In this process interstitial inflammation of the muscle is excited, and gradually an ovoid capsule develops about the parasite. Two, and occasionally three or four, worms may be seen within a single capsule. This process of encapsulation has been estimated to take about six weeks. Within the muscles the parasites do not undergo further development. Gradually the capsule becomes thicker and ultimately lime salts are deposited within it. This change may take place in man within four or five months. The trichinae may live within the muscles for an indefinite period. They have been found alive and capable of developing as late as twenty or twenty-five years after their entrance into the system. These calcified capsules appear as white specks in the muscles. In many instances however these worms are completely calcified. In the hog the trichinae cause few if any symptoms. An animal, the muscles of which are swarming with living trichinae, may be well nourished and healthy looking. An important point also is the fact that in the hog the capsule does not readily become calcified, so that the parasites are not visible as in the human muscles.

Modes of Infection.--The danger of infection depends entirely upon the mode of preparation of the flesh. Thorough cooking, so that all parts of the meat reach the boiling point, destroys the parasites; but, in larger joints, the central portions are not often raised to this temperature. The frequency of the disease in different countries depends largely upon the habits of the people in the preparation of pork. In North Germany, where raw ham and wurst are freely eaten, the greatest number of instances have occurred. In South Germany, France, and England cases are rare. Salting and smoking the flesh are not always sufficient, and the Havre experiments showed that animals are readily infected when fed with portions of the pickled or the smoked meat as prepared in this country.

Symptoms.--The eating of trichinous flesh is not always followed by this disease.

In the course of a few days after eating the infected meat there are signs of disturbance of the stomach and bowels, and pain in the abdomen, loss of appetite, vomiting and sometimes diarrhea; and yet, these preliminary symptoms do not always occur, for in some of the large epidemics cases have been observed in which they have been absent. Pain in different parts of the body, general debility and weakness have been noted in some of the epidemics. In some instances the stomach and bowel disturbances have been so marked from the outset that the attack resembled our cholera. The invasion symptoms develop between the seventh and tenth day. Sometimes not until the end of the second week, and they are marked by fever, a chill in some cases and pain and swelling and tenderness along the muscles involved. The migration of the parasites into the muscles excites a more or less intense inflammation of these muscles, which is characterized by pain on pressure and movement, and by swelling and tension of the muscles, over which the skin may be swollen. The limbs are placed in some position in which these muscles are more at rest. Difficulty in chewing and swallowing is caused by the involvement of the muscles controlling these acts. In severe cases the involvement of the diaphragm and intercostal muscles may lead to difficult breathing (Dyspnoea) which sometimes proves fatal. Watery swelling, a feature of great importance, may be seen early in the face, particularly about the, eyes. Later it develops in the extremities when the swelling and stiffness of the muscles are at their height. Profuse sweats, tingling and itching of the skin and in some instances hives (Urticaria) have been described.

There are emaciation and anemia. In the severe cases the appearance may be like that in the third week of typhoid fever. In mild cases the fever and muscular symptoms subside in ten to fourteen days, in others only after two or three months. The mortality, from one to thirty per cent, seems to depend upon the virulence and number of parasites.

PHYSICIANS' TREATMENT.--If discovered within twenty-four to thirty-six hours, thoroughly empty the bowel with purgatives. Rhubarb and senna, or an occasional dose of calomel may be given. Relieve the pains afterwards and support the strength.

DISEASES OF THE SKIN.

The skin is divided into three layers. Beginning with the outer one and naming inward, they are named as follows: The outer layer is called the epidermis or cuticle (near or upon the skin). The second layer is called the corium, derma cutis vera, or true skin. The third layer is called the sub-cutaneous (under the skin) (fatty or connective) tissue. This last layer contains the sweat glands, the lower end of the deep-seated hair follicles, (little sacs containing the roots of the hair)

and larger branches of the lymphatics, blood vessels and nerves, and serves in general as a bed for the true skin to rest upon, and by which the true skin is connected with the deeper parts, muscles, etc. The appendages of the skin are the hair, nails, sebaceous and sweat-glands. The discharge from the sweat-glands form a little or larger tumor. The contents of a wen are from sebaceous glands--fat secretions--fat tumor. The following names are frequently mentioned in the skin diseases:

Macule. (Spots, patches). Skin is altered in color, but the skin is not raised or depressed; freckle, etc.

Papule. (Pimple). Elevated piece of skin, varying in size from a pin-head to a coffee bean.

Tubercle. (Node-lump). A solid elevation of the skin, varying in size from a pea to a cherry.

Tumors. These are soft or firm elevations of the skin, like a wen or hard lump. They are always deep-seated.

Wheel. A round flat, white or pink elevation of the skin; such as hives, mosquito bites, etc.

Vesicle. This is a pin-head or pea-sized elevation of the outer layer (epidermis) filled with a watery fluid.

Bleb. (Bulla). A circumscribed elevation of the skin and contains a watery fluid, such as a burn, etc.

Pustule. A rounded elevation of the outer layer (epidermis) of varying size, containing pus (matter).

A vesicle, bleb, and pustule are hollow; macule, papule, and tubercle are solid.

Scale. (Squama). This is a dry attached or unattached thin piece from the skin as a result of disease of the skin.

Crust. This is a dried mass as a result of fluid oozing from a diseased skin.

Excoriation. Like a scratch mark.

Fissures. This is a crack, like that found on chapped hands.

Ulcer. (Sore). Eating away of the parts.

Scar. Ulcer healed leaving a mark, like from a healed cut.

Pigmentation. Discoloration.

ACNE. (Simple Acne).--This is an inflammation of the sebaceous (fatty, cheesy) glands. It forms these pimples or pustules and these are intermingled with black-heads (comedones), flesh-worms. They vary from a pin-head to a split-pea in size, and are of a bright or dark red color. They occur for the most part on the face; also on the back, neck and chest.

Condition.--An over secretion, or alteration and retention of the fatty (sebaceous) matter, and this is followed by inflammation involving the glands, ducts of the glands, and hair follicles. Pus often forms and tissue may be destroyed.

Causes.--These skin glands are active at the time of puberty. The active cause may be the stomach troubles, constipation, womb disorders, and poor general nutrition.

PHYSICIANS' TREATMENT for Acne.--All stomach troubles, constipation, and womb troubles should be looked into and remedied. The diet and hygiene must be regulated. Food that stimulates and is hard to digest should be prohibited. When there is dyspepsia and constipation, bitter tonics, like compound tincture of gentian, one dram before meals, or pepsin (five grains) and loosening medicines like salts should be given.

Tincture of Nux Vomica is a good stomach and bowel tonic given in doses of one to two drops before meals.

Calomel, one-half grain at night for a few nights, followed in the morning by epsom salts or some mineral water like Abilena or Hunjadi is useful. The following is a good combination by Dr. Schalek:

Tincture of Nux Vomica	2 drams
Dilute Nitro Muriatic Acid	4 drams
Sherry Wine enough for	3 ounces

Mix and take one teaspoonful three times a day.

Diet.--See diet for dyspepsia and constipation. All fatty, greasy, rich foods are prohibited.

Local Treatment.--If the skin is quite red and tender, mild soothing applications should be used. Most cases require vigorous treatment. First wash the parts with warm water and the best soap, rinse with hot water and then dry carefully. Remove the black-heads by careful pressure of the fingers, or with black-head extractor; the pimples and pustules should be freely cut, to allow the matter to escape and all the matter taken out.

External Medication, Ointment and Lotions.--Lotions are to be preferred in cases of oily discharge. If the skin becomes rough and chapped, soap should not be used in washing, and a soothing ointment should be applied. Drugs used are for stimulating the skin and healing the lesions.

1. Soothing Ointment.--

Precipitated Sulphur	1 dram
Benzoinated Lard	1/2 ounce
Lanolin	1/2 ounce

For local use but not in oily cases. (Dr. Schalek.)

2. The following used as a soothing lotion:

Washed Sulphur	2-1/2 drams
Spirits of Camphor	3 drams
Biborate of Sodium	2 drams
Glycerin	6 drams
Distilled water enough for	4 ounces

Mix and shake well and apply freely so as to leave a film on the face. (Dr. Schalek.)

3. Dr. Duhring's Lotion, following:

Precipitated Sulphur	2 drams
Glycerin	2 drams
Alcohol	1 ounce
Lime water	1 ounce
Rose water	2 ounces

Mix and shake before using and apply.

4. Kummerfield's Lotion. "Oriental Lotion."

Precipitated Sulphur	4 drams
Powdered Camphor	10 grains
Powdered Tragacanth	20 grains
Lime water	2 ounces
Rose water	2 ounces

Mix; shake well and apply every few hours.

5. Stimulating preparations.

Corrosive sublimate	1/2 to 2 grains
Emulsion bitter almonds	4 ounces

Mix thoroughly and use to stimulate the skin.

6. Ointment of white precipitate (five to fifteen per cent strength) can be used in place of one above.

7. The Following Hebra Lotion (I give as written).

Hydrarg. Bichlor	1 dram
Aqua Distill	4 drams
Ov. Albuminis	3 drams
Succi Citri	3 drams
Sacchari	1 ounce

Mix and apply as directed.

Caution.--Sulphur and mercury preparations should not be used at the same time, nor immediately succeeding each other, as they will stain the skin.

BALDNESS. (Alopecia). Causes.--Hereditary and diseases. Congenital and senile (old age) baldness is incurable. Congenital (born without hair) baldness is rare.

MOTHERS' REMEDIES. 1. Baldness, Well Recommended for.--"A first class hair restorative is made of sage tea and whisky in equal parts with a dash of quinine in the bottle."

2. Baldness, Vaseline and Quinine for.--

"Vaseline	1 ounce
Quinine	1/2 ounce"

Mix together and apply to the scalp.

3. Baldness, Good Canadian Remedy for.--"Strong sage tea. Rub the scalp frequently. I have used this with great success."

PHYSICIANS' TREATMENT for Baldness.--Persons who have an hereditary tendency to baldness should pay close attention to the hygiene of the scalp, as this is very important. The hair should be shampooed two or three times a week, to remove sebaceous accumulations and other foreign materials. After the scalp has been thoroughly rinsed with clean water and dried, some oil or (tube) Vaseline should be rubbed in, Fine-toothed combs should never be used, The daily wetting of the hair is injurious, Rats should be light and well aired, When the hair begins to fall, stimulating applications should be used, in the form of ointments or lotions. The following are among the best with the author's name given but in English instead of Latin.

Dr. Schalek. 1.

Bichloride of Mercury	3 grains
Tinct. of Cantharides	1/2 ounce
Oil of Sweet Almonds	1 dram
Spirits of Rosemary	1 ounce
Rectified Spirits of Wine	2 ounces
Distilled water enough to make	6 ounces

Mix; shake bottle well; rub thoroughly into the scalp every morning.

2.	Carbolic add	15 grains
	Glycerin	2 drams
	Cologne water	1 ounce

Mix, and apply to the scalp once daily.

3.	Precipitated Sulphur	1 dram
	Lanolin	2-1/2 drams
	Glycerin	2-1/2 drams
	Rose water enough to make	1 ounce

Mix well. Part the hair in different places and rub ointment into the scalp.

4. Ihle's Mixture.--

Resorcin	1-1/2 drams
Castor Oil	1-1/2 ounces
Spirits of Wine	5 ounces
Balsam Peru	10 drops

Mix. Rub into the scalp daily with a piece of flannel.

5. Bulkley's Lotion.--

Tincture Cantharides	1/2 ounce
Tincture Capsicum	1/2 ounce
Castor Oil	1 dram
Cologne Water	1 ounce

Mix and apply daily to the scalp.

6. Lassar's Ointment.--

Pilocarpine Muriate	30 grains
Vaseline	5 drams
Lanolin	2 ounces
Oil of Lavender	20 drops

Mix and apply to the scalp.

BALD PATCHES. (Alopecia Areata).--These appear rather suddenly. They are circular bald patches which may appear on any hairy part of the body, but more frequently on the scalp. It is considered a chronic trouble, but tends to final recovery.

Cause.--Occurs usually between the ages of ten and forty. It may be from a parasite.

PHYSICIANS' TREATMENT.--Cod-liver oil, elixir quinine, iron and strychnine one dram three times daily. Arsenic, Fowler's solution, four drops three times daily.

Local Treatment.--Stimulating remedies, like sulphur, tar, tincture of cantharides, capsicum, in various strength in combination such as given for baldness. In old persons it may become permanent.

ANIDROSIS. (Lessened Sweat Secretion).--This means a diminution of the sweat secretion. The patient does not sweat enough, especially in certain skin diseases like psoriasis, etc.

Treatment.--Hot water, vapor baths, friction, massage, etc., should be used to increase the sweat secretion. Treat the accompanying skin disease.

FOUL SWEATING. (Bromidrosis). Symptoms.--The odor may be very disagreeable, or resemble the odor of certain flavors or fruits. It is generally found in the arm-pit and genital organs.

MOTHERS' REMEDIES. 1. Offensive Sweating, Alum Water for.--"A wash made with a teaspoonful of alum and a quart of water will prevent offensive sweating. We all know how disagreeable it is to sit near a person in a street car or any crowded place, who has an odor of perspiration about them, How easy it would be to use this wash and rid yourself of this difficulty,"

2. Sweaty Feet, Borax and Alcohol for.--"Dissolve a tablespoonful of powdered borax in half a pint of diluted alcohol (half alcohol, half water) and rub the feet at night, You will find this a splendid remedy." I

3. Sweating, Simple Home Remedy to Produce.--"Place a rubber sheet or blanket under the patient. Have a simple blanket soaking in hot water and when all is ready, wring blanket as dry as possible and wrap about the patient up to the neck. After this a dry blanket is wrapped around the patient. Care should be taken not to have the blanket hot enough to burn the patient, but not too cool. After a few minutes the patient is taken out, rubbed dry gently and left to rest and sleep." This treatment will be found very beneficial and inexpensive.

PHYSICIANS' TREATMENT for Foul Sweating.--Frequent bathing, dressing powders of boric and salicylic acids, etc.

1.	Salicylic Acid	1/2 ounce
	Powdered Starch	1/2 ounce

Mix and dust on the parts.

2. **Boric acid** powdered may also be used.

3. Powdered Boric Acid and Salicylic Acid; Equal parts.

To be used as a dusting powder on the sweating parts.

3. One per cent solution of potassium permanganate or permanganate of potash is good applied to the parts.

CALLOSITY or Callositas.--This is circumscribed yellowish-white, thickened and horny patches of one of the layers of the cuticle (epidermis).

Causes--They come as the result of the occupation or pressure, and sometimes without any seeming cause.

Symptoms.--They occur mostly on the hands and feet and are usually sensitive.

PHYSICIANS' TREATMENT, for Callosity or Callositas.--Remove the cause of the horny masses. The latter is done by soaking them with prolonged hot water baths and scraping off the mass afterwards. This should be continued and done frequently.

Salicylic Acid	30 grains
Collodion	4 ounce

Mix and apply with a camel's hair pencil.

CORNS. (Calvus).--A small, flat, deep-seated, horny growth, mostly on or between the toes.

Cause.--Usually the result of too tight or too loose shoes. Due to pressure and rubbing.

MOTHERS' REMEDIES.--Corns, one of the Surest Remedies.--"Take salicylic acid, make a thick paste with flour, put on absorbent cotton and apply, leaving same on several days; soak well and corn will come out." This is a thoroughly tried remedy and a good one. This is about as good a cure as there is for corns. After this paste has been on the corn for three days, it should be removed and the feet soaked well, and the corn scraped off.

2. Corns, Turpentine and Kerosene for.--"A very simple remedy is to apply turpentine or kerosene oil to the affected part on going to bed." It is always a good plan to soak the feet well before treating the corn, as the turpentine will penetrate more quickly.

3. Corns, to Remove Without Pain.--

"Alcohol	1/2 ounce
Muriatic Acid	1 dram
Nitric Acid	1 dram
Oil of Rosemary	1 dram
Chloroform	2 drams
Tincture Iron	2 drams

Mix the above, and apply freely to the corn with little brush or feather until it can be removed with thumb lance. It may require several applications."

4. Corns, Onion a Cure for.--"Soak a small onion in vinegar four hours, then cut in two and bind on the corn at night. In the morning (if the onion has remained over the corn) the soreness will be gone and you can pick out the core. If not cured in first application repeat."

5. Corns, Castile Soap an Effective Remedy for.--"Rub the corn night and morning with castile soap, as often as possible shave it, being careful not to cut deep enough to make it bleed." Be faithful in soaping it thoroughly night and morning for several days until it disappears. This is a very simple but effective remedy.

6. Hard Corns, Iodine a Successful Remedy for.--"Paint the corns with iodine every night for three nights, stop three nights, then apply three nights again, and so on for two weeks." Have tried this and know it to be very successful, especially good for hard corns.

7. Corns, Castor Oil for.--"Apply castor oil; rub it thoroughly, then soak feet. It will soften and remove corns."

8. Corns, Vinegar and Bread for.--"Take bread and soak in vinegar for twenty-four hours, put a plaster on for three or four nights. If not cured on first application, repeat."

PHYSICIANS' TREATMENT for Corns.--Remove the cause; soften them by prolonged soaking in hot water, and then gently scrape off the softened particles, continue this for several days; then put a narrow strip of rubber or salicylated plaster (adhesive plaster) over to protect them from pressure. The following is good to soften them:

1.

Salicylic Acid	1-1/2 dram
Extract of Cannabis indica	10 grains
Collodion	1 ounce

Mix and paint on the corn for several days and after soaking corn scrape it off with a sharp knife.

2. A Good but Weaker Remedy:-

Salicylic Acid	30 grains
Extract of Cannabis indica	5 to 10 grains
Collodion	1/2 ounce

Both of these prescriptions are good, the first being stronger with salicylic acid.

3. When the corns are soft with inflammation, wash and dry the foot and apply a solution of nitrate of silver, sixty to one hundred and twenty grains to the ounce of water, to every part every four or five days.

Ulcerating Corns.--Cauterize with nitrate of silver in stick form.

CARBUNCLE. (Anthrax).--A carbuncle is an acute circumscribed inflammation of the skin and tissues beneath, of the size of an egg, orange, or larger. It is a hard mass and ends in local death of some of the tissue and formation of pus, which empties upon the surface through several sieve-like openings.

Symptoms.--There is a feeling of general sickness, chilliness and some fever. The skin over the sore part is hot and painful. The several dead parts may run together until the entire mass separates in a slough. In favorable cases it proceeds to heal kindly, but in severe cases it may spread to the surrounding tissues and end fatally, sometimes by the absorption of putrid materials, or by the resulting weakness. It runs usually from two to five weeks.

Causes.--It comes in middle or advanced life, usually oftener in men than in women. It occurs frequently in patients suffering from diabetes, in whom it is usually fatal.

MOTHERS' REMEDIES. Carbuncles, Poppy Leaves to Draw and Ripen.--"A poultice of poppy leaves is very efficacious to draw or ripen a carbuncle." A poultice made from these leaves is very quieting and soothing, and at the same time will cause the carbuncle to ripen.

2. Carbuncle, Slippery Elm and Sassafras Root for.--"Sassafras root and slippery elm bark boiled together and the decoction thickened with cornmeal." This should be changed as often as it becomes cool.

3. Carbuncle, Sheep Sorrel Poultice for.--"Gather a bunch of sheep sorrel leaves, wrap them in a cabbage leaf and roast in the oven. Apply to the carbuncle, and it will soon ripen and break."

4. Carbuncle, Bread and Milk Poultice for.--"Keep warm bread and milk poultice on until the core comes out, then put on salve or Vaseline and keep covered until all healed."

5. Carbuncle, the Common Scabious for.--"Take scabious, the green herb and bruise it. Apply this to the affected part. This has been found a very effectual remedy." The common field scabious have many hairy, soft, whitish green leaves, some of which are very small and rough on the edges, others have hairy green leaves deeply and finely divided and branched a little. Flowers size of small walnut and composed of many little ones. Sometimes called "Morning Bride," "Devil's Bit," etc.

6. Carbuncle, Snap Bean Poultice for.--"Apply snap bean leaves beat up fine. Bruise the leaves until they are real fine, then apply as a poultice."

PHYSICIANS' TREATMENT for Carbuncles.--Keep up the strength by a nourishing diet and in some cases, stimulants.

Local.--Cut it open thoroughly by a cross (crucial) cut, like this (x). The cut must reach through the mass to sound tissue beneath and beyond it. Then scrape out all the dead tissue. Dress with iodoform or sterile gauze. An antiseptic like listerine, glyco-thymoline, etc., can be used to wet the gauze, put on as a dressing afterwards and then more dry gauze above, strapped with adhesive plaster. Water and instruments must be boiled, hands must be absolutely clean. Everything around it must be clean. Sometimes it is necessary to go slowly and take out at each dressing only what can be easily removed, It is not always possible to get the whole mass away at once. Opening the carbuncle and giving free drainage afford great relief from the fever and often general symptoms. When the part feels as if it needed redressing, it should be done, for it then gives much relief. The dressings frequently become hard and do not absorb all of the material ready to be discharged. It is usually proper and prudent to dress a carbuncle two or three times a day. There is no danger if the one who dresses it is clean with the instruments, hands and gauze or cotton.

LIVER SPOTS, Moth Patch, Chloasma, etc.--This is a discoloration of the skin of a yellowish to a blackish tint of varying size and shape.

Causes.--It may be due to external agencies, such as rubbing, scratching, heat (tanning and sunburn) blistering; or due to diseases such as tuberculosis, cancer, malaria, Addison's disease, disease of the womb, pregnancy.

PHYSICIANS' TREATMENT for Liver Spots.--Remove all causes if possible.

Local.--This must be carefully used, find out first how sensitive the skin is. Dr. Bulkley recommends this lotion:

Corrosive Sublimate	5 grains
Dilute Acetic Acid	2 drams
Borax	40 grains
Rose water enough for	4 ounces

Shake bottle, mix and apply to the part night and morning.

If the skin becomes too scaly, a mild soothing ointment should be substituted for the above. White suggests the following:

Hydrarg. Ammon. Chlar	2 drams
Subnitrate Bismuth	2 drams
Starch	1/20 ounce
Glycerin	1/2 ounce

Mix and apply twice daily.

The application of peroxide of hydrogen has only a temporary effect.

BLACK-HEADS. Flesh Worms, Comedones, Pimples, etc.--This is a disorder of the sebaceous glands in which the sebaceous (fatty, cheesy) secretions become thickened; the excreting ducts, appearing on the surface, as yellowish or blackish points. They appear chiefly on the face, neck, chest, and back and are very unsightly.

Symptoms.--They are easily pressed out, and appear then as thread-like, whitish masses which contain fatty material. The black point may be due to pigment or to dirt from without. Comedones may exist with acne and seborrhoea and excessive secretion of sebum.

Causes.--Want of tone to the skin, which performs its functions sluggishly. Stomach-bowel disorders, menstrual disturbances and anemia are other causes and assist in making them worse. Improper care of the skin and dusty air may be other assistant causes.

MOTHERS' REMEDIES. For Pimples and Black-heads.--l. Pimples on the face, effective yet harmless remedy for:

Camphor	10 grains
Acacia (pulverized)	20 grains
Sulphur (precipitated)	2 drams
Lime water	2 ounces
Rose water	2 ounces

Apply on the face with a soft cloth at bedtime. Allow to dry and brush off the excess of the powder."

Anyone suffering from these eruptions is usually willing to try every known remedy. The above is excellent and very effective and is harmless.

2. Pimples, Alum Water for.--"Take a teaspoonful of alum to a quart of water and use as a wash, say three times a day. This will cure ordinary pimples on the face."

3. Skin Blotches, Cream of Tartar and Sulphur for.--"Two ounces cream tartar and one ounce of powdered sulphur (from the lump). Mix. Dose:--Teaspoonful in a little water three times a day will cure."

4. Rough Skin, Healing Cream for.--"One-fourth cup tallow melted, one teaspoonful glycerin, small lump camphor, dissolved. Mix all together by warming sufficiently." Rub in thoroughly as you do any face cream.

PHYSICIANS' TREATMENT for Pimples.--Remove the cause if possible. The diet should be like that given under dyspepsia and constipation. Menstrual disorders should be remedied.

Local.--Remove the plugs (of sebum) and stimulate the skin glands. For this purpose prolonged (ten minutes at a time) bathing of the face with hot water and soap; tincture of green soap in the more indolent, sluggish cases, should precede the pressing out of the black-heads: Lateral pressure with the fingers or with the comedone extractor, especially contrived for this purpose, will express the black-heads. After they are out, the skin dried and cleaned, various stimulating remedies can be applied in ointments and lotions such as following:

1.	"Precipitated Sulphur	1 dram
	Ointment of Rose water	1 ounce

Mix and rub on at night.

2.	Beta-Naphthol	1/2 dram
	Resorcin	1/2 dram
	Lanolin	1 ounce

Mix and apply locally.

INFLAMMATION of the Skin. (Dermatitis).--This is due to many causes. It can come from injuries, for instance the rubbing or pressure of ill-fitting clothes, bandages, bites of insects and from scratching.

Varieties.--Dermatitis ambustionis, (burning). This is due to excessive heat upon the skin.

PHYSICIANS' TREATMENT for Inflammation of the Skin.--Relieve the pain; protect the parts; exclude the air. Paint the burned part with a one to five per cent solution of cocaine, according to the severity of inflammation. Then apply soothing lotions of equal parts of lime-water and olive or linseed oil; cover the whole with absorbent cotton. Dusting powder of soda bicarbonate may also be used, or common soda. In burns with vesicles, etc., open them and then cover with carbolized oil, gauze and adhesive to hold the dressing. The parts can be washed with a solution of boric acid, one teaspoonful to a cup of water; then dust upon the parts sugar of lead once or twice a day. Some use it in solution; I like the powder better. Infusion of lobelia, one ounce to pint of hot water, is good. Also lead and laudanum wash.

ECZEMA. (Humid Tetter-Salt Rheum-Dry Tetter). Definition.--Eczema is an inflammatory disease of the skin, characterized at its commencement by redness, pimples, vesicles, pustules and their combinations, with itching and burning. It terminates in a watery or pus-like discharge with the formation of crusts or scaling.

Varieties.--There are many varieties, red, scaly, fissured, watery looking and hard skin.

Symptoms.--Itching is almost always a symptom of this disease. There is more or less pouring out of liquid (serum). The dry, scaly type, and the weeping type, may alternate with each other. There are six cardinal symptoms; inflammation, itching, moisture, crusting, infiltration (liquid filling of the tissues), fissuring or cracking. Dr. Fox says that nearly one-third of all skin diseases are eczema in some of its stages or varieties. In one kind there is red spot (macule). The skin is dry, of a bright or dull red color, with intense itching or burning, more or less watery swelling in the acute stage. In the chronic stage, the skin becomes thick and covered with fine dry scales, usually in the face (Eczema Erythematosum).

Eczema Vesiculosum. (Vesicular Eczema).--This is preceded by a feeling of heat and irritation about the part. In a short time pinhead sized vesicles appear. These frequently run together and form patches. They rupture rapidly; the liquid is poured out, dries up and forms crusts. The discharge stiffens linen, a characteristic of this variety.

Eczema Pustulosum. (Pustules). Pustular Kind.--This is nearly like the preceding. The vesicles have pus in them from the start or develop from the vesicles. When the pustules rupture, their contents dry up to the thick greenish-yellow crusts. The scalp and face, in children especially, are the favored spots for this kind. It occurs in poorly nourished children.

Eczema Papulosum. (Papular Variety).--This is characterized by flat or sharp pointed reddish pimples (papules), varying in size from a small to a large pin-head. They are usually numerous, run or crowd together and form large patches. The itching is usually very intense. This causes much scratching, rawness and crusts. The pimples may continue as such, or change into vesicles. In chronic cases they run together, and finally form thick scaly patches, and may run into a scaly eczema.

Eczema Rubrum (red).--The skin looks red, raw, and "weeps." It is most commonly found about the face and scalp in children, and the lower parts of the legs in the old.

Eczema Squamosis. (Scaling).--This may follow any of the other varieties, but usually follows the red and pimple (papule) variety. They are various sized and shaped reddish patches, which are dry and more or less scaly. Thickening is always present, also a tendency to cracking of the skin, especially if it affects the joints. There are other varieties but these are the most important.

RECOVERY.--Eczema has a tendency to persist and rarely disappears spontaneously.

Causes.--Gout, diabetes, rheumatism, Bright's disease, dyspepsia, constipation, nervous trouble, heat, cold, strong soaps, acids, alkalies, rubbing, scratching, etc.

MOTHERS' REMEDIES. 1. Eczema, Lemon or Vinegar for.--"Rub the spots with sliced lemon. This will sometimes relieve the itching. Bathing with vinegar water is better for some as it destroys the germs." The bowels should be kept open, and then constitutional faults removed as the eruption of the skin is but a local manifestation of a functional fault.

2. Eczema, Olive Oil and Powder for.--"Bathe with olive oil and sift over the skin a powder composed of equal parts of fine laundry starch and oxide of zinc powder." Do not bathe with water until healed.

3. Eczema, Herb Tea for.--"A good wash for eczema is made of an ounce of bruised blood-root and yellow dock, steeped well in a pint of alcohol, and half pint of vinegar." Apply gently to the affected parts.

4. Eczema, Potato and Camphor for.--"Make a poultice of a cold potato with a small quantity of camphor. This is very good and relieves the trouble very soon."

5. Eczema, Sulphur and Lard for.--"An excellent eczema cure is made by applying a paste made of sulphur and lard to the affected parts." This is very easily prepared, and has been known to cure many cases.

6. Skin Diseases, Burdock Tea a Standard Remedy for.--"Take a handful of the freshly bruised burdock root to two quarts of water and boil down one-half; drink from a half to one pint a day." This is considered one of the best home remedies for skin diseases that is known and is perfectly harmless.

7. Skin Disease, Blood Purifier for.--

"Iodide Potash	192 grains
Fluid Extract Stillingia	1 ounce
Fluid Extract Prickly Ash Bark	1/2 ounce
Fluid Extract Yellow Dock	1 ounce
Compound Syrup Sarsaparilla to make	8 ounces

Mix."

8. Tetter, Reliable Remedy for.--"Turpentine 1 ounce, red precipitate 3 drams, Vaseline 4 ounces. Mix, rub on the affected parts several times a day." This is a splendid ointment for a severe case of tetter.

PHYSICIANS' TREATMENT for Eczema.--Water is likely to make acute cases worse. In order to cleanse the parts use water softened by starch or bran. Use oily preparations to soften the crusts and then they can be removed with water and good soap.

In Chronic Sluggish Cases.--Water and strong soaps may be used. Cloths wrung from hot water and applied, will frequently relieve the itching. Use lotions in *moist* and salves in *dry* eczema. For the acute kind the remedy should be soothing, and more or less stimulating for the chronic forms.

Local Treatment for the acute and sub-acute (between acute and chronic) eczema.

In acute cases, with much pouring out of liquid (serum), lotions have a cooling effect. They should be frequently renewed.

1. Black Wash.

Calomel	1 dram
Mucilage Tragacanth	1 dram
Lime water	10 ounces

Mix. Can be used full strength or diluted. Bathe the affected parts several times daily for fifteen or twenty minutes with this lotion and apply oxide of zinc ointment afterwards.

2. Lead and Laudanum wash.--When the parts discharge moisture with burning feeling, and are very sensitive the following is good:

Laudanum	1/2 ounce
Solution of Sugar of lead	7-1/2 ounces

Mix and apply externally with gauze saturated with it.

3. A solution of boric acid is also a good remedy.

4. Apply the following soothing application frequently, allowing the sediment to remain on the skin:

Powdered Calamine	1 dram
Oxide of Zinc	1 dram
Glycerin	1 dram
Lime water	6 ounces

5. Dusting powders.--Corn, potato or rice starch powders. Mennen's baby powder is also good. Borated kind is the best for this.

6. Oxide of Zinc ointment alone, applied night and morning, is valuable in many cases.

The Black wash should be used twice a day just before the oxide of zinc ointment is applied. In other cases powdered oxide of zinc is dusted over the part if the discharge is watery or profuse.

7. McCall Anderson's Ointment.--

Oxide of Bismuth	1 ounce
Pure Oleic Acid	8 ounces
White Wax	3 ounces
Vaseline	9 ounces
Oil of Rose	5 drops

Make an ointment and apply. The proportions of each ingredient call be reduced one-half, for smaller amount.

8. Pastes are often borne better than ointment. The following is a good one. Lassar's paste:

Starch	2 drams
Oxide of Zinc	2 drams
Vaseline	4 drams

Mix and make a paste, apply to the part and cover with soft gauze.

9. For the Itching.--

Powdered Oxide of Zinc	1/2 ounce
Powdered Camphor	1-1/2 dram
Powdered Starch	1 ounce

Mix and dust on as needed.

When the disease is not so acute (sub-acute) applications of a mildly stimulating character are needed. For this purpose, resorcinal in the proportion of two to thirty grains to the ounce of lard, according to the severity and amount of hardness existing. Apply to the part. Stimulant and soothing.

External Treatment of Chronic Eczema.--Applications for chronic and lasting sluggish eczema.

1. Tincture of green soap used with hot water until the skin is bared and then dress with oxide of zinc ointment.

2. Tar in the form of the *pure Official tar ointment.*

3. Salicylic acid thirty to sixty grains to an ounce of lard and applied for stimulating purposes.

4. Dr. Schalek uses the same remedies in part and the following for a fixed dressing, especially on the eyes. They do not need to be changed often.

Glycogelatin Dressing.--

Gelatin	10 drops
Oxide of Zinc	10 drops
Glycerin	40 drops
Water	40 drops

Mix and apply to the part.

The above may be made in any quantities,--using drops, spoonfuls, etc. Dress the parts in a thin gauze bandage, over which the melted preparation is painted. I have given many different prescriptions, but those who treat skin diseases know that a great many are needed, for they act differently upon different persons.

Special Varieties of Eczema and what to do for them.--

Eczema of Children.--This is generally acute of the vesicular (watery) or vesicular pustular (pus forming) variety. The parts commonly affected are the scalp and the face.

PHYSICIANS' TREATMENT for Eczema.--Remove the causes, watch the feeding. Keep the folds of the skin dry and free from friction. To prevent scratching, masks must be applied to the scalp and face, or the hands must be tied in bad cases. The local treatment is the same as above except the strength of the drugs used must be reduced in proper proportion.

Eczema of the Scalp, Milk Crust.--Remove the crusts by soaking the scalp with some bland oil for twelve hours, followed by a shampoo, (the hair should be cut in children) then the lotions and thin ointment (see above) should be applied.

Eczema of the Face.--A mask of soft linen with holes cut out for the eyes, mouth and nostrils may be used.

Eczema of the Scrotum.--A well fitting suspensory should be worn, sponge the parts with very hot water and follow with the anti-itching lotion and dusting powders for the itching.

Eczema of the Hands in Adults.--Keep the hands out of water as much as possible. Dry them thoroughly and then anoint. Greatly thickened patches may be softened by soap plasters or bathe the parts in ten or twenty per cent solutions of caustic potash and followed by a salve application. The internal treatment must be given for the cause.

Diet in Eczema.--Avoid salty foods, such as salted fish or pork and corned beef; greasy foods such as bacon and fried dishes; pastry and cheese.

MOTHERS' REMEDIES for Salt Rheum. 1. Alum Wash and Cathartic for.--"Use an astringent wash as alum, tablespoonful in pint of water, and keep bowels opened by cooling medicines, as cream tartar, rochelle salts, etc." The alum solution will be found very cooling and by keeping the bowels open you will carry off all the impurities thus cleansing the blood, which is one of the essential things to do in salt rheum.

2. Salt Rheum, Ammonia and Camphor for.--"Apply ammonia and camphor to the cracks. Have used this successfully when everything else failed." Care should be taken not to have the ammonia too strong, as it may irritate the skin more. If used properly, it is a good remedy.

3. Salt Rheum, Cactus Leaf Cure for.--"From one large cactus leaf take out the thorns, add one tablespoon of salt, three tablespoons lard, stew out slowly, and grease with this at night. Remarks:--This cured my hand that had been in an awful condition for years."

4. Salt Rheum, Pine Tar for.--"Apply pine tar as a paste." This is an excellent remedy but care should be taken in using it, as pine tar is very irritating to some people, and should be used very cautiously.

BOIL. (Furunculus, Furuncle). Causes.--Boils may appear in a healthy person, but they are often the result of a low condition of the system; they are frequently seen in persons suffering from sugar diabetes.

MOTHERS' REMEDIES. 1. Boil, My Mother's Poultice for.---"Poppy leaves pounded up and bound on are good. My mother has used this recipe and found it to be good." This remedy not only makes a good poultice, but is very soothing, as poppies contain opium. The leaves may be purchased at any drug store.

2. Boil, Soap and Sugar Poultice for.--"Poultice made of yellow or soft soap and brown sugar, equal parts. Spread on cloth and apply faithfully." This makes a good strong poultice, and has great drawing powers and would be apt to create a good deal of pain, but would draw the boil to a head. The above remedy was sent in by a number of mothers, all of whom said they had tried it with success when other remedies failed.

3. Boil, Vinegar or Camphor for.--"May be cured by bathing in strong vinegar frequently when they first start. When it stops smarting from the vinegar cover with vaseline or oil." Bathing the boil in vinegar seems to check the growth and does not allow them to become as large as they would ordinarily. If you do not have vinegar in the house, camphor will answer the same purpose.

4. Boil, Bean Leaf Poultice for.--"Apply snap bean leaves, beat up fine." Bruise the leaves so that they are real fine, and apply to the boil. This acts the same as a poultice.

5. Boil, Another Vinegar Remedy for.--"If taken at first a boil can be cured by dipping the finger in strong vinegar and holding on the boil until it stops smarting. Repeat three or four times then apply a little oil to the head of boil."

PHYSICIANS' TREATMENT for Boils.--Tonics such as iron, quinine, and strychnine are good. Elixir, iron, quinine and strychnine from a half to one teaspoonful three times a day is a good tonic for an adult. Sulphide of calcium one-tenth grain four times a day is good. Paint the inflamed spot when it first begins, with a solution of gun cotton (collodion) and renew it every hour until a heavy contractile coating is formed. Poultices, if used, should contain sweet oil and laudanum. Alcohol and camphor applied over the skin in the early stages is recommended by Ringer. This I know is good. Another, wipe the skin and use camphorated oil. When boils occur in the external ear, the canal should be washed out with hot water. If it is ripe it should be opened. The following is good for the pain of a boil:

Iodoform	4 grains
Menthol	2 grains
Vaseline	1 dram

Mix and smear a cotton plug and insert in the ear two or three times a day.

ABSCESS.--An accumulation of pus (matter) in any part of the body.

External Abscess.--Boil the knife, wash your hands in clean, hot, soapy water. Wash the abscess and surrounding parts in hot water and good soap, and rinse off with alcohol, a salt solution, or listerine, etc. Then make a good deep clean cut and scrape out if necessary. Dress with a clean linen gauze or absorbent cotton, Poultices may be used if you are careful. Such an abscess should be dressed twice a day. The inner dressing should be soft and thick enough to absorb all the secretion given out between dressings.

MOTHERS' REMEDIES. 1. Abscess, Beech Bark Poultice for.--"Poultice made of red beech bark and wheat bran," A poultice made of the bark will cause a drawing feeling, and the wheat bran will retain the heat. The proportions for making the poultice should be about half and half.

2. Abscess, Milk and Salt Poultice for.--"Make a poultice of one cup of hot milk and common salt three teaspoonfuls; salt added gradually so it will not curdle. Cook until smooth and creamy, then add enough flour so it will spread but not be dry. Divide this into four poultices and apply in succession every half hour. This will remove the soreness and it should be kept oiled until healed."

3. Abscess, More Good Poultices for.--"Take equal parts of rosin and sugar, mix well and apply for several days until the abscess is broken. If this does not cause the abscess to break, poultice hourly with flaxseed meal."

FELON. (Whitlow).--An inflammation of the deeper structures and frequently it is under the covering of the bone, (periosteum). If under the latter it must be opened soon or the resulting pus will burrow and destroy bone, joints, etc. The pain is intense, and after the patient has passed one sleepless night walking the floor and holding his finger it should be opened.

How? Place the hand with the fingers extended with the palm up (it is usually under the finger or in the palm of the hand) upon the table; stand by the side of the arm. Attract the patient to something else; have a curved two-edge knife ready and put the point, one-half inch, toward the palm, away from the felon part, press hard and the patient will jerk his hand and the cut will be made down to the bone, the membrane and tissues all opened freely, a vent given for the pus and in ten minutes very little pain. Dress as for an abscess. If opened this way, it need not be reopened.

If in the Palm.--This needs a doctor, and must be opened with care. There are too many blood vessels to be careless there and one who understands it must do it. Open a true felon early before it has time to destroy the bone.

SUPERFICIAL FELONS. Mothers' Remedies. 1. A Cure if Taken in Time.--"If taken in time a felon may be cured without lancing, but if poultice or liniment is used it is important that they should be bound on tightly as the mechanical compression is more essential than the application. A good remedy is finely pulverized salt, wet with spirits of turpentine bound tightly and left two or three days, wetting with the turpentine when dry without removing the cloth."

2. Felon, Treatment until time to Lance.--"If the felon has succeeded in getting a good start and pains considerably, it is well to paint it with iodine; in a few days it will become very painful, the pain being so intense that you cannot sleep. See a physician at once then, and have it lanced as the sac of pus on the bone must be opened. Then apply flaxseed poultices. Care should be taken not to have it lanced too early, as this is dangerous.

3. Felon, Strong Remedy for.--"Turpentine, yellow of egg and salt, equal parts, bind on." This is very strong and should only be allowed to remain on the finger a short time.

4. Felon, Lemon to draw inflammation from.--"Take a lemon, make a little hole, put finger in it and hold there a number of hours." Lemons have a great many healing qualities in them, and seem to be very good for felons. The acid in the lemon seems to help draw out the inflammation and serves as a poultice.

5. Felon, Hot Water Cure for.--"When you first feel it coming put the finger in a cup of hot water, just so it does not blister, keep adding more hot water as it cools for one hour. This has been tried several times and it has always stopped them."

6. Felon, Soap and Cornmeal Poultice for.--"Poultice with soft soap and cornmeal. This never fails if taken in time."

7. Felon, Smartweed Poultice for.--"Apply the bruised leaves of smartweed and bind on tight as can be borne." This makes a very good poultice applied in this way.

8. Felon, Hot Application for.--"When a felon first starts, soak the finger in equal parts of alcohol and hot water; keep it as hot as the finger will bear it."

9. Felon, an Old, Tried Remedy for.--"Put wood ashes, covered with warm water in a dish on the stove, hold the affected part in this, allowing it to get as hot as can be borne."

10. Felon, Turpentine Cure for.--"Soak the finger for one hour in turpentine. This has been known to cure a great many cases of felon."

11. Felon, Weak Lye Application for.--"Stick your finger in weak lye (can lye). Have water just as hot as you can stand your finger in. Hold it in as long as possible."

12. Felon, Rock Salt and Turpentine for.--"Rock salt dry and pounded fine. Mix equal portions with turpentine. When dry change. This cured a felon on my father." As much of our Canadian salt is rock salt, it is the most common salt to use.

PHYSICIANS' TREATMENT for Superficial Felons.--Such may be averted perhaps. I have heard of that but have never seen it done. They are not the genuine, true blue, terrible felons, but even these can give much pain. They do not need such a deep opening, and they are not so dangerous to the structures. They are superficial and abscesses, perhaps, might be the better term. For these many applications have been made.

1. Some hold the finger in hot lye. That is a good poultice.

2. Yolk of an egg and salt (equal parts) make a salve as a drawer.

3. The membrane within the shell of an egg is another good drawing remedy.

Dr. Chase gives this definition of a felon in his first edition: "This is on one of the fingers, thumb or hand and is very painful. It is often situated at the root of the nail." The latter is the kind, and also that of the structures above the covering of the bone that are eased by local treatment. Especially the superficial, about the nail, etc. Steaming with herbs will do such good, or any hot poultice will do good. Dr. Chase says in another place, "Whitlow resembles a felon, but it is not so deeply seated. It is often found around the nail. Immerse the finger in strong lye as long and as hot as can be borne several times a day." Such felons are curable by local treatment. I prefer the salt and yolk of the egg to the lye. If you cannot stand this all the time, steam in the intervals with strong herbs or use hot poultices, and then open when it points.

ULCERS. An Eating Away of the Parts, Causes.--Diseases like syphilis, tuberculosis, leprosy. Disturbances of nutrition, constitutional ulcers, local conditions. Ulcers are acute and chronic. An acute ulcer is a spreading ulcer, in and about which acute destructive inflammation exists.

Treatment.--Keep them thoroughly clean (aseptic) and use soothing applications, mild lotions and salve.

Chronic Ulcer.--This is one which does not tend to heal, or heals very slowly. Sometimes such ulcers need to be stimulated like the application of nitrate of silver and then healing applications. Carbolated oxide of zinc ointment is a good healing ointment.

MOTHERS' REMEDIES. 1. Sores and Ulcers, the Potato Lotion for.--"Take the water you boil potatoes in and in one quart of it boil one ounce of foxglove leaves for ten minutes, then add one ounce tincture of myrrh to the lotion, bathe the affected parts with the lotion warm, then keep a cloth wet with it on the sore, if possible, until cured."

2. Sores and Ulcers, Chickweed Ointment for.--"Chop chickweed and boil in lard, strain and bottle for use." This makes a fine green cooling ointment, It is surprising to see the relief obtained by this simple ointment.

3. Old Sores and Wounds, Healing Ointment for.--

"Honey	4 ounces
Spirits of Turpentine	1/2 ounce
Beeswax	4 ounces
Oil of Wintergreen	1/2 ounce
Tincture of Opium	1 ounce
Fluid Extract Lobelia	1/4 ounce
Lard	3/4 pound

Mix by the aid of gentle heat, stirring well at the same time. This is a very useful ointment for healing wounds and old sores."

4. Sores and Ulcers, Excellent Salve for.--"One tablespoon of melted mutton or even beef tallow while warm; add some spirits of turpentine and one teaspoonful of laudanum, stir well."

5. Ill-Conditioned Sores, an Old German Remedy for.--"Wash or syringe the sore with weak saleratus water, and while wet fill with common black pepper. Remarks:-- This is a highly recommended German remedy, and has been tried by my mother with good, results."

6. Sores, Cuts, Antiseptic Wash for; Also Tooth Wash.--"Peroxide of hydrogen. Should always be kept in the house." If you are cut by anything that might cause infection or if scratched by a cat, in fact wherever there is chance for infection and blood poison, peroxide of hydrogen may be used by moistening well the wound with it as soon as you can. As a mouth wash put a little in a glass of water. Directions usually on the bottle.

7. Indolent Ulcers and Boils, Chickweed and Wood Sage Poultice for.--"Equal parts of chickweed and wood sage pounded together make a good poultice for all kinds of indolent ulcers and boils."

8. Ulcers, Proud Flesh, Venereal Sores and all Fungus Swellings, Blood Root and Sweet Nitre for.--"Two ounces pulverized blood root; one pint of sweet nitre; macerate for ten days, shake once or twice a day."

9.

Rosin	1 ounce
Beeswax	1 ounce
Mutton Tallow	4 ounces
Verdigris	1 dram

Melt the rosin, tallow and wax together, then add the verdigris. Stir until cool and apply.

Add a few drops of carbolic acid to the above and you will have the carbolated salve which is quite expensive when bought prepared and under the manufacturer's label.

10. Sores and Chapped Hands, Sour Cream Salve for.--"Tie thick sour cream in a cloth and bury in the ground over night. In the morning it will be a nice salve. Excellent for chapped hands or anything that requires a soft salve."

11. Old Sores, A Four-Ingredient Remedy for.--"Soften one-half pound of Vaseline, stir into it one-half ounce each of wormwood, spearmint and smartweed. This is good for old and new sores. My people near Woodstock, Canada, used this and found it very good."

12. Ulcers and Sores, Carrots will heal.--"Boil carrots until soft and mash them to a pulp, add lard or sweet oil sufficient to keep it from getting hard. Spread and apply; excellent for offensive sores. Onion poultice made the same way is good for slow boils and indolent sores." This makes a very soothing poultice and has great healing properties.

13. Ulcers and Sores, a Remedy that Cures.--"To one-fourth pound of tallow add one-fourth pound each of turpentine and bayberry and two ounces of olive oil. Good application for scrofulous sores and ulcers." This makes a good ointment, but should not be continued too long at a time as the turpentine might have a bad action on the kidneys.

14. Ulcers and Old Sores, Bread and Indian meal for.--"Take bread and milk or Indian meal, make to consistency of poultice with water, stir in one-half cup of pulverized charcoal. Good to clean ulcers and foul sores." The bread and Indian meal make a good poultice while the charcoal is purifying and a good antiseptic.

PHYSICIANS' TREATMENT for Ulcers.--Keep them thoroughly cleaned. A mild, weak, hot solution of salt water is good in chronic, slow healing, indolent ulcers. Carbolated salve applied afterwards is healing. Sometimes a stimulating poultice is necessary, like salt pork followed by soothing salves. If an ulcer looks red and angry, it needs soothing. If there is any "proud flesh" powdered burnt alum applied directly upon it and left on for an hour or two is good. Then soothing salves.

Balsam of Peru is good for chronic ulcers. It stimulates them to a little activity.

A salve made by boiling the inner bark of the common elder, the strained juice mixed with cream or Vaseline is a good healing application for ulcers.

Poultice an irritable, tender, painful ulcer with slippery elm bark. Repeat when necessary.

Indolent Sluggish Ulcer.--This kind needs stimulating, salt solution, or salt pork applied.

Poultice made of sweet clover is well recommended for ulcers. As before stated, the *active* kind should have soothing treatment. The *chronic* indolent kind, should be stimulated occasionally and *then* soothing applications applied.

SHINGLES (Herpes Zoster). Definition.--This is an acute inflammatory disease of the skin, characterized by groups of vesicles upon the inflamed base, distributed along the course of one or more cutaneous (skin) nerves.

Symptoms.--The eruption is preceded by a great deal of neuralgic pain and is almost always one-sided. They first appear as red patches and upon these patches vesicles soon develop (skin elevations with liquid in them); these are separate, size of a pin-head to a coffee bean, swollen with a clear fluid, and clustered in groups of two to a dozen. They may dry up in this stage, or they may fill with pus or run together, forming larger patches; new crops may appear, while the others fade. The vesicles rarely rupture of themselves, but dry into brownish crusts, which drop off leaving a temporary colored skin. It follows the course of a nerve. The most common seat of this disease is over one or more intercostal (between the rib) nerves, extending from the backbone to the breastbone. It also occurs along the side of the face and temple.

Causes.--It is a self-limited disease, runs its course in a few weeks, of nervous origin and may be produced by exposure to weather changes, blows and certain poisons.

MOTHERS' REMEDIES. Shingles, Herb Remedy for.--1. "Make a solution of yerba rheuma, one ounce to a pint of boiling water, and apply freely to the part several times a day." The yerba rheuma has an astringent action and contracts the tissues, relieving the inflammation of the skin. It also relieves the itching.

2. Shingles, Mercury Ointment for.--"Apply night and morning an ointment from the oleate of mercury." This preparation will be found effective, but care should be taken not to use too much of it, as oleate of mercury is very powerful. It relieves the burning and itching.

PHYSICIANS' TREATMENT for Shingles.--Protect the vesicles from rupture or irritation and relieve the pain. Paint the surface with a solution of gun cotton (collodion). Tonics to keep up the strength.

EXCESSIVE SWEATING. (Hyperidrosis).--This is a disorder of the sweat glands in which sweat is thrown out in excessive quantities.

Symptoms.--It may be great only in the armpit where it stains the clothing. When it comes on the hands and feet they may be wet, clammy and have an offensive odor. They may be soaked, inflamed and painful.

Causes.--The local forms may be due to a nervous condition; it is often the result of general debility.

Treatment.--General tonics are needed and those given under anemia, which see.

Applications for the local treatment.--Solution of alum applied to the part will act as an astringent.

White oak bark tea is good as anything. It should not be used so strong as to stop sweating entirely. Then follow it with dusting powders of starch or boric acid, containing salicylic acid (two to five per cent). When it occurs upon the feet use the Diachylon ointment. It must be made up fresh in a drug store. This is applied on strips of lint or muslin after the parts have been thoroughly washed and dried; it should be renewed twice daily, the parts being dried with soft towels and then covered with dusting powder, followed by the ointment.

FRECKLES. (Lentigo).--Freckles are an excessive deposit of pigment in the skin.

Causes.--Exposure to the sun's rays aggravates this condition.

MOTHERS' REMEDIES for Freckles. 1. Freckles, Buttermilk for.--"Buttermilk on the face every night." This is a very simple remedy, and as buttermilk is very easily obtained, anyone troubled with freckles can try this remedy without very much expense. This simple remedy has been known to cure many cases.

2. Freckles, to Remove.--"Nitrate of potash applied to the face night and morning is very good, and the freckles will soon disappear."

3. Freckles, Alcohol and Lemon Juice for.--"Use alcohol and lemon juice freely at night." Lemon juice is very good for the skin if applied frequently.

4. Freckles, Excellent Lotion for.--

"Rose Water	4 ounces
Alcohol	1/2 ounce
Hydrochloric Acid	1/2 dram

Mix and apply with sponge or cloth three times daily.

5. Freckles, Borax Water for.--"Rain water eight ounces, borax one-half ounce. Mix and dissolve; wash parts twice daily."

6. Freckles, Canadian Remedy for.--"Glycerin, lemon juice, rosewater, equal parts. Apply at night with a soft cloth,"

PHYSICIANS' TREATMENT for Freckles.--They are apt to return on exposure to the sun. The following ointment may be of service. Care should be taken not to blister:

Ammoniated Mercury	1 dram
Subnitrate of Bismuth	1 dram
Glycerin Ointment	1 ounce

Mix and apply every other night.

PRICKLY HEAT RASH.--An acute inflammatory disease of the sweat glands; minute pimples and vesicles develop.

Symptoms.--It occurs upon the body and consists of many pinhead sized bright red pimples and vesicles which are very close together. It appears suddenly, and is usually accompanied by much sweating and subsides in a short time with slight scaling following. There is itching, tingling and burning usually present.

Cause.--Excessive heat in summer in children and weak people.

MOTHERS' REMEDIES. 1. Prickly Heat, Soda Water for.--"Bathe with saleratus (baking soda) water, dry carefully and apply good talcum powder freely."

2. Prickly Heat, Relief from pain of.--

"Borax Powder	6 drams
Menthol	10 grains
Rose Water	6 ounces

Bathe the parts and between applications dust on lycopodium powder."

The borax powder will be found good to cover the parts and muriate of morphia relieves the pain. The rose water is simply put in to dissolve the other ingredients.

3. Prickly Heat, a Hamilton, Ontario, Mother Found Burnt Cornstarch good for.--"Dust with browned cornstarch. This acts like talcum powder and is not so expensive."

4. Rash, Soothing Ointment for. l.--"Make an ointment of one dram of boric acid powder to one ounce of vaseline. First wash the affected parts with a strong solution of saleratus, then apply the ointment

and dust talcum powder over this." The washing with saleratus is very important as this is a good antiseptic and thoroughly cleanses the parts.

PHYSICIANS' TREATMENT for Prickly Heat.--It disappears usually in a few days. Tonics for the weak, light clothing, a light nourishing diet and frequent cold bathing. Alcoholic drinks are prohibited. White oak bark tea as a wash for the sweating, followed by dusting powders of starch, oatmeal, and zinc oxide, etc.

MOTHERS' REMEDIES. 1. Chafing, Fuller's Earth Eases.---"Wash parts well with boracic acid water, then dust with fuller's earth," The boracic water is cleansing and fuller's earth is very healing. This is a very simple but effective remedy.

2. Chafing, Good Home Remedy for.--"Usually all that is required is washing the parts well with castile soap and cold water, and anointing with plain Vaseline," This remedy is always at hand, and is one to be relied upon. Vaseline, as we all know, is very healing.

3. Chafing, Borax and Zinc Stops.--"Wash parts frequently with cold water and use the following solution:

Pure Water	2 gills
Powdered Borax	1 teaspoonful
Sulphate of Zinc	1/2 teaspoonful

Apply by means of a soft rag several times daily. After drying the parts well, dust with wheat flour, corn starch or powdered magnesia;"

The above combination is excellent as the water cleanses the parts and the borax and zinc are very soothing and healing.

4. Chafing, Common Flour good to stop.--"Burn common wheat flour until brown. Tie in rag and dust chafed parts."

MOLE. (Naevus).--Mole is a congenital condition of the skin where there is too much pigment in a circumscribed place. It varies in size from a pin-head to a pea or larger. The face, neck and back are their usual abiding place.

PHYSICIANS' TREATMENT for Moles.--They should be removed by knife or by electricity. The last is the best, especially for the hairy variety.

Causes.--If they are subject to too much irritation they develop into malignant growth.

ENLARGED NAIL. (Onychauxis).--The nail may become too long, thick or wide.

Treatment.--Remove the cause. Trim away the excessive nail tissue with a knife or scissors. In paronychia, inflammation around the nail, pieces of lint or cotton should be inserted between the edge of the nail and the inflamed parts, and wet solution of antiseptics, like listerine or salt water, applied with cloths.

INFLAMMATION OF THE NAIL. (Onychia). Treatment.--Cut into the back part if it needs it. That will relieve the tension and pain. Sometimes the nail must be removed. The inflammation is at the base (matrix) of the nail.

LOUSE, Disease of the Skin Produced by.--This is a disease of the skin produced by an animal parasite, the pediculus or louse. There are the head louse, pediculus capitis; the body louse, pediculus corporis; the pubis, (about the genitals) pediculus pubis. The color of lice is white or gray. They multiply very fast, the young being hatched out in about six days and within eighteen days are capable of propagating their same species. The nits are glued to the hair with a substance which is secreted by the female louse.

HEAD LOUSE or Pediculus Capitis. Treatment.--The symptoms are very apparent. Apply pure kerosene, rub it into the hair thoroughly. It can be mixed with an equal part of balsam of peru. It should be left on the scalp for twelve to twenty-four hours and then removed by a shampoo. Other remedies that can be used are, tincture of staphisagria (stavesacre), this can be made into an ointment; or ointment of ammoniated mercury. The dead nits are removed from the hair by dilute acetic acid or vinegar. Cutting the hair is not usually required. An infusion of quassia is good as a wash.

Body Louse or Clothes Louse (Pediculus Corporis).--This parasite lives in the clothes. It is apt to be found in the folds or seams, especially where the clothes come in close contact with the skin, as about the neck, shoulders and waist. This creature visits the body for its meal. They may produce different kinds of skin troubles like eczema, boils, etc.

PHYSICIANS' TREATMENT for Lice.--Destroy the lice and their eggs (ova) by thoroughly baking or boiling the clothing. The irritated skin can be healed by soothing applications like Vaseline, and oxide of zinc.

(Pediculus Pubis).--Lice on the hair of the pubis or about the genitals. This is the smallest parasite of the three varieties, and it attaches itself firmly to the hair with its head buried in the follicular openings, and it is removed with great difficulty.

PHYSICIANS' TREATMENT for Lice.--1. Ointment of mercury, blue ointment. This is to be used frequently. It is rather unclean and may create a severe inflammation so be careful of it.

2. Solution of corrosive sublimate, from one to four grains to one ounce of water. This is good and can be used once or twice a day; rub thoroughly into the parts. It will cause redness and inflammation may follow if too much is used. It is very effective. Kerosene with an equal quantity of balsam of peru is a good remedy.

BLISTER DISEASE, (Pemphigus).--This is an acute or chronic skin disease in which there are blisters of various sizes and shapes, and these usually occur in crops.

Symptoms.--The disease may attack any part of the body. The blisters range from the size of a pea to a large egg. They contain at first a clear fluid, which soon becomes cloudy and looks more or less like pus. They last several days and then dry up. They do not rupture of themselves very often. It is not catching.

Causes.--These are obscure and not understood. A low state of the system is usually found.

PHYSICIANS' TREATMENT for Blister Disease.--General treatment should be given. Arsenic is the best remedy and can be given in the form of Fowler's solution, five drops after meals at the beginning far an adult. This should be increased until some poisonous symptoms, such as bloating in the face is produced.

Elixir Quinine, Iron and Strychnine is good as a tonic, one teaspoonful after meals. Regulate the diet, give nourishing and easily digested food.

Local Treatment.--Puncture the blisters. Then put on a mild ointment like Vaseline; bran and starch baths can be given in some cases. The length of the time of the disease is uncertain.

THE ITCH DISEASE. (Psoriasis) *(*not Common Itch). Definition.--This is a chronic inflammatory disease of the skin, in which there appear upon the skin thick, adherent, overlapping, scales of a shiny, whitish color, and these are situated upon a reddish, slightly raised and sharply outlined (defined) base.

Symptoms.--They begin as small reddish spots, sharply defined against the healthy skin. They may be elevated slightly and soon became covered with whitish pearl colored scales. If the scales are picked off, there is left a smooth red surface, and from this, small drops of blood ooze out. No watery or pus-like discharge escapes at any period of this disease. These spots extend at the circumference (periphery), reaching the size of the drops, or of the coins, or they may run together and form ring-shaped, or crooked wavy lines of patches, with a center that is healing up. A few scattered spots may be present, or large areas may be involved. In rare cases the whole skin is affected. These spots or patches may occur an any part of the body, but involve the extending part of the limbs, especially the elbows and knees. There may be slight itching present at times.

Course of the Disease.--It is chronic; patches may continue indefinitely or they may disappear in one place, while new crops appear elsewhere. This disease usually appears far the first time between the ages of ten and fifteen; it may then return at various intervals during a lifetime. It is usually worse during the winter.

Causes.--Are usually unknown, it may occur in all classes and kinds of people.

PHYSICIANS' TREATMENT for Itch Disease.--Remedies for the general symptoms are demanded. The general health must be looked after. Stimulating foods and drinks and the use of tobacco are forbidden.

Arsenic in the form of Fowler's solution from three to ten drops three times a day; or the arsenious acid in pills of 1/50 of a grain three times a day. This medicine must not be used in the acute form, but only in chronic cases.

Local Treatment.--1. Remove the scales first and follow this by stimulating applications unless there is much inflammation. In such cases soothing lotions should be applied. Dr. Schalek of New York, recommends the following:

2. Remove the scales thoroughly with hot water and soap and then apply:

Chrysarobin	1 dram
Ether, Alcohol	Equal parts of each and enough to dissolve the first remedy
Collodion	1 ounce

Mix and apply with a brush to the parts affected.

This solution may cause inflammation and great swelling, and on that account it should not be used on the face, it stains the skin. Dr. Hare recommends a bath only before the application. In that way some scales remain and there is not so much inflammation and swelling resulting. The stain can be removed with a weak solution of chlorinated lime.

3. Tar Remedy.--Tar is also a good remedy in ointment forms. The skin should be closely watched to find out how sensitive it is to the tar's action, not only in this but in all skin diseases. Drugs should be changed occasionally, for they lose their efficiency.

4. Tar and Sulphur Remedy for.--Never use tar on the face, it stains.

	Ointment of Tar	1 ounce
	Ointment of Sulphur	1 ounce
	Mix thoroughly and apply at night.	
5.	Precipitated Sulphur	6 drams
	Tar	6 drams
	Green Soap	2 ounces
	Lard	2 ounces
	Powdered Chalk	4 drams
	Apply frequently.	

If necessary more lard can be used, especially if the skin is very tender.

6. Another good local application. It is composed of the following ingredients:

Resorcinol	1 dram
Zinc Oxide	1 dram
Rose Water Ointment	10 drams
Apply twice a day to the part affected.	

After mixing the ointment heat it until the resorcinol crystals melt to prevent any irritation of the skin from them.

Ichthyol	2-1/2 drams
Salicylic Acid	2-1/2 drams
Pyrogallic Acid	2-1/2 drams
Olive Oil	1 ounce
Lanoline	1 ounce
Mix thoroughly and apply.	

The result of the disease is always favorable as to life and general health. It yields to treatment, but it has a tendency to recur.

ITCH. Common Itch (Scabies).--Itch is a contagious disease, due to the presence of an animal parasite. There is intense itching in this disease. The parasite seeks the thin, tender regions of the skin, the spaces between the fingers, wrists and forearms, the folds in the armpit, the genitals in men and the breasts in women.

Cause.--It is always transmitted by contagion. An intimate and long contact is usually needed. A person occupying the same bed with one who has it is liable to take it. The female parasite lives from six to eight weeks, during which time she lays fifty eggs, which, when hatched out, become impregnated in their turn.

MOTHERS' TREATMENT for Common Itch. 1. Mustard Ointment for.--"Make an ointment of cup of fresh lard (without salt) and a tablespoonful of dry mustard, work to cream and apply." This is very soothing.

2. Itch, Grandmother's Cure for.--"Sulphur and lard mixed; rub on at night, then take a good bath, using plenty of soap, every day." The above ingredients are always easily obtained and anyone suffering with this disease will find relief from the itching by using this remedy. It is very soothing.

3. Itch, Herb Ointment for.--"Mix the juice of scabious with fresh lard and apply as an ointment. A decoction made from the same herb might be taken at the same time to purify the blood. It is always well to take some blood tonic together with any outward application you may use." Some who read the above may know scabious by other names as the "morning bride" or "sweet scabious" or "devil's bit," etc.

4. Itch, Elecampane Root Ointment for.--"Boil elecampane root in vinegar, mix with fresh lard, beating thoroughly." This is an excellent remedy for itch, having a very soothing effect and relieving the itching.

5. Itch, Oatmeal for.--"A poultice of oatmeal and oil of bays; cures the itch and hard swellings." Oatmeal poultices are more stimulating and draw more rapidly than those made of linseed meal.

6. Itch, a Mother at Parma, Michigan, Sends the Following.-- "Make a salve of sulphur and lard and each night apply it to the whole body; also one tablespoonful internally for three mornings, then skip three and so on. This is the only thing I know of that will cure itch. I have tried it with success."

7. Itch, Kerosene for.--"Apply kerosene oil, undiluted, to the parts several times a day. Apply nitrate of mercury ointment to the body."

8. Itch, Splendid Ointment for Common Itch.--

"Lac-Sulphur	160 grains
Napthaline	10 grains
Oil Bergamot	4 drops
Cosmoline	1 ounce

Rub lac-sulphur into fine powder. Sift it into the melted cosmoline and stir until nearly cool, then add napthaline and oil bergamot. Stir until cool."

PHYSICIANS' TREATMENT for Itch.--If the skin is much inflamed or irritable, soothing baths and ointments should be used at first. There are three indications to be met in the treatment; first, to destroy the cause, the parasite; second, to cure the result of their work; third, to prevent a return or transmission to others.

First Thing to Do.--Soak the body thoroughly with soap (green soap if you have it) and water, this softens the outer layer (epidermis). This layer covers the female parasite which burrows under it. The male does not burrow and it is therefore easier to kill. Rub the skin thoroughly with a rough towel after the soaking. This rubbing will remove the outer skin scales and with it some of the parasites. The towel should be boiled at once to prevent it from conveying the parasite to others. Then apply the ointment, which, if thoroughly applied, relieves the patient at once. The skin should be well softened and rubbed in order to open every track (burrow) of the parasite. Allow the ointment to remain on all night and use it for three or four nights successively.

Ointments.--1. Simple sulphur ointment alone.

2.	Oil of Cale (from Juniper)	1 dram
	Sulphur Ointment	2 drams
	Lanolin	5 drams
3.	Flowers of Sulphur	6 ounces
	Oil of Fagi	6 ounces
	White Chalk	4 ounces
	Green Soap	16 ounces
	Lard	16 ounces

Apply at night. This is not so strong.

4. For children the following can be used:

Sulphur	1 dram
Balsam Peru	1 dram
Lard	1 ounce

Apply as usual.

5. The following for adults:

Precipitated Sulphur	2 drams
Carbonate of Potash	1 dram
Lard Ointment	1-1/2 ounces

Rub well into the skin.

Second:--Heal the resultant sores with soothing applications like Vaseline and a little camphor in it.

Third:--Boil and disinfect all underwear and bedding or any article liable to give an abiding place to the parasite. It is easily cured with proper treatment.

DANDRUFF (Seborrhoea).--The scurfs or scales (dandruff) upon the scalp are formed from seborrhoea.

Definition.--The word seborrboea means to flow suet or fatty fluids. Seborrhoea is a functional disorder of the sebaceous gland (fatty, suet matter) and this secretion is somewhat altered in character.

Varieties.--There are three varieties. These depend upon the character of the material excreted.

1. Oily seborrhoea (seborrhoea oleosa).

2. Dry seborrhoea (seborrhoea sicca).

3. Mixed type of both.

Oily seborrhoea.--Symptoms.--This appears most frequently upon the nose and forehead and sometimes upon the scalp. The skin looks oily, glistening, with the appearance of dust adhering to it. Small drops of oil are seen to ooze out of the follicles and when wiped off it reforms at once. The ducts of the follicles appear gaping or they are plugged with black-heads (comedones). The hair is rendered unusually oily, when it appears on the scalp, and it is especially noticeable on bald heads. It is very common in the negro, almost natural or physiological.

Dry Seborrhoea.--This is a more common form and occurs upon the hairy or non-hairy parts, but chiefly upon the scalp (dandruff). The affected parts are covered with grayish, greasy scales, which are easily dislodged, the skin underneath is oily and slate gray in color. This type of the disease forms one type of dandruff. When it is of long standing the hair becomes dry and falls out.

Mixed type.--This type is common upon the scalp. The surface is covered, more or less, with scales and crusts. If the disease continues long the hair becomes dry, lusterless and falls out. Permanent baldness may result.

Causes.--These may be constitutional and local. "Green sickness" (chlorosis), disorders of the stomach and bowels are often the cause.

Local.--Uncleanness, lack of care of the scalp, heavy and airtight hats may cause it. Some writers claim parasites are the cause.

MOTHERS' REMEDIES.--1. Dandruff, Home Preparation from New York State Mother.--"Into one pint of water drop a lump of fresh quick-lime, the size of a walnut; let it stand all night, pour off the clear liquid, strain, and add one gill of the best vinegar, wash the roots of the hair with the preparation. It is a good remedy and harmless."

2. Dandruff, a Barber's Shampoo for.--"Shampoo with the following:

Sassafras	5 cents worth
Salts of Tartar	10 cents worth
Ether	10 cents worth
Castile Soap	5 cents worth

Dissolve the above in one gallon of soft water. Rinse the hair thoroughly and repeat as often as necessary. This recipe was given me by a barber and I find it very good,"

3. Dandruff, Lemon Juice for.--"Cut a lemon in two, loosen the hair and rub the lemon into the scalp. Do this in the evening before retiring, for about a week, then stop for a few nights, then use for another week, and so on until cured."

4. Falling Hair, a Brook, Ontario, Lady Prevents.--"Garden sage, make a quart sage tea, add equal parts (a teaspoonful) of salt, borax and rosewater, and one-half pint of bay rum. Wet the head with this every night."

5. Hair Restoratives, Simple and Harmless.--"A simple and harmless "invigorator" is as follows:

Cologne Water	2 ounces
Tincture of Cantharides	2 drams
Oil of Lavender	10 drops
Oil of Rosemary	10 drops

Use twice daily. If it makes the scalp a tittle sore, discontinue for a short time."

6. Dandruff, Talcum Powder an Excellent Remedy for.--"Take talcum powder and sprinkle in the hair thoroughly, then brush," This is a very good remedy.

PHYSICIANS' TREATMENT for Dandruff.--If there are general diseases, they should be treated.

Local--In mild cases, shampooing with hot water and a good soap may be sufficient when the scales and crusts are thick and abundant; first soften them with olive oil and then remove them with hot water and green soap.

After the scalp has been cleaned, the remedies should be applied. The remedies should be thoroughly rubbed in and applied in the form of ointments or lotions and used once daily. Cutting the hair may be necessary. The odor of sulphur may be overcome by the use of perfume. If the scalp becomes too dry after shampooing some oil should first be applied, whatever application is used afterwards.

Remedies.--Resorcin, sulphur, salicylic acid, in combination with other ingredients. Some favorite prescriptions are now given:

1.	Resorcin	1 to 2 drams
	Pure Castor Oil	1 dram
	Alcohol	2 ounces
	Mix and rub well into the scalp.	
2.	Precipitated Sulphur	1 dram
	Salicylic Acid	15 grains
	Ointment Petrolatum	1 ounce
3.	Washed Sulphur	4 drams
	Castor Oil	10 drams
	Oil of Cocoa	1 ounces
	Balsam of Peru	1/2 ounce
	Apply twice daily.	
4.	Carbolic Acid	20 drops to 1 dram
	Oil of Almonds	4 drams
	Oil of Lemon	1 dram
	Distilled Water, enough to make	2 ounces
	Apply after washing.	

The oily type is best treated with lotions and powders. The disease is very obstinate, but generally gets well.

WEN (Sebaceous Cyst. Steatoma).--A wen varies in size from a millet seed to an egg, and it is due to the distention of a sebaceous gland by its retained secretions. They occur most commonly on the scalp, face and back. They cause no pain, grow slowly, and after they have grown to a certain size remain stationary for an indefinite time. Sometimes they become inflamed and ulcerate.

Treatment.--Make a free cut and take the mass out. Its covering (capsule) or sac must be removed at the same time, for if any of this membrane (capsule) is left it will fill up again. Equal parts of fine salt and the yolk of an egg beaten together and applied continuously will eat the skin open and the mass can then be taken out. This is quite painful and takes several days, while with the knife there is little pain if cocaine is injected and it will all be over in a few minutes.

RINGWORM (Tinea Trichophytina).--Ringworm is a contagious disease of the skin, produced by the presence of a vegetable parasite. The disease affects the hair follicles of the scalp and the beard, and also of the portions of the body that, seemingly at least, have no hair.

Varieties.--Ringworm affecting the body called Tinea Circinata. Ringworm affecting the scalp called Tinea Tonsurans. Ringworm affecting the beard, etc., Tinea Barbae (barbers' itch).

Ringworm of the Body.--This type of ringworm usually begins as one or several round, somewhat raised and very small, defined congested spots and these are covered with a few branny scales. The disease extends from the circumference and, while healing in the center, assumes a shape like a ring and these rings may become as large as a silver dollar and remain the same size for months or years, or they may go together (coalesce) to form circle (gyrate) patches. Vesicle and pimples frequently crop out at the circumference.

Mothers' Remedies for Ringworm.--1. Gunpowder and Vinegar for.--"Make a paste of gunpowder and vinegar and apply. Sometimes one application will be sufficient; if not, repeat."

2. Ringworm, Cigar Ashes for.--"Wet the sore and cover with cigar ashes. Repeat frequently. This will cure if taken in time." This is a very simple and effective remedy. Cigar ashes are always easy to obtain and if applied to the ringworm at the very beginning, the nicotine in the tobacco will draw out the soreness and relieve the inflammation.

3. Ringworm, Kerosene for.--"Apply kerosene with the finger or a cloth several times a day."

4. Ringworm, Ontario Mother Cured Boy of.--"Wash head with vinegar and paint with iodine to kill germ. Cured a neighbor's boy."

5. Ringworm, Another from a Mother at Valdosta, Georgia.--

"Burdock root and vinegar." Take the dock root and steep it the same as any ordinary herb tea, then add your vinegar, making the proportions about half and half. Apply this to the affected part.

6. Ringworm, Egg Skin Remedy for.--"Take the inner skin of an egg and wrap around it, and cover with a piece of cloth."

7. Ringworm, from a Mother at Owosso. Michigan.--"Take gunpowder and wet it and put it on the sores," This remedy has been tried a great many times and always gives relief when taken right at the beginning. So many people will wait, thinking the ringworm will disappear of its own accord, instead of giving some simple home remedy like the above a trial.

PHYSICIANS' TREATMENT for Ringworm.--1. For infants and children simpler remedies should be used at first. Scrub each patch with tincture of green soap, or merely good soap and water may be employed. Then apply tincture of iodine to the patches, once or twice a day, enough to irritate the patches. Dilute acetic acid, or dilute carbolic acid will do the same work. A ten per cent solution of sodium hyposulphite is a good remedy also.

2. Corrosive sublimate, one to four grains to the ounce of water, is very good to put on the patches. For children the strength should be about one-half grain to the ounce.

3. Ammoniated mercury is also very good to put on. Sometimes a combination of remedies will do better, as follows:

	Milk of Sulphur	2-1/2 drams
	Spirits of Green Soap	6 drams
	Tincture of Lavender	6 drams
	Glycerin	1/2 dram
4.	Pure Iodine	2 ounces
	Oil of Tar	1 ounce
	Mix with care gradually.	
5.	Creasote	20 drops
	Oil of Cadini	3 drams
	Precipitated Sulphur	3 drams
	Bicarbonate Potash	1 dram
	Lard	1 ounce
	Mix, to be used in obstinate cases in adults.	

Ringworm of the Scalp.--Cautions and Treatment.--Be careful that others do not catch it from you. Separate the child affected. Cleanse the diseased parts from time to time by shampooing with a strong soap. The hair over the whole scalp should be clipped short and the affected parts shaved, or if allowed, the hairs in the affected parts pulled out. The remedies are then applied if possible in the shape of ointments, which are thoroughly rubbed in. Vaseline and lanolin are better as a base for the medicine, as they penetrate deeper. Following remedies are the most valuable:

1. **Carbolic acid,** one to two drams to glycerin one ounce.
2. **Oleate of mercury**, strength ten to twenty per cent.
3. **Sulphur Ointment,** ten to twenty per cent strength.
4. **Tincture of Iodine.**

This variety lasts longer than the ringworms on the body, months sometimes are required to cure it.

BARBER'S ITCH (Ringworm of the Beard).--Mother's Remedies. 1. Standard Remedy for.--"Plain Vaseline two ounces, venice turpentine one-half ounce, red precipitate one-half ounce. Apply locally. Great care should be taken not to expose affected parts to cold and draughts while ointment is in use, especially if affected surface is large." The above is a standard remedy and will be found very effective in all cases of barber's itch. The Vaseline will assist in healing the sores and softening up the scabs.

2. Barber's Itch, Healing Ointment for.--"Plain Vaseline four ounces, sulphur two ounces, sal-ammoniac powder two drams. Mix and apply daily after cleansing the parts thoroughly with castile soap and soda water. This is also an almost infallible cure for common itch." The Vaseline is very good and healing, while the sulphur has a soothing effect and is a good antiseptic.

3. Barber's Itch, Reliable Remedy for.--"Citrine ointment one dram, Vaseline or cosmolin one ounce. Mix thoroughly. Wash the affected parts clean and apply this ointment on a soft rag three times a day." This is a standard remedy and one to be relied upon. It is very soothing and has great healing properties.

4. Barber's Itch, Sulphur and Lard for.--"Sulphur and lard mixed together and applied three or four times a day. Have found this to be the best of anything ever used for barber's itch." This remedy will be found very good if the case is not very severe. If the face is covered with sores, filled with pus and of long standing a stronger treatment should be used. See other Mothers' Remedies, also Doctors' Treatment.

5. Barber's Itch, Cuticura Ointment for.--"Apply cuticura ointment to the sores, and as it draws out the water press a clean cloth against the sore to absorb the water. This will generally draw the water out in three or four days."

PHYSICIANS' TREATMENT for Barber's Itch.--Pulling out the hairs or close shaving every day. Keep the affected parts soaking with olive oil for two successive days. The evening of the third day the shampoo is employed, the skin is washed free from crusts and scales, shave cleanly. After shaving bathe the parts for ten minutes with borated water, as hot as can be borne; while this is being done, all pustules or points where there is a mucous fluid coming out to the surface are opened with a clean needle. Sponge freely over the affected surface with a strong solution of hyposulphite of sodium for several minutes and not allow it to dry; this solution may contain one dram and perhaps more to the ounce. After a thorough and final washing with hot water, the tender skin is carefully dried and gently smeared with a sulphur ointment containing one to two drams of sulphur to the ounce of Vaseline, often with the addition of from one-quarter to one-half grain of mercuric sulphide. In the morning wash the ointment off with soap and water, the sodium solution is reapplied and a borated or salicylated powder is thoroughly dusted and kept over the parts during the day and apply ointment at night. The shaving must be repeated at least the next day. As soon as there are no pustules (lumps), or they have diminished in size, the ointment at night is superseded by the use of the dusting powder. The washing with very hot water and with the solution hyposulphite is continued nightly, when the inflammation excited by the parasite is limited to the follicles that are invaded. Continue the dusting powder after the ointment is discontinued.

WART (Verucca). Mothers' Remedies.--1. An Application for, also Good for Cuts and Lacerations.--"Make a lotion of ten drops tincture of marigold to two ounces of water and apply." This is also good for severe cuts and lacerations. It may be applied by cloths or bandages if the case requires.

2. Warts, Match and Turpentine Wash.--"Dissolve matches in turpentine and apply to wart three or four times," This preparation helps to eat them away and if kept on too long is apt to produce a sore; care should therefore be taken in using this remedy.

3. Warts, Muriate of Ammonia for.--"Take a piece of muriate of ammonia, moisten and rub on the wart night and morning; after a week's treatment the wart, if not extra large, will disappear."

4. Warts, Turpentine for.--"Rub frequently with turpentine for a few days and they will disappear. This is a very simple remedy, but a good one, and worth trying if you are afflicted with warts."

5. Warts, to Remove.--"The juice of the marigold frequently applied is effectual in removing them. Or wash them with tincture of myrrh."

6. Warts, Milkweed Removes.--"Let a drop of the common milkweed soak into the wart occasionally, the wart will loosen and fall out. This can be applied as often as convenient; here in Canada we do not have to go far to get a plant."

7. The following is a good application:

Salicylic Acid	1/2 dram
Cannabis Indicia	5 grains
Collodion	1 ounce

Mix and apply to the wart.

Tincture of thuja is very good in some cases when applied daily.

HIVES, Nettle Rash (Urticaria). Causes.--Foods such as shell fish, strawberries, cheese, pickles, pork and sausages.

Medicines that may cause it.--Quinine, copaiba, salicylic acid, etc. Disorders of the stomach and bowels. Insects, like mosquito, bedbug, etc.

MOTHERS' REMEDIES.--1. Hives or Nettle Rash, Slippery Elm.--"Slippery elm used as a wash and taken as a drink." Slippery elm is especially good for any skin disease, as it is very soothing to the parts and relieves the itching. If taken as a drink it acts on the kidneys and bowels, throwing off all the impurities.

2. Hives or Nettle Rash, External and Internal Home Medicine for.--"Bathe with weak solution of vinegar. Internal remedy; sweet syrup of rhubarb with small lump of saleratus (size of a pea) dissolved in it. This dose was given to a two-year-old child." The rhubarb helps to rid the stomach and bowels of its impurities, relieving the disease, as hives are usually due to some disorder of the kidneys and bowels.

3. Hives or Nettle Rash, Tea and Powder for.--"Rub with buck-wheat flour; this will relieve the itching almost immediately. Sassafras tea is a good internal remedy."

4. Hives or Nettle Rash, Catnip Tea for.--"Boil catnip leaves to make a tea, slightly sweeten and give about six or eight teaspoonfuls at bed time and keep patient out of draughts." The tea can be taken throughout the day also. If taken hot on going to bed it causes sweat-ing and care should be taken not to catch cold while the pores are opened.

5. Hives or Nettle Rash, Mother from Buckhorn, Florida, says following is a sure Cure for.--"Grease with poplar bud stewed down until strong; take out buds, add one teaspoonful lard, stew all the water out. Grease and wrap up in wool blanket."

6. Hives or Nettle Rash, from a Mother at New Milford, Pennsylvania.--"One tablespoonful castor oil first. Then put one table-spoonful salts and cream tartar in glass of water; take one spoonful before eating. Have used this and found it excellent." The castor oil acts on the bowels and the cream of tartar on the blood.

7. Hives or Nettle Rash, Buttermilk for.--"Buttermilk applied two or three times a day. Found this to be good for nettle rash." Buttermilk is very soothing and will relieve the itching. This is an old tried remedy.

8. Hives or Nettle Rash, Baking Soda Wash for.--"Make a strong solution of common baking soda, about three teaspoonfuls to pint of water. Sponge or bathe body thoroughly." Any mother who has a child in the house knows how valuable baking soda is in case of burns, on account of its cooling properties. For this same reason it will be found excellent for above disease, as it will relieve the itching and is very soothing. Good for children if used not quite as strong.

9. Hives or Nettle Rash, Canada Blue Clay for.--"Mix up blue clay and water to make a paste. Leave until dry and then wash off."

PHYSICIANS' TREATMENT for Hives or Nettle Rash.--Remove causes. Bowels and kidneys should act freely. Abstain from eating for a day or two if necessary.

For the Itching.--Diluted vinegar, applied is effective. Also camphor.

Cream of Tartar	2 ounces
Epsom Salts	2 ounces

Take three or four teaspoonfuls to move the bowels, or one teaspoonful every three hours if the bowels are regular enough. For a child one year old, give one teaspoonful in water every three hours until the bowels move freely.

SUNBURN.--When severe, sunburn may present the symptoms of inflammation of the skin. Then there will be redness, swelling and pain followed by deep discoloration of the skin.

MOTHERS' REMEDIES for Sunburn.--1. Lemon Juice and Vinegar for.--"An application of the juice of a lemon or vinegar."

2. Sunburn, Ammonia Water for.--"Ammonia will remove sunburn in one night." Care should be taken in using this remedy. The ammonia should be diluted half with water and not used too often.

3. Sunburn, Relief from Pain and Smarting of.--"Benzoated zinc ointment or Vaseline applied to the affected parts is sure to give relief and avoid much pain and smarting."

4. Sunburn, Preparation for.--"I have found nothing better than mentholatum." Mentholatum is simply a mixture of Vaseline or cosmolin and menthol. They are both very healing, and will be found beneficial.

PHYSICIANS' TREATMENT for Sunburn.--Soothing ointments and dusting powders are generally sufficient for sunburn. Talcum powder (Mennen's borated), rice powder, oatmeal powders are good and healing. The following are good:

1.	Oxide of Zinc Powder	1/2 ounce
	Powdered Camphor	1-1/2 dram
	Powdered Starch	1 ounce

Mix. Dust on the parts.

2.	Powdered Starch	1 ounce
	Powdered Camphor	1 dram

Well mixed and applied is soothing to the parts.

3. The following is a good combination:

Carbonate of Lead	1 dram
Powdered Starch	1 dram
Ointment of Rose Water	1 ounce
Olive Oil	2 drams

Mix and apply to the inflamed skin.

GANGRENE.--This is the death of a part of the body in mass. There are two forms, moist and dry.

Dry Gangrene.--This is a combination produced by a loss of water from the tissues. The skin becomes dark and wrinkled and is often hard, like leather. Senile or old age gangrene, and really due to the arterial sclerosis, usually occurs in the lower extremities, involving the toes. A slight injury may first start up the trouble. The pain in this variety is not usually great.

MOTHERS' REMEDIES.--1. Gangrene, Remedy from New York that cured a Gangrenous Case.--"A man aged 74 years had a sore below the knee for fifteen years; at last gangrene appeared in his foot and three physicians pronounced his case hopeless on account of his age. I was called as a neighbor and found the foot swollen to twice its natural size, and the man in pain from head to foot. I ordered cabbage leaves steamed until wilted, then put them over the limb from knee to foot and covered with a cloth. In about fifteen minutes they were black, so we removed them and put on fresh ones, repeating the change until the leaves did not turn black. Then the sore was thoroughly cleansed with a weak solution of saleratus and while wet was thickly covered with common black pepper and wrapped up. The saleratus water and pepper was changed night and morning until the sore was entirely healed. After the third day this man had no pain, and in four weeks was entirely healed. A year later he said he had never had any trouble with it or with rheumatism which he had had for years before."

PHYSICIANS' TREATMENT for Gangrene.--The skin should be treated. Poultices sometimes may be good, or bottles of hot water around the parts. A general tonic should be given.

Moist Gangrene. Causes.--Wounds, fractures, injuries, pressure from lying in bed and frost bite.

PHYSICIANS' TREATMENT for Moist Gangrene.--Remove

the cause if possible. This kind is more dangerous, and a physician should be called as the best treatment that can be given is none too good.

BLISTER.--This is a watery elevation of the outer skin. It is caused by rubbing, for instance of a shoe, friction from anything, or from burns. It frequently appears on the hands after working for some time at manual labor, when the hands are not accustomed to work. It is the common blister which hardly needs much describing.

MOTHERS' REMEDIES for Blister.--1. Linseed Oil for.-- "Linseed oil used freely." This is a very good remedy because it is soothing. Any good soothing lotion or salve that will draw out the soreness and pain is helpful.

2. Blister. A Method of Raising a Blister.--"If a blister is needed take an ordinary thick tumbler, rub alcohol inside and around the rim, then invert over a piece of cotton, saturated with alcohol and ignited; after a few minutes the glass may be removed and clapped on the surface of the body. As the glass contains rarified air the flesh will be drawn up into it and a blister formed."

IVY POISONING.--The parts usually affected are the hands, face, the genitals, the arms, the thighs and neck.

Symptoms.--These usually appear soon. Red patches, with scanty or profuse watery pimples, with a watery discharge after bursting. There is swelling, intense burning and itching. The parts sometimes swell very much and look watery. The person can hardly keep from scratching.

MOTHERS' REMEDIES.--1. Ivy Poisoning, Buttermilk and Copperas for.--"Wash in copperas and buttermilk three or four times a day. Have seen this used and it helped." The copperas and buttermilk is very good when applied to the parts immediately after the poison is discovered. The copperas acts very much like sugar of lead and in some cases is very much more effective.

2. Ivy Poisoning, Cure for.--

"Bromine	10 to 20 drops
Olive Oil	1 ounce

Mix. Rub the mixture gently into the affected parts three or four times a day. The bromine being volatile the solution should be freshly made."

This remedy is frequently used by physicians, and is very effective.

CHAPPED HANDS AND FACE. Mothers' Remedies.--1. Chapped Hands, Quince Seed Cream for.--"Soak one teaspoonful of quince seeds in one cup warm water over night. Strain through a cloth and add one ounce glycerin, five cents' worth bay rum, and perfume if you choose."

2. Chapped Hands, Soothing Lotion for.--"Bathe them in soft water using ivory soap and Indian meal; when dry bathe in vinegar. Have tried this treatment and my hands feel soft and easy after treatment." It would be best to dilute the vinegar with water one-half.

3. Chapped Hands, Glycerin for.--"Use glycerin freely." Glycerin is very irritating to some people, then again it works like a charm. You can tell only by trying it.

4. Chapped Hands, Carbolic Salve for.--"We always use a good carbolic salve for these, as we have found nothing better for sores of any kind." A few drops of carbolic acid added to any good salve will give you the above.

5. Chapped Hands, Glycerin and Lemon Juice for.--"Two-thirds glycerin, one-third lemon juice, mix well together; apply nights."

6. Chapped Hands, Camphor Ice for.--"Camphor ice." Apply frequently after thoroughly washing and drying the hands.

7. Chapped Hands, Remedy from a New York Lady.--

Glycerin	4 ounces
Cologne	2 ounces
Benzoin	1/2 ounce
Rain water	1 pint

Mix thoroughly and apply to the hands after washing.

This remedy has also been used for years by a friend, and we have proved it good. If applied frequently during the winter the hands will not chap."

8. Chapped Hands, Rose Cream for.--"Get ten cents' worth of rose water, five cents' worth of glycerin and the juice of one lemon. Mix and rub on the affected parts,"

9. Chapped Hands, Preventive for.--"A little diluted honey or almond oil will restore softness and prevent chapping."

10. Chapped Hands or Face, from a Twin Falls Idaho, Mother.---"One-fourth ounce gum tragacanth dissolved in one and half pints of soft water; then add ounce each of alcohol, glycerin and witch-hazel, also a little perfume. I find this one of the best remedies I ever used for sore or chapped hands."

PHYSICIANS' TREATMENT for Chapped Hands.--

1.	Subnitrate of Bismuth	3 drams
	Oleate of Zinc	3 drams
	Lycopodium	2 drams

Mix. Apply to the parts three times daily.

2. Powdered camphor mixed with Vaseline is healing.

3. Ointment of water of roses (cold cream) is a soothing application. It can be improved by adding a little glycerin and benzoic acid--this keeps it sweet in warm weather.

4. Powdered zinc oxide, or starch as a dusting powder.

FACE CREAMS, Mothers' Preparations.--l. Cream of Pond Lilies.--"This agrees especially well with oily skins; will keep indefinitely.

Orange Flower Water, triple	6 ounces
Deodorized Alcohol	1-1/2 ounces
Bitter Almonds, blanched and beaten in a mortar	1 ounce
White Wax	1 dram
Spermaceti	1 dram
Oil of Benne	1 dram
Shaving Cream	1 dram
Oil of Bergamot	12 drops
Oil of Cloves	6 drops
Oil of Neroli Bigrade	6 drops
Borax	1/5 ounce

Dissolve the borax in the orange flower water, slightly warmed. Mix the wax, spermaceti, oil of benne and shaving cream in a bainmaire, at gentle heat. Then stir in the perfumed water and almonds. Strain through a clean muslin strainer, place in a mortar and while stirring gradually work in the alcohol in which the oils have been previously dissolved."

2. Face Cream, When Facing our North Winds, in Canada, I Use this.--"Honey, almond meal, and olive oil to form paste. Use after getting skin cleaned. I used it myself and find it good when going out driving."

3. Face Cream, Lanolin Cream.--

Lanolin	1 ounce
Sweet Almond Oil	1/2 ounce
Boric Acid	40 drops
Tincture of Benzoin	10 drops

This is a good skin food to be rubbed into the skin with the tips of the fingers."

4. Face Cream, Cucumber Lotion.--

"Expressed Juice of cucumbers	1/2 pint
Deodorized Alcohol	1-1/2 ounces
Oil of Benne	3-1/4 ounces
Shaving Cream	1 dram

Blanched Almonds 1-3/4 drams The preparation of this is the same as for almond lotion. It is an excellent cosmetic to use in massaging the face and throat, as it not only tones any relaxed tissues, but also may he used to cleanse the skin during the day. A complexion brush is an excellent investment; one should be chosen that has fine camel's hair bristle's. It should be used in connection with good soap."

5. Face Cream, Almond Lotion to Whiten and Soften the Skin.--

Bitter Almonds, blanched and beaten	4 ounces
Orange Flower Water	12 ounces
Curd Soap (or any fine toilet soap)	1/2 ounce
Oil of Bergamot	50 drops
Oil of Cannelle	10 drops
Oil of Almonds	20 drops
Alcohol (65% solution)	4 ounces

Powder or break up the soap; dissolve in the orange flower water by heating in a bain-maire, gradually work almonds into the soap and water. Strain and finish as directed above. This is a bland lotion, very cleansing, whitening and softening."

6. Face Cream. the Cold Ontario Wind Harmless When Using this.--"Wash in warm water, rub face dry with corn-meal. This takes place of bottle cream."

FROST BITES.--Keep the patient in a cold atmosphere, or put into a cold bath and the frozen part rubbed with snow or ice until sensation is felt and color returns; then discontinue the rubbing and apply ice water compresses. Stimulants such as brandy, coffee and hot drinks are given, but external heat is only gradually permitted, for the circulation returns very slowly to the frost-bitten parts, and in trying to hasten it, we run the risk of producing or, at least, increasing the tendency to gangrene of the frozen parts.

MOTHERS' REMEDIES.--l. Frost Bites. Remedy from Northern New York.--"Soak the parts affected in kerosene oil; this will soon draw out the frost."

2. Frost Bites, Roasted Turnips for.--"Roasted turnips bound to the parts frosted." This is a very soothing application, but should not be put on warm. Cold applications are what are needed in frost bites.

[Transcriber's Note: From the Mayo Clinic (2005): 1. Get out of the cold. 2. Warm hands by tucking them into your armpits. If your nose, ears or face is frostbitten, warm the area by covering it with dry, gloved hands. 3. ***Don't rub the affected area, especially with snow***. 4. If there's any chance of refreezing, don't thaw out the affected areas. If they're already thawed out, wrap them up so they don't refreeze. 5. Get emergency medical help if numbness remains during warming. If you can't get help immediately, warm severely frostbitten hands or feet in warm--not hot--water.]

BUNIONS.--This is a lump over a joint usually of the big toe, usually due to pressure and a wrong position of the surfaces of the joint.

MOTHERS' REMEDIES.--1. Bunions, Remedy from Your Flower Garden.--"Peel the outside skin from the leaf of 'Live Forever' and apply as a poultice. Repeat until cured. This is a very good remedy and one that should be tried if you are troubled with bunions or corns."

2. Bunions, A Cure for.--

"Tincture of Iodine	2 drams
Tincture of Belladonna	2 drams

Apply twice a day with camel's hair brush."

This mixture when applied will have a drawing effect, and care should be taken not to leave it on too long, as it will irritate the parts and make it very sore.

3. Bunions, Iodine for.--"Apply tincture of iodine to the bunion night and morning. This will reduce size; if used at first will entirely remove."

4. Bunions, Tested Remedy for.--"Take about one teaspoonful salicylic acid in two tablespoons of lard, and apply night and morning. Before doing this apply adhesive plasters to the affected parts." This is a standard remedy.

PHYSICIANS' TREATMENT for Bunions.--Rest of the part, cold applications and liniments.

CHILBLAINS. (Erythema Pernio).--This occurs usually in people with a feeble circulation or scrofulous constitution, usually seen in the young or very old. The redness shows most, as a rule, on the hands and feet. The redness may be either a light or dusky shade. It itches and burns especially when near artificial heat. The redness disappears on pressure, and the parts are cool rather than hot. It is an inflammation that follows freezing or a frost-bite. It may return for years at the return of cold weather.

MOTHERS' REMEDIES. 1. Chilblains, a Cure for.--"Equal parts of extract of rosemary and turpentine. Apply night and morning until cured." The rosemary is very soothing, and the turpentine creates a drawing sensation. It has cured many cases of chilblains.

2. Chilblains, Witch-hazel for.--"Bathe feet in lukewarm water and soda and apply carbolized witch-hazel." This remedy is very soothing, and always give relief.

3. Broken Chilblains, Ointment for.--

"Sweet Oil	1/2 pint
Venice Turpentine	1-1/2 ounce
Fresh Lard	1/4 pound
Beeswax	1-1/2 ounce

Simmer gently together in a pan water bath until the beeswax is melted, stirring until cool. When it is ready for use apply on going to bed on a soft rag."

4. Chilblains, Vinegar Cure.--"Soak the feet in a weak solution of vinegar, then rub good with Vaseline or oil."

5. Chilblains, Home-made Salve for.--

Fresh Lard	2 ounces
Venice Turpentine	1/2 ounce
Gum Camphor	1/2 ounce

Melt together, stirring briskly. When cold it is ready for use.

6. Chilblains, Common Glue for.--"Put a little common (dissolved) glue in hot water and soak the feet in it. Repeat if necessary." This is very good and gives relief."

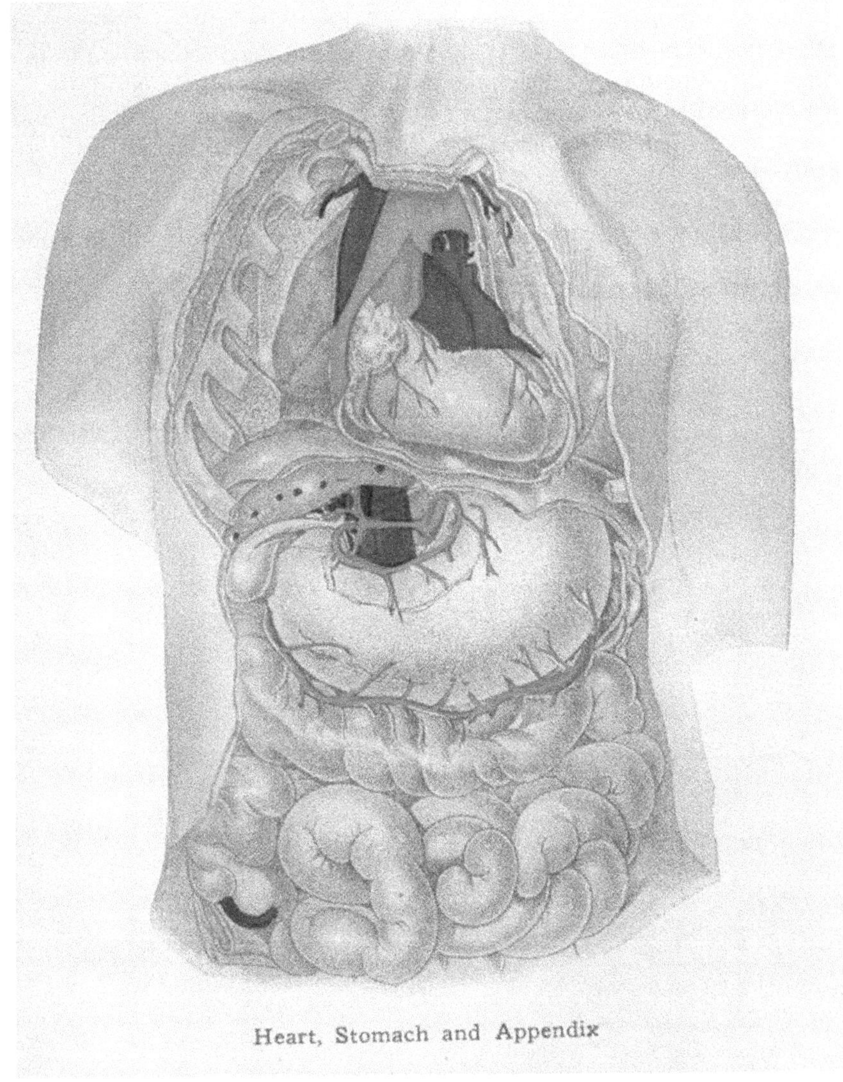

Heart, Stomach and Appendix

7. Chilblains, the Onion Cure for.--"Raw onion rubbed on chilblains every night and morning." The onion seems to have a very soothing effect upon the chilblains, and this remedy has been known to cure many stubborn cases. It is always well to soak the feet well before applying this treatment, as the juice from the onion will penetrate more quickly.

8. Chilblains, the Hemlock Remedy for.--"Hemlock twigs mixed with lard and pounded until it is green, then bound on."

PHYSICIANS' TREATMENT for Chilblains.--Thick woolen stockings, mittens and ear protections should be worn. Daily cold baths, especially of such parts, should be taken. Alcohol applied to the parts, full strength, will harden the tissues. Camphor also is good.

Internal.--Iron should be given to establish a better circulation and give strength. Tincture of iron, five drops three times a day, is good.

External.--1. Alum as a wash applied to the parts.

2. **Ointment of ichthyol**, one-half strength, is very good in some cases.

3. Rosin made in an ointment is also good to relieve some cases.

4. Lard and iodine ointment is excellent for some.

5. The following is also good:

Prepared Chalk	1 ounce
Powdered Camphor	10 grains
Linseed Oil	2 ounces
Balsam of Peru	20 drops

Mix and apply.

DIGESTIVE ORGANS, DISEASES OF.

CANKER SORE MOUTH. (Aphthous Stomatitis.)--This is a variety of inflammation of the mouth where there are one or more vesicles (cankers) upon the edges of the tongue, the cheek or the lips.

Causes.--They are most common in children between two and six years of age; but are not rare in adults. Predisposing causes are spring and autumn, tuberculosis, teething, poor nutrition, stomach and bowel disorders.

Symptoms.--The vesicles soon rupture and leave the ulcer (canker). There may be a few or many, pin-head or split pea in size, along the edges of the tongue, inside the cheeks. They are very tender.

MOTHERS' REMEDIES.--1. Canker Sore Mouth, Raspberry Leaf for.--"Infuse a handful of raspberry leaves in a half pint of boiling water for fifteen minutes; when cold strain and add two ounces tinc. of myrrh, rinse the mouth with a little of it two or three times a day, swallow a little each time until relieved. This is also good for spongy gums, loose teeth, bad breath and for gently correcting and cleansing the stomach."

2. Canker Sore Mouth, Oak Bark Tea for.--"Red Oak bark, a little salt and pepper." The bark should be boiled down to make a good strong tea, according to age of person. The salt has an astringent effect upon the mouth and is also a good antiseptic. The pepper should not be used when the parts are very red and inflamed. It should be used only when they are rather sluggish.

3. Canker Sore Mouth, Boracic acid for.--"Rinse the mouth with a solution of boracic acid and put some of the dry powder on the canker," This is a very good remedy as the boracic acid is a good antiseptic and is especially good for children and mild cases of canker sore mouth.

4. Canker Sore Mouth, Canker Weed Tea for.--"Apply canker weed found in the woods. A small plant with dark green leaves spotted with white." Make a tea of the canker weed by steeping it, then strain and apply to the affected parts. This is a very good remedy.

5. Canker Sore Mouth, Honey and Borax for.--"Honey and borax used as a mouth wash or swabbing is excellent." The honey is very soothing and the borax is a good antiseptic.

6. Canker Sore Mouth, Wild Turnip for.--"Dried wild turnip grated fine and put in mouth. I know this is excellent."

7. Canker Sore Mouth, Alum for.--"Take a piece of alum, rub on the canker often."

8. Canker Sore Mouth, Borax Water for.--"Rinse the mouth well with a weak solution of borax water, then put a little dry borax on the canker. They will generally heal after one or two applications."

9. Sore Mouth, Common and Effective Remedy for.--"Make an infusion of sumach bobs (not the poison ones, of course). Good for sore throat when used as a gargle and a little swallowed frequently." This is a very effective remedy and is also good for sore mouth.

10. Sore Mouth, Shoemaker Root and Borax good for.--"Take the inside bark of shoemaker root and steep it; strain, add a little borax; have known it to take off canker where doctors failed." If the above cannot be secured make a tea from common strawberry leaves. You can use this for a baby by swabbing the mouth, and I have known some mothers to throw in a small piece of alum making it stronger for an older person.

1. PHYSICIANS' TREATMENT for Canker Sore Mouth.--If from the diseases mentioned treat them. In the meantime to relieve the local conditions keep the mouth clean and use as a mouth wash boric acid, one teaspoonful to a cup of warm water.

2. Burnt alum applied directly to the part is good.

3. Nitrate of silver pencil applied directly to the canker until it turns whitish, cures in a few applications. Use twice a day.

4. A wash of sage tea is good also, but it must be strong.

5. The juice of a ripe tomato is good applied locally.

Sore mouth should be kept absolutely clean. Thrush frequently comes from uncleanness.

GANGRENOUS STOMATITIS.--This is a rapidly spreading gangrenous affection of the cheeks and forms a rare occurrence and ending fatally in most cases. The trouble may extend to the jaws and lips.

Causes.--It is more common in girls and boys and usually appears between the ages of two and five years. It is worse in the low countries like Holland, but it is not contagious. It is more likely to attack the sickly children suffering from the effects of overcrowding. It may follow diseases like scarlet fever, typhoid fever, smallpox, etc.

Symptoms.--It usually affects first the mucous membrane of one cheek, near the corner of the mouth, as a dark, ragged, sloughing ulcer and spreads for two or three days before the substance of the cheek is infected. If you grasp the cheek between the thumb and finger you can then feel a hard and sensitive lump. The cheek may be eaten through by the third day, though a week generally passes before this happens. There is a burning watery discharge from the unhealthy wound. The breath smells terribly and it is almost unbearable. The gangrene may spread over one half of the face of the side affected.

TREATMENT.--The death rate is eighty to ninety per cent. This is a very dangerous disease and a doctor must be in attendance. Cut, away all the dead tissue by using burning caustics, such as fuming nitric acid, solid zinc chloride, nitrate of silver, carbolic acid on the actual canker. Sometimes mild applications like sub nitrate of bismuth, chloride of potash or the following do well:--

Sulphate of copper	2 drams
Powdered cinchona	1/2 ounce
Water enough to make	4 ounces

Mix and apply. Peroxide of hydrogen is good as a disinfectant or boric acid solution, etc., may be used. Keep up the patient's strength. Fortunately this disease is rare. I have never seen a case in practice.

Salivation.--Stop the mercury, keep the bowels open and use the same antiseptic washes as directed for sore mouth.

Chlorate of Potash Solution, Soda Solutions, Boracic Acid Solutions.--Brush the ulcers with nitrate of silver sticks. Keep the mouth clean with hot water washes and some of the antiseptics put in the water as boric acid, soda, glycothymotine, listerine, etc.

ACUTE DYSPEPSIA.--(Acute Indigestion, Acute Gastritis). "Gaster" is the Greek for stomach; "itis" means inflammation,--thus acute inflammation of the stomach. It may be acute or chronic. When acute it may be called acute gastritis, acute gastric catarrh, acute dyspepsia or acute indigestion. When chronic it may be called chronic gastritis, chronic catarrh of the stomach, chronic dyspepsia or chronic indigestion.

Causes.--This is a very common complaint and is usually caused by eating foods that are hard to digest, which either themselves irritate the stomach, or remain undigested, decompose, and so excite an acute dyspepsia, or indigestion, or it may be caused by eating or taking in more than the stomach can digest. A frequent cause is eating decomposing food, particularly in hot weather. Alcohol is another great cause.

Symptoms.--In mild cases. Distress in the stomach, headache, weary feeling, thirst, nausea, belching of wind, sour food, and vomiting; the tongue is heavily coated and the saliva increased. In children there are loose bowels and colicky pains. It lasts rarely more than twenty-four hours. Vomiting usually relieves the patient.

Severe cases.--These may set in with a chill; fever 102 or 103. The tongue is much coated, breath foul and frequent vomiting, loss of appetite, great thirst, tenderness in region of the stomach; repeated vomiting of food at first, then of bile stained fluid with mucus; constipation or diarrhea. Attacks last one to five days.

MOTHERS' REMEDIES.--1. Indigestion or Dyspepsia, Mustard and Molasses for.--"Mustard is an excellent household remedy kept in every home. A tablespoonful of white mustard mingled with two ounces of molasses and then taken once a day will act gently on the bowels and is a beneficial remedy in dyspepsia." By acting upon the bowels it relieves the stomach of any food that may have caused a disturbance and relieves the dyspepsia.

2. Flatulent Dyspepsia, Wormwood tea for.--"Wormwood, one to two teaspoonfuls, water one pint. Make a tea and take from one to four teaspoonfuls daily." This is an old tried remedy and one that should be given a trial if affected with dyspepsia.

3. Indigestion or Dyspepsia, Dry salt for.--"One-half teaspoon dry salt taken before each meal. Knew a gentleman who was nearly worn out with this trouble and entirely cured himself with this simple remedy." It is always well to give these simple remedies a fair trial, before resorting to strong drugs. Salt is a good stimulant.

4. Indigestion or Dyspepsia, Chicken Gizzard Skin for.--"Four ounces good brandy, one-fourth pound of loaf sugar, one tablespoonful pulverized chicken gizzard skin, one teaspoonful Turkish rhubarb dried on paper stirring constantly; this prevents griping; the chicken gizzard skin is the lining of the gizzard which should be thoroughly cleaned and dried then pulverized. To prepare put brandy and sugar together (crush the sugar), light a paper and set fire to the brandy; let burn until sugar is dissolved, then add the gizzard skin and rhubarb, stir together and if too thick add a little water and boil up. Dose :-- Infant, one-half teaspoonful every four hours; child, one teaspoonful every four hours; adult, one tablespoonful every four hours. Have used this remedy for a great many years and given it to a great many people who have worn out all other remedies."

5. Indigestion or Dyspepsia, an Excellent Tonic for.--

Tincture Gentian Compound	2 ounces
Tincture Rhubarb	2 ounces
Tincture Ginger	1/2 ounce
Essence Peppermint	2 ounces
Bicarbonate Soda	1/2 ounce
Water to make	8 ounces

Mix.

For acute cases of indigestion where the stomach and bowels are full and distended, or sour stomach, spitting up of food. This will often relieve at once and with continued use relieves entirely."

6. Indigestion or Dyspepsia, Fruit Diet Cure for.--"Persons afflicted with this disease would find great relief if they would confine themselves to a diet of fruit only for several days." This gives the stomach an opportunity to rest up and get back to its natural state.

7. Indigestion or Dyspepsia, Hickory Ashes for.--"Take a swallow of hickory limb ashes and water three times a day."

8. Indigestion or Dyspepsia, Salt and water for.--"Drink sal and water before eating breakfast."

9. Indigestion or Dyspepsia, Slippery Elm for.--"Chew slippery elm; it aids digestion."

10. Indigestion or Dyspepsia, Cold Water for.--"A glass of cold water half hour before eating."

11. Indigestion or Dyspepsia, Hot Water for.--"Sip a cup of boiling hot water before eating anything."

12. Indigestion or Dyspepsia, Yolk of Egg and Salt for.--"A very simple but good remedy is the yolk of one egg, with a small quantity of common salt before breakfast. This treatment has been tried and known to cure in many cases."

13. Indigestion or Dyspepsia, Lemon Remedy for.--"Drink a half glass of water into which has been put the juice of a lemon (no sugar) morning and evening. This is a fine remedy."

14. Indigestion or Dyspepsia, Hops Excellent for.--"Pour one quart of boiling water over one-half ounce of hops, cover this over and allow the infusion to stand for fifteen minutes; the tea must then he strained off into another jug. A small cupful may be drank in the morning, which will create an appetite and also strengthen the digestive powers. It is an excellent medicinal drink." Hops does its work by the soothing and quieting action on the whole system, and should be taken regularly for some time.

15. Indigestion or Dyspepsia, Tested Remedy for.--"A good digestive is made as follows:

Tincture of Leptandrin	1 ounce
Tincture of Hydrastis	1 ounce
Tincture of Colombo	1 ounce
Wine of Pepsin	1 ounce

Mix. Dose, two teaspoonfuls after each meal."

The leptandrin acts on the liver, the colombo is a bitter tonic and hydrastis is a good tonic for the stomach.

16. Indigestion or Dyspepsia, Chamomile Tonic for Aged Persons also for Children.--"Put about one-half ounce chamomile flowers into a jug, pour a pint of boiling water upon them, cover up the tea, and when it has stood about ten minutes pour it off from the flowers into another jug; sweeten with sugar or honey. A cupful in the morning will strengthen the digestive organs, a teacupful in which is stirred a large dessert spoonful of moist sugar and a little grated ginger is an excellent thing to give to aged persons a couple of hours before dinner," It is remarkable to see how this treatment aids the digestion, especially in chronic cases. It may also be given to fretful children in small doses.

PHYSICIANS' TREATMENT in mild cases of acute Dyspepsia.--These recover by themselves by giving the stomach rest, and taking a dose of castor oil. Hot water is good to help to clean out the stomach.

Treatment in severe forms.--Promote vomiting by drinking large amount of warm water. This cleans the stomach of the sour, foul, decomposing food. If warm water does not cause vomiting, give any simple emetic you may have at your hand, such as mustard, etc., one teaspoonful. If the stomach tastes very sour, take some baking soda; subnitrate of bismuth (ten grains) is good, if you have it. If the bowels are constipated you should take an enema (injection) or salts. Soda water can be drank freely. Rest the stomach for a day from food. For the thirst cracked ice is relished. As the patient is usually very thirsty the mouth should be rinsed frequently with cool water and some can be swallowed. As stated before for nausea and sour belching, baking soda or bismuth subnitrate can be used when there is much gas, sour belchings; crust coffee is very good. Burn the toast and make a hot coffee of it.

DIET.--Given us by the Lady Superior of one of the largest Catholic Hospitals in Ohio.

May take--

Soups--Clear thin soups of beef, mutton or oysters.

Fish--Oysters raw, shad, cod, perch, bass, fresh mackerel.

Meats--Beef, mutton, chicken, lamb, tripe, tongue, calf 's head, broiled chopped meat, sweetbread, game, tender steak.

Eggs--Boiled, poached, raw.

Farinaceous--Cracked wheat, hominy, rolled oats, rice, sago, tapioca, crackers, dry toast, stale bread, corn bread, whole wheat bread, graham bread, rice cakes.

Vegetables--Spinach, string beans, green peas, lettuce, cresses, celery, chicory, asparagus.

Desserts--Rice, tapioca or farina pudding, junket, custards, baked apples, apple snow, apple tapioca, ripe fruits--raw or stewed.

Drinks--One cup of milk and hot water equal parts, or one glass of pure cool water, sipped after eating, Panopepton or cracked ice.

Must Not Take--Rich soups or chowders, veal, pork, hashes, stews, turkey, potatoes, gravies, fried foods, liver, kidney; pickled, potted, corned or cured meats; salted, smoked or preserved fish; goose, duck, sausage, crabs, lobster, salmon, pies, pastry, candies, ice cream, cheese, nuts, ice water, malt or spirituous liquors.

CHRONIC DYSPEPSIA (Chronic Indigestion--Chronic Gastritis--Stomach Trouble).--A chronic digestive disorder characterized by increased secretion of mucus, changes in the gastric juice, weakening of the stomach muscles and diseased changes in the mucous membrane.

Causes.--The use of unsuitable and improperly prepared food, too much fat, starchy foods, New England pie, and hot meals, biscuits, cakes, etc., greasy gravies, too strong tea or coffee, and too much alcohol. Eating too much food, eating too fast, and eating between meals. Drinking of ice and cold water during or after meals. Chewing, especially, and smoking tobacco.

Symptoms.--Almost every bad feeling can be put under this head, both physical and mental. It has been coming on gradually for some time and the warnings have not been heeded; The appetite is variable, sometimes good and often poor. Among the early symptoms are feelings of distress or oppression after eating, and they may amount to actual pain; great or small. Sometimes feels sick at the stomach, belching of gas and bitter liquids and vomiting of food immediately after eating or some hours later.

Stomach tender and painful to the touch. Stomach and abdomen are distended, especially after meals, with costive bowels or diarrhea.

Feels weary, blue, tired, discouraged, poor sleep, bad dreams, bitter taste in the mouth, tongue coated especially on the back part, craves different things, much wind on the stomach, acid stomach, heavy feeling in the stomach, sometimes as if a stone lay there. Stomach feels weak, it is hard to sit up. Frequently must lie down after meals. Urine may have sand in it, Stomach feels full after eating only a little, must open up the clothes across the stomach. Persons are cross, irritable, discouraged, gloomy, nervous, generally look thin, haggard and sallow. The dreams are of horrid things, nightmare.

MOTHERS' REMEDIES, Stomach Trouble, Spice Poultice for,--1. "Take all kinds of ground spices and make a poultice. Heat whisky and wet the poultice with it, then apply to the stomach and bowels." This will always give relief. Wetting the poultice with whisky will be found very beneficial as it will retain the heat longer.

2. Stomach Trouble, Oil of Hemlock for,--"The Oil of Hemlock is a superior remedy in gastric irritation of the stomach. Dose:--One to two drops in sweetened water every ten or twenty minutes until relief is afforded, for an adult."

3. Cramps in Stomach, Ginger and Soda for.--"One teaspoonful of ginger stirred in half glass of hot water in which a half teaspoonful of baking soda has been dissolved." The ginger is very beneficial, as it warms up the stomach and thereby relieves the cramps, and the baking soda relieves any gas in the stomach that may be causing the trouble.

4. Cramps in Stomach, Oil of Peppermint for.--"Put a few drops of peppermint in a glass of warm water. Take a teaspoonful every few minutes until relieved." This is an old time-tried remedy our grandmothers used to use and can be relied upon.

5. Cramps in Stomach, Mustard Poultice and Eggs for.--"Make a mustard poultice with whites of eggs instead of water, and apply same to bowels. Give a teaspoonful of blackberry tea every fifteen or twenty minutes until relieved." The poultice acts as a counter irritant and will almost always relieve the cramps without further medicines.

6. Pains in Stomach, Hot Plate for.--"Hot plate laid on stomach. Use the heavy English made plates, common to us in Canada, as they will hold heat longer."

PHYSICIANS' TREATMENT for Chronic Gastritis.--Most cases can be cured if the patient is willing to do the proper thing in eating and drinking and regulating the habits. It takes time to cure such cases, and plenty of grit and courage and "stick" on the patient's part. Remember it has been a long time coming, longer than it will be going if the patient does right. Diet and habits must be corrected. You cannot help the trouble if you put into the stomach what has caused it. We eat too much fat and too much improper and improperly cooked foods, our bread, etc., is half baked. Gravies are rich and greasy, everything is highly seasoned, very much like the life we lead.

Diet.--A regular time for eating and no eating between meals. Do not eat too much or too fast, or anything that you know disagrees with you. Fried foods are generally harmful, pies, cakes, hot breads, strong tea and coffee and alcohol, gravy and highly spiced foods; vinegar pickles, preserves, etc., are generally bad. If there is acid belching gas on stomach, the starch foods should be restricted, particularly potatoes and the coarser vegetables. Potatoes fried in lard or butter are always bad unless you are a hard physical worker. Dr. Osler, England, says breads, pancakes, pies, and tarts, with heavy pastry and fried articles of all sorts, should be strictly prohibited. As a rule, white bread toasted is more readily digested than bread made from the whole meal. Sometimes graham bread is better. Sugar and very sweet articles of food should be used in great moderation or avoided altogether. Ice cream frequently aggravates it. Soda water is a great dyspepsia producer. Fats, except a little good butter, very fat meats, and thick greasy soups and gravies should be avoided.

Ripe fruits are good in some cases. Bananas generally are not digested. Berries are frequently harmful. Milk is splendid diet for some people.

Cautions.--The bowels must be kept "moving" every day, try to do it by dieting, rubbing the abdomen and exercise. Bathing the abdomen in cool water is good. Go to the closet at a regular time every day and try to have a passage, as this helps. Never put off going to stool when nature calls. Dyspepsia is frequently made worse by constipation. Seek good cheerful company. Do not worry over your condition. By care and diet you will soon be all right.

Home Treatment.--1. Drink a glass of cold water an hour before breakfast, or hot water if it agrees better with you.

2. Do not eat much meat.

3. If the stomach wants tone, bitter tonics, like quassia, gentian, cardanum are good, even if drank as teas. When the tongue is coated with a white thick fur, golden seal is good. Medicines are not as essential as care and diet.

4. Charcoal in small doses is good for' a "gassy" stomach.

5. If a bitter tonic is needed the following is good:

Bicarbonate of Soda	1 dram
Tincture of Nux Vomica	1 to 2 drams
Compound tincture of Gentian, enough for	

Mix and take one teaspoonful to a dessert spoonful before meals.

NERVOUS DYSPEPSIA.--This is acquired from over work, worry, excitement, hurried or irregular meals, or inherited. It shows itself in all sorts of symptoms and they must be met as they come. Diet the same as for general dyspepsia, never eat when you are tired, rest after eating.

ULCER OF THE STOMACH AND DUODENUM (Upper part of bowel).--Round or perforating ulcer. The stomach ulcer is most common in women of twenty or thirty; servant girls, shoemakers, and tailors are frequently attacked. Ulcer of the duodenum is usually in males and may follow large superficial burns. The ulcer in the stomach is usually situated near the pylorus (small end) and in the first portion of the duodenum.

Symptoms.--Pain, local tenderness, vomiting and bleeding. These may not show until perforation or bleeding occurs. Distress after eating, often nausea and vomiting of very acid fluid, loss of weight and lack of blood.

Pain in the region of the stomach and the back is the most constant symptom. It is usually sharp, increased at once by food, relieved by vomiting. The tender spot can be located. Bleeding occurs in about one-half the cases and is usually profuse, bright red and fluid; if retained in the stomach the blood becomes clotted and brown. Tar-like stools when there is blood in the bowels. They usually recover under treatment, but may recur.

PHYSICIANS' TREATMENT FOR ULCER OF THE STOMACH.--1. Rest in bed most of the time for several months.

2. Feed by the rectum at first in severe cases, then peptonized or plain milk or buttermilk (three to four ounces) every two hours, some adding eggs, chicken, scraped beef and farinaceous food, made of: rice, flour, corn, potatoes, etc.

CANCER OF THE STOMACH.--Usually occurs after the age of forty.

Symptoms.--Indigestion for a few months; lack of blood and loss of weight. Well marked case shows the following symptoms:--Distaste for food, nausea, irregular vomiting, especially in cases where it is located near the pylorus--the opening between the stomach and the small intestine--usually one hour or more after eating; bleeding rarely profuse, usually of "coffee-ground type," dragging, gnawing or burning pain in the region of the stomach, back, loins or shoulders, usually increased by food; progressive loss of weight and strength; peculiar sallow look, skin pale or yellowish.

Course.--The person usually dies in twelve to eighteen months, sometimes in three to four months.

PHYSICIANS' TREATMENT of Cancer of the Stomach and Bowels.--There is no cure for this trouble except by an operation. This must be done early; even this may not cure but it, at least, prolongs life and makes the patient more comfortable while life does last.

In the line of medicine the only thing to do is to give only such remedies as will ease the symptoms.

Diet.--Attend to this also and you will save pain and distress. Every case should be treated as it needs and no special directions can be given here.

BLEEDING FROM THE STOMACH.--(Haematemesis).

Causes.--Cancer and ulcer of the stomach are main causes of excessive bleeding; poisons also cause it; injuries also.

Symptoms.--The vomited blood may be fluid or clotted; it is usually of dark color. The longer it remains in the stomach the darker it becomes. There may be great weakness and faint feeling on attempting to rise before a vomiting of blood. The contents of the bowels when passed look "tarry."

PHYSICIANS' TREATMENT for Bleeding of the Stomach.--- Absolute rest in bed is necessary. The bowels should be moved by an enema and it can be repeated carefully as often as necessary. Cracked ice in bag over the stomach. If the patient vomits much medicine is useless. They generally recover with rest. The extremities can be bandaged if there is great weakness and also external heat can be applied if there is a tendency to faintness.

Caution.--A person so afflicted, if he has ulcer, must be careful of his diet for months after an attack. He should be careful not to lift, over work, over eat or worry.

NEURALGIA OF THE STOMACH (Cardialgia, Gastralgia, Gastrodynia).--This is a severe pain in paroxysms in the region of the stomach.

Causes.--The patients are of a nervous type. They may have anemia, exhaustion from sickness and bleedings, the menstruation be at fault. Grief, worry and anxiety.

Symptoms.--The attack comes suddenly as a rule. The pains are agonizing in the stomach region, they may dart to the back or pass around the lower ribs. The attack lasts from a few minutes to an hour or two. It does not depend upon the food taken.

PHYSICIANS' TREATMENT for Neuralgia of the Stomach.- -The causes should be understood and especial treatment given for them. The patients are usually run down and a tonic treatment is needed. Constipation and menstrual troubles should be cured, worry, trouble and anxiety, if possible, be removed. The following is good for nervous patients:--

Valerianate of zinc	18 grains
Valerianate of quinine	18 grains
Iron Arsenate	2 grains

Mix and make into eighteen pills and take one after meals.

Bitter tonics can be taken such as gentian, columbo, quassia. Change of air and scene may be needed. Sometimes morphine must be given for the attack. A physician should do this. If there is much gas, soda and peppermint are good.

DIARRHEA:--Causes.

(a) Improper or excessive food, including green or over-ripe fruit.

(b) Poison substances; such as decomposed milk or meat either fresh or canned: or caused by arsenic, mercury or colchicum.

(d) Exposure to cold, wet or draughts.

(c) Stomach disorder, preventing thorough digestion.

(e) Extension of inflammation from other organs.

Symptoms.--Sudden colicky pain in the bowels, moving about with rumbling noises. The pain is not constant and is followed at intervals with a sudden extreme desire to empty the bowels. The stools may be four to twenty a day, watery or gruel-like in appearance and they sometimes contain mucus or undigested food. The stools usually relieve the pain for the time. It usually lasts two or three days or longer.

MOTHERS' REMEDIES.--Diarrhea.--1. "Wild Sage Tea." Wild sage tea is a very good remedy for bowel trouble because of its astringent virtues. Before the sage is used, however, the bowels should be thoroughly cleansed with castor oil or salts.

2. Diarrhea, Egg and Nutmeg for.--"Beat up an egg, grate in half a nutmeg and sweeten to taste. Repeat two or three times during the day. Remarks: Has been known to help in chronic cases when doctors' medicine failed."

3. Diarrhea, Scorched Flour and Sugar for.--"Scorched flour in boiled milk or scorched flour and sugar eaten dry is very good. This is a simple but a never failing remedy if taken right at the beginning of the trouble."

4. Diarrhea, Excellent Compound for.--

"Paregoric	1 ounce
Tincture of Camphor	1/2 ounce
Tincture of Ginger	1/2 ounce
Tincture of Red Pepper	1/2 ounce
Essence of Peppermint	1/2 ounce
Ether	1/2 ounce

Mix.--Dose for adult, one teaspoonful to four of water every two hours if necessary. This is an excellent remedy."

5. Diarrhea, Spice Poultice for.--"Make a poultice of all kinds of ground spices, heat whisky and wet the poultice, apply to the stomach and bowels."

6. Diarrhea, Blackberry Root Tea for.--"One-half ounce blackberry root boiled in one pint water fifteen minutes, strain. Dose.--One teaspoonful every hour or two until relieved."

7. Diarrhea, Hot Milk, for.--"A glass of sweet milk that has been boiled well. Drink hot; use several times daily until checked."

8. Diarrhea, Castor Oil for.--"Castor oil. Dose.--One to four teaspoonfuls according to age. Wrap warm flannel around abdomen."

9. Summer Complaint, Former Canadian's Remedy for.--"Eat one blossom of the May weed every hour or two until relieved. This remedy came from Port Huron and has been used by my father with success."

10. Summer Complaint, a Goderich Lady Found this Good for.--"Powdered rhubarb, cinnamon, baking soda (one tablespoonful of each), dissolve in one pint of boiling water, add one tablespoonful of peppermint; take every hour one teaspoonful in water."

11. Summer Complaint, Inexpensive Remedy for.--

"Paregoric	2 ounces
Brandy	1 ounce
Jamaica Ginger	1 ounce

Have used this and found it excellent." Dose: 1/2 dram every 3 hours.

12. Summer Complaint, Fern Root Good to Relieve.--"A decoction is made with two ounces of the sweet fern root boiled in one and one-half pints water to one pint. Dose.--A tablespoonful several times a day as the case requires. Most useful in diarrhea," This may be purchased at any drug store and will be found a very good treatment for diarrhea.

13. Summer Complaint, Milk and Pepper a Common Remedy for.--"Sweet milk and black pepper once or twice a day. Dose.--Three or four swallows. Mother used to use this for us children." The milk should be warmed, for in this way it relieves the diarrhea while the pepper is stimulating.

PHYSICIANS' TREATMENT for Diarrhea.--1. Rest in bed is the best. Abstain from food, especially at first, and then only give a little milk and boiled water or milk and lime water every two hours for two days. Cracked ice is good for the thirst.

2. A dose of one-half to an ounce of castor oil to an adult is of great benefit, as it removes all the irritating matter from the bowels. This often cures a light diarrhea. Follow by a blackberry wine or blackberry cordial if it is more severe.

3. For children.--An infusion of path weed is an excellent remedy for this trouble in children; after castor oil in one to two teaspoonful doses has been given. If castor oil is too bad to take, you can use what is called "spiced syrup of rhubarb," one to two teaspoonfuls to a child one to two years old, and then follow with blackberry wine.

4. For infants.--An infusion of chamomile is good for the green diarrhea of teething babies.

5. Another for infants.--For infantile diarrhea the root of geranium maculation or cranesbill, boiled in milk in the proportion of one or two roots to the pint, will be found of great service and is tasteless.

6. Ginger tea is frequently of good service, especially when the stomach needs "toning."

7. Infants of six months.--Chalk and bismuth mixture by Dr. Douglass, of Detroit.

"Subnitrate of Bismuth	2 drams
Paregoric	2 fluid drams
Chalk mixture	2 fluid drams

Mix and shake bottle. Give one-half to one teaspoonful for loose bowels in a child six months old, every two to four hours as needed."

DIET IN DIARRHEA.--From the Head Nurse of a Large Hospital.

May Take--

Soups.--Milk soup well boiled, clam juice, beef tea.

Meats.--Scraped fresh beef or mutton well broiled, sweetbread, beef juice from freshly broiled steak (all sparingly).

Eggs.--Lightly boiled or poached on dry toast.

Farinaceous.--Rice, sago, macaroni, tapioca, arrowroot, dry toast, milk toast, toasted crackers.

Desserts.--Milk puddings, plain, with sago, rice, tapioca or arrowroot (no sugar).

Drinks.--Tea, toast water, boiled peptonized milk, Panopepton.

Must Not Take--

Oatmeal, wheaten grits, fresh breads, rich soups, vegetables, fried foods, fish, salt meats, lamb, veal, pork, brown or graham bread, fruits, nuts, pies, pastry, ice cream, ice water, sugars, sweets, custards, malt liquors, sweet wines.

Infants.--Bottle-fed infants should stop milk and use egg albumen, etc. This is prepared by gently stirring (not to a froth) the white of one egg in a cup of cold water and one-fourth teaspoonful of brandy and a little salt mixed with it. Feed this cold.

If it causes foul or green stools it must be stopped. Dr. Koplik, of New York, recommends stopping the feeding of breast and bottle-fed infants in severe diarrhea or cholera infantum and to use the following:--Albumin water, acorn cocoa, or beef juice expressed and diluted with barley water. The white of one egg is equal in nourishing value to three ounces of milk and is well borne by infants. The albumin water can be used alternately with the solution of acorn cocoa or beef juice or barley water. Liebig's soup mixture is better liked by older children. Meat juice is made from lean beef, slightly broiled, then cutting it in squares and squeezing these in a lemon press. Rice or barley water can be added to this if the meat juice causes vomiting. Add only one or two teaspoonfuls of barley or rice water and increase, if it agrees well, in a day or two.

CHOLERA MORBUS (Acute Inflammation of Stomach and

Upper Bowel).--This is most common in young people in late summer, after indiscretion in eating.

Symptoms.--Sometimes the patient feels tired, then nausea, etc. The attack though is usually sudden, with nausea, vomiting, and cramp-like pains in the abdomen. The contents of the stomach are vomited. The bowel discharge at first is diarrhea and later like rice water. Repeated vomiting and purging, with severe cramps. It looks like true cholera.

MOTHERS' REMEDIES, Cholera Morbus.--Castor Oil for.--"Castor oil one tablespoonful for an adult, one-half tablespoonful for children." This is an old, tried remedy and very good.

2. Cholera Morbus, Blackberry Root and Boiled Milk for.--"Steep the root of the long blackberry, give in one-half teaspoonful doses; alternate with teaspoonfuls of well boiled sweet milk, one-half hour apart."

3. Cholera Morbus, Blackberry Cordial for.--"Take a quantity of blackberries, strain out all of the juice. To each pint of juice add a pint of sugar. Then put in a little bag or cloth one-half ounce of cinnamon, one-fourth ounce of mace, two teaspoonfuls of cloves. Place this little bag with spices in the berry juice and boil for about two minutes, after which remove bag of spices and add one large cup of brandy or whisky to each pint of juice."

4. Cholera Morbus, Tincture Cayenne Pepper for.--"Tincture cayenne pepper, five to ten drop doses in a little hot water. Before giving this medicine it is well to drink a quantity of tepid water and produce vomiting. This can be made more effective by adding five or ten drops of camphor."

5. Cholera Morbus, Nutmeg and Jamaica Ginger for.--"Grate one teaspoonful nutmeg, put few drops Jamaica ginger in three or four tablespoonfuls of brandy, add little water." The writer says this is one of the finest remedies she has ever known for summer complaint.

6. Cholera Morbus, Home Remedy for.--"To a pint of water, sweetened with sugar, add chalk one-half dram, anise, two drams, cayenne pepper, ten grains; boil this down to one-half pint. Give a teaspoonful every hour or two until relieved. Kerosene may be applied to the abdomen with cloths. This is a very good remedy and easily prepared."

7. Cholera Morbus, Old Reliable Remedy for.--

Tincture Rhubarh	4 ounces
Spirits Camphor	2 ounces
Paregoric (Tinct. opii camph.)	3 ounces
Spirits Ammonia	4 ounce
Essence Peppermint	1 dram

Take a half teaspoonful every two hours. This is a tested recipe; have known of its being used the last fifty years."

The camphor and paregoric will relieve the pain, while the rhubarb and pepper are stimulating and laxative.

8. Cholera Morbus, Common Remedy for.--"To check vomiting and purging, the following mixture is excellent:

Essence of Peppermint	1 ounce
Water	1 ounce
Carbonate of Potash	20 grains
Paregoric	1 teaspoonful
White Sugar or Honey	2 teaspoonfuls

Mix and shake well. Dose.--One teaspoonful every ten or twenty minutes until the patient becomes quiet. If necessary keep up bodily heat by means of hot flannels or bricks to extremities. Keep the patient quiet."

This is an excellent remedy for this trouble and may be used by anyone. The above mixture is for an adult.

PHYSICIANS' TREATMENT for Cholera Morbus.--l. Heat to the bowels and to the extremities. Give plenty of hot water to aid vomiting and to wash the stomach. It is always well to keep on drinking hot water and frequently the vomiting stops. If not, the camphor, laudanum and water can be given.

2. Morphine by hypodermic method. A doctor must give this.

3.

Tincture of Camphor	15 drops
Laudanum	15 drops

Mix in one-third of a cup of hot water. This is a good remedy. Mustard poultice to the stomach and bowels benefits.

CHOLERA INFANTUM, Symptoms.--Usually begins with a diarrhea, which is often so mild as to attract but little attention, but should be a warning. If a weakly baby has a diarrhea which persists, or is foul smelling and especially if there is a marked loss of flesh and dullness of mind, there is ground for worry. If a bright child loses interest in things and has diarrhea something is wrong. The two essential features are vomiting and diarrhea, and the vomiting is persistent. First it vomits food, then the mucus and bile. The thirst is great, but anything taken to relieve it is instantly thrown up. The stools are frequent, large and watery. They may be painless and involuntary. They may look like dirty water, but later they loose all color. They are sometimes so thin and copious as to soak through the napkin and saturate the bed. They may be without odor, and again the odor is almost over-powering. The prostration is great and rapid. The fontannelles, openings in the head, are depressed, the face becomes pale and pinched, and the eyes are sunken. It occurs usually during the summer months, oftener in babies under eighteen months and still more under a year old.

Cautions.--This book will probably find its way into homes many miles from a drug store and possibly a long distance from a physician. Should a child in that home show symptoms of cholera infantum it would be imperative for that mother to begin at once home treatments. We, therefore, give below a number of remedies which a mother can either prepare in her home or can take the precaution to have filled at some convenient time and keep constantly at hand, properly labeled so she can turn to them at any moment. On the other hand, should you have to wait even three or four hours for a physician begin one of the treatments below until he comes; you may save the child's life by doing so. Cholera infantum and pneumonia claim so many of our little ones each year, and in many cases snatch them away within a few hours of the first noticeable symptoms that we must advise you to call a physician as soon as you suspect it is serious. Cases vary and only a trained eye can detect the little symptoms and changes that may weigh in the balance the life of baby.

MOTHERS' REMEDIES for Cholera Infantum.--l. Castor oil and warm applications for.--"Give the child one teaspoonful of castor oil, then wring woolen cloths out of warm whisky and apply to the abdomen. This will most always give relief, especially after the castor oil has acted upon the bowels."

2. Cholera Infantum, First Thing to Do.--"The first thing to do is to give a teaspoonful of castor oil, so as to thoroughly clean out the bowels. Then add one tablespoonful of turpentine to one quart of hot water and wring cloths out of this and apply to the bowels to relieve the pain that is always present in this disease. The turpentine is especially good for the bowels when they are bloated and have much gas in them."

3. Cholera Infantum, White of Egg and Cathartic for.--"One teaspoonful castor oil every two hours, until the movements are natural. Give no food except albumen water, which is composed of the white of one egg (slightly beaten) and a small pinch of salt in a glass of cold water which has been previously boiled. Feed this by spoonfuls."

4. Cholera Infantum, Olive or Sweet Oil for.--"One teaspoonful sweet or olive oil three times a day and an injection of one tablespoonful of the oil at night, to be retained in the bowels. If continued this will completely cure."

5. Cholera Infantum, Spice and Whisky Poultice for.--"Take all kinds of ground spices, make a poultice. Heat whisky and wet the poultice. Apply to the stomach and bowels."

6. Cholera Infantum, Cabbage Leaf Poultice for.--"Take a cabbage leaf, hold it over the stove until warm as can be stood on back of hand; lay it across the child's abdomen. Repeat if necessary."

7. Cholera Infantum, Herb Remedy for.--"Strawberry root, blackberry root and raspberry root, equal parts, steeped together. I have used this remedy and found it good, but it should be used in time." Make a tea of these roots and take one teaspoonful every hour until relieved. This is a mild astringent.

8. Cholera Infantum, Tomatoes Will Relieve.--"Make a syrup of peeled tomatoes well sweetened with white sugar. Give one teaspoonful every half hour." This syrup is very soothing and the tomatoes are especially good if there is some ulcerated condition of the bowels. This preparation should always be strained before using.

9. Cholera Infantum, Injection for.--"For infant one year old inject into the bowels one pint of thin starch, in which is mixed from three to five drops of laudanum; cool, repeat night and morning. Plenty of water or cold barley water may be given and the food for a time may consist of egg albumen with a few drops of brandy. When the symptoms first appear apply a spice plaster or hot application over the abdomen; and keep child as quiet as possible." This is a remedy recommended and used by a number of physicians and has cured many severe cases.

Diets and Drinks.--Stop ordinary feeding at once. A little cream and water, or barley water and cream may do. If the breast milk excites the stomach and the bowels, stop it for a few hours. You can give a few drops of raw beef juice or a little brandy and water. To satisfy the thirst, wrap up a small bit of ice in a linen cloth and let the baby mouth it. Dilute the milk or stop entirely and give only water, or lime water and milk, barley water. Give all the water the child can drink boiled and cooled.

PHYSICIANS' TREATMENT for Cholera Infantum.--1. Washing out of the bowel frequently by injection controls the diarrhea. Use water of a temperature of 107. Elevate the tube about two feet above the bed, use one-half pint at one time. As the half pint flows in disconnect the funnel attached to the tube and the contents of the bowel are allowed to escape. Then allow another one-half pint to flow in. Some may escape and this is not an unfavorable sign. Keep on until a quart is given. This treatment is to wash and clean out the gut and stimulate the heart. The salt solution should be used, if necessary. Give only two daily.

2. For Vomiting.--Wash out the stomach through a tube or by giving a great deal of water.

3. Subcarbonate of bismuth for the vomiting and straining; two or three grains in powder every two or three hours. If there is much colicky pain, add one-half grain of salol to the bismuth powder.

4. Castor oil; one teaspoonful may be needed if the bowels have any fecal matter in them.

5. Mustard poultice or spice poultice on the belly is useful.

Vomiting.--This is simply a symptom; many diseases cause it, as scarlet fever, tuberculosis, meningitis, acute dyspepsia, biliousness, chronic dyspepsia, indigestion, neuralgia of the bowels, appendicitis, ulcer and cancer of the stomach, pregnancy, etc. Many persons with dyspepsia vomit their food.

MOTHERS' REMEDIES for Vomiting.--1. Spice Poultice to Stop.--"Make a poultice of one-half cup of flour and one teaspoonful of each kind of ground spice, wet with alcohol or whisky. Apply over the stomach." This acts as a counter irritant and has the same action on the system as a mustard plaster, only not so severe and can be left on for hours, as there need be no fear of blistering. This kind of a poultice should always be used when it is necessary to leave one on any length of time.

2. Vomiting, Mustard Plaster to Stop.--"Plaster of mustard on pit of stomach." Be very careful not to allow the plaster to remain on too long, as it will blister, and this would be worse to contend with than the vomiting.

3. Vomiting, Parched Corn Drink to Stop.--"Take field corn and parch it as brown as you can get it without burning. When parched throw in boiling water and drink the water as often as necessary until vomiting is stopped."

4. Vomiting, Peppermint Leaves Application for.--"Bruise peppermint leaves and apply to the stomach." This can be found in any drug store in a powder form, and is easily prepared by crushing the leaves and applying to the stomach. If you have the essence of peppermint in the house, that will answer about the same purpose taken internally and rubbed over abdomen.

5. Vomiting, to Produce, Mustard and Water for.--"To produce vomiting take two tablespoonfuls dry mustard, throw luke warm water over it and let stand a minute, then drink." This is an old, tried remedy that we all know about.

6. Vomiting, to Produce, Warm Water for.--"Drink a quart of warm water and you will easily find relief at once." The warm water remedy is very good as the water helps the patient by removing all decomposed food.

PHYSICIANS' TREATMENT for Vomiting.--The only way to treat it is to treat the disease that causes it. Here I may mention a very simple remedy; a tea made from wood soot is frequently helpful. It is the creosote in the wood soot that gives it its medical virtue.

2. For nervous vomiting; two to five drops of garlic juice is good. Dose of syrup for a child [is] one teaspoonful. Dose of syrup for an adult is four teaspoonfuls.

3. A little brandy on cracked ice is often good.

4. Oil of cloves, one-half to one drop, helps in some cases.

5. Lime water added to milk is good in babies.

6. Vinegar fumes, saturate a cloth and inhale the fumes.

7. Seidlitz powder often settles the stomach, soda also.

8. Mustard plaster over the stomach is good in all cases.

9. One-tenth of a drop of ipecac is good for nausea and vomiting.

10. One-half of a drop of Fowler's solution every two hours is useful in nausea following a spree. So also one drop dose of nux vomica every half hour.

APPENDICITIS.--Inflammation of the vermiform appendix is the most important of acute bowel troubles. Sometimes the appendix may contain a mould of feces, which can be squeezed out readily. Sometimes foreign bodies like pins are found there; in about seven per cent of cases foreign bodies are found.

It is a disease of young persons. Fifty per cent occur before the twentieth year. It is most common in males. Persons who do heavy lifting are quite subject to the disease. Some cases follow falls or blows. Indiscretions of diet are very apt to bring on an attack, particularly in those who have had it before. Pain in the appendix in such persons, frequently follows the eating of food hard to digest. Gorging with peanuts is also a cause.

Symptoms.--In a large proportion of cases the following symptoms are present:--Sudden pain in the abdomen, usually referred to the right groin region. Fever often of moderate form or grade. Disturbances of the stomach and bowels, such as nausea, vomiting and frequently constipation. Tenderness or pain in the appendix region. The pain in fully one-half of the cases is localized in right lower part of the abdomen, but it may be in the central portion, scattered, or in any part of the abdomen. Even when the pain is not in the region of the appendix at first, it is usually felt there within thirty-six or forty-eight hours. It is sometimes very sharp and colic-like; sometimes it is dull. The fever follows rapidly upon the pain. It may range from 100 to 102 and higher. The tongue is coated and moist usually,--seldom dry. Nausea and vomiting are commonly present. It rarely persists longer than the second day in favorable cases. Constipation is the rule, but the attack may start with diarrhea.

Local Signs.--Tenderness of the rectus muscle (to the right of the centre of the abdomen) and tenderness or pain on deep pressure. The muscle may be so rigid that a satisfactory examination cannot be made. Sometimes there is a hardness or swelling in the appendix region. Tenderness, rigidity and actual pain on deep pressure; with the majority of cases, a lump or swelling in the region of the appendix.

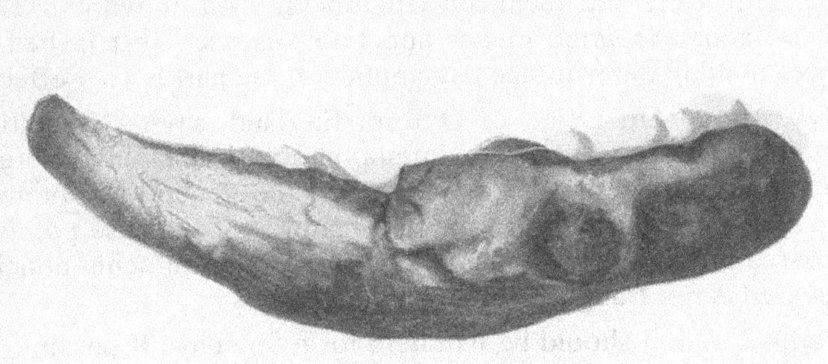

VERMIFORM APPENDIX.
When Affected by Inflammation and Gangrene
Necessitating an Operation.

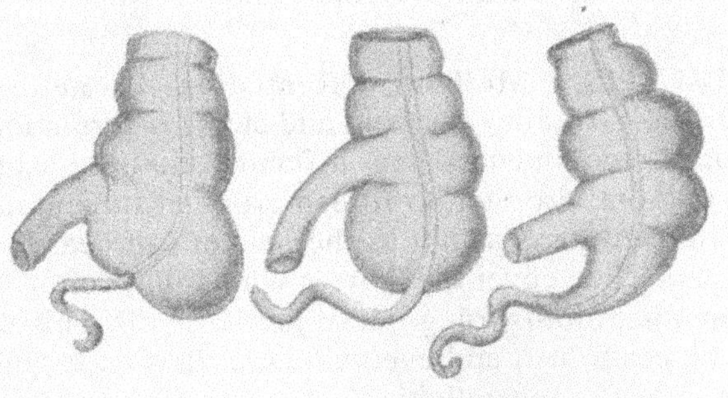

VERMIFORM APPENDIX.
Showing Different Types.

Vermiform Appendix.when Affected by Inflamation and Gangrene
necessitating an Operation
Vermiform Appendix showng Different Types.

Recovery.--Recovery is the rule. It frequently returns. General peritonitis may be caused by direct perforation of the appendix and death in appendicitis is usually due to peritonitis.

Surgeons have declared that sudden pain in the region of the appendix, with fever and localized tenderness, with or without a lump almost without exception means appendix disease. Rest in bed, take measures to allay the pain; ice bag applied to the part is very effective.

Operation.--Dr. Osler, of Oxford, England, says.--"Operation is indicated in all cases of acute inflammatory trouble in this region, whether the lump is present or not, when the general symptoms are severe, and when by the third day the features of the case points to a progressive (condition) lesion. An operation after an acute attack has disappeared is not fraught with much danger."

Diet.--All food should be withheld for a few days if possible. Liquids, such as egg albumen, weak tea, thin broth, barley or rice water, or milk diluted with lime water may be given in small quantities if necessary. When the acute symptoms have subsided, milk may be taken undiluted, and eggs may be added to the broth. When the pain and fever have disappeared entirely, gruels made of rice or barley, soft--boiled egg, scraped beef, stewed chicken, toast, and crackers may be added to the list; still later, mashed potatoes and vegetables, finely divided and strained, may be allowed and, finally, when well, usual diet resumed.

APPENDICITIS, Mothers' Remedies.--Home Treatment Found Good for.--"To allay the pain and stop the formation of pus in appendicitis it is recommended that a flannel cloth be saturated with hot water, wrung out, drop ten to fifteen drops of turpentine on it and apply to the affected parts as hot as the patient can bear. Repeat until relief is obtained. Then cover the bowels with a thin cotton cloth, upon which place another cloth wrung out of kerosene oil. This sustains the relief and conduces to rest and eventual cure. It is an essential part of the absorbent cure for appendicitis, and since its adoption doctors do not resort to a surgical operation half so often." The above is a standard remedy and will most always give relief.

PHYSICIANS' TREATMENT for Appendicitis.--The bowels should at first be moved by an enema, The patient should be perfectly quiet in bed. The ice-bag should be applied to the part, but wrapped in flannel and flannel also on the skin, It must not be allowed to make the flesh too cool. This coolness relieves the inflammation of the part. Small doses, from one-tenth to one drop, of aconite can be given for the fever and inflammation the first twenty-four hours. Dose every one to three hours. But little medicine is now given in appendicitis.

Caution.--Keep the bowels regular, especially if you have ever had appendicitis before, also be careful of your eating. This disease will attack high livers, hearty eaters and those with constipated bowels more quickly than others.

INFLAMMATION OF THE BOWELS. Mothers' Remedies.--1.--Inflammation of the Bowels, Excellent Remedy for.--"First bathe the abdomen with warm salt water, then lay over the navel a piece of lard the size of black walnut. Hold the hand over this until it softens; then rub well into the bowels. This often relieves when pills and powders fail." The massaging brings about action of the bowels without a cathartic usually. Sweet oil or olive oil instead of lard, will do as well.

2. Inflammation of the Bowels, Red Beet Poultice for.--"Take red beets; chop up, put in bag, warm a little and put across the stomach. This will draw out the inflammation quickly and makes a very good poultice."

3. Inflammation of the Bowels, Hop Poultice for.--"Take hops, strain them and put in a sack. Lay across the stomach and bowels."

4. Inflammation of the Bowels, Griddle Cake Poultice for.--"Apply hot griddle cakes on bowels. This acts as a poultice, and should be replaced as soon as cold." This remedy saved my life when I was seventeen years of age. Am now fifty. This remedy will be found very good, but care should be taken not to burn the patient.

5. Cold or Pain in the Bowels, Spice Poultice for Child or Adult.--"Take a cloth sack large enough to cover abdomen; take all kinds of ground spices, put in the bag and tie up, sprinkle bag lightly with alcohol, just enough to dampen spices; lay this on abdomen." This serves as a poultice and is an excellent remedy for this trouble. This may be used for a child as well as an adult.

6. Inflammation of the Bowels, Simple Remedy Always at Hand for.--"Apply hot woolen cloths to abdomen as hot as can be wrung out, change every few minutes. My life was saved twice when I was several hundred miles from a doctor by this treatment." This simple but never failing remedy is easily prepared and, as we all know, heat is the most essential thing for this trouble, especially moist heat.

7. Inflammation of the Bowels, a Rather Unique Remedy for.--"Cut the head off of a hen, cut open down the breast, take out the inwards, pound flat and roll with rolling pin and apply to the bowels. This will draw out all inflammation, but must be done in as little time as possible." The above remedy can do no harm. Many people use it. Perhaps other poultices would be easier to prepare, just as effective and save the hen.

8. Inflammation of the Bowels, Marshmallow Leaves, a Canadian Remedy for.--"Green marshmallow leaves (dry will do). Wet flannel and apply hot." Make a strong tea of the marshmallow leaves and while hot dip flannels and apply to abdomen.

9. Inflammation of the Bowels, Syrup of Rhubarb for.--"Add to three pints of simple syrup one and three-fourths ounces of crushed rhubarb, one-fourth ounce each of crushed cloves and cinnamon, one dram of bruised nutmeg, one pint of diluted alcohol, evaporate liquid by a gentle heat to one-half pint. Excellent in bowel complaint in one-half dram (one-half teaspoonful) doses every hour until it operates." The rhubarb moves the bowels and casts out all irritating matter. The oil of cloves stimulates the membranes of the bowels and the cinnamon and nutmeg are astringents.

MOTHERS' REMEDIES for Toothache, Dry Salt and Alum for.--1. "Equal parts. Take common salt and alum. Mix and pulverize these together, wet a small piece of cotton and cause the mixture to adhere to it and place in the hollow tooth. At first a sensation of coldness will be produced, which will gradually disappear, as will the toothache. This is an excellent remedy and should be given a trial by any person suffering with this trouble."

2. Toothache, Oil of Cloves Quick Relief for.--"If the tooth has a cavity take a small piece of cotton and saturate with oil of cloves and place in tooth, or you may rub the gum with oil of sassafras." These are both good remedies, and will often give relief almost instantly.

3. Toothache, Home-Made Poultice for.--"Make a poultice of a slice of toast, saturate in alcohol and sprinkle with pepper and apply externally. This will give almost instant relief."

4. Toothache, Clove Oil and Chloroform for.--"Clove oil and chloroform, each one teaspoonful. Saturate cotton and apply locally."

5. Toothache, Sure Cure for.--

"Peppermint water	1/2 ounce
Nitre	1/4 ounce
Chloroform	1 dram
Ether	1 dram
Oil of mustard	10 drops

Remark: This remedy will give relief where all others fail. Not only for toothache, but for neuralgia pains in any part of the body, apply with cloth moistened and lay on the parts affected. Continue until relieved."

6. Toothache, Salt and Alum Water for.--"Fill a bottle of any size half full of equal parts of pulverized alum and salt, then fill up the bottle with sweet spirits of nitre. Shake and apply it to the tooth and gums. Apply it freely, as there is nothing to hurt or injure you."

7. Toothache, Oil of Cinnamon for.--"A drop of oil of cinnamon will frequently relieve very serious cases of toothache. Apply to the tooth with a little cotton. This will at least give temporary relief until you can see your dentist and have the tooth treated."

8. Toothache, Reliable Remedy for.--"Chloroform, clove oil, alcohol, one half ounce of each. Mix together and saturate a piece of cotton and place it in the tooth. This is sure to give relief."

9. Toothache, From Decayed Teeth.--"If the tooth is decayed take a small piece of raw cotton, saturate with chloroform and place in cavity."

MOTHERS' TOOTH POWDERS.--1. "The ashes of burnt branches of the common grape vine make a very superior tooth powder. It will clean the blackest of teeth, if continued for a few mornings, to that of pure white."

2. Tooth Powder.--"Precipitated chalk four ounces, powdered orris root eight ounces, powdered camphor one ounce; reduce camphor to fine powder moistening with very little alcohol, add other ingredients. Mix thoroughly and sift through fine bolting cloth." Have used this with great success.

3. Tooth Powder.--"All tooth powders, or anything that has a grit will, with the friction of the brush, scour loose from the enamel of the teeth; and this is far superior to any of them in every respect.

Soap tree bark	1 pound
Turpentine	2 ounces
Powdered orris root	2 ounces
Alkanet root	1/2 ounce

Diluted alcohol, half water, sufficient to make the whole into one gallon. Let it stand in an earthen jar to macerate for fourteen days; stir occasionally, then strain and filter through filtering paper. The alcohol will have no injurious effect. This is an excellent tooth remedy."

4.--Tooth Wash.--"One teaspoonful of boracic acid in a pint of boiling water.

Tincture Myrrh	1/2 teaspoonful
Spirits of Camphor	1/2 teaspoonful
Essence of Peppermint	1/2 teaspoonful

Use in the water in which you brush your teeth. Let boracic acid water cool, then add last three ingredients."

5. Tooth Powder.--"Precipitated chalk four ounces, pulverized sugar two ounces, powdered myrrh one ounce, pulverized orris root one ounce. Mix and sift through fine bolting cloth. This is fine."

6. Tooth Powder, Commonly Used.--

"Precipitated Chalk	12 drams
Rose Pink	2 drams
Carbonate of Magnesia	1 dram
Oil of Rose	5 drops

Mix all well together and after using it you will find the following mouth-wash fine for rinsing out the mouth."

Antiseptic Mouth Wash.--

"Boric Acid	10 grains
Resorcin	4 grains
Salol	2 grains
Thymol	1/2 dram
Glycerin	1/2 dram
Pure water	1 ounce

This sweetens and cleanses the mouth."

7. Tooth Powder, Simple and Unsurpassed.--

Cream of Tartar, powdered	3 ounces
Cochineal	1 dram
Alum, powdered	4 drams
Myrrh	1 dram
Cinnamon	1 ounce
Sugar	1 ounce

Mix and pass through a sieve. This is a preparation that has no superior for cleaning, preserving and whitening the teeth.

PHYSICIANS' TREATMENT for Toothache.--1. Chloretone dissolved in oil of cloves and applied on a cotton wad is very good for toothache.

2. Creosote.--Put on a piece of cotton and put this in the hollow tooth.

3. Toothache in an ulcerated or hollow tooth, caused from wet feet, etc. Take a hot foot bath and drink a hot lemonade, hot ginger, or hot pennyroyal tea, and go to bed and take a good sweat. Aching tooth needs the care of a dentist. It pays to retain your natural teeth in good shape.

INTESTINAL OBSTRUCTION.--Causes.--This may be caused by strangulation, telescope (intussusception) of the bowels, twists and knots, strictures and tumors, abnormal contents.

1. Strangulation is the most frequent cause; this is caused by adhesions and bands from former peritonitis, or following operations. The strangulation may be recent and due to adhesion of the bowels to the abdominal cut or wound, or a coil of the bowel may be caught between the pedicle of a tumor and the wall of the pelvis. These cases are rather common after some operations.

2. Intussusception.--This means that one portion of the bowel slips into an adjacent portion. These two portions make a cylindrical lump varying in length from one-half inch to a foot or more. Irregular worm-like motion of the bowel is a cause of intussusception.

3. Twists and knots.--Most frequent between thirty and forty. (There is an unusually long mesentery.)

4. Strictures and tumors.--These are not very important causes.

5. Abnormal contents.--Fruit stones, coins, pins, needles, false teeth, round worms rolled in a mass. Coins rarely cause inconvenience.

Symptoms of Acute Obstruction.--Constipation, pain in the bowels, and vomiting are the three most important symptoms. Pain sets in early, and may come on abruptly when walking or more commonly when working. It is at first colicky, but soon becomes continuous and very intense, vomiting soon follows and is constant and very distressing. First the stomach contents are vomited, and the greenish bile-stained material, and soon the material vomited is a brownish-black liquid, with a bowel odor. This peculiar vomiting is a very characteristic symptom. Constipation may be absolute, without the discharge of either feces or gas. Very often the contents of the bowel below the obstruction are discharged. The abdomen is usually distended and when the large bowel is involved this is extreme. If it is high up in the small intestine, it may be very slight. At first, the abdomen is not tender, but later it becomes very sensitive and tender. The face is pale and anxious and finally collapse symptoms intervene. The eyes are sunken, the features look pinched and a cold, clammy sweat covers the skin. The pulse becomes rapid and weak. There may be no fever, and it may go below normal. The tongue is dry, parched, and the thirst is incessant.

Recovery.--The case terminates as a rule in death in three to six days, if aid is not given.

Treatment.--Purgatives should not be given. For the pain, hypodermics of morphine are needed. Wash out the stomach for distressing vomiting. This can be done three to four times a day. Thorough washing out of the large bowel with injections should be practised, the warm water being allowed to flow in from a fountain syringe and the amount carefully estimated. Hutchinson recommends that the patient be placed under an anesthetic, the abdomen kneaded, and a copious enema given with the hips placed high or patient in inverted position. Then the patient should be thoroughly shaken, first with the abdomen held downward and subsequently in the inverted position. If this and similar measures do not succeed by the third day surgical measures must be resorted to.

For bloating, turpentine cloths should be used, and other hot, moist applications.

Diet.--Should be very light, if any, for a day or so.

RUPTURE (Hernia).--Hernia means a protrusion of an organ from its natural cavity, through normal or artificial openings in the surrounding structures. But by the term hernia, used alone, we mean the protrusion of a portion of the abdominal contents through the walls, and that is known by the popular term of "rupture."

The most common forms of rupture protrude through one of the natural openings or weak spots in the abdominal walls, as for instance, the inguinal (groin) and femoral canals. The femoral canal is located at the upper and inner part of the thigh, and this place is a seat of rupture, especially in women. Rupture may also occur at the navel, when it is called umbilical hernia or rupture. The contents of a hernia are bowel and omentum (a covering of the bowel) separately or together. The bowel involved in a rupture is usually the lower portion of the small bowel, but the large bowel is sometimes affected. A sac covers the bowel or omentum in a rupture. This sac consists of the protruded portion of peritoneum, which has been gradually pushed through one of the canals (inguinal or femoral) or of the process of peritoneum, which has been carried down by the testicle in its descent, and the connection of which with the peritoneum of the abdomen still continues, not having been obliterated, as it usually is before birth. The former is called an acquired rupture sac; the latter is a congenital rupture sac, and it is found only in groin (inguinal rupture).

Causes.--Rupture is more common in men than in women. It may occur at any time of life. The majority of cases occur before middle age, and the largest number during the first ten years of life, owing to the want of closure of the peritoneum which is carried down by the testicles before birth. Rupture is most frequently strangulated between the ages of forty and fifty.

Location.--The great majority of cases of rupture are groin or inguinal rupture.

Symptoms.--A fullness or a swelling is first noticed in the groin, which is made worse in standing, coughing and lifting. This disappears on lying down and reappears on rising in many cases, even at first; coughing makes the lump or swelling harder. It may come on both sides, when it is called double rupture or hernia.

MOTHERS' REMEDIES.--Rupture, Poultice for.--"Take equal parts of lobelia and stramonium leaves; make a poultice and apply to the parts. Renew as often as necessary. This combination makes a very effective poultice and is sure to give relief."

PHYSICIANS' TREATMENT.--A person should wear a truss (support) that fits perfectly, and this should not cause any pain or discomfort. The truss should be worn all day, taken off at night after going to bed and put on before rising, when still lying down. If it is put on after rising a little of the gut may be in the canal and pressed down by the support. There are many kinds of supports.

Operations now performed for rupture are very successful if the patient takes good care for months afterwards until the parts are thoroughly healed. The operation simply closes a too large opening. The testicles descending through the groin canal from the abdominal cavity before birth and in congenital rupture, left too big an opening. In acquired rupture, these natural openings were enlarged by lifting, falls, etc. The round ligament of the womb goes down through this canal and sometimes there is too large an opening left or acquired by accident.

Irreducible Rupture.--This is when the rupture cannot be returned into the abdominal cavity, and it is without any symptoms of strangulation. They are of long standing and of a large size. This condition is often due to carelessness of a patient in not keeping in a reducible rupture with a proper support. Adhesions form, holding the rupture. Even if it is small, it gives rise to much discomfort and the patient is always in danger of strangulation of the rupture.

Operation for radical cure is generally a success.

Strangulation Hernia or Rupture.--This means the rupture is so tightly constricted that it cannot be returned into the abdominal cavity, and its circulation is interfered with; then there is not only obstruction to the passage of the feces, but also an arrest of circulation in the protruded portion of bowel which, if not relieved, results in gangrene and death. This occurs more often in old than in recent ruptures and more often in congenital than in acquired rupture.

Symptoms.--Sudden and complete constipation with persistent vomiting. The lump may be tense, hard and irreducible. Then there is faintness, collapse; severe abdominal pain, complete constipation, with no gas passing, then vomiting, at first of food, then of the bile-stained fluid and finally of fluid with a bowel odor. All these symptoms increase and the patient gradually sinks from exhaustion in eight or nine days, though in very acute cases the patient may die within forty-eight hours.

MOTHERS' REMEDIES.--Strangulated Hernia, Hop Poultice for.--"A large warm poultice of hops over the abdomen will be found one of the best known means of relieving strangulated hernia."

PHYSICIANS' TREATMENT.--It must be reduced or an operation must be performed and soon.

To reduce.--The patient is put under an anesthetic and placed on his back with the hips (pelvis) raised and the thigh of the affected side flexed, bent up and rotated inward if the rupture be inguinal or femoral. This motion relaxes the parts. The neck of the sac is then seized with the thumb and fingers of one hand, and thus fixed, while with the other hand, the operator endeavors to return the strangulated gut by gentle pressure in the proper direction. In femoral rupture, this is at first downward, to bring the gut opposite the opening then backward and then upward. In groin (inguinal) rupture it is usually slightly upward and outward. It must be coaxed, kneaded and squeezed carefully. Care must be taken. If it cannot be returned in from five to ten minutes no further time should be wasted, but an operation should be performed immediately. This consists in cutting down to the constriction and through it, thus allowing the rupture to he reduced.

The patient should be kept in bed and treated the same way as for other abdominal operations.

Caution.--Persons with rupture must be very careful not to lift or fall. If a support is worn it must fit perfectly and be worn with comfort.

INTESTINAL COLIC. (Enteralgia).--Causes.--Predisposing; poor general condition, worry, over-work, nervous disposition. Exciting causes; exposure, gas in the bowels, mass of feces, undigested or irritating food, cold drinks, green fruit, ice cream when a person is very warm.

Symptoms.--Intermittent pain usually in the umbilical (navel) region, moving from place to place, dull or sharp pain, relieved by pressure or bending forward. Abdomen is distended or drawn back. It lasts a few minutes or many hours, ending gradually or suddenly, after a passage of gas or movement of the bowels.

PHYSICIANS' TREATMENT.--1. Remove cause first if possible. Mild cases; put heat to the abdomen by hot water bag, wring cloths out of hot water and put in them ten drops of turpentine and place over the bowels hot. Give dose of peppermint water or ginger tea.

2. Severe case.--Morphine hypodermically, if necessary, in a severe case; mustard poultice is good, also a spice poultice.

3. Tincture of Colocynth (bitter cucumber) is an excellent remedy for this trouble. I have often used it with great success. Put five drops of it in a glass half full of water and give two teaspoonfuls every fifteen minutes until relieved. A few doses generally relieve the patient.

THE LIVER.--The liver is the largest gland in the body, and is situated in the upper and right part of the abdominal cavity. The lower border of the liver corresponds to the lower border of the ribs in front and to the right side. It weighs fifty to sixty ounces in the male; in the female, forty to fifty ounces. It is about eight to nine inches in its transverse measurement; vertically near its right surface it is six to seven inches, while it is four to five inches thick at its thickest part. Opposite the backbone from behind forward it measures about three inches. The left lobe, the smallest and thinnest, extends to the left, over what is called the pit of the stomach.

BILIOUSNESS.--This condition presents different symptoms in different cases, but it always includes languor, headache or dizziness, perhaps some yellow color of the skin and conjunctiva, and a general sense of want of tone, depression of spirits and discomfort.

Causes.--The liver does not perform its function well, or there is a retention of bile in the bile ducts. Most of the symptoms do not depend directly upon the changes in the bile, but upon failure of proper digestion in the stomach and intestines. Certain poorly prepared foods or improper food for stomach digestion, quickly cause the development of active fermentation and its results irritate the stomach mucous membrane bringing about a faulty stomach secretion of mucus, which causes further trouble. It may end in a sick headache.

TREATMENT. Prevention.--Normal, easily digested food, open bowels. Active exercise, horseback riding, massage of the liver region. Stooping over and bending from side to side and bending back with feet close together are good aids.

Diet.--Do not over-eat. Avoid alcohol in any form. Stimulating foods such as spices, mustard salads, concentrated meat extracts and meat broths, pepper, horseradish are not to be used. Do not use too much salt; strong coffee and tea are harmful. In severe cases milk either diluted with water or lime water or peptonized should alone be used.

Gruels, albumen water, kumiss, buttermilk and oyster broth may be allowed. Orange juice as well as lemonade may generally be given. Fasting is good in biliousness. No one will starve in a few days of fasting.

MOTHERS' REMEDIES.--1. Biliousness, Lemons for.--"One lemon squeezed in a glass of water with a very little sugar, repeat for several days." Lemon is a very good medicine, and it is surprising to know how few people realize what medical properties the lemon contains. This is a good, simple, but very effective remedy.

2. Biliousness, Salt and Water for.--"Take a teaspoonful of salt to a cup of water and drink before breakfast for a few mornings." It is a well-known fact that a little salt in warm water before breakfast is laxative and also cleanses the system and bowels on account of its purifying action.

3. Biliousness, (chronic) Dandelion Tea for.--"Dandelion root is highly recommended for this." The root should be collected in July, August or September. Dose:--A strong tea may be taken freely two or three times a day, or the fluid extract may be purchased at any drug store.

4. Biliousness, a cheap and very safe plan.--"Drink plenty of cold water and exercise freely in the open air." Following the above advice is often better than medicines and spring tonics, also unless doing hard physical labor, cut down on the meat eating. In fact, eat less generally for a time.

5. Biliousness, Salt Lemonade for.--"Hot salt lemonade night and morning. Juice of one lemon and teaspoonful salt to as much hot water as you can drink."

6. Biliousness, Boneset Tea for.--"Pour hot water on boneset and let stand until it is cold. Take a swallow occasionally." This is very good.

PHYSICIANS' TREATMENT. Medicines.--1. Nitro-hydrochloric acid three drops three times a day in half a tumblerful of water is valuable.

2. Twenty drops of fluid extract of Queen's root three times a day.

3. The following combination forms a good pill to be taken every night:

Extract of Chirata	40 grains
Podophyllin	4 grains
Wahoo	8 grains
Culver's root	8 grains
Creosote	10 grains

Mix and make into twenty pills. Take one every night.

4. For the Attack.--Take calomel one-sixth grain tablets; one every fifteen minutes until six are taken, and then follow with two to four teaspoonfuls of epsom salts.

JAUNDICE (Icterus).--A symptom consisting in discoloration by bile pigment of the skin, whites of the eyes, other mucous membranes and secretions.

Causes.--Obstruction of the gall ducts, from gall stones, inflammation, tumor, strictures, from pressure by tumors, and other enlarged abdominal organs.

Symptoms.--The skin and the conjunctiva (red membrane of the eyes) are colored from a pale lemon yellow to a dark olive or greenish black. The itching may be intense, especially in a chronic case. The sweat may be yellow. The stools are a pale slate color, from the lack of bile, and are often pasty and offensive. The pulse is slow. Recovery depends upon the cause. Plain, simple jaundice cases recover in a few days or weeks.

MOTHERS' REMEDIES.--1. Jaundice, Sweet Cider Sure Cure for.--"New cider before it ferments at all. Drink all you can." This is a very simple remedy, but a sure one if taken in the early stages of jaundice. It causes the bowels to move freely and carries off any impurities in the system.

2. Jaundice, Lemon Juice for.--"Take a tablespoonful of lemon juice several times a day." This disease is produced by congestion of the liver, and as lemon is excellent as a liver tonic it is known to be an excellent remedy for jaundice.

3. Jaundice, Peach Tree Bark for.--"Take the inner bark of a peach tree, and make a strong tea, and give a teaspoonful before each meal for five days, then stop five days, and if the patient's indications do not warrant a reasonable expectation that a cure is effected repeat the medicine as above. I never knew of a case in which the above medicine failed to cure. Keep the bowels open with sweet oil."

MOTHERS' REMEDIES for Liver Complaint. Mandrake Root for.--1. "Dry and powder the mandrake root (often called may-apple) and take about one teaspoonful." This dose may be repeated two or three times a day, according to the requirements of the case. This is a stimulant, a tonic and a laxative, and is especially good when the liver is in a torpid and inactive condition.

2. Liver Trouble, Dandelion Root Tea for.--"Steep dandelion root, make a good strong tea of it; take a half glass three times a day." This is a very good remedy as it not only acts on the liver, but the bowels as well. This will always cure slight attacks of liver trouble.

3. Torpid Liver, Boneset Tea for.--"Drink boneset tea at any time during the day and at night. It is also good for cleansing the blood." This is a very good remedy, especially for people who live in a low damp region.

4. Liver Trouble, Mandrake Leaves for.--"A very good remedy to use regularly, for several weeks, is to use from one to three grains of may-apple (mandrake) seed, night and morning, followed occasionally by a light purgative, as seidlitz powder or rochelle salts." This is sure to give relief if kept up thoroughly.

5. Liver Trouble, Mullein Leaf Tea for.--"Mullein leaves steeped, and sweetened. Drink freely." This acts very nicely upon the liver.

PHYSICIANS' TREATMENT for Liver Trouble.--1. For the itching, hot alkaline baths with baking soda in water, or dust on the following:--

Starch	1 ounce
Camphor, powdered	l-1/2 drams
Oxide of Zinc	1/2 ounce

Mix and use as a powder, or use carbolic vaselin locally. Move the bowels with salts and do not give much food for a few days. Use nothing but milk.

2. The following is good to move the bowels when the stool is yellow and costive in a child one year old:

Sulphate of Magnesia	2 ounces
Cream of tartar	2 ounces

Mix and give one-half teaspoonful in water every three hours until the bowels move freely. Phosphate of soda in one dram doses every three hours is good.

3. Severe Type and Epidemic Form.--Give one to two drops of tincture myrica cerifera (barberry) every two hours for an adult. This I know to be very good.

4. The common simple kind of jaundice will get well readily by moving the bowels freely and keeping the patient on light food.

CATARRHAL JAUNDICE. (Acute catarrhal angiocholitis).--Jaundice caused by obstruction of the terminal portion of the common duct, by swelling of the mucous membrane.

Causes.--This occurs mostly in young people. It follows inflammation of the stomach or bowels, also from emotion, exposure, chronic heart disease. It may be epidemic.

Symptoms.--Slight jaundice preceded by stomach and bowel trouble. Epidemic cases may begin with chill, headache and vomiting. There may be slight pain in the abdomen, the skin is light or bright yellow, whites of the eyes are yellowish, pain in the back and legs, tired feeling, nausea, clay colored stools. Pulse is rather slow, liver may be a little enlarged. It may last from one week to one to three months.

PHYSICIANS' TREATMENT for Catarrhal Jaundice.--1. Restrict the diet if the stomach and bowels are diseased. Sodium phosphate may be given one teaspoonful every three hours to keep the bowels open. Drink large quantities of water and with it some baking soda one-half to one teaspoonful in the water.

2. If you have calomel you may take one-tenth of a grain every hour for four hours, and then follow with the sodium phosphate in one-half teaspoonful doses every two to three hours, until the bowels have fully moved, or epsom salts, two to four teaspoonfuls. Keep in bed if there is a fever or a very slow pulse say of forty to fifty.

GALL STONES. (Biliary Calculi, Cholelithiasis).--Cases of gall stones are rare under the age of twenty-five years. They are very common after forty-five, and three-fourths of the cases occur in women. Many people never know they have them. Sedentary habits of life, excessive eating and constipation tend to cause them. They may number a few, several, or a thousand, or only one.

Symptoms.--There are usually none while the stones are in the gall bladder, but when they pass from the gall bladder down through the (channel) duct into the bowel they often cause terrific pain, especially when the stone is large. Chill, fever, profuse sweating and vomiting, which comes in paroxysms or is continuous. The pain may be constant or only come on at intervals. The region of the liver may be tender, the gall bladder may be enlarged, especially in chronic cases and very tender. In some cases the pain comes every few weeks and then may be scattered, sometimes seeming to be in the stomach, and then in the bowels, or in the region of the liver. When a person has such pains and locates them in the stomach or bowels, and they come periodically, every week or two or more, he ought to be suspicious about it being gall stones, especially if the symptoms do not show any stomach trouble. If the stone is large and closes the common duct, jaundice occurs; the stools are light colored; the urine contains bile. The attacks of pain may cease suddenly after a few hours, or they may last several days or recur at intervals until the stone is passed. The stones may be found in the bowel discharges after an attack. Death may occur from collapse during an attack.

MOTHERS' REMEDIES.--1. Gall Stones, Sweet Oil for.-- "Massaging the part over the region of the liver lightly night and morning is very good, following by drinking a wineglassful of sweet oil at bedtime." The patient should take some good cathartic the next morning, such as a seidlitz powder or cream of tartar. Teaspoonful in glass of water each morning. This treatment should be continued for several weeks and is very effective.

9

2. Gall Stones, Tried and Approved Remedy for.--"Drink about a wineglass of olive oil at bedtime followed in the morning by a cathartic, as seidlitz powder, or cream of tartar and phosphate of soda; teaspoonful each morning in wineglass of water. This treatment to be pursued several weeks. Massage the part over the liver lightly night and morning. If the suffering is intense use an injection of thirty drops of laudanum to two quarts of water." In many cases the cathartic may not be needed as the olive oil will move the bowels freely. Massaging the parts over the liver will cause it to work better and has proven successful in many cases.

PHYSICIANS' TREATMENT for Gall Stones.--1. For the pain. Morphine must be used and by the hypodermic method; one-fourth grain dose and repeated, if necessary, and chloroform given before if the pain is intense, until the morphine can act. Fomentations can be used over the liver.

2. Soda.--The bowels must be kept open by laxatives, Sodium Phosphate or Sodium Sulphate, (Glauber's) salt.

3. Olive Oil.--Olive oil is used very extensively. I do not know whether it does any good; some people think it does. From two to ten ounces daily, if possible. The phosphate or sulphate of sodium should be taken daily in one to two teaspoonfuls doses each day. Some claim these salts prevent formation of gall stones.

4. Powder for the Itching.--For the intolerable itching you may use the following powder, dust some of it over the skin:

Starch	1 ounce
Zinc Oxide	1/2 ounce
Camphor	1-1/2 drams

Mix into a powder.

Diet.--This must be thoroughly regulated. The patient should avoid the starchy and sugar foods as much as possible. He or she should also take regular exercise. If a person afflicted with gall stones keeps the stomach and bowels in good condition, they will be better. Pure air, sunshine, exercise, and diet are big factors in the treatment of chronic diseases. A woman so afflicted should not wear anything tight around the stomach and liver, corsets are an abomination in this disease; olive oil if taken must be continued for months.

Surgery.--The operation is indicated when the patient is suffering most of the time from pain in the liver region or when the person is failing in health, or during an acute attack. When there are symptoms of obstruction or when there is fever, sweating shows that there is pus in the gall bladder. Also an operation is then necessary, and in most cases it results satisfactorily.

CANCER OF THE GALL BLADDER, AND BILE DUCTS. Causes.--It usually occurs between forty and seventy years of age. The cases that originate here show no percentage in either sex; but those that appear here as secondary cancers are three times as frequent in women as in men. Chronic irritation by gall stones is an important cause. They are hard to diagnose and, of course, fatal in the secondary kind. For the primary kind early complete removal may cure if you can get at them.

CIRCULATORY DISTURBANCES OF THE LIVER. (Acute Hyperemia or Congestion).--This occurs normally after meals, and in acute infections, diseases, etc.

CHRONIC CONGESTION OR NUTMEG LIVER.--This is due to an obstruction of the blood circulation in the liver by chronic valvular heart disease with failure of heart action. Lung obstruction in the trouble called Emphysema, Chronic Pneumonia, etc., may cause it. The cut section of a liver shows an appearance like a nutmeg, due to a deeply congested central vein and capillaries. In a later stage the liver is contracted, central liver cells are shrunk and the connective tissue is increased.

ACUTE YELLOW ATROPHY. (Malignant Jaundice).--This is fortunately a rare disease. There is rapid progress, and it is fatal in nearly all cases. The liver is very small and flabby. The symptoms are many and are hard to differentiate. You must depend upon your physician. The only thing for him to do is to meet the symptoms and relieve them if possible.

CIRRHOSIS OF THE LIVER. (Sclerosis of the Liver, Hobnail Liver, Gin Drinkers Liver, Hard Liver).--This occurs most often in men from forty to sixty years old. It is not uncommon in children.

Cause.--It is usually due to drinking of alcohol to excess, especially whisky, brandy, rum or gin. The liver is small and thin; hard, granular, white bands run through it and press on the liver cells and destroy them.

Symptoms.--These are few as long as proper circulation in the heart is maintained. Fatty cirrhosis is often found in post-mortems. The first symptoms are the same as those accompanying chronic gastritis, dyspepsia, They are:--Appetite is poor, nausea, retching and vomiting, especially in the morning; distress in the region of the stomach, constipation or diarrhea. These increase and vomiting of blood from the stomach may occur early and late. Bleeding from the stomach and bowels, etc., cause the stools to look like tar. Nosebleed and piles are common and profuse; bleeding may cause severe lack of blood. The epigastric and mammary veins are enlarged. Ascites (dropsy in the abdomen) usually occurs sooner or later and may be very marked, and it recurs soon after each tapping. The feet and genital organs may be oedematous (watery swelling), jaundice is slight and does not occur until late. During the late stage the patient is much shrunken, face is hollow, the blood vessels of the nose and cheeks are dilated, abdomen is greatly distended. Delirium, stupor, coma or convulsions may occur at any time.

PHYSICIANS' TREATMENT for Cirrhosis of the Liver.--It is usually fatal; sometimes even after temporary improvements. No coffee or alcohol; simple diet, bitter tonics, keep bowels open, A physician must handle such a case.

ABSCESS OF THE LIVER. Hepatic Abscess: Suppurative Hepatitis.--This is a circumscribed collection of pus in the liver tissue. If there is only one abscess it is in the larger lobe in seventy per cent of the cases. The amount of fluid contained in such an abscess may be two or three quarts and its color varies from a grayish white to a creamy reddish-brown; when the abscess is caused by a type (amebic) of dysentery, there is generally only one abscess, occurring more often in the right lobe, whereas other forms due to septic infection give rise to many abscesses.

Causes.--This disease is rare even in tropical climates. When it is excited by gall stones, it is invariably septic in character and the infecting material reaches the interior through the liver vessels or bile passages. Stomach ulcers, typhoid fever, appendicitis, may bring on such an abscess. Pus wounds of the head are sometimes followed by a liver abscess. The most common method of infection is through the portal vein. Other causes that may be mentioned are foreign bodies traveling up the ducts, as round-worms and parasites.

Symptoms.--Hectic temperature, pain, tenderness, and an enlarged liver, and often slight jaundice. In acute cases the fever rises rapidly, reaching 103 or 104 in twenty-four hours. It is irregular and intermittent, and it may be hectic, that is, like the fever of consumption. Shakings or decided chills frequently are present with the rise of fever and when the fever declines there may be profuse sweating. The skin is pale and shows a slight jaundice, the conjunctiva being yellowish. Progressive loss of strength with disturbance of the stomach and bowels is present. The bowels are variable and constipated and loose. Dropsy of the abdomen (Ascites) may develop, on account of pressure on the big vein, inferior vena-cava. Lung symptoms, severe cough, reddish-brown expectoration are often present.

THE ABSCESS.--May break into the pleural cavity, bronchial tubes, lungs and stomach, bowels, peritoneum or through the abdominal wall.

Recovery.--The result is unfavorable as it generally goes on to a rapid termination. The abscess should be opened and evacuated when its location can be detected. The death rates ranges from fifty to sixty per cent.

Treatment.--Open it if you can, Sponge liver region with cool water. For the pain, mustard poultices, turpentine stupe or hot fomentations prove beneficial. Keep up strength by stimulation and quinine.

Diet in Liver Troubles sent us from Providence Hospital (Catholic), Sandusky, Ohio:

May Take--

Soups--Vegetable soups with a little bread or cracker, light broths.

Fish--Boiled fresh cod, bass, sole or whiting, raw oysters.

Meats--Tender lean mutton, lamb, chicken, game, (all sparingly).

Farinaceous--Oatmeal, hominy, tapioca, sago, arrowroot (well cooked), whole wheat bread, graham bread, dry toast, crackers.

Vegetables--Mashed potato, almost all fresh vegetables (well boiled), plain salad of lettuce, water-cress, dandelions.

Desserts--Plain milk pudding of tapioca, sago, arrowroot or stewed fresh fruit (all without sugar or cream), raw ripe fruits.

Drinks--Weak tea or coffee (without sugar or cream), hot water, pure, plain or aerated water.

Must Not Take--

Strong soups, rich made dishes of any kind, hot bread or biscuits, preserved fish or meats, curries, red meats, eggs, fats, butter, sugar, herrings, eels, salmon, mackerel, sweets, creams, cheese, dried fruits, nuts, pies, pastry, cakes, malt liquors, sweet wines, champagne.

ACUTE GENERAL PERITONITIS. (Inflammation of the Peritoneum, Lining of the Abdominal Cavity).--Causes. Primary; Occurs without any known preceding disease, and is rare. Secondary; Occurs from injuries, extension from inflamed nearby organs, such as appendicitis or infection from bacteria, without any apparent lesion (disease of the bowel). Perforation causes most of the attacks of peritonitis. Peritonitis may accompany acute infections or accompany chronic nephritis, rheumatism, pleurisy, tuberculosis and septicemia. Peritonitis occurs from perforation of the bowel in typhoid fever also, and it frequently occurs after appendicitis and sometimes after confinement.

Symptoms.--This is often the history of one of the causes mentioned above, followed in cases with perforation or septic disease by a chill or chilly feeling and pain, varying at first, with the place where the inflammation begins. The patient lies on his back, with the knees drawn up, and the body bent so as to relax the muscles of the abdomen, which are often rigidly contracted,--stiff at first on the side where the pain starts. The pain may be absent. The abdomen becomes distended, tympanitic (caused by gas). An early symptom is vomiting and it is often repeated. There is constipation; occasionally diarrhea occurs. The temperature may rise rapidly to 104 or 105 and then become lower; it is sometimes normal. The pulse is frequent, small, wiry and beats 100 to 150 per minute; the breathing is frequent and shallow. The tongue becomes red and dry and cracked. Passing the urine frequently causes pain; sometimes there is retention of urine. The face looks pinched, the eyes are sunken, the expression is anxious, and the skin of the face is lead colored or livid. Hiccoughs, muttering, delirium or stupor may be present.

Recovery, Prognosis, etc.--The action of the heart becomes weak and irregular, respiration is shallow, the temperature taken in the rectum is high, the skin is cold, pale and livid, death occurs sometimes suddenly, usually in three to five days; less often thirty-six to forty-eight hours; or even after ten days. The results depend mainly upon the cause of the inflammation, and the nature of the infection, infectious disease that produces it, being usually very bad after puerperal sepsis (after confinement), induced abortion, perforation of the bowel or stomach, or rupture of an abscess.

LOCAL PERITONITIS.--This may come from local injury, but it is usually secondary to empyema, tuberculosis, or cancer, abscess, perforation of the stomach or bowel, ulcer, etc.

Symptoms.--Onset is usually sudden. There is sudden local pain, increased by any movements; tenderness, and vomiting; then chills, irregular fever, sweating, difficult breathing, emaciation.

TREATMENT OF THE ACUTE PERITONITIS.--There must be absolute rest, morphine by hypodermic method, one-fourth to one--half grain to relieve the pain. Ice cold and hot fomentations with some herb remedy like hops, smartweed, etc.; or cloths wrung out of hot water with five to ten drops of turpentine sprinkled on them. This is very good when there is much bloating from gas.

The turpentine should be stopped when the skin shows red from it. The cloths should not be heavy or they will cause pain by their weight. Ice water can be used when cold cloths are needed.

For vomiting.--Stop all food and drink for the time and give cracked ice.

Diet.--Should be hot or cold milk with lime water or peptonized milk if necessary. If the feeding causes vomiting, you must give food by the rectum. For the severe bloating enemas containing turpentine should be given, one to two to six ounces of water used with ten to thirty drops of turpentine in it; sometimes it is necessary to resort to surgery.

TUBERCULAR PERITONITIS.--This may occur as a primary trouble or secondary to tuberculosis of the bowels, lungs, and Fallopian tube. It is most frequent in males between twenty and forty.

Symptoms.--These are variable. It may occur like acute peritonitis with sudden onset of high fever, pain, tenderness, bloating, vomiting and constipation; these symptoms passing into those of chronic peritonitis. Often there are gradual loss of strength and flesh, low and irregular fever; frequently the temperature goes below normal with a little ascites tympanites, constipation, diarrhea and masses in the abdomen which consist of the omentum (apron covering the bowels) rolled up and matted into a sausage-shaped tumor in the upper part of the abdomen, or of thickened or adherent coils of the bowel, enlarged mesentric lymph nodes, etc. Spontaneous recovery may occur, or the course of the disease may resemble that of a malignant tumor.

Treatment.--If there is effusion and few adhesions, cutting in and removing the fluid may help. In other cases good nourishing diet with cod liver oil is best.

ASCITES. (Hydroperitoneum. Abdominal Dropsy).--This is an accumulation of serous fluid in the peritoneal cavity. It is but a symptom of disease.

Local Causes.--Chronic peritonitis, obstruction of the portal (vein) circulation as in cirrhosis of the liver, cancer or other liver disease, from heart disease, tumors, as of the ovaries or enlarged spleen. All these mentioned may produce this dropsy.

General Cause.--Heart disease, chronic nephritis, chronic malaria, cancer, syphilis, etc.

Symptoms.--Gradual increasing distention of the abdomen, causing sometimes a sense of weight, then difficulty of breathing from pressure. The abdomen is distended, flattened at the sides unless it is very full. The skin may be stretched tense, superficial veins are distended. The navel may be flat or even protrude and around it the vessels may be greatly enlarged. There is fluctuation when you tap sharply at one side, while holding your hand on the other side you feel a wavy feeling.

PHYSICIANS' TREATMENT for Ascites.--First treat the disease causing it. Sometimes it is necessary in order to prolong life to repeatedly tap the patient as in cirrhosis of the liver. When it is caused by the heart or kidneys, give cathartics that carry away much liquid, hydragogue cathartics. One dram of jalap at night followed by a big dose of salts before breakfast. Cream of tartar and salts are good, equal parts. Or cream of tartar alone, one to two drams, with lemon juice in water in repeated doses. Digitalis and squill, of each one grain to cause great flow of urine. Infusion of digitalis is also good to increase flow of urine, when the heart is the real cause of the ascites. These treatments take the liquids away through the proper channels, the bowels and kidneys.

Ascites caused by an Ovarian Tumor.--The tumor must be removed. I am not in favor of indiscriminate operating, but operations often save lives. I remember one case in which I very strongly urged the lady to have an operation performed. It was a case of ascites, caused, as I was sure, by a tumor of the ovary. The lady, as almost all people do,--and I do not blame them for it,--dreaded even the thought of an operation, but she was finally compelled to have an operation or die. She filled so full that it was almost impossible for her to breathe. She went away from home in terrible shape, almost out of breath, and returned home a well woman and has remained so. Such cases formerly died. But not all cases of ascites can be cured by an operation, it depends upon the cause. In many cases all one can do is to doctor the cause, if that cannot be removed, make the patient's remaining days as comfortable as possible.

DISEASES OF THE RECTUM AND ANUS.--The lower part of the alimentary canal is called the rectum, originally meaning straight. It is not straight in the human animal. It is six to eight inches long. The anus is the lower opening of the rectum. In health it is closed by the external **Sphincter** (closing muscle). Disease may wear this muscle out and then the anus remains open, causing the contents of the bowel to move involuntary.

CONSTIPATION. Causes.--1. Mechanical obstruction.

2. Defective motion of the bowels.

3. Deficient bowel secretions.

4. Other causes. Mechanical obstruction.--Anything that will hinder the free and easy passage of the feces (bowel contents). Too tight external sphincter (rectum) muscle, stricture, tumors, etc. Bending of the womb on the bowel.

Defective Worm-like Bowel Movement.--Irregular habits of living head the list causing this defective action. Everyone should promptly attend to Nature's call. Some people wait until the desire for stool has all gone, and in that way the "habit" of the bowels is gradually lost. Everyone should go to stool at a certain regular time each day, and at any other time when Nature calls. If a person heeds this call of Nature, the call will come regularly at the proper time, say every morning after breakfast. If these sensations (Nature's calls) are ignored day after day, the mucous membrane soon loses its sensitiveness and the muscular coat its tonicity, and as a result, large quantities of fecal matter may accumulate in the sigmoid (part of the bowel) or in the rectum without exciting the least desire to empty the bowels. Again, irregular time for eating and improper diet are liable to diminish this action also. Foods that contain very little liquid and those that do not leave much residue are liable to accumulate in the bowel and at the same time press upon the rectum hard enough to produce a partial paralysis.

Deficiency of the Secretions.--Many of the causes that hinder worm-like motion are also likely to lessen the normal secretions of the bowel. Some kinds of liver diseases tend to lessen the secretions of the bowel, because the amount of bile emptied into the bowel is lessened. Sometimes the glands of the intestine are rendered less active by disease and other causes.

Sundry Causes.--Diabetes, melancholy, insanity, old age, paralysis, lead poisoning and some troubles of local origin, like fissure of the rectum, ulceration, stricture and polypus.

Symptoms.--Headache, inattention to business, loss of memory, melancholy, sallow complexion, indigestion, loss of appetite, nervous symptoms. Spasmodic muscular contraction of the external sphincter. The bowel contents press upon it; spasm of this sphincter muscle is frequently brought on by the presence of a crack in the mucous membrane, caused by injury inflicted during expulsion of hardened feces. Instead of aiding a bowel movement, the muscles now present an obstruction beyond control of the will and aggravate the condition. The most frequent cause of disease of the rectum is constipation and anyone of the following local diseases of the rectum and anus may be a symptom of constipation. (1) Fissure or crack of the anus. (2) Ulceration. (3) Hemorrhoids (piles). (4) Prolapse (falling). (5) Neuralgia. (6) Proctitis and periproctitis.

Fissure of the anus is a common local symptom of constipation. The feces accumulate when the bowels do not move for a few days, the watery portion is absorbed; they become dry, hard, lumpy, and very difficult to expel, frequently making a rent (tear) in the mucous membrane and resulting eventually in an irritable fissure. Ulceration of the rectum and the sigmoid (part of the bowel) is a symptom of persistent constipation, because the pressure exerted upon the nourishing blood vessels by the fecal mass causes local death of the tissues.

Hemorrhoids (Piles) may be produced by constipation in several ways; first by obstruction to the return of the venous (dark) blood. Second, by venous engorgement (filling up) of the hemorrhoidal veins during violent and prolonged straining at stool. Third, as a result of the general looseness of the tissues in those suffering from constipation.

Prolapse (Falling of the Bowel).--This falling of the rectum may be partial or complete, and may be caused by straining or by the downward pressure exerted by the fecal mass during the emptying movement of the bowel. It may also be the result of a partial paralysis of the bowel caused by pressure of the feces upon the nerves.

Proctitis and Peri-Proctitis.--Inflammation of the rectum and surrounding tissue that may or may not terminate in an abscess and fistula, sometimes follows injury to the very sensitive mucous membrane by the hardened feces.

Neuralgia of the Rectum.--This may sometimes result from the pressure of the fecal mass upon the nearby nerves causing pain in the sacrum coccyx (bones).

MOTHERS' REMEDIES.--1. Constipation, a Good Substitute for Pills and Drugs.--"Two ounces each of figs, dates, raisins, and prunes (without pits) one-half ounce senna leaves. Grind through meat chopper, and mix thoroughly by kneading. Break off pieces (about a level teaspoonful) and form into tablets. Wrap each in a wax paper and keep in covered glass jars, in a cool place. Dose.--One at night to keep the bowels regular. Very pleasant to take."

2. Constipation, Substitute for Castor Oil.--"Take good clean figs, and stew them very slowly in olive oil until plump and tender, then add a little honey and a little lemon juice, and allow the syrup to boil thick. *Remarks.*--Keep this in a covered glass jar and when a dose of castor oil seems necessary, a single fig will answer every purpose. Not unpleasant to take."

3. Constipation, Hot Water for.--"A cup of hot water, as hot as one can drink it, a half an hour before breakfast." The hot water thoroughly rinses the stomach and helps the bowels to carry off all the impurities.

4. Constipation. Excellent Nourishment for Old People.--"A tablespoonful of olive oil three times a day internally for weak or very old people: it can be injected,--used as an enema." Olive oil will be found very beneficial for young people as well as old. It acts as a food for the whole system and is very nourishing.

5. Constipation, Salt and Water for.--"A pinch of salt in a glass of water taken before breakfast every morning. I have found it a very good remedy." This is a remedy easily obtained in any home and will be found very helpful. Few people seem to realize how valuable salt is as a medicine. It acts as a stimulant and loosens the bowels.

6. Constipation, Water Cure for.--"Drink a quantity of water on retiring and during the day." This simple home remedy has been known to cure stubborn cases of constipation if kept up faithfully.

7. Constipation, Tonic and Standard Remedy for.--"Calomel one ounce, wild cherry bark one ounce, Peruvian bark one ounce, Turkish rhubarb ground one ounce, make this into one quart with water, then put in sufficient alcohol to keep it." Dose:-- Take a small teaspoonful each morning when the bowels need regulating, or you need a stimulating tonic.

8. Constipation, Glycerin and Witch-Hazel Remedy Where Castor Oil Failed--"Equal parts of glycerin and witch-hazel." Dose :-- One teaspoonful every night at bedtime. In severe cases where you have been unable to get a movement of the bowels by the use of other cathartics, take a teaspoonful every two hours until the bowels move freely. This remedy has been known to cure when castor oil and other remedies have failed.

9. Constipation, Well-known Remedy for.--

"Fluid Extract Cascara Sagrada	1 ounce
Syrup Rhubarb	1 ounce
Simple Syrup	2 ounces
Mix."	

One teaspoonful at night or fifteen drops four times a day for an adult.

10. Constipation, Effective Remedy, in the most Stubborn Cases of.--

"Fluid Extract Cascara Sagrada	1 ounce
Fluid Extract Wahoo	1 ounce
Neutralizing Cordial	2 ounces
Mix."	

Adults may take a teaspoonful of this mixture before retiring, this will be found very effective in the most stubborn cases of constipation.

11. Constipation, Remedy from a Mother at Lee, Massachusetts.--

"Senna Leaves	1/2 pound
English Currants	1/2 pound
Figs	1/4 pound
Brown Sugar	1 large cup

Chop all together fine. Dose:--One-fourth to one-half teaspoonful every night. Do not cook. The best remedy I know."

12. Constipation, Fruit and Hot Water Cure for.--"Drink a pint of hot water in the morning before eating. Eat fruit, plenty of apples, eat apples in the evening, and they will loosen the bowels. Chew them fine, mix with saliva."

13. Constipation, Herb Tea for.--"One ounce senna leaves steeped in one-half pint of hot water, with a teaspoonful of ginger powdered; strain. This is a most certain and effective purge, and mild in its action upon the bowels. Dose:--A cupful at bedtime. This is far superior to salts."

14. Constipation, Purshiana Bark Tea Without an Equal for.-- "An infusion of one ounce of purshiana bark to one pint of boiling water; infuse for one hour and strain. It stands without an equal in the treatment of constipation in all its varied forms. Dose:--One teaspoonful, morning and evening according to symptoms or until the bowels are thoroughly regulated." This is fine for constipation, especially if of long standing. It may be used in connection with cascara. This will give relief when other remedies fail.

PHYSICIANS' TREATMENT for Constipation.--Too much reliance has been placed upon medicine in the treatment of this disease and too little attention given to diet, and the establishment of regular habits in eating, exercising, sleeping and attending to the calls of Nature. Also, local disease of the rectum has been overlooked until of late years. Remedies of a laxative and cathartic nature soon lose their power and the dose must be repeated or a new remedy must be given. This method of treatment is well recommended and is very good.

1--Stretching of the sphincter.

2--Frequent rectal and abdominal massage.

3--Copious injection of warm water (in the beginning only).

4--Application of electricity over the abdomen and in the rectum.

In addition to this treatment which must be carried out by a physician the patient must observe the following rules: Go to stool daily, and as near the same time as is convenient, correct errors of diet. Drink an abundance of water and eat sufficient fruit. Take plenty of outdoor exercise; take a cold bath every morning followed by a thorough rubbing. Dress warmly in winter and cool in summer. Change of temperature or climate if the case demands it. Be temperate in all things affecting the general health. Stretching the sphincter must be done carefully, but in a thorough manner. It can only be done properly by an experienced person. Stretching of the sphincter closes the opening so that the feces are not passed at all times. It is circular in shape. Sometimes this grows larger, stiffer, or it acts spasmodically. The opening is often so tight in some people that it is difficult to introduce even a finger, and it frequently produces a spasm of pain in the bowels, stomach and head to do so. This kind will produce constipation or make it worse. In such cases it should be stretched thoroughly but carefully so that the muscle will be able to close the opening and the bowel contents will not pass at any time unhindered. There are two methods of stretching the muscle--forcible or gradual. The forcible method is generally done by inserting the two thumbs into the anus and stretching the muscle thoroughly in every direction until there is no resistance. (Dilators are made for this purpose, but unless they are very carefully used they will tear the muscle). The forcible method should be done under an anesthetic. Gradual stretching is done when an anesthetic cannot be used. It is better to do too little than to do too much at the first sitting. The muscle is very stubborn sometimes, and it requires careful handling or the irritability will be increased. An instrument in the hands of a careful man is all right. They can be stretched by the fingers or the Wales' bougie, thus: Patients should come to the office two or three times a week, the instrument (bougies) are introduced and allowed to remain within the bowel until the muscle resistance is overcome, and many times their withdrawal will soon be followed by a copious stool. Forcible stretching is seldom required more than once, if a large sized instrument is used from time to time afterward, just as in gradual stretching; when thorough dilatation has been accomplished, the muscle instead of acting as an impassable barrier to the discharge of the feces, now offers only passive resistance, but sufficiently strong, however, to prevent any unpleasant accidents, yet not strong enough to resist the power of the expulsory muscles when the latter are brought into full play during stool. Large quantities of feces do not now accumulate; consequently the pressure upon the mucous membrane and neighboring nerves is eliminated, and the bowel regains its normal sensibility and strength. There are now sold dilators in sets for self use in almost every drug store. These when used continuously do good and successful work.

Abdominal Massage. (Kneading, Rubbing, etc.).--This is an essential feature in the treatment. It was practiced by Hippocrates hundreds of years ago. Place the patient in the recumbent position upon a table which can be so manipulated that the head may be raised or lowered, the body rolled from side to side. Gentle but firm pressure is then made with the palm of the hand and the ball of the thumb over the large intestine beginning in the lower right groin region. Then go up to the ribs on the right side, then over the body to the same place on the left side and down to the left lower side and center, accompanying the pressure by kneading the parts thoroughly with the fingers. Repeat this several times for about ten to twelve minutes. At first this should be practised every day; later twice a week. Special treatment should be given the small intestines and liver when the bile and intestinal secretion are lessened. In children gentle rubbing of the abdomen with circular movements from right to left with a little oil for ten minutes daily will help to increase the action of the bowels and often bring on a normal movement.

Copious Warm Water Injections.--This is good at the beginning of the treatment when the feces become packed. They soften the mass and aid its discharge. The water must go above the rectum into the colon. To do this a colon tube from eighteen to twenty-four inches long, a good syringe (the Davidson bulb) hard rubber piston or a fountain syringe, the nozzle of which can be inserted into the tube, are required. The patient is placed in the lying down position on the left side with knees drawn up, with the hips elevated. Oil the tube and pass it gently and slowly up the bowel for a few inches until it meets with a slight obstruction. A few ounces of water are then forced through the tube and at the same time pressure is made upward with the tube; by these means the obstruction will be lifted out of the way each time the tube meets with resistance; the procedure must be repeated until the tube is well within the colon. Attach the syringe to the tube and allow the water to run until the colon is distended. A quart to a gallon of warm water can be used depending upon the age and amount of feces present. The water should be retained as long as possible.

The injections should be continued daily until all the feces has been removed. They should not be used for weeks as has been recommended. If soap suds are used in the enema, green or soft soap should be used, not the hard soap.

Electricity.--One pole may be placed over the spinal column and the other moved about over the course of the colon, or one over the spine and the other over the rectum.

Again constipation is caused by the womb lying upon the rectum. Change this condition. (See diseases of women).

Rules.--Patients should go to stool daily at the same hour, usually after the morning meal. You can educate the bowel to act daily at the same hour or after breakfast; or on the other hand not more than once in two or three days in those who are careless in their habits. Some patients need to have two or three movements daily in order to feel well. It may take time to educate the bowels to do this, but it can be done in many cases and many persons become constipated because they put off attending to the educated bowel's call, and often produce constipation by carelessness. It is surprising how many educated people put off this duty; Nature neglected, soon ceases to call. If constipated persons will persevere in going to the closet at or near the same time every day and devote their entire time while there to the expulsion of the fecal contents, and not make it a reading room, they will bring about the desired result. Patients are apt to become discouraged at first; they should be informed that the final result of the treatment is not influenced by the failure of the bowel to act regularly during the first few days. Do not strain to expel the stool.

Corrections of Errors in Diet.--This is one of the necessary features in the treatment. All kinds of foods known to disagree should be discarded. The foods should be easily digested. In children the diet should be rich in fats, albuminoids and sugar, but poor in starches. A reasonable amount of fruits such as apples, oranges, and figs should be allowed. Meals should be at regular hours. Foods that can be used:

May Take--

Soups.--Meat broths, oyster soup.

Fish.--Boiled fish of all kinds, raw oysters.

Meats.--Almost any fresh tender meat, poultry, game, not fried.

Farinaceous.--Oatmeal, wheaten grits, mush, hominy, whole wheat bread, corn bread, graham bread, rye bread.

Vegetables.--Boiled onions, brussels sprouts, spinach, cauliflower, potatoes, asparagus, green corn, green peas, string beans, salads with oil.

Desserts.--Stewed prunes, figs, baked apples with cream, ripe peaches, pears, oranges, apples, melons, grapes, cherries, raisins, honey, plain puddings, fig puddings, apple charlotte.

Drinks.--Plenty of pure water, cold or hot, new cider, buttermilk, orange juice, unfermented grape juice.

Must Not Take--

Salt, smoked, potted or preserved fish or meats, pork, liver, eggs, new bread, puddings of rice or sago, pastry, milk, sweets, tea, nuts, cheese, pineapple, spirituous liquors.

Foods classed as laxatives are honey, cider, molasses, and acid fruits, such as apples, pears, peaches, cherries, and oranges. Berries are effective laxatives on account of the acids and seeds they contain. (Huckleberries are constipating). Prunes, dates and figs are good and effective, also fruit juices.

Drinks.--There are few laxatives better than a glass of cold water or preferably hot water, taken upon an empty stomach before breakfast; water prevents the feces from becoming dry and massed, and stimulates the intestinal movements. A pinch of salt added to the water increases its effectiveness.

Out-door Exercise.--This should be taken regularly and freely.

Bathing.--The best time is before breakfast, and in as cold water as possible. The bath should be followed by a thorough rubbing of the skin with a Turkish towel.

Clothing.--Warm clothing in winter; cool clothing in summer. Cold weather induces constipation, and warm weather diarrhea. Moderate manner of living is everything.

PHYSICIANS' TREATMENT for Constipation. 1. One year to three years.--For infants one teaspoonful or less of black molasses or store syrup, or of olive oil; and Mellin's food eaten dry, is good for babies a year and older.

2. Small Children.--Increase cream in the milk, give oatmeal or barley water. Castile soap suppository, enema, massage, castor oil, or citrate of magnesia if drugs are needed.

3. Older Children.--In older children, fruit, oatmeal, etc. Black molasses is good for children, one to two teaspoonfuls.

4. Fluid Extract of Cascara Sagrada.--Dose: ten to sixty drops at night. This is good for a great many cases and sometimes it cures the trouble, but on the other hand it seems to injure some people.

5. The Aromatic Cascara is also good; doses are larger and pleasant to take. This is more agreeable for children.

6. The Compound Licorice Powder is a mild, simple laxative and effective. It is composed of senna eighteen parts, licorice root powder sixteen parts, fennel eight parts, washed sulphur eight parts, sugar fifty parts. Dose:--One to two teaspoonfuls.

7. For one dose, or one capsule, the proportions would be:

	ONE CAPSULE	AMOUNT FOR ONE DOZEN
Aloin	1/4 grain	3 grains
Extract of Belladonna	1/8 grain	10 grains
Extract Nux Vomica	1/4 grain	3 grains
Powdered Gentian	3 grains	36 grains

Mix and put up in twelve capsules and take one at night.

There are many tablets and pills made that can be bought at any drug store. No doubt some of them are first class, though perhaps not attaining to that high degree of virtue claimed in their advertising columns.

ITCHING OF THE ANUS. (Itching Piles) (Pruritus ani).Causes.--

An inherited or an acquired nervous constitution. Disease of the colon, rectum or anus. Improper diet. Skin affections in that region. Operations about the rectum and anus with resulting discharge sometimes.

Diseases in the neighboring organs. Disease of the general system. Diarrhea, discharge of mucus and pus, fissure, etc. Irregular habits and dissipation. Over-seasoned foods such as lobster, salmon, shell-fish and foods containing much grease or starch are especially conducive to it; the same is true of tea, coffee, cocoa, strong alcoholic drinks. Skin diseases, lice, pin worms often cause it.

After Operations.--Some part has not healed, and there is left an irritating discharge.

Symptoms.--There is intense itching at the anus, increased by warmth, and contact of the buttocks. The itching grows worse after the patient becomes warm in bed. It may spread and extend to the scrotum, down the limbs and sometimes over the lower back.

PHYSICIANS' TREATMENT FOR ITCHING OF ANUS. Preventive and Palliative.

DIET.--May Take.--Strong drink must be prohibited; tea, coffee, cocoa, if used at all should be sparingly used. A light diet such as bread, milk, eggs, nourishing soups, kumiss and a little fresh fish, broiled steak, etc., may he used.

May Not Take--Hot cakes, pastry, parsnips, cheese, pickles, beans, cucumbers, cabbage, oatmeal, pork, shell-fish, salmon, lobster, salt fish, confectionery and starchy or highly seasoned foods are to be prohibited. Regular meals, no lunches between meals, and the patient must not over-eat at any time. Long course dinners and over-indulgence in highly seasoned foods and wines aggravate it.

Remedies for Bath.--The bowels should move daily and the parts should be kept clean. The parts should be bathed with hot water or weak solutions of carbolic acid, alcohol or listerine, the heat being especially soothing. Bathing the parts with bran, oatmeal, flaxseed, salt, rice, slippery elm teas, or tar water adds much comfort to these parts. Do not wash much with soapy water.

1. Separate the Buttocks with Gauze, a thin layer of cotton or a piece of soft cloth. This eases the soreness, pain and itching by absorbing the secretions and preventing irritations while walking. The patient should not scratch the parts. Direct pressure over the itching parts with a soft cloth, or by drawing a well oiled cloth across the sore parts several times gives relief.

2. Dr. Allingham Recommends the introduction of a bony or ivory nipple-shaped plug into the anus before going to bed. It is self retaining, about two inches in length, and as thick as the end of the index finger. He claims it prevents the night itching by pressing upon the many veins and terminal nerve fibres of the parts. When the rawness is extensive and the parts are highly inflamed, the patient should be kept to bed and kept on his back with the limbs separated until the irritation is allayed.

3. Local Applications.--Soothing remedies: These can be used when the parts are inflamed and raw. Lead and opium wash, or boric acid, or linseed oil, or starch, or cocaine, and zinc stearate with boric acid. This form of zinc adheres to the parts when rubbed on, and is thus more valuable.

4. The following is good to dust in the parts:--

Boric Acid	2 drams
Stearate of Zinc	2 drams
Talcum	1 dram

Apply as a dusting powder.

5. The following is good for the raw parts:--

Carbolic Acid	1 scruple
Menthol	10 grains
Camphor	10 grains
Suet enough to make	1 ounce

Mix. Apply freely two or three times daily after cleansing the parts. Melt the suet and when partially cold, add the other ingredients.

6. The following is good for the itching and to heal the raw surfaces:--

Carbolic acid	1 dram
Zinc oxide	1 dram
Glycerin	3 drams
Lime water	8 ounces

Mix and apply once or twice daily to relieve the itching.

7.

Carbolic acid	1 dram
Calamin prep	2 drams
Zinc oxide	4 drams
Glycerin	6 drams
Lime water	1 ounce
Rose water enough to make	8 ounces

Mix. Keep in contact with the itching area by means of gauze or cotton while the itching is intense.

8. For injections into the rectum for rawness of the mucous membrane, the following is well recommended. Use three drams of this at one time.

Fluid extract Witch Hazel	2 ounces
Fluid extract Ergot	2 drams
Fluid extract Golden Seal	2 drams
Compound tincture Benzoin	2 drams

Carbolized Olive or Linseed Oil 1 ounce
Carbolic acid 5 per cent
Mix and shake well before using.

9. For the same purpose:--
Ichthyol 1 dram
Olive oil 1 ounce
Mix and apply in the rectum on a piece of cotton.

PILES. (Hemorrhoids).--Hemorrhoid is derived from two Greek words, meaning blood and flowing with blood. "Pile" is from

10

a Greek word meaning a ball or globe. Hemorrhoids, or piles, are varicose tumors involving the veins, capillaries of the mucous membranes and tissue directly underneath the mucous membrane of the lower rectum, characterized by a tendency to bleed and protrude. They were known in the time of Moses.

Varieties.--There are the external (covered by the skin) and the internal (covered by mucous membrane).

Causes.--Heredity. More frequent in males. Women sometimes suffer from them during pregnancy. Usually occurs between the ages of twenty-five and fifty. Sedentary life, irregular habits, high-grade wines and liquors, hot and highly seasoned and stimulating foods. Heavy lifting. Those who must remain on their feet long or sit on hard unventilated seats for several hours at a time. Railway employees, because they take their meals any time and cannot go to stool when Nature calls, causing constipation. Purgatives and enemata used often and for a long time. Constipation is perhaps the most frequent cause: when a movement of the bowels is put off for a considerable time the feces accumulate and become hard and lumpy and difficult to expel. If this hard mass is retained in the rectum, it presses upon the blood vessels interfering with their circulation and by bruising the vessels may induce an inflammation of the veins when the hardened feces are expelled; straining is intense, the mass closes the vessels above by pressure and forces the blood downward into the veins, producing dilatation when the force is sufficient. One or more of the small veins near the anus may rupture and cause a bloody (vascular) tumor beneath the mucous membrane or skin.

External Piles.--Two kinds, venous piles and skin or simple enlarged tags of skin. Venous piles usually occur in robust persons. They come on suddenly and are caused by the rupture of one or more small veins during the expulsion of hardened feces. There may be one or more, and may be located just at the union of the mucous membrane and the skin. Their size is from a millet-seed to a cherry, livid or dark blue in color, and appear like bullets or small shots under the skin. At first they cause a feeling of swelling at the margin of the anus; but as the clot becomes larger and harder, there is a feeling of the presence of a foreign body in the lower part of the anal canal (or canal of the anus). The sphincter muscle resents this and occasionally contracts, spasmodically at first, producing a drawing feeling; later these contractions become longer and more frequent, and there is intense suffering caused by the pile being squeezed, and this suffering may be so great that sleep is impossible without an opiate. Because of the straining, irritation of the rectum and pain in the sphincter, the piles soon become highly inflamed and very sensitive. The clot may be absorbed without any treatment. Occasionally it becomes ulcerated from the irritation, infection takes place and an abscess forms around the margin of the anus terminating in a fistula.

Skin Piles. (Cutaneous).--These are enlarged tags of the skin. They frequently follow the absorption of the clot in the venous piles where the skin is bruised and stretched. There may be one or many and usually have the skin color. These cause less suffering than the venous variety, and sometimes they exist for years, without any trouble, providing care is taken; but when bruised from any cause, such as a kick or fall, sitting on a hard seat, stretching of the parts during stool, or when they become irritated by discharges from the rectum or vagina, they become inflamed and cause much annoyance and pain. When they are acutely inflamed they swell greatly, are highly colored, swollen, painful, and extremely sensitive to the touch and cause frequent spasmodic contractions of the sphincter muscle and may finally result in an abscess. The pain is usually confined to the region of the anus, but may go up the back, down the limbs or to the privates.

MOTHERS' REMEDIES FOR PILES. Sulphur and Glycerin for.--"Equal parts of sulphur and pure glycerin. Grease parts." This preparation is very healing, and will often give relief even in severe cases.

2. Piles, Strongly Recommended Remedy for.--

Extract Belladonna	15 grains
Acetate lead	1/2 dram
Chloretone	1 dram
Gallic acid	15 grains
Sulphur	20 grains
Vaseline	1 ounce

Mix.

In protruding, itching and blind piles, this ointment will give you almost instant relief. If kept up several days it will promote a cure."

3. Piles, Good Salve for.--"Red precipitate two and one-half drams, oxide of zinc one dram, best cosmoline three ounces, white wax one ounce, camphor gum one dram." It is much better to have this salve made by a druggist, as it is difficult to mix at home. This it a splendid salve and very good for inflammation.

4. Piles, Smartweed Salve for.--"Boil together two ounces of fresh lard and half an ounce smartweed root. Apply this to the piles three or four times a day." This is very healing, and has been known to cure in many cases when taken in the early stages.

5. Piles, the Cold Water Cure for.--"Take about a half pint of cold water and use as an injection every morning before trying to have a movement of the bowels." This simple treatment has cured many cases where the stronger medicines did not help.

6. Piles, Simple Application and Relief from.--"Mix together one tablespoonful plain vaselin and one dram flower of sulphur. Apply three times daily and you will get relief."

7. Piles, Steaming with Chamomile Tea for.--"A tea made of chamomile blossoms and used as a sitz bath is excellent; after using the sitz bath use vaselin or cold cream and press rectum back gently."

PHYSICIANS' TREATMENT for Piles.--What to do first.-- The palliative treatment of both varieties of external piles is the same. In all cases the patient should lie flat on his back in bed and remain there for a few days. Highly seasoned foods and stimulants, tea, coffee, whisky, wine, etc., must be discarded. Secure a daily half liquid stool by the use of small doses of salts, Hunyadi or Abilena water. Cleansing the parts with weak castile soap water is essential to allay the pain, reduce the inflammation and soothe the sphincter muscle; cold, or if it is more agreeable, hot applications may be kept constantly on the parts. Hot fomentations of hops, smartweed, wormwood, or poultice of flaxseed, or slippery elm, or bread and milk give almost instant relief in many cases; while in others soothing lotions, and ointments or suppositories are needed.

The lead and laudanum wash is always reliable.

Lead and Laudanum Wash.--

Solution of Subacetate of Lead	4 drams
Laudanum	20 drams
Distilled water enough to make	4 ounces

Mix thoroughly and apply constantly ice cold on cotton to the sore parts.

The following ointments, lotions, and suppositories to be used freely within the bowels and to the piles, are effective in relieving the pain, reducing inflammation and diminishing pain and spasm in the sphincter.

1.	Ointment of Stramomium	1-1/2 drams
	Ointment of Belladonna 2-1/2 drams	
	Ointment of Tannic Acid	1/2 ounce

Mix thoroughly and apply inside and outside the anus.

2. Camphor Gum 1 dram
Calomel 12 grains
Vaselin 1 ounce

This must be thoroughly mixed. Apply freely within the anus and to the piles. Good for the pain.

3. For External Piles cleanse them well with a sponge dipped in cold water, and then bathe them with distilled extract of witch hazel.

4. If there is much itching with the piles use the following salve:--
Menthol 20 grains
Calomel 30 grains
Vaselin 1 ounce

Mix and apply to the piles.

5. I use quite frequently the following for sore external piles:

Chloroform and Sweet oil in equal parts

Apply freely with cotton or on to the piles. Ten cents will buy enough to use.

Operation for Piles.--When these measures do not relieve the pains or the piles become inflamed from slight causes and often, it is best to operate. This can be done in a few minutes with a local anesthetic and the patient frequently goes to sleep afterward, almost free from pain. Inject a three per cent solution of eucaine, or six per cent solution of cocaine. Thoroughly cleanse the part and hold the buttocks apart, pierce the pile at its base with a thin sharp-pointed curved knife, laying it open from side to side. Remove the clot with a curette, cauterize the vessel and pack the cavity with gauze to prevent bleeding and to secure drainage.

Cutaneous (skin) piles are operated upon as follows.--Each one is grasped in turn with a pair of strong forceps and snipped off with the scissors, or removed with a knife. Close the wound with sutures, if necessary, and dress it with gauze. Small ones need no sutures. Be careful not to remove too much tissue. Much after-pain can be prevented by placing in the rectum a suppository containing one-half grain of opium or cocaine before either of the above operations are performed. The after treatment is quite simple. Keep the patient quiet, cleanse the parts frequently, and secure a soft daily stool. Cleanse with tepid boiled water with clean sterilized gauze and give salts in small doses, one to two drams to produce a stool.

INTERNAL PILES. Symptoms.--The two prominent symptoms are bleeding and pain. The bleeding is usually dark. It may be slight and appear as streaks upon the feces or toilet paper; it may be moderate and ooze from the anus for some time after a stool, or it may be so profuse as to cause the patient to faint from loss of blood while the "bowels are moving." Death may follow in such a case unless the bleeding is stopped. The blood may look fresh and fluid or if retained for some time, it looks like coffee grounds, sometimes mixed with mucus and pus. Patients who bleed profusely become pale and bloodless, and are very nervous and gloomy and they believe they are suffering from cancer or some other incurable trouble. The first the patient notices he has internal piles is when a small lump appears at the end of the bowel during a stool and returns spontaneously; afterwards the lump again protrudes after the stool and others may appear. They become larger and larger, come down oftener and no longer return spontaneously, but must be replaced after each stool. As a result of this handling, they grow sensitive, swollen, inflamed and ulcerated, and the sphincter muscle becomes irritable. Later on one or more of the piles are caught in the grasp of the sphincter muscle and rapidly increases in size. It is then hard to relieve them, and when returned they act as foreign bodies, excite irritation and they are almost constantly expelled and the same procedure goes on at each stool. The sphincter muscle contracts so tightly around them as to cause strangulation and unless properly treated they become gangrenous and slough off.

Recovery, Pain, etc.--The pain is not great in the early stages, but when the muscle grasps and contracts the pile or piles it becomes terrible and constant. Piles rarely end fatally. Palliative treatment does not afford a permanent cure. They frequently return, but by care and diet many can be kept from returning so frequently. They should be treated upon their first appearance when the chances of a permanent cure without an operation are much better.

PHYSICIANS' TREATMENT for Internal Piles.--What to do first. The cause should be removed. Restore a displaced womb. Regulate the bowels, liver, diet, and habits. Much can be accomplished by these measures if properly used, in allaying inflammation diminishing pain and reducing the size of the piles. These measures will not cure them if they are large, overgrown and protruding. When the piles are inflamed, strangulated or ulcerated, the patient should remain in bed in a recumbent position and hot fomentations of hops, etc., and hot poultices, of flaxseed, slippery elm, bread and milk, the ice bag, or soothing applications and astringent remedies, should be applied to the parts. In some cases cold applications are the best. The cold or astringent applications give the best results where the piles are simply inflamed and the sphincter muscle does not act spasmodically, jerkily. But when the piles are strangulated, "choked tight" by the sphincter muscle, hot fomentations, poultices and soothing remedies give the most relief, because they reduce spasmodic contractions of the muscle and allay the pain. Instead of the poultices and fomentations, the "sitz" bath can be used. Put in the steaming water, hops, catnip, tansy, pennyroyal, etc., and the steam arising will frequently give great relief. This can be given frequently; ten to twenty drops of laudanum can be added to the poultices when the piles are very painful.

1. For inflamed piles, the following combinations may be used:--

Gum Camphor	1 dram
Calomel	12 grains
Vaselin	1 ounce

Mix thoroughly and apply freely around the anus and in the rectum on the piles.

The external parts should always be bathed with hot water, thoroughly, before using.

2.

Gum Camphor	2 drams
Chloretone	1 dram
Menthol	20 grains
Ointment of Zinc Oxide	1 ounce

Mix and apply directly to the piles.

3. When there is a slight bleeding, water of witch-hazel extract, one to two ounces to be injected into the rectum. This witch-hazel water freely used is good for external piles also. This is good and well recommended.

4. If the protruded pile is inflamed and hard to push back, the following is good and recommended highly:--

Chloretone	1 dram
Iodoform	1 dram
Gum Camphor	1 dram
Petrolatum	1 ounce

Mix and use as a salve.

5. An ointment composed of equal parts of fine-cut tobacco and raisins, seedless, chopped fine and mixed with enough lard, makes a good ointment to apply on both external and internal piles.

6. Tea of white oak bark, boiled down so as to be strong, and mixed with lard and applied frequently, is good as an astringent, but not for the very painful kind. It will take down the swelling.

7. Take a rectal injection of cold water before the regular daily stool. This will soften the feces and decrease the congestion.

Preventive Treatment.--This is very important and includes habits and diet and other diseases. If the patient is thin and pale give tonics. Correct any disease of any neighboring organ. Attend to any disease that may be present.

For Constipation.--Take a small dose of salts or hunyadi water so as to have one semi-solid stool daily. If necessary remove any feces that may even then be retained, by injections of soap suds or warm water containing oil. Discontinue injections as soon as a daily full stool can be had without it.

Habits.--Full-blooded people should not use upholstered chairs as the heat of the body relaxes the tissues of the rectum. A cane seated chair is best or an air cushion with a hollow center. It is best to rest in bed, if possible, after stool for the rest relieves the congestion and soreness. An abundance of out-door exercise, when the piles are not present, or bad, consisting of walking or simple gymnastics may usually be indulged in; violent gymnastics and horseback riding must be avoided. A daily stool must be secured.

Diet.--Such patients should avoid alcoholic beverages, spiced foods, strong coffee, and tea, cheese, cabbage, and old beans.

Foods Allowed.--Potatoes, carrots, spinach, asparagus, and even salads, since they stimulate intestinal action and thus aid in keeping the stool soft. Stewed fruits, including grapes, oranges, pears, and apples. Water is the best to drink. Meats: tender broiled, boiled or baked beef--do not eat the inside part to any great amount. Other meats, but no pork or ham, fresh fish, chicken. The foods should not be too highly seasoned; vinegar is not to be used to any extent and this excludes pickles, etc.

PERIPROCTITIS. Abscess Around the Anus and Rectum. (Ano-rectal) (Ischio-rectal Abscess).--This is an inflammation of the tissues around the rectum which usually terminates in the above named abscess. It occurs mostly in middle-aged people. Men are affected more often than women.

Causes.--Sitting in cold, damp hard seats; horseback riding, foreign bodies in the rectum such as pins, fish-hooks, etc., blows on the part, kicks, tubercular constitution, etc.

Symptoms.--Inflammation of the skin, like that of a big boil, some fever, throbbing pain, swelling of the part, heat and fullness in the rectum, these symptoms increase until the pus finds an outlet into the rectum.

PHYSICIANS' TREATMENT for Periproctitis.--Little can be done in a palliative way. It generally terminates in an abscess. Make the patient as comfortable as possible, by applying cold or hot things to the part, rest in bed, mild laxatives to keep the bowels open. Cut it open as soon as possible, and it should be laid wide open, so that every part is broken up. Then it should be thoroughly washed and scraped out. Sometimes it is necessary to use pure carbolic acid to burn out the interior. The dressing should be as usual for such wounds and removed when soiled and the wound washed out with boiled water and then gauze loosely placed in the bottom and in every corner of the wound. The dressing should be continued until all has been healed from inside out. Be sure to leave no cotton in to heal over it. Such patients should be built up with nourishing foods, and should remain quietly in bed. Cod liver oil is good for some patients. Iron, etc., for others. Keep the bowels regular. Outdoor life and exercise. If treated right it should not return.

FISTULA IN ANUS.--This usually follows the abscess. It has two openings, one upon the surface of the body near the anus, and the other in the rectum. There are a great many varieties of fistula, but it is unnecessary to name them. What can be done for them?

PHYSICIANS' TREATMENT.--If the general health is good an operation is the best thing to do, but patients in the last stage of consumption, nephritis, diabetes, or organic heart disease, are not apt to receive much benefit from an operation. The patient in poor condition should be given the treatment suitable to his condition, according to the advice of a trusted physician.

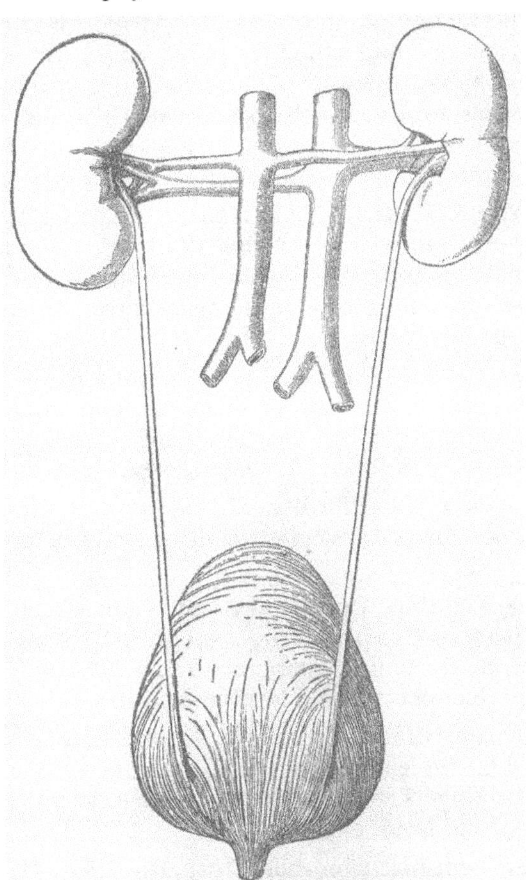

Kidneys, Ureters and Bladder.

DISEASES OF THE KIDNEYS AND BLADDER.

KIDNEYS.--The kidneys are deeply placed and cannot be felt or distinctly identified when normal. They are most accessible to pressure just below the last rib, behind. The right kidney usually lies lower than does the left, but even then, the lower part of this kidney is an inch above the upper part of the hip bone, or an inch above a line drawn around the body parallel with the navel. The kidney is about four inches long. The long axis of the kidneys corresponds to that of the twelfth rib; on an average the left kidney lies one-half inch higher than the right.

As stated before, each kidney is four inches long, two to two and one-half in breadth, and more than one inch thick. The left is somewhat longer, though narrower, than the right. The kidney is covered with what is called a capsule. This can be easily stripped off. The structure of the kidney is quite intricate. At the inner border of each kidney there is an opening called the pelvis of the kidney, and leading from this, small tubes penetrate the structure of the kidney in all directions. These tubes are lined with special cells. Through these tubes go the excretions (urine) from the body of the kidneys, to the pelvis, and from the pelvis through the ureters, sixteen inches long, to the bladder.

KIDNEY TROUBLE. MOTHERS' REMEDIES.--1. Kidney Trouble and Inflammation of the Bladder, Cornsilk for.--"Get cornsilk and make a good strong tea of it by steeping slowly, and take one ounce three or four times a day. This acts well on the kidneys, and is a harmless remedy to use."

2. Kidney Trouble, Flaxseed and Lemons for.--"Make a tea by placing the flaxseed in a muslin or linen bag, and suspend it in a dish of water, in the proportion of about four teaspoonfuls for each quart of water. After allowing the seeds to soak for several hours remove the same and tea will be ready for use. The addition of a little lemon juice will improve the flavor. Give in quantities as may be found necessary."

3. Kidney Trouble, Temporary Relief for.--"Rub witchhazel on stomach and back; use freely." This is an old-time remedy, and can be relied upon to at least give temporary relief. The witch hazel has a very soothing effect upon the parts affected.

4. Kidney and Bladder Trouble, Buchu Leaves for.--"Get five cents' worth of buchu leaves at any drug store, and make a good strong tea of it by steeping. This acts nicely on the kidneys. This remedy is easily prepared, and is not expensive."

5. Kidney Trouble, Common Rush Root for.--"Take a handful of the root of common rush in one and one-half pints of water, boil down to one pint. Dose:--One tablespoonful every two or three hours.

For a child ten years, give one teaspoonful four times a day. For a child of four to six years, one-half teaspoonful four times a day."

6. Kidney Trouble, Effective and Easy Cure for.--

"Fluid Extract of Cascara Sagrada	1 ounce
Fluid Extract of Buchu	2 ounces
Fluid Extract of Uva Ursi	2 ounces
Tincture Gentian Comp	1 ounce
Simple Syrup	1 pint

Mix the above ingredients and give a teaspoonful four times a day. This is a very good remedy, as the cascara sagrada acts on the bowels and the buchu and uva ursi acts on the kidneys, carrying off all the impurities that would otherwise be retained in the system and cause trouble."

7. Kidney Trouble, Sheep-Sorrel Excellent for.--"Make a decoction of sheep sorrel, one ounce to pint of water; boil, strain and cool. Give wineglassful, three or four times a day. If necessary apply the spinal ice bag to kidneys." The sheep sorrel is a good kidney remedy, and the ice bag by continuous application will relieve the congestion.

MOVABLE KIDNEY. (Floating Kidney. Nephroptosis).--Causes.--This condition is usually acquired. It is more common in women than in men, possibly due to lacing and the relaxations of the muscles of the abdomen from pregnancy. It may come from wounds, lifting too heavy articles, emaciation.

Symptoms.--They are often absent. There may be pain or dragging sensation in the loins, or intercostal neuralgia; hysteria, nervousness, nervous dyspepsia and constipation are common. The kidney can be felt. A dull pain is caused by firm pressure. Sometimes there are attacks of severe abdominal pain, with chill, fever, nausea, vomiting and collapse. The kidney becomes large and tender. The urine shows a reddish deposit and sometimes there is blood and pus in the urine.

Treatment.--If the symptoms are not present, it is best for the patient not to know the true condition, as nervous troubles frequently follow a knowledge of its presence. If the symptoms are present, replace the kidney while the patient is lying down and retain it by a suitable belt. Also treat the nervous condition. If the symptoms are of the severe kind an operation may be needed to fasten the kidney in its proper condition. This is quite generally successful, and does away with much suffering and pain. The pain may be so severe at times as to require morphine. Sometimes the pain is due to uric acid or oxalates in the urine. For this regulate the diet.

Diet for Movable Kidney.--The diet should be such as to produce fat. Milk is excellent where it is well borne; if not well borne give easily digested meats, such as chicken, roast beef, broiled steak and lamb chop; fish of various kinds and vegetables, such as spinach, carrots, asparagus and cauliflower; of fats, butter, cream, and chocolate; for constipation, cider, buttermilk, grape-juice, fruits and honey.

ACUTE CONGESTION OR HYPEREMIA OF THE KIDNEYS.--This occurs at the beginning of acute nephritis; in acute infectious diseases, after taking turpentine, chlorate of potash, cantharides, carbolic acid, alcohol, etc.; after one kidney has been removed.

Kidney.--The kidney is enlarged, dark red, while the covering is very tight (tense). The urine is scanty, and there is increased specific gravity (normal is 1015 to 1020) and contains albumin and a few casts.

Treatment.--The cause should always be removed if possible. Rest in bed, and as a diet use only milk; if the congestion is bad, use dry cupping over the kidneys and inject large quantities of hot normal salt solution in the bowels. Hot fomentations of wormwood or smartweed are of benefit. If you can get the patient into a sweat the congestion will be somewhat relieved by it.

CHRONIC CONGESTION OF THE KIDNEYS. Causes.--Diseases of other organs and obstruction to the return of the circulation in the veins. Cirrhosis of the liver causes it. The kidney is enlarged dark red, the urine is diminished, with albumin and casts and sometimes blood.

Treatment.--Remove the cause if possible. Fluid diet, like milk, broths, etc. Dry cupping or sweating materials can be used. Rest in bed if possible. The bowels should be kept open, and the kidneys should rest.

BLOOD IN THE URINE. (Haematuria). Causes.--The congestion of the kidneys, pernicious malaria, etc., nephritis, tuberculosis, kidney stones. The urine looks smoky and dark, or bright red.

Treatment.--This depends upon the cause. The patient must rest in bed and the kidneys should not be stimulated. Cold applications to the loins. Hot applications would injure.

URAEMIC TOXAEMIA.--This means poison in the blood occurring in acute and chronic nephritis (inflammation of the kidneys). The cause is unknown. The disease is acute and chronic.

ACUTE URAEMIA. Symptoms.--The onset may be sudden or gradual. The headache is severe, usually on the back top of head (occipital) and extending to the neck; there is persistent vomiting with nausea and diarrhea attending it. This may be due to inflammation of the colon. Difficulty in breathing, which may be constant or comes in spells. This is worse at night, when it may resemble asthma; fever if persistent, is usually slight until just before death. General convulsions may occur. There may be some twitching of the muscles of the face and of other muscles. The convulsions may occur frequently. The patient becomes abnormally sleepy, before the attack, and remains so. One-sided paralysis may occur. Sudden temporary blindness occurs sometimes. There may be noisy delirium or suicidal mania. Coma (deep sleep) may develop either with or without convulsions or delirium, and is usually soon followed by them; sometimes by chronic uraemia or recovery.

CHRONIC URAEMIA.--This develops most often in cases of Arterio-sclerosis or chronic interstitial nephritis, (one kind of Bright's disease). The symptoms are less severe than those of acute uraemia, but similar, and of gradual onset, sometimes with symptoms of the acute attack. There is often constant headache and difficult breathing; the tongue is brown and dry, sometimes there is nausea, vomiting, diarrhea, sleeplessness, cramps of the legs and much itching may be present. It may last for years. Death may occur when the patient is in coma (deep sleep). There may have been mania, muscular twitchings or convulsions before death.

Treatment.--Found under "Chronic Interstitial Nephritis."

ACUTE BRIGHT'S DISEASE. (Acute Inflammation of the Kidneys. Acute Nephritis).--This occurs chiefly in young people and among grown men. Exciting causes are exposure to cold, wet, burns, extensive skin tears (lesions), scarlet fever, diphtheria, typhoid fever, measles and acute tuberculosis, poisons; and pregnancy is one cause when it occurs in women.

Symptoms.--After exposure or scarlet fever the onset may be sudden, sometimes with chills or chilliness, variable fever, pain in the loins, watery swelling of the face and extremities, then of other portions of the body like the abdomen, then general dropsy. Sometimes there is nausea, vomiting, headache, delirium, or very deep sleep. The urine is scanty, dark colored, of increased "specific gravity" and contains albumin, cells and casts. Anemia is marked. After some fever disease, the onset is gradual with anemia, swelling of the eyelids, face and extremities; scanty thickish urine containing casts, then headache, nausea, vomiting, little or no fever, dry skin. In these cases there may be gradual recovery, attack of uraemia, or they may end in chronic nephritis.

Diagnosis.--Examine the urine often in pregnancy, scarlet fever, etc., and especially when watery swelling is noticed.

Recovery.--The result in your children when it comes with scarlet fever is not so good. It may run into chronic nephritis. In adults when it is due to exposure the rule is recovery.

Treatment.--The patient must be kept in bed until there is complete recovery. He should be clothed in flannel.

Diet and Nursing.--This must be of milk, water or mineral water in large quantities; milk or buttermilk should be the main article of food. You can give gruels made of arrowroot or oatmeal, barley water, beef tea and chicken broth. But it is better to stick strictly to milk. As the patient gets better, bread and butter, lettuce, watercress, grapes, oranges, and other fruits may be given. The return to a meat diet should be gradual. The patient should drink freely of mineral waters, ordinary water or lemonade, these keep the kidneys flushed and wash out the "debris" from the tubes. One dram of cream of tartar in a pint of boiling water, add the juice of half a lemon and a little sugar; this when taken cold is a pleasant satisfactory diluting drink. Cream of tartar one dram, juice of lemon, sugar sufficient, water one pint, may be given whenever desired. There should be hot water baths daily or oftener; or you can produce sweating by placing hot water jars around the patient, and watch to see whether it is too weakening. It can also be done by introducing steam underneath the bedding, that is then lifted a little, so that the steam vapor can circulate about the patient. Be careful not to burn the patient with the hot steam. This, of course, is done through a hose attached to a steaming kettle. Also see treatment of dropsy under "scarlet fever."

Bowels, Attention to.--They should be moved every morning by a saline (salt) cathartic, if necessary, especially if the dropsy continues. This produces watery stool. Cream of tartar and epsom salts, equal parts, is good remedy; one-half teaspoonful every three hours for a child one year old until the bowels move freely; one-half to one ounce can be given to an adult.

CHRONIC BRIGHT'S DISEASE. (Chronic Parenchymatous Nephritis. Chronic Diffuse Desquamative or Tubal Nephritis. Chronic Diffuse Nephritis with Exudation). Causes.--Young adult life and most common in males. It may come from acute inflammation of the kidneys that was due to exposure, pregnancy, or scarlet fever, or follow excessive use of alcohol, etc. In children it usually follows acute inflammation of the kidneys or scarlet fever.

Condition.--The kidneys may be enlarged, with thin capsule, white surface, cortex thickened and yellowish, or whitish (large white kidney). The epithelium of the tubules is granular, or fatty or the tubules are distended and contain casts. Cells of the "Glomeruli" and their capsules are swollen. There is moderate increase of interstitial tissue. In other cases, the "small white kidney," the kidney is small and pale either at first or as a later stage of the large white kidney. The surface is pale, rough and granular; the capsule is thickened and partially adherent; the surface is thin with white and yellowish areas of fatty degenerations. The interstitial tissue is much increased; epithelial degeneration in the tubules extensive. There is also the large red kidney, and with any of these types the left heart may be enlarged and the arteries thickened.

Symptoms.--If it occurs after acute nephritis the symptoms of acute nephritis subside, but anemia and the changes in the urine persist. Usually there is a gradual onset with paleness and puffiness of the eyelids, ankles or hands in the morning. Later there is difficult breathing, increased watery swelling of the face, extremities and dependent portions of the body; worse in the morning. There is a pasty yellowish pallor, afterwards dropsy of the abdominal and chest cavities. The urine is diminished, high colored, specific gravity usually 1020 to 1025 with much albumin. Many casts which are named hyaline, granular, epithelial and fatty. The action of the heart is bad. There may be trouble with the stomach and bowels, constipated, etc. The digestion is poor and the patient frequently suffers with much gas. Recovery is rare after it has lasted one year.

Treatment. Diet.--Milk or buttermilk should be the main article of food. You can give gruels made of arrowroot or oatmeal, barley water, beef tea, and chicken broth, but it is better to keep strictly to milk. As the patient gets better, bread and butter, lettuce, watercress, grapes, oranges and other fruits may be given. The return to the meat diet should be gradual. The patient should drink freely of mineral water, ordinary water, or lemonade. These keep the kidneys flushed and wash out the "debris" from the tubes. One dram (teaspoonful) of cream of tartar in a pint of boiling water, add the juice of a half a lemon and a little sugar. This when taken cold is a pleasant, satisfactory drink. Medical treatment is not satisfactory. The only thing to do is to give medicines to meet the indications; fifteen to twenty grain doses of lactate of strontium. Diuretin also is used. Basham's mixture for anemia is of help in some cases. It can be bought at any drug store.

CHRONIC INTERSTITIAL NEPHRITIS. (Sclerosis or Cirrhosis of the Kidneys. Granular, Contracted or Gouty Kidney).--This is met with, (a) as a sequence of the large white kidneys forming the so-called pale granular or secondary contracted kidney; (b) as an independent primary affection; as a sequence of arterio-sclerosis.

Causes.--The primary form is chronic from the onset, and is a slow creeping degeneration of the kidney substance, and in many respects an anticipation of the gradual changes which take place in the organ in extreme old age. Families in which the arteries tend to degenerate early are more prone to this disease. Doctor Osler says: "Among the better classes in this country Bright's disease is very common and is caused more frequently by over-eating than by excesses in alcohol."

Arterio-Sclerotic Form.--This is the most common form in this country, and is secondary to arterio-sclerosis. The kidneys are not much, if at all, contracted; very hard, red and show patches of surface atrophy. It is seen in men over forty who have worked hard, eaten freely, and taken alcohol to excess. They are conspicuous victims of the "strenuous life," the incessant tension of which is felt first in the arteries. After forty, in men of this class, nothing is more salutary than to experience the shock brought on by the knowledge of albumin and cast tubes in the urine.

Symptoms.--Perhaps a majority of the cases are latent (hidden) and are not recognized until the occurrence of one of the serious and fatal complications. There may have been no symptoms to suggest to the patient the existence of a dangerous malady. In other cases the general health is disturbed. The patient is tired, sleepless; he must get up two or three times at night to pass urine; the digestion is disordered, the tongue is coated; the patient complains of a headache, failing sight, and gets out of breath by exercising. There may be vomiting, headache, neuralgia, and increase of the quantity of urine is common. This is light in color, of low specific gravity, 1005 to 1012; frequently there is a trace of albumin and a few casts of the hyaline and granular kind. In the late stages the albumin may be increased with high specific gravity and a less quantity of urine. The disease often lasts for a year.

In the arterio-sclerotic variety the urine may be normal or diminished in quantity, specific gravity normal or increased, the casts are more numerous, and the albumin is usually more abundant. There is an enlargement of the heart; the pulse is increased in tension; the wall of the artery is thickened. The skin is usually dry, with eczema common, but dropsy is rare, except when it is due to heart failure. There may be bronchial and lung troubles; attacks of uraemia, or hard breathing caused by the heart, frequently occurs. There may be hemorrhage of the brain or hemorrhage of the membranes, and these are often fatal.

Recovery.--Chances are unfavorable, but life may be prolonged for years, especially with care and especially if it is discovered early.

Treatment.--A quiet life without mental worry, with gentle but not excessive exercise, and residence in a climate that is not changeable should be recommended. A business man must give up his worry; his rush; his hurried eating, and rest. The bowels should be kept regular; there should be a tepid water bath daily, and the kidneys should be kept acting freely by drinking daily a definite amount of either distilled water or some pleasant mineral water. Alcohol, tobacco, excessive eating and improper food must not be allowed. Weak tea and coffee may be allowed. The diet should be light and nourishing. Meat should not be taken more than once a day. If it is possible, the patient should be urged to move to a warm equable climate during the winter months, from November to April, like that of southern California. Medicines must be given to meet the indications. No special directions can be given. The heart, stomach, and bowels must be watched.

DIET as Allowed by a Prominent Hospital.--

May Take:--

Soups.--Broths with rice or barley, vegetable or fish soup.

Fish.--Boiled or broiled fresh fish, raw oysters, raw clams.

Meats.--Chicken, game, fat bacon, fat ham (sparingly).

Farinaceous.--Hominy, oatmeal, wheaten grits, rice, stale bread, whole wheat bread, toast, milk toast, biscuits, maccaroni.

Vegetables.--Cabbage, spinach, celery, water-cresses, lettuce, mushrooms, mashed potatoes, cauliflower, onions.

Desserts.--Rice and milk puddings, stewed fruits, raw ripe fruits.

Must Not Take:--

Fried fish, pork, corned beef, veal, heavy bread, hashes, stews, battercakes, lamb, beef, mutton, gravies, peas, beans, pastry, ice cream, cakes, coffee, tobacco, malt or spirituous liquors.

PYELITIS.--This is an inflammation of the pelvis of the kidney and may be caused by bacteria from the blood, or by ascending pus, infection or tuberculous infection from the lower tracts like the ureter, bladder and urethra.

Symptoms.--There is pain in the back, with tenderness and pressure, cloudy-looking urine, either acid or alkaline, containing pus, mucus, and sometimes red blood cells; chills, high fever, and sweating occur. This may become chronic and then it becomes quite serious.

Anemia and emaciation are then marked. Mild cases usually recover; pus cases may end in other diseases or death from exhaustion.

Treatment. Diet.--In mild cases fluids should be taken freely, particularly the alkaline mineral water to which citrate of potash can be added. Tonics should be given when called for, and milk diet and buttermilk may be taken freely. When a tumor has formed, and even before, it is perceptible, if the symptoms are serious and severe, an operation may be necessary.

KIDNEY STONE. (Renal Calculus. Nephro-Leithiasis).-- Forming of a stone or gravel in the kidney or its pelvis may occur in intra uterine, (before the child is born), in the womb, or at any age. A family tendency, sedentary life, excesses in eating and drinking and very acid urine predispose. They vary in size from that of fine sand to that of a bean.

Symptoms.--Patients may pass gravel for years without having an attack of renal (kidney) colic, and a stone may never lodge in the ureter. A person may pass an enormous number of calculi. Dr. Osler speaks of having had a patient who had passed several hundred kidney stones (calculi) with repeated attacks of kidney colic. His collection filled an ounce bottle. A patient may pass a single stone and may never be troubled again. A stone remaining in the kidney may cause dull aching pain in the affected kidney, or the pain may be referred to the other side and sometimes there may be blood or pus in the urine, with chill and fever due to pyelitis. Kidney (renal) colic comes on when a stone enters the ureter, if it is at all large. At attack may set in abruptly, without any apparent reason, or it may follow a strain in lifting. The pain may be agonizing in character, which starts in the flank of the affected side, passes down along the course of the ureter and is felt in the testicle and along the inner side of the thighs. The testicle is drawn back. The pain may also go through the abdomen and chest, and be very severe in the back. In severe attacks nausea and vomiting are present and the patient is collapsed; sweating breaks out in his face and the pulse is feeble and weak. The pain lasts from an hour to several days, until the stone reaches the bladder, partial suppression of the urine during the attack occurs, but a large quantity of urine is usually passed after it and a feeling of soreness may, be present for several days. The stone may again cause pain in passing through the urethra, or it may remain in the bladder as a nucleus for a bladder calculus (stone). Dr. Osler gives Montaigne's description as follows; "Thou art seen to sweat with pain, to look pale and red, to tremble, to vomit well nigh to blood, to suffer strange contortions and convulsions, by starts to let tears drop from thine eyes, to urine thick, black and frightful water, or to have it suppressed by some sharp and craggy stone that cruelly pricks and tears thee."

Treatment.--Great relief is experienced in the attacks by the hot baths or fomentations which sometimes are able to cause the spasm to

relax. If the pain is very severe morphine should be given by the hypodermic method and inhalations of chloroform given until morphine has had time to act. Local applications are sometimes grateful,--hot poultices or cloths wrung out of hot water may be helpful. Cloths wrung out of steaming hop, wormwood, or smartweed teas, are of benefit sometimes. Change of position often gives relief; when the stone is large an operation may be needed. The patient should drink freely of hot lemonade, soda water, barley water. When the patient is free from the attack, he should live a quiet life and avoid sudden exertion of all kinds. There should be a free passage of urine always. The patient should drink daily a large but definite quantity of mineral, or distilled water which is just as satisfactory. You may take the citrate or bicarbonate of potash. Mineral springs are good to visit, such as Saratoga, Hot Springs, Arkansas, etc. Abstain from alcohol and eat moderately. Live an open-air life with plenty of exercise and regular hours. The skin should be kept active; a cold friction bath in the morning is good, if one is strong; but if he is weak and debilitated the evening warm bath should be substituted. The patient should dress warmly, avoid rapid alterations in temperature, and be careful not to allow the skin to become suddenly chilled.

Diet.--Most persons over forty eat too much. One should take plenty of time to eat, and not too much meat should be eaten.

"Queen of the Meadow."--The Indians used this medicine quite frequently in the treatment of kidney and bladder troubles. A lady, whom I know well, told me that she had a cousin who was affected with the kidney stone colic. At one time, when he was suffering from an attack, an Indian happened in their home and saw him suffering. He went into the meadow and dug some of this remedy and made a tea of it. It seemed to do the work, for while he gave it, the pain was eased and he never had any more attacks. I give this for what it is worth. The remedy will certainly do no harm for it is a good diuretic.

INFLAMMATION OF THE BLADDER. (Cystitis). Causes.--It may occur from injury from passing a catheter, etc., from the use of drugs like cantharides, from the presence of a stone, from stricture of the urethra and from gonorrhea or cold.

Symptoms.--The urine is passed more frequently, sometimes the desire to pass the urine is almost constant. The distress is relieved for only a few minutes by passing the urine; sometimes only a few drops are passed, and it gives no relief from the desire for passing urine. The straining is extremely severe. Sometimes the patient will lean over the vessel quivering with the muscular effort to pass urine. The bowels often move at the same time from the straining. The urine becomes thick with much mucus, then scanty, and then tinged with blood.

BLADDER TROUBLE. Mothers' Remedies. 1. English Oil of Sandal Wood for.--"Get one ounce of the pure English oil of sandal wood, take four drops three times a day in a little water. As you urinate more freely reduce the dose. This is a splendid remedy."

2. Bladder Trouble, Effective Herb Teas for.--"Make a tea of half ounce of buchu leaves, half ounce of uva ursi leaves (barberry leaves), one pint of boiling water. Dose: Two or three tablespoonfuls three times a day, or may drink quite freely." A tea made of cornsilk is a common and standard remedy.

Treatment.--Remove cause if possible. Fomentations of hops, smartweed, wormwood are good, even hot water over the bladder. Hot hip bath is good, and also the warm foot bath. The bowels should be kept open with saline laxatives. Buchu tea is very good. Use about one-half ounce of the leaves to a pint of warm water and let it steep, not boil. Drink freely of this. Pumpkin seed tea or watermelon seed tea is good, also flaxseed tea. Dr. Hare recommends the following at the beginning if there is fever:

Tincture of Aconite	3 drams
Sweet Spirits of Nitre	1 ounce
Solution of Citrate of Potash	enough to make 6 ounces

Mix.

Give a dessertspoonful every four hours until all fever ceases and the pulse is quiet. The patient should be kept quiet.

Diet.--Should be milk only.

CHRONIC INFLAMMATION OF THE BLADDER.--Causes.--It follows repeated attacks; partial retention of urine in the bladder, decomposing there; Bright's disease, inflammation of the urethra, injury, etc.

Treatment.--Wash out the bladder with pure warm water or water containing about one to two teaspoonfuls of boric acid to the pint of warm water. This should be given once or twice a day; or enough permanganate of potash can be put into the water to give the water a tinge of the color. An injection of golden seal, one teaspoonful to the pint of warm water, is good if there is much mucus. The best way to give the irrigation is to attach a small funnel to a soft rubber catheter and fill the bladder by raising the funnel when full of water above the patient's belly; or you can attach the rubber tube of a fountain syringe to a catheter at one end and to a funnel at the other and raise the funnel to the desired height; or you can attach a catheter to the rubber tube of a fountain syringe (clean one) and raise syringe high enough to allow the water to run into the bladder gently. The patient will stand just about so much water. The rubber can then be detached from the catheter and the water allowed to run out.

DISEASE OF THE PROSTATE GLAND.

The prostate, which both in structure and in function is rather a muscle than a gland, is situated at the neck of the bladder and around the first inch of the urethra. It is divided into two lateral (side) lobes (parts) by a deep notch behind and a furrow at the upper and lower surfaces. The so-called middle or third lobe is the portion which is between the two side lobes at the under and posterior part of the gland, just beneath the neck of the bladder. The urethra (the channel for the urine to pass through from the bladder out through the penis) usually passes through the gland at about the junction of its upper and middle third.

HYPERTROPHY OF THE PROSTATE.--This is a general enlargement of the gland in all directions. All the three lobes may enlarge and in about one-third of the men who have passed middle life some enlargement takes place, and in about one-tenth of all men over fifty-five this enlargement becomes of importance in regard to the size.

The middle lobe may enlarge so much that it may extend up into the bladder and block the opening into the urethra; the side lobes may compress the urethra into a mere slit, or may lengthen it so that the prostatic portion measures three or four inches, or may twist and distort it so that the most flexible instrument can only be made to pass through it with difficulty.

Symptoms.--The earliest symptom may be increased frequency in passing urine, especially at night. Soon some urine is retained in the bladder, and this may increase so much that only an ounce or two can be passed spontaneously, although the bladder contains one pint or more. The stream of urine is feeble, and will drop perpendicularly towards the feet of the patient. In some cases an inflammation of the prostate and bladder is set up, and then the symptoms felt are very distressing. There is an almost constant desire to pass urine; there is much pain and straining with it; a slight bleeding may follow and night rest is broken; the general strength fails from the continual suffering; the urine becomes foul, smells like ammonia, and is reduced in quantity; inflammation of the kidneys develops also; general poisoning occurs; and the patient dies of uraemia and in a "coma" condition.

Treatment. Preventive.--The patient should avoid taking cold in this disease. Light and easily digested diet is necessary. The bowels must be kept regular. Alcohol of any kind should not be used. The bladder should be emptied at regular intervals. Some patients keep a catheter and "draw" their own urine. Unless the patient takes great care, the bladder and urethra will be irritated and perhaps infected through neglect of cleanliness. Medicines are not very useful in severe cases. Operation is the only reliable cure especially when some urine is always retained.

URINARY PASSAGE. Mother's Remedy.--1. Dandelion Root Will Clean.--"A decoction made of the sliced root of dandelion in white wine is very effectual for cleansing and healing inward ulcers in the urinary passage. If the fresh root cannot be obtained, buy extract of dandelion and give two teaspoonfuls in water once in two or three hours as the case requires. It also acts on the liver, gall and spleen."

DROPSY.--Dropsy should be regarded as a symptom, which may arise from many causes, such as heart disease, lung disease or kidney disease, or it may depend upon obstruction to the normal flow of blood and lymph through the vessels and tissues.

From Heart Disease.--In heart disease dropsy is due to a weak heart. The heart is unable to supply the arteries with enough blood to maintain the normal pressure, or to damming up of blood in the venous system as the result of imperfect emptying of the heart cavities. In kidney trouble the dropsy depends more on the lack of proper nourishing processes in the capillary walls and upon changes in the blood and blood pressure. If the kidneys are diseased, they may not be able to eliminate the proper amount of liquids which accumulate and finally escape into the tissues. Liver troubles cause dropsy by producing pressure upon the large blood-vessels going to the liver, and consequently the fluid is generally confined to the lower limbs and abdomen.

MOTHERS' REMEDIES. Dropsy, 1. Juniper Berries Fresh or Dry for.--"The berries of the juniper tree are regarded as excellent home remedies in dropsy. They may be eaten fresh or dry, or make a decoction and drink. Two teaspoonfuls of the berries two or three times a day is considered a dose. It is well to bruise them thoroughly by breaking the seeds with a hammer before taking." The decoction is more effective. This helps the dropsy by acting on the kidneys.

2. Dropsy, Wild Milkweed for.--"Steep the root of the wild milkweek and drink the tea in doses of a wineglass three times a day. This is a sure cure if taken in early stages."

3. Dropsy, White Bay Buds for.--"White bay buds steeped in water." The white bay buds can be secured at any drug store, and are easily prepared. Make a tea of these the same as you would make green tea for the table, only stronger. Take several times a day. This is an excellent remedy.

4. Dropsy, Canada Thistle for.--"Steep dwarf elder root, or Canada thistle root, and drink the tea." This is an old tried remedy that our grandmothers used to use, and can be depended upon. We all know that in olden times mothers had to use these herb remedies, as doctors could not be secured as easily as they can in these days.

5. Dropsy, Very Effective Remedy for.--"Make a decoction of fresh dandelion root slices, one ounce to one pint of water boiled down to one-half pint, strain, adding two drams of cream of tartar. Dose: A wine glassful two or three times a day."

6. Dropsy, Common Herb Remedy for.--"One gallon white beech bark, after the rough bark is removed, good big handful of blackberry root, cut fine, and also of sassafras root. Cover with cold water and steep to get the strength; then strain. When cool, not cold, add one pint bakers' yeast and one cup of sugar. Let it stand twenty-four hours in a warm place. Then strain and set in a cool place. Take a wineglassful three times a day before meals. This has been highly recommended to me by a friend in Kalkaska, Michigan."

7. Dropsy, "Queen of the Meadow" for.--"Is a symptom of morbid conditions existing in the system, therefore nutritious diet, alkaline baths and a general hygienic regulation of the daily habits are of the greatest importance. Take one teaspoonful of powder of "Queen of the Meadow" in a cupful of water three or four times a day as the case may require. Either use tea or powder."

PHYSICIANS' TREATMENT for Dropsy.--Treat the disease that causes it. Remedies should be given that will cause an outpouring of the liquids. Salines, such as epsom salts in large doses. Cream of tartar and epsom salts (equal parts) taken freely is effective. If the kidneys are inactive owing to heart trouble, the following may be used: An infusion of digitalis in one to four teaspoonful doses every three to four hours. This pill is good.

Powdered Digitalis	20 grains
Powdered Squills	20 grains

Mix into twenty pills and take one every five hours.

INFECTIOUS DISEASES.

INFECTION AND CONTAGION.--These words are often used in such a way that a wrong impression is made. A disease may be infectious but not contagious. Malaria is an instance. Infection means an ability to enter the body from any source, wind, water, food or other persons and produce a characteristic disease. The agency doing this is known as a germ. Contagion is properly a poisoning of one individual from contact with a diseased individual in some way known or unknown. It may be conveyed indirectly through clothes, etc., or other person; but always comes from some person sick with the same disease. Diseases may be both infectious and contagious. Nearly all the epidemic diseases of infancy are both infectious and contagious and accompanied by fever. In nursing children, suffering from infectious diseases the mother or nurse should avoid their breath and handle them as little as possible. All secretion from bowels and kidneys should fall in a vessel containing a disinfecting solution of Copperas, bichloride of mercury, etc., and should be emptied into the sewer or buried. Following are the solutions as made. **Copperas:**--Put a lump as big as a walnut in the chamber with one-half pint of water, to receive feces, urine, sputum and vomited matter from infectious and contagious patients.

2. Solution of chlorinated soda, four fluid ounces; water ten ounces, useful for hands and dishes, not silverware. Dissolve eight corrosive sublimate tablets, also called bichloride, in a gallon of water.

This is used to disinfect floors, woodwork, rubber, and leather, but not metal parts. Great care must be taken to have the hands washed after handling such a patient, so as not to infect the food, eyes, mouth, or any small skin sores.

Diet in Infectious Diseases.--Foods that can be used: Milk, milk-water, milk and lime-water, Mellin's food, malted milk, imperial granum, albumin water, rice water, oatmeal water, barley water, egg (white part), and barley water, arrowroot water, whey, whey and cream mixture, cream and rice mixture, beef tea, beef extract, mutton broth, beef juice. Chewing broiled steak and only swallowing the juice, dry toast and soft boiled eggs, milk toast, dried beef broth, soups, rice, cornstarch, tapioca, etc. The diet must not consist of solid food in any severe case of fever. Small quantities of cold drinks can be given, frequently repeated if there is no vomiting. Frequent washing with tepid water or cool water lessens the fever and produces sleep. The bowels should be kept open at least once a day, and castor oil or salts usually can be given. (See Nursing and Dietetics department.)

Table of Infectious Diseases.

	Incubation lasts	*Date of characteristic symptom.*	*Whole duration.*
Mumps	*7 to 20 days*	*1st day*	*7 days or less*
Whooping Cough	*2 to 7 days*	*7 to 14 days*	*2 months*
Diphtheria	*1 to 12 days*	*1 to 2 days*	*1 week to 1 month*
Erysipelas	*2 to 8 days*	*1 to 2 days*	*1 week to 3 weeks*
Varioloid	*10 to 13 days*	*1 day*	*1 to 3 weeks*
Chicken Pox	*12 to 17 days*	*1 day*	*4 to 7 days*
German Measles	1 to 3 weeks	1 day	3 to 4 days
Measles	12 to 14 days	4 days	7 to 9 days
Scarlet Fever	1 to 7 days	1 to 2 days	7 to 12 days
Typhoid Fever	1 to 14 days	7 to 8 days	3 to 5 weeks
Smallpox	10 to 14 days	3 to 4 days	2 to 4 weeks

SCARLET FEVER. Definition.--Scarlet fever is an acute infectious disease, with a characteristic eruption.

Modes of Conveying.--The nearer a person is to a patient the more likely one is to take or convey the disease. Clothing, bedding, etc., may retain the poison for months. Scales from the skin of a patient, dried secretions, the urine if inflammation of the kidneys (nephritis) exists, the discharges (feces) from the bowels, are all means of infection. The longer a person remains near the patient the more likely he is to convey the disease. Foods handled by those sick of the disease, or by those who may have been near patients may convey the disease. This is especially true of milk. Epidemics of scarlet fever have been started by dairy-men who had scarlet fever in their family. I once attended a family where the only known cause for it in that family was a long-haired dog of a neighbor who had scarlet fever in the family. The dog was in the room with the sick ones, and visited the neighbor's family and played with the children who afterwards came down with the fever. Discharges from the ear, caused by scarlet fever, are said to be capable of giving it.

Remains in the Room, how long?--It may remain for months in a room, and extend over two years as recorded by Murchison. We do not yet know how the poison obtains entrance to the body. Hence, the need for thorough disinfection.

Age, Occurrence, Susceptibility.--All children exposed to the disease do not contract the disease. It is less contagious than measles. A person who is exposed once, and does not take it, may take it at a future exposure. It occurs at any age and in all countries. It occurs oftener in autumn (September) and winter (February). Isolated cases occur, and then it is called sporadic. This disease attacks nursing children less frequently than older children. It is not often seen during the first year of life.

How Often?--As a rule, it attacks a person only once; yet there are recorded cases of well observed second and third attacks, but fortunately these are very rare. I once attended a family where they had it and claimed to have had it before, but very lightly.

Incubation.--The vast majority of cases develop within three to five days after exposure. If eleven days elapse without the appearance of symptoms we may reasonably expect that the danger is past, at least in the great majority of cases exposed.

Contagiousness.--There is danger of catching the disease during the stages of incubation, eruption and scaling. It is most contagious in the last two stages.

Onset.--Sometimes the onset is sudden; there may be a convulsion, preceded by a sharp rise in the temperature. An examination in such cases may reveal a marked sore throat or a membranous deposit on the tonsils preceding the eruption, and nothing more. A chill followed by fever and vomiting ushers in a large number of cases. These may be mild or severe. The severity of these symptoms usually indicates the gravity of the attack.

Rash.--The rash or eruption appears from twelve to thirty-six hours after the onset, usually on the second day, and looks like a very severe heat rash, but is finer and thicker. It consists of a very finely pointed rose-colored rash. In mild cases it is hardly noticeable. Usually it first appears on the upper part of the chest around the collar bones, spreads over the chest and around upon the back. Also it is now seen on the neck, beneath the jaw, behind the ears and on the temples, thence spreads over the body. There is a paleness about the mouth and wings of the nose, while the cheeks are flushed with a flame-like redness. There is much itching if the rash is severe. It attains the full development at the end of two or three days, and then gradually declines. In some cases the rash is seen only twenty-four hours.

Fever.--The fever rises rapidly in the first few hours to 104 or 105-8/10 degrees. It remains high except in the morning, until the eruption reaches its full development and falls with the fading eruption, and in uncomplicated and typical cases, within six days becomes normal.

Sore Throat.--This we find on the pillars of the fauces, uvula, tonsils, and pharynx, reddened and inflamed. Sometimes it is very severe, and a membrane comes on one or both tonsils and pillars of the fauces. There is, generally a severe sore throat, and this makes swallowing difficult.

Tongue.--The tongue is covered with a coating at the onset, and may present a slightly reddened appearance at the borders and tip. The papillae are prominent and covered and look like a strawberry sometimes, or like the tongue of a cat. In fatal poisonous cases it becomes dry and cracked.

Scaling.--As the disease subsides the outer layer of the skin dries and peels off. The extent of this depends upon the severity of the attack. In some cases the scaling is hardly perceptible, and sometimes it appears only on certain parts, such as on the toes and inner parts of the thighs. There is always some scaling. This is called "desquamation." Generally speaking, scaling begins where the eruption first appeared on the upper part of the chest and neck. The scales may be fine and branny or as is most common, the skin peels in large particles. Some scaling is always present. The length of the scaling time is variable. It usually lasts from three to four weeks, but often longer. This stage is considered by many as the most contagious, as the fine scales fly in the air.

Complications. Nose.--The nose is affected at the same time if the "sore throat" is very severe. A membrane may also form in the nose.

Ear.--This may be affected in as high as one-fifth of the cases and needs careful watching and attention. Both ears may be diseased and deafness frequently results from it. Ten per cent of those who suffer from "deaf-mutism" can trace their affliction to scarlet fever. The ears usually become afflicted in the third week. The fever rises and there is pain in the ears or ear. The onset may not appear alarming and not be suspected until the discharge makes its appearance This is unfortunate; these complications are serious, as meningitis and abscess of the brain may result. The ear trouble (otitis) usually occurs during the scaling. The patient may be up and around. There is a rise of the temperature to 103 or 104 degrees, the patient begins to vomit food and has a headache. At night the child starts from its crib and cries as if in pain. They do not always locate the pain in the ear. The face and hands may twitch. The fever may fall to normal and rise sharply again. Such symptoms should call for a thorough examination.

Eye.--Inflammation of the (conjunctiva) red membrane of the eyes, often occurs.

Kidneys.--There may be a mild form of inflammation in the earlier stages. The severe form comes, if at all, usually in the third week. It occurs in five to seven per cent of the cases. It may occur in the mildest case, as such cases are not so closely watched. The first symptom is a slight bloating of the eyes and face and spreads over the whole body. Sometimes the swelling is very slight; at other times it is extreme. The urine diminishes early and sometimes is wholly suppressed. It may be light colored, smoky or straw colored. This trouble usually runs for weeks. The patient may get uremia and result fatally.

Heart.--This also may be affected as the valves may become diseased.

Joints.--Rheumatism also may occur, and other complications.

Chorea.--Follows scarlet fever also, especially in girls from twelve to fifteen years.

Diagnosis.--In most cases it is easy to distinguish from other diseases. Dermatitis, inflammation of the skin ("Itis" always means inflammation). In dermatitis the throat symptoms and strawberry tongue are absent.

From Measles.--By the rapid onset, absence of cold symptoms of the nose, eyes, and bronchial tubes, blotchy eruptions that occur in measles. There is no strawberry tongue in measles and no coughing at beginning.

Recovery.--The prognosis is favorable in uncomplicated cases. It also depends upon the character of the epidemic type of the disease. In England it varies from thirteen to fourteen per cent. In this country it is sometimes as low as two to four per cent. The kidney trouble is always feared for it may result in uremia and death, or the acute may be followed by chronic nephritis or Bright's disease, which will ultimately prove fatal.

Sanitary Care of Room and Patient.--If you are exposed to this disease what can you do? If a child, it must be put in a room by itself. If several children have been exposed they should be put in separate rooms. These rooms should have no carpet, curtains, rugs, etc., or any unnecessary furniture, for everything must be disinfected afterward, and sometimes destroyed. The clothes worn just before the sickness should be sterilized in steam or boiled and then aired in the sun. Anyone suffering from sore throat who has been about the patient should not be allowed to be near the healthy. All the children must be kept from school. It is well for them to spray their throats with a simple cleansing solution morning and night, with a full teaspoonful of boric acid to a glass full of warm water; or you can use common salt, but not strong enough to irritate the throat, about one teaspoonful to a glass of water. If you have listerine or glyco-thymoline or any such disinfectant use them, one teaspoonful to sixteen spoonfuls of water. Hot water itself is a very good gargle, very healing and cleansing. Anyone who enters the sick room and comes out again should wear a sheet all over him. On coming out, he or she should leave this sheet outside the window of another room. If the person has a beard he should wash his face with a 1 to 2000 solution of corrosive sublimate, and the hands also, before leaving the sick room. The one who waits upon the sick one should remain there, but everyone can not do so. They must stay away from the healthy if possible.

City and State Supervision.--If you live in the city your physician should notify the health board who will probably send someone to instruct you regarding cautions and some cities have private rules, laws, etc., for them to follow while under quarantine. A copy is usually furnished also to your close neighbors. Also some of the state departments of health have made up pamphlets which are circulated free on request dealing with the sanitary science of infectious and contagious diseases. Some colleges use these same pamphlets in their study of sanitary science. Much valuable information is contained in them. Comparatively few people learn of these pamphlets. For the benefit of those who have not read or seen them we quote from their scarlet fever subjects as follows:

HOW TO AVOID AND PREVENT SCARLET FEVER.

Do not let a child go near a case of scarlet fever. This is especially important to be observed.

Children are in much greater danger of death from scarlet fever than are adults; but adult persons often get and spread the disease, and sometimes die from it. Mild cases in adults may cause fatal cases among children. Unless your services are needed keep away from the disease yourself. If you do visit a case, bathe yourself and change and disinfect your clothing and hair, beard, if any, and hands before you go where there is a child. Do not permit any person or thing or a dog or cat, or other animal to come from a case of scarlet fever to a child. No cat or dog should be permitted to enter the sick room.

Do not permit a child to wear or handle clothing worn by a person during sickness or convalescence from scarlet fever.

Beware of any person who has sore throat. Do not kiss or come near to such a person. Do not drink from the same cup, blow the same whistle, or put his pen or pencil in your mouth. Whenever a child has sore throat and fever, and especially when this is accompanied by a rash on the body, the child and attendant should immediately be isolated until the physician has seen it and determined whether it has scarlet fever. Strict quarantine should be established and maintained throughout the course of the disease. Exposed persons should be isolated until such time has elapsed as may prove that they are not infected. The period of incubation, that is the interval of time between exposure to the contagion of scarlet fever and the first sign of the disease in the person so exposed, varies. In many cases it appears in seven days, in some cases in fourteen days, and in some cases twenty-one days; the average period is about nine days. Quarantine of persons exposed should not be raised under four weeks.

Children believed to be uninfected may be sent away from the house in which there is scarlet fever to families in which there are no persons liable to the disease, or to previously disinfected convalescent wards in hospitals; but in either case they should be isolated from the public until the expiration of the period of incubation. This time may vary, but for full protection to the public isolation should be observed for four weeks.

Persons who are attending upon children or other persons suffering from scarlet fever, and also the members of the patient's family, should not mingle with other people nor permit the entrance of children into their house.

SANITARY CARE OF INFECTED AND SICK PERSONS AND ROOMS.

All persons known to be sick with this disease (even those but mildly sick) should be promptly and thoroughly isolated from the public and family. In ordering the isolation of infected persons, the health officer means that their communication with well persons and the movement of any article from the infected room or premises shall be absolutely cut off.

Except it be disinfected, no letter or paper should be sent through the mail from an infected place. That this is of more importance than in the case of smallpox is indicated by the fact of the much greater number of cases of sickness and of deaths from scarlet fever,--a disease for which no such preventive as vaccination is yet known.

The room in which one sick with this disease is to be placed should previously be cleared of all needless clothing, drapery and other materials likely to harbor the germs of the disease; and except after thorough disinfection nothing already exposed to the contagion of the disease should be moved from the room. The sick room should have only such articles as are indispensable to the well-being of the patient, and should have no carpet, or only pieces which can afterwards be destroyed. Provision should be made for the introduction of a liberal supply of fresh air and the continual change of the air in the room without sensible currents or drafts.

Soiled clothing, towels, bed linen, etc., on removal from the patient should not be carried about while dry; but should be placed in a pail or tub covered with a five per cent solution of carbolic acid, six and three-fourths ounces of carbolic acid to one gallon water. Soiled clothing should in all cases be disinfected before sending away to the laundry, either by boiling for at least half an hour or by soaking in the five per cent solution of carbolic acid.

The discharges from the throat, nose, mouth, and from the kidneys and bowels of the patient should be received into vessels containing an equal volume of a five per cent solution of carbolic acid, and in cities where sewers are used, thrown into the water closet; elsewhere the same should be buried at least one hundred feet distant from any well, and should not by any means be thrown into a running stream, nor into a cesspool or privy, except after having been thoroughly disinfected. Discharges from the bladder and bowels may be received on old cloths, which should be immediately burned. All vessels should be kept scrupulously clean and disinfected. Discharges from the nose, ears, etc., may be received on soft rags or pieces of cloth and which should be immediately burned.

All cups, glasses, spoons, etc., used in the sick room, should at once on removal from the room, be washed in the five per cent solution of carbolic acid and afterwards in hot water, before being used by any other person.

Food and drink that have been in the sick room should be disinfected and buried. It should not be put in the swill barrel.

Perfect cleanliness of nurses and attendants should be enjoined and secured. As the hands of the nurses of necessity become frequently contaminated by the contagion of the disease, a good supply of towels and basins, one containing a two per cent solution of carbolic acid (two and three-fifths ounces of carbolic acid to a gallon of water) and another for plain soap and water should always be at hand and freely used.

Persons recovering from scarlet fever, so long as any scaling or peeling of the skin, soreness of the eyes or air passages or symptoms of dropsy remain, should be considered dangerous, and, therefore, should not attend school, church or any public assembly or use any public conveyance. In a house infected with scarlet fever, a temporary disinfection after apparent recovery may be made, so as to release from isolation the members of the household who have not had the disease.

Diet and Nursing.--Food should be given every two to four hours. Only water can be given as long as there is nausea and vomiting, and sometimes not even that. After they have stopped you can give milk and water and then milk. You should give it to a child every two to three hours, about one-fourth of a glass full and warm if possible. A child can take at least one quart in twenty-four hours. Watch the stomach and bowels for bad symptoms; if necessary you can put in one teaspoonful of lime water after the milk has been heated. If the child will not take milk, use one of the prepared foods. Mellins' malted milk, Borden's malted milk, peptonized milk, Imperial Granum, and follow the directions on the bottle. The different food waters mentioned above are to use when milk and other food preparations cannot be given. Albumen (white of an egg and water, not whipped) can be given and always cold. Cold milk also tastes better.

During the Sickness, etc.--The linen, bedding, etc., of the patient should be put into a one to five-thousand solution of corrosive sublimate (you can buy that strength tablet) before being boiled, dried and aired in the sun. The sick room must be kept well ventilated, but no drafts should be allowed to go over the patient. The temperature is better at 68 degrees F. The patient should be kept in bed during all the feverish stage and during the scaling stage also.

Care must be taken lest the patient take cold. During this time there is a great danger of ear and kidney trouble. It would be safer to keep the patient in bed until the peeling is done. Children are naturally lively, risky, and a little careless. To keep the scales from flying you can grease the patient with cold cream, vaselin, lard, etc. This will also help to ease the itching. The peeling is aided by bathing the patient every day with warm, soapy water.

Special Treatment.--In ordinary cases little treatment is needed except to keep the throat and nose free from excessive secretions. The urine should be examined daily, and the bowels should move once or twice a day. Cold water should be given frequently after the nausea has passed away. Milk is the usual food, but must not be given during the vomiting stage. Equal parts of milk and water can be given after the vomiting stage, if the patient will not take pure milk.

During the vomiting stage very little water even can be given. The greatest danger in scarlet fever comes from the throat complications and the high fever.

When the fever is high the patient suffers from delirium. A temperature of 105 is dangerous and such patients must be bathed well in water, commencing at 90 degrees and rubbed well all over while in the water, allowing the temperature of the bath to fall to 85 or 80 degrees while so doing; bath to last five to fifteen minutes. Bathe the head with water, at the temperature of 50 degrees, all the time the temperature is at 103 degrees or higher. Always use the thermometer to determine the temperature of the water. Weakly children often do not stand the bath well, so you must exercise discretion in giving it often. The temperature must be kept down to 102 to 103-1/2, and baths must be used often to do so. Where baths cannot be used, frequent washing with water at 60 to 70 degrees must be adopted without drying the child afterwards. A mother should always remember that a feverish, restless child needs a bath or a good washing with cool soap and water. If the bowels and kidneys do not act freely enough give the following:

a175Epsom Salts	2 ounces
Cream of Tartar	2 ounces

Mix and give one-half teaspoonful in water every three hours until the bowels move freely.

This is the dose for a child one year old.

Dropsy in Scarlet Fever.--In this case you must have a doctor. A simple way to make a dropsy patient sweat is to place the patient upon a cane seated chair, pin a blanket around the neck, covering the whole body. Under the chair place a wooden pail half full of cool water and into this put a brick baked as hot as possible; or you can introduce steam under the blanket while the patient is sitting on a chair, or lying in bed, taking care not to scald the patient. This will cause sweating, and relieve the dropsy and also congested kidneys.

How Soon May a Scarlet Fever Patient Associate with the Healthy?--It is best to wait a few weeks after scaling ends. Give the patient a bath in a one to 10,000 corrosive sublimate solution first.

Caution.--An ordinary case of scarlet fever does not need much medicine. Nursing and care are essential. Even the slightest case should be watched. There is always danger of the eyes, ears and kidneys becoming affected. If the child complains of pain in the head the ear must be examined. If the urine passed is small in quantity, or if there are any signs of dropsy, treatment must be given at once. You have heard very much lately about the sting of the honey bee for rheumatism. I often use a preparation of this for the kidney troubles in scarlet fever. The name is Apis Mel. I use the second or third homeopathic attenuation in tablet form and give one to two about every two hours. I have found this effective in such cases where the urine is small in quantity, and there is some dropsy. The lightest cases can have dropsy, especially if special care is not taken when scaling goes on.

I was once attending three children for scarlet fever. The one that had it in a mild form became affected with dropsy. For this I steamed her. In her case I placed her in a cane-seated chair, pinned a blanket tightly around her so as to thoroughly cover her, put a pail of cool water under her chair and dropped into the pail a hot baked brick. The hot brick caused steam to rise from the water and enveloped the child, producing sweating. This was done frequently, and the child considered it a joke, but it relieved her of the bloat. It was in the country and these crude means produced the desired result. By attaching a rubber tube to a steaming kettle and introducing the steam under the covering the same result can be produced. Sometimes you may not have all things you wish, then you must make use of what is handy. You would be surprised perhaps to know how much can be done to relieve sickness by what can be found in every house. (For disinfectants see chapter on nursing.)

MEASLES.--Measles is an acute infectious disease, distinguished by a characteristic eruption on the mucous membranes and skin. It is very contagious and spreads through the atmosphere. Almost everyone is susceptible to measles and suffers at least one attack. The disease is not frequent during the first year of life. It prevails in all countries.

Incubation.--This varies from thirteen to fifteen days. In calculating this period we include the time from exposure to the appearance of the eruption. One attack generally protects the person from another attack. The period of the greatest danger of taking it extends through the period of the eruption. It diminishes as the eruption fades. From this we learn that the infection in measles takes place generally in the incubation stage.

Symptoms and Description of Ordinary Type.--The first symptoms may be only a headache or a slight disturbance of the stomach. There may be some fever in the evening. There is now a redness and watery condition of the eyes, and general feeling of weariness. The cold symptoms (coryza) are not yet marked, but if we look in the mouth we may see a few spots on the mucous membrane of the cheek. Then follow the sneezing, running at the nose, sore and red eyes; running water, sensitiveness to the light, cough and fever. The eruption now appears, and is first noticed on the side of the head and the wings of the nose, as a red spotted eruption, which soon looks like a pimple, and then "blotchy." Older people feel quite sick. The aching all over, and headache are sometimes almost unbearable, especially when there is much coughing. The face, eyes and scalp are soon covered by the red rose irregularly shaped pimples, which next appear rapidly on the back of the hands, fore-arms, front of the trunk, on the back and lower extremities. This order is not always maintained. Sometimes it first appears on the back.

The eruptive stage generally lasts three or four days, during which time the symptoms are all aggravated, especially by any strong light, on account of the sore eyes for the measles are also in them. We have active cold symptoms like sneezing, running at the nose, snorting, snuffling, hawking. The cough is terribly severe, annoying, making the lungs and stomach very sore. The head feels as if it would split. The patient holds his chest and "stomach" while coughing. Symptoms of acute bronchitis develop. Sometimes there is much diarrhea. Pneumonia often develops through carelessness. The fever reaches its height when the eruption is fully developed. The eruption fades after it has been out for three or four days, and then all the symptoms decrease, the fever lessens and becomes normal by gradual morning remissions.

Scaling begins when the pinkish hue of the rash has disappeared and continues until the last vestige of reddish spots has disappeared. As a rule it is completed in two to four weeks after the first eruption has appeared. Sometimes the scaling is difficult to see, but it is never absent in measles: It is best seen on the front part of the chest, shoulders, and the inner surface of the thighs. The temperature may reach 104 to 105-8/10 without complications. This description gives a picture of a typical case. The eruption that appears in the mucous membrane of the mouth appears three to four days before the skin rash. It is accompanied by redness of the pharynx and of the front and back pillars of the fauces. The soft palate is studded with irregular shaped, rose colored spots or streaks and the hard palate presents small whitish vesicles. They are also found on the colored mucous membrane of the cheeks and on that opposite the gums of the upper and lower teeth. The rash of measles is a characteristic eruption of rose colored or purple colored papules (pimples). As a rule the whole face is covered with the eruption and is swollen. Diphtheria may complicate measles. Bronchitis and brancho-pneumonia also may occur, especially if the patient is careless and takes cold. Diarrhea is frequently present.

Eyes.--Following severe cases fear of light, spasm of the orbicularis muscle, inflammation of the lachrymal duct, conjunctivitis, ulceration of the cornea and amaurosis (general blindness) may result. Hence the necessity of careful attention to the eyes. Never read anything during the attack of the measles. The ear may also become afflicted. There are other complications, but these mentioned are the important ones.

Mortality in Measles.--The mortality in childhood and infancy is about eight per cent. Mortality is greatest for number of cases during the first year. Six per cent between fifth and eighth years.

Diagnosis.--Presents few difficulties in a typical case. The mode of onset is cold symptoms of the nose and eye, cough; appearance of the mouth, throat and the blotchy eruptions are very characteristic.

Treatment. Prevention.--As soon as you know it to be the measles, separate the case and put the patient in a well-aired room where you can have air without a draft and where the room can be made and kept dark. Those persons who must go in the room should put over them a linen robe, and hang it outside of the sick room. It should thoroughly cover them. When not in use hang it in the open air. An attendant who wears a beard should disinfect his beard, face, head and hands before mingling with the well.

MOTHERS' REMEDIES.--1. Measles, Lemon Remedy from a Canadian Mother.--"Give child all cold lemonade it can drink and keep in warm room. This acts just as well as if the drinks are hot. We tried both on our children and cured both ways." Don't give so much of the cold as to chill. The cold drink makes child sweat, just as hot does. Also helps to carry off impurities by flushing bowels, just as clear water would.

2. Measles, Elder Blossom Tea to Drive Out.--"Elder blossom tea is good for a cold or fever. Gather the blossoms, and make a tea. Pleasant to take. Sweeten if desired. This is also good to drive out the measles." This remedy should be taken warm and is especially good to bring out the rash in children. Take a teaspoonful every hour.

General Treatment.--An ordinary case of measles does not need much treatment. If the patient has a high fever and is very hot and restless, bathe with tepid or cool water every two or three hours, till the patient becomes quite restful. Sometimes they have too much covering and that makes them hot and restless. Remove a little at a time. Bathing will not hurt the rash, for it can be done under the clothes and without any danger to the patient.

Cold Drinks.--These are refreshing and beneficial, if not given too freely. One-third of a glass of water is enough at one time, but it can be given often, if it does not chill the patient. After the feverish days have passed, diluted milk or plain milk can be given in greater amount.

Cough in Measles.--It is likely to be severe, straining and barking and hard to relieve. If it is too severe you can give, for a child one year old:

Acetanelid	1/2 dram
Dover's Powder	1/2 dram

Mix and make into thirty powders.

Give one-half powder every two hours when awake or restless.

2. For a child two years old:

Paregoric	2 to 5 drops
Syrup Ipecac	3 drops

Mix.

Give every three hours, according to age, one to three hours for a child two years old.

3. For Irritation of the Skin.--Sponge once a day with water at 100 degrees F. containing a little alcohol or a pinch of sodium bicarbonate or soda.

4. For Scaling.--Use ointment of benzoinated lard, combined with five per cent of boric acid.

Diet.--The food should be light; milk, broths, and when the fever is gone chicken and soft boiled eggs, jelly, toasted bread, crackers, cereals, with cocoa for drink. Orange juice or lemon juice may be given in moderation. Milk, one pint per day for every fifty pounds in weight of the patient, during a fever sickness, is a safe and liberal allowance. Smaller children in proportion. Mothers will be apt to give too much and it may then prevent rest and steep. When the fever subsides you can give more milk and some of the above foods. Water, as before stated, can be given for the thirst quite frequently.

Teas.--The laity gives lots of these to bring out the rash. It seems to me before the rash is out the patient is feverish and chilly and the skin is dry, and a small amount of tea given every hour or two might do good unless the patient is made warmer. There are many varieties given. Elder blossom seems to have the call. For some time after the patient is well he may be bothered with a cough;

it better be looked after if it continues, for there might be bronchitis or some lung trouble left and unknown.

Caution.--A person who has had the measles or German measles, should be very careful about taking cold, for if they do they are liable to have serious trouble, especially in the chest. It is very easy to take bronchitis or pneumonia during and after an attack of measles. The mucous membrane of these parts is left somewhat swollen and it remains susceptible to disease for some time. "An ounce of prevention is worth a pound of cure." Remain in the house three or four days longer than may seem necessary and you will be paid for so doing by having good bronchial tubes and lungs,--as good as before if you were careful during the attack.

GERMAN MEASLES.--This is an acute self-limited disease and contagious. It has a mild fever, watery eyes, cough, sore throat and enlargement of the glands of the neck, not seen in the common measles. It has an eruption that may come the first day to the fourth.

Incubation Period Runs.--From fifteen to twenty days.

Rash.--Just before the rash appears there is a headache, nausea and irritation of the bronchial tubes. The eruption is so similar to that of measles at the outset that it is hard to differentiate between them. The eruption in the mouth, however, is not so characteristic. Before the appearance of the eruption, the glands on the back of the neck and angles of the jaw may be enlarged. At the time of its appearance the glands in the armpits and groin become enlarged to the size of a bean and bigger, and they remain enlarged for weeks after the eruption has disappeared.

Treatment.--Similar to the measles if any is needed.

CHICKEN POX (Varicella).--This is an acute infectious disease, characterized by a peculiar eruption. Children are the ones usually attacked. It generally occurs before the tenth year. It is transmitted through the atmosphere. The period of coming on is usually fourteen days, but it may extend to nineteen days. It is perhaps the simplest and mildest disease of childhood. It occurs but once, is contagious, is very common, and resembles varioloid. It has a mild light fever and large vesicles almost the size of a split pea, scattered over the body. There may be few and there may be hundreds. They are reddish gray and appear first on the head and face, then on the body, one crop following another on the body. They are filled at first with a clear liquid, which soon turns yellowish, then breaks and dries up. They leave no scar unless they are scratched or are very large. The patient is usually well in a week, but the scars last longer.

MOTHER'S REMEDY.--1. Chicken Pox, Catnip Tea and Soda Water for.--"Put the patient to bed and give catnip tea. A daily bath of saleratus water is good and the bowels should be kept open." One of the most essential things is to keep the patient warm.

PHYSICIANS' TREATMENT FOR CHICKEN POX.--Exclude other children. The child should be lightly fed and on ordinary food. Large vesicles on the face, when yellow, should be pricked with a needle that has been boiled, then wash them with a disinfecting lotion twice daily.

The following is a good lotion:

Boric Acid	1/2 ounce (4 teaspoonfuls)
Boiled Water	1 pint

Mix thoroughly and use twice a day on the eruption.

The child should not pick the sores on his face, as this may cause delay in healing and leave a mark.

MUMPS (Parotitis).--This is an acute infectious disease of one or both of the parotid glands, located at the angle of the jaw, and extending up to the ear, and, also, to other salivary glands. It appears only once. One attack gives immunity. It may come at any age; but appears mostly before the age of fifteen. It comes on one side first and may pass over to the other side in a few days, as it usually does, and gives the face a broad appearance, under the ears, or ear, and makes chewing and swallowing almost impossible. There is no soreness of the throat in mumps. In well-marked cases there is considerable fever and pain. It may last from a few days to a week. The usual length of time the disease lasts is one week. There is no tendency to form pus, even when the face is very hard and swollen and tender. It will occasionally leave the face and appear in the breasts and ovaries in the females or in the testicles of the males, and in both places it causes much pain.

Treatment.--The patient should be kept in the house and isolated in bed as long as the symptoms last. When there is much pain, laudanum diluted one-third with water may be applied continually with a soft warm cloth. Oil of hyoscyamus applied twice daily to the sore parts is good if laudanum is not used. When the swelling goes down I know of nothing as good as a hot bean poultice, which must be changed often so as to keep hot. Bean poultice.--Simply boil the beans in water until they are soft and thick enough to use as a poultice. The bowels should be kept open with salts. The food must be liquid, such as milk, soups and gruels. If there is not much fever, soft boiled eggs and milk toast from the beginning. Do not use vinegar, acids or astringents.

WHOOPING-COUGH (Pertussis).--Whooping cough is an acute specific infectious, disease caused by a micro-organism. It is characterized in a majority of cases by a spasmodic cough, accompanied by a so-called whoop. It is not only infectious, but very contagious. It is propagated through the atmosphere in schools and public places; the air of which is contaminated with the specific agent of the disease. This agent is thought to reside in the sputum and the secretions of the nose and air passages of the patient. It is very contagious at the height of the attack. The sputum of the first or catarrhal stage is thought to be highly contagious. The sputum in the stage of decline is also thought to be capable of carrying the disease. It prevails in all countries and climates. During the winter and spring months it is most frequent. At times it prevails as an epidemic. It occurs most frequently in infancy and childhood, but a person can take it at any age. Second attacks are rare. It is most frequent between the first and second year; next most frequent between the sixth and twelfth month. After the fifth year the frequency diminishes up to the tenth year, after which the disease is very infrequent. Not everyone who is exposed contracts the disease. It seems that whooping-cough, measles, and influenza frequently follow one another in epidemic form. This is one of the diseases much dreaded by parents. It is very tedious and endangers the life of weak and young children by exhaustion. It is a terrible thing to watch one with this disease, day in and day out. It can be known by the impetuous, continuous and frequent coughing spells, following each other rapidly until the patient is out of breath, with a tendency to end in vomiting. When it comes in the fall or winter months there will likely be spasmodic coughing until summer through the usual colds contracted. Summer is the best time to have it.

Symptoms.--There is an incubation stage, but it is hard to determine its length. After the appearance of the symptoms there are three stages; the catarrhal, the spasmodic, and the stage of decline.

The First Stage.--This is characterized by a cough which is more troublesome at night. One can be suspicious, when instead of getting better in a few days, it gets worse and more frequent, without any seeming cause. After four or five days the cough may be accompanied by vomiting, especially if the cough occurs after eating. There may be some bronchitis, and if so there will be one or more degrees of fever. Fever is present as a rule, only during the first few days, unless there is bronchitis. As the case passes into the spasmodic or second stage, the paroxysms of coughing last longer, the child becomes red in the face and spits up a larger amount of mucus than in ordinary bronchitis. This period of the cough without a whoop, may last from five to twelve days. In some cases there is never a whoop. The child has a severe spasmodic cough, followed by vomiting. Usually at the close of this stage the incessant cough causes slight puffiness of the eyelids and slight bloating of the face.

Spasmodic or Second Stage.--The peculiar whoop is now present. The cough is spasmodic. The child has distinct paroxysms of coughing which begin with an inspiration (in-breathing) followed by several expulsive, explosive coughs, after which there is a deep, long-drawn inspiration which is characterized by a loud crowing called the "whoop." This paroxysm may be followed by a number of similar ones. When the paroxysm is coming on the face assumes an anxious expression, and the child runs to the nearest person or to some article of furniture and grasps him or it with both hands. It is so severe sometimes that the child will fall or claw the air, convulsively. In the severest and most dangerous types, a convulsion may come on in a moderate degree, the face is red or livid, the eyes bulge and when the paroxysm ends a quantity of sticky tenacious mucus is spit up. In other cases there is vomiting at the end of the paroxysm. There is frequently nose-bleed. In the intervals the face is pale or bluish, eyelids are puffy and face swollen. There is little bronchitis at this period in the majority of cases. In some cases the number of paroxysms may be few. There are generally quite a number during the twenty-four hours.

Stage of the Decline.--In this stage the number and severity or the paroxysms lessen. They may subside suddenly or gradually after four to twelve weeks. The whoop may reappear at times. The cough may persist, more or less, for weeks after the whoop is entirely gone.

Complications.--Bronchitis is common, it may be mild or severe. It may run into capillary bronchitis and this is dangerous.

Diagnosis.--Continued cough, getting worse and spasmodic, worse at night, livid face when coughing, causes great suspicion as to its being whooping-cough. The whoop will confirm it.

Mortality is quoted as twenty-five per cent during the first year. Between first and fifth year about five per cent, from fifth to tenth year about one per cent. Rickets, or wasting disease (marasmus) and poor hygienic surroundings makes the outlook less favorable.

MOTHERS' REMEDIES. 1. Whooping-Cough, Chestnut Leaves for.--"Steep chestnut leaves, strain, add sugar according to amount of juice and boil down to a syrup; give plenty of this. A friend of mine gave this to her children. She said they recovered rapidly and the cough was not severe." They are not the horse-chestnut leaves.

2. Whooping-Cough, Chestnut Leaves and Cream for.--"Make an infusion of dry chestnut leaves, not too strong, season with cream and sugar, if desired. The leaves can be purchased at a drug store in five cent packages."

3. Whooping-Cough, Mrs. Warren's Remedy for.--

"Powdered Alum	1/2 dram
Mucilage Acacia	1 ounce
Syrup Squills	1/2 ounce
Syrup Simple, q. s	4 ounces

Mix this.

This is one of the best remedies known to use for whooping - cough. It has been used for many years, and some of our best doctors use it in their practice. I do not hesitate to recommend it as a splendid remedy."

4. Whooping-Cough, Raspberry Tincture for.--"Take one-half pound honey, one cup water; let these boil, take off scum; pour boiling hot upon one-half ounce lobelia herb and one-half ounce cloves; mix well, then strain and add one gill raspberry vinegar. Take from one teaspoonful to a dessertspoonful four times a day. Pleasant to take."

PHYSICIANS' TREATMENT for Whooping-Cough.--The patient should be isolated and sleep in a large, well ventilated room. In spring and summer weather, the child is better in the open air all day. In the winter the child should be warmly clothed. Pine wood and a fairly high altitude are probably the best. The greatest care should be taken in all seasons to keep from taking cold, or bad bronchitis or pneumonia may result. All complications are serious, especially in nursing children. There should be no appreciable fever, and when the paroxysm of cough is over the child should sleep or play quite well, until the next one returns. So if there is much fever the case needs watching.

Medical Treatment.--Medicines have little effect in controlling the disease. The severity can be lessened. If the child is much disturbed at night, the following is good:

1.	Acetanelid	1/2 dram
	Dover's Powder	1/2 dram

Mix thoroughly and make up into thirty powders; for one year old one-half a powder every two hours while awake or restless.

2.	Syrup of Dover's Powder	1 fluid dram
	Tincture of Aconite	10 drops

Simple Syrup enough to make two ounces.

Mix and give one-half teaspoonful every two hours for a child one year old. Shake bottle.

3. But the best treatment I know is the following: Go to any good drug store and get a fifty-cent bottle of vapo-cresolene. Burn this, according to the directions given on the bottle in the evening. Use a small granite cup, put about one-third of an inch of the medicine in this, set cup on a wire frame above a lamp, (can buy a regular lamp with the medicine) close windows and let the child inhale the fumes. This will give the patient a good night's sleep. I have used this for years, and know it is good and effective. A tea made of chestnut leaves is said to be good, and is often used as a home remedy. The leaves of the chestnut that we eat, not the horse-chestnut.

Diet.--This is an extremely important part of the treatment. As the child vomits frequently, especially after eating, the food is generally vomited, so there should be frequent feeding in small quantities. The food should be digestible and nourishing. Milk is a good food for older children. In nursing infants they should be nursed oftener, especially if they vomit soon after nursing. In older children, you must not feed too heavy and hearty foods; meat and potatoes should not be given to young children having the disease. When vomiting is severe the food should be fluid and given often. The child must be nourished. If this disease occurs in the winter the person attacked, after he is seemingly well, must be careful not to take cold. The condition of the mucous membrane of the air tube after an attack of this disease, makes it very easy for the person to contract inflammation of that part and have in consequence laryngitis, bronchitis, or pneumonia. Thc cough in very many cases will last all winter without any additional cold being added.

DIPHTHERIA.--Diphtheria is an acute disease and always infectious. There is a peculiar membrane which forms on the tonsils, uvula, soft palate and throat and sometimes in the larynx and nose. It may form in other places such as in the vagina, bowels, on wounds or sores of the skin. I once cut off the fingers for a child under the care of another doctor. The child came down with diphtheria, and the membrane formed on the fingers. Also it is often epidemic in the cold autumn months. Its severity varies with different epidemics. Children from two to fifteen years old are most frequently attacked with it. Catarrhal inflammations of the respiratory mucous membrane predisposes to it.

Cause.--The exciting cause is a bacillus called after the discoverers--Klebs-Loeffler--and this may be communicated directly to another person from the membrane or discharges from the nose and mouth, secretions of convalescents, or from the throat of normal persons. The local condition (lesion) may be a simple catarrhal inflammation, or a greenish or gray exudate, involving chiefly the tonsils, pharynx, soft palate, nose, larynx and trachea, less often the conjunctiva and alimentary tract. It is firmly adherent at first and leaves a bleeding surface when detached; later it is soft and can be removed.

Symptoms.--Incubation period usually lasts from two to seven days after exposure, usually two, generally there is chilliness, sometimes convulsions in young children, pain in the back and extremities and a fever of 102-1/2 to 104 degrees.

PHARYNGEAL DIPHTHERIA.--In typical cases this begins with slight difficulty in swallowing, and reddened throat (pharynx), then there is a general congestion of these parts, and membrane is seen on the tonsils. It is grayish white, then dull or yellowish; adherent and when removed it leaves a bleeding surface upon which a fresh membrane quickly forms. If the disease runs on, in a few days the membrane covers the tonsils and pillars of the fauces, often the uvula. The glands around the neck often enlarge. Temperature 102 to 103 degrees. Pulse 100 to 120. The constitutional symptoms are usually in proportion to the local condition, but not always. The membrane frequently extends into the nostrils and frequently there is a burning discharge. In malignant cases all the symptoms are severe and rapidly progressive ending in stupor and death in three to five days. Death may occur from sudden heart failure or complications.

LARYNGEAL DIPHTHERIA, Formerly Called Membranous Croup.--Diphtheria in the larynx may occur alone or with the pharyngeal kind, and was formerly called "Membranous Croup."

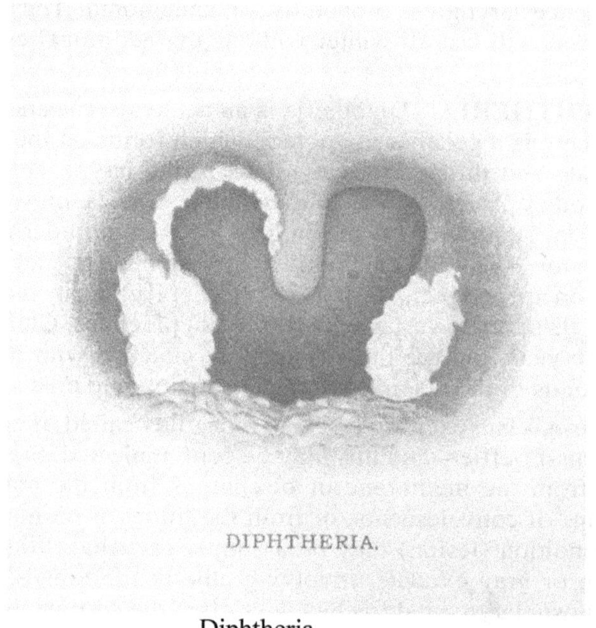
DIPHTHERIA.

Diphtheria

After several days of hoarseness and coughing the breathing suddenly becomes hard, generally at night, and it is at first in paroxysms, but later it is constant. The space above the breast bone (sternum) is depressed and there is a drawing in of the spaces between the ribs during inspiration accompanied with a husky voice and blue look. The fever is slight. If the obstruction in the larynx is severe the cyanosis,--blueness,--and difficulty of breathing increase, and gradual suffocation leads to (coma) deep sleep and death.

Diagnosis.--Diagnosis can only be made certain by proper chemical tests. The presence of membrane on a tonsil and a small patch streak, or speck of membrane, on the adjacent surface of the uvula or tip of the uvula; a patch of membrane on the tonsil and an accompanying patch on the posterior wall of the pharynx; the presence of a croupy cough and harsh breathing with small patches of membrane on the tonsil or epiglottis. These symptoms are very suspicious and warrant separation of the patient. If such conditions are seen in any one, it will be the part of prudence to send for your doctor immediately. You give the patient a better chance by sending early, protect yourselves and also your neighbors.

Recovery.--Chances in mild cases are good. Antitoxin has brought the death rate down from forty to twelve per cent. Death may occur from sudden heart failure, obstruction in the pharynx, severe infection, complications or paralysis.

MOTHERS' REMEDIES.--Diphtheria is such a dangerous disease and so rapidly fatal that the family physician should be promptly called. Until he arrives the following may be used to give some relief:

2. Diphtheria, Kerosene Good for.--"Kerosene oil applied to the throat of child or adult is very good."

3. Diphtheria, Hops and Hot Water Relieves.--"Make two flannel bags and fill with hops which have been moistened with hot water; place bags in a steamer and heat. Keep one bag hot and the other around the throat. Change often, relief in short time." Mrs. Shaw has tried this in a case of diphtheria and other throat trouble and recommends it as an excellent remedy.

PHYSICIANS' TREATMENT for Diphtheria. Prevention.--The patient should be isolated as soon as the spots or membrane are seen. Other children who have been with the sick one should at once be given "immunizing" doses of antitoxin, and the furniture of the sick room such as hangings, carpets. rugs, etc., should be removed and disinfected, only the necessary articles being kept in the room. The room should be kept well ventilated, but no draught should get to the patient. The one nursing the patient should not come near the other members of the family. All articles of clothing worn by the patient should be dipped in a 1 to 2000 solution of corrosive sublimate before they are removed from the sick room. (Other solutions may be used; see Nursing Department). Dishes, etc., should be treated in the same way and foods left over should be put in a vessel containing an antiseptic solution, and then burned. Everyone going into the sick room should cover their head with a cap and wear a robe-covering over their clothes, and on leaving the room should gargle or rinse their mouth with a solution of boric acid, about one or two teaspoonfuls to a glass of water, The infant should not be nursed at the breast lest the breast become infected; the milk should be pumped out and fed to the infant with a bottle. If the infant has diarrhea milk must be stopped, the bowels irrigated, and no milk given until all danger from this source is past. The nurse must be careful of the discharges from the nose, mouth and bowels. Discharges from the bowels and the urine must be received in a vessel with an antiseptic solution in it like copperas, lime, etc. Cloths used to receive the discharge from the nose and mouth should be thrown in a vessel containing a solution of 1 to 2000 of corrosive sublimate and then burned. The nurse should wear a gauze protection over her nose and mouth when she is near the patient, and glasses, so that no sputum or discharge from the patient can enter these organs. When the nurse leaves the sick room for a rest or walk, she should change her clothes in an unused room and put them where they can air, wash her hands, face and hair in an antiseptic solution. Great care must be taken by the nurse, or she will carry the disease. The doctor also must take the same care.

PHYSICIANS' MEDICAL TREATMENT.--Antitoxin is the best. 1/100 grain of corrosive sublimate or more according to age is frequently given in the severe cases and is beneficial.

Local Treatment.--In older persons, inhaling steam may benefit. Gargling the throat or spraying the nose and throat is cleansing and helpful; but in children it is sometimes hard to do this, for they may struggle and thus injure and weaken themselves more than they can be benefited by the spraying or gargling. Swab the throat if you can with solution of corrosive sublimate, 1 to 1000. Peroxide of hydrogen, one-sixth to one-half to full strength, is good in many cases, used as a gargle and a swab. Wash out the nose with a normal salt solution. One dram to a pint of water. The persons doing this must take great care or the patient will cough and the discharge will go over them.

When in the Larynx.--Steam inhalations without or with medicine in them and the application of cold or hot to the neck are good. Compound tincture of benzoin is good to use in the water for steaming; one-half to one tablespoonful to a quart of water. A tent can be made by putting a sheet over the four posts of the bed and steam vapor introduced under this covering.

Diet.--The main food is milk, albumin water, broths, eggs given every two hours. Some doctors give stimulants with the food.

Cautions.--Members of the family have no idea how much they can aid the physician in this terrible disease. Pay particular attention to the directions the doctor gives you, if you are doing the nursing, watch so that you may detect any bad symptom, and immediately inform the physician. A harsh cough with increased difficulty in breathing may mean that the disease has extended to the larynx. If such symptoms are first noticed in the physician's absence, he should be sent for at once so he can treat it properly at the start. If the kidneys do not act properly he should be informed. One may take nephritis in diphtheria also. I was called one morning at 3 a. m., to see a case I was attending; she seemed to the parents to be worse; she was, but today she is living, and I believe her life was really saved by her parents. I would rather a loving mother and father nurse a case any time than a selfish, lazy professional nurse. Good nurses are a blessing; selfish ones are a curse; I have met both kinds. After an attack of this disease the patient is left "weak" in many organs. He should be careful, not only of taking cold, but of over-doing. The heart and nervous system in some cases have been terribly wrecked. Take life easy for some time, for you may be thankful that you are alive.

ACUTE TONSILITIS. (Follicular Inflammation of the Tonsils). Causes.--Authors regard this as an infectious disease. It is met with more frequently in the young; infants may take it. Some authors state it can be communicated either through the secretions or by direct contact, as in the act of kissing (Koplik). It is frequent in children from the second to the fourth year, but it is more common after than before the fourth year. Sex has no influence. In this country it is more common in the spring. The predisposing causes are exposure to wet and cold and bad hygienic surroundings. One attack renders a person more susceptible. It spreads through a family in such a way that it must be regarded as contagious. The small openings (Lacunae) of the tonsils become filled with products which form cheesy-looking masses, projecting from the openings of the (Crypts) hidden sacs. These frequently join together, the intervening tissue is usually swollen, deep red in color and sometimes a membrane forms on it in which case it may look like diphtheria.

Symptoms.--Chilly feelings or even a chill and aching pains in the back and limbs may precede the onset. The fever rises rapidly and in the young child may reach 105 degrees in the evening of the first day. The infant is restless, peevish and wakeful at night; it breathes rapidly, and there is high fever and great weakness. Nursing is difficult, not only on account of the pain in swallowing, but because in the majority of cases there is more or less inflammation of the nose. The bowels are disturbed as a result of swallowing infectious secretions from the mouth with the food. The tonsils are enlarged and studded with whitish or yellowish white points. The glands at the angle of the jaws may be enlarged. In older children the tonsils are enlarged and the crypts plugged with a creamy deposit. The surface is covered with a deposit and the pillars of the fauces, uvula and pharynx may all be inflamed. The tongue is coated, the breath is bad, the urine high colored, swallowing is painful; the pain frequently runs to the ear and the voice sounds nasal, as if one had mush in his mouth when talking. In severe cases the symptoms all increase, and the parts become very much swollen. Then the inflammation gradually subsides, and in a week, as a rule, the fever is gone and the local conditions have greatly improved. The tonsils, though, remain somewhat swollen. The weakness and general symptoms are often greater than one would suppose. The trouble may also extend to the middle ear through the eustachian tubes.

Diagnosis Between Acute Tonsilitis and Diphtheria.--Follicular form. "In this form the individual, yellowish, gray masses, separated by the reddish tonsilar tissue are very characteristic, whereas in diphtheria the membrane is of ashy gray and uniform, not patch."--Osler. A point of the greatest importance in diphtheria is that the membrane is not limited to the tonsils, but creeps up the pillars of the fauces or appears on the uvula. The diphtheric membrane when removed leaves a raw, bleeding, eroded surface; whereas, the membrane of follicular tonsilitis is easily separated as there is no raw surface beneath it.

MOTHERS' REMEDIES. 1. Tonsilitis, Raw Onion and Pork for.--"Take a raw onion and some salt pork, chop together, make a poultice on which put a little turpentine and wrap around the throat." This is a very good remedy and should be used for some time. Change as often as necessary.

2. Tonsilitis, Peppermint Oil Good for.--"Apply peppermint oil thoroughly on the outside of the throat from well up behind the ear nearly to the chin, also just in front of the ear. This will soon penetrate through to the tonsils; apply freely if the case is severe and later apply hot cloths if relief does not follow without."

3. Tonsilitis, Borax Water for.--"One-fourth teaspoonful borax in one cup of hot water, gargle frequently." This may be used for ordinary sore throat not quite so strong.

4. Tonsilitis, Salt and Pepper Will Relieve.--"Apply salt pork well covered with pepper to the swollen parts; will often give relief."

5. Tonsilitis, Peroxide of Hydrogen Will Cure.--"Tonsilitis and contagious sore throats are just now extremely popular. Persons having a tendency to them will seldom be sick if they gargle daily with a solution of peroxide of hydrogen and water in equal parts for adults. Peroxide diluted with five parts of water and used as a head spray will prevent catarrhal colds." Children, are often sent to school immediately after an attack of tonsilitis, when they should be at home taking a tonic and building up by a week of outdoor play.

6. Tonsilitis, a Remedy Effective for.--"Rub the outside of the throat well with oil of anise and turpentine, and keep the bowels open." Care should be taken not to take cold. The anise is very soothing and the turpentine will help to draw out the soreness. This would be a good remedy for children.

PHYSICIANS' TREATMENT for Tonsilitis. 1. First Home Treatment.--Put the patient to bed alone in a pleasant room, comfortably warm; for this disease is recorded as contagious in this form. Cold applied externally around the sore spot is good. Use an ice bag if you have it; or wring cloths out of cold water and put just under the jaw and a flannel over that, bound around the neck. It must be changed often to keep cold.

2. Smartweed.--Cloths wrung out of smartweed tea are very good when applied under the jaw.

3. Salt Pork.--Salt pork, well salted and peppered, sewn to a cloth and applied on both sides, if both are diseased, directly to the lumps is very good. These can be kept on indefinitely. I have used them.

4. Liniment.--A strong blistering liniment applied externally where the lumps are is also good. These applications tend to withdraw some of the blood from the sore tonsils, and of course, that relieves them. There are many such that can be used. Poultices should not be applied for this form as they tend to hasten formation of pus.

5. Internally.--Dip your clean moistened finger tip into dry bicarbonate of soda (baking soda), rub this gently on the sore tonsil and repeat it every hour. You can also put one teaspoonful of it in one-half glass of very hot water and gargle if you do not use it locally.

6. Hot Water.--Gargling frequently with very hot water is splendid. If you wish you can use one teaspoonful of some antiseptic, like listerine, in it.

7. Thyme.--You can make a tea of the common garden thyme and gargle or rinse your mouth and throat with it every half to one hour. This is not only healing and soothing, but it is also antiseptic. This is a constituent of many of the antiseptic preparations.

8. Steaming With Compound Tincture of Benzoin.--Tincture of benzoin is splendid. Put one tablespoonful in a quart of hot water and inhale the steam. Put a sheet over your head and pitcher; or put it in a kettle, and roll white writing paper into a funnel, tie one part over the spout and put the other end in your mouth if possible; or you can inhale simple steam in the same way. I know this is excellent and often recommended; everyone has it, and it costs literally nothing, except to heat the water.

9. For the Pain.--Dissolve two drams of chloral hydrate in an ounce of water, use a camel's hair pencil if you have it, or a soft piece of cloth tied on a smooth stick, and apply directly to the diseased parts. This is for older persons, relieves the pain very much. There are many other simple remedies that can be used in this way.

10. MEDICINES. Parke, Davis & Co., Anti-Tonsilitis Tablet No. 645 is very good. This can be bought at any drug store. For a child give one-half a tablet every two hours for four doses, then every three hours. An adult can take one to two every one to three hours according to the severity of the case.

11. Aspirin.--Aspirin is another good remedy; five grains every four hours for an adult; but used only under doctor's directions.

12. Dr. Hare of Philadelphia, uses 1/200 grain mercurius biniodide (pink powder) every four to six hours to abort tonsilitis. I would recommend the following:--Give one-tenth drop dose of a good tincture of aconite and 1/200 grain of the mercury biniodide (one to two tablets a dose) every hour, alternately, one of them one hour and the next, etc. If there is much deposit I would put ten tablets of mercury protoiodide (one-tenth of a grain in a tablet) in one-half glass of water and give two teaspoonfuls every hour until the bowels move freely, then every three to four hours. The aconite can be used if there is much fever, with hot, dry skin, alternately everyone-half hour. I prefer the pink powder when there is no deposit or membrane. These I have used for years, and know them to be excellent. For children the dose is about one-half. After twelve hours the remedies should be given only every three to four hours.

QUINSY. (Suppurative Tonsilitis).--In from two to four days the enlarged gland becomes softer and finally may break, sometimes in the pharynx; the breaking gives the patient great relief. Suffocation has sometimes followed the rupture of a large abscess and the entrance of the pus into the larynx. This form of tonsilitis was formerly called quinsy. By this term now is meant an abscess around the tonsils, (Peritonsilar abscess). The structures are very much swollen.

Causes are somewhat similar to what has produced the regular tonsilitis. It may follow exposure to cold and wet, and is very liable to recur. It is most common between fourteen and twenty-five years. The inflammation here is more deeply seated. It involves the main tissue of the tonsil and tends to go on to suppuration.

Symptoms.--The general disturbance is very great. The fever goes to 104 or 105 degrees; the pulse 110 to 120. Delirium at night is not uncommon. The weakness may be extreme. The throat is dry and sore, hurts terribly to swallow, this being the first thing of which the patient complains. Both tonsils may be involved. They become large, firm to the touch, dusky red and swollen, and the surrounding parts are also much swollen. The swelling may be so great that the tonsils may touch each other or one tonsil may push the uvula aside and almost touch the other tonsil. There is much saliva. The glands of the neck enlarge, the lower jaw is almost immovable and sometimes it is almost impossible to open the mouth at all.

QUINSY. Mothers' Remedies. 1. Willow Gargle for.--"Steep pussy willow and gargle throat with it. This remedy if taken in time, will cure quinsy and it will not return."

2. Quinsy, Liveforever Root Good Poultice for.--"Get the root of liveforever, pound it up and bind on throat as you would a poultice." We have tried this, and it has always given relief, if done in time.

3. Quinsy, Plaster of Lard and Salt for.--"Take one tablespoonful lard and stir into as much table salt as possible making it about like mortar. Spread on a cloth and apply." Splendid for sore throat and quinsy.

4. Quinsy, Oil of Anise Effective for.--"Rub inside of throat with oil of anise."

5. Quinsy, Quick Remedy for.--"In severe cases of quinsy where the tonsils are inflamed and almost meet, a third of a grain of mercury and chalk, or "gray powder," acts very quickly. Cold compresses used nightly to harden the throat is very good. At night use a gargle made of a teaspoonful tincture of cayenne pepper to half pint of water." This remedy is very good and is sure to give relief.

6. Quinsy, Pleasant Peppermint Application for.--"There is nothing better for this disease than oil of peppermint applied externally to the neck and throat." This is an excellent remedy.

7. Quinsy, Kerosene Good for.--"A cloth wet with kerosene oil applied to the throat is very good; also gargling with kerosene oil." Repeat the application of the wet cloths every two or three hours.

8. Quinsy, Raw Beef Has Cured.--"Bind raw beefsteak over the tonsils on one or both sides of the throat as required." The beefsteak acts as a poultice and counter-irritant, drawing the inflammation out in a short time. This is very good, and is easily prepared.

9. Quinsy, Easy and Simple Remedy for.--"Strong sulphur water. Broke up two cases I know."

PHYSICIANS' TREATMENT for Quinsy.--The external applications used should now be hot. Hot water; hot poultices, cloths wrung out of smartweed hot, and thyme tea or golden seal teas. The same steaming process and hot water gargles can be used as given under follicular tonsilitis. But if it continues the tonsils or tonsil must be opened to save pain and life. Just as soon as there is suppuration they should be opened. It will feel softer to the finger touch when ready for opening.

Prevention of Attacks.--By taking care a good many attacks of tonsilitis can be avoided. A person subject to this trouble must be careful about taking cold. He should not sit down with wet clothes, or feet, or shoes that are wet. Girls should wear rubbers and keep dry feet and skirts. Sleeping in damp unused beds is bad. Putting on underwear that has not been dried thoroughly and aired, and the use of bedding, pillows, etc., in the same condition should not be tolerated. Sleeping on the first floor is generally unhealthy for such persons, for it is generally damp.

Do not get chilled; wear sufficient clothing. Drying clothes in a kitchen is an abomination and terrible to one subject to this disease or rheumatism. You can keep from having it so often by proper care. It is likely to return, and repeated attacks will cause permanently enlarged tonsils and they will become so diseased that they, will not only be annoying, but dangerous to health and life. You will go around with your mouth open, "talk through your nose." The tonsil must then be removed, also the adenoids in the throat, to enjoy proper mental and physical health. Enlarged tonsils with pus in them are a menace to anyone. A person who has had these troubles should be careful not to expose himself to the danger of taking cold after an attack.

The parts are still tender and in danger of a return upon the least error in your daily life. I once had a friend who had a return of tonsilitis brought on through going out too soon, and the second attack was worse than the first, a genuine "hummer."

What to do with enlarged tonsils.--Moderate enlargement of the tonsils giving rise to no symptoms or inconvenience need not be interfered with. When, however, the enlargement is great, or when with moderate sized tonsils there are resulting troubles, such as liability to inflammatory rheumatism attacks, active local treatment will be called for; especially is this true when the tonsils contain pus and interfere with the breathing. They should be removed. An anaesthetic is not usually necessary, as the pain is not severe.

INFLUENZA (La Grippe).--La Grippe is an acute infectious disease caused by a germ. It may be epidemic, attacking a large number of persons at one time, or it may continue in the same region for some time and is then called endemic. It is caused by a germ, discovered by a man named Pfeiffer.

The Onset.--The onset may be from one to four days and is usually sudden with a chill and all the symptoms of an active fever due to a general infection, varying according to the location. If in the organs of respiration it begins like a severe cold; active fever, severe pains in the eyes, back, arms, legs, and in the bones; "aches all over" and great prostration. After the fever subsides there is usually a general sore feeling. Symptoms of bronchitis, pleurisy or pneumonia may develop. Then there is the nervous type, generally with a bad headache, neuralgia, pains in the head, backache, legs and arms ache and prostration. May also have inflammation of nerves. Then again the stomach and bowels may be the main seat, for La Grippe has no respect for any organ. We have then symptoms of acute indigestion with fever, nausea, vomiting, stomach pains or acute bowel trouble with fever, colicky pain in the abdomen; diarrhea; or we may have the febrile (fever) type. This may be the only symptom. The fever may be continuous or remittent, and last several days or several weeks and often with pains accompanying it.

In all forms convalescence is often gradual on account of the bodily and mental prostration with general soreness for several days. Many persons never fully regain their health, especially if they are careless during the attack, and almost any disease like bronchitis, kidney disease, pleurisy, pneumonia, etc., may follow.

LA GRIPPE, Mothers' Remedies.--1. Pepper, Red or Cayenne for.--"Make a tea of red pepper or cayenne, and take a tablespoonful in a cup of hot water, drink slowly, before each meal and on retiring. Larger doses in proportion to the intensity of the disease." Sponging the face, temples and neck with water as hot as can be borne relieves the headache of la grippe, which is often very painful and annoying.

2. La Grippe, Easy Remedy for.--"Plenty of good physic with hot teas of any kind has helped my own family."

3. La Grippe, Pleasant and Effective Remedy for.--"Use the oil of peppermint freely; rubbing it on the forehead, in front and back of the ears and each side of the nose. Inhale through each nostril separately. If the throat is affected pour two or three drops in small dish of hot water. Invert a funnel over the dish with the small end in the mouth and draw long breaths. Soak the feet in hot water at bedtime and take a good sweat, if possible."

4. La Grippe, To Allay Fever in.--"To produce sweating and to act on the kidneys and to allay restlessness in fever use the following: Lemon juice and water equal parts, enough to make four ounces; bicarbonate of potassium, one dram; water, three ounces. Make and keep in separate solutions to be used in tablespoonful doses several times daily and taken while effervescing, that is, foaming and bubbling up."

5. La Grippe. Poor Man's Herb Vapor Bath for.--"Give a Turkish or vapor bath every other day. A pail of hot water, with a hot brick thrown into it and placed under a cane-seated chair is the poor man's vapor bath. The patient should be covered. Then take the following herb tea:

Yarrow	2 ounces
Vervain	2 ounces
Mullein	2 ounces
Boneset	1 ounce
Red Sage	2 ounces

Add two quarts of water and boil down to three pints; strain, and then add one ounce fluid extract of ginger; sweeten with honey or syrup; take a wine glassful three times a day, hot. Keep the bowels open and let the diet be light."

6. La Grippe, Red Pepper Treatment From Canada for.-- "Take a bottle of alcohol and put enough red peppers in it so that when four drops of this liquid are put in a half cup of water it tastes strong. This is what I always break up my grippe with." Peppers thus prepared stimulates and warms up the stomach and bowels, and increases the circulation.

PHYSICIANS' TREATMENT for La Grippe.--All discharges from the nose, throat and lungs should be disinfected, for the disease is contagious. Go to bed and stay there. You have no business to be around if you value your health. I am not writing of common cold. A great many people say they have had this disease when they have not had it. One who has had this disease is sick enough to go to bed, and there is where he should be. For the chill a sweat should be produced by putting hot water in fruit jars, wrapping them and placing them around the patient's feet, legs and body. Hot tea drinks can be given; hot lemonade, teas made from hoarhound, ginger, hops and catnip are good.

Corn Sweat.--The corn sweat can be used. Put from ten to twenty-five ears of corn in a boiler, boil thoroughly until the boiled corn smell appears, then put the corn ears into five packs, putting from two to five ears in a pack, according to the age of the patient. Use cloths or towels, but do not put the ears in contact, wrap the cloth between them. Put one pack to the feet and one at each side of the hips, and in each armpit. This will soon cause sweating and restore the external (capillary) circulation. It will generally produce a grateful sweat. Keep the clothes on the patient. After the patient has perspired enough you can remove one pack at a time. Have fresh aired sheets and night dress ready, and after bathing the patient slowly and carefully under the clothes with tepid water and drying all of the body put on the new night-dress and sheets. This remedy is also good for colds and inflammatory diseases of all kinds and when used carefully and thoroughly is always good. Of course, if there is great weakness it cannot be used, for it weakens a patient somewhat. I have saved lives with this sweat, and I know I have cut short many colds and inflammatory diseases. After the sweat the patient should have enough covering to keep comfortably warm and care must be taken to keep from the cold.

Fever.--If the disease goes on and there is high fever, so that the patient suffers from it, it is better to reduce it by cool sponging than by the coal tar products like antipyrin, acetanilid, etc. They are weakening and this is a weakening, prostrating disease. Good, careful cool sponging generally relieves the excessive fever and restlessness. The fever does not continue so long in this disease and it is not, therefore, so harmful. Delirium is present in some cases when the fever is not high.

Irritating Cough.--This can frequently he controlled by steam inhalations as directed under tonsilitis. You can also put in the steaming water one teaspoonful to one tablespoonful of compound tincture of benzoin for this disease. Hoarhound tea can be put in the water and the steam inhaled. If such measures do not stop the cough, medicine will be needed.

Sore Throat.--Spraying the throat with a solution of boric acid, one dram to one pint of hot water, is good. Listerine is good in the same way and dose.

Bowels.--They should be kept open from the first. Salts are usually handy and good.

Medicines.--Ten grains Dover's powder at night is good; unless there is much weakness. Some give quinine, some salol. Quinine, one to two grains, is given one to three hours. Salol, five grains, every three hours, especially for the backache.

Aspirin in five-grain doses for an adult every four hours is given very much now. The bowels should be kept open with salts.

Diet.--Children should take milk if there is no vomiting or diarrhea. If there is vomiting and diarrhea, give only water or diluted milk, or nothing if they continue. Water can generally be given.

For adults a good, nourishing diet when convalescence commences is necessary. During the sickness, milk, eggs,--raw and soft boiled, broths, soups, milk toast, can be given. A person must be very careful after an attack of the grip. He should remain in the house for some time, a week after he is well and thinks he can go out.

TYPHOID FEVER.--Typhoid fever is an acute infectious disease caused by a (Bacillus) germ, named after the discoverer (Eberth). This germ enters into the system, as stated below, locates itself in different organs, especially in the small intestine. It does its worst work in Peyer's glands, situated in the small intestines. They enlarge, ulcerate, break down and their structure is cast off into the bowel. This eating goes so far, in some cases, that it eats through the tissue to the blood vessels and other bleeding follows. Sometimes it goes through all the coats, the peritoneal being the last one. If this occurs we have what is called perforation of the bowel and the peritoneum around this perforation inflames and there is the dread complication of peritonitis. This is very fatal, as the patient is weakened from the inroads of weeks of fever and from the effects of the poison germ. Typhoid fever is also characterized by its slow (insidious), slyly, creeping onset, peculiar temperature, bloating of the abdomen, diarrhea, swelling of the spleen, rose-colored spots and a liability to complications, such as bleeding from the bowels, peritonitis, bronchitis and pneumonia. Its average duration is three to four weeks, often longer. In order to take this disease there must first be the poison germ and then this enters into the system, generally through water that contains the germ, milk, oysters and other foods, etc.

Cause.--The typhoid bacillus (typhoid). This enters into the alimentary canal usually through contaminated water or with milk directly infected by the milk or by water used in washing cans. Also through food to which the germs are carried from the excreta (discharges) by flies, occasionally through oysters by freshening.

Filth, improper drainage and poor ventilation favor the preservation of the bacillus germ and lower the power of resistance in those exposed.

Time.--It occurs most frequently between August and November and in those of from fifteen to twenty years of age. The Peyer's patches and solitary glands of the bowel enlarge, become reddish and are somewhat raised. These go on and ulcerate until the blood vessels may be eaten into and bleeding sometimes results, it eats through the bowel, then there is perforation and peritonitis. The spleen is enlarged, the liver shows changes, the kidney functions are also deranged.

Symptoms.--The symptoms are variable. The following gives the symptoms in a typical case:

Incubation.--The period of incubation lasts from eight to fourteen and sometimes to twenty-three days. During the period the patient feels weak, is almost unable to work, has chilly feelings, headache and tiring dreams, does not know what is the matter with him, constipation or diarrhea, has no appetite, may have some pain in the abdomen which is occasionally localized in the right lower side. Soreness on deep pressure is often found there. In some cases there is nosebleed.

First Week.--After the patient is obliged to take to his bed: During the first week there is in some cases a steady rise in the fever each evening showing a degree or degree and one-half higher than the preceding evening, reaching 103 to 104, and each morning showing higher fever than the preceding morning. The pulse is characteristically low in proportion to the temperature, being about 100 to 110, full of low tension, often having double beat. The tongue is coated;

there is constipation or diarrhea; the abdomen is somewhat distended and a little tender to the touch in the lower right portion. There may be some mental confusion at night. Bronchitis is often present. The spleen becomes enlarged between the seventh and tenth day and the eruption usually appears during this period on the stomach and abdomen.

Second week.--All the symptoms are intensified in the second week, the fever is always high and the weakening type; the pulse is more frequent; the headache is replaced by dullness; the bowel symptoms increase and we have the "pea soup" discharge if there is diarrhea; there is a listless, dull expression on the face; the tongue is coated in the center, red along the edges and the tip, becomes dry and sometimes cracked and almost useless. It is hard to put it out of the mouth, it sticks to the teeth or lips and curls there, and sometimes the patient allows it to remain partly out of the mouth. There may be bleeding from the bowels and perforation of the bowel, producing peritonitis.

Third week.--The temperature is lower in the morning with a gradual fall; the emaciation and weakness are marked. Perforation of the bowel or bleeding may occur. Unfavorable symptoms now include low muttering, delirium, shakings of the muscles, twitching of the tendons, grasping at imaginary things, lung complications and heart weakness.

Fourth week.--In a favorable case: The fever gradually falls to normal, the other symptoms disappear. Death may occur at any time after the second week from the disease or complications. The convalescence is very gradual and the appetite is very great.

Special symptoms and variations.--It may come on with a chill sometimes it is observed by nervous symptoms only.

Walking type.--In this type the patient is able to be around and can walk. The temperature is as high, but some of the other symptoms are not so violent. This is a dangerous kind because the patient is able to walk and thinks it foolish to remain quiet in bed. Walking and being around are likely to injure the bowels, and there is then more danger of bleeding from the bowels. A typhoid fever patient should always go to bed and remain there until he has fully recovered.

Digestive Symptoms.--The tongue is coated, white and moist at first, and in the second week it becomes red at the tip, and at the edges. Later it is dry, brown and cracked. The teeth and lips are covered with a brown material, called sordes.

Diarrhea.--In some cases constipation is prominent, in others diarrhea is a prominent symptom. Bloating is frequent, and an unfavorable symptom, when it is excessive. Bleeding from the bowel occurs usually between the end of the second and the beginning of the fourth week. A sudden feeling of collapse, and rapid fall of the temperature mark it. It is not always fatal.

Perforation of the bowel is usually shown by a sudden sharp pain coming in paroxysms generally localized in the right lower side. The death rate varies very much; in hospitals it is seven to eight per cent. Unfavorable symptoms are continued high fever, delirium and hemorrhage. Persons who are hard drinkers do badly and very many of them die.

TREATMENT. Prevention. Sanitary Care.--Do away with the causes. Keep your cellars clean; do not have them damp, filthy, and filled with decaying matter, as these all tend to weaken the system and make you more susceptible to the poison. In the country, no drainings should come near the wells or springs. Not all water that looks clear and nice is pure. The "out-houses" must be kept clean, and emptied at least twice each year. In the small cities, especially, the water should be boiled during the months when the supply is limited and the wells are low. If more attention was paid to our water supply to make certain that it was not contaminated, and to our foods, especially milk, and to keeping our cellars and drains in a good clean and dry condition, we would have little typhoid fever. Carelessness is the real cause of this terrible disease. The milk should be boiled as well as the water when there is an epidemic of typhoid.

Sanitary Care of the Household Articles.--Dishes must be isolated, washed, dried separately and boiled daily. Thermometers must be isolated, kept in a corrosive sublimate solution one to one thousand, which must be removed daily. Linen when soiled must be soaked in carbolic acid, one cup of carbolic acid to twenty of water, for two hours before being sent to the laundry. Stools must be thoroughly mixed with an equal amount of milk of lime and allowed to stand for one hour. Urine must be mixed with an equal amount of carbolic acid, one to twenty, and allowed to stand one hour. Bed pans, urinals, must be isolated and scalded after each time of using. Syringes and rectal tubes must be isolated, and the latter boiled after using. (See Nursing Department). Tubs should be scrubbed daily, canvasses changed daily and soaked in carbolic acid as the linen is. Hands must be scrubbed and disinfected after giving tubs or rubbing over typhoid fever patients. Blankets, mattresses, and pillows must be sterilized after use in steam sterilizer. I know some people have not all the necessary conveniences, especially in the country, but the greatest care must be taken. A professional nurse was once taking care of a very severe case of typhoid for me. I was continually cautioning her to be more careful of herself. She did not heed it, and finally took the disease and battled eight long weeks with it, before there was much improvement. Careful nursing and a well regulated diet are the essentials in a majority of cases. Put the patient in a well ventilated room, and confine him to the bed from the beginning, and have him remain there until well. The woven wire bed with soft hair mattress, upon which there are two folds of blanket, combines the two great qualities of a sick bed, smoothness and elasticity. A rubber cloth should be placed under the sheet. An intelligent nurse should be in charge; when this is impossible, the attending physician should write out special instructions, regarding diet, treatment of the discharges and of the bed linen.

Much of the above on typhoid is from the world-wide authority, Dr. Osler, and should be-followed in all cases if possible.

Diet and Nursing in Typhoid Fever.--Milk is the most suitable food. Three pints every twenty-four hours may be given when used alone, diluted with water or lime-water.

The stools will show if the milk is digested. Peptonized milk, if not distasteful, may be used. Curds are seen in the stools if too much milk is given and is undigested. Mutton or chicken broth or beef juice can be used; fresh vegetable juices can be added to these, instead of milk. The animal broths are not so good when diarrhea is present. Some patients will take whey, buttermilk, kumiss, when ordinary milk is distasteful. Thin barley gruel well strained is an excellent food for this disease. Eggs may be given, either beaten up in milk or better still, in the form of albumin water, This is prepared by straining the whites of eggs through a cloth and mixing them with an equal quantity of water, which may be flavored with lemon. Water can be given freely; iced tea, barley water, or lemonade may be used, and there is no objection to weak coffee or cocoa in moderate quantities. Feed the patient at stated intervals. In mild cases it is well not to arouse the patient at night. When there is stupor, the patient should be aroused for food at the regular intervals night and day. Do not give too much food. I once had a case in which I did not give more than one quart of liquid food in four weeks, as it distressed her. She made a good recovery on plenty of water.

Cold Sponging.--The water may be warm, cool, or ice cold, according to the height of the fever. A thorough sponge bath should take from fifteen to twenty minutes. The ice cold sponging is quite as formidable as the full cold bath, for which there is an unsuperable objection in private practice.

The Bath.--This should be given under the doctor's directions, and I will not describe it.

Medical Treatment.--Little medicine is used in hospital practice. Nursing is the important essential in typhoid fever.

Management of the Convalescent.--An authority writes, My custom has been not to allow solid food until the temperature has been normal for ten days. This is, I think, a safe rule, leaning perhaps to the side of extreme caution; but after all with eggs, milk toast, milk puddings, and jellies, the patient can take a fairly varied diet. You cannot wait too long before you give solid foods, particularly meats, They are especially dangerous. The patient may be allowed to sit up for a short time about the end of the first week of convalescence, and the period may be prolonged with a gradual return of strength. He should move about slowly, and when the weather is favorable should be in the open air as much as possible. Keep from all excitement. Constipation now should be treated with an enema. A noticeable diarrhea should restrict the diet to milk and the patient be confined to the bed. There are many who cannot have a professional nurse. Good nursing is necessary in typhoid fever. Any sensible person who is willing to follow directions can do well. But she must do as the doctor directs.

These are some things you need to do: Look out for bad symptoms; twitching of the tendons, grasping at imaginary things are bad symptoms. Inform the doctor and soon. Never allow the patient to sit up in bed. The stool must be passed lying flat and you must place the bed pan without the patient's aid. Bleeding may be started by the least exertion. I knew of one woman who lost her life through necessity of getting up and passing the stool sitting on a chamber. Bleeding came on suddenly, and before the doctor could get there she was nearly gone. Cough and sudden pain in the lungs need prompt attention. I dismissed a boy on one Wednesday as convalescent. That night it became suddenly cold and he became chilled. The mother sent for me the next day, and we pulled him through pneumonia. Suppose she had waited another day? She was not that kind of a mother. Your greatest trial will come in convalescence, when the patient is so hungry. Be careful or you will kill the patient by kindness. A minister I knew killed himself by going against the doctor's orders and eating a hearty dinner. The doctor was rather profane, and when he went to see the preacher, after the relapse caused by the dinner, he relieved his mind in no gentle manner. Again allow no visitors in the sick room or one adjacent. They are an abomination. Many people are killed by well-intentioned ignoramuses. Do not whisper; the Lord save the patient who has a whisperer for a nurse. I cannot urge too strongly proper nursing in this disease. It is an absolute necessity. A nurse to be successful must have good sense and also must obey all directions. A diet is a necessity in this disease. The patient must not move any more than is absolutely necessary for his comfort. He must never try to help move himself. The muscles of the abdomen must remain lax and quiet. The danger, I think, is in the bowels. The mucous covering in the interior is inflamed and ulcerated, and there is always some danger of the ulceration eating through the coating into the blood vessels, causing more or less bleeding and even eating the bowel enough to cause an opening (perforation) and the escape of the bowel contents into the abdominal cavity causing inflammation of the peritoneum (peritonitis) and almost certain death. Walking typhoid is dangerous for that reason. The food must be of such nature that it is all digested. It must not leave lumps to press upon the sore places in the bowels causing more trouble there and more diarrhea.

TYPHUS FEVER, (Filth Disease).--Typhus fever is an acute, infectious disease, characterized by a sudden onset, marked nervous symptoms, and spotted rash and fever ending quickly after two weeks. Also called jail, camp, hospital, or ship fever. Filth has a great deal to do with its production. There is no real characteristic symptom except the eruption.

Symptoms.--It generally lasts two weeks. Incubation period of twelve days or less, marked at times by slight weary feeling. The onset is usually sudden, by one chill or several, with high fever, headache, pain in back and legs, prostration, vomiting, and mild and active delirium. Pulse does not have the double beat, often there is bronchitis.

Eruption.--"This appears on the third to fifth day; the fever remaining high. During the second week all the symptoms increase and are weakening with marked delirium and coma vigil" (unconscious, delirious, but with the eyes open). When death occurs it usually comes at the end of the second week from exhaustion. Favorable cases terminate at this time by crisis; the prostration is extreme; but convalescence is rapid.

Fever.--Sudden onset to even 104 to 105 degrees; steady rise for four or five days with slight morning remissions; terminating by crisis on the twelfth to fourteenth day, falling in some cases below normal; in fatal cases there is a rapid rise to 108 or 109 degrees. The eruption appears on the abdomen on the third to fifth day.

Treatment like Typhoid.--Mortality, twelve to twenty per cent.

SMALLPOX or Variola.--Smallpox is an acute infectious disease. It has a sudden onset with a severe period of invasion which is followed by a falling of the fever, and then the eruption comes out. This eruption begins as a pimple, then a watery pimple (vesicle) which runs into the pus pimple (pustule) and then the crust or scab forms. The mucous membrane in contact with the air may also be affected. Almost all persons exposed, if not vaccinated, are almost invariably attacked. It is very contagious. It attacks all ages, but it is particularly fatal to young children.

Cause.--An unknown poison in the contents of the pustules or crusts in secretion and excretion, apparently, and in the exhalations of the lungs and skin; one attack does not always confer immunity for life. It is contagious from an early period. Direct contact does not seem to be necessary, for it can be carried by one who does not have it.

Symptoms.--Incubation lasts from ten to fourteen days, and is usually without symptoms. Invasion comes suddenly with one or more chills in adults, or convulsions in children, with terrible headache, very severe pain in the back and extremities, vomiting, the temperature rising rapidly to 103 or 104 degrees.

Eruptions.--This usually appears on the fourth day as small red papules on the forehead, along the line of the hair and on the wrists, spreading within twenty-four hours over the face, extremities, trunk and mucous membrane.

Symptoms of fever diminish with the appearance of the rash, which is most marked on the face and ripens first there. The papules become hollowed vesicles and a clear fluid fills them on the fifth or sixth day. They fill with pus about the eighth day, and their summits become globular, while the surrounding skin is red, swollen and painful. The general bodily symptoms again return and the temperature rises for about twenty-four hours. Drying of the eruption begins the tenth or eleventh day. The pustules dry, forming crusts, while the swelling of the skin disappears and the temperature gradually falls. The crusts fall off, leaving scars only where the true skin has been destroyed.

Confluent form.--All the symptoms are more severe. The eruption runs together and all the skin is covered.

Varioloid.--This is smallpox modified by vaccination. The invasion may be sudden and severe. It is usually mild and gradual, but with severe pain in the back and head. A scanty eruption of papules, often only on the face and hands, appears on the third or fourth day, with disappearance of constitutional symptoms.

Treatment.--Vaccinate the children the second or third month, and all persons about every six years, and always after exposure to the disease or during epidemics. Put the patient in a room cleared of all furniture, carpets, curtains, rugs, etc.; keep the patient thoroughly clean, and the linen should be frequently changed. The bed clothing should be light. Disinfect and sterilize everything thoroughly that has been in contact with the patient. Get a good experienced nurse, and one who has been around the disease.

Diet.--Give the supporting diet early. During the first stage give milk, broths of different kinds, albumin water. Relieve the intense thirst by water and lemonade. When the first (initial) fever subsides and the patient feels improved, give milk, eggs, chops, steak, or rare roast meat, bread or toast; vegetables, such as potato, spinach, celery, asparagus tips, cauliflower tops. When the second fever returns go back to the liquid diet again, and give regularly and as much as possible every two or three hours during the day, and every three or four hours during the night. Milk, plain or peptonized; milk punch, raw eggs, broths, beef juice. If swallowing is difficult, give food cold and oftener, and in less quantity. Increase the diet rapidly during convalescence.

Cold drinks should be freely given. Barley water and oatmeal water are nutritious and palatable. Milk broths, and articles that give no trouble to digest.

Nursing.--Nursing is the main thing. The bowels should be kept open with salts. There is no special medicine we can claim will do good. Aconite may be used for the fever at first, in drop doses every hour for twenty-four hours. But the least medicine that is given the better it will generally be.

There is, I believe, something in protecting the ripening papules from the light. The constant application on the face and hands of lint soaked in cold water, to which antiseptics such as carbolic acid or bichloride may be added, is perhaps the most suitable treatment. It is very pleasant for the patient at least, and for the face it is well to make a mask of lint which can be covered with oiled silk. When the crusts begin to form, the chief point is to keep them thoroughly moist, which may be done with oil or glycerin; vaselin is particularly useful, and at this stage can be freely used upon the face. It frequently relieves the itching also. For the odor, which is sometimes so characteristic and disagreeable, the diluted carbolic acid solutions are probably the best. If the eruption is abundant on the scalp the hair should be cut short. During, convalescence frequent bathing is advisable. It should be done daily, using carbolic soap freely in order to get rid of the crusts and scabs. There is danger to others as long as the skin is not smooth and clean, and not free from any trace of scabs. As you must have a physician, I give but little medical treatment. Nursing is the main thing in this disease.

General Rules for Disinfection.--The walls, woodwork, and ceiling may be cleaned by washing with one to one thousand solution of corrosive sublimate solution, or a five per cent carbolic acid solution, Or by rubbing with bread if solutions would injure. All dust must be removed. Plastered walls and ceilings may be white-washed. Woodwork must then be scrubbed with soap and thoroughly wiped. Then fumigate, at least three pounds of sulphur should be burned in the room for each 1,000 cubic feet of space. Placing it in a pan supported in another containing water to guard against fire. After scrubbing or fumigating, the room and its contents should be freely aired for several days, admitting sunlight if possible. All useless articles and badly soiled bedding should be burned. Such pieces of clothing as will not be injured may be boiled or soaked in a one to one thousand formaldehyde solution (one ounce of twelve per cent solution in one gallon of water), or two per cent carbolic acid solution. Clothing, bedding, etc., may be disinfected in the steam sterilizer.

Hands, Body, etc.--Special outer garments may be worn while in the sick room and removed, and clothing aired before leaving. Hands of the attendant should be washed in one to one thousand corrosive sublimate solution.

Vaccination and Re-vaccination and its Prevention of Smallpox. We quote in part from an article prepared by the State of Michigan. It is well known that smallpox can be prevented or modified by vaccination; and a widespread epidemic of the disease can be attributed only to an equally widespread ignorance or willfulness concerning smallpox and its prevention by vaccination and re-vaccination.

A Good Time to be Vaccinated.--Smallpox is usually most prevalent in the winter and spring months, reaching the highest point in May. The rarity of smallpox in Michigan for several years led to a feeling of security and to neglect vaccination, resulting in an increased proportion of inhabitants not protected by recent vaccination. This made possible a widespread epidemic. The proper preventive of such an epidemic is general vaccination and re-vaccination of all persons not recently thus protected. There is no better settled fact than that vaccination does protect against smallpox. But after a time the protection is weakened, therefore after a lapse of five years there should be re-vaccination.

Why Vaccinate.--Because vaccination is a preventive of all forms of smallpox, and because by traveling, or by travelers, by articles received in the mail or from the stores or shops, or other various ways anyone at any time, may, without knowing it, be exposed to smallpox, it becomes important so far as possible without injury to health to render every person incapable of taking the disease. This may be done so perfectly by vaccination and re-vaccination with genuine bovine vaccine virus that no question of ordinary expense or trouble should be allowed for a day to prevent the careful vaccination of every man, woman and child in Michigan, and the re-vaccination of every one who has not been vaccinated within five years. It is well established that those who have been properly vaccinated are far less likely to take smallpox if exposed to it, and that the very few who have been properly vaccinated and have smallpox have it in a much milder form and are much less disfigured by it than those who have not been thus vaccinated. The value of vaccination is illustrated by the following facts: On March the 13th, 1859, Dr. E. M. Snow, of Providence, R. 1., found in a cluster of seven houses twenty-five families, and in these families ten cases of smallpox, all apparently at about the same stage of the disease. In the same families there were twenty-one children, who had never been vaccinated. The ten cases and the remaining members of the families, including the twenty-one children, were quarantined at home, and the children were all vaccinated and compelled to remain with the sick. Several other cases of smallpox occurred in the persons previously exposed, but not one of the twenty-one children referred to had the slightest touch of the disease.

In Sweden, the average number of deaths in each year from smallpox per million inhabitants was:

Before the introduction of vaccination (1774-1801), 1,973;

During the period of optional vaccination (1802-1816), 479;

And during the period of obligatory vaccination (1817-1877), 189.

Vaccination was introduced in England near the beginning of the nineteenth century, and since 1853 compulsory vaccination has been attempted. In England the number of deaths in each year from smallpox per one million inhabitants was:

At the close of the eighteenth century, 3,000.

From 1841 to 1853 (average), 304.

From 1854 to 1863 (average), 171.

Smallpox entirely prevented by re-vaccination.--In the Bavarian army re-vaccination has been compulsory since 1843. From that date till 1857, not even a single case of unmodified smallpox occurred, nor a single death from smallpox. During the year of duty, Dr. Marson, physician of the London Smallpox Hospital, has never observed a single case of smallpox in the officers and employees of the hospital, who are re-vaccinated when they enter the service, and who are constantly exposed to the infection.

"Out of more than 10,000 children vaccinated at Brussels with animal lymph, from 1865 to 1870, and who went through the terrible epidemic of smallpox, which in 1870 and 1871 frightened the world, not a single one was to my knowledge reported as being attacked by the disease. The same immunity was shared by those, a much larger number, whom I had re-vaccinated and who at the same time were living in epidemic centers."--*Dr. Warlemont, of Brussels.*

Who should be Vaccinated.--Everybody, old and young, for his own interest, and that he may not become a breeding place for the distribution of smallpox to others, should seek that protection from smallpox which is afforded by vaccination alone. It is believed that all persons except those mentioned in the following paragraph may, if the operation is properly performed, at the proper time, and with pure bovine virus, be vaccinated with perfect safety to themselves. Even those who have had smallpox should be vaccinated, for otherwise they may take the disease; and it seems to be proved that a larger proportion, of those who have smallpox a second time, die than of those who have the disease after vaccination.

Who should not be Vaccinated.--Unless exposure to smallpox is believed to have taken place or likely to take place, teething children, pregnant women, persons suffering from measles, scarlet fever, erysipelas, or susceptible to and recently exposed to one of these diseases, persons suffering with skin diseases or eruption, and in general feeble persons not in good health, should not be vaccinated. In all cases in which there is any doubt as to the propriety of vaccinating or postponing vaccination the judgment of a good physician should be taken. The restriction, as to vaccinating teething children makes it important that children should be vaccinated before the teething process has begun, because smallpox is very much more dangerous than vaccination. Smallpox is exceedingly dangerous to pregnant women.

When should a person be Vaccinated.--The sooner the better as a rule, and especially whenever there is much liability of exposure to smallpox. Children should be vaccinated before they are four months old; those who have never been vaccinated, should, except teething children, be vaccinated at once. Because the vaccination often loses its protective power after a time, those who have been vaccinated but once or twice should, in order to test and to increase the protective power of the former vaccination, be vaccinated again, and as often as the vaccination can be made to work. In general, to insure full protection from smallpox, one should be vaccinated as often as every five years. It has been found that of those who have smallpox the proportion of deaths is very much less among those who have three or four good vaccination scars than among those who have but one scar.

Vaccination after exposure to Smallpox.--Vaccination as late as the second day after known exposure to smallpox is believed to have prevented the smallpox; vaccination the third day after exposure has rendered the disease much milder than usual, and in a case in Iowa, vaccination on the seventh or eighth day after exposure to smallpox ran a partial course and was believed to have modified the attack of smallpox, which, however, it did not wholly prevent. A recent case in Michigan was vaccinated three days after exposure, as were also the wife, mother, and two children, both under five years of age; all vaccinated again six days after the exposure. The health officer reported as follows: "The results were gratifying. During the first week of the eruption it was evidently aborting and without doubt as the result of vaccination eight days before the eruption. A complete and fine recovery. Certainly an aborted course, with scarcely a mark left, and not another case in the above family, whom necessity compelled to occupy the same house, the same rooms, continual contact with the contagion, scores one more big credit mark for vaccination."

With what should one be Vaccinated.--Because the potency of virus depends largely upon its being fresh, and it is so easy to obtain pure and fresh bovine virus, and because such bovine virus is efficient it is better in all cases to use only the pure and fresh bovine virus.

Where should Vaccination be Performed.--In a room or place free from persons suffering from disease, and from dust which may convey to the scratched surface germs of any communicable disease; certainly not in or near a room where there is erysipelas or consumption, nor in the presence of one who has just come from a person sick with erysipelas, diphtheria, or scarlet fever.

By whom should one be Vaccinated.--The operation of vaccination should be performed always by a competent and responsible physician. To try to vaccinate one's self or one's family is poor economy, for it often results not only in a waste of money and of time, but in a false and dangerous feeling of security. To trust to vaccination by nurses and midwives is equally foolish. A well-educated and experienced physician has the skill, and the special knowledge necessary to the best judgment on all of the questions involved, without which the operation may be a failure or worse than a failure. In work of this kind the best is the cheapest, whatever it costs.

After Vaccination.--Let the vaccinated place alone. Do not scratch it or otherwise transfer the virus where it is not wanted. Protect it by a bandage, or cloth which has been boiled and ironed with a hot iron. Try to keep the pustule unbroken, as a protection against germs of diseases and against unnecessary discomfort. A bad sore arm may not be and probably is not true vaccination, but may be due to lack of care during and after vaccination to keep out septic germs.

Common appearances after Vaccination.--For a day or two nothing unusual should appear. A few days after that, if it succeeds regularly, the skin will become red, then a pimple will form, and on the pimple a little vesicle or blister which may be plainly seen on the fifth or sixth day. On the eighth day the blister (vesicle) is, or should be, plump, round, translucent, pearly white, with a clearly marked edge and a depression in the center; the skin around it for about half an inch is red and swollen. This vesicle and the red, inflamed circle about it (called the areola) are the two points which prove the vaccination to be successful. A rash, and even a vesicular eruption, sometimes comes on the child's body about the eighth day, and lasts about a week; he may be feverish, or may remain quite well. The arm may be red and swollen down as far as the elbow, and in the adult there will usually be a tender or swollen gland in the arm-pit, and some disturbance of sleep for several nights. The vesicle dries up in a few days more, and a crust forms which becomes of a brownish mahogany color, and falls off from the twentieth to the twenty-fifth day. In some cases the several appearances described above may be delayed a day or two. The crust or scab will leave a well-marked, permanent

scar.

What to do during and after Vaccination.--Do nothing to irritate the eruption, do not pull the scab off, when it drops off throw it in the fire. When the eruption is at its height show it to the doctor who performed the vaccination. If it is satisfactory, ask him for a certificate stating when and by whom you were vaccinated, whether with bovine or humanized lymph, in how many places and with what result at each place. When the arm is healed, if the vaccination did not work well, be vaccinated again as soon as possible, and in the best manner possible. This will be a test to the protection secured by the former vaccination, and will itself afford increased protection. Do not be satisfied with less than four genuine vaccine scars, or with four if it is possible to secure more than four. This vaccination a second or third time in close succession is believed to be hardly less important than vaccination the first time, and hardly less valuable as a protection against smallpox. Without doubt many persons are living in a false sense of security from smallpox because at some time in their lives they have had a little sore on their arm caused by a supposed or real vaccination, or because an imperfect vaccination failed to work, or because they were successfully vaccinated, or had the varioloid, or the unmodified smallpox many years ago. Until smallpox is stamped out throughout the world so that exposure of the disease shall be practically impossible, the only personal safety is in such perfect vaccination that one need not fear an exposure to smallpox through the recklessness of the foolish.

Make a record of your Vaccination.--Do not fail to procure and preserve the certificate mentioned in the preceding paragraph, and also to make a personal record of the facts with regard to any vaccination of yourself or in your family. From it you may sometime learn that it is ten years since you or some member of your family was vaccinated, when you thought it only five.

Lives saved from smallpox in Michigan.--Since the State Board of Health was established, many thousands of people in Michigan have been vaccinated because of its recommendations; and the statistics of deaths, published by the Secretary of State, show that at the close of the year 1906, the death rate from smallpox in Michigan had been so much less than before the board was established as to indicate that over three thousand lives had been saved from that loathsome disease.

The average death rate per year, for the five years, 1869-1873, before the board was established, was 8.5 per 100,000 inhabitants, and since the board was established, for the thirty-three years, 1874-1907, it was only 1.5. Since 1896 an uncommon mild type of the disease has prevailed very extensively, but the death rate has been exceedingly low, being for the eleven years, 1897-1907, slightly less than one death for each 100,000 inhabitants. The great saving of life from smallpox in civilized countries has been mainly because of vaccination and revaccination.

VACCINATION, Symptoms.--At first a slight irritation at the place of vaccination. The eruption appears on the third or fourth day as a reddish pimple surrounded by a reddened surface. On the fifth or sixth day this pimple becomes a vesicle with a depressed center and filled with clear contents. It reaches its greatest size on the eighth day. By the tenth day the contents are pus-like and the surrounding skin is more inflamed and often quite painful. These symptoms diminish, and by the end of the second week the pustule has dried to a brownish scab, which falls off between the twenty-first and twenty-fifth days, and leaves a depressed scar. Fever and mild constitutional symptoms usually go with the eruption and may last until about the eighth day.

Reliable lymph points should always be used. Clean the skin near the insertion of the deltoid muscle on the arm, and with a clean (sterile) knife or ivory point, a few scratches are made, deep enough to allow a slight flow of liquid, but *no bleeding.* The vaccine virus moistened, if dried on a point, is rubbed into the wound and allowed to dry. A piece of sterile gauze, or a "shield," is used as a dressing. This shield can be bought at any drug store. One vaccination may give immunity for ten to twelve years, but it is better to be vaccinated every six years at least.

DENGUE. Break-bone Fever, Dandy Fever.--This is an acute infectious disease characterized by pains in the joints and muscles, fever, an initial reddish swollen eruption and a terminal eruption of variable type. It occurs in the tropical regions and the warmer portions of the temperate zone. The disease appears in epidemics, rapidly attacking many persons.

Symptoms.--Incubation lasts from three to five days without any special symptoms. The onset is marked with chilly feelings, an active fever with temperature gradually rising. There is severe pain in the muscles and in the joints which become red and swollen. There is intense pain in the eyeballs, head, back and extremities. Face looks flushed, eyes are sunken, the skin looks flushed and mucous membrane looks red. This is the beginning rash. The high fever falls quickly after three or four days, sometimes with sweating, diarrhea or nose bleed. The patient feels stiff and sore then, but comparatively well. A slight fever returns after two to four days, although this sometimes remains absent. Pains and eruptions, like scarlet fever or hives, appear. An attack usually lasts seven to eight days. Convalescence is often long and slow, with stiffness and pain in the joints and muscles and great weakness. A relapse may return within two weeks.

PHYSICIANS' TREATMENT for Dengue.--An anti-plague serum is sometimes used, though with doubtful results. The pain is controlled by doses of morphine of one-eighth to one-fourth of a grain every four or five hours. Hyoscin, one hundredth of a grain, is also given for the pain. The high temperature can be relieved by cold and tepid sponging. Tonics are given during the convalescence and continued for some time.

CEREBRO-SPINAL MENINGITIS.--This is an acute infectious disease. It comes in epidemics, when there are many cases, or appears here and there as a separate case (sporadic). It is caused by a specific organism (germ) and the disease attacks the membranes of the brain and spinal cord.

Of late years great progress has been made by patient investigation, and a serum is now prepared for the treatment of this disease. The results of this treatment are better than the treatments formerly used, and there is good reason to believe that in a few years this treatment will be as effective in this disease as antitoxin is in diphtheria.

Cause.--Young adults and children are affected most often. Bad surroundings and over-exertion are predisposing factors.

Conditions.--There is congestion of the membranes of the brain and spinal cord which are covered with an exudate confined on the brain, chiefly to the base.

Symptoms. Ordinary Form.--Incubation is of unknown length and occasionally marked by want of appetite, headache, and pain in the back. The invasion is usually sudden, chill, projectile vomiting, throwing forward, severe headache, pain and rigidity of the back of the neck, pain in various parts of the body, skin over-sensitive, irritable, and temperature about 102 degrees, with all symptoms of an active fever. Later, pains are very severe, especially in the head, neck and back; the head is drawn back; often the back is rigid; the muscles of the neck and back are tender and attempts to stretch them cause intense pain. The vomiting now is less prominent. Temperature is extremely irregular, 99 to 105 degrees or more. Pulse is slow, often 50 to 60, and full and strong at first. The delirium is of a severe and variable type in common, alternating with partial or complete coma, the latter predominating toward the close of fatal attacks. Stimulation of nerve centers causes cross-eyed look, drooping of upper eyelid, movement of eyeballs unequal, contracted, dilated, or sluggish pupils; acute and painful hearing, spasmodic contractions of the muscles followed by paralysis of the face muscles, etc. The disease may last several hours or several months. Many die within five days. In fatal cases the patient passes into seemingly deep sleep with symptoms of a very prostrating and weakening fever, and often retention of urine. Mild cases occur with only a little fever, headache, stiff muscles of the neck, discomfort in back and extremities. The malignant type occurs epidemically or sporadically.

Malignant type.--Sudden invasion with severe chills, slight rise in temperature, pain in the back of the neck, headaches, stupor, muscular spasms, a slow pulse, often purple bleeding, eruption, coma and death within hours, rather than days. This is a terrible disease, and a physician is needed from the first. The death rate varies from twenty to seventy-live per cent. Treatment must be given by a physician.

Spinal meningitis is inflammation of the membrane of the spinal cord along with the accompanying back and extremity symptoms, while the head remains clear and free from complications.

MENINGITIS.--This is an inflammation of the membranes covering the brain alone, and generally commences with fever and severe headaches, with avoidance of light and noise as these are painful. In some cases we have delirium, stupor and coma.

Treatment.--Treatment must be given by a physician, but cold applications to the head and back are generally good. The bowels also must be kept open.

MENINGITIS. Tubercular, (Basilar Meningitis).--This affection which is also known as acute hydrocephalus (meaning water on the brain), is essentially an acute tuberculosis in which the membranes of the brain, sometimes of the cord bear the brunt of the attack. It is more common in children than in adults. It is more frequent between the second and fifth years, than in the first year. It is caused by the tubercular infection, and follows the usual course of this disease. Ordinary meningitis is rapid and well defined in its course, with "high fever," severe pains in the head, intense nervousness, avoidance of light and sound, loss of appetite and constipation. These symptoms are easily understood and are generally clearly read by those around the patient. Unfortunately in tubercular meningitis the clearly defined symptoms are absent in the beginning, and when the physician is called the condition is dangerous. Usually the patient complains but little. There is a slight headache, low fever, no heat in the head, patient is pale most of the time, has little appetite, vomits occasionally and desires to sleep. He is nervous, stupid and lies on his side curled up with eyes away from the light. This disease appears mostly in delicate children, who are poor eaters and fond of books; usually in those inheriting poor constitutions. The mortality is very high. Parents who have thin, pale sallow children with dainty appetites, who frequently complain of headaches and are fond of books, should be afraid of infection from tuberculosis and make the little ones live in the open air and keep away from school. But earlier in the lives of these children care must be taken. A child with that pale, thin, sallow, delicate face and poor body should be fed with the best of food and live in the open air. I once had a family who lost their only two babies through this disease. After the first one died I instructed them carefully how to treat the second child. However, they loved their child foolishly and not wisely and fed it everything it wanted, and you know the children take an advantage of their parents. Give plenty of good, wholesome digestible food. Dress them comfortably and warm and keep them out in the open air. No cakes, candy, peanuts or any food that is not nourishing and easy to digest.

TUBERCULOSIS. (CONSUMPTION).--Tuberculosis is an infectious disease caused by the bacillus, tuberculosis, and characterized by the formation of nodules or diffuse masses of new tissue. Man, fowls and cows are chiefly affected.

Indians, negroes and Irish are very susceptible. The disease is less common at great altitudes. Dark, poorly ventilated rooms, such as tenements and factories and the crowding of cities favors infection, as do in-door life and occupations in which dust must be inhaled. Certain infections such as measles, whooping-cough, chronic heart, kidney and liver diseases and inflammation of the air tract are predisposing factors. Inhalation is the chief mode of transmission. Hereditary transmission is rare.

Forms. The Lungs.--Consumption. This is caused by a germ. Some have the form called galloping consumption. This person is attacked suddenly, wastes away and dies, in a very short time. There is rapid loss of strength and weight, high fever, night sweats, fast breathing, pains in the chest, cough and profuse expectoration, and rapid loss of strength.

Ordinary Consumption.--Begins slowly and the patient is not aware of the danger. He may have loss of appetite, dyspepsia, diarrhea and distress after meals. He looks pale, is weak and loses flesh. Soon he has a hacking cough, worse in the morning, with a scanty, glairy sputum. His weight continues to decrease, his heart is weak and beats faster. He has pain in his chest below the shoulder blades. He may have a slight bleeding from the lungs. His cough becomes worse, the expectoration gets thicker and more profuse, with night sweats, high fever, and shortness of breath. The eyes are bright; the cheeks are pale or flushed. Chronic looseness of the bowels may be present. Bleeding from the lungs may occur at any time, but it is most frequent and profuse during the last stages. The patient becomes very weak, thin and pale, emaciated. The brain action remains good, and he remains hopeful almost until the last. Tuberculosis may exist in almost every part of the body and we have many forms. It is not necessary to discuss all. It would tend to confusion. I will name the most of them:

1. **Acute Miliary Tuberculosis.**
    - **(A.) Acute General Miliary Tuberculosis.**
    - **(B.) Pulmonary (lung) type.**

(C.) Tubercular Meningitis.

2. **Tuberculosis of the lymph nodes (glands).** This was formerly called Scrofula. This is more curable and will be treated more fully elsewhere.
3. **Tuberculous Pleurisy.**
4. **Tuberculous Pericarditis.**
5. **Tuberculous Peritonitis.** (Of this there are a good many cases.)
6. **Tuberculosis of the Larynx.**
7. **Acute Pneumonia (Pulmonary Tuberculosis) or "Galloping Consumption."**
8. **Chronic Ulcerative Pulmonary Tuberculosis.**
9. **Chronic Miliary Tuberculosis.**
10. **Tuberculosis of the Alimentary Canal.**
11. **Tuberculosis of the Brain.**
12. **Tuberculosis of the liver, kidneys, bladder, etc.**
13. **Tuberculosis of joints,** this will be treated more fully elsewhere.

CERVICAL, TUBERCULOSIS (Scrofula).--This is common in children that are not well nourished, living in badly ventilated and crowded houses, and in the negroes. Chronic catarrh of the nose and throat and tonsilitis predispose to it. The glands under the lower jaw are usually the first involved. They are enlarged, smooth, firm and often become matted together. Later the skin may adhere to them and suppuration occurs, that is, pus forms. An abscess results that breaks through the skin and leaves a nasty looking sore or scar. The glands in the back of the neck may enlarge also; or in the arm pit or under the collar bone and also the bronchial glands. There is usually secondary anemia. A long course and spontaneous recovery are common. Lung or general miliary tuberculosis may occur.

Mesenteric Kind.--Symptoms are loss of flesh and strength, anemia, distended abdomen (pot-belly) and bloated, with offensive diarrhea.

MOTHERS' REMEDIES.--1. Consumption, Simple Home Method to Break up.--"A cloth saturated with kerosene oil, bound around the chest at night and frequently repeated, will remove lung soreness, and it may be taken inwardly with advantages, eight to ten drops three or four times a day in sarsaparilla. It has been tried efficaciously as a cure for consumption."

2. Consumption, Physicians' Remedy for.--

Arsenic Acid	1 part
Carbonate of Potash	2 parts
Cinnamyllic Acid	3 parts

Heat this until a perfect solution is obtained, then add twenty-five parts cognac and three parts of watery extract of opium which has been dissolved in twenty-five parts of water filtered. Dose:--At first take six drops after dinner and supper, gradually increasing to twenty-two drops.

Mild cases are cured in two months, but the severe cases may require a year or two. This treatment should be given under the care of a physician, as it is poisonous and needs close watching.

PHYSICIANS' TREATMENT for Consumption.--Tuberculous peritonitis is often present. General better hygienic measures; fresh air, nourishing food; cod-liver oil. The glands are now often cut.

Sanitary Care. Prevention of Tuberculosis.--The sputum of consumptives should be carefully collected and destroyed. Patients should be urged not to spit about carelessly, but always use a spit cup and never swallow the sputum. The destruction of the sputum of consumptives should be a routine measure in both hospitals and private practice. Thorough boiling or putting in the fire is sufficient. It should be explained to the patient that the only risk, practically is from this source.

The chances of infection are greatest in young children. The nursing and care of consumptives involves very slight risks indeed, if proper precautions are taken.

Second.--A second important measure, relates to the inspection of dairies and slaughter houses. The possibility of the transmission of tuberculosis by infected milk has been fully demonstrated, and in the interest of health, the state should take measures to stamp out tuberculosis in cattle.

Individual Prevention.--A mother with pulmonary tuberculosis should not nurse her child. An infant born of tuberculosis parents or of a family in which consumption prevails, should be brought up with the greatest care and guarded most particularly against catarrhal affections of all kinds. Special attention should be given to the throat and nose, and on the first indication of mouth breathing or any affection of the nose, a careful examination should be made for adenoids. The child should be clothed in flannel, and live in the open air as much as possible, avoiding close rooms. It is a good practice to sponge the throat and chest night and morning with cold water. Special attention should be paid to the diet and to the mode of feeding. The meals should be given at regular hours, and the food plain and substantial. From the onset the child should be encouraged to drink freely of milk. Unfortunately in these cases there seems to be an uncontrollable aversion to fats of all kinds. As the child grows older, systematically regulated exercise or a course of pulmonary (lung) gymnastics may be taken. In the choice of an occupation, preference should be given to an out of door life. Families with a predisposition to tuberculosis should, if possible, reside in an equable climate. It would be best for a young person belonging to such a family to remove to Colorado or Southern California, or to some other suitable climate before trouble begins. The trifling ailments of children should be carefully watched. In convalescence from fevers, which so frequently prove dangerous, the greatest care should be exercised to prevent from catching cold. Cod-liver oil, the syrup of iodide of iron and arsenic may be given.

Enlarged tonsils should be removed. "The spontaneous healing of local tuberculosis is an every-day affair. Many cases of adenitis (inflammation of the glands) and disease of the bone or joints terminate favorably. The healing of pulmonary (lung) tuberculosis is shown clinically by the recovery of patients in whose sputa elastic tissue and bacilli have been found."

General Measures.--The cure of tuberculosis is a question of nutrition; digestion and assimilation control the situation; make a patient grow fat, and the local disease may be left to take care of itself. There are three indications:

First, to place the patient in surroundings most favorable for the greatest degree of nutrition; second, to take such measures as in a local and general way influence the tuberculosis process; third, to alleviate the symptoms. This is effected by the open air treatment with the necessary feeding and nursing.

At Home.--In the majority of cases patients must be treated at home. In the city it has many disadvantages. The patient's bed should be in a room where he can have plenty of sunshine and air. Two things are essential--plenty of fresh air and sunshine. While there is fever he should be at rest in bed. For the greater part of each day, unless the weather is blustering and raining, the windows should be open. On the bright days he can sit out-doors on a balcony or porch, in a reclining chair. He must be in the open air all that is possible to be. A great many patients spend most of the time out in the open air now. In the country places this can be easily carried out. In the summer he should be out of doors from eleven to twelve hours; in the winter six to eight at least. At night the room should be cool and thoroughly ventilated. "In the early stages of the disease with much fever, it may require several months of this rest treatment to the open air before the temperature falls to normal." The sputum is dangerous when it becomes dry. As long as sputum is moist the germs are held in the sputum; but when it is dry they are released and roam at will in the atmosphere and are inhaled. They are then ready to lodge themselves in suitable soil. Always keep the sputum (expectoration) moist, and then there is no danger.

Diet. Treatment.--The outlook in this disease depends upon the digestion. Nausea and loss of appetite are serious obstacles. Many patients loathe foods of all kinds. A change of air or a sea voyage may promptly restore the appetite. When this is not possible, rest the patient, keep in the open air nearly all day and feed regularly with small quantities either of buttermilk, milk, or kumiss, alternating if necessary with meat juice and egg albumin. Some cases which are disturbed by eggs and milk do well on kumiss. Raw eggs are very suitable for feeding, and may be taken between meals, beginning with one three times a day, and can be increased to two and three at a time. It is hard to give a regular diet. The patient should be under the care of a physician who will regulate the kind of diet, amount and change. When the digestion is good there is less trouble in feeding. Then the patient can eat meat, poultry, game, oysters, fish, animal broths, eggs. Nothing should be fried. Avoid pork, veal, hot bread, cakes, pies, sweet meats, rich gravies, crabs, lobsters.

Diet in Tuberculosis furnished us by a Hospital.--

May Take.--Soups.--Turtle or oyster soup, mutton, clam, or chicken broth, puree of barley, rice, peas, beans, cream of celery or tomatoes, whole beef tea; peptonized milk, gruel.

Fish.--All kinds of fresh fish boiled or broiled, oysters or clams, raw, roasted or broiled.

Meats.--Rare roast beef or mutton, lamb chops, ham, fat bacon. sweetbreads, poultry, game, tender steaks, hamburger steak rare.

Eggs.--Every way except fried.

Farinaceous.--Oatmeal, wheaten grits, mush, hominy, rice, whole wheat bread, corn bread, milk toast, biscuits, muffins, gems.

Vegetables.--Potatoes baked, boiled, or creamed, string beans, spinach, onions, asparagus, tomatoes, green peas, all well cooked, cresses, lettuce, plain or with oil dressing, celery.

Desserts.--Farina, sago, tapioca, apple or milk pudding, floating island, custards, baked or stewed apples with fresh cream, cooked fruits, rice with fresh cream.

Drinks.--Fresh milk, cool, warm, or peptonized, cocoa, chocolate, buttermilk, pure water, tea, coffee, panopepton.

Must Not Take.--Fried foods, salt fish, hashes, gravies, veal, pork, carrots, parsnips, cabbage, beets, turnips, cucumbers, macaroni, spaghetti, sweets, pies, pastry, sweet wines.

WHAT EVERY PERSON SHOULD KNOW ABOUT TUBERCULOSIS, WHETHER HE HAS THE DISEASE OR NOT.

Tuberculosis is caused by a germ.

Tuberculosis is communicable and preventable.

Consumption of the lungs is the most common form of tuberculosis.

Consumption of the bowels is the next most common form.

The germ causing tuberculosis leaves the body of the person who has the disease by means of the discharges; by the sputum coughed up from the lungs, by nasal discharge, by bowel excrement, by urine, by abscesses.

If the sputum of the consumptive is allowed to dry, its infected dust floats in the air, and is breathed into the lungs.

Any person breathing such air is in danger of contracting tuberculosis. It is best not to stand near a person suffering with tuberculosis who is coughing, because in this act finely divided droplets of saliva are thrown from the mouth, and may be carried for a distance of three feet. These may contain large numbers of the bacilli. They are also sometimes thrown out in forcible speaking. The ordinary breath of a consumptive does not contain them.

If the bowels or other discharges from the tuberculous person are not disinfected, but are thrown into a sewer, privy, river or buried they are a source of danger, and may pollute a source of drinking water.

Impure milk, that is, milk from a tuberculous cow or milk exposed to infected dust is a common source of tuberculosis. Milk from suspected sources should be boiled. The all-important thing to do to prevent tuberculosis from spreading from one person to another, and from one part of the body to another, is immediately to destroy all discharges from the body of a person who has tuberculosis.

Destroy by fire or by disinfectant all sputum, all nasal discharges, all bowel excrement, all urine as soon as discharged. For such a purpose use a five per cent solution of carbolic acid (six and three-fourths ounces of carbolic acid to one gallon of water).

No person, well or sick, should spit in public places or where the sputum cannot be collected and destroyed.

Flies carry sputum and its infection to food, to your hands, your face, clothes, the baby's bottle, from which the germs are taken into the mouth, and thus gain access to the stomach or lungs.

Spitting on the sidewalk, on the floor, on the wall, on the grass, in the gutter, or even into a cuspidor containing no disinfectant is a very dangerous practice for a consumptive to indulge.

The person infected with tuberculosis should protect himself, his family, his associates and the public by not spitting in public places, and by promptly destroying all discharges.

The well person should defend himself by insisting that the tuberculous person shall destroy all discharges.

Well persons should set the example of restraint and themselves refrain from spitting promiscuously. A person may appear quite healthy and yet be developing tuberculosis without knowing it.

Such a person, if he spits where he pleases, may be depositing infected sputum where it can endanger the health and lives of other persons.

Do not sleep with a person who has tuberculosis, nor in the room occupied by a tuberculous person, until that room has been thoroughly disinfected.

Any person is liable to contract tuberculosis, whether he is well or not. Sickly persons, or those having bad colds, influenza bronchitis or pneumonia or any general weakness are much more liable to contract tuberculosis than a perfectly well or robust person. If you have a cough that hangs on consult at once a reliable physician who has ability to diagnose tuberculosis.

Prevention is possible; it is cheaper and easier than cure.

Any person having tuberculosis can recover from the disease if he takes the proper course in time.

Advanced cases of tuberculosis, that is, those cases where the disease is well developed, are the most dangerous to the public and the most difficult to cure.

Every advanced case of tuberculosis should be in a sanatorium.

Sanatoria offers the best chance, usually the only chance, of cure to an advanced case.

They also protect well citizens from danger of infection from advanced stages of tuberculosis. There are fewer deaths from tuberculosis in those localities where sanatoria are established for the care of tuberculous persons.

One person out of every seven who die, dies from tuberculosis.

One child out of every ten dies from tuberculosis.

Homes and school-houses greatly need more fresh air supplied to their occupants.

Day camps are city parks, vacant lots or abandoned farms where the tuberculous persons of a community may go and spend the entire day in rest, receiving instructions in proper hygiene and skillful treatment. Such camps are supplied with tents, hammocks, reclining chairs, one or more nurses, milk, eggs and other nourishment.

Dispensaries are centers of sanitary and medical instruction for local tuberculous persons.

Every locality should establish and maintain a dispensary for the benefit of tuberculous persons; for their instruction how to prevent the disease from spreading, and how to conduct themselves to insure relief and cure.

Householders are required by law to report a case within their households to the local health officers. The local health officer has certain duties to perform under the law, and co-operation with him by the householder and tuberculous person, works for the suppression of this disease.

Do not consider a tuberculous person an outcast, or one fit for the pesthouse. Your crusade is against tuberculosis, not against the person suffering from the disease.

Give the freedom of a well person to the tuberculous who is instructed and conscientious in the observance of necessary precautions. Be very much afraid of the tuberculous person who is ignorant or careless in the observance of necessary precautions.

PNEUMONIA (Lobar) Lung Fever.--Inflammation of the lungs. This is an acute infectious disease characterized by an exudative inflammation of one or more lobes of the lungs, with constitutional symptoms due to the absorption of toxins (poison), the fever terminating by crisis (suddenly). In speaking of pneumonia you frequently hear the expression "the lungs are filling up." This is the real condition. The structures surrounding the air cells are inflamed and from the inflamed tissues a secretion exudate is poured out into the cells. This is expectorated, thrown out, by coughing; but it is poured out into the cells faster than it can be spit up and consequently it remains in some of the cells and fills them up.

The air does not get into such cells and they fill, with many others, and make that section solid. When the patient is improving he keeps on spitting this up, until all is out and the air cells resume their normal work. Sometimes they remain so and we have chronic pneumonia.

Causes of Pneumonia.--Pneumonia occurs frequently as a complication of other diseases, such as typhoid fever and measles. Yet the majority of cases occur spontaneously. Many times the disease seems to be induced by exposure to the cold, and there can be no doubt that such exposure does at least promote the development of this affection. It seems, however, probable that there is some special cause behind it without which the exposure to cold is not sufficient to induce this disease. Pneumonia may occur at any period of life, and is more common among males than females. It occurs over the entire United States, oftener in the southern and middle, than in the Northern States; it is more frequently met with during the winter and spring months than at other times in the year.

Symptoms.--The onset is usually abrupt with a severe chill and chills lasting from fifteen minutes to an hour, with the temperature suddenly rising and an active fever. There is usually intense pain in a few hours, generally in the lower part of the front of the chest, made worse by breathing and coughing. The patient lies on the affected side so as to give all chance for the other lung to work, cheeks are flushed, with anxious expression; the wings of the nostrils move in and out with each breath. The cough is short, dry and painful. Rapid, shallow, jerky breathing, increasing to difficult breathing. On the first day the characteristic expectoration mixed with blood appears (called rusty). Pulse runs from 100 to 116, full bounding, but may be feeble and small in serious cases. After three or four days the pain disappears, the temperature keeps to 104 or 105, but falls quickly the seventh, fifth, eighth, sixth and ninth day in this order of frequency. In a few hours, usually twelve, the temperature falls to normal or below, usually with profuse sweating and with quick relief to all symptoms. This relief from distressing symptoms is, of course, a time of rejoicing to both patient and friends and the patient and nurse may feel inclined to relax a little from the strict observance of rules followed up to this time. Do not, under any circumstances, yield to such folly. Keep patient properly covered, as he is weak from the strain and the pores are open.

Convalescence is usually rapid. A prolonged rise of temperature after the crisis may be regarded as a relapse. Death may occur at any time after the third day from sudden heart failure, or from complications such as pleurisy, nephritis, meningitis, pericarditis, endocarditis, gangrene of the lungs.

MOTHERS' REMEDIES.--1. Lungs, Salt Pork for Inflammation of.--"Salt pork dipped in hot water, then covered thick with black pepper. Heat in the oven and lay or bind on the throat and lungs."

2. Lungs, Raspberry Tincture for Inflammation of.--"Take one-half pound of honey, one cup water; let these boil; take off the scum; pour boiling hot upon one-half ounce lobelia herb and one-half ounce cloves; mix well, then strain and add one gill of raspberry vinegar. Take from one teaspoonful to a dessertspoonful four times a day. Pleasant to take."

3. Lungs, Herb Ointment for Congestion of.--

"Oil of Turpentine	1/2 ounce
Oil of Hemlock	1/2 ounce
Oil of Peppermint	1/2 ounce
Oil of Feverweed	1/2 ounce

Mix this with one cup warm lard."

Rub this ointment on throat or lungs and apply a flannel over it. Heat it through thoroughly with hot cloths. If used thoroughly and the cold is taken in time will prevent pneumonia.

4. Lungs, Mullein for Congestion.--"The mullein leaves may be purchased at any drug store or gathered in the fields. Make a tea of the leaves by steeping them. Add enough water to one tablespoon mullein to make a pint, which will be three doses, taken three times a day." This is a very good remedy.

5. Lungs, Salve for Weak.--

"Bees Wax	1 ounce
Rosin	1 ounce
Camphor Gum	1 ounce
Lard about the size of an egg."	

The beeswax forms sort of a coating and may remain on for several hours. This is very good.

PHYSICIANS' TREATMENT FOR LUNGS.--The home treatment should be to put the patient to bed and try to produce sweating. This will cause the blood to leave the congested lung and return to the full regular circulation. By doing this, you not only relieve the congested lung, but also the pain. If the patient is stout and strong, give him the "corn sweat" under La Grippe (see index); or you can put bottles of hot water about the patient. Use fruit jars, wrap cloths around them so that you will not burn the patient. Always put one to the feet. If you have a rubber water bag, fill that and put it to his affected side over the pain. After you get him into a sweat you can remove a little, of the sweating remedy at a time and when all are removed give him a tepid water sponging. By this time the physician will be at hand. If you give medicine you can put fifteen drops of the Tincture of Aconite in a glass one-half full of water and give two teaspoonfuls of this every fifteen minutes for four doses. Then give it every one-half hour. Water can be given often, but in small quantities; plain milk alone, or diluted, or beaten with eggs will make a good diet and keep up the strength.

Fomentations.--Cloths wrung out of hot hop tea are often applied to the affected part with good effect. Be careful about wetting the patient. Flaxseed poultices are used.

If used they must be moist and hot. Some doctors are opposed to them. An antiphlogistine poultice is good. Apply it hot. For children you can grease the whole side of the chest, back and front, with camphor and lard and put over that an absorbent cotton jacket. In the early life of the country, home treatment was necessary. Men and women were posted on herbs, etc. Teas made of them were freely and successfully used. A great mistake made was the indiscriminate use of lobelia in too large doses. We have learned that the hot herb drinks in proper doses are of help. Teas made of boneset, hoarhound, pennyroyal, ginger, catnip, hops, slippery elm, etc., were good and are now. They produced the desired result--sweating--and relieved the congestion of the internal organs and re-established the external or (peripheral) circulation. So in the home treatment of pneumonia, etc., if you are so situated that you cannot get a physician use teas internally for sweating, fomentations upon the painful part and if done properly and not too excessively, they will accomplish the desired result. With the corn sweat, I have saved many lives.

ERYSIPELAS.--Erysipelas is an infectious disease, and it is usually caused by a germ which we call "streptococcus pyogenes." The disease shows itself by its local symptoms, pain, swelling, etc., and also by general or constitutional symptoms such as fever, headache, etc., as hereafter given.

Causes.--It is a disease that occurs at any time, and is sometimes epidemic, that is, attacks many persons at a time, like La Grippe. It occurs more often in the spring; it is contagious, and can be carried by a third person or in bedding, etc.

Symptoms.--The type that appears upon the face is the most common. The incubation lasts from three to seven days and it usually comes suddenly with a chill, followed by an active fever and with the local inflammation. In some cases the local condition appears first. There is at first redness, usually of the bridge of the nose and it rapidly spreads to the cheeks, eyes, ears, etc. It is red, shiny hot, drawing, but with a distinct margin at its edges, showing how much skin is inflamed. It may take the form of vesicles. The eyelids may be so swollen as to close, the face and scalp greatly swollen with watery swelling of the eyelids, lips, eyes, ears, etc. The glands under the jaw may become enlarged. The general or constitutional symptoms may be severe. The fever may rise to 104 to 106 and terminates suddenly. The parts that were first affected become pale and more normal, as other parts are involved. It occurs also on other parts of the body. A sting of an insect sometimes looks like it at first; but it does not spread like erysipelas. It seems to me to be more dangerous around the head.

MOTHERS' REMEDIES. 1. Erysipelas, Slippery Elm Bark for.--"Slippery elm used as a wash and taken as a drink." Slippery elm is a very good remedy for this on account of its soothing effect to the affected parts. It is very good to take internally, as it cleanses the system by acting on the bowels and kidneys.

2. Erysipelas, Bean Poultices for.--"White navy beans boiled soft and applied as a poultice to the affected parts and renewed frequently is a sure cure for erysipelas if taken in time." This is a very good and effective poultice, but care should be taken not to use it too long, as the parts will become too soft and might slough.

3. Erysipelas, Soda Wash for.--"Put about a tablespoonful of baking soda in one pint of water and bathe parts several times a day," This is an extremely simple remedy for such a serious disease, but has been known to do good in many cases. The baking soda is soothing.

4. Erysipelas, Easy Remedy for.--"Keep parts well bathed with witch-hazel." A good preparation should be bought. By applying this freely to the affected parts it will be found to have a very soothing effect.

5. Erysipelas, Copperas Liniment for.--"A few cents' worth of common copperas. Make a solution and keep applying it. This kills the poison as it comes on and relieves the pain. I knew of a very bad case to be cured by this treatment."

6. Erysipelas, Cranberry Poultice for.--"Take cranberries and stew them and make a poultice of them." This is a remedy that cannot be beaten for this disease. It gives relief in a very short time and saves the patient a great deal of suffering. If the whisky is used to wet the poultice it is much better, as it keeps the poultice moist longer. All that is necessary is simply to put on more whiskey and it will not be necessary to change the poultice so often.

PHYSICIANS' TREATMENT for Erysipelas.--It is best to separate the patient from the others in the family. Some people very easily take this disease. I know one who cannot be in the room where such a patient is for even five minutes without contracting it.

Local Treatment.--1. Wash the parts with a solution of boric acid, one-half teaspoonful to eight teaspoonfuls of tepid water, put this on the inflamed parts. Then apply a poultice of bruised cranberries. Wash the face each time with the solution before applying the cranberry poultice afresh.

2. Paint thoroughly with tincture of iodine outside of the margin of the disease where the skin shows no sign of the trouble. This is very effective. If done freely it produces a slight inflammation. The stain made by it remains for some time and that is the objection to it on the face, but do not hesitate on that account if the other remedies do not work well or are not at hand.

3. The following is a splendid local application.--Cleanse thoroughly the inflamed part with pure castile soap and water, and then wash this off with one to one thousand corrosive sublimate solution. Dry the skin with a soft towel and apply a thick coating of equal parts of Ichthyol and vaselin, and over this place antiseptic gauze or sterilized absorbent cotton. Keep this in place with adhesive straps. If the diseased surface is small it may not be necessary to use the gauze, etc.

4. Tincture Chloride of Iron in dose of ten to twenty drops and more if necessary four times a day, well diluted with water. This is very hard on the teeth and should be taken through a glass tube.

Diet.--Milk, broths, etc., liquid diet or foods. (See Nursing Dept. under liquid diet.)

Nursing.--When you nurse any infectious patient, you must be not only careful of your patient, but of yourself. It is not necessary in order to do good nursing to endanger yourself; and a nurse who does not know how to care for herself, cannot successfully nurse the sick. In erysipelas I always watch the eruption closely. Sometimes it recedes, and the patient, of course, is worse. Then there are some people who believe in "pow-wowing." They have that done and then do not take care of themselves. I have attended such cases. One case was especially striking. The "pow-wow" person did his work and then the patient thought himself well and proceeded to enjoy himself and caught cold. The result was the "going in" of the eruption and a beautiful cough. I succeeded in my efforts and the next day he had the erysipelas going along nicely, but no cough. I write this so you will take proper care of yourself and shun conjurers and their "pow-wow."

TOXEMIA, SEPTICEMIA; PYEJMIA.--Toxemia refers to the group of symptoms and lesions caused by the presence in the blood of toxins (poison) usually resulting from bacterial growths.

Septicemia refers to the condition caused by the presence in the blood of bacteria (microbes) as well as toxin.

Pyemia refers to the same condition as septicemia with the development of fresh places of suppuration.

Sapremia is a septic intoxication, the result of the absorption of toxins.

SEPTICEMIA.--The presence of bacteria in the blood, introduced from a local lesion (wound, injury, etc.) or with no obvious local infection.

Symptom.--If there is a local infection, symptoms of this precede the septicemia. The invasion may be sudden or gradual, with chill or chilly feelings, followed by symptoms of active fever and later of an asthenic (absence of strength and feeling) fever, with dry tongue and dullness or delirium. Death may occur in one to seven days.

PYEMIA.--This means the presence in the blood of bacteria with resultant foci (places) of suppuration.

Symptoms.--They are local at first where the lesion is. The invasion of the general infection is marked by a severe chill, then high fever and sweating, repeated daily or at irregular intervals.

Fever is variable with sudden falls. In some cases the fever assumes very weakening type and the patient looks like a case of typhoid fever in the third week, and death soon occurs.

In other cases the chills, fever and sweating are repeated at irregular intervals. The patients are emaciated and the skin has a sallow color. Death usually occurs eventually from exhaustion in a few days or months.

Local Treatment.--This should be attended to from the beginning. If you injure your finger or any part and it soon looks red, and feels sore, open it up thoroughly with a clean instrument and cover it with a clean gauze or cotton. It must not be covered too tightly so that the discharge, if any, can leave the wound. Enough dressing must be put on to absorb that. Then keep the wound clean, and so it can "run" if necessary. If you neglect this or do it carelessly and admit dirt you will make it worse.

See treatment of wounds, etc.

General Treatment.--Keep the strength up in every way. The strength should be kept up by giving nourishing diet that will suit that special case and medicine that will produce a tonic effect, such as quinine and strychnine.

ASIATIC CHOLERA.--This is an acute infectious disease caused by a specific organism and characterized by profuse watery discharges from the bowels and great prostration.

Causes.--Some inherit a weakness, making them more susceptible than others to this disease. Other causes are intemperance, general debility, unhygienic surroundings, exciting causes. The spirillum (cholera asiaticus) found in the stools, watery discharges and intestines of affected cases and its transmission by infected food and water.

Symptoms.--After an incubation period of about one to five days, the invasion is marked either by simple diarrhea with some general ill-feeling and prostration, or by abdominal pains, vomiting and diarrhea. Mild cases may recover at this time. In the stage of collapse, there are frequent watery movements resembling rice water, with vomiting, great thirst, abdominal pains and eruptions on the legs. There is sudden collapse and temperature that is below normal; nearly all secretions are greatly diminished. In the so-called cases of cholera sicca (dry) death occurs before the diarrhea begins, although a rice water fluid is found in the intestines after death. After two to twenty-four hours those who have not died may recover or pass into the stage of reaction in which the signs of collapse and purging disappear. After improvement, with slight rise of temperature at times, there may be a relapse or the patient may have inflammation of some of the viscera (cavity organs) and suppression of the urine with delirium, coma and death.

The prognosis is worse in infancy, old age and debilitated persons, and in cases of rapid collapse, low temperature and great blueness.

Death rate from thirty to eighty per cent.

Treatment.--Isolate the patient and disinfect all discharges and clothing.

Use boiled water during an epidemic.

For pain, morphine hypodermically, and apply hot applications to the abdomen.

For vomiting.--Wash out the stomach and give cocaine, ice, coffee, brandy or water by the mouth. Intestines may be irrigated with a two per cent solution of tannic acid.

During collapse.--Hypodermic of camphor, hot applications to the body. Good nursing and careful diet.

YELLOW FEVER.--Yellow fever is an acute infectious disease characterized by jaundice, hemorrhages, albuminuria (albumin in the urine).

Cause.--It is common in the West Indies and epidemic in nearby countries. It is most common in crowded, dirty, poorly drained portions of sea coast cities. It is probably caused by a specific organism which is conveyed from one person to another by mosquitoes and not in clothing, as formerly believed. One attack usually confers immunity.

Symptoms.--Incubation is about three to four days. There may be a fore-warning period, but the attack is usually sudden, with chills, headache, backache, rise in fever, and general feverish symptoms, vomiting, and constipation. Early in this disease the face is flushed, while the conjunctiva and the mucous membrane lining the eyelids is congested and slightly jaundiced. Fever is 102 or 103 degrees, and falls gradually after one to three days. Pulse is slow, and while the temperature rises, it again falls. The stage of calm follows the fall of the temperature with increased jaundice and vomiting of dark altered blood, the "black vomit." Hemorrhages may also occur into the skin or mucous membranes. Brain symptoms are sometimes severe. Convalescence is usually gradual. The disease varies from great mildness to extreme malignancy. Mortality from fifteen to eighty-five per cent.

Treatment.--Prevent spread of the infectious mosquitoes; use screens and netting in infected districts. Careful nursing, food by rectum while vomiting is frequent. For the hemorrhage opium is given; frequent bathing will keep down the fever; and for the vomiting cocaine is given and cracked ice.

PLAGUE (BUBONIC PLAGUE).--Plague is an infectious disease characterized by inflammation and suppuration of the lymph nodes and cutaneous (skin) hemorrhages. It has long been known as the Plague or "Black Death," on account of its "flea-bite looking eruptions." This disease is becoming a serious matter on our western coast, especially in and around San Francisco. The disease exists in India all the time, and there is now danger of it becoming epidemic (existing all the time) in San Francisco, according to today's, Jan. 10th, *Detroit Free Press.* Mr. Merriam, chief of the U. S. Bureau of Biological Survey, recently appeared before congress and asked for more money to investigate this and other conditions, and how to stamp out the carriers of this dreadful disease. European wharf rats, introduced about San Francisco, have spread the plague to the ground squirrels, and the gophers, rabbits, field mice, and other rodents are now being infected. In India, fleas on the native squirrel, perpetuate the plague. The way to stop the plague is to kill the carriers.

Causes.--The bacillus pestis (pests) is transmitted through insects, small animals, like rats, through the air, or in clothing, bedding, and is contained in the feces and urine. The poor in unhygienic districts are most often attacked.

Bubonic Type.--In this type the lymph nodes, particularly in the arm-pit, and groins show inflammatory lesions with marked overgrowth of new tissue. Sometimes there is suppuration, hemorrhage and local death of the part. The bacilli are formed in great numbers in the affected nodes and secondary lesions.

Septicemic Type.--In this type all lymph nodes and nodules show signs of toxemia and the bacilli are formed in the primary (first) lesions and in the blood.

Pneumonic Type.--In this type there are areas of broncho-pneumania, with lesions of the bronchial lymph nodes. The bacilli occur in these situations and in the sputa.

Symptoms.--In the bubonic plague (the usual form) the invasion is marked by headache, depression, pain in the back, stiffness of the extremities and fever. This rises for three or four days, then falls several degrees and is followed by a more severe secondary fever of the prostrating type. At about the third to the fifth day the lymph nodes usually become enlarged most often in the inguinal (groin) region. This is followed by a resolution (getting better) suppuration formingpus or necrosis (local death of the part). "A flea bite looking eruption and hemorrhages from the mucous membrane often occur. The mild cases, which often occur at the beginning of an epidemic, and at its close, are marked only by slight fever and glandular swelling, which may terminate in the forming of pus in the part. In these cases the symptoms are slight and last only a few days."

Septicemic Plague.--This is characterized by symptoms of severe general infection, with hemorrhages, rapid course, and death in three or four days, without the development of swelling of the lymph nodes. Cultures from the blood show bacteria.

Pneumonic Plague.--The symptoms are those of a severe "lobular" pneumonia, with bloody sputum containing many bacilli. It is usually rapidly fatal. Death rate may reach ninety per cent.

Treatment. Prevention.--Prolonged isolation, disinfection of the discharges, cremation of plague victims, destruction of rats, and preventive inoculation of healthy persons with sterilized cultures of the bacillus pestis.

Immunity following this procedure is said to last from one to eighteen months.

For pain, morphine; for weakness, stimulation; for fever, bathing; for buboes, application of ice, injection of bichloride and excision have been advised.

DYSENTERY.--A group of inflammatory intestinal affections, either acute or chronic, and of infectious origin, characterized by frequent painful passages, (containing mucus and blood) or by loose movements.

Acute Catarrhal Dysentery.--This is the most common form in the temperate climate The colon is congested and swollen with a covering of blood-tinged mucus on its mucous membrane.

Symptoms.--The invasion: This is usually marked by diarrhea, then cramp-like general pain in the abdomen and frequent mucous, bloody stools, accompanied by hard straining at stool. The temperature may reach 102 to 103 degrees. After one or two days the stools consist entirely of bloody mucus and are very frequent. The thirst is great. In about one week the stools may become normal.

MOTHERS' REMEDIES. 1. Dysentery, Sweet Cream for.--"One or two teaspoonfuls of thick cream every hour. Three doses is usually sufficient. (This remedy proved successful with my baby when all others failed)."

2. Dysentery, One Ounce Dewberry Root for.--"Boil in one quart of water one ounce of dewberry root. This should be boiled down to one-half pint and a half wineglassful given to patient two or three times a day, or in severe cases, a half wineglassful every two or three hours until discharge diminishes."

3. Dysentery, "Colt Tail" Remedy for.--"The herb called "Colt Tail," steep and drink the tea. It's a tall weed and grows in damp places. It is one of the best herbs for this." This is especially good when the discharge from the bowels is bloody or contains mucus.

4. Dysentery, Sugar and Brandy for.--"Two tablespoonfuls brandy poured into a saucer. Set fire to the brandy and hold in flame lump of sugar on fork. This is a very good remedy, and has cured cases when doctors' remedies failed. This sugar will melt and form a syrup. Dose:--One-half teaspoonful every two hours or oftener if necessary."

5. Dysentery, Herb Remedy for.--"Take four ounces poplar bark, four ounces bayberry bark and three ounces tormentil root, simmer gently in four quarts of water, down to three, strain and add two pounds granulated sugar; let it come to boiling point, skim and add one-half pound blackberry or peach jelly and one-half pint best brandy. Keep in a cool place, take one-half wineglassful three or four times a day or more often if required."

6. Dysentery, New Method to Cure.--"A hot hip bath will often relieve distressing sensations of dysentery or itching piles." This is a very simple remedy and will have a very soothing effect upon the whole system, relieving any nervousness that may be present and usually is with this disease.

7. Dysentery, Starch Injection for.--"Use injection of one cup thin boiled starch, and one-half teaspoonful laudanum. Repeat every 3 to 4 hours."

8. Dysentery, To Cure Bloody.--"Put a teaspoonful of salt into a quart of warm water and inject into the bowels to wash them out thoroughly."

PHYSICIANS' TREATMENT for Dysentery.--Remain in bed on fluid diet, and give a free saline cathartic or castor on, one-half ounce, followed by salol five grains in capsules every three hours.

2. Bismuth subnitrate, one-half to one dram every two to three hours.

3. Irrigation of the colon with normal salt solution or weak solution of silver nitrate at about one hundred degrees with a long rectual tube. Dr. Hare, of Philadelphia, recommends one two-hundredth grain of bichloride of mercury every hour or two (in adults), if the stools are slimy and bloody and if much blood is present, and high rectal injections of witch-hazel water and water, half and half. I know this last is good, and also the following; Oil of fireweed, five drops on sugar every two to three hours.

4. Ipecac.--In acute dysentery ipecac is one of the best remedies, Dr. Hare says; "When the passages are large and bloody and the disease is malignant as it occurs in the tropics, ipecac should be given in the following manner: The powdered ipecac is to be administered on an empty stomach in the dose of thirty grains with thirty drops of the tincture of deodorized opium, which is used to decrease the tendency to vomit. Absolute rest is essential for its success. Finally a profuse gray, mushy stool is passed." This is a favorable sign.

Nursing and Diet.--The patient should always remain in bed and use bed-pan. He must be given a bland, unirritating diet, composed of milk, with lime-water, beef peptonoids, broth, egg albumin, etc., in acute cases.

MALARIA FEVER.--Malarial fever is a group of diseases characterized by intermittent, quotidian (daily), tertian (every other day) or quartan (every fourth day) fever or remittent fever; there are also several pernicious types of this disease and chronic malarial condition of the system with enlargement of the spleen.

Causes.--It occurs most frequently in low lands, along sea coasts, and swamps, particularly in the tropics and warmer portion of the temperate zone. The exciting cause it what is called the plasmodous malarial, a parasite developing in the body of all species of anopheles, a common form of mosquito and transmitted to man, its intermediate host, by the bite of the infected mosquitoes.

INTERMITTENT MALARIAL FEVER. (a) Tertian. (b) Quartan. (c) Quotidian. Symptoms.--The symptoms of all these are the same, except that in tertian fever, the paroxysms occur every third day; in quartan they occur every fourth day. Quotidian occurs daily.

The incubation time is unknown. It consists usually of three stages, cold, hot, and sweating, and they usually occur in the morning. "The cold stage is ushered in by yawning, lassitude and headache, and rapid rise of temperature; sometimes nausea and vomiting followed by shivering and rather violent shaking with chattering of the teeth." It may last from ten minutes to two hours. The internal temperature may rise to 104 to 106 degrees, while the surface is blue and cold, with severe headache, often nausea and vomiting. Hot stage: this may last from one-half to five hours; the temperature may increase somewhat, the face is flushed, the skin is red and hot, great thirst, throbbing headache and full bounding pulse. Sweating stage lasts two to four hours, and entire body may be covered; fever and other symptoms abate and sleep usually follows. The patient feels nearly well between attacks.

REMITTENT OR CONTINUOUS MALARIAL FEVER (Aestivo-Autumnal Fever).--This form occurs in the temperate zone regions, especially in the summer and autumn. The symptoms vary greatly. The fever may be irregularly intermittent, but at longer intervals than the Tertian variety. The cold stage is often absent, and in the hot the temperature falls gradually. The appearance is often like typhoid for there may be then hardly any remission of fever.

PERNICIOUS MALARIAL FEVER.--This is a very dangerous disease. The chief forms are the comatose, algid and hemorrhagic.

(a) Comatose form is characterized by delirium or sudden coma (deep sleep) with light temperature.

(b) The algid or asthenic form begins with vomiting and great prostration. The temperature is normal or below normal. There may be diarrhea and suppression of the urine.

(c) The hemorrhagic form includes malarial hemoglobinuria, hemoglobin in the urine. Haemoglobin is the coloring matter of the red corpuscles.

Treatment. Prevention.--Destroy mosquitoes and protect from them by screens. Small preventive doses of quinine for persons in malarious regions, three grains three times a day. Five grains three times a day will nearly always cure tertian and quartan cases, especially if the patient is kept in bed until the time for one or two paroxysms has passed. Attacks often stop spontaneously for a time when the patient is kept in bed, even without the administration of quinine.

In Remittent Fever larger doses are necessary. For pernicious forms: Hydrochlorate of quinine and urea ten to twenty grains, given hypodermically, every three or four hours until improvement occurs, when the sulphate of quinine by the mouth may be substituted.

AGUE. (See Malarial Fever.)--By ague is meant the cold chills and fever; or dumb ague where there is little chill, mostly chilly and fever. These attacks may come on every day, every other day, or every third day.

MOTHERS' REMEDIES. 1. Ague and Fever, Dogwood Good for.--"Take one ounce of dogwood root and one quart of water. Make an infusion by boiling down to one-half pint. Strain and give one-half wineglassful every two or three hours."

2. Ague in Face, Menthol and Alcohol Effective Remedy for.--"After making a solution of teaspoonful of menthol crystals, dissolved in two ounces of alcohol, apply several times a day to the face. Care should be taken that this solution does not enter the eyes, as it would be injurious,"

3. Ague, Simple Remedy for.--"Give purgative and follow with quinine. Give large 4 grain capsule every four hours.

MOTHERS' REMEDIES. 1. Chills and Fever, Peruvian Bark and Rhubarb for.--

"Pure Rye Whisky	4 ounces
Pulverized Peruvian Bark	1 dram
Pulverized Rhubarb	1 ounce

Mix.

Put in bottles. Dose for adults:--One tablespoonful three times a day. This is an excellent remedy."

2. Chills and Fever, Horse-radish for.--"Take fresh green horseradish leaves, bruise and mash them to the consistency of a poultice and bind on the bottom of the feet. This will tend to reduce the fever and is a reliable remedy. I have often used this with great satisfaction."

3. Chills and Fever, Dogwood Known to be Good for.--"Make a decoction of one ounce of dogwood root, boiled in one quart of water down to one pint; strain, and give half wineglassful every two or three hours." This remedy has been used by our grandmothers for many years, and is one to be depended upon. The dogwood root can be purchased at any drug store.

Treatment.--For acute cases quinine in various doses. I usually prescribe two grains every two hours until the ears ring, and then take only enough to keep them in that condition.

It is well always to see that the bowels and liver are active before taking quinine. The medicine acts better when the patient remains quiet in bed. If the chill and fever comes on every day, the quinine should be taken every hour between the paroxysms.

MALTA FEVER.--This occurs in the Mediterranean countries, India, China, the Philippines and Porto Rico. The fever is irregular or marked by intervals of "no fever" for two or more days with febrile relapses lasting one to three weeks. Constipation, anemia (scarcity of blood), joint symptoms and debility exist. Ordinary cases may last three months to two years. Mortality two per cent.

Treatment.--Like that for typhoid. Change climate, if possible.

BERI-BERI.--Beri-beri is a disease rarely occurring in the United States. It is usually found in the warmer climates and peculiar to certain regions such as India, and Japan.

It is characterized by paralysis and fatal effusion, also neuritis, which is an inflammation of the nerves. It seems to be undecided among the medical profession as to whether the disease is infectious or not. Some claim it is brought on by the eating of bad rice or certain raw fish. Young men in those climates seem to be most susceptible to beri-beri.

Treatment.--There is very little known about this disease. Fortunately it does not often occur here. It is necessary to keep up the strength by food and tonics and relieve the pain.

ANTHRAX. (Charbon, Wool Sorters' Disease, Splenic Fever).--This is "an acute infectious disease of animals, transmitted to man by inoculation into the wounds, or by inhalation of, or swallowing the germs." Butchers, tanners and shepherds are most liable to it. The exciting cause is the bacillus anthracis (anthrax bacillus). The local skin condition is a pustule containing the bacilli, which may also invade the general circulation. If the germs are inhaled, there is bronchopneumonia; if swallowed, areas of inflammation and local death occur in the intestines. The spleen and lymph nodes are enlarged.

Symptoms. 1. External anthrax, malignant pustule. This begins in a papule (pimple) at the point of inoculation turning into a vesicle and then a pustule, (blister-like pimple) surrounded by an inflammatory area (space) with marked watery swelling. The nearby glands are enlarged and tender. At first the temperature rapidly rises; later it may be below normal. The fever symptoms may be severe. Recovery takes place slowly. Death occurs in three to five days.

MALIGNANT ANTHRAX (swelling).--In this lesion is a pustule, with very marked swelling. It most frequently occurs on the eyelid and face and the swelling may terminate in fatal gangrene.

2. Internal anthrax.--(a) Internal anthrax is caused by the introduction of the bacteria into the alimentary canal in infected meat, milk, etc. The invasion is marked by a chill, followed by moderate fever, vomiting, diarrhea, pain in the back and legs and restlessness. Sometimes convulsions occur and hemorrhages into the skin from the mucous membranes. The spleen is swollen. Prostration is extreme and it often ends in death.

(b) Charbon or Wool Sorter's disease occurs among those employed in picking over wool or hair of infected animals--the germs being inhaled or swallowed. The onset is sudden with a chill, then fever, pain in the back and legs, and severe prostration. There may be difficulty of breathing and signs of bronchitis, or vomiting and diarrhea. Death is a common termination, sometimes within a day. Death rate is from five to twenty-six per cent. Greatest when the swelling is near the head.

Treatment.--The wound or swelling should be cauterized and a solution of carbolic acid or bichloride of mercury injected around it and applied to its surface. Stimulants and feeding are important.

LOCKJAW. (Tetanus).--Tetanus or lockjaw, as it is commonly called, is an infectious disease and is characterized by painful and violent contractions of the voluntary muscles; it may be of the jaw alone or of a considerable part of the body.

Causes.--The intelligence and mental faculties are not impaired. In most cases it follows a wound or injury, although in others there seems to be no exciting causes. Fourth of July celebrations furnish a great many of our lockjaw cases. Ten to fifteen days usually elapse after the wound before lockjaw really sets in.

Symptoms.--It comes on occasionally with a chill or chilly feelings; usually by rigidity (stiffness) of the neck, jaw and face. On arising in the morning there is sometimes a stiffness of the muscles at the back of the head. It is not unusual on taking a slight cold to have a stiff neck and often the patient's attention is not attracted by this symptom. Sometimes this stiffness begins or soon extends to the muscles of the lower jaw; the throat becomes dry and is painful and gradually the stiffness increases to a continuous contraction, spasm, and extends to the muscles of the trunk and extremities. The body becomes rigid in a straight line or bent backward, forward or sidewise. This spasm occurs after any slight irritation and is extremely painful. Temperature is usually low. During the first spasms the patient may attempt to open his mouth as he may naturally be suspicious of the trouble that is coming; he succeeds with difficulty and even finds it hard to swallow; soon the jaws may be firmly closed, and it is from this feature of the disease that it gained the name of lockjaw. The contractions in some cases do not extend beyond the neck and face muscles. During the contractions the face may be drawn into frightful contortions. Food can be given only through such spaces as may exist between the teeth, as often the patient cannot open his mouth himself, nor can it be pried open by any force that would be allowable. When the muscles of the trunk are affected the abdomen may be drawn inward, become very hard and stiff, chest movements are affected, making it difficult to breathe, sometimes almost to suffocation. Sometimes the body becomes bent like a bow, as in some cases of spinal meningitis, so that only the head and heels support the weight of the body. The body may become so rigid that it can be lifted by a single limb as you would a statue. It is fortunate that there are few cases, comparatively, of lockjaw as the distorted face and general contractions of the body are painful to witness.

Recovery.--The mortality in lockjaw cases runs about eight per cent. Sometimes death is caused by exhaustion from the muscular exertions; the patient is seldom able to sleep and sometimes wears out in a few days. Sometimes suffocation brings a sudden end to his sufferings and usually one or two days to ten or twelve days is the limit. Among the lower classes where sanitary science is seldom observed, and even among the better classes, lockjaw has been known to occur in infants. It usually comes on, in ten to fifteen days after birth, and the child seldom lives more than a few days, It is hard to account for such cases which may come on suddenly from the slightest excitement such as sudden noises, etc.

MOTHERS' REMEDIES.--l. Lockjaw, Successful Remedy for.--"A very good and successful remedy for this disease, is to apply a warm poultice of flaxseed meal, saturated with laudanum and sugar of lead water, to the jaws and neck."

2. Lockjaw, Smoke as a Cure for.--"Smoke the wound for twenty minutes in the smoke of burnt woolen cloths. This is considered a never failing remedy."

PHYSICIANS' TREATMENT.--If from a wound cut open and use antiseptics. Isolate the patient and have absolute quiet. Antitoxin is used with success in some cases of lockjaw, but this and other remedies or measures must be handled by a physician, Opium is sometimes given and stimulants such as brandy, whisky, etc. As it is a case of life or death in a very short time, we cannot advise depending upon home treatment. A preventive caution that must always be observed is the use of antiseptics and the strictest care of all injuries and wounds that might result in lockjaw. This is a disease where an ounce of prevention is worth a thousand pounds of cure, because by the time the disease is recognized as lockjaw and has really made an appearance, it may be too late for medical skill. While you are waiting for the doctor you may apply cold cloths or even an ice bag to the spine. If the spasms are severe let the patient inhale chloroform to kill the pain and quiet him. In the meantime secure the best physician within your reach, and follow his directions carefully, be calm and self-possessed when in the presence of the patient, for you must remember that he has full possession of his mental faculties and will notice every evidence of fear or worry in the faces of those who are nursing him. This will only add to his sufferings, affect his nervous system and undermine his general vitality. Read carefully the nursing department in this book and you will gain some valuable hints and knowledge regarding the sick room.

GLANDERS.--This is an acute disease of the horse and occasionally of man. It is called "glanders" when the affection appears in the nostrils, and is called "farcy" when in the skin.

Causes.--The bacilli is usually introduced from infected horses through the nose, mouth and cheek, mucous membranes or skin abrasions (rubbing off of the skin). There are large or small lumps in the skin, mucous membrane of the nose and mouth.

Symptoms. Acute Glanders.--1. Incubation lasts from three to four days. There are signs of inflammation at the site of infection and general symptoms. In two or three days, small lumps appear on the mucous membrane of the nose, and ulcerate, with a discharge of mucus and pus. Sometimes these nodules die locally, and their discharge is then foul. The glands around the neck are enlarged. An eruption appears over the face and joints. Inflammation of the lungs may occur. Death may take place in eight to ten days.

2. Chronic Glanders.--This may last for months. It acts like chronic cold with ulcer in the nose. Some recover.

3. Acute Farcy.--The local and general signs are those of an infection, with necrosis (local death) at the site (in the skin) of inoculation; nodules, (lumps) known as "farcy buds" form along the lymphatics (glands) and form pus. There may be pus collections in the joints and muscles. Death often occurs in one to five days.

Chronic Farcy.--Tumors in the skin of the extremities, containing pus. The process is local, the inflammatory symptoms light, and the duration may be months or years.

Treatment of Glanders.--This disease does not often occur in man; it is an awful affliction. All infected horses must be killed, it is dangerous for man to be around one. If seen early, the wound should be cut out or burned out with caustics, and afterwards dressed like any wound.

The "farcy buds" should be opened early. There is very little hope in acute cases of glanders. In chronic cases recovery is possible, but it will be after a long tedious time. There must be proper nourishing food and tonic medicines. Each case should be treated according to the indications. It is safe to say the parts should be thoroughly cut or scraped out and then treated with antiseptics and the general system built up, by tonics and stimulating remedies, if needed. As stated before, acute glanders and acute farcy are almost always fatal.

BIG-JAW OR LUMP-JAW. (Actinomycosis).--This is an infectious disease of cattle, less frequently of man, and it is caused by what is called the "ray fungus." This grows in the tissues and develops a mass with a secondary chronic inflammation.

This disease is widespread among cattle, and also occurs in the pig. In the ox it is called the "big jaw." The infection may be taken in with the food, and it locates itself often in the mouth or surroundings. Oats, barley, and rye may carry the germ to the animals. The fungus may be found even in decayed teeth.

Alimentary Canal Type.--The jaw has been affected in man. One side of the face is swollen or there may be a chronic enlargement of the jaw, which may look like a sarcoma (tumor). The tongue also is sometimes affected and shows small growths. It may also occur in the intestines and liver. There is at first a tumor (lump), and this finally suppurates.

In the Lungs.--They also can be affected. It is chronic here and there is cough, fever, wasting and an expectoration of mucus and pus, sometimes of a very bad odor (fetid). It sometimes acts like miliary tuberculosis of the lungs, and this is quite frequent in oxen. Other diseases of the lungs and bronchial affections occur and abscesses and cavities are formed that may be diagnosed during life.

Symptoms.--If in the jaw there may be toothache, difficulty of swallowing and of opening the jaw. The adjacent muscles may be hardened (indurated). A swelling appears at the angle of the jaw and this quickly passes into suppuration; later it opens first outside, then inside--into the mouth and discharges pus containing little yellow masses. It will extend down even into the bowels unless it is properly treated. Then there will be stomach disturbances and diarrhea. It may ulcerate through the bowels and cause peritonitis. The liver, spleen and ovaries may also become affected.

The Skin.--There may be chronic suppurating ulcers of the skin and the "ray fungus" can be found in them.

Diagnosis.--The "ray fungus" can be found. There is a wooden hardness of the tissues beyond the borders of the ulcers; there are the little yellow granules in the pus. The course is chronic. Mild cases recover in six to nine months or earlier, the mouth form being the most favorable.

Treatment.--Surgical. Remove the parts involved. Internally, iodide of potash in large doses is recommended. The food should be plenty and nourishing. In this case we must recommend you to a physician instead of the home treatments.

GONORRHEA (Urethritis).--This can be called an infectious inflammation of the urethra, caused by the gonococcus, a microbe or germ, causing a specific inflammation of the mucous membrane of the urethra or vagina.

Incubation.--The time that elapses between the exposure and development of the symptoms in the urethra is variable, extending from a few hours to twelve or fourteen days. In the great majority of cases, however, the disease appears during the first week. The patient notices a drop of milk-like fluid at the opening of the urethra, which is slight, red and puffed or turned out; a tickling sensation is often felt in this locality, and the next time urine is passed it is attended with a feeling of warmth at the end of the canal, or with actual scalding. After this the symptoms increase rapidly in number and severity, so that within forty-eight hours, or even sooner, the disease may be described as having passed its first or increasing stage, the characteristic phenomena of which are as follows:

Changes in the meatus (opening). There are redness, eversion (turning out), ulceration and eating away and often erosion of the lips of the opening of urethra. Sometimes, but rarely, so much swelling that the person can hardly pass the urine, which drops away. The other symptoms are too well-known by those who have had this disease to need a description.

Prognosis.--It is now considered more than a cold, and it is the cause of terrible sickness in both sexes, among the innocent as well as the guilty.

Treatment.--It may be cured perhaps in a short time, and yet no one can be certain of its absolute cure. This disease is better understood now, and the treatment is entirely different from formerly. The strong injections are now considered not only useless but dangerous to the future health of the patient. The best treatment is mild antiseptic injections, irrigation carefully done by an expert person; remaining quietly in bed, being careful to use food and drink that are not stimulating, keeping the bowels open by proper diet and mild laxatives and the urine mild by soothing diuretic remedies. Unfortunately those affected want quick work and they get it, frequently to their future sorrow. The following are good injections. Before each injection the urine should be passed and an injection of an antiseptic like listerine, etc., one dram to an ounce of boiled water, to cleanse the canal. You can use twice a day the following:

Fluid Extract Hydrastis (colored)	1 dram
Water	1 ounce

Use one dram of this for each injection. It stains the clothes so you must be careful. This is good and healing.

GONORRHEAL ARTHITIS. (Gonorrheal Rheumatism, Inflammation of the Joints).--This is more common in men than women. Occurring during, and at the end of or after inflammation of the urethra. It usually involves many joints, such as the temporal, maxillary and collar bone. The effusion in the joints is usually serious.

Symptoms.--Variable joint pains may be the only one. The attack may resemble an acute articular rheumatism of one joint, or a subacute rheumatism of one or more.

Sometimes there is a chronic one-jointed inflammation usually of the knee. The tendon sheaths and bursae may be involved alone, or with the joints. Gonorrheal septicemia may result from arthritis. This is protracted. Iritis is a most frequent complication. The urethra source of the infection must be cured.

Treatment.--Keep the joint quiet and you can use an ice cap for the pain. Tonic treatment with quinine, iron, and arsenic in chronic cases is needed. The joints should be kept at rest in acute cases. In chronic cases massage and slight motion. The tonics must be chosen for each individual case. One afflicted with this must be under treatment for a long time.

HIP JOINT DISEASE. (Morbus Coxarius).--This is more common in children than in adults.

Cause.--It is usually tubercular.

Symptoms. First stage.--It may be overlooked; slight lameness, a little stiffness is noticed at times. The muscles begin to dwindle.

Second stage.--Child limps very perceptibly, dwindling is more apparent. Pain appears.

Treatment.--Absolute rest. Lying down treatment if begun early arrests this disease often. Build up the system. Splints and brace are needed sometimes.

KNEE JOINT DISEASE. (White Swelling).--This is simply a tuberculous knee.

Treatment.--Rest. Stop motion of the joint by some form of splint or plaster of Paris cast. Get a good physician at the beginning in these cases and you will save lots of after worry and blame for yourself. It does not pay to wait. These joint diseases will progress, and often treatment is begun months after trouble is seated. It ought to be criminal negligence and dealt with accordingly to neglect such diseases. Parents should never forget that they have endowed their children with such a constitution, and they should be glad and willing to correct it as far as they can.

LEPROSY. Definition.--Leprosy is a chronic infectious disease, caused by what is called the "Bacillus Leprae," and is characterized by the presence of tubercular nodules in the skin and mucous membranes (tubercular leprosy), or by changes in the nerves (anaesthetic leprosy). These forms are separate at first, but ultimately they are combined and there are disturbances of sensation in the characteristic tubercular form.

History.--Leprosy is supposed to have originated in the Orient, and to be as old as the records of history. It appears to have prevailed in Egypt even so far back as three or four thousand years before Christ. The Hebrew writers make many references to it, and it is no doubt described in Leviticus. The affection was also known both in India and China many centuries before the Christian era. The old Greek and Roman physicians were familiar with its manifestations, ancient Peruvian pottery represent on their pieces deformities suggestive of this disease. The disease prevailed extensively in Europe throughout the middle ages and the number of leper asylums has been estimated at, at least, 20,000. Its prevalence is now restricted in the lands where it still occurs while once it was prominent in the list of scourges of the old world.

It is now found in Norway and to a less extent in Sweden, in Bulgaria, Greece, Russia, Austro-Hungary and Italy, with much reduced percentage in middle Europe; it is the rarest of diseases in England where once it existed. In India, Java, and China, in Egypt, Algiers, and Southern Africa, in Australia and in both North and South America, including particularly Central America, Cuba, and the Antilles, it exists to a less extent. It has been recognized in the United States chiefly in New Orleans, San Francisco, (predominantly among the Chinese population of that city). The disease has steadily decreased among the latter colonists in Minnesota, Wisconsin and Iowa. Isolated cases have been recognized in almost every state, and leprous cases are presented at the public charities of New York, Philadelphia, Boston, etc. The estimated number of lepers a few years ago in the United States varied between two hundred and five hundred. It is represented as diminishing in frequency in the Hawaiian Islands, Porto Rico and the Philippines. In the Hawaiian Islands it spread rapidly after 1860, and strenuous attempts have been made to stamp it out by segregating all lepers on the island of Molokai. There were 1,152 lepers in that settlement in 1894. In British India, according to the leprosy commission, there were 100,000 lepers in 1900.

Cause.--The bacillus, discovered by Hansen, of Bergen, in 1874, is universally recognized as the cause of leprosy. It has many points of resemblance to the tubercle bacillus. These bacilli have been found in the dwellings and clothing of lepers as well as in the dust of apartments occupied by the victims.

The usual vehicle by which the disease is transmitted is the secretions of a leprous patient containing bacilli or spores. The question of inheritance of leprosy is regarded now as standing in the same position as that relating to the inheritance of tuberculosis; no foetus, no new-born living child, has been known to exhibit the symptoms of either disease. Several cases have been cited where infants but a few weeks old exhibited symptoms of leprosy. It affects men more than women. Infection is more common after the second decade, though children are occasionally among its victims. When it occurs in countries where it had not previously existed, its appearance is invariably due to the infection of sound individuals by lepers first exhibiting symptoms where the disease is prevalent.

Neisser states this: "The number of lepers in any country bears an inverse ratio to the laws executed for the care and isolation of infected persons. The disease appears to spread more rapidly in damp and cold, or warm and moist, climates than in temperate countries. It is not now regarded as contagious. The leprosy of the book of Leviticus not only includes lepra, as that term is understood today, but also psoriasis, scabies and other skin affections," The leper, in the eye of the Mosaic law, was ceremoniously unclean, and capable of communicating a ceremonial uncleanness. Several of the narratives contained in the Bible bear witness to the fact that the Oriental leper was seen occasionally doing service in the courts of kings, and even in personal communication and contact with officers of high rank.

Symptoms.--Previous symptoms: Want of appetite, headache, chills, alternating with mild or severe feverish attacks, depression, nosebleed, stomach and bowel disturbances, sleeplessness. The durations of these symptoms is variable. Some patients will remember that these symptoms preceded for years the earliest outbreak of lepra (leprosy). In other cases only a few weeks elapsed. These earlier skin lesions are tubercular, macular (patches), or bullous elevations of the horny layer of the skin. It may then be divided into three varieties tuberculous, macular and anaesthetic.

LEPRA TUBEROSA. (Tuberculated, Nodulated or Tegumentary (skin) Leprosy).-- This nodular type comprises from ten to fifty per cent of cases. After the occurring of the symptoms just mentioned spotted lesions appear, which are bean to tomato in size, reddish brown or bronze-hued patches, roundish, oval or irregular in contour, well defined, and they occur upon the face, trunk and extremities. The skin covering them is either smooth and shining, as if oiled, or is infiltrated, nodulated and elevated. The surface of the reddened spots is often oversensitive.

After a period ranging from weeks to years, tubercles rise from the spots described, varying in size from a pea to that of a nut, and they may be as large as a tomato. They are in color, yellowish, reddish-brown, or bronzed, often shining as if varnished or oiled, are covered with a soft, natural, or slightly scaling outer skin, roundish or irregular in shape and are isolated or grouped numbers of very small and ill-determined nodules may often be seen by careful examination of the skin in the vicinity of those that are developed. They may run together and cause broad infiltrations and from this surface new nodules spring. They may be in the skin or under the skin and feel soft or firm. The eruption of these tubercles is usually preceded at the onset by fever, as well as by puffy swelling of the involved region, eyelids, ears, etc. These leprous tubercles choose the face as their favored site. They mass here in great numbers, and thus produce the characteristic deformity of the countenance that has given to the disease one of its names, Leontiasis (lion face).

In such faces the tubercles arrange themselves in parallel series above the brows down to the nose, over the cheeks, lips and chin, and as a result of the infiltration and development of the conditions the brows deeply over-hang; the globes of the eyes, and the ears, are so studded with tubercular masses as to stand out from the side of the head. The trunk and extremities, including the palms of the hands and soles of the feet, are then usually involved to a less degree. The armpit, genital and mammary regions, and more rarely the neck and the palms of the hands and soles of the feet, may be invaded. In occasional cases when the development of tubercles upon the face and ears is extensive, there may not be more than from five to fifty upon the rest of the body, and these either widely scattered and isolated or agglomerated in a single hard, flat, elevated plaque of infiltration upon the elbow or thigh. When the tubercles run together (become confluent) large plaques of infiltration may form, which are elevated and brownish or blackish in color.

The soft palate and larynx are often involved when the skin lesions are present. The voice may sound gruff and hoarse, and the tongue, the larynx and soft palate have been found studded with small sized, ashen-hued tubercles. These tumors or tubercles may degenerate and form into irregularly outlined, sharply cut, glazed ulcers, with a bloody or sloughing floor, or they may disappear and leave behind pigmented, shrunken depressions, or they lose their shapes from partial resorption. A large plaque may flatten in the center until an annular disk is left to show its former location. Coincident symptoms are disturbance in the functions of the sweat and sebaceous secretion, thinning and loss of hair in the regions involved, especially the eyebrows, and disorders of sensibility. Later results, are a nasal catarrh, atrophy of the sexual organs in both sexes, with impairment or loss of procreative power, hopeless blindness. However the course of the disease is very slow, and years may elapse before these several changes are accomplished. Often the disease appears quiescent for months at a time, after which fever occurs and with it acute or sub-acute manifestations appear, including gland disease, orchitis, ulcerative processes, slow or rapid, followed by gangrene and a relatively rapid progress is made toward a fatal conclusion.

Toward the last the mutilations effected by the disease may result. Parts of the fingers or toes, whole fingers or toes, and entire hand or foot may become wholly or partially detached by the ulcerative and other degenerations. This stage of this type of the disease may extend through ten or more years. After it has fully developed the dejected countenance of the leper, with his leonine expression and general appearance is highly characteristic.

LEPRA MACULOSA.--This form is more common in tropical countries and is distinguished chiefly by its macular (spotty) lesions. In size they vary from a small coin to areas as large as a platter. They are diffused or circumscribed, roundish or shaped irregularly, yellowish, brownish or bronzed in color, often shiny or glazed. They may be infiltrated and may be elevated, or on a level with the adjacent tissues. The patches are usually at first very sensitive, but they finally become insensitive, so that a knife can be thrust deeply into them without being felt. The regions chiefly affected by this type are the back, exposed parts, the backs of the hands and wrists, the forehead, the cheeks, ears, back of the feet, and ankles. The eruptions may be scanty or general; conspicuous or insignificant. The eruptive symptoms are associated commonly, early or late, with the serious phenomena described below.

LEPRA ANAESTHETICA. (Nerve Leprosy. Atrophic Leprosy. Lepra Trophoneurotica).--Before the development of this form of leprosy there may be one or two years of ill-health. Usually the skin at this time becomes in localized patches over-sensitive, sometimes there is over-sensitiveness and special nerves, because of their enlargement, become accessible to the touch. Those named later become tender, and the seat of lancinating or shooting pains. This clinical variety may be commingled in its symptoms with each of the other types. With or without such commingling, however, there commonly is noted, after exposure to cold or after being subject to chills first an eruption, red (erythematous) patches, or of "bullae," size of a bean on cheeks, ears, back of the feet, and ankles. The eruption may be outer skin covering (epidermis) and filled with a clear tinted or blood-mixed serum, and usually occurring upon the extremities. The scars that follow are shrunken (atrophic) patches, each often greater in extent than the base of the original trouble, color whitish, shiny, glazed, or better described as a tint suggesting the hue of mica; their outline is circular and form also the dumb-bell figure by running (coalescing) together, or juxtaposition. These scars are always without sensitiveness (anaesthetic), and they may exist together with spotted and non-sensitive patches upon the trunk or other parts such as the face, hands, feet, ankles, thighs, but rarely on the palms and soles. Neither those of the one class nor of the other, however, are disposed over the surface of the body in lines, bands or curves, corresponding with the distribution of the skin (cutaneous) nerves. Sometimes the ulnar and other nerves (median, posterior tibial, peroneal, facial and radial) that are accessible to the touch are swollen, tender, insensitive or as rigid as hardened cords. Reddish-gray swellings may be recognized by the eye along the nerve tract. General shrinking skin symptoms follow. The skin becomes dry and harsh; there is little or no sebaceous product and the skin of the face seems tightly drawn over the bones. As a consequence of deforming shrinking (atrophy) of the eyelids, a persistent overflow of tears, consequent eye changes follow, and a constant flow of saliva escapes from the parted lips. The fingers are half drawn into the palm of the hands; the nails are distorted and ulceration occurs later. These ulcers are irregular, oval, roundish or linear in form covered with thin blackish, flattened, tenacious crusts with soft bases, and their floors covered with a soft debris mixed with blood, the whole insensitive to every foreign body, and external application. At last the symptoms of mutilating lepra (leprosy) may occur, digits or portions of the wrist, part of hand (meta carpus) or corresponding portions of the foot may be detached from the body. Death may occur at any time during the course of the disease. In this form it is said to last from eighteen to twenty years and is thus not so rapidly fatal as the tubercular variety.

Treatment.--The main treatment is the isolation and segregation of all lepers from contact with the well; wholesome laws are enforced in some countries where leprosy prevails, and provision is made not only for the isolation and segregation, but also for their care. On account of its relative variety America has not yet awakened and legislation only forbids the entry of infected persons. At Molokai, in the Hawaiian Islands, provision is made for the care of lepers. Many of the public hospitals for the care of the sick poor refuse to receive lepers. The child of a leprous woman should be removed from the mother after birth and not nursed by another woman. No medicines are known to have any curative effect. An immediate change of residence and climate should be made if the patient happens to live in a district where the disease prevails. A highly nutritious diet should be taken.

The outlook.--The future is in general dark for the leper. It is often of a malignant character, and a fatal result is the rule. A change of climate and conditions may help. Scandinavian lepers who have removed to the United States have been greatly benefited by the change, but there is no known cure. The isolation should be as effective as that for tuberculosis. It is not contagious but infectious.

HYDROPHOBIA.--Rabies and hydrophobia are two different terms, meaning the same disease, the former meaning to rage or become mad. This term applies more especially to the disease as it exists in the maniacal form in the lower animals, while hydrophobia comes from the Greek, meaning "dread of water." As we occasionally find this dread of water only in the human subject, the term is properly used in such a case. The lower animals frequently attempt to drink water even though the act brings on a spasmodic contraction of the swallowing (deglutitory) muscles. Hydrophobia is an acute infectious disease communicated to man by the bite of an animal suffering from rabies. It is due to a definite specific virus which is transmitted through the saliva by the bite of a rabid animal. Its natural habitat (location) is the nervous system, and it does not retain its virulence when introduced into any other system of organs. It is essentially a nervous disease and transmitted by the saliva of rabid animals. When inoculated into a wound this virus must come in contact with a broken

nerve trunk in order to survive and reproduce itself. If by accident it attacks the end of the broken nerve trunk, it slowly and gradually extends to the higher nerve centers and eventually produces the disease.

The incubation, or the time it takes for the disease to develop, varies, but usually is from three to six months. There is a recorded case where the person began to show symptoms of the disease thirteen days after having received a severe wound on the head. The incubation period is seldom longer than six months. The symptoms of the disease in the human being vary within narrow limits. There are three classic symptoms usually encountered, and these are fear, apprehension or excitement, together with deglutitory (swallowing) spasms, terminating in general paralysis. The patient remains conscious of his agony to the end, but the period of illness is of short duration, lasting from one to three days.

The bites of rabid dogs cause ninety per cent of the cases in man and animals. The cat is the next important factor in spreading the disease and about six per cent of the cases are caused by this animal. For other cases four per cent come from bites of horses, wolves, foxes, etc. The wolf in Russia, or other animals like it, may be the chief cause there; but dogs cause ninety per cent, taking all the cases found. Man, dog, cat, horse, cattle, sheep, goat, hog, deer, etc., are subject to the disease either naturally or experimentally. The disease is confined commonly to dogs, because the dog naturally attacks animals of his own species and thus keeps the disease limited mainly to his own kind. Naturally the dog follows this rule, but on the other hand, in the latter stages of the disease he usually goes to the other extreme and even attacks his own master, etc. The dogs that are the most dangerous and do the greatest damage are of the vicious breeds.

The rabbit or guinea pig is used for demonstration in the laboratory. Guinea pigs respond to the virus more rapidly than do other animals and therefore they are especially useful in diagnostic work. Rabbits, however, on account of the convenient size and ease with which they are operated upon, are usually the choice in the production of material used in treating patients.

The director of one Pasteur Institute says, "We have two classes of patients to deal with in the Pasteur institute. The larger class, of course, are those inoculated by the bite of rabid animals, but we also have a few who are infected by the rabid saliva accidentally coming in contact with wounds already produced. In these accidental eases the disease is almost as likely to result as in those to whom the virus is directly communicated by the bite." The wounds considered most dangerous are the recent fresh wounds. The possibility of infection decreases with the formation of the new connective tissue which protects the ends of the broken nerve fibres. One must remember, however, that wounds over joints, especially on the hands, are likely to remain open for some time. A dog ill of this disease can give the disease to man through licking a wound. Such a case has been recorded. This dog licked the child's hands before it was known to be mad. The child died from the disease. As stated before ninety per cent of the cases are inoculated by the bites of rabid animals.

The wounds are considered according to their severity and location. Lacerating, tearing wounds upon uncovered surfaces, especially the head, are the most dangerous. This is due to the fact of the closeness of the brain and the large amount of infection in such a wound, and for this reason treatment should be immediately given. But smaller wounds should also be treated for the smallness of the wound furnishes no sure criterion as to the future outcome of the disease. All possible infections should be regarded as dangerous when considering the advisability of taking the Pasteur Treatment. The small wound has usually a longer period of incubation, because of the small amount of infection, still it may cause a fatal termination. A dog never develops rabies from a lack of water or from being confined or overheated during the summer months. A spontaneous case of rabies has never been known. It must be transmitted from animal to animal and the history of the case will point to a previous infection by a diseased animal.

Where rigid quarantine rules exist the disease does not occur. In Australia they quarantine every dog, that comes to that country, for six months, and in consequence they have never had a case of rabies. In Russia they have had many cases. In Constantinople the disease frequently "runs riot." France has lost as many as 2,500 dogs in one year. Before the Pasteur Treatment was instituted (in 1885) there was an average of sixty deaths in human beings in the Paris hospitals.

Belgium and Austria average one thousand dogs annually. There was a yearly average in Germany of four hundred dogs, dying of rabies, until the law requiring the muzzling of dogs was strictly enforced and since that time the disease is practically unknown. We do not have strict quarantine laws against dogs, and the result is death from hydrophobia in many states annually. It was formerly believed that rabies was a hot weather disease. The number of cases during the winter months of late years has disproved that belief, for the records of the institute for treatment of hydrophobia at Ann Arbor have shown a decrease of cases during the summer months. This was before 1908. This shows that rabies is not a hot weather disease.

Ordinarily cases of rabies occur here and there (sporadic), but if the conditions are favorable epidemics break out. One dog may bite several dogs and these dogs bite others and thus spread the disease to many. Not every animal bitten by a mad dog develops the disease. The disease does not always follow the bite. Only about forty per cent of all animals bitten by a mad dog contract the disease. This is given by a noted authority. Statistics also show that in man the disease develops in only about twenty per cent of the cases in those who have been bitten by rabid dogs. But in dealing with those who have been bitten such measures should be taken as would be if they were certain of developing the disease; one cannot tell how much poison enters the system in such cases and preventive procedures should be taken. There are reasons why everyone who is bitten does not contract the disease.

The location and character of the bite must be considered. Bites on the head, neck and hands have been recognized as more dangerous, from early times, and such bites produce fatal results quicker than do bites on other parts of the body, and the reason is largely due to the fact that the other parts of the body are more or less protected by the clothing, and this clothing prevents the entrance of so much poison into the system. Bites on the head give a high mortality rate and are rapidly fatal. The close proximity to the brain is one reason.

The part the clothing plays in protection is clearly shown by the following quotation from an eminent authority: "In India where the natives dress very scantily, the mortality was exceedingly high up to a few years ago, at which time the British introduced the Pasteur laboratories. The clothing protects the body and it holds back the saliva and can be looked upon as a means of filtering the saliva of the rabid animal, most of the saliva is held back as the teeth pierce the clothing, so that upon entering the flesh the teeth are practically dry, and only a portion of the virus is introduced. Upon entering the wound this small amount of virus is further diluted by the tissue juices to the non-infectious point. We know from actual experimental work in the laboratory that the higher dilution will not kill."

If a portion of the brain of an animal dead from street virus is taken and made up in a dilution of one to five hundred, and this is injected, we find that it does not produce death. But a dilution of one to three hundred will invariably kill. This is practically what very often happens when one is bitten through the clothing. The saliva may be filtered and held back so that a small amount is introduced; perhaps a dilution of one to five hundred of the virus may get into the wound, but this is usually not enough to cause the disease. There is no possible way of estimating the amount of the inoculation. In such cases one's chances of never contracting the disease are only decreased; that is all we can say.

The treating of individuals, bitten by rabid animals, in the Pasteur Institutes, is simply the practical application of results obtained by Pasteur from his original work on rabies virus. Pasteur was a French chemist living in Paris, and he began his search for the cause and cure of rabies in 1880. He hoped to find a sure method of preventing the development of the dread disease, even if he could not find a cure for it after it had developed. While he was pursuing this research Pasteur had access to the cases of rabies in the Paris hospitals, and these numbered sixty each year. He had practically an unlimited supply, for France could furnish him with twenty-five hundred more mad dogs, and a large number of other animals each year.Pasteur devoted the remainder of his life to the study of this subject. He collected some saliva from the mouth of a child, on December 11, 1880, who had died at the Hospital Trousseau four hours before. This saliva he diluted with distilled water, and this mixture he injected into rabbits, and they all died, and the saliva taken from these rabbits when injected into other rabbits caused their death with rabies. He found also that saliva from rabid dogs almost always caused the disease. The incubation period varied within wide limits, and very often the animals lived. He then used the blood of rabid dogs for inoculation, but these blood inoculations always failed to produce the disease. Pasteur was convinced after careful study of rabid animals during the many months necessary to complete his experiments, that rabies was a disease of the nervous system, and that the poison (virus) was transmitted from the wound to the brain by the way of the nerve trunks. Then to prove his theory Pasteur removed a portion of the brain of a dog that had died of rabies. A part of this was rubbed up in sterile water and used to inoculate other animals; and subcutaneous inoculations with this material almost always produced death.

After this Pasteur tried a new method and injected directly into the nervous system, either into the nerve trunk or directly into the brain, after trephining, and all such injections produced rabies in the injected animal and death. He also found that rabbits inoculated in the brain always died in the same length of time. When he injected into the nerve trunk the inoculation period was longer, depending upon the distance from the brain. Two problems now remained for Pasteur to solve, and these were, how could he obtain the definite virulence and how could he reduce the virulence regularly and gradually, so that it could be used by inoculation safely as a vaccine to produce immunity to rabies in healthy animals, and also to prevent the development of rabies in animals bitten by rabid animals. He first tried successive inoculations. These inoculations were made, after trephining, directly to the brain, and he used a portion of the brain as a virus each time. He inoculated rabbit number one with a portion of brain taken from a rabid dog, and this rabbit died on the fifteenth day. He then inoculated rabbit number two with a portion of the brain of rabbit number one; from the brain of rabbit number two the virus was supplied for inoculating rabbit number three, and thus the brain of each inoculated rabbit was taken, after its death, for material to inoculate the next rabbit in the series. This experimentation showed him that each rabbit in the series died a little sooner, showing that the virus was becoming more virulent, till no increase in activity of the poison was shown after the fiftieth successive inoculation. "Rabbits inoculated with a brain suspension of rabbit number fifty all died in seven days." This caused Pasteur to name the virus of number fifty "virus fixe," a virus of definite length. He now had obtained a virus of definite strength and the next question was, how could the virulence be gradually and definitely reduced.

This he accomplished after many experiments. He proved that pieces of the "medulla oblongata" suspended in sterile tubes which contained fragments of caustic potash, steadily and gradually reduced their virulence as they dried, till the fourteenth day, when they were practically inert. New specimens were prepared each day and cords which had dried in one day Pasteur called "one-day virus;" cords which had dried in two days, "two day's virus," and so on up to the fourteenth day. With this graduated virus he now experimented on dogs, and the injection he used on the first day consisted of an emulsion of fourteen-day virus; for the second day, the thirteen-day virus, thus using a stronger virus each day, until on the fourteenth day he used the full strength virus. This treatment produced what is called immunity in the dog, and even the direct inoculation into the brain of the strong virus would not produce death.

After Pasteur had thoroughly satisfied himself by repeated trials, he announced his wonderful discovery, and it was in 1886 that Pasteur considered the preventive inoculation in human beings as resting upon a satisfactory experimental basis. During these five years this eminent man proved that it was possible to protect or immunize the lower animals, rabbits and dogs, against inoculation with the virulent virus.

The efficiency of this immunity was given trials by different methods of inoculation. It was found that sixty per cent of dogs inoculated under the "dura" (a membrane of the brain) were saved if treatment was given the second day. This test is more severe than is required to meet the ordinary infection of rabies. Pasteur, after a series of these final tests were so convincing, prescribed the preventive inoculations in human beings and on July 6th, 1886, the first human patient received the first treatment of his series of inoculations.

The method of obtaining the attenuated virus used in the treatment is as follows: A rabbit is inoculated by the brain method before described, each day, with suspension of the fresh, fixed virus. These rabbits die in six days after the inoculation. In this way a rabbit dies each day; the spinal cord is removed, divided into sections, and suspended in a flask containing potassium hydrate. The action of potassium hydrate is drying (desiccating). A series of these cords, which have been hung on fourteen successive days, are always kept in stock for the treatment of patients. The virus becomes less active with each successive day of exposure to drying (desiccation) and finally the virulence is altogether lost.

When the patient comes for treatment the fourteenth and thirteenth-day cords are used for the first inoculation, and on each successive day the patient receives inoculation, the strength of which has been regulated by the number of days the cord has been hanging. During the first four days patients receive injections of six cubic centimeters of emulsions made from cords aging from fourteen to seven days, and from the fifth day until the completion of the course of treatment patients receive emulsions from cords of higher immunizing properties, but no cords desiccated for less than four days are used.

Death rate from 1878-1883 before Pasteur treatment was instituted taken from documents in the department of the Seine:

1878	143 bitten.	24 deaths.
1879	76 "	12 "
1880	68 "	5 "
1881	156 "	22 "
1882	67 "	11 "
1883	45 "	6 "

Average of one death to every six bitten, or seventeen per cent mortality.

Incubation period from eleven days to thirteen months, average one hundred and twenty days, depending upon location of bite. Pasteur Institute records during the years 1886-1887 and first half of 1888, show that Pasteur had under his supervision 5,374 persons bitten by animals either proven or thought to have been mad. Mortality for 1886 was 1-34 per cent, during 1887 it was 1-12 per cent, during 1888 it was 77/100 per cent. With the later treatment the mortality has decreased to 3-10 per cent in 1908. The Pasteur method of treatment is a process of immunization which must be completed before the development of the disease. It is of no value after the symptoms have appeared.

Those who have not been affected can be immunized the same as those who have been bitten. The individual who has been bitten by a mad dog realizes when and how severely he has been bitten, and were it not for the so-called period of latent development of the virus, it would not be possible to carry out the Pasteur treatment. The patient may, if he will, take advantage of this fact and be immunized by treatment before the disease has developed. Deep and severe bites are most dangerous, but the disease may develop simply from a rabid dog licking a scratch of the skin. As before stated bites on exposed or uncovered surfaces, are more dangerous than those through clothing. There is a very easy access of the saliva to the wound in the unprotected part, while in the protected parts the teeth in passing through the protection, clothing, are freed of their saliva at least partially. The virus is conveyed from the bitten part or inoculation to the central nervous system through the nerve trunk, and the rapidity of extension depends upon the resistant powers of the patient, the virulence and the amount of virus deposited in the bitten part at the time the person was bitten. This disease develops only in nerve tissues. Virus can be found in the nerves of the side bitten, while the corresponding nerves on the opposite side are free from it. It can be ascertained that the virus is present in the medulla oblongata before the lower portion of the cord.

Comparative danger.--A wound of the hand after a delay of three weeks is as dangerous as a bite on the head exposed only a few days. There is always a possibility of an accumulative action and extension of the virus along the nerve trunk to the central nervous system during the interval of exposure, and this should be always borne in mind. It is stated by authority that the virus is not transmitted by the bite of a rabid animal until two days previous to the appearance of the first symptoms. It is with some difficulty that a decision is reached in advising patients who are bitten to take treatment early in the course of the disease. The symptoms are often so very obscure and slight that they are not recognized. If a dog which is not naturally vicious suddenly bites without any cause it should be tied securely and watched for seven days; and should it develop symptoms of the disease during this period the bite should be considered dangerous.

Immediate treatment of the wound.--A temporary measure is the cauterization of the wound; do not neglect this because a few hours have passed since the person was bitten, for wounds may be cauterized with advantage even after two or three days have elapsed. Of course the earlier it is done the better. If they are thoroughly laid open and scrubbed it is more effective. Nitric acid used freely is the best method to use. Wash the wound freely with boiled water after the acid has been applied; ninety-five per cent carbolic acid may be used if nitric acid cannot be obtained.

If carbolic acid is used it is necessary that it be washed from the wound by the free use of absolute alcohol, followed by boiled water and a dressing of bichloride of 1-7000. This prevents the ulceration of the wound by the carbolic acid. Cauterization thoroughly done destroys a part of the inoculated virus. Thorough cauterization is especially necessary with large wounds in which large quantities of the virus is inoculated.

When to send patients to an Institute.--Send them immediately, if there is good reason to believe the animal had rabies. It is not wise to wait until the animal dies; it is very important that treatment is begun as soon as possible, especially in severe bites.

What to send for examination.--The entire head may be sent by express, or better, the health officer should bring it in person. This saves time and relieves anxiety; or a portion of the brain may be removed under thoroughly clean conditions and placed in a sterilized twenty per cent solution of glycerin and water. In this way the virus retains its virulence and putrefaction is diminished. The first method is the best, taking the head directly. The head after it reaches the laboratory is examined microscopically for "negri bodies," and if there is no contamination the microscopic findings are verified by animal inoculations. The presence of negri bodies in a specimen is of great value owing to the rapidity with which a diagnosis can be made. In one case a positive diagnosis was reported within twenty minutes after the specimen entered the laboratory and within the next hour and a half the patient bitten by the dog the same day had begun her course of protective injections and was saved.

Protection.--To stamp out this disease city authorities, etc., can enact laws. All ownerless dogs should be killed, and the keeping of useless dogs should be discouraged by taxation. All dogs should be thoroughly muzzled where the disease prevails. This article is made up from an article written by an acknowledged authority on this disease, a man in charge of a Pasteur Institute.

Cities where Pasteur Institutes are located:

Ann Arbor, Michigan.
Chicago, Illinois.
Minnesota.
New York City.
Baltimore, Maryland.
Austin, Texas.
Toronto, Ont.

DISEASES OF THE BLOOD AND DUCTLESS GLANDS.

Anaemia, or Anemia.--This may be defined as a reduction of the amount of blood as a whole or of its corpuscles, or of certain of its more important constituents, such as albumin and haemoglobin. *Primary* or *essential* anemia includes chlorosis and pernicious anemia; secondary anemia results from hemorrhages, poor nourishment or intoxications, poisons. Chlorosis, a primary anemia chiefly of young girls, characterized by marked relative decrease of haemoglobin.

Causes.--It usually occurs in blondes of from twelve to twenty years of age and most often from fourteen to seventeen years of age, when the menstrual function is being established and during which time they are rushed with their school work. There may be a family history of chlorosis or tuberculosis. Poor food, hard, unhealthy work, confinement in close unventilated rooms are other causes.

Symptoms.--Rounded fleshy appearance may continue. There is some difficulty of breathing, palpitation of the heart on slight exertion, from a fright or from excitement, tendency to faint feeling or even fainting, headache, a tired feeling, hard to stir or do anything, irritable temper, poor or changeable appetite, the digestion is disturbed, there is constipation, coldness of the hands and feet, difficult menstruation, irregular menstruation, leucorrhea, amenorrhea, and sometimes there is a slight fever. The color is often of a yellowish-green tinge, and this is more noticeable in the brunette type, though the cheeks may be flushed; the whites of the eyes bluish white in color. The heart sounds are not right. The blood is pale in color. The red cells are diminished, but usually are not below eighty per cent of the normal;

the haemoglobin is greatly reduced, sometimes to thirty-five or forty per cent. The age, greenish tint of pallor, bluish whites of the eyes, poor nutrition, etc., aid in making the diagnosis.

Treatment.--Fresh air, good food, care of the bowels and rest if the symptoms are severe. When it is not so severe, plenty of outdoor exercise is necessary and beneficial. That takes them away from their cramped sedentary life and gives the sunshine, good pure air, and change of the scene. Horseback riding is a very good form of exercise, but it should be slow riding. "Tending" the horse is also good, and sleeping in the open air is excellent. Automobile riding is too straining and should not be indulged in.

1. Blaud's pills are very much used. The formula follows:

Dried Sulphate of Iron	2 drams
Carbonate of Potash	2 drams
Syrup	Sufficient

Mix thoroughly, and make forty-eight pills. Take

one to three pills, three times a day after meals.

2. Fowler's solution of arsenic is also very good remedy; three to four drops three times a day. It must be watched for bad symptoms and should only be taken under a physician's supervision.

Diet.--This should be good and varied to suit the special taste, and as the stomach and bowels are usually disordered such food should be chosen as will best agree. Diet plays a very important part.

PERNICIOUS ANAEMIA.--This is characterized by great decrease of the red cells of the blood with a relatively high color index and the presence of large number of germs. The causes are unknown.

Condition.--The body is not emaciated. A lemon color of the skin is usually present. The muscles are a dark red, but all the other organs are pale and fatty. The heart is large and fatty. The liver and spleen are normal in size, or only slightly enlarged with an excess of iron in the pigment. The red cells may fall to one-fifth or less of the normal number. The rich properties of the blood are fearfully decreased.

Symptoms.--Stomach and bowels, dyspepsia, nausea and vomiting, or constipation, may precede other symptoms or they may last throughout the case. The onset is gradual and unknown, with gradually increasing weary feeling, paleness and some difficulty in breathing and palpitation of the heart on exertion. There is paleness of the skin and the mucous membranes, the lips look pale, no color. The paleness becomes extreme, the skin often having a lemon yellow tint. The muscles are flabby; the ankles are swollen, you can see the arteries beat. Hemorrhages may occur into the skin, mucous membrane and retina of the eye. Nervous symptoms are not common. The pallor and weakness become extreme, sometimes with intervals of improvement and death usually occurs. The following is Addison's description given by Dr. Osler:

It makes its approach in so slow and insidious a manner that the patient can hardly fix a date to the earliest feeling of that languor which is shortly to become extreme. The countenance gets pale, and white of the eyes become pearly, the general frame flabby rather than wasted. The pulse perhaps larger, but remarkably soft and compressible, and occasionally with a slight jerk, especially under the slightest excitement. There is an increasing indisposition to exertion, with an uncomfortable feeling of faintness or breathlessness in attempting it; the heart is readily made to palpitate; the whole surface of the body presents a blanched, smooth and waxy appearance; the lips, gums and tongue seem bloodless, the flabbiness of the solid increases, the appetite fails, extreme languor and faintness supervene, breathlessness and palpitation are produced by the most trifling exertion, or emotion; some slight oedema (swelling) is probably perceived about the ankles; the debility becomes extreme. The patient can no longer rise from the bed; the mind occasionally wanders; he falls into a prostrate and half torpid state and at length expires; nevertheless, to the very last, and after a sickness of several months' duration, the bulkiness of the general frame and the obesity (fat) often present a most striking contrast to the failure and exhaustion observable in every other respect. The disease is usually fatal.

Treatment.--The patient should remain in bed and should use a light nourishing diet, taking food in small amounts and at stated intervals. Rest in bed is essential. Dr. Osler treated a case in the following way: I usually begin with three minims (drops) of Fowler's solution of arsenic three times a day and increase the dose to five drops at the end of the first week; to ten at the end of the second week; to fifteen at the end of the third week, and if necessary go up to twenty or twenty-five. Symptoms of an overdose are rare; vomiting and diarrhea occur. Then the medicine must be discontinued for a few days.

SECONDARY ANEMIA. Causes.--Hemorrhage form (bleeding). (a) Rapid bleeding from the rupture of an aneurism, from a blow, or eating into the blood vessels by an ulcer. **(b)** Slow bleeding as from nose-bleed, flow from the womb, piles or in "bleeders" people who bleed readily.

2. Inanition form.--Not nourished because of interference in taking food or assimilating food, from cancer of the gullet, or disease of the stomach.

3. Toxic poison cases; from acute and chronic diseases, such as typhoid fever, tuberculosis, rheumatism, syphilis, malaria, nephritis; or chronic lead poisoning, mercury, arsenic, and copper poisoning.

Symptoms.--There is pallor, dizziness, headache, palpitation and dyspnoea, difficult breathing on exertion; there is weakness, tendency to fainting, poor appetite, dyspepsia and constipation. The red blood cells are diminished, also the haemoglobin. Death may occur from a single hemorrhage.

Treatment.--Remove the cause and rest. Good fresh air, good easily digested food. The bowels must be kept regular. Iron and arsenic are good remedies if necessary. It is not possible to give special directions. A person in this condition needs a good physician. There is no time to waste. Iron and arsenic are good remedies, but they must be used intelligently and in proper doses. Blaud's pill is good in some cases. It contains iron. Also Fowler's solution of arsenic.

LEUKAEMIA.--An affection characterized by persistent increase in the white blood corpuscles, associated with changes, either alone or together, in the spleen, lymphatic glands and bone-marrow.

1. Spleen and Bone-Marrow, (Spleen-Medullary) type.--The changes are especially localized in the spleen and in the bone-marrow while the blood shows a great increase in elements which are derived especially from the latter tissue.

2. Lymphatic Type.--The changes in this type are chiefly localized in the lymphatic apparatus, the blood showing an especial increase in those elements derived from the lymph glands.

Causes--Unknown. It is most common before middle age.

Symptoms.--Either type may be acute or chronic. The invasion may be gradual, sometimes with disturbance of the stomach and bowels, or nose-bleed. (a) The first type is the common one. The spleen generally becomes enlarged; it is sometimes tender and painful, it may occupy over half of the abdominal cavity and varies in size after a hemorrhage, diarrhea or after a meal. There may be paleness of the face, etc., early and late nausea, vomiting, diarrhea, and dysentery are common, as is also ascites (dropsy in the abdomen). The pulse is rapid, full and soft. Fever is usual. Hemorrhages occur in the skin, retina, pleura, peritoneum, etc. Headache, dizziness, short breathing, and fainting may occur from the anemia. The liver may be enlarged. The blood shows a great increase in the white cells. Sometimes they are more numerous than the red blood cells. (b) Lymphatic type is rare, various groups of the lymph glands are enlarged, usually separate, but sometimes matted together; others, such as the tonsils may become large. The blood shows an increase of the white cells, but less than in the other form. The spleen is usually somewhat enlarged. Recovery is rare; the lymphatic cases may last only six or eight weeks. The course is usually progressive for two or three years.

Treatment.--The same as for Pernicious Anaemia.

FALSE LEUKAEMIA. (Pseudo-Leukaemia).--Also called Hodgkin's disease, malignant lymphoma, and general lymphadenoma. This is a progressive anemia and enlargement of the lymph glands and the skin, with secondary lymphoid growth in the liver, spleen and other organs.

Causes.--Males are more affected than females, and usually young persons. Continual local irritation causes a local enlargement of the gland, but the actual cause is unknown.**Symptoms.**--The lymph glands of the neck, arm-pit or groin are enlarged and without any pain, followed by anemia, loss of strength and slight fever. The glands enlarge slowly or rapidly, forming large masses, while the growth extends to other regions. The spleen may be felt; the skin may be bronzed. In cases with involvement of deep seated nodes the first symptoms may be those of pressure on blood vessels, nerves, trachea, bronchial tubes or other structures.

Treatment.--Cut them out if they are small and localized. Arsenic, quinine, cod-liver oil are good medicines.

PURPURA.--This is not strictly a disease, but a symptom. This includes a group of affections characterized by hemorrhages into the skin.

Symptoms.--There are hemorrhages into the skin, and this takes the form of small blood spots underneath the skin, (petechia) and spots like the bursting of a blood vessel shows vibices or ecchymoses. The first are in small minute points and appear, as a rule, in the hair follicles and unlike the erythemas (redness) do not disappear upon pressure. Another kind occurs as streaks, while the ecchymoses are larger, but similar in nature to the first kind. They may be larger than a split pea, and they range from a deep red to a livid bluish tint. They assume a yellowish brown, then a yellow color, as they fade away and finally disappear. This eruption appears in a series of crops and the legs are the usual seat.

1. Symptomatic Purpura. (a) Infectious. Occurs in typhus fever, endocarditis, cerebro-spinal meningitis, typhoid fever, etc. **(b) Toxic;** from snake bites, iodide of potash, quinine, copaiba, bella donna, ergot, etc., and with jaundice. **(c) Cachectic;** with cancer, tuberculosis, leukaemia, false leukaemia, scurvy, etc. **(d) Neurotic;** with hysteria, neuralgia, and some organic disease. **(e) Mechanical;** due to violent effort and poor venous circulation.

2. Type arthritic purpura. (a) Simple Purpura. A mild form usually occurring in children, sometimes with pains in the joints, rarely any fever. There is anemia, disturbance of the stomach and purpuric spots on the legs, often on the arms and trunks. **(b) Rheumatic purpura;** this usually occurs in men from twenty to forty years old. There is usually pain and swelling of several joints, temperature 101 to 103 degrees, purpuric eruption chiefly on the legs and about the affected joints, often with hives and digestive disturbances: **(c) Henoch's purpura;** usually in children and is sometimes fatal. There are recurrent joint pains and swelling, disturbances of the stomach and bowels, skin troubles resembling it, and hemorrhage from mucous membrane.

PURPURA HAEMORRHAGIC.--This is a severe form, usually seen in delicate girls. The cause is unknown.

Symptoms.--Weakness, extensive purpuric spots (small blood spots in the skin), eruption, hemorrhages from the mucous membranes which may cause secondary anemia, slight fever, slow clotting of the blood. The duration is from ten to fourteen days. Death may occur within a day in cases marked by profuse bleedings into the skin and prostration.

Treatment.--Remove the causes. Fresh air, food and tonics, etc. This disease is serious and needs careful treatment from a physician.

HAEMOPHILIA. "Bleeders."--This is a hereditary disorder characterized by a tendency to persistent bleeding, spontaneously or even after a slight injury.

Causes.--Usually hereditary through many generations. It is transmitted through daughters, themselves usually not "bleeders," to their male children. It is found most often in the Anglo-German races.

Condition.--The blood vessel walls are thin; the skin is delicate, clotting of the blood is usually retarded.

Symptoms.--It comes spontaneously or after only slight wounds; the person is extremely delicate. The bleedings occur from the skin, or mucous membrane, or from wounds, but rarely during menstruation or confinement. They vary from small spots to bleeding which may end fatally, or in recovery with marked anemia. There may be pain and swelling of the joints, etc., and this may leave deformities resembling deformed arthritis. The result is worse the earlier the disease shows itself. They may live to old age.

Treatment.--Avoid, as much as possible, wounds and operations in "bleeding" families. Marriage of the women should be discouraged. For bleeding: rest, ice, tannic or gallic acid or adrenalin locally if the bleeding points can be reached. Plug the nostrils for nose-bleed both behind and in front.

SCURVY. (Scorbutus).--A constitutional disease characterized by weakness, anemia, sponginess of the gums and tendencies to bleeding.

Causes.--This disease has been called "The calamity of sailors." It has been known from the earliest times, and has prevailed particularly in armies in the field and among sailors on long voyages. It has become a very rare disease in the United States.

Predisposing Causes.--Overcrowding; dark unhealthy rooms; prolonged fatigue; mental depression.

Exciting Cause.--The lack of fresh vegetables, poisoning from slightly tainted food, or an infection. The gums are swollen, sometimes ulcerated, skin is spotted, bluish, etc,

Symptoms.--It comes on gradually (insidiously). There is loss of weight, progressively developing weakness and pallor, very soon the gums are swollen and look spongy and bleed easily. The teeth may become loose and fall out. The breath is very foul. The tongue is swollen, but it may be red and not coated. The skin becomes dry and rough and (ecchymoses) dark spots soon appear, first on the legs, and then on the arm and trunk and particularly about the hair follicles. These are spontaneous or follow a slight injury. In severe cases hemorrhages under the periosteum (the covering of the bones) may cause irregular swelling, especially in the legs, and these may break down and form ulcers. The slightest bruise or injury causes hemorrhages into the injured part. Extravasion under the skin, especially in the lower extremities may be followed by permanent hardness (induration) and stiffness due to connective tissue infiltration (scurvy sclerosis). There may be pains in the joints and often watery swelling (oedema) of the ankles. Bleeding from internal mucous membranes is less common than from the skin. The appetite is poor, palpitation of the heart and feebleness and irregularity of the pulse are prominent symptoms. Owing to the sore gums the patient is unable to chew the food. The urine often contains albumin and is scanty and concentrated. There are weariness, depression, headache and finally delirium or coma, or symptoms due to hemorrhages within the brain; or day and night blindness may be present.

Recovery.--The patient will recover if the cause can be removed, unless it is far advanced. Death may result from complications.

Treatment. Preventive.--Fresh or canned vegetables or fruit must be eaten.

Treatment for the attack.--Dr. Osler, of England, says: "I think the juice of two or three lemons daily and a diet of plenty of meat and fresh vegetables will cure all cases unless they are far advanced. For the stomach small quantities of scraped meat and milk should be given at short intervals, and the lemon juice in gradually increasing quantities. As the patient gains in strength you can give a more liberal diet, and he may eat freely of potatoes, cabbage, water cresses, and lettuce. A bitter tonic may be given. Permanganate of potash or dilute carbolic acid forms the best mouth-wash. Penciling the swollen gums with a tolerably strong solution of nitrate of silver is very useful. Relieve the constipation by enemas."

ADDISON'S DISEASE. Diseases of the Suprarenal (above Kidneys) Bodies.--A constitutional disease characterized by great weakness, stomach and bowel symptoms, heart weakness, and dark coloring of the skin.

Causes.--It usually occurs in men from twenty to forty years old. The skin and mucous membrane and sometimes the serous, like the pleura, etc., membranes are pigmented (darkened).

Symptoms.--There is a gradual onset of weakness, changeable symptoms in the stomach and bowels and darkening of the skin. There is great feeling of fatigue and feeble irregular action of the heart; nausea and vomiting and often absence of appetite and some diarrhea. The abdomen may be painful and drawn back in the course of the disease. The pigmentation (coloring of the skin) varies from the light yellow to dark brown, olive or black. It usually begins on the skin or regions naturally pigmented; or where pressure is exerted by the clothing. The mucous membranes are also pigmented. Death may occur from fainting, extreme weakness, convulsions or delirium or through tuberculosis. Usually death occurs within one year, though this may occur in a few weeks to two years, sometimes after intervals of improvement.

Treatment.--This must be to meet the indications as they arise. It is a serious disease and should be under the supervision of a competent physician.

DISEASES OF THE SPLEEN. 1. Rupture of the spleen.--This may occur spontaneously from no apparent cause, or from hurts received in cases of typhoid or malaria.

Symptoms.--Severe pain, and signs of intestinal hemorrhages.

2. Acute inflammation of the spleen (splenitis).--This occurs in acute infections after injuries.

Symptoms.--They are pain, tenderness, and enlargement of the spleen.

Treatment.--Treat the cause and relieve the pain. As this is a serious and painful affection a physician should be called. The pain is often relieved by a mustard poultice or hot fomentations. The patient should remain in bed for acute inflammation of the spleen no matter what the cause.

3. Chronic Splenitis. Causes.--It comes from malaria, syphilis or leukaemia, etc.

Symptoms.--There is the feeling of weight and symptoms of pressure on the lungs or bowel.

Treatment.--Remove the cause. If it comes from malaria, attend to that, etc.

MOTHERS' REMEDIES. 1. Blood Purifier, Molasses and Sulphur as a.--"Take a pint of molasses to five cents' worth of sulphur, and mix well." A teaspoonful four times a day in the spring will do wonders towards purifying the blood.

2. Blood Purifier, Sassafras Tea, Known all over as.--"Sassafras tea made from the root and boiled to extract the strength." Drink freely of this for a few days in the spring. It thins the blood, and is a good tonic.

3. Blood Purifier, Herb Tea Used as.--

Burdock Root	2 ounces
Yellow Dock	2 ounces
Slippery Elm Bark	1 ounce
Mezeron Root	1 ounce
Licorice Juice	1 ounce

Simmer gently in three pints of water down to one quart; when cold, strain and add one-fourth ounce of iodine potassium." A wineglassful may be taken three times a day. This preparation is a fine blood purifier and can be relied upon.

4. Blood Purifier, Sweet Fern for.--"Make a tea of this and drink freely. This is very good to take in the spring of the year, as it thoroughly cleanses the system."

5. Blood Purifier, Doctor Recommends Senna and Salts for:-- "Five cents' worth of senna leaves, one tablespoonful of epsom salts in one quart of cold water; cover and let stand over night, then strain and put in bottles. Take a wine-glass full every morning until you feel well." This is from Mrs. Jonathan Shaw, she has used it with good results in her family. A physician in England told her if people would use this the year round they would seldom need a doctor.

6. Blood Purifier, Remedy Easy to Make for.--"We always use one teaspoonful of cream of tartar, two spoonfuls of sulphur, and mix with syrup. Any size spoon will do. Take a teaspoonful at a dose." This is an excellent remedy, and should be taken before retiring; about three times a week would be sufficient.

7. Blood Purifier, Beech Bark and Blackberry Root a Good.-- "One gallon white beech bark (after the rough bark is removed), good big handful of blackberry root (cut fine), and also of sassafras root. Cover with cold water and steep to get the strength, then strain. When cool (not cold) add one pint baker's yeast and one cup sugar. Let it stand twenty-four hours in a warm place. Then strain and set in a cool place. Take a wineglassful three times a day before meals. This has been highly recommended to me by a friend from Kalkaska, Michigan."

8. Blood Purifier, from a Madison, Connecticut, Mother.-- "Take blackberry root, black cherry bark, spruce boughs, wintergreens: sarsaparilla roots; steep in a large vessel, till all the goodness is out; strain and when lukewarm put in a cup of yeast, let work and bottle up."

9. Blood Purifier, How to make, Celery Compound for a.--

"Celery Compound	2 ounces
Chamomile Flower	1 ounce
Sassafras Root	1 ounce
Senna Leaves	1 ounce
Mandrake	1 ounce
Wintergreen Essence	1 ounce
Whisky	1 gill
White Sugar	1 pound
Hops	2 handfuls

Steep three hours in four quarts of water, strain, add sugar, when cold add wintergreen and whisky. Dose:--One teaspoonful before meals and at bedtime."

10. Blood Purifier, Another Effective Herb Remedy.--"Pour boiling hot water on four ounces of gentian root with two ounces of dried orange peel, a sufficient amount of water should be used to exhaust the strength in the root and orange peel; then boil in a porcelain pot until there is left one-half pint of the concentrated infusion to every ounce of gentian root used. Then to every one-half pint add one

17

half ounce alcohol. The effect of the alcohol is to coagulate it from a quantity of jelly looking substance which must be separated by straining. This is one of the best strengtheners of the human system. Dose:--One teaspoonful in an ounce of water."

11. Blood Purifier, Burdock for.--"The root is the part employed eliminating very rapidly the specific poison from the blood. Best administered in decoction by boiling two ounces of the root in three pints of water, to two pints. Dose:--One tablespoonful four times a day." Burdock is a splendid blood purifier and is not expensive. It can be purchased at any drug store for a reasonable amount.

DISEASES OF THE THYROID GLAND.--Inflammation of the thyroid gland, (Thyroiditis),--Acute inflammation of the gland, simple or suppurative. It may develop in a patient with goitre, or acute infectious diseases, or from other parts, or from wounds. The gland is enlarged and soft and may contain abscesses.

Symptoms.--Pain, tenderness, and enlargement of the part or of all the gland. Fever may be present even in cases without signs of pus forming (suppuration). If there is great enlargement, there may be symptoms of compression of vessel, nerves or the windpipe.

Treatment.--If there is pus it must be carefully opened. The patient must remain quiet in bed. Sometimes cold applications relieve. Do not use warm applications. This disease is not frequent and the patient needs care and watching more than medicine.

GOITRE (BRONCHIAL). Causes.--No satisfactory explanation can be given for this disease. It seems to be more prevalent where lime-stone water is used. Heredity plays a part. This is an enlargement of the thyroid gland. Chronic enlargement of the thyroid is sporadic. Cases are scattered and endemic in certain mountainous regions. It affects young women most often. A great excess in lime drinking water may be the cause. It is very prevalent about the eastern shore of Lake Ontario and in parts of Michigan. It is a common complaint in this country.

Symptoms.--There is a gradual painless enlargement of the whole gland or one lobe, etc. It may press on the windpipe, and cause difficult breathing, also on the blood vessels and nerves.

Recovery.--This is usually favorable as to life, but not so favorable as a cure. It becomes chronic. A sudden fatal ending may come.

GOITRE, MOTHERS' REMEDIES,--1. Three Ingredient Remedy for.--"The following treatment is excellent, but must be continued for several months:

Extract of Belladonna	1/2 dram
Compound Ointment Iodine	1/2 dram
Vaselin	1/2 ounce

Apply this to the affected parts several times a day." If this treatment is kept up faithfully it is sure to help.

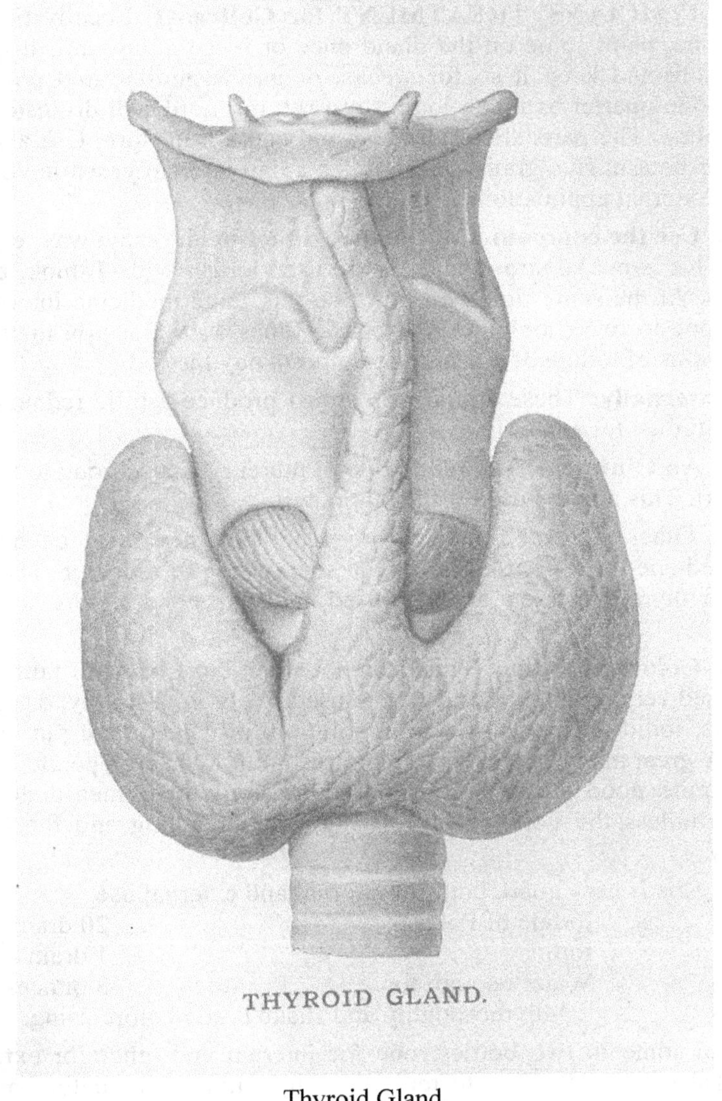
THYROID GLAND.

Thyroid Gland.

2. Goitre, Simple Remedy for.--"Wring a cloth from cold water and bind it around the neck every night when retiring. This is a sure cure if continued for some time."

3. Goitre, Inexpensive Remedy for--"Apply the following several times a day: Extract of belladonna one-half dram, compound ointment of iodine two drams; this treatment must be kept up several months." The above treatment will be found very beneficial and is not an expensive one.

PHYSICIANS' TREATMENT for Goitre.--1. Locally tincture of iodine; paint some on the gland once or twice a day until it gets a little sore and keep it so for weeks, or use cosmoline and put in it about one-quarter as much iodine and rub on. Lard will do instead of cosmoline. The parts should be kept red and a little sore. Use also iodide of potash, five grains, three times a day internally, while you are using external applications.

2. Use the compound of tincture of iodine the same way, externally. This is not so strong and can he used longer with, I think, better results. At the same time you may use this same medicine internally. Take one to two drops internally three times a day; or you may take five grains of iodide of potash three times a day instead.

Externally: These applications must produce a little redness and be continued for some time.

3. An Ointment. The red iodide of mercury is also good to rub on the part. This may be used if the others fail.

4. Other medical remedies are used, but they must be closely watched and must be used under the supervision of a doctor. The thymus or thyroid extracts are thus used and with good results in many cases.

5. Colorless Iodine: This does not stain, but I have no faith in it. It is used very much now and can be used freely. It is simply, druggists tell me, iodide of potash made in solution, dissolved, and put on the part. A great many cases of large goitres are now being operated upon with quite good success. It is not done until other measures have failed, unless the goitre is interfering with breathing and the blood supply.

6. This is very good, both for internal and external use.

Iodide of Potash	20 drams
Iodine	1 dram
Water enough for	3 ounces

Mix thoroughly and shake bottle before using.

Put some in two bottles; one for internal and other for external use. Take internally five to ten drops in a little water before meals. Externally, put on the enlarged neck, night and morning, unless it feels too sore, when you can use it once a day or less.

EXOPHTHALMIC GOITRE. (Parry's, Graves or Basedows Disease).--It is characterized by exophthalmos (bulging of the eyes), Goitre, fast beating of the heart, trembling and nervousness.

Causes.--It is most common in women from twenty to thirty. Several cases may occur in the same family. The exact cause is unknown.

Symptoms.--Acute cases. Sudden onset, vomiting, diarrhea, the heart beats fast with throbbing arteries, bulging of the eyes, enlarged thyroid gland. Death may occur in a few days.

Chronic Cases.--There is usually a gradual onset of tachy cardia,--fast beating of the heart,--pulse being 100 to 180 or more, if excited. Later there are throbbing of the arteries and of the thyroid glands.

Bulging of the eyeball is sometimes extreme. There may be fever and usually is anemia, emaciation, weakness, nervousness, perspiration, difficult breathing, dark color of the skin. It usually lasts several years. Spontaneous recovery may occur in six months to a year and is not common. Recovery is rare in advanced cases.

Treatment.--Prolonged rest in bed, with an ice bag constantly over the heart, or better over the lower part of the neck and upper breast bone. Avoid all worry and excitement. Drugs are uncertain. Surgery is sometimes resorted to. The thyroid extract has been used.

MYXOEDEMA.--This is a constitutional disease due to atrophy (wasting away) of the thyroid gland and characterized by swollen condition of the tissue under the skin, wasting of the thyroid and mental failures. Three forms exist, myxoedema proper, cretinism and operative myxoedcma.

Causes of Cretinism.--This may exist at birth (congenital) or it may develop at puberty, and is due to the absence or loss of function of the thyroid gland. Sporadic (here and there) cretinism may follow an acute infectious disease or it may be congenital. Myxoedema may be hereditary and is most common in women.

Symptoms, (a) Cretinism.--Mental and bodily development is slow. There is extraordinary disproportion between the different parts of the body. The condition is sometimes not recognized until the child is six or seven years old, then the slow development is noticed. The tongue looks large and hangs out of the mouth. The hair may be thin, the skin very dry. Usually by the end of the first year and during the second year the signs of the cretinism become very marked and should be recognized. The face looks large, looks bloated, the eyelids are puffy and swollen, the nose is flat and depressed and thick. Teething is late, and the teeth that do appear decay. The fontanelles are open. The abdomen is swollen, the legs are short and thick, the hands and feet are not developed and look pudgy. The face is pale and has a waxy, sallow tint. The muscles are weak and the child cannot support itself. Above the collar bone there are pads of fat. The child does not develop mentally and there may be one of the grades of idiocy and imbecility (feeble-minded).

(b) Myxoedema, proper--The skin is infiltrated, causing loss of the lines of the facial expression, skin is dry and harsh, much thickened, especially in the region above the collar bone. The face is broad, with coarse features, the nose is broad and thick, the mouth is large, lips thick, hair scanty and coarse, slowness of motion and thought, weak memory, irritability, headache, suspiciousness, followed sometimes by hallucinations, delusion and dementia (insane). The disease may progress for ten or fifteen years. Death may occur early.

Operative type.--This rarely develops except the thyroid glands have been entirely removed and then only if no extra glands are present.

Symptoms.--Are the same as that of cretinism.

Treatment.--An even, warm climate. Thyroid extract, to be given by a physician, is the remedy. After the recovery occasional small doses still may be necessary for some, or in cretinism for life.

DISEASES OF THE NERVOUS SYSTEM.

NEURALGIA.--Pain occurring in the course of the nerves and in their area of distribution. The pain has remission and intermissions, and is due to some morbid affection of the nerves of sensation or their spinal or (brain) centers.

Causes.--The affection may depend upon some functional disturbance alone; or it may be due to some organic disease of the nerve or to some disease or diseased state outside of the nervous system. It occurs more frequently in women past the middle-age, in those of a nervous tendency. As stated, it affects women more than men. Debility is a frequent cause. Neuralgia is frequently associated with the various forms of anemia. It may occur at the onset of acute diseases like typhoid fever. Exposure to cold causes it in susceptible persons. Decayed teeth may cause neuralgia of the fifth nerve. It also occurs in rheumatism, gout, lead poisoning, and diabetes. Persistent neuralgia may be a feature of hidden Bright's disease.

Symptoms.--Pain is the chief and characteristic symptom. It may develop suddenly and without warning, or soreness or stiffness in the tissues surrounding may precede it. There is a burning or violent sensation in the course of the affected nerve, increased on exertion in acute cases. In other cases the pain comes intermittently or in paroxysms, and is of a darting, stabbing character, or accompanied by tingling sensations. There may be a want of sensation of the skin in the affected region or over-sensitiveness over the entire nerve-trunk with certain painful points. The attacks of pain may come only at long intervals of time, but usually they occur every few minutes and last for some hours. Pain may be continued for hours or days in severe cases. In rare cases it may persist for months or years, being worse at a certain time each day, especially in cases where malaria exists. There is paleness or congestion of the part affected, various

eruptions, and changes in the color of the hair occur and, in advanced chronic cases, symptoms of interference with the general nutrition also occur. Spasms of the adjacent muscles may accompany the severe paroxysms.

Varieties.--Neuralgia may be classified according to its causes, as neurotic, toxic, rheumatic, etc.; or according to its location as trifacial, intercostal, sciatic, and so on, Exposure to cold, mechanical irritations, tumors, pressure on the nerves, and wounds may lead to neuralgia. It is more frequent in cold and damp climates than in dry and warm locations; everyone should remember the causes.

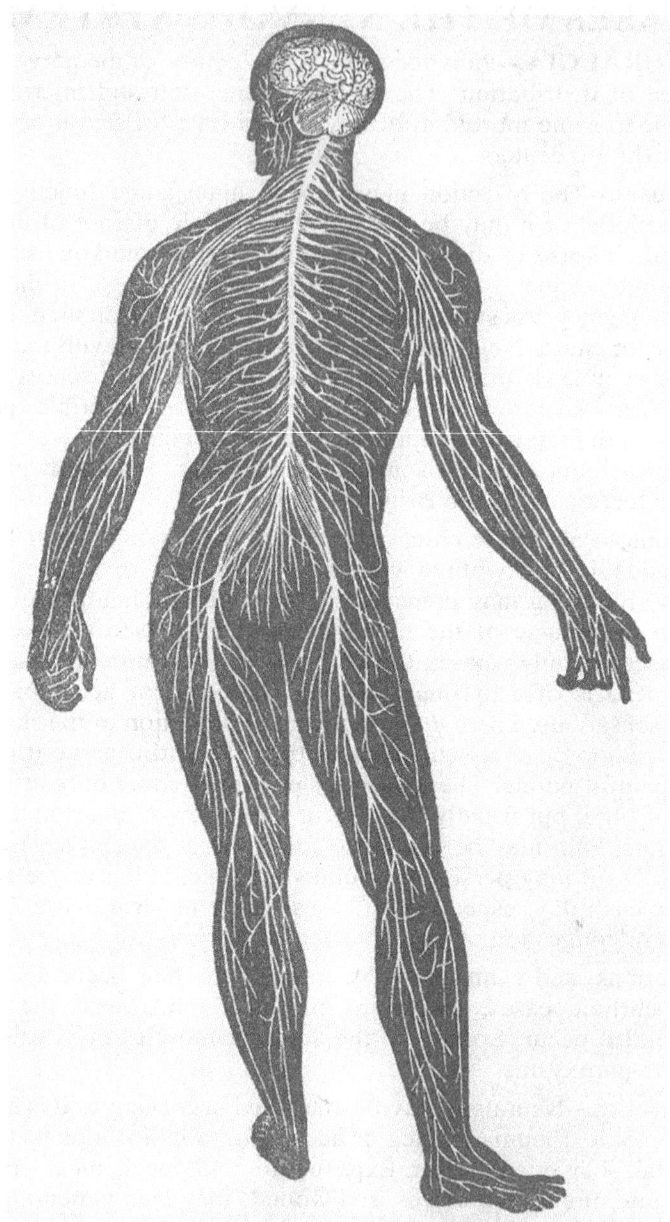
The Nervous System.

MOTHERS' REMEDIES. Neuralgia.--1. Lemon Juice as Liniment for.--"Cut a lemon in two and squeeze juice on parts afflicted and rub in, then place hot cloths over it. I know this will cure the pain." This is very good.

2. Neuralgia, Salt and Vinegar Will Relieve.--"A small sack of hot salt applied to the pain, or steam with vinegar." The heat from the salt is very effective and the moisture of the vinegar is also very good. This simply produces a counter irritation.

3. Neuralgia, Quinine Will Cure.--"Use quinine three times a day." It is well in taking quinine to take two grains three times a day for two days, then take some good cathartic, so as not allow the quinine to remain in the system. This is very beneficial, especially when neuralgia is due to malarial conditions.

4. Neuralgia, Four Ingredient Remedy for.--

"Oil of Peppermint	1 ounce
Oil of Mustard (strong)	1/4 ounce
Vinegar	1 pint
White of one egg.	

Beat egg and stir all together."

5. Neuralgia, Good Liniment for.--

"Essential Oil of Mustard	1 dram
Tincture Aconite	1 dram
Glycerin	1 ounce
Alcohol	4 ounces

Mix and shake well before using."

This remedy is a valuable external preparation for all nervous and neuralgia pains, rub twice a day until relieved.

6. Neuralgia, Menthol Liniment for.--"One dram of menthol liniment, two ounces of alcohol. This makes a very excellent liniment for many purposes. For rheumatism, neuralgia, headache, etc." This liniment will be found very beneficial as the menthol is soothing and quieting, and we all know that alcohol is very good to be applied for any of the above mentioned diseases.

7. Neuralgia, Belladonna Plaster for.--"Melt three ounces of rosin plaster and add one-half ounce of extract of belladonna. An excellent application in neuralgia and rheumatism."

PHYSICIANS' GENERAL TREATMENT for Neuralgia.--Remove the cause if possible. If from anemia, give tonics for that and try to cure that disease. Tonics with good nourishing food, and proper surroundings are needed for anemia. In malaria, syphilitic or gouty patients, constitutional treatment must be given for those diseases before the neuralgia will be better. The systematic use of galvanic electricity, properly used, is the most valuable means at the physician's disposal, especially in the descending current, beginning with the mild current and gradually increasing in strength. Internally: Arsenic, bromine, ergotinc, aconite, gelsemium, valerian, ether, cannabis indica and quinine are recommended. Opium may be used in the very severe forms, but it must be used with caution, or you will make your patient a drug fiend, and his latter state will be worse than the first condition. Wet compresses, vapor baths, cold affusions, wet cloths, are highly recommended.

1. For the Cure of an Attack--

Antipyrine 30 grains
Citrate of Caffeine 20 grains

Make into ten powders. Take one everyone-half hour until 3 doses are taken. Three (3) doses at least should relieve the neuralgia.

2. Antipyrine 30 to 60 grams

Bromide of Potash 3 drams

Mix: and make into ten powders; one every thirty minutes until relieved or until six doses have been taken; this is better than the first prescription when there is much nervousness with the neuralgia or neuralgic headaches.

3. If caffeine in first prescription causes nervousness, give this one:

Antipyrine 30 to 60 grains

Citrate of Caffeine 10 grains
Bromide of Potash 3 drams

Mix and make ten powders. Take one every half hour until relieved or until six doses have been used.

These are very effective prescriptions, but if a person has any heart trouble I would not advise their use except under a physician's care. (Sometimes a patient with neuralgia gets desperate, and he will even resort to morphine). Antipyrine is one of the simplest coal tar remedies, and most persons can safely take it. Persons who are subject to neuralgia or headaches need to take good care of themselves. Get plenty of rest and sleep. Neuralgia at first can be cured, but when it once becomes chronic, especially neuralgia of the face, it is hard to cure and frequently makes life a constant misery. Plenty of outdoor life is essential. In that way the system will be built up, and when the body is strong the disease can be thrown off much easier. A great many people depend too much upon strong medicines. Medicines are all right in their place, but all the medicine in the world cannot cure a person unless that person does his or her part.

SPECIAL DISEASES. Facial Neuralgia. (Neuralgia of the fifth pair of Cranial Nerves. Also known as Trifacial Neuralgia. Neuralgia of the Trigeminus. Tic doloureux, etc.).--This form is more frequent than all other forms combined, this nerve being peculiarly susceptible to functional and organic disorders. All three branches are very rarely affected together, the ophthalmic (eye) branch being most often involved. The symptoms depend upon the branch involved.

1. Ophthalmic Neuralgia Pain, (eye neuralgia pain).--This pain is above the eye, or frontal kind, with a special painful point at the supraorbital (above the eye) notch. Sometimes the pain is very severe in the eye-ball.

2. Supramaxillary Neuralgia.--In this the pain is along the infraorbital (nerve beneath the eye) nerve, and there is a marked tender point at the opening in the bone (infraorbital foramen) beneath the eye. A toothache-like pain in the upper teeth is common in this variety.

3. Inframaxillary (lower maxillary) Neuralgia.--This is characterized by a scattered (diffused) pain along the inferior dental (teeth) branch, and extends from the temporal (side forehead) region over the side of the face to the chin, with pain in the lower teeth and side of the tongue. The pain in this nerve may come on without any special cause, or it may come after excitement of a physical or mental nature. Disorders of nutrition occur. The circulation is interfered with and the face, at first pale, becomes red. Eruptions may appear along the course of the nerve, while salivation and "running" (lachrymation) of the eyes are often prominent symptoms. Spasms of muscles of the face (tic doloureux) may accompany the paroxysms and this is the most terrible form of nerve pain. The attacks may be mild or very severe and sometimes sudden. This is a terrible disease, especially when it has existed for some time. A person with severe pain in the face should always attend to it immediately, before it becomes chronic.

Treatment.--It is directed towards removing the cause, if possible. Chronic cases are difficult to cure. The patient should be careful not to take cold, keep strong and healthy by regular hours for sleep, good sufficient clothing. The general health must be improved. These directions apply to all kinds of neuralgia.

INTERCOSTAL NEURALGIA.--A neuralgia of one or more of the intercostal nerves. These nerves run in a groove in the lower edge of the ribs.

Causes.--It may develop without any special cause. It comes in anemia, after exposure to cold, from affection of the vertebrae, ribs, spinal cord, or from the pressure of tumors, or aneurism of the aorta. This is next in importance to neuralgia of the fifth nerve, and occurs more often in women and very common in those who have hysteria. It is more common on the left side and mostly in the nerves situated from the fifth to the ninth intercostal space. If it is located in the nerves distributed to the mammary glands it gives rise to neuralgia of the mammary gland. The flying darts of pain in the chest (pleurodynia) are to be regarded as neuralgic in character.

Symptoms.--The pain is usually very severe, especially on movement of the intercostal (between the ribs) muscles. With this pain, as a rule, an eruption (herpes) appears along the course of the affected nerve and this is supposed to be due to the extension of the inflammation from the nerve-ends to the skin. Pain, when pressed upon, is most marked near the spinal vertebral, the breastbone (sternal) end and the middle part of the nerve. The trouble may continue a long time after the eruption (herpes) has disappeared, for it is very obstinate.

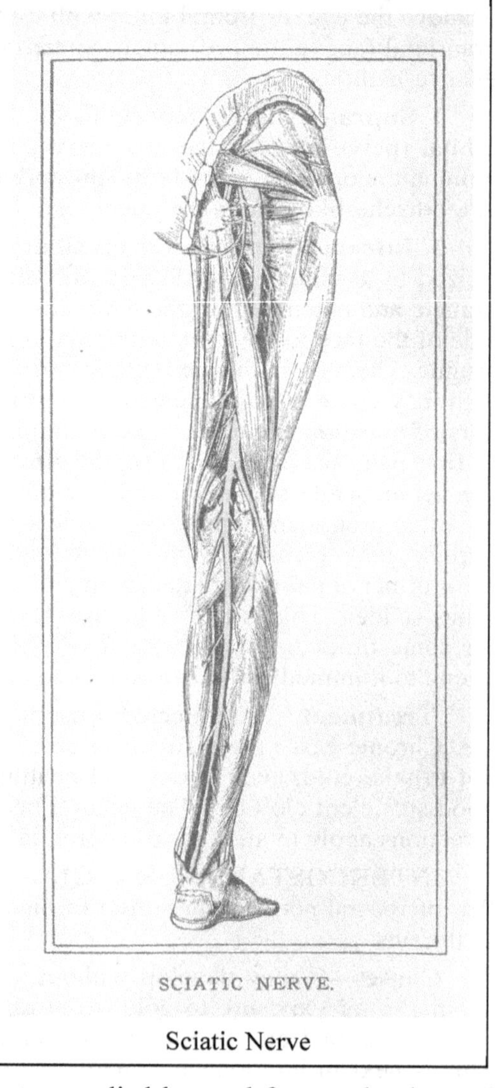
SCIATIC NERVE.

Sciatic Nerve

PHYSICIANS' TREATMENT for Intercostal Neuralgia.--This consists in using remedies that will cause counter-irritation. Electricity and pain destroying (anodynes) remedies are indicated in chronic cases. Apply heat for pain in the "breasts." For the eruption an ointment like oxide of zinc can be used.

Local Treatment.--A mustard plaster is frequently good to use. It produces the counter-irritation desired. Application of dry heat from hot cloths; a hot sand bag may help in some cases. A rubber bag containing hot water can also be used. Fomentations of hops, etc., applied hot and frequently changed to keep them hot are beneficial in some cases. I have found in some cases that an adhesive plaster put over the sore parts relieves the severe pain. Porous plasters are also good. Tincture of ranunculus bulbosus (buttercup) is a good remedy. Put ten drops in a glass half full of water, and take two teaspoonfuls every hour.

SCIATICA.--This is as a rule a neuritis of the sciatic nerve or of its cords of origin. It is characterized by pain chiefly along the course of the sciatic nerve.

Causes.--It occurs most commonly in adult males. The person may have a history of rheumatism or gout in many cases. Exposure to cold after heavy muscular work or exertion, or a severe wetting are common causes. The nerves in the pelvis may be compressed by large tumors of the ovaries or womb, by other tumors, or by the child's head during confinement. Occasionally hip joint disease causes it. The nerve, as a rule, is swollen, reddened, and in a condition of "interstitial neuritis." The pain may be most severe where the nerves emerge from the hip bone, behind, or in the inner back, and middle part of the thigh.

Symptoms.--Pain is the most constant and troublesome. It is sometimes very severe. The onset is usually gradual, and for a time there is only a slight pain in the back of the thigh; soon the pain becomes more intense, extends down the thighs, and leg and reaches to different parts of the foot. The very sensitive spots can often be pointed out by the patient, and on pressure these spots are very painful. It is gnawing and burning in character, usually constant, but sometimes it comes in paroxysms, and is often worse at night. Walking usually causes great pain. The knee is bent and the patient treads on his toes. As a rule it is an obstinate trouble, and it may last for months, or even with slight remissions for years. In the severer forms the patient must remain in bed and such cases are very trying for both patient and doctor.

(See **Mothers' Remedies** under Neuralgia above).

PHYSICIANS' TREATMENT. Cautions for Sciatica.--Remove all causes if you can. Rheumatism and gout, if the patient have them, should be treated. The patient should not overwork or expose himself to wet, damp weather. Keep every part dry. Rest in bed with the whole leg fixed is a valuable mode of treatment in many cases. Hot water bags from the hip to the knee placed along the painful nerve, sometimes gives great relief. Mud baths are beneficial. Hot Springs baths relieve many cases. Fly blisters placed along the track of the nerve relieve the pain in many cases. Fomentations of smartweed and hops are good, but they must be changed often so as to be hot. Wet or dry cupping is a help in many cases. It draws the blood from the inflamed nerve. Morphine given hypodermically will relieve the pain, but it is a dangerous medicine to use in a chronic case. The patient will be very likely to form the habit, and that is worse than the sciatica. By care and treatment most cases can be greatly helped and cured. Rhus tox (poison ivy) is very good in minute doses in cases where it is impossible to remain in one position for any length of time. Ten drops of the tincture in a glass two-thirds full of water and two teaspoonfuls given every hour. I have helped many cases with this remedy. The hot iron along the track of the nerve is helpful. Electricity is better in a chronic case where there is wasting of the legs, and it should be combined with massage. The galvanic current should be used.

MOTHERS' REMEDIES. Nervousness. 1. Catnip Tea for.--"A tea made of catnip will quiet the nerves. This is good for women when they are apt to be nervous."

2. Nervousness, Hops Will Stop.--"Purchase a small package of hops at any drug store, and make a tea of it, drinking frequently in tablespoonful doses." It is a harmless remedy, and should be used more freely by nervous people. The hops are very soothing. Nervous mothers should never be without this. It is surprising to see how few people know the value of some of these simple home remedies.

3. Nervousness, Effective Remedy for.--

"Spirits of Camphor	1/2 ounce
Comp. Spirits of Lavender	1/2 ounce
Tincture of Valerian	1 ounce
Sulphuric Ether	1/2 ounce

Mix. Dose, one or two teaspoonfuls every three hours."

The foregoing remedy is very effective, as spirits of camphor and the tincture valerian quiet the nerves. The sulphuric ether also has a soothing effect. This combination makes a fine tonic, but should not be taken too long, as it is quite strong.

4. Nervousness, Five Ingredient Remedy That Relieves.--"In extreme nervous debility with tendency to fainting fits, use the following:

Spirits of Camphor	1/2 ounce
Aromatic Spirits of Ammonia	1/2 ounce
Spirits of Lavender Compound	1 ounce
Tincture Valerian	1 ounce
Tincture Castor	1 ounce

Mix. Dose.--From one to three teaspoonfuls at intervals of from fifteen minutes to three hours, according to urgency of symptoms. This mixture should be kept on hand by all persons subject to fainting fits."

Spirits of camphor and aromatic spirits of ammonia stimulates the heart, while the tincture of valerian quiets the nervous system.

5. Nervousness, "Lady's Slippers" Breaks up.--"A decoction is made with two ounces of the root, sliced, to two pints of water, boiled to one and one-half pints. Dose: One tablespoonful four times a day. Has been used with marked success in epilepsy and in other various nervous diseases." This is used very extensively for nervous people, and has proven very successful.

HEADACHE.--This term means a pain in the head, all over the head, or at one particular spot. It may be only a symptom of a general constitutional derangement, some disease of some other organ, a temporary inability of some organ like the stomach, liver, bowels, etc., to do work, or it may be due to some local affection depending upon some trouble with the skull and its contents. It is frequently but a symptom of some other trouble. It occurs in fevers, infectious diseases, brain disease, etc. There are different varieties depending upon the causes.

Sick Headache.

Nervous Headache.

Catarrhal Headache.

Congestive Headache.

Neuralgic or Gastric (stomach) Headache.

Bilious Headache.

"Bowel" Headache.

"Womb" Headache.

Rheumatic Headache.

CATARRHAL HEADACHE and RHEUMATIC HEADACHE may be treated together. This is due to exposure to a draught of air, walking against the sharp and keen wind, by getting the feet or other parts of the body wet, sudden suppression of perspiration about the head, or by some other exposure such as might result from cold, influenza or attack of rheumatism. There may be aching pains and a feeling of heavy weight in the forehead; tearing, stitching pains above the eyes, in the cheek bones; sometimes the skull feels as if it would fall to pieces. In the rheumatic variety the scalp is sore and tender, tearing throbbing pains or hard aching pains. There is some fever, dry skin, the pulse is faster.

Treatment.--Get into a sweat by hot drinks of lemonade and hot foot baths. Apply cold or warmth to the head, lie down and keep quiet.

Medicine.--Aconite in doses of one-tenth of a drop to an adult every hour will frequently abort it: open the bowels with salts. Remain in bed.

NERVOUS HEADACHE.--This may occur as a sick headache or be simply a nervous headache: This occurs oftenest in a nervous person, or in persons who are run down by different causes, such as diseases, overwork, worry, trouble, etc. It is not periodic, and has no fixed type, but breaks out at indefinite intervals, and is excited by almost any special cause such as motions, mental exertions, menses, excitement, overdoing, over-visiting, want of sleep. It is often due to eye strain in persons who have poorly fitted, or who do not wear glasses. It appears in any part of the head, usually one-sided, or it may be all over the head, which feels enlarged and sometimes as if a band was around it. The least mental effort makes it worse. Sometimes there is a feeling as if a nail was being driven into the head; head is too big; eyes feel heavy and the lids droop; sees double; hard to keep eyes open. This kind of headache, or sick-headache, can be brought on suddenly by womb trouble, especially if the womb has fallen from a jar, fall, etc. The patient often moans and cries, laments and simply cannot stand thc pain. In some cases the menses cause it, and it appears at every menstrual period.

Treatment.--The patient should be quiet and remain in bed in a darkish room. Womb troubles and other diseases that cause it such as protruding piles, etc., should be attended to. Tincture gelsemium is a good remedy. Put ten drops in a glass half full of water, and take two teaspoonfuls every half hour until better. A tea made from lady's slipper is also effective in some cases, used freely. Bromide of potash in ten-grain doses one-half hour apart, for three doses, if necessary, is quieting in many attacks. Mustard plaster to back of the neck.

CONGESTIVE HEADACHE.--In this kind there is or seems to be too much blood in the head. The patient may be stupid, with a flushed face. If conscious, the brain feels as if it was rising or falling, especially upon the motion of the head. The top of the head sometimes feels as if it would fly off. The head throbs and beats violently. The hands and feet may be cold, the face flushed or pale, the eyes bright, the pulse is generally heavy, full and fast, or it may be feeble, slow and intermittent.

Treatment.--1. The patient should remain in bed in a dark room, with the head usually high. Cold should be applied to the head and heat to the hands and feet. Move the bowels with salts and, if necessary, give an enema also. It is well to give the foot-bath before going to bed. If these things do not relieve the headache a doctor should be called, for it may mean something serious. A hot mustard foot-bath and a mustard plaster applied to the nape of the neck are of great value. In severe cases an ice bag or very cold water, applied to the forehead and temples will very often give great relief.

2.	Spirits of Camphor	1 ounce
	Spirits of Lavender	2 ounces
	Alcohol	2 ounces

Wet the top of the head with it.

3.	Camphor	1 dram
	Oil of Peppermint	1 dram
	Chloroform	1-1/2 ounces
	Alcohol enough for	3 ounces

Shake the bottle and apply a little of the liquid to the place. Horseback riding and walking are good for nervous girls and women.

NEURALGIC HEADACHE.--This commonly comes periodically, usually, one-sided. It may occur at the same hour for several days in succession. The pains are of all kinds. It may start in the morning or at any time. It involves more especially the eyes, side of the head, face, and goes into the teeth and neck. It comes in persons subject to neuritis in other parts or neuralgia.

Treatment.--Build up the system with tonics in the interval. Lead a quiet restful life. Acetanilid in five-grain doses frequently relieves it. This is a dangerous medicine to use, except under a doctor's supervision. Spigelia in doses of one-twelfth of a drop of the tincture is good for left-sided attacks; two doses are enough, one-half hour apart.

STOMACH OR GASTRIC HEADACHE.--This, as the name indicates, is due to some acute or chronic trouble with the stomach. It is caused by over-loading the stomach, or eating food that does not agree, such as fat meat, gravies, starchy food, warm bread, pastry, etc., or it may be due to dyspepsia. The tongue is generally coated, the mouth tastes bitter. If it is acute and the stomach is full, take a common emetic like warm water, salt water or mustard water. If it is due to decomposed food, drink lots of warm water and take an enema and also a dose of salts. If there is much gas in the stomach, take some baking soda in a glass of warm water; one drop doses of tincture of nux vomica every half hour for three hours often relieves.

HEADACHE FROM CONSTIPATION.--This is frequent. There is generally a dull, heavy feeling in the forehead, the head feels full and sometimes dizzy, the patient feels blue and morose, the tongue is coated on its back part, mouth tastes bitter, patient is drowsy and stupid and work goes hard. A free passage from the bowels relieves the headache.

Treatment.--Cure the constipation as directed in another part of the book. Take a good full enema of warm soap suds and water, and one drop of tincture of nux vomica every hour for six hours during the attack.

BILIOUS HEADACHE.--This is so-called because the bilious symptoms are the most prominent. It may be caused by violent anger, disputes, excessive eating causing congestion of the liver; abuse of spirits; some persons are of a bilious constitution and the least error in diet and habit produces such an attack. The pain may be violent or dull, the head may throb terribly; the whites of the eyes have a yellowish look, and the face may be of a dark brown hue, the patient may vomit bile. The vomiting causes more brain distress. The mouth is bitter, the tongue coated yellowish, the breath smells badly. Bowels may be irregular.

Treatment.--A free movement of the bowels often relieves. First take an enema and then one-half ounce of epsom salts. Do not eat anything but drink all the water you may wish. A tea made of blue flag is often of benefit. The diet should be regulated so as not to overload the stomach and liver and the bowels should move freely daily.

WOMB HEADACHE.--Women who suffer from womb troubles such as leucorrhea, torn cervix, falling womb displacements and diseases of the inner womb, ovaries and tubes, suffer from all kinds of headache. The pain may be in the nape of the neck, the back part of the head and on the top behind (occiput). It may come on suddenly when the womb is displaced by a sudden fall or over-lifting, etc. The woman should then go to bed and lie down with her arms crossed over her chest, with the knees drawn up and weight resting upon them and chest with the buttocks elevated, (knee-chest-position). This replaces the womb. The other troubles should be corrected or these headaches will keep on. The womb and its appendages are the cause of many kinds of headaches, neuralgias, dyspepsia, and constipation; correct the troubles and the headache will disappear.

MENSTRUAL HEADACHES.--These are very common. They may be regular every month, and they are then caused by some trouble with the womb or ovaries, or may be due to a run-down condition or heredity. It comes sometimes from suppression of the menses as a consequence of some violent emotion, fright, anger, grief, or by exposure to wet, draughts of air, privations, over-fatigue, etc. It may last for several days. The headache may be mild or severe.

Treatment.--A foot bath or sitz bath is very good, with free drinking of pennyroyal tea after the bath, and when in bed. Place warmth to the feet, moist heat over the abdomen, such as a hot water bag or fomentations. Remain quietly in bed. If constipated, take an enema. Frequently a free bowel movement gives much relief in this trouble. During the interval doctor the patient for the trouble causing the headache for which see another part of this book, "Diseases of Women."

MOTHERS' REMEDIES, 1. Headache, Paregoric and Soda for.--"A teaspoonful of paregoric, with one-half teaspoonful of baking soda in a tumbler of water, May be taken all at once or sipped slowly."

2. Headache, Hops Good for.--"Make a strong decoction of hop tea, and take a wineglassful every half hour until relieved." This is an old tried remedy and a good one.

3. Headache, Mustard Excellent for.--"Place a mustard plaster on the back of the head, also bathe the feet in mustard water and stay in a darkened room, and avoid all excitement and noise." The one essential thing is to get the nerves quieted; take as little food as possible for twenty-four hours, giving the stomach an opportunity to rest, as most of the headaches come from a disordered stomach.

4. Headache, Peppermint Beneficial for,--"Bathe the head in strong peppermint. Then apply cloths wrung from water as hot as can be endured." Hot or cold applications are known to be very beneficial. After the cloths are taken off, the soothing effect can be further enhanced by gentle rubbing of the forehead.

5. Headache, Cold Application in Case of.--"Apply cold applications on the forehead and over the eyes." These cold applications have been known to give relief in a very few minutes to many people suffering with severe headaches. It is well to continue the treatment; even after relief has been obtained, for at least a half hour. Gentle rubbing of the head is very good, also.

6. Headache, Castor Oil Will Relieve.--"One tablespoonful of castor oil. Have used this and found relief." This remedy gives relief as the castor oil carries off the food that is distressing the stomach. It is well to take two tablespoonfuls of lime-water in a glass of milk three times a day for about a week after the castor oil has operated.

SICK HEADACHE. (Migraine. Hemicrania).--Migraine is a peculiar form of severe paroxysms of unilateral (one side) headache often associated with disorders of sight.

Causes.--It is frequently hereditary, and it has occurred through several generations. Women and members of nervous families are usually attacked. Many of the headaches from eye-strain are of this type, It is often inherited, and may last from puberty to the menopause. Some authors claim that decay of the teeth without toothache will cause it. Adenoid growths in the pharynx and particularly abnormal conditions of the nose will cause it. Many of the attacks of severe headaches in children are of this nature, and the eyes, nose and throat should be examined when children or older persons suffer from this complaint. Mental emotion, physical or mental fatigue, disorders of the female genital organs, eye-strain, etc., loud noises, toothache, act as predisposing causes. Some think it a poisonous condition due to the absorption of poisons from the stomach and intestines, and others regard it as a nervous condition due to anemia and all conditions which weaken the resistance of the nervous system.

Symptoms.--The premonitory symptoms, which may last a few hours or a day or more, are sleepy feelings of discomfort, uneasiness, weariness, chills, vertigo (dizziness), disturbance of the sight or disturbances of the senses. The real attack may follow quickly, beginning with the characteristic headache, at first one sided, located in one spot in the temple, eye or back of the head, but spreading, as it increases in severity, until it involves all of one side of the head and occasionally both sides. The pain is usually constant and of great severity and it is increased by motion, noises, light, or mental strain. The skin over the painful part is very sensitive. There are loss of appetite, nausea and vomiting. If the stomach has a great deal of food in it, vomiting relieves the pain sometimes. In the spasmodic form the affected side is painful, the skin is cool, the pupil is dilated, and the flow of saliva is increased. In the paralytic form the affected side is flushed, hot, the vessels are dilated and the pupils are contracted. There is great weakness, prostration and depression. The urine may be abundant or suppressed, temporarily. The results of treatment in this disease are uncertain, as the attacks are likely to occur in spite of treatment. They usually cease in old age, and in women they may stop after the menopause. The attacks in women are likely to occur at or near the menstrual periods.

First Thing to do in Sick Headache.--It is well to remain in a darkened room away from noise, etc. If the head throbs and beats very hard, either a cold ice bag or hot applications often bring relief. A mustard plaster at the base of the brain with a hot foot-bath often helps. Some people by stroking the forehead and temples have the power to ease the pain, producing quiet and sleep. If the bowels are costive, salts should be taken to move them, or they can be moved by an enema, if salts are not at hand. If the stomach is full, or tastes sour, drink a lot of warm water and vomit, or produce vomiting by tickling your throat with your finger, after having taken a large quantity of warm water for sometimes warm water thus taken fails to cause vomiting. If there is no food in the stomach, but there is sour and bilious vomiting, the warm water will frequently help. For a sour stomach or when it is full of gas, a teaspoonful of baking soda in some hot water will often feel very pleasant and grateful. The patient should keep absolutely quiet after these are done, and often they fall into a refreshing sleep.

EMERGENCY MEDICINES.--If anemia is the cause, give tonics such as iron and arsenic. If the patient feels faint and nauseated, a small cup of strong hot coffee gives relief, sometimes. Antipyrin, given early in doses of two and one-half grains often relieves. Take another dose in one-half hour if necessary. But such remedies are hard on the heart.

TREATMENT. Preventive in Sick Headache.--The patient is often aware of the causes that bring on an attack. Such causes should be avoided. A great many people who are afflicted with this trouble are not only careless in their eating, eating anything and everything and at all times--at meal time and between meals--but also careless in their habits of life. Patients should avoid excitement, like card parties, etc., staying up late, or reading exciting books. The meals should be regular, no food taken that is hard to digest. Pies, cakes, puddings, gravies, ham, pork, sausage, and fried foods must be avoided. Rich, greasy foods will not do for such persons to eat. Strong tea and coffee are bad. Plenty of water should be taken between meals. At meals it is better to take no water unless it is hot water. Every morning on arising it is well to drink a large quantity of either cold or hot water. This washes out the stomach, bowels and kidneys, and stimulates them to better perform their functions. The bowels must be kept regular, one or more passages a day and at a regular hour. Sometimes, especially in younger persons, the eyes are at fault and may need glasses. Frequently it is caused by overwork in school in young girls, especially during their menstrual periods. Social duties cause them in many women, and then strong tea or coffee, or headache powders, or tablets, are taken to keep up or to stop the pain, making the patient more liable to the attacks in the future; and then still more tea, coffee, and headache remedies are taken until the patient is a slave to the remedies taken to help her. A great many of these headaches can be helped by simple measures, and the time between the attacks, in about all cases, made longer if the patient will but work with the physician, not only at the time of the attack, but in the interval. The clothing should be comfortable. The feet should always be kept dry. This applies especially to neuralgia. In fact the above measures of prevention and care apply to all kinds of headaches and neuralgias. Prevention is worth more than the cure.

MOTHERS' REMEDIES. 1. Sick Headache, Hop Tea Will Relieve.--"Hop tea is very good if a good strong decoction is made. A wineglassful may be taken every half hour or hour until relieved." This is very easily prepared, as the hops may be purchased at any drug store.

2. Sick Headache, a Favorite Remedy for.--"Aconite liniment or aconite rubbed on the forehead will relieve the pain in the head almost instantly. One drop of the tincture of nux vomica in a teaspoonful of water every five or ten minutes will quickly relieve." Nux vomica is good only when the headache comes from constipation and stomach trouble and too high living.

3. Sick Headache, Aromatic Spirits of Ammonia for.--"For a nervous headache there is nothing better for immediate relief than fifteen or twenty drops of the aromatic spirits of ammonia." This relieves the pain and quiets the nerves and stimulates the heart.

4. Sick Headache, Camphor Application for.--"A very simple but effective remedy is a cloth wet with spirits of camphor and sprinkled with black pepper applied to the head gives almost instant relief."

5. Headache, Soda and Peppermint for.--"One teaspoonful (level) of soda in two-thirds glass of hot water, add five or eight drops of oil of peppermint and a little sugar. Drink quite warm. This has been often tried and proven to be a success." The soda will relieve any gas in the stomach and the peppermint aids digestion and relieves sickness of the stomach.

6. Sick Headache, Lemon Good for.--"One lemon before breakfast will help to keep off sick headache. Have never found a remedy to cure sick headaches. A sack of hot salt will always help the pain." The lemon will help to tone up the stomach and the salt applied to the head will help the pain by relieving the congestion. It is always well to take a good cathartic after a spell of sick headache.

PHYSICIANS' TREATMENT for Sick Headache.--

1.	Antipyrine	25 grains
	Citrate of Caffeine	10 grains
	Bromide of Potash	25 grains

Mix and make into five powders. One powder as needed. (You might take second one in three hours.) This is not good when it is bilious sick headache. In fact, it would make it worse. It is good for sick headache and neuralgia due to eye or nerve strain, but then the first remedy, antipyrine, can be left out. It is not needed. I would then put twice as much of the bromide of potash, fifty grains, and take a powder every two hours until better.

2.	Citrate of Caffeine	1/2 dram (30 grains)
	Phenacetine	60 grains
	Bicarbonate of soda	60 grains
	Aromatic powder	12 grains

Mix and make twelve powders. Take one every three hours. This is good. Sometimes it is depressing on the heart for some people, due to the phenacetine. Acetanilid can be substituted in same dose.

(The homeopathic treatment is very successful in relieving spells of sick headache. See chapter on Homeopathy.)

3. Sodium Phosphate, taken every morning, about one-half to one teaspoonful in hot water. It is good for the bowels and liver.

4. Prescription for the Liver and Bowels in Sick Headache.--

Sulphate of soda	30 grains
Salicylate of soda	10 grains
Sulphate of Magnesia	1 grain
Benzoate of Lithia	5 grains
Tincture of Nux Vomica	3 minims
Distilled water	4 ounces

This mixture should be made up in large quantity and placed in a siphon by one of the concerns which charge soda water, and from one-quarter to one-half a glass of this water, at ordinary temperature, is to be taken every morning at least one-half an hour before breakfast; enough being taken to insure an adequate bowel movement during the forenoon. This ought to be a good combination to use regularly.

5. Dr. Hare gives the following recommendations. Probably no single source of pain compares in its frequency to headache, chiefly because it is essentially a symptom of diseases or functional disturbances.

It may come from constipation or eye strain, from brain disease, anemia, uremia, too much blood in the head, etc. In many cases a mild laxative to thoroughly empty the bowels is necessary. Sometimes the urine will be deficient in solids and liquids, so that the effete and poisonous material are retained in the blood, which produce headache. For such cases if the urine is acid, the frequent use of Vichy water, to which is added a little bicarbonate of potassium, about five grains to a drink, as a diuretic will prove of great service. If the urine is alkaline (and this you can tell by using a red litmus paper which will turn blue if it is alkaline) ten grain doses of benzoate of ammonium three (3) times a day are often useful.

NERVE TUMORS (Neuroma).--A morbid increase in the tissue-elements of the peripheral (the external surface) nerves.

Varieties. True and False Nerve Tumors.--True nerve tumors (neuromata) are composed of nerve-fibres provided with a medullary (marrow) sheath or of nerve tissue; false nerve tumors are composed of other structure than nerve tissue, are usually of secondary origin, extending to the nerve from nearby structures.

Symptoms.--The true nerve tumors may be hereditary or due to wounds or blows and amputation. They may give rise to no symptoms, or may cause intermittent pain. Pressure increases this pain, when the condition of the nerve fibre is interfered with. Loss of local sensation and power may develop. It is sometimes possible to feel the little nodular growths, and they can be seen when they are superficial. They may give no pain, or they may become very sensitive. They may become chronic and they are very liable to do so. Some of them may disappear.

PHYSICIANS' TREATMENT for Nerve Tumor.--The severe forms should be cut out; others can be let alone.

NEURITIS (Inflammation of the Nerves. Neura-Nerves; Itis--Inflammation. Inflammation of the Bundles of Nerve Fibres).--Nagel describes it as "an inflammation of the nerves of an acute or chronic nature, associated with more or less degeneration, change in the nerve fibrils of the affected nerves."

Causes.--An injury to the nerves, frequent muscular strains, exposure to cold. Inflammation can extend to the nerve from adjacent inflamed structures. Pressure can cause it. Fractures of bones cause it by compression and it is also caused by infectious diseases, such as rheumatism, typhoid fever, syphilis, etc. In some cases it simply appears without apparent cause.

When the disease process involves the nerve sheaths and connective tissue structures in particular, an interstitial neuritis results; when the disease locates itself in the nerve fibrils it gives rise to "parenchymatous neuritis" (main part of the nerve is inflamed).

Simple Neuritis.--This means that a single nerve of a group of adjacent nerve trunks is affected. If a number of nerves are affected at the same time it is called Multiple Neuritis or Polyneuritis.

Causes.--(a) Exposure to cold. This is a very frequent cause, as for example, in the facial (face) nerve. (b) Traumatism,--that is, wounds, blows, injuries caused by fractures and dislocations; pressure from tumors, sleeping with the head resting on the arms. Pressure from crutches, "crutch paralysis." (c) Diseases involving the nerves due to extension of inflammation from nearby structures, as in neuritis of the facial nerve due to decay of the temporal bone.

Symptoms.--The constitutional or general symptoms are usually slight. The pain is the most important symptom, being of a boring in the parts to which it is distributed. This pain may be very distressing, or of a stabbing character, and is usually felt in the course of the nerve; or it may cause little inconvenience. Sometimes the skin is red and swollen over the affected parts. There is impaired nerve function and as a result of this the muscles supplied by these nerves become weak, and occasionally paralyzed. In severe cases they may become atrophied and an eruption often appears along the course of the nerve. Sometimes the hair and nails are not properly nourished, causing falling out or grayness of the hair and loss of the nails. This neuritis may extend from the peripheral (external) nerves and involve the larger nerve trunks or even reach the spinal cord. This rarely occurs in neuritis from cold, or in that which follows fevers; but it occurs most frequently in neuritis caused by blows, wounds, etc., (traumatic).

Duration.--This varies from a few days to weeks or months. If the primary cause can be remedied it usually ends in full recovery. Sometimes it is followed by the chronic form.

PHYSICIANS' TREATMENT for Neuritis.--The first thing to do is to try to remove the cause. Then absolute and continued rest of the affected part. If one has a sore hand it will be rested, if possible; so it must be with the sore and inflamed nerve.

For the Attack.--After having placed the part in absolute rest, moist heat applied to it frequently brings great relief. Sometimes a mustard plaster applied along the sore part does good. This produces a counter irritation and thus draws some of the congestion from the congested, inflamed nerve. Ice is more effective in some cases than heat. The bowels should be kept open daily with salts. Build up the general health with tonics; no alcohol can be used. If it shows a tendency to become chronic, use massage, electricity or change of climate. Atrophy (shrinking) of the muscles is likely to follow if the disease continues long and for this massage and electricity must be given.

Treatment. Preventive.--A person who has once had neuritis must exercise all care to keep from taking cold or exposing themselves to severe cold winds and storms. Wet clothing will be apt to cause its return. Damp houses are bad. The climate should be dry and not changeable. There should be enough and proper kind of clothing to keep the body heat at the normal point. Plenty of rest and sleep are required. These cautions also apply to rheumatism and neuralgias.

Multiple Neuritis.--Other names: Polyneuritis, Disseminated Neuritis, Peripheral Neuritis. **Meaning**--Multiple neuritis is an inflammatory disease of the peripheral (toward the end of the nerves or external nerves) nervous system. It varies much in extent and intensity and affects symmetrical parts of the body.

Varieties.--These arise from differences in the nature, causes, severity and location of the disease process.

Causes.--They are many. (1.) The poison that comes from infectious diseases such as typhoid fever, diphtheria, smallpox, leprosy, la grippe, etc. (2) From poisons such as alcohol, lead, arsenic; phosphorus, mercury, coal gas, etc. (3) From anemia, cancer, tuberculosis, syphilis, septicemia, diabetes. (4) From cold, over-exertion, etc.

Symptoms.--Acute febrile multiple neuritis. A typical case: This comes on from exposure to cold, over-exertion, or in some cases spontaneously. There are chills, headaches, pains in the back, limbs and joints, and the case may be called rheumatism. Loss of appetite, coated tongue, constipation, and other symptoms of stomach and bowel trouble. The temperature rises rapidly, and may go to 103 to 104 degrees. The limbs and back ache, but intense pain in the nerves are not always constant. The pain is usually sharp, severe, and located in the limbs, and is worse from moving and pressure. There are tingling feelings in the hands, feet and body, and a feeling as if ants or insects were crawling over them, and there is also increased sensitiveness of the nerve trunks or entire limb. There is loss of muscular power, first marked, perhaps, in the legs, and it extends upwards and reaches the arms. Sometimes it first begins in the arms. In typical cases the extending muscles of the wrist and ankles drop. (Wristdrop and foot-drop). In severe cases there is a general loss of muscular power, producing a flabby paralysis. This may extend to the muscles that control speaking, swallowing and hearing resulting in impairment of these functions.

The muscles soften and waste away rapidly. Disorders of nutrition are frequent, like watery swelling (oedema), glossy looking skin, sweating, hives, etc.

Recovery.--The course of the disease varies considerably. In mild cases the symptoms disappear very soon. In the worst form the patient may die in a week or ten days. As a rule, in moderately severe cases after persisting for five or six weeks, the condition remains about the same for a few months, and then improvement slowly begins and recovery takes place in six to twelve months. In neuritis from alcohol drinking there is a rapid onset as a rule, with delirium and delusions. The result is usually favorable and after persisting for weeks or months improvement gradually begins, the muscles regain their power, and even in the most desperate cases recovery may follow. The mental symptoms are very severe in alcoholic cases. Delirium is common. It takes much longer for such cases to regain what they call their normal condition.

Neuritis following diphtheria and other infectious diseases. The outlook in cases from these diseases is usually favorable, and except in diphtheria, fatal cases are uncommon. It is most common from diphtheria. Recovery, in neuritis from diphtheria, takes place in about three months, but some cases are fatal.

Neuritis from lead.--The first symptoms are those of intestinal colic, lead line on the gums, "dropped-wrist." The recovery is quite gradual and the poison may be cast out in three to four months.

In Neuritis from Arsenic.--We have disturbance of the stomach and bowels first, then the legs and arms are about equally affected, weakened; may recover in two to six months.

Treatment for acute kind.--The first thing to do is to rest in bed and control the pain and acute symptoms. Hot applications help to relieve the suffering. Patient must be kept comfortably and constantly warm and quiet. Hot applications of lead water and laudanum.

Medicines.--It may be necessary to use morphine to control the pain. Remedies such as antipyrine or aspirin are often used. A physician must be called. When the disease is caused by arsenic and lead and alcohol, of course you must remove the cause before you can hope for any improvement.

Caution.--Any one can readily understand from reading this description that the thing to do is to be careful not to needlessly expose yourself to taking cold. One subject to rheumatism or neuritis, even in small degree, should take care not only not to take cold but not to overdo in laboring; cold, wet and over-exertion cause the majority of the acute attacks. But some are caused by diseases, such as diphtheria, typhoid fever, etc., and a great many cases of neuritis following these and other infectious diseases can be avoided if proper care is taken during and after these diseases. Such care can easily be taken. Keep your rooms warm and comfortable, and the patient in bed or in a comfortable room until all danger is past. How often I have heard a doctor blamed for such results when in most cases it is the patient's or nurse's fault. Certain results will follow certain diseases and only proper care can keep such results from following. Dropsy frequently follows even a light case of scarlet fever. Why? Simply because, on account of being a light case, the child is left to roam at will about the rooms and catches cold, takes la grippe. If people would only take care of themselves this disease would not leave so many lifelong victims. I have seen men and women who have just recovered from this disease stand on the street corners on a cold, damp day, and talk an hour, and the next day they wondered how they could possibly have taken cold. We cannot disobey the laws of nature safely. Persons who are subject to neuritis or rheumatism should be especially careful on cold, damp, wet days and of over-exertion.

GENERAL AND FUNCTIONAL BRAIN DISEASES. NERVOUS PROSTRATION. NERVOUS EXHAUSTION. NEURASTHENIA.

NERVOUS PROSTRATION.--Is a condition of weakness or exhaustion of the nervous system, giving rise to various forms of mental and bodily inefficiency.

Causes. 1. Hereditary causes.--Some children are born of parents who are weak themselves, and who have led fast lives through business or pleasure and these parents have given their offspring a weakened body, and the children are handicapped with a nervous predisposition and furnish a considerable proportion of "nervous" patients.

2. Acquired.--It is acquired by continual worry and overwork, sexual indiscretion, excesses, irregular living and indiscretion in diet. A great many business men, teachers and journalists become "neurasthenics." It may follow infectious diseases, particularly influenza, typhoid fever and syphilis. It also follows operations sometimes. Alcohol, tobacco, morphine may produce a high grade of the disease, if their use is abused.

Symptoms.--These are varied. The most prominent symptom is fatigue. The patient feels so tired and complains of being unable to do any mental labor. It is almost impossible to put the mind on one subject for any length of time. There are headache, dizziness, want of sleep, and there is great depression of spirits; patient is gloomy, irritable in temper with manifestations of hysteria. Sometimes there are marked symptoms of spinal trouble. Pain along the spine with spots or areas of tenderness. Pains simulating rheumatism are present. There is frequently great muscular weakness, great prostration after the least exertion, and a feeling of numbness, tingling, and neuralgic pains. In spinal symptoms, there is an aching pain in the back, or in the back of the neck, which is a quite constant complaint. Then there are the anxiety symptoms in many cases. There may be only a fear of impending insanity or of approaching death, or of apoplexy, in simple cases. More frequently the anxious feeling is localized somewhere in the body, in the heart region, in the head, in the abdomen, in the thorax (chest, etc.). In some cases the anxiety becomes intense. They are so restless they do not know what to do with themselves. They throw themselves on the bed, complain, and cry, etc. Sometimes the patients become so desperate they commit suicide. Some patients do not wish to see anyone. Some patients cannot read, reading wearies them so much, or they get confused and dizzy and must stop. Some are very irritable. They complain of everything. Remember they cannot help it, usually. Some are easily insulted and claim they are misunderstood. The circulation may be disturbed in some cases. Then there is palpitation of the heart, irregular and very rapid pulse, pains, and feeling of oppression around the heart, cold hands, and feet. The heart's action may be increased by the least excitement and with the fast pulse and palpitation there are feelings of dizziness and anxiety and such patients are sure they have organic disease of the heart. No wonder. Flashes of heat, especially in the head, and transient congestion of the skin are distressing symptoms. Profuse sweating may occur. In women, especially, and sometimes in men, the hands and feet are cold, the nose is red or blue, and the face feels "pinched." Nervous dyspepsia is present in many cases. The digestion is poor and slow and constipation accompanies it. Sometimes there is neuralgia of the stomach. The sexual organs are seemingly affected, many men are "almost scared to death" and they use all sorts of quack remedies to restore their sexual vigor. Spermatorrhea is their bugbear. They usually get well if they stop worrying. In women there is the tender ovary and the menstruation may be painful or irregular. The condition of the urine in these patients is important. Many cases are complicated with lithaemia (sand-stone in the urine). It is sometimes also increased in quantity.

PHYSICIANS' TREATMENT for Nervous Prostration.--The patient must be assured and made to believe that the disease is curable, but that it will take time and earnest help on the part of the patient. Much medicine is not needed, only enough to keep the system working well. Encouragement is what is needed from attendants. Remove the patient from the causes that produce the trouble, whether it be business, worry, over-study, too much social duties, or excesses of any kind. The patient must have confidence in the physician, and he must be attentive to the complaints of the patient. It is the height of foolishness and absurdity for a physician to tell such a patient before he has thoroughly examined him or her that the troubles are imaginary. I believe that is not prudent in the majority of cases. I have heard physicians talk that way to such patients. I thought, what fools! The patient needs proper sympathy and sensible encouragement. You must make them believe they are going to get well. If you do not wish to do this, refuse such cases, or you will fail with them.

If there are any patients that need encouragement and kindly, sympathetic, judicious "cheering up," these patients are the ones, and they generally are "laughed at and made fun of" by people who should know better. Remember their troubles are real to them, and are due to exhaustion or prostration of the nervous system and this condition, as before described, produces horrid feelings and sensations of almost every part of the body. The patient must be made to believe that he may expect to get well; and he must be told that much depends upon himself, and that he must make a vigorous effort to overcome certain of his tendencies, and that all his power of will will be needed to further the progress of the cure.

First, then, is rest.--Both mental and physical diversions, nutritious though easily digested food, and removal of baneful influences as far as possible. Physical exercise for the lazy. Rest for the anemic and weak. For business or professional men the treatment is to get away and far off, if possible, from business. It will often be found best to make out a daily programme for those that must remain at home, something to keep the mind busy without tiring, and then times of rest. The patient, if it is possible, should be away from home if home influences and surroundings are not agreeable. Dr. S. Weir Mitchell, of Philadelphia, has devised and elaborated a cure, called a rest cure, for the relief of this class of patients, and it is wonderfully successful especially in thin people. "Be the symptoms what they may, as long as they are dependent upon nerve strain, this 'cure' is to be resorted to, and if properly carried out is often attended with surprising results." "A bright, airy, easily cleaned, and comfortable room, is to be selected, and adjoining it, if possible, should be a smaller one for an attendant or nurse. The patient is put to bed and kept there from three to six weeks, or longer as may be necessary, and during this time is allowed to see no one except the nurse and doctor, since the presence of friends requires conversation and mental effort. The patient in severe cases must be fed by the nurse in order to avoid expenditure of the force required in the movement of the arms. No sitting up in bed is allowed and if any reading is done it must be done by the nurse who can read aloud for an hour a day (I have seen cases where even that could not be done). In the case of women, the hair should be dressed by the nurse to avoid any physical effort on the part of the patient. To take the place of ordinary exercise, two measures are employed, the first of which is massage or rubbing; the second, electricity. By the kneading and rubbing of the muscles and skin the liquids in the tissues are absorbed and poured into the lymph spaces, and a healthy blush is brought to the skin. This passive exercise is performed in the morning or afternoon, and should last from one-half to an hour, every part of the body being kneaded, even the face and scalp. In the afternoon or morning the various muscles should be passively exercised by electricity, each muscle being made to contact by the application of the poles of the battery to its motor points, the slowly interrupted current being used. Neither of these forms of exercise call for any expenditure of nerve force; they keep up the general nutrition. The following programme for a day's existence is an example of what the physician should order:

7:30 a. m.--Glass of hot or cold milk, predigested, boiled or raw as the case requires.

8:00 a. m.--The nurse is to sponge the patient with tepid water or with cold and hot water alternately to stimulate the skin and circulation, the body being well wrapped in a blanket, except the portion which is being bathed. After this the nurse should dry the part last wetted, with a rough towel, using some friction to stimulate the skin.

8:30 a. m.--Breakfast. Boiled, poached or scrambled eggs, milk toast, water toast, or a finely cut piece of mutton chop or chicken.

10:00 a. m.--Massage.

11:00 a. m.--A glass of milk, or a milk punch, or egg-nog.

12:00 m.--Reading for an hour.

1:00 p. m.--Dinner. Small piece of steak, rare roast beef, consomme soup, mutton broth, and any one of the easily digested vegetables, well cooked.

3:00 p. m.--Electricity.

4:30 p. m.--A glass of milk, a milk punch or egg-nog.

6:30 p. m.--Supper. This should be very plain, no tea or coffee, but toast and butter, milk, curds and whey, or a plain custard.

9 :30 p. m.--A glass of milk or milk punch.

In this way the day is well filled, and the time does not drag so heavily as would be thought. If the stomach rebels at over feeding, the amount of food must be cut down, but when all the effort of the body is concentrated on respiration, circulation, and digestion a large amount of nourishment can be assimilated by the exhausted body, which before this treatment is undertaken may have had its resources so shattered as to be unable to carry out any physiological act perfectly. For the treatment to be successful the rules laid down should be rigidly followed, and the cure should last from three to six weeks or longer."

HYSTERIA.--A state in which ideas control the body and produce morbid changes in its functions.

Causes.--It occurs mostly in women, and usually appears first about the time of puberty, but the manifestations may continue until the menopause or even until old age. It occurs in all races. Children under twelve years are not very often affected. A physician writes: One of the saddest chapters in the history of human deception, that of the Salem witches, might be headed, "Hysteria in Children," since the tragedy resulted directly from the hysterical pranks of girls under twelve years of age. During late years it has been quite frequent among men and boys. It seems to occur oftener in the warm and mild climates than in the cold. There are two predisposing causes that are very important--heredity and education. Heredity acts by endowing the child with a movable (mobile) abnormally sensitive nervous organization.

Cases are seen most frequently in families with marked nervous disease tendencies, whose members have suffered from various sorts of nervous diseases.

Education.--The proper home education is neglected. Some parents allow their girls to grow up accustomed to have every whim gratified, abundant sympathy lavished on every woe, however trifling, and the girl reaches womanhood with a moral organization unfitted to withstand the cares and worries of every-day life. And between the ages of twelve and sixteen, the most important in her life, when the vital energies are absorbed in the rapid development of the body, the girl is often "cramming" for examinations and cooped in close schoolrooms for six or eight hours daily; not only that, but at home she is often practicing and taking lessons on the piano in connection with the full school work. The result too often is an active bright mind in an enfeebled body, ill-adapted to subserve the functions for which it was framed, easily disordered, and prone to act abnormally to the ordinary stimuli of life.

Direct Influences.--Those influences that directly bring on the attack are fright, anxiety, grief, love affairs, and domestic worries, especially in those of a nervous nature. Diseases of the generative organs and organic diseases in general, and of the nervous system especially, may be causes of hysteria.

Symptoms.--These may be divided into two classes: 1. Interparoxysmal or time between the paroxysms (spells). 2. Paroxysmal. During the time of the attack. *First variety*--The will power seems defective. In bad cases self-control is lost. The patient is irritable, and easily annoyed by the slightest trifle; is very excitable and easily moved to laughter or tears without any apparent cause for either. Easily discouraged and despondent. She wants lots of sympathy. *Second*--Loss of sensation is frequently present, and it is most commonly one-sided; it may involve certain parts, as one or two limbs, the trunk escaping, or part of one limb. Various spots of want of sensation (feeling) may exist. The skin of the affected side is frequently pale and cool and a pin prick may not cause bleeding. In some cases they feel the touch of the hand, but there is no feeling from heat. There may also be oversensitiveness to pain and of the skin. It may be one-sided or both, or only in spots. The left ovarian region is a common sensitive point; also over the breasts, lower positions of the ribs, on top of the head and over many portions of the backbone. Pain in the head is a very common and distressing symptom, and is usually on the top. Pain in the back is common. Abdominal pains may be very severe and the abdomen may be so tender as to be mistaken for peritonitis. Various parts of the body may have neuralgic pains. There may be intense pain around the heart. There may be complete blindness, the taste and smell may be disturbed or complete loss of hearing. *Third*--Paralysis is frequently present. It may be one-sided or only of the lower extremities, or only one limb. The face is usually not involved when it is on one side. The leg is more affected than the arm. Sensation is lessened or lost on the affected side. Paralysis of the lower extremities is more frequent than one-sided paralysis. The power in the limbs hardly ever is entirely lost; the legs may usually be moved, but the legs give way if the patient tries to stand. The affected muscles do not waste. The feet are usually extended and turn inward. Sudden loss of voice occurs in many cases. The paralysis is generally paroxysmal, and is frequently associated with contractures, shortening of the muscle. The contractures may come on suddenly or slowly, and may last minutes, hours, or months, and some cases even years. Movements of the hands, arms, etc., like the motions in chorea are often seen in the young. A trembling (tremor) is sometimes seen in these patients. It most commonly involves the hands and arms, more rarely the head and legs. These movements are small and quick. *Fourth*--Swallowing may be difficult on account of spasms of the muscles of the pharynx. The larynx may be involved and interfere with respiration. Indigestion in some form is often present. The stomach and bowels may be very much bloated with gas. There may be a "phantom tumor" in the intestine (bowel). Constipation may be very obstinate, vomiting may be present and persistent and hiccough present. The action of the heart may be irregular, and rapid heart action is common. The least motion may cause difficult breathing and false Angina Pectoris (heart pang); the urine is retained not infrequently in female patients.

Symptoms of the Paroxysms.--Convulsive seizures are common manifestations of hysteria, and frequently present a great similarity to epilepsy. The prodromal (fore-running) symptoms are frequently present and may begin several days before the convulsion occurs. In milder forms, in which the cause may be due to a temporary physical exhaustion, or emotional shock, the fore-running symptoms are of short duration. The patient may become very nervous, irritable, impatient, have fits of laughing and crying, alternately, or have a feeling of a chill rising in the throat. The convulsion follows these symptoms. The patient generally falls in a comfortable place; consciousness is only apparently lost, for she frequently remembers what has taken place; the tongue is rarely bitten, In the milder forms the movements are apt to be disorderly. In the severe forms the movements are apt to be a lasting contraction of the muscles and the patient may have the head and feet drawn back and the abdomen drawn front. There then may follow a condition of ecstacy, sleepiness, catalepsy, trance, or the patient may show symptoms of a delirium with the most extraordinary sights of unreal things. These convulsions may last for several hours or days. Firm pressure over the ovaries may bring on a convulsion, or if made during a convulsion may arrest it. The disease is rarely dangerous to life, yet death has followed exhaustion induced by repeated convulsions or prolonged fasting. The duration of hysteria is very uncertain.

DURING A CONVULSION. The first thing to do is not to be frightened. A patient in a convulsion from hysteria very seldom injures herself during the convulsions. If you are sure it is hysteria, give a nasty tasting medicine, asafoetida is a splendid remedy, but not in pill form, for there is no taste or smell to them. Sometimes a convulsion may be arrested by the sudden use of ice to the backbone or abdomen or by dashing cold water in the face and chest, or by pressing upon the ovaries. When the hysteria is of a mild form it is sometimes a good plan, when the convulsion comes on, to place the patient in a comfortable position and then leave her, and when the patient comes to and finds herself alone and without sympathy, the attacks are less likely to be repeated. Sometimes if you watch a patient closely when she is seemingly unconscious, you will see, if you look at her very guardedly, that one eyelid is not entirely closed, and that the patient really sees much that is occurring around her. I am writing of real genuine hysteria, in which the patient is not quite right, not only physically but mentally,--especially the latter,--during the attack at least. For that and other reasons such patients should not be treated cruelly.

Preventive Treatment of Hysteria.--In order to be successful in this line of treatment the cause must be found and treated. An English physician writes: "It is pitiable to think of the misery that has been inflicted on these unhappy victims of the harsh and unjust treatment which has resulted from false views of the nature of the trouble; on the other hand, worry and ill-health, often the wrecking of the mind, body and estate, are entailed upon the near relatives in the nursing of a protracted case of hysteria. The minor manifestations, attacks of the vapors, the crying and weeping spells are not of much moment, and rarely require treatment. The physical condition should be carefully looked into and the mode of life regulated, so as to insure system and order in everything. A congenial occupation offers the best remedy for many of these manifestations. Any functional disturbance should be attended to and a course of tonics prescribed. Special attention should be paid to the action of the bowels. The best preventive treatment is the one that is given early, when the girl is growing from childhood to girlhood. It should be begun even earlier. A weakly baby should be built up by proper food and outdoor life. Dainties should not be given to such a child. When the child is old enough, as some mothers think, to go to kindergarten school, keep the little one at home. It is plenty early enough to send such a child to school when she is seven years old. This early school work rushes the child, makes it nervous. If you should happen to listen to the heart of many young school children you would find it pounding away at a furious rate. Do not hurry a weakly child. Do not hurry or rush a young girl even though she is strong, from the ages of twelve to sixteen years. Our school system does just that. Instead of taking life easy when she is nearing the crisis (puberty) or is in that period, she is hurried and rushed and crammed with her school work; the girl frequently goes to school during this period, even when she is unwell and sits there for an hour or more with wet skirts and sometimes wet shoes and stockings. Every day I see girls of all ages go past my office here in this cultured city of Ann Arbor, without rubbers, treading through the slush and water. Is it any wonder they become sickly, become victims of hysteria and suffer from menstrual disorders? Dysmenorrhea must follow such carelessness, and the parents are to blame in many cases. Be careful of your children, especially girls at this age, care less for their intellectual growth, and pay more attention to their body development, even if it should happen to be at the expense of their intellectual development. A healthy body is better than all the knowledge that can be obtained, if it goes, as it too often does, with a body that is weak and sick. Outdoor life is necessary. Horseback riding is splendid; walking is also good exercise at a regular time each day."

PHYSICIANS' TREATMENT for Hysteria.--If there is any womb trouble, it must be attended to. There is frequently trouble with the menses in cases of hysteria. It sometimes comes from anemia or simply comes without any special reason. Tonics like arsenic, iron, strychnine and cod-liver oil are needed for anemia. Iron valerate is good, in one grain doses, three times a day, in this disease, when the patient is not fleshy.

1. The following is recommended by Dr. Goodell:

Of each one scruple (20 grains).

Quinine Valerate
Iron Valerate
Ammonia Valerate

Make into twenty pills. Take one or two pills three times a day. (This is a good tonic in such cases.)

2. Fowler's Solution of Arsenic in three to five drops doses is frequently used (three times a day) and is a good lasting tonic in cases where the patient has a very pale white looking skin.

3. Asafoetida in three to five-grain pills is a splendid tonic in such cases, and in that form is pleasant to take. Take three during the day, before meals.

4. Sumbul or musk root is a good remedy. Tincture in one-half dram doses three times a day. This is good when the patient is very nervous.

5. The following is good when anemia is prominent:

Dried Sulphate of Iron	20 grains
Alcoholic extract of Sumbul	20 grains
Asafoetida	10 grains
Arsenious acid	1/2 grain

Mix thoroughly and make twenty pills, one after each meal.

6. Tincture of hops in doses of one-half to two teaspoonfuls is good for nervousness and sleeplessness, taken at bedtime. It can also be taken regularly four times a day in from one-half to one teaspoonful doses.

7. General Cautions.--Proper, easily digested foods must be taken. Keep the bowels open daily. Let trash and dainties alone. Pies, cakes, and rich foods are an abomination for such patients. Candy is not to be eaten. Let novels alone. Go to bed at nine and sleep until six or seven. Bathe five or ten minutes every morning or evening in tepid water or cool water. The patient should be warmly clothed. Sleep in a pleasant, sunshiny and airy room. In severe forms of the disease the "Rest Cure" and feeding described under Nervous Prostration should be used.

EPILEPSY. (Falling Sickness).--This is an affection of the nervous system, characterized by attacks of unconsciousness, with or without convulsion.

Causes.--In a large proportion of cases the disease begins before puberty. It rarely begins after twenty-five. It is more liable to attack females than males. Heredity is thought by some to play a big role. Dr. Osler says: "In our figures it appears to play a minor role." Another doctor says: "Heredity plays an important role in the production of the disease. Besides epilepsy, insanity, migraine, alcoholism, near relationship of parents (consanguinity) and hysteria are among the more common ancestral taints observed." All factors which impair the health and exhaust the nervous system are predisposing causes. Injury to the head often causes it. Teething, worms, adherent foreskin and clitoris, closing of the internal opening of the womb, delayed menstruation, are sometimes the cause.

Symptoms.--There are two distinct types. The major attacks--or "grand mal"--in which there are severe convulsions with complete loss of consciousness, etc.; and the minor attacks or "petit mal," in which the convulsive movements are slight and may be absent, and in which the loss of consciousness is often but momentary or practically absent. In some the attacks occur during the day; in others during the night, and they may not be noticed for a long time.

Characteristic paroxysm of the Major attacks.--This may be ushered in by a localized sensation, known as the Aura, in some part of the body; but it may come without any warning and suddenly. The convulsions begin suddenly and at first are tonic, that is, it does not change but holds on. Thc patient falls unconscious regardless of the surroundings, and the unconsciousness may be preceded by an involuntary piercing cry. The head is drawn back and often turned to the right. The jaws are fixed (tonic spasm). The fingers are clenched over the thumb and the extremities are stiff. The breathing is affected and the face looks blue. The urine and bowel contents may escape; but this occurs oftener in the next stage. This tonic spasm usually lasts from a few seconds to a half minute when it is succeeded by the clonic spasm stage.

Clonic spasm stage.--In this the contraction of the muscles is intermittent. (Tonic spasm is the opposite condition.) At first there is trembling, but it gradually becomes more rapid and the limbs are jerked and patient tosses violently about. The muscles of the face are in intermittent motion, the eyes roll, the eyelids are opened and closed convulsively. The jaws move forcibly and strongly, and the tongue is apt to be caught between the teeth and bitten. The blue look now gradually decreases. A frothy saliva, which may be bloodstained from the bitten tongue, escapes from the mouth. The urine and bowel contents may escape involuntarily. The length of time of this stage is variable. It may last two minutes. The contraction becomes less violent and the patient gradually sinks into the condition of deep sleep, when the breathing is noisy and stertorous, the face looks red and swollen, but no longer bluish. The limbs loose their stiffness and unconsciousness is profound. The patient, if left alone, will sleep for some hours and then awakes and complains only of a dull headache. His mind is apt to be confused. He remembers nothing or little of what has occurred. Afterwards the patient may be irrational for some time and even dangerous.

The minor attack or "petit mal."--There is a convulsion; a short period of unconsciousness, and this may come at any time, and may be accompanied by a feeling of faintness or vertigo. Suddenly, for example, at dinner time the person stops talking and eating, the eyes are fixed and staring and the face is slightly pale. The patient usually drops anything he may be holding. The consciousness returns in a moment or two and the patient resumes conversation as if nothing had happened. In other instances there is a slight incoherency or the patient performs some almost automatic action. He may begin to undress himself, and on returning to consciousness find that he has partially disrobed. He may rub his beard or face, or may spit about in a careless way. An eminent physician states: "One of my patients, after an attack, was in the habit of tearing anything he could lay his hands on, particularly books; violent actions have been committed and assaults made, frequently giving rise to questions which come before court. In the majority of cases of "petit mal" (light attacks) convulsions finally occur, at first slight, but ultimately the grand mal (major attacks) becomes well developed, and the attacks may then alternate."

Recovery.--The authority above goes on to say: "This may be given today in the words of Hippocrates: 'The prognosis in epilepsy is unfavorable when the disease is congenital (that is, existing at birth), when it endures to manhood, and when it occurs in a grown person without any previous cause. The cure may be attempted in young persons but not in old.' " Death rarely occurs during the fit,

19

but it may happen if the patient is eating. If the attacks are frequent and the patient has marked mental disturbance the conditions are unfavorable. Males have a better outlook than females.

PHYSICIANS' TREATMENT.--What to do during the Attack of Epilepsy.--Keep the patient from injuring himself, loosen the clothing, take off the collar or anything tight about the neck. Place a cork or spool or tooth-brush handle between the teeth to keep the patient from biting his tongue, but attach a stout cord to the object and hold it in that way.

Preventive and general treatment.--In the case of children the parents should be made to understand that in the great majority of cases epilepsy is incurable. The patients need firm but kind treatment. It does not render a person incapable of following some occupations. "Julius Caesar and Napoleon were subjects of epilepsy." The disease causes gradual impairment of the mind, and if such patients become extremely irritable or show signs of violence, they should be placed under supervision in an asylum. A person with this disease should not marry.

Diet.--Give the patient a light diet at regular hours, and the stomach should never be overloaded. There are cases in which meat is injurious, and it should not be eaten more than once a day and at noon time. A vegetable diet seems best. The patient should not go to sleep until the digestion is completed in the stomach.

Causes.--Should be removed if possible. Circumcision should be done, especially in the young. In case of a female child the "hood of the clitoris" should be kept free. Undue mental and physical excitement should be avoided. Systematic exercise should be taken. Baths in cold water in the morning, if possible, as the skin should be in good working condition.

Medicines.--The bromides are the best, and should always be given under proper supervision of a physician or nurse.

Caution.--I wish to add that parents should always attend to the seemingly harmless "fits" in their young children. It will not do to say they are due to teething or worms. If they are, the worms at least can be treated and that cause removed. They may be due to too tight opening in the penis. If that opening is small, or if the foreskin is tight it will make the child irritable and cause restless sleep. Attend to that immediately. The same advice applies to female children. The "cover" of the "clitoris" may be tight, making the little one nervous; loosen it. If your child keeps its fingers rubbing its private organs there is reason for you to have the parts examined and the cause removed as masturbation often starts in that way. The parts itch and the child tries to stop the itching. These little things often cause "big things" and I am sure "fits" can be stopped very often by looking after the private organs in both sexes.

SHAKING PALSY. (Paralysis Agitans).--This is a chronic affection of the nervous system, characterized by muscular weakness, trembling and rigidity.

Causes.--It usually occurs after the fortieth year, and is more common in men than in women. The exciting causes are exposure to cold and wet, business worries, anxieties, violent emotional excitement and specific fevers.

Symptoms.--The four prominent symptoms are trembling, weakness, rigidity, and a peculiar attitude. It generally develops gradually, usually in one or the other hand. There is at first a fine trembling, beginning in the hands or feet, gradually extending to the arms, the legs and sometimes the whole body. The head is not involved so frequently. This trembling (tremor) consists of rapid, uniform "shakings." At first it may come in spells, but as the disease advances it is continuous. Any excitement makes it worse. It is very marked in the hands. The trembling generally ceases during sleep. The muscles become rigid and shortened; the head is bent and the body is bent forward; the arms are flexed (bent) and the thumbs are turned into the palms and grasped by the fingers; the legs are bent, movement soon becomes impaired and the extremities show some stiffness in motion. There is great weakness of the muscles and it is most marked, where the trembling is most developed. There is no expression on the face, and the person has a slow and measured speech. The walk is very peculiar, and in attempting to walk the steps are short and hurried. The steps gradually become faster and faster, while the body is bent forward and the patient must keep on going faster to keep from falling. It is difficult to go around in a short circle. The patient cannot change his position in bed easily. The mind is rarely affected.

Recovery.--It is an incurable disease. It may run on for twenty years or more. There may be times of improvement, but the tendency is to grow, gradually worse.

PHYSICIANS' TREATMENT for Shaking Palsy.--This is simply to make the patient as comfortable as possible. Regulate the diet. The patient should not worry or have much exercise. Frequent warm baths are sometimes beneficial with gentle massage of the muscles.

APHASIA.--A partial or total inability to express thoughts in words or to interpret perceptions.

Varieties.--Motor and sensory aphasia.

Causes.--Softening of the brain, tumors of the brain, lesions in syphilis especially, hemorrhage in the brain, blows on the head, and inflammation of the brain and its covering.

Symptoms of Motor Aphasia.--The patient cannot make the muscles of the larynx, tongue, palate and lips perform their functions and produce speech. The patient knows what he wishes to say, but cannot pronounce it. This may be complete or partial. Complete, when the patient can only utter separate sounds. Partial, when the words are only slightly mispronounced and when some certain words cannot be pronounced at all. In some cases, nouns only or verbs cannot be pronounced. Agraphia, means inability to write down the thoughts. Sensory aphasia: word deafness. This is an inability to interpret spoken language. The sound of the word is not recognized and cannot be recalled; but sounds such as that of an engine whistle, or an alarm clock, are heard and recognized. Word-blindness: the person cannot interpret written language. Pharaphrasia: cannot use the right word in continued speech; the patient uses words but misplaces them.

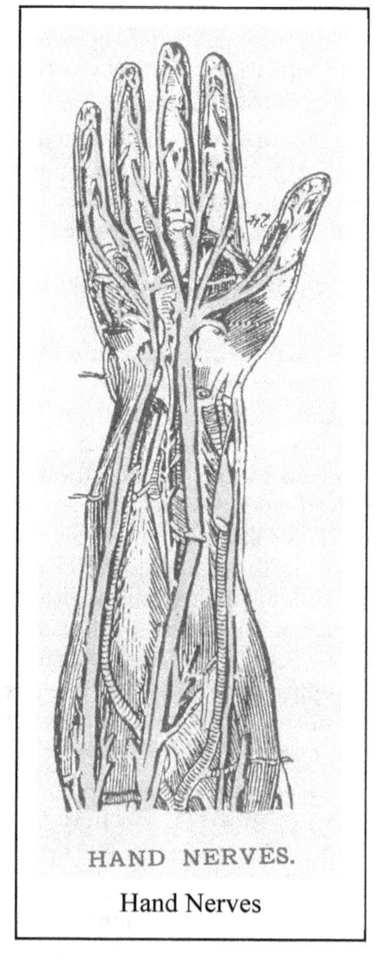

HAND NERVES.

Hand Nerves

Recovery depends a great deal upon the cause.

Treatment.--Treat the cause. If from syphilis, iodide of potash and mercury. If from an injury or tumors, operate if possible. Teach the patient how to speak, read and write. The result of this often gives you a pleasant surprise.

WRITERS' CRAMP. Causes.--This occurs much oftener in men than in women, and usually between the ages of twenty-five and forty. The predisposing causes are a nervous constitution, heredity, alcoholism, worry, etc. The chief exciting cause,--excessive writing, especially when it is done under a strain.

Symptoms.--It usually begins with fatigue, weight, or actual pain in the affected muscles. In the spasm form the fingers are seized with a constant or intermittent spasm whenever the person grasps the pen. The neuralgic form is similar in symptoms but severe pain and fatigue comes with writing. The tremulous form: In this the hand when used becomes the seat of the decided tremor. The paralytic form: The chief symptoms are excessive weakness and fatigue of the part and these disappear when the pen is laid aside.

Recovery.--If taken in time and if the hand is allowed perfect rest, the condition may improve rapidly. There is, however, a tendency to recur.

PHYSICIANS' TREATMENT for Writers' Cramps.--There must be absolute rest of the hand. General tonics, such as iron, strychnine, arsenic, and cod-liver oil may be needed to tone up the system.

APOPLEXY. (Cerebral Hemorrhage). (Brain Hemorrhage). Causes.--Bleeding (hemorrhage) into the brain substance is almost always due to an affection of the walls of the large or small arteries of the brain, producing rupture and subsequent bleeding. Persons of fifty or over are more subject to it, and it is more common in men than in women. Any disease that will cause degeneration of the arteries, helps to cause it, such as nephritis, rheumatism, syphilis, gout and alcoholism. Nephritis is one of the most certain causes, because arteriosclerosis (hardening and decaying of the walls of the arteries) and hypertrophy of the heart are associated with nephritis, etc.

Direct Causes.--Straining at stool, heavy lifting, anger, rage, fright, etc.; paroxysm of whooping-cough or convulsions may cause it in children.

Symptoms.--Sometimes the patient experiences headache, dizziness, paleness or flushing of the face, fullness in the head, ringing in the ears, etc., temporary attacks of numbness or peculiar tingling in one-half of the body. When the bleeding takes place there is usually loss of consciousness. In the attack:--If the bleeding is extensive the patient falls suddenly into coma, and this may soon prove fatal. If the bleeding is slight at first and gradually increases, the patient is delirious at first, then one arm, then one side, and finally the whole body may become paralyzed, and unconsciousness, and even death may come from the paralysis of the heart and breathing nerve centers. In many cases the patient falls unconscious without previous warning. The face is red, the eyes injected, the lips are blue, the pulse is full and slow, and the breathing is slow and deep. The head and eyes may be strongly turned to the injured side. The pupils may be unequal. The paralysis may not be noticed while the patient is unconscious and is quiet. The urine and the bowels contents may pass involuntarily or the urine may be retained. Sometimes when the case is very grave the patient does not awake from his deep sleep (coma); the pulse becomes very feeble, respiration becomes changed, mucus collects in the throat, and death may occur in a few hours or days. In other cases the clot in the brain is gradually absorbed, and the patient slowly returns to consciousness. Sometimes relapses occur. In mild cases instead of deep coma, there may be only headache, faintness, nausea and vomiting.

Subsequent Symptoms.--When the patient improves, consciousness returns, but there remains a half-side paralysis, hemiplegia, on the side and opposite to that of the seat of the injury in the brain. It may not take in the whole side, only a part. The gait is peculiar. In walking the patient supports the paralyzed arm. In many cases the paralyzed parts gradually regain their functions in a few weeks, but not always complete. The leg improves more than the arm. There is danger of other attacks. When the sleep (coma) is very deep, the breathing is embarrassed, with vomiting and prolonged half-consciousness and extension and complete paralysis, the danger to life is great.

What can I do at once? Loosen the clothing around the neck and waist. Raise the head and shoulders and put cold to the head (ice bag if you have it) and warmth to the feet, legs and hands. Watch the bladder closely. The urine must be drawn frequently in this disease, especially if there is much paralysis. It may dribble away, but that is not enough. Look out for bed sores, especially if the sickness is a long one.

APOPLEXY. 1. Mothers' Remedies, Simple yet Effective Remedy for.--"Place the feet of the patient in hot water and mustard," This is a very simple treatment for such a serious disease, but very often will relieve as the hot bath will cause a reaction, take the pressure of blood from the brain and by this means has been known to save many lives.

2. Apoplexy, Simple Injection for.-"Place dry salt on the tongue and give an injection as follows:

Warm water	1 quart
Common salt	2 teaspoonfuls
Brandy	1/2 ounce

This injection is recommended for any kind of a shock which affects the circulation."

The injection of the bowels will relieve the congestion by drawing the blood away from the brain.

Medical treatment must be to regulate the diet, bowels, kidneys, and stomach. Restore the general health.

Caution.--A person who has had an attack of this kind may have another. The mode of life must be changed in most cases. The patient must take things easy. The bowels, kidneys, stomach, and liver must work naturally and the stomach must not be overloaded. Too much meat must not be eaten; alcohol must be let alone; rich foods are prohibited. Hurry, worry, anger, fright, excitement, etc., are bad. Be lazy, take life easy, do not get over-heated, and sleep, *sleep,* SLEEP,--in a room where there is plenty of good air. Do not lift or strain to have a passage of the bowels. Stooping is injurious. The blood must be kept from the head. Take proper care and you are likely to live years longer. And now you may wonder why I give such cautions. Apoplexy is directly due to a breaking of the wall of a blood vessel, large or small; due to a weakening, or decay, or degeneration of the wall. This lets the blood into the substance of the brain and presses upon the nerve centers, causing the trouble and paralysis. Any wrong action tends to fill the blood vessels very full and the weakened wall bursts.

PALSY. Paralysis.--A loss of movement, entire or partial, in the voluntary muscles of the body. When this loss of power is complete it is called paralysis; when it is not complete, paresis.

Causes.--Inflammation of the brain and spinal cord, tumors in these parts, accidents and injuries, poisons, apoplexy, etc.

Symptoms.--The patient cannot make all the usual motions of the part. The affected muscles may waste after a time.

Different Varieties.--

(a) Paralysis of the ocular (eye) muscles.--The vision becomes double, the eyelids do not act normally, may droop. The eye may not move in every direction as it should.

(b) Paralysis of the muscles of mastication (eating). Symptoms.--If paralysis is only on one side, it is difficult to chew; if on both sides, chewing is impossible. The jaw hangs down.

(c) Paralysis of the facial (face) muscle.--This is a rather common occurrence, and is due to exposure to wet, and cold, diseases of the middle ear, tumors, etc. Symptoms:--The eyelids do not close tightly, and tears are continually trickling over the cheek; the corner of the mouth droops and the saliva runs out, etc. The mild cases last two or three weeks; the severe form from four to six weeks; the worst cases usually recover in a long time.

(d) Paralysis of the muscles of the upper extremity.--There are various and many symptoms, but with all there is the same loss of the usual motion. That particular muscle does not do its special work; for instance, if the paralysis is of the deltoid muscle of the arm and shoulder, it is not possible to raise the arm, usually pain in the shoulder. The muscle soon wastes and the head of the arm bone (humerus) falls away from the shoulder, etc.

(e) Paralysis of the muscles of the lower extremities.--Paralysis of the "Gluteus Maximus and Minimus." (Hip muscles). Lifting up of the thigh is difficult and so is walking up hill or rising from sitting position. The toes are turned out. The other muscles may be paralyzed and simply cannot do their usual duty.

(f) Toxic (poison) paralysis. Lead paralysis.--It is hard to extend the fingers. The lead line is shown on the gums.

PHYSICIANS' TREATMENT for Palsy.--Remove the cause. Give salts and iodide of potash. Paralysis from arsenic, mercury, zinc or copper:--The symptoms are those of neuritis and are greatly similar in each kind. The spongy gums show mercury; the puffy face and diarrhea show arsenic poison. Remove the cause.

CONGESTION OF THE BRAIN. (Diseases of the Cerebral (Brain) Circulation). (Hyperaemia).--The brain is too full of blood.

Causes. For Active Congestion.--Over-exertion in study, etc.; chronic pletbora (too much blood in the blood vessels); from constant use of alcohol, tobacco, amyl nitrite, and from the stomach.

For passive congestion.--Local obstruction to the return of blood from the brain. Prolonged mental and physical exertion with excesses and irregular living may cause it.

Symptoms of active kind.--Head feels warm, face is red, the arteries in the neck beat hard, violent headache, ears ringing, very restless and does not sleep well.

Symptoms of the passive form.--The headache is not so great; there may be stupor, drowsiness and dull intellect and very sleepy.

Recovery.--Favorable if the cause is removed.

Treatment for active congestion.--Keep the patient absolutely quiet in a dark, well aired room, with the head and shoulders raised, an ice bag or cold cloths to the head and warm applications to the hands and feet. A warm foot bath will aid in drawing the blood away from the head. Give salts (salines) to move the bowels. These take away a great deal of water from the blood and aid in relieving the congestion of the head.

Treatment for passive congestion.--Remove the cause if possible. Give a light nutritious diet; prohibit alcohol in any form; keep the bowels regular.

CEREBRAL ANEMIA. (Too little blood in the brain). Causes.--Heart disease, general anemia, and mental excitement.

Symptoms.--"Fainting spells," dizziness, the ears ring and there are spots before the eyes; nausea and vomiting may go ahead of the fainting spells. The face is pale, the pupils are dilated, the pulse is small and feeble, and there may be cold sweating on the body. If you can remove the cause the result is favorable.

Treatment.--For the fainting fits:--Place the patient in the "lying down" position and this frequently restores consciousness; loosen any tight clothes, corset, waist, collar, etc. Give plenty of fresh air and do not crowd. Keep quiet yourself; do not get excited. In mild cases, mild stimulants may be necessary. Let the patient smell of camphor, put a cloth with camphor or ammonia near the nose. In other cases amylnitrite and strychnine may be necessary. Small doses of whisky or brandy frequently help. Remove the cause. Give tonics for general anemia.

TUMORS OF THE BRAIN AND INFLAMMATION, Abscess, etc. Abscess. Causes.--This is always secondary and comes from some other part of the body. It comes often in young and middle life and is more common in males than in females. The most frequent cause is inflammation of the ear and the next is from fracture of the skull bones. It may be large or small.

Symptoms.--May come slowly or quickly. After an injury to the head the symptoms may come on suddenly such as intense headache, delirium, vomiting, chills, high fever, and sometimes convulsions, and a very deep seeming sleep (coma). In chronic cases the symptoms are not so severe.

Treatment.--An operation if the abscess can be reached. If not, an ice bag should be applied to the head; quiet the distress with narcotics.

TUMORS OF THE BRAIN.--Varieties in order of their frequency. Gumma, tuberculous tumors, glioma, sarcoma, cancer, etc.

Causes. Predisposing.--Men are about twice as often affected as women until fifty and then it is about equal. It is more frequent in early adult life. The exciting causes are blows and severe emotional shock.

Gumma (in third stage of Syphilis) appear as a round, yellow, cheesy mass, usually beginning in the membranes and are usually seen between thirty and fifty. They come from syphilis.

Tuberculous tumors. These appear as hard masses and vary in size. They may be single or many, and are situated in any part of the brain. More than half of the tumors appearing in children are of this variety.

Glioma. "Glue-tumor." They come from tissue forming the basis of the supporting framework of the nervous tissue. This kind occurs often in the young.

Sarcoma and Cancer are rare.

Symptoms.--The most of the growths start in the membranes of the brain, and by compressing a certain part of the brain they produce their special symptoms such as headache, vomiting, inflammation of the nerves of the eye, double vision, blindness, the memory impaired, dullness and apathy, an irritable temper, and sometimes become demented. There is often vertigo or a sense of giddiness. There may be convulsions, and paralysis of some muscles. A general tuberculosis tendency or history of syphilis will help to make the diagnosis. In children it is more likely to be tuberculous. The result is more favorable in tuberculous growths in children and syphilitic tumors in adults. It may last from a few months to three years in a bad case.

Treatment.--For gumma, caused by syphilis, iodide of potash and mercury should be given. In both kinds, syphilitic and tuberculous, a nutritious diet and general tonic treatment, such as cod-liver oil, iron, arsenic, and quinine should be given. The bowels must be kept open and special attention given to the digestion.

For headache.--Ice bags, cold to the head, mustard to the nape of the neck.

For Vomiting.--Mustard over the stomach.

Surgery is necessary for some tumors that can be reached. You will naturally depend upon your attending physician for advice and treatment.

SYPHILIS OF THE BRAIN. Causes.--The symptoms of syphilis of the brain, belong to the third stage of the disease, and are rarely ever observed until at least one year or longer from the time of the first lesion (chancre). It may be from ten to twenty years coming on. Both sexes are equally liable, and it may come at any age. Syphilis may produce a circumscribed tumor, a disease of the arteries or a general hardened infiltration of the brain. The tumors are small, yellowish, and cheesy in the center. They originate in the "Dura Mater" (covering) and spread to the brain structure proper. The disease of the arteries causes a thickening of these vessels, a narrowing of the blood channel in them, thus producing a clot.

Symptoms.--Of gumma (syphilis tumors) at the base of the brain, are persistent headache, worse at night; sleeplessness, depression of the mind, memory impaired, vertigo, sometimes vomiting and paralysis of some of the nerves (third and sixth pairs). Violent convulsions, like epilepsy, appear in some cases.

Symptoms when arteries are diseased.--Temporary loss of speech, numbness or weakness in one limb, the sight is disturbed, or vertigo; and, when the clot (thrombus) appears, symptoms of apoplexy, This is a common variety of syphilis of the brain.

How to tell what the disease is.--The history of the patient will help. An apoplexy in a young person would suggest syphilis.

Recovery.--The chances are better when the disease forms gumma (tumors) than when the blood vessels are diseased.

Treatment.--Should be begun and properly carried on when the person has the primary sore (chancre), and then these after troubles may not follow. This is one of the diseases where the victim reaps a big harvest on account of the sexual sin, and in order to escape the bad results for himself, etc. he should go through a regular course of treatment when he first contracts the disease, perhaps for a year or more, This treatment should last as a rule for some years. It is late to begin when the brain symptoms show brain involvement. For this there must be radical and careful treatment with mercury and iodide of potash; with tonics and general building up treatment, and then even if the patient lives he may be a nuisance to himself and others.

GENERAL PARESIS. (Paretic dementia. General Paralysis of the Insane. Softening of the Brain).--This belongs under diseases of the mind, but there are so many cases that a description of this disease may be instructive and interesting. One author says: "General paresis is a chronic, progressive, diffuse, encephalitis (inflammation of the brain), resulting in structural changes in the cerebral (brain) tissue, with involvement of the cortical, and meningeal, (covering) blood and lymph vessels, presenting characteristic symptoms, with progressive course and fatal termination usually within three years." There are three stages:--1. The period of incubation (the prodromal stage). 2. A stage of pronounced mono-maniac activity with symptoms of paralysis. 3. Stage of extreme enfeeblement with diminution and final loss of power. These stages run into each other. First stage in a typical case:--There are tremblings and slight trouble in speech and expression of the face. The mind has exalted and excited spells, etc.

Symptoms.--The patient is irritable. The mental and moral character is unstable. His affairs are in confusion. He uses bad language, neglects his family, goes with drunkards and bad women, makes indecent proposals to respectable women of his acquaintance without realizing that it is improper. He cannot keep his mind on one thing. Speech is a little thick, indistinct and hesitating. Syllables are dropped or repeated, speech finally becomes undistinguishable. He is very excited; he thinks he is persecuted. He is a big fellow generally. He is a king, he is rich and mighty. This is the usual run. As the disease progresses he becomes feeble-minded more and more so continually. Persistent insomnia comes on early and frequently recurring, one-sided headache often goes with it. Sometimes there is an uncontrollable desire to sleep. Loss of consciousness is an early symptom. After severe attacks there may be one-sided paralysis (hemiplegia) which usually disappears in a few hours or days. Convulsions like epilepsy may appear early, but usually occur in the later stages. The pupils are mostly dilated, rarely contracted, and they are often unequal and react slowly to light. When the tongue is protruded it trembles and is put out in a jerky manner. The hands tremble, in the advanced stage. The speech is jerky and slow. Syllables are dropped and repeated. One early symptom is retention of the urine. There is another annoying symptom--a constant grinding of the teeth. The walk is very spasmodic, but in advanced stages it becomes slouching or dragging. The skin may be red or blue. When the feeble-mindedness is fully developed the mind does not perceive anything accurately. He sees imaginary things, and things that he does see do not appear to him as they are. Finally he has no mind.

Treatment.--The end is sure. You can relieve the distress partly. Personal attention by a physician is needed.

INSOMNIA.--Insomnia is not a disease, but a symptom of disease. It may, however, become so active, prominent, and important a symptom as to constitute a condition which merits individual management and treatment.

Definition.--Insomnia is the term employed to denote actual or absolute sleeplessness, and also lack of fully restful sleep, which might be termed relative sleeplessness.

Causes.--Organic causes. Disease of the brain and spinal cord. Toxic causes due to poison circulating in the blood which by irritation of the brain and cord (axis) and especially of the brain, cause such diseases as nephritis (chronic), jaundice, typhoid fever and consumption.

Primary causes. Depend upon insanity.

Nervous or simplest causes.--These are present in nervous persons and comprise the two conditions of congestion and anemia of the brain. The brain congestion is typified by the nerve-tire of the student; over-study and anxiety bring too much blood to the brain and necessarily too much activity and then insomnia. Anemia of the brain acts in the opposite manner. The brain cells are not properly nourished and hence irritated, and sleeplessness follows.

SLEEPLESSNESS. Mothers' Remedies. 1. Hop Pillow Stops.--"People affected in this way will be very much benefited by the use of a pillow composed of hops, or cup of warm hop tea on retiring. The hops have a very soothing effect upon the nerves."

2. Sleeplessness, Easy and Simple Remedy for.--"On going to bed, take some sound, as a clock-tick or the breathing of some one within hearing, and breathe long breaths, keeping time to the sound. In a very short time you will fall asleep, without any of the painful anxieties attending insomnia."

3. Sleeplessness, Ginger at Bedtime for.--"Ginger tea taken at bedtime soothes one to sleep," This is a very good remedy when the stomach is at fault. It stimulates this organ and produces a greater circulation, thereby drawing the blood from the head. This will make the patient feel easier and sleep will soon follow.

4. Sleeplessness, Milk Will Stop.--"Sip a glass of hot milk just before retiring. This is very soothing to the nerves, and a good stimulant for the stomach,"

PHYSICIANS' TREATMENT.--Remove the cause and be careful in using drugs. In the organic kind the treatment is not very successful. In the toxic kind drugs must be given to correct other diseases and also tonics given. For brain congestion and anemia kind other means must be used first, and the drugs as the last resort.

Treatment of the congestive insomnia.--1. Hot or warm general body-baths are very advantageous to stimulate the circulation and restore its balance alike in congestion and anemic cases. After such baths the patient must go to bed at once and not get chilled in cold rooms or by drafts. They must be properly covered and kept warm.

2. Cold spongings, cold shower baths, or cold plunge baths are given when the hot or warm bath does not produce the correct result. If this does not depress it is better than the warm bath. The person should be rubbed with warm rough towels until the skin is aglow. If he feels rested and quieted, the reaction is proper; if depressed, the treatment is too vigorous and not suitable.

3. The patient should stand ankle deep in a tub of hot water and a "drip sheet," from water at 75 to 80 degrees temperature, thrown over him. Then rub the patient's back and abdomen hard and a general brisk rub-down immediately after leaving the tub. This treatment should quiet, not excite or depress.

4. The cold abdominal pack is valuable. Flannel is wrung out in water, 75 to 80 degrees temperature and laid in several thicknesses upon the abdomen; place a dry towel over this, cover all with oiled silk, overlapping widely in order to protect the bed. Tie or bandage all this firmly. The effect of this work is first that of a cold then of a warm poultice.

5. Exercise. This should be in the open air when possible. A fast walk, horseback ride or ride on bicycle for a half hour before bedtime, followed by a rub-down will frequently give a good sleep. Dumb-bell, Indian club exercise, chest weight, are good in some cases.

Diet.--A light easily digested supper is often better than a heavy meal. Sometimes a little eaten before bed-time will give sleep. A piece of toast, for instance. It draws the blood from the brain and more to the stomach.

Medicines. If you must use them.-- The bromides are the best. Sodium and strontium bromide are first choice. Twenty to thirty grains in water one-half hour before retiring. Chloral hydrate should not be used often. Sulphonal, trional, etc., should always be given with a little food-never alone. Sometimes bread pills do just as well.

ANEMIC CONGESTION. Diet.--A light supper before retiring, like hot milk, broths, milk punch, etc., will very frequently promote sleep by removing the cause and quickening the circulation. Give nutritious, easy food to digest. The baths are not so valuable for this kind of insomnia. A cold sponge bath or plunge may be of service.

Medicines.--Tonics are needed here as in regular anemia. The patient must be carefully treated, and very many of these cases can be cured. The patient must render all the aid he can give, and the physician should gain his confidence. If he does he will not need to give much medicine to put the patient to sleep, and if he does give it he can frequently use a Placebo with the same effect. Mind has an influence over mind. By "Placebo" is meant any harmless substance, as bread-pills, given to soothe the patient's anxiety rather than as a remedy.

SLEEP WALKING.--There is a tendency to sleep walking in some families, often more than one child will do this to a greater or less extent. It is very extreme in some cases, and the next morning they do not know anything about it. The person is very seldom hurt and he can do some dizzy things. Many persons walk about in their sleeping room or simply get out of bed. Fatigue, worry, poor sleep, restlessness, nervousness, a hearty late dinner are aggravating causes. As age advances and the person becomes stronger, the patient will do less of it.

Treatment.--Avoid over-eating, worry, over-study. The evening should be spent quietly. Such persons had better drop parties, late hours or anything that tends to cause worry, fatigue or nervousness.

STAMMERING.--This may be inherited to some extent; excitement, nervousness, bodily fatigue, want of rest, etc., make it worse.

MOTHER'S REMEDY. 1. Stammering, Easy Cure for.--"Read aloud in a room an hour each day. Repeat each word slowly and distinctly."

PHYSICIANS' TREATMENT.--The person should be taught early to talk slowly, and to do everything to control himself and not get nervous. There are schools for this trouble, and they seem to do good work. They teach the patients how to speak slowly, distinctly and to keep their minds off of themselves.

HICCOUGH.--This is caused by intermittent, sudden contraction of the diaphragm; obstinate hiccough is a very distressing symptom and sometimes it is hard to control.

Causes.--Inflammatory causes. It is seen in gastritis, peritonitis, hernia, appendicitis, and in severe forms of typhoid fever. Irritative causes. Swallowing hot substances, local disease of the gullet near the diaphragm, and in many cases of stomach trouble and bowel disorder, especially when associated with gas (flatus). Specific causes: Gout, diabetes or chronic Bright's disease. Nervous (Neurotic) causes. Hysteria, epilepsy, shock, or brain tumors.

MOTHERS' REMEDIES. 1. Hiccough. Vinegar for.--"One teaspoonful vinegar sipped carefully (so it will not strangle the patient) will stop them almost instantly."

2. Hiccough, Sugar and Vinegar Stops.--"A few drops of strong vinegar dropped on a lump of sugar and held in the mouth until dissolved, will stop most cases of hiccoughs."

3. Hiccough, Sugar Will Relieve Patient of.--"Place a little dry sugar on the end of the tongue and hold the breath. I have tried this remedy after others have failed and obtained instant relief."

4. Hiccough, Simple Remedy for.--"Have patient hold both ears closed with the fingers, then give them three swallows cold water while they hold their breath."

5. Hiccough, Home Remedy to Stop.--"Take nine swallows of cold water while holding the breath."

6. Hiccough. Vinegar Stops.--"One teaspoonful of vinegar thickened with sugar and eaten slowly."

7. Hiccough, Cinchona Bark in Peppermint Stops.--"Put about one-fourth teaspoonful of cinchona bark, powdered in two ounces of peppermint water, and give one teaspoonful every five or ten minutes until relieved, or three drops of camphor and aqua ammonia in wineglassful of water," These remedies are very good when the stomach is at fault, as they have a stimulating effect.

PHYSICIANS' TREATMENT.--Sudden start may check it in the light forms. Ice, a teaspoonful of salt and lemon juice may be tried. Inhalations of chloroform often relieve. Strong retraction of the tongue may give immediate relief. Spirits of camphor, one teaspoonful. Tincture of cayenne pepper one to two drops in water. Ten grains of musk by the rectum. Hoffman's anodyne one teaspoonful in ice water is very good.

INJURIES TO THE HEAD. Concussion or Laceration of the Brain.--The brain may be injured by a blow on the head, or indirectly by falling fully upon the feet or sitting down hard upon the buttocks.

Symptoms.--The person who is injured may lose his balance and fall, become pale, confused, and giddy, may have nausea and vomiting and recover. If the injury is more severe and there is a tear of the membranes of the brain or the brain itself, the patient will fall and lie quietly with a feeble and fluttering heart, cold, clammy skin, and apparent unconsciousness; he can be roused by shouting but will not reply intelligently. He will be able to move his limbs. The urine and contents of the bowels will be passed involuntarily. As he gets better he may vomit. He may soon return to entire consciousness, but still suffer from some headache, feel wearied, and tired, and not feel like exerting himself. This may continue for some time. Occasionally the results are more serious even after a long time has passed, and an abscess of the brain should be watched for, sometimes epilepsy or insanity follows. If the patient grows worse instead of recovering, either deep seeming sleep sets in or symptoms of inflammation of the covering (meninges) or the brain itself follows. Such injuries must be carefully watched, for you can not tell at first how severe they may prove to be.

TREATMENT. What to do First.--Put the patient to bed without any pillow, and put around his body hot water bottles or bags, suitably covered. He should be kept quiet and free from excitement, and sleep should be encouraged. Hot water or ice water, when awake, as is most agreeable to the patient, may be given. Aromatic spirit of ammonia, during the shock is better for the patient to take than alcohol, for alcohol excites the brain; dose, one-half to two drams; the former can be given every ten minutes in a little water for about three doses. Surgical treatment may be necessary at any time.

INJURIES OF THE SPINAL CORD. Concussion of the Spine.--A severe jarring of the body followed by a group of spinal symptoms supposed to be due to some minute changes in the cord, of an unknown nature.

Causes.--Severe concussion may result from railway accidents or violent bending of the body, fall from a house, blow on the back, jumping, etc.

Symptoms.--May come on suddenly, when it is due to a jar of the brain as well as the cord. Loss of consciousness, complete paralysis, small pulse, collapse, and within a few hours death may follow. In other cases improvement, though very slow, follows. Walking is difficult and the upper extremities are weak in these cases. There are pain and tenderness along the spine. Brain symptoms, such as headache, dizziness and fainting, may be present or absent.

Treatment.--Absolute rest from the beginning, stimulants if necessary, electricity is useful.

TRAUMATISM OF THE CORD. (Blows, etc.).--(Fractures and dislocations, gun-shot and stab wounds, etc.).

Symptoms.--They differ according to the place where the cord is injured. The motion and feeling power may be disturbed. There may be sudden complete paralysis of the upper and lower extremities depending on how severely the cord is injured, and how high up the injury is. The bladder and rectum may not act properly. The contents may be retained or "run-away." Death follows sooner or later if the injury is extensive. In some cases the symptoms are slight in the beginning, but increase in a few days, or they may suddenly increase a few months afterwards. In other cases, bad symptoms at first may gradually abate which is due to the blood clot having been absorbed.

Recovery depends upon the extent of the injury and the constitution of the patient. It is always well to be careful about expressing an opinion about this injury.

Treatment. Immediate.--Surgical treatment is necessary. Absolute rest is a necessity, and must be had for weeks according to the severity of the case. It may seem long and become tedious, but the case must have rest for a long time.

ORGANIC DISEASES OF THE SPINAL CORD. Caisson Disease; Divers' Paralysis. Causes.--This affection occurs in divers, bridge builders, and others who are subject to increased atmospheric pressure. The symptoms develop on coming suddenly to the surface when the atmospheric pressure is greatly lessened.

Symptoms.--They usually occur on the return to the surface of the water, or after a few hours have passed. There are pains in the ears and joints and nose-bleed. The pulse is slow and strong. Neuralgia of the stomach and vomiting often occur. Paralysis of one side, or of the lower extremities may occur. Brain symptoms may develop and death may follow in a few hours. In most cases recovery takes place in a few days or weeks.

Treatment.--Persons who are engaged in such work should change very gradually from a great depth to the surface, and should not go into the outer air suddenly.

MYELITIS.--Myelitis is an inflammation of the spinal cord.

Causes.--It may occur at any age, and is more common in male than in female. The exciting causes are prolonged exposure to severe colds, too great mental and physical exertion, sexual excess, blows, bleeding into the cord, alcoholic excess, acute infectious diseases, syphilis, etc.

Symptoms.--These depend upon the location of the inflammation and the severity. The onset may be sudden or gradual--when it is sudden, there may be a chill followed by a fever of 101 to 103 degrees--general feeling of illness, loss of appetite, with coated tongue and constipation. There may be over-sensitiveness to pain and touch. Pain may radiate from the back into the limbs, with numbing and tingling of the limbs. The urine may be retained or may dribble away. Usually there is obstinate constipation. There is frequently the feeling of a band around the body. Paralysis may follow in the lower extremities and higher up, sometimes, depending upon how high up in the cord the inflammation exists. This paralysis may cause no motion of the limbs or produce an exaggerated contracting of the affected muscles, the knees being drawn up on the abdomen and the heels touching the buttocks.

Recovery.--Chances for recovery depend upon the cause. Most cases are chronic and may last for years.

Treatment.--Treatment depends also upon the cause. Rest in bed; counter-irritation, wet cupping, with care on account of bed sores. A water-bed from the first may prevent bed-sores. The urine must be drawn if it is retained. The medical treatment must be carefully given and a physician of experience should be obtained.

LOCOMOTOR ATAXIA. Tabes dorsalis. Posterior Spinal Sclerosis).--A hardening (sclerosis) affecting the posterior parts of the spinal cord and characterized by incoordination, which means a condition where a person is unable to produce voluntary muscular movements; for instance, of the legs, etc., loss of deep reflexes to bend them back; disturbances of nutrition and sensation, and various affections of sight.

Causes.--This is a disease of adult life, persons under twenty-five being rarely affected, and is more common in men than women (ten to one). Sometimes children suffering from hereditary syphilis have it. The chief predisposing cause is syphilis which precedes it in from seventy to eighty-five of the cases according to various authorities. Exposure to cold and wet, sexual and alcoholic excesses, mineral poisoning, and great physical exertion also exciting causes.

Symptoms.--These are numerous. They appear in succession and with the same regularity.

Stages.--Stages of pain; the stage of ataxia, peculiar gait; and the state of paralysis.

1. Prodromal or forerunning; the stage of pain.--This consists of lightning-like pains in the lower extremities, numbness, formication (feeling of ants, etc., crawling), sensation of dead extremities; pins and needles in the soles of the feet and fingers, coldness, itching of arms and scrotum or other parts, a sensation of constriction around the chest, headache, pain in the small of the back and loins of an aching character may occur. These symptoms may constitute the only evidence of locomotor ataxia and last for years; but sooner or later there are added absence of knee cap bone reflex (knee jerk), and immobility of the pupil. The loss of the knee jerk is always observed in time. The pupil fails to respond to light while it still accommodates for distance, called Argyll Roberston pupil. There may be imperfect control of the bladder with slow, dripping or hasty urination. Later the control is not imperfect, but it may be painful. Inflammation of the bladder may occur which is dangerous. There is usually obstinate constipation and loss of sexual power. These symptoms may last for several months and years, and then the second stage symptoms appear.

2. Stage of Ataxia (Disturbance of motion).--The disturbance of motion (ataxia) is very marked, especially in the lower extremities; the walking becomes difficult and uncertain; there is difficulty in rising or rapid turning;

the legs are wide apart; feet lifted too high and come down too forcibly; the length of the steps is irregular, and the body is imperfectly balanced. If the patient stands with his feet together and eyes closed he begins to sway, (Romberg's symptom), which is due to a defect in controlling the muscles from impairment of sensation. There may be imperfect use of the hands in dressing, writing, etc.; lancinating pains are marked in all cases and come on in paroxysms. The pains are mostly in the legs, but also occur in the arms, head, loins, back, and trunk. Then the sense of touch is partially lost. The prick of a pin may not be felt until a few seconds after being applied. This stage may last for years and remain at a "standstill;" but it is usually progressive, and advances to the third stage.

3. The stage of paralysis is marked by a gradual change to the worse, and the patient must remain in bed, because he cannot get out. The lower and sometimes the upper extremities have lost a great deal of their power of sensation: The joints, mostly the knee and hip joints show on both sides of the body a painless swelling, owing to the great quantities of watery liquid there. Dislocations and fractures occur simultaneously. Bed-sores and peculiar ulcers on the sole of the foot also occur. The urine dribbles away constantly, for all control of the bladder is lost. Death occurs from exhaustion; bedsores, inflammation of the bladder, or pneumonia coming on as a complication.

Treatment;--The only thing to do when the patient has this disease is to make him comfortable and arrest the progress of it, if possible. It is incurable, but treatment sometimes arrests the progress and at least lessens the suffering and prolongs life as long as it is worth living to them. I have given a longer description than was necessary, for I wanted men who live such fast lives to understand what it brings them for most cases are caused by syphilis. The description could have been made longer and other symptoms and complications put in. I think enough has been given and perhaps this description may deter some one from going the same road.

The Diagnosis is made at first by the fatigue, peculiar pains, loss of the knee jerk, the peculiar pupil and history of syphilis. Later it is made from the ataxia; the peculiar walk, etc., and the bladder disturbances.

HEREDITARY ATAXIA. Friedrich's Disease.--This peculiar disease is due to a degenerative disease of the posterior and lateral columns (parts) of the spinal cord, occurring in childhood, and often in several children of the same family.

Causes.--More in boys than in girls and oftener in the country districts. Heredity is frequently a cause and it is traced to syphilis, epilepsy, alcoholism, and insanity in the ancestors. Several children of the same family may have it.

Symptoms.--In very young children it is noticed that they are slow in learning to walk; the child staggers in trying to stand or to walk; it uses its hands clumsily, and has difficulty in speaking. The movements of the hands are peculiar, the hands move like in chorea, the speech is slow and drawling.

Recovery.--Very doubtful, but they may last for years.

INFANTILE PARALYSIS. (Acute Anterior Polio Myelitis).--This is an acute disease occurring almost exclusively in young children with paralysis, followed by rapid dwindling of the muscles of the parts affected by the paralysis.

Causes.--Found in children under three years old. It is more common in summer than in winter. It often follows scarlet fever, measles, and diphtheria.

Symptoms.--The onset is usually sudden; often the child is put to bed at night seemingly well and in the morning is found paralyzed in one or more limbs. High fever or chills, general feeling of illness, pain all over the body, decided brain symptoms, like delirium or convulsions and intermittent contractions of the muscles may usher in the disease. These forerunning symptoms may last a short time or for several weeks, after which the paralysis is noticed, being extensive as a rule, and affecting one, two, or all of the extremities and sometimes the muscles of the trunk. This general paralysis soon disappears being left permanently in only one extremity, chiefly in one leg. The other symptoms disappear. The paralyzed part atrophies (wastes) rapidly. The disease is very rare in adults. If the paralysis does not show a decided change within the first few months, full recovery is doubtful.

Treatment.--During the acute stage there must be absolute quiet and rest with a diet that is not stimulating, one that is easily digested; ice to the head or cold cloths, counter-irritation to the spine; electricity should be used after a few weeks. There is quite a good deal of this paralysis, and the case should receive careful attention from the start.

TASTE.--Taste-Buds.--There are three kinds of papillae or eminences on the human tongue,--the circumvallate, the fungiform and the filiform. The circumvallate are from seven to twelve in number and lie near the root of the tongue, arranged in the form of a V, with its open angle turned forward. Each one is an elevation of the mucous membrane, covered by epithelium and surrounded by a trench. On the sides of the papillae, embedded in the epithelium, are small oval bodies called taste-buds. These taste-buds consist of a sheath of flattened, fusiform cells, enclosing a number of spindle-like cells whose tapering ends are prolonged into a hair-like process. As the filaments of the gustatory nerves terminate between these rod-like cells, it is probable that they are the true sensory cells of taste.

In the human tongue taste-buds are also found in the fungiform papillae, often seem as red dots scattered over its surface; and to an area just in front of the anterior pillar of the fauces. It is also possible that single taste-cells are scattered over the tongue, as the sense of taste exists where no taste-buds can be found.

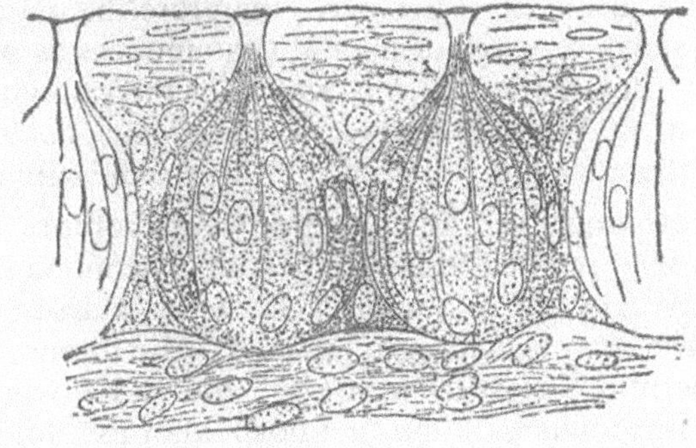

Taste Buds.

Many so-called tastes are really smells. This is easily proved by compressing the nostrils and attempting to distinguish by taste different articles of food.

The taste sensation is greatest when the exciting substance is at the temperature of the body. There is no perceptible sweetness to sugar when the tongue has been dipped for a half-minute in water either at the freezing temperature or warmed to 50 degrees C. Neither is there any sense of taste until the substance is dissolved by the natural fluids of the mouth, as will be seen by wiping the tongue dry and placing sugar upon it.

The four primary taste-sensations are bitter, sweet, sour and salt. These probably have separate centers and nerve fibers. Sweet and sour tastes are chiefly recognized at the front and bitter and alkaline tastes at the back of the tongue. The same substance will often excite a different sensation, according as it is placed at the front or back of the tongue.

There are also laws of contrast in taste sensations. Certain substances will enhance the flavor of another and others will destroy it. Again, certain tastes may disguise others without destroying them, as when an acid is covered with a sweet.

INSANITY. History.--The earliest reference to insanity is found in the book of Deuteronomy. Another reference is in Samuel where it speaks concerning David's cunning and successful feigning of insanity. "And he changed his behavior before them and feigned himself mad in their hands, and scrabbled on the door-posts of the gate, and let his spittle fall down upon his beard," Feigning insanity under distressing circumstances has been one of man's achievements throughout the centuries. It is spoken of in Ecclesiastes. Jeremiah says in regard to the wine cup: "And they shall drink and be moved and be mad." Nations also were poisoned by the wine cup, for Jeremiah says, "Babylon has been a golden cup in the Lord's hands, that made all the earth drunken. The nations have drunken of her wine, therefore the nations are mad." Greek writers speak of cases of mental unsoundness as occurring with some frequency in Greece. The inhabitants of the Roman Empire were afflicted with mental unsoundness and Nero was considered crazy. In ancient Egypt there were temples and priests for the care of the insane.

Hippocrates, who lived four hundred years before Christ, was the first physician who seemed to have any true conception of the real nature of insanity. For many centuries later the masses believed that madness was simply a visitation of the devil. The insane, in the time of Christ, were permitted to wander at large among the woods and caves of Palestine. The monks built the first hospital or asylum for the insane six centuries after Christ.

A hospital for the insane was established at Valencia in Spain in 1409. In 1547 the hospital of St. Mary of Bethlehem was established near London and was known as "Bedlam" for a long time.

The first asylum to be run upon reform principles was St. Luke's of London, founded in 1751. About 1791 Samuel Hahnemann established an asylum for the insane at Georgenthal, near Gotha, and the law of kindness was the unvarying rule in the institution. Hahnemann says in his Lesser Writings: "I never allow any insane persons to be punished by blows or other corporeal inflictions." Pineli struck the chains from the incarcerated insane at the Bicetre, near Paris in 1792 or 1793.

There has been a gradual tendency during the last century toward better things in the behalf of the insane. A hundred years ago they were treated with prison surroundings and prison fare. Then asylum treatment began to prevail. This means close confinement, good food, sufficient clothing and comfortable beds. Asylum care means the humane custody of dangerous prisoners. "From the asylum we move on to the hospital system of caring for the insane and this system recognizes the fact that the lunatic is a sick man and needs nursing and medical treatment in order to be cured. Hospital treatment has been gradually introduced during the past thirty years or more," and in time it will eventually supercede asylum treatment and prison or workhouse methods in the management of the insane everywhere.

Causes of Insanity.--There are many and various causes. One author states: "Mental abnormality is always due to either imperfect or eccentric physical development, or to the effects of inborn or acquired physical disease, or to injurious impressions, either ante-natal or post natal, upon the delicate and intricate physical structure known as the human brain." Some physical imperfections, more than others, give rise to mental derangements, and some persons, more than others, when affected by any bodily ailment, tend to aberrated conditions of the mind. Some impressions more than others, are peculiarly unfortunate by reason of their crowding effects upon the brain tablets of a sensitive mind. To these natural defects and unnatural tendencies, we apply, in the general way, the term "Insane Diathesis." This diathesis may be inherited or acquired. Those who are born to become insane do not necessarily spring from insane parents or from an ancestry having any apparent taint of lunacy in the blood. But they do receive from their progenitors oftentimes certain impressions upon their mental and moral, as well as upon their physical being, which impressions, like iron molds, fix and shape their subsequent destinies."

The insane diathesis in the child may come from hysteria in the mother. A drunken father may impel epilepsy, madness or idiocy in the child. Ungoverned passions, from love to hate, from hope to fear, when indulged in overmuch by the parents, may unloose the furies of unrestrained madness in the minds of the children. "The insane may often trace their sad humiliation and utter unfitness for life's duties back through a tedious line of unrestrained passion, of prejudice, bigotry, and superstition unbridled, of lust unchecked, of intemperance uncontrolled, of avarice unmastered, and of nerve resources wasted, exhausted, and made bankrupt before its time. Timely warnings by the physician and appeals to his clients of today, may save them for his own treatment, instead of consigning them to an asylum where his fees cease from doubling, and the crazed ones are at rest." The causes of the insane diathesis (constitution) are frequently traceable to the methods of life of those who produce children under such circumstances and conditions that the offspring bear the indelible birthmark of mental weakness. Early dissipations of the father produce an exhausted and enfeebled body; and a demoralized mind and an unholy and unhealthy existence in the mother, are causes. Fast living of parents in society is a fruitful cause of mental imperfections in their children. "The sons of royalty and the sons of the rich, are often weak in brain force because of the high living of their ancestry."

The fast high livers of today are developing rapidly and surely, strong tendencies to both mental and physical disorders. Elbert Hubbard says of those who live at a certain hotel and waste their substance there, that they are apt "to have gout at one end, general paresis at the other, and Bright's disease in the middle."

Drunkenness, lust, rage, fear, mental anxiety or incompatibility, "if admitted to participation in the act of impregnation will each, in turn or in combination, often set the seal of their presence in the shape of idiocy, imbecility, eccentricity, or absolute insanity."

Diogenes reproached a half-witted, cracked-brained unfortunate with this remark, "Surely, young man, thy father begat thee when he was drunk."

Burton in his anatomy of melancholy states that: "If a drunken man begets a child it will never likely have a good brain," Michelet predicts: "Woe unto the children of darkness, the sons of drunkenness who were, nine months before their birth, an outrage on their mothers."

Children of drunkards are often "sad and hideous burlesques upon normal humanity." Business worry may cause unsoundness in the offspring generated under such conditions.

One father had two sons grow up strong and vigorous, mentally and physically, while a third son was weak, irresolute, fretful, suspicious and half demented. The father confessed to his physician that on account of business troubles he was half crazy and during this time the wife became pregnant and this half-crazy son was born and the father states that "he inherits just the state of mind I was then in." Many such cases could be mentioned. "A sound body and a cheerful mind can only be produced from healthy stock." Mental peculiarities are produced by unpleasant influences brought to bear upon the pregnant mother. The story is told of King James the Sixth of Scotland, that he was constitutionally timid and showed great terror at a drawn sword. His father was murdered in his mother's presence while she was pregnant. Children born under the influence of fear may be troubled with apprehensions of impending calamity, so intense that they may become insane at last. An instance is given of "an insane man who always manifested the greatest fear of being killed and constantly implored those around him not to hurt him." His mother lived with her drunken husband who often threatened to kill her with a knife.

Other Causes of Insanity. Imperfect Nutrition.--Whatever tends to weaken the brain or exhaust the central forces of life must favor the growth of insanity. The brain is not properly nourished.

Blows and Falls upon the Head.--Sometimes such injuries are forgotten, but they result infrequently in stealthily developed, but none the less dangerous, conditions, which may result in the derangement of all mental faculties. A child should not be struck on the head. Teachers or parents should not box a child's ears. One author says such a person "is guilty of slow murder of innocents."

Fright is Another Cause.--Punishing a child by locking it in a dark room or by "stories of greedy bears or grinning ghosts produces, oftentimes, a mental shock that makes a child wretched in early life, and drives him into insanity at a later date." Overtaxing the undeveloped physical powers is another cause.

Insanity is most Prevalent among the Working Classes.--Our factories, shops and stores frequently employ the young of both sexes and they are overtaxed by day and night and they become feeders of our hospitals for the insane. Another cause is forced education in the young. Our present school system tends to break down the body. The work may not be too hard, but the amount of anxiety and worry, which this work causes in the minds of sensitive children, tends to enfeeble them. Many children are sensitive, with nervous temperaments, and they are easily affected by the strain of mental toil. Delicate children should be kept in the open air and their physical condition should be considered more than their mental. Girls, especially, at the age of puberty, should be built up instead of rushed through a heavy routine of study. Herbert Spencer says: "On old and young the pressure of modern life puts a still increasing strain. Go where you will, and before long there comes under your notice cases of children, or youths of either sex, more or less injured by undue study." Here, to recover from a state of debility thus produced, a year's vacation has been found necessary. There you will find a chronic congestion of the brain that has already lasted many months and threatens to last much longer. Now you hear of a fever that has resulted from the over excitement, in some way, brought on at school. And, again, the instance is that of a youth who has already had to desist from his studies, and who, since he has returned to them is frequently taken out of his class in a fainting fit.

Social pleasure also tends to weaken the system of parents who produce nervous and weakened children. Another great cause of insanity is the unnatural, improper and excessive use of the sexual organs, and diseases that often come from indiscriminate sexual relations. General paresis is very often caused by specific disease. I might go on and enlarge upon these causes, but enough has been written to give warning to those who are breaking nature's laws.

Classification.--There are many classifications. I will mention only the leading names, such as Melancholia, Mania. Dementia, General Paresis.

MELANCHOLIA (Sad Mania).--Melancholia is a disease characterized by great mental depression.

Causes--Predisposition, physical disease, dissipation, work and worry, shock, brooding. In simple melancholia the mildest attack may be called the "blues."

ACUTE MELANCHOLIA.--Is generally the result of some mental shock.

CHRONIC MELANCHOLIA is the end of all other forms of

mental depression. All these have their own peculiar manifestations and need a special line of treatment.

MANIA.--This type of insanity means a raving and furious madness. There are many cases of this kind. The causes are many and may be the same as those which produce melancholia. In melancholia the shock, etc., causes depression, while in the mania the causes of mental injury tend to produce irritation and excitement. In dementia, the causes of insanity tend to exhaust the body and to mental failure, while in general Paresis "the shock of disease comes after long and unwise contact with worry, wine and women." Insufficient sleep often causes mania. It often follows after exhausting and irritating fevers. Long continued ill health, together with worry, etc., may cause it.

To sum up, "mania" may result from any unusual shock or strain upon the nervous system; or it may come after any unusual mental excitement in business, politics or in religion. Such are the exciting or stimulating causes, but we must go back of the presence of worldly misfortune and trace the tendency to mental disorder through channels of hereditary influence. "Infants are born every day whose inevitable goal is that of insanity." What is said in the Bible about sins of the parents is true.

DEMENTIA.--This term literally means "from mind," out of mind, and such a person is in a state of the most deplorable mental poverty. We all have seen such cases and some cases are not only very sad but disgusting.

PRIMARY DEMENTIA comes on independently of any other form of insanity.

SECONDARY DEMENTIA follows after some other form of insanity,--chiefly melancholia or mania. Dementia may be acute or chronic.

SENILE (OLD AGE) DEMENTIA may be Primary.--Acute dementia attacks both sexes, but it occurs most often in females, though in a milder degree. It is a disease of youth, being rarely seen beyond thirty years of age. It seems to depend often upon exhausting influences operating at a period of rapid growth. Monotony of thought and feeling or want of mental food can also induce it. Children who are sent at an early age into factories often pass into the condition of acute dementia. Prison life also tends to produce such a condition. Acute diseases such as typhoid and other fevers are sometimes followed by acute dementia. Persons frequently go "out of their mind" suddenly in this age, and upon recovering from acute dementia, the patient finds a great "vacancy of memory."

Chronic Dementia.--Shakespeare says, "Last scene of all, that ends this strange, eventful history, is second childishness and mere oblivion; sans teeth, sans eyes, sans taste, sans everything."

"The Sans Everything."--Is the sad and hopeless obscuration by time or disease of the once bright, vigorous, scintillating mental powers of exhuperant and lusty youth. Everyone has seen such people who are partially or hopelessly demented. It may come from diseases, such as epilepsy and syphilis; alcohol produces it.

Senile dementia is the result of old age and of acquired brain disease. It is different from simple old age or dotage. In old age the mind is weakened, but the patient is conscious of it, such a person forgets a name or date and gropes about in his memory to find it.

The demented person is not conscious of loss of memory, but applies wrong names to persons, and serenely thinks he is right.

The senile demented person does not realize his condition, and if there is any mental power left he cherishes delusions or false beliefs.

The victim of old age is unconscious of his weakness.

GENERAL PARESIS.--Wine, worry and women produce a great many cases of this disease. The doctors claim a notorious criminal now committed to one asylum and about whom we have read so much, is a victim of this disease.

First stage.--There is worry, anxiety, sleeplessness and melancholy.

Second stage.--Stage of mania, wealth, power, and grandeur, alternating in some cases with attacks of temporary depressions.

Third stage.--Patient passes into a condition of subacute or chronic mania, with a slow tendency to decadence of all the powers, idiotic.

Fourth stage.--Stage of physical and mental failure and of death. Syphilis causes most cases. It usually develops between twenty-five and fifty years. The outlook for such cases is very unfavorable, as the patient usually dies from one to eight or ten years after the beginning of the disease.

TREATMENT.--There have been great advances made in recent years in the treatment of persons mentally unsound. They should be placed under proper treatment at an early stage. The causes have been given so that preventive measures may be taken.

CONSTITUTIONAL DISEASES.

RHEUMATIC GOUT. (Rheumatic Arthritis. Arthritis Deformans).--Cause.--It occurs most often from thirty to fifty-five, usually in women, generally at or after the change of life, and most frequently in those who have not had children. The involvement of the joints is most common in adult males.

Exciting cause may be: Exposure to cold and wet, improper food, unhygienic surroundings, worry, blows and acute infections.

Conditions.--Several joints are usually involved symmetrically. At the edge of the joints there is formation of new bone covered with cartilage, causing the enlargement of the bone and often partial loss of motion in that joint.

Symptoms.--Several distinct types exist. 1. General progressive types which may be acute or chronic.

Acute.--This occurs usually in women from twenty to thirty and at the change of life. It comes on like acute joint rheumatism, many joints being affected, permanent enlargement appearing early, redness of the joints rarely existing, the pain being very severe, some fever, feel very tired, with anemia, loss of flesh and strength. The first and later attacks are often associated with pregnancy, confinement or nursing.

Chronic Type.--There is a gradual onset of pain or stiffness in one or more joints, usually of the fingers, then of the corresponding joints of the other side and then other joints. The swelling at first may be in the soft parts of the joints with effusion in the joints and tenderness. The pain varies from slight to severe. Periods of improvement and getting worse alternate; the joints becoming enlarged and deformed, often nearly stiff in partial bending on account of the thickened bone and soft tissues. The muscles that move the joint dwindle and there may be changes in the skin and nails of the parts affected due to the want of proper nourishment. Disturbances of the stomach and anemia are common. The heart is not affected. There may be only a few joints affected, or many, with great deformity, before the disease reaches the period of inactivity.

2. Monarticular or one joint type.--This usually occurs in males over fifty; one joint or a few large joints may be affected, generally with shrinking of the corresponding muscles. If it occurs in the hip it is called Morbus Coxae Senilis,--Hip joint disease in the aged.

Recovery.--The disease usually goes on with intervals of improvement and often results in great crippling and disability. In some cases it becomes permanent.

General Treatment.--The climate should be warm and dry. The patient should avoid exposing himself; lead a general hygienic life, with as nourishing food as his digestion will permit. The chief line of treatment should be to improve the general health and relieve the pain. The stomach, bowels, and kidneys should be kept working well. Nourishing food should be taken, but its effect must be watched. Cod-liver oil to build up the system, iron and arsenic may be of value. Sometimes iodide of potash is good. Early and thorough treatment at Hot Springs offers the best hope of arresting its progress, the Hot Springs in Bath County, Va., and in Arkansas. Much can be done at home by hot air baths, hot baths, and compresses at night to the tender joints.

Local.--Massage carefully given is helpful. The hot air treatment is good. Baking the joints is now frequently done.

GOUT (PODAGRA).--A disorder of nutrition characterized by excess of uric acid in the blood, attacks of acute arthritis (inflammation of joints) with deposit of urate of sodium in and around the joints; with various general symptoms.

Causes.--Heredity; male sex, usually appears from thirty to fifty and rarely under twenty; from continued use of alcoholic liquors, especially fermented, with little or no exercise; too much meat. Unhygienic living with poor food, and excessive drinking of ale and beer may be followed by the "poor man's gout." It is common in lead workers.

Symptoms. Acute Type.--There is often a period of irritability, restlessness, indigestion, twinges of pain in the hands and feet; the urine is scanty, dark, very acid, with diminished uric acid and deposit when it is cooled. The attack sets in usually early in the morning with sudden intense pain in a joint of the big toe, generally the right; less often in an ankle, knee, wrist, hand or finger. The part swells rapidly, and is very tender, the overlying skin being red, glazed and hot. The patient is usually as cross as a wounded bear. The fever may be 103. The pain may subside during the day, and increase again at night. There is no suppuration (pus forming). The symptoms usually decrease, gradually, the entire attack may last from five to eight days. Scaling of the skin over the sore part may follow.

After the attack, the general health may be improved, and the joint may become normal or but slightly stiff. It recurs at intervals of a few months commonly.

Retrocedent Gout.--This is a term applied to serious symptoms which sometimes go with rapid improvement of the local joint conditions. There are severe pains in the stomach, nausea, vomiting, diarrhea, pain in the heart, difficult breathing, palpitation, irregular and feeble action of the heart with brain symptoms, probably from uraemia. These attacks often cause death.

Chronic Gout, Causes, etc.--Frequent acute attacks; many joints, beginning with the feet, become stiff and deformed, perhaps with no motion. The overlying skin may ulcerate, especially over the knuckles. Dyspepsia, arterio-sclerosis, enlargement of the left ventricle of the heart and a great quantity of urine with low specific gravity are common. The patient is morose and irritable. Eczema, chronic bronchitis, frequently complicate the case.

Death often occurs from uraemia, meningitis, pleurisy, pericarditis or peritonitis.

Treatment, Preventive.--Live temperately, abstain from alcohol, eat moderately, have plenty of fresh air and sunshine, plenty of exercise and regular hours. These do not counteract the inherited tendency. The skin should be kept active, if the patient is robust, by the morning cold bath with friction after it; but if he is weak and debilitated, the evening warm bath should be substituted. The patient should dress warmly, avoid rapid alternations in temperature, and be careful not to have thc skin suddenly chilled.

Diet in Gout.--Most persons over forty eat too much. Eat reasonably and at regular hours and take plenty of time to eat. Do not eat too freely of meats and avoid too much starchy and sugary foods. Fresh vegetables and fruits may be used freely, except cranberries and bananas.

Dr. Osler of England says.--

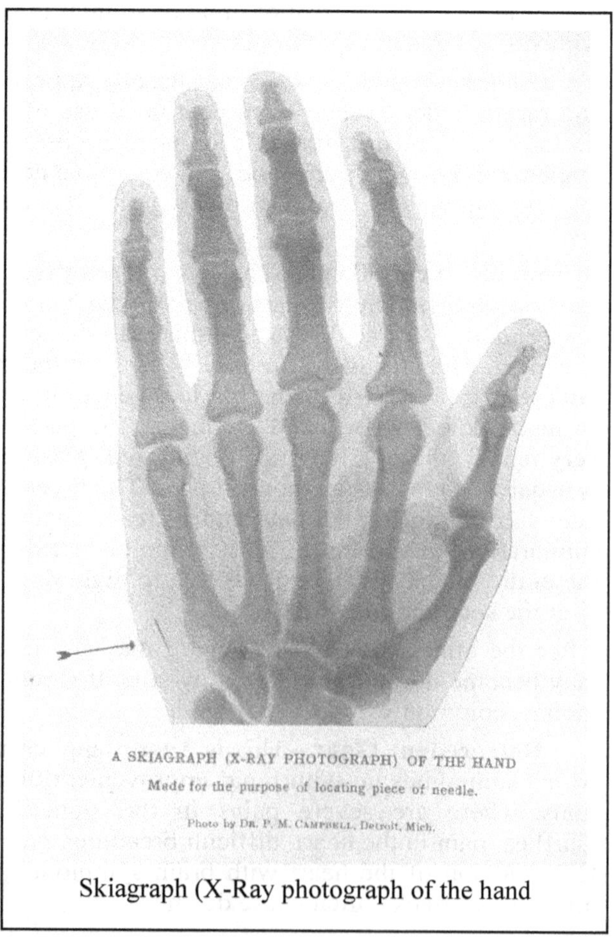

A SKIAGRAPH (X-RAY PHOTOGRAPH) OF THE HAND
Made for the purpose of locating piece of needle.
Photo by Dr. P. M. Campbell, Detroit, Mich.

Skiagraph (X-Ray photograph of the hand

While all stimulants are injurious to these patients some are more so than others, particularly malted liquors, champagne, port and a very large proportion of all the light wines. Take large quantities of water on an empty stomach, mineral waters are no better than others, but treatment of chronic and irregular gout at springs gives the advantage of regular hours, diet, etc.

Diet from a prominent hospital for gout patient:--

May Take--

Soups.--Fresh fish soups, vegetable broths clear.

Fish.--Raw oysters, fresh fish, boiled.

Meats.--Fat bacon, boiled or broiled chicken, game (all sparingly).

Farinaceous.--Cracked wheat, oatmeal, rice, sago, hominy, whole wheat bread, or biscuits, rye bread, graham bread or rolls, crackers, dry toast, milk toast, macaroni.

Vegetables.--Mashed potatoes, green peas, string beans, spinach, cabbage, cucumbers, cresses, lettuce, celery.

Desserts.--Plain milk pudding, junket, rice and milk, sago and milk, stewed fruits, all without sugar.

Drinks.--Weak tea (no sugar), milk, buttermilk, toast water, pure water, cold or hot.

Must Not Take--

Veal, pork, goose, duck, turkey, salted, dried, potted or preserved fish or meat (except fat bacon), eels, mackerel, crabs, salmon, lobster, eggs, rich soups, gravies, patties, tomatoes, sweet potatoes, asparagus, mushrooms, rhubarb, lemons, pickles, vinegar, fried or made dishes, rich puddings, spices, pies, pastry, sweets, nuts, dried fruits, tobacco, coffee, cider, malt liquors, sweet wines, champagne.

Treatment.--In an acute attack raise the affected limb and wrap the "sick" joint in cotton wool; warm fomentations may be used. The wine or tincture of colchicum in doses of twenty to thirty drops may be given every four hours in combination with the citrate of potash, fifteen grains, or the citrate of lithium five to ten grains. Stop the tincture of colchicum as soon as the pain is relieved and then you can give wine of colchicum ten drops every four hours, watching for irritation of the stomach, bowels and kidneys.

Dr. Hare of Philadelphia says.--For hospital practice a very useful mixture is made by adding one part of bicarbonate of sodium to nine parts of linseed oil. The joint is then wrapped in a piece of lint soaked with this concoction. In some cases oil of peppermint has been recommended. In chronic gout Dr. Hare also gives for diet milk and eggs, the white meat of chicken; fruits, cooked without sugar being added, are allowed. Tea and coffee being used only in moderation. If any wine is taken it must be followed by copious draughts of pure water and the last article should be used ad libitum. On the other hand, pastries and, more than all, sweet wines, are the worst things that such a patient can take, and must be absolutely prohibited.

RHEUMATIC FEVER (Articular Rheumatism).--Causes. This may be acute or chronic. It is an infectious disease characterized by inflammation of several joints. The joints are held in place by ligaments and are inclosed by a thin membrane. In this acute rheumatism these parts become congested and inflamed, there is redness and swelling, heat and pain. Fluid is passed into the joint sometimes and then the parts look watery (oeclematous). The inflammation and swelling cause great pain in the joint.

Predisposing.--A damp climate, winter and spring, young adults and persons who are exposed to damp, wet and cold.

Condition.--There is congestion of the soft parts of the joints and effusion into the joint cavities of a watery fluid. Endocarditis, pericarditis, myocarditis, pleurisy and pneumonia may complicate it. The first named, endocarditis, is very common and as the mitral valves become inflamed it is likely to leave valvular trouble unless carefully watched and treated at the time.

Symptoms.--The invasion may be gradual, with a very tired feeling and often tonsilitis; but it is usually sudden, with pains, soreness in one or more joints and fever. The knees, ankles, elbows and wrists are much affected, but it frequently goes through almost every joint in the body and sometimes repeats the terrible dose. I know, for I had it twice. The suffering, torture and pain sometimes are simply indescribable and almost too hard to bear. The joints become hot, red, painful, swollen and tender to touch and motion. It seems to hurt worse when anyone comes near, for the patient is afraid of careless handling.

Fever.--This runs from 102 to 104 and is modified by profuse perspiration with bad odor and, generally, it does not afford any relief. The urine is very acid, very thick and looks like thick, strong coffee. The symptoms frequently disappear partially from one joint or joints as they begin in other joints, attacking several in rapid succession, the fever varying and changing with the degrees of joint involvement.

We may see the shoulder and hip, the elbow and wrist, knee and ankle, etc., all affected at once: Heart complications are frequent and bear close watching, for they are dangerous to life and the future health of the patient. The patient becomes very anemic and this progresses rapidly. When improvement does begin it is gradual; or the disease may become chronic. Care must be taken not to be too active when improvement sets in or you will cause a return by using the joints before they have become thoroughly well. I did the same thing in my anxiety to get out, but would never be as reckless again. Pain and stiffness of the joints often last long after convalescence has set in. One who has had this disease once is liable to another attack if he is not careful.

MOTHERS' REMEDIES. 1. Articular Rheumatism.--A gentleman sends us the following treatment for articular rheumatism and writes as follows: "I send you the following treatment for articular rheumatism because I used it myself and was cured in a very short time, in fact, about ten days. It was a number of years ago in the early spring when my knee joints, ankles and wrists began to pain me and continued to become worse for about a week, at the end of which time both my knees were perfectly stiff. I sent for my physician; he wrapped my knees with common baking soda; taking long wide bandages he was enabled to have the baking soda a fourth of an inch thick around the knee, raising the bandage as he laid the soda on; after this was completed I had heavy wet hot cloths laid around my knee and renewed every fifteen or twenty minutes for probably eight or ten hours. In the meantime I was taking the salicylate of soda and the cathartic, veronica water, as directed below. The following day I sat up with my legs resting on a chair, straightened out, and hot flat irons at my knees. I began this treatment on Saturday, and the following Thursday was able to walk about and go out of town, and never had rheumatism since, but at two or three different times I suspected it was coming on and used the salicylate of soda and veronica water as a successful preventive; at least the rheumatism did not materialize.

Veronica Water.--Dose:--Glassful every two and one-half hours till bowels are free, then one dose a day.

Also

Salicylate of Soda	1 ounce
Water	6 ounces

Large teaspoonful every two hours with a quinine pill every other dose."

2. Rheumatism, Cotton Excellent for Inflammatory.--"Take a roll of cotton batting and wrap the limb, or part of the body affected, as firmly and tightly as possible, without tearing the cotton, let it remain "twenty-four hours, then tighten it up by unwinding and rewrapping the cotton as tight as possible, as on the first application, and so continue every twenty-four hours until cured, which, in my case, was three days. I had been troubled with rheumatism for a long time, and was unable to walk. I tried everything, doctors and all, but nothing helped me. A lady from Cincinnati, who was visiting at a neighbor's, called at my house one day and learning what was the matter with me, advised me to put cotton on as stated above. I had no faith in it, but I had tried everything else and concluded I would try that, with the result that it cured me. Possibly if a case should require a longer time for a cure than mine it might be necessary, or be better, to replace the cotton with a fresh roll. The rewrapping every twenty-four hours is intended to keep the cotton batting firmly and tightly around the part affected as the swelling recedes."

Prevention.--Wear flannel late and early. Keep from taking cold. Put off wet things of every kind immediately upon getting home and dry your body and put on dry well-aired clothes. Never sleep in a damp bed, under damp unaired clothes. When you go away from home do not sleep in a room or bed that has been unoccupied for any length of time, especially if there is no furnace in the house. Do not sit down in wet damp clothes, stockings, shoes, etc. Do not sit down anywhere to "cool off." It is inviting trouble and sickness. Do not lie on the damp ground, do not sleep on the first floor of an old damp house. Have plenty of sunlight and air in your sleeping room. These directions apply to the chronic cases also. It does not matter so much if one is wet or sweating as long as he keeps moving or working. On wash day do not dry your clothes in the kitchen or sitting room, or put them on your bed, unless they have been thoroughly dried, aired and warmed before using. These little things mean much in real life.

PHYSICIANS' CAUTION for Articular Rheumatism.--Go to bed and remain there and do not get up too soon, for remember the parts are still tender when they may not be painful.

Local Treatment.--1. There must be absolute rest. Remove the sheets from the bed and wrap woolen cloths or blankets about the patient and protect the inflamed joints from the weight of the coverings. Cover the joints with gauze or absorbent cotton, after putting on the parts a thick coating of ichthyol ointment.

2. Sometimes hot fomentations are helpful in relieving the suffering; sometimes cold cloths are best.

3. The following is good. Apply with cloths wrung out of it:

	Carbonate of Soda	6 drams
	Tincture Arnica	10 ounces
	Glycerin	2 ounces
	Water	9 ounces
4.	Oil of Wintergreen	1 ounce
	Compound Soap Liniment	8 ounces
	Mix.	

Rub the affected parts with oil of wintergreen and then wrap the parts in cotton wool and soak with the solution.

5. "A layer or two of gauze saturated with methyl-salicylate is wrapped around the painful joints and covered with paraffin paper, or other impervious dressing, held in place by a bandage. This is renewed once or twice daily until the pain in all the joints is relieved."

6. Internal.--Sodium salicylate or aspirin given until the pain and temperature are relieved; usually five to ten grains of sodium salicylate every three hours for an adult; or five grains of the aspirin every three hours.

7. Dr. Hare recommends for the beginning in a strong, healthy individual, ten drops of the tincture of aconite at once in a little water, and follow it by a teaspoonful of a mixture containing fifteen drops of tincture of aconite and two ounces of water everyone-half hour, until perspiration on the skin betokens the circulatory depression through the action of the drug. I use aconite in this disease very often, but not in such doses as the first one. It seems to me that it is uselessly large. I use about one-tenth of a drop at a dose everyone to two hours during the first twenty-four hours.

Nursing.--The nurse must have the patience of Job to attend a patient sick with this disease; but you must remember the suffering is awful. The patient may be very restless and the pillows may need rearranging every few minutes. Also be careful how you handle the patient. It hurts terribly to be even touched. A rough, hearty person has no business to care for such a patient. I allow patients to say anything they wish, for this is a painful disease. They may swear at me if they wish. I know how it is, for I was there twice, the last time for six long weeks. Have patience and courage and cheer your patient. Do not look cross or scold.

Diet.--Milk mainly, broths, gruels, albumen water, oyster or clam broth, milk toast, buttermilk, kumiss. Do not give solid food. Water, lemonade, vichy or carbonated water.

CHRONIC RHEUMATISM.--Causes.--Heredity may predispose to it. It is most common in those who are exposed to hard labor in the cold and wet; especially in women about middle age. It occasionally follows sub-acute, but rarely acute rheumatism.

Symptoms.--Many large joints are usually affected; sometimes it may be only one joint; at times, the small joints only are affected. It may be only on the one side. It usually persists in the joints involved, but may attack others. The chief symptoms are stiffness of the joints, especially after a rest and this diminishes after some motion, also pain, which grows worse in damp weather. The joints may be tender to the touch, slightly swollen, rarely red. They may in time become entirely stiff and deformed. The general health may be good or there may be anemia, dyspepsia and valvular disease due to sclerosis,--hardening of the valves of the heart.

Prognosis.--This is good as to life, but the disease is often progressive.

Treatment. Preventive.--A warm, dry, unchangeable climate, good surroundings, good food; keep the stomach and bowels and kidneys in good condition, avoid taking cold. Do not sit down in a draft to "cool off." Do not go into a cool room in summer when you are warm or sweated. Do not sleep in a bed that has not been used for months and kept for "company." Do not dry your clothes in the kitchen and in that way make the whole house steamy and damp. Do not sleep under unaired damp covers or in a damp night dress. Always air and dry your bedding and night dress before using. Do not take a hot bath and go into a cool room to cool off, but wrap yourself up so as to be warm and cool off gradually. Any additional cold will cause more rheumatism.

Sleeping rooms on the first floor are an abomination for rheumatic persons. Do not sit down in wet clothes, stockings or shoes. Take them off immediately on getting home, wipe yourself dry and put on dry garments. Care in such little seemingly foolish things will do wonderful things for a rheumatic person. I had two rheumatic attacks in my first year of practice. Since then I have learned caution and through a hard and busy life I have kept myself reasonably well by looking after such little aids and cautions as, the above. I never sit down for any length of time in damp or wet clothes, and if I can do that, persons that are not driven like doctors can do the same. These cautions apply to not only this kind of rheumatism, but to all kinds of rheumatism, neuralgias, and to inflammatory diseases, such as neuritis, tonsilitis, pneumonia, pleurisy, etc. Hot air baths, Hot Springs, massage will be more effectual in this disease than in the former. Iodide of potash also is very useful. Flannel underwear, heavy and light weight, is very beneficial in rheumatism. Great benefit can be derived at home by wrapping the affected joints in cold cloths, covering with a thin layer of flannel and protected by oiled silk. A great many cases are helped by using hot fomentations of hops, wormwood, smartweed, etc. Turpentine applied locally to the joints is effective, but it is very likely to injure the kidneys when used freely and in these days when there are so many diseases of the kidneys one must be careful or they will produce an incurable and serious disease in the place of one that is painful, but not necessarily dangerous. Many of the simple remedies have a good effect on the rheumatic troubles.

PHYSICIANS' TREATMENT for Rheumatism.--Dr. Hare gives the following to rub on large joints:

1.	Ichthyol	1/2 to 1 ounce
	Lard	1 ounce
2.	Tincture of Aconite	6 drams
	Tincture Arnica	1 ounce
	Oil of Turpentine	1 ounce (1 or 2)
	Soap Liniment enough for	8 ounces

Use as a liniment three times a day. This can be used for some weeks.

3.	Strong Water of Ammonia	6 drams
	Oil of Cajeput	1 dram
	Tincture of Belladonna	1 to 2 ounces
	Camphor Liniment enough for	8 ounces

Use as a liniment.

4.	Tincture of Aconite	1 ounce
	Tincture Belladonna	2 drams
	Strong Ammonia Water	4 drams
	Chloroform Liniment	6 drams

Used as a liniment on chronic or inflamed muscles or joints.

5.	Iodide of Potash	1/2 ounce
	Compound Syrup of Sarsaparilla	3 ounces
	Distilled Water	3 ounces

Mix and take a dessertspoonful in a glass of water two hours after meals for chronic rheumatism.

6. This is prepared by Parke, Davis & Co., and made into a syrup:

Red Clover	32 grains
Queen's Root	16 grains
Barberry	10 grains
Prickly Ash Bark	4 grains
Burdock Root	16 grains
Poke Root	16 grains
Honduras Bark	16 grains
Iodide of Potash	8 grains

This portion to each fluid ounce of the syrup.

7. The following is good:

Equal parts of each of the following:

Blue Cohosh Root
Black Cohosh Root
Poke Root
Yellow Dock Root
Blue Flag Root
Prickly Ash Root
Burdock Root
Dandelion Root

Bruise them thoroughly or grind them coarsely, steep and make a tea and drink freely of it. If you wish you can take three to five grains of Iodide of Potash to each dose. This may in time disorder the stomach and you may then stop it for a time. All these can he used in muscular rheumatism also. The food should not be rich or highly seasoned. Spices are bad for such patients. Pickles, mustard, etc., are best let alone.

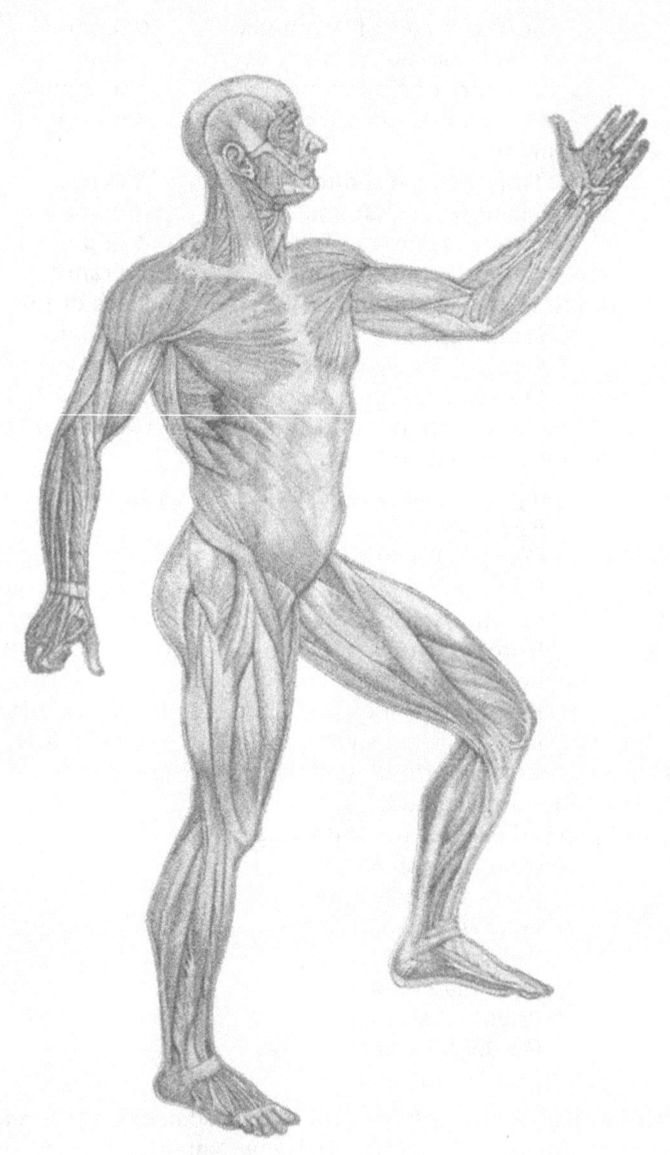

MUSCULAR SYSTEM.

Muscular System.

MUSCULAR RHEUMATISM.--This is a very painful affection of the voluntary muscles, called also neuralgia, or according to its location, torticollis (stiff neck, wry neck), pleurodynia, lumbago (rheumatism in the back).

Causes.--Predisposed to it by previous attacks, having a rheumatic or gouty constitution (diathesis). It follows sudden exposure, hence it is most common in men.

Symptoms.--Local pain in the muscles, sharp or dull, aching constant, or caused by certain movements and is usually relieved by pressure. It lasts from a few days to several weeks and frequently recurs. The common forms are: **Lumbago**. This affects the muscles of the back, and usually comes on suddenly with a sharp stich-like pain, and is chiefly seen in those who labor hard, often completely disabling them for a time.

Torticollis (stiff or wry neck).--It is usually on the side or back of the neck. Comes from a draught of cold wind on the neck, etc.

Pleurodynia, pain in the chest muscles, etc.--With pain in all movements of the chest, resembling intercostal neuralgia or pleurisy.

Diet for Rheumatism from the Head Nurse of a Prominent Hospital:--

May Take--

Soups.--Mutton broth, chicken or beef tea, in small quantities.

Fish.--Raw clams or oysters, fresh fish (whiter kinds) boiled.

Meats.--Chicken, calf 's head, sweetbread, tripe, broiled fat bacon or broiled ham (all sparingly).

Farinaceous.--Whole wheat, corn or brown bread, arrowroot, rice, dry toast, milk toast.

Vegetables.--Spinach, green peas or cabbage (well boiled), celery, lettuce, cresses, radishes.

Desserts.--Milk, rice or arrowroot pudding, (all without sugar), junket.

Drinks--Tea (without sugar), buttermilk, pure water, plain with lemon or lime juice (no sugar).

Must Not Take--

Pork, veal, turkey, goose, duck, fried fish or salt meats, cooked oysters or clams, salted, dried, potted or preserved fish or meats (except fat bacon or ham), crabs, salmon, lobster, eggs, rich made dishes, gravies, potatoes, tomatoes, beans, asparagus, mushrooms, candies, rich puddings, pies, pastry, nuts, cheese, coffee, cider, malt liquors, wines.

Treatment for Stiff Neck.--Wry Neck, (torticollis).--Warmth applied either dry or moist as hot salt bag or fomentations of hops, etc. Parke, Davis & Co., Detroit, now make a preparation called capsicine. This is very good for this trouble, rubbed on thoroughly as directed. It can be bought at most drug stores. It is also good for headaches and neuralgias. The same line of treatment, hot and cold applications, can be given for pain in the chest muscles (pleurodynia) and lumbago.

A MOTHERS' REMEDY for Stiff Neck.--Hot Salt and Oil of Sassafras.--"If troubled with stiff neck, fill a bag with hot salt and sleep on it, or rub the neck with oil of sassafras which, by the way, is also excellent for lumbago and to scatter, not cure, rheumatism pains."

PHYSICIANS' TREATMENT for Rheumatism.--Preventive.--Avoid exposure as stated for other rheumatism. Rest the chest by strapping with adhesive plaster as in pleurisy. Porous plasters are good and liniments; sometimes help is obtained by rubbing freely with camphor. Hot dry or wet applications are frequently useful. Mustard plaster is very good when the space is not too great. Mix the mustard with the white of an egg and after it is taken off grease the part and keep on warm cloths. Hot foot baths and hot drinks of lemonade or teas, after which the person should go to bed and sweat and remain there for some hours.

Liniment.--

Oil of Wintergreen	1/2 to 1 ounce
Compound Soap Liniment	8 ounces

Mix and rub on thoroughly.

MOTHERS' REMEDIES.--Lumbago, Menthol Liniment for.--Apply the menthol liniment, cover with a thick cloth and put the hot water bottle next to it and go to bed. If up through the day have a cotton batting sewed to cloth and keep affected parts warm, using the liniment freely." The menthol liniment will be found an excellent remedy for lumbago, The menthol absorbs quickly and by applying the hot water bottle relief is sure to follow.

1. Weak Back, Vinegar and Salt for.--"One tablespoonful of salt and one tablespoonful of vinegar to a quart of hot water. Bathe the back, then rub well with sweet oil and relief will soon follow,"

2. Weak Back. Simple Remedy for.--"Aching may be relieved by taking a large pinch of buchu leaves, steep and drink. Sweeten if desired. Use a pint of water for steeping the leaves," This is a good remedy for a weak back, resulting from kidney trouble. The buchu leaves acts quickly on the kidneys and it is surprising to see how quickly the backache will disappear. You can purchase a two ounce package for five cents at any drug store.

3. Weak Back, Good Liniment for.--

"Tincture of Aconite	1 ounce
Oil of Wintergreen	1/2 ounce
Tincture of Belladonna	1 ounce
Tincture of Arnica	1 ounce
Aqua Ammonia	2 ounces

Mix and use as a liniment."

This is a very good liniment.

4. Lameness, Chloroform Liniment for.--"Chloroform liniment is the best for all lameness and sore limbs."

5. Lameness, Plantain Leaves and Cream for.--"Make ointment from plantain laves, simmered in sweet cream or fresh butter. This is very cooling."

MOTHERS' REMEDIES.--1. Rheumatism, Saltpetre Good in Cases of.--"One ounce of saltpetre to one pint of water. Take one teaspoonful of the above in a large glass of water, about six times daily." The saltpetre acts on the kidneys, carrying off the impurities in this way. Care should be taken not to continue this treatment too long at a time, as continued use would result in injury to the kidneys.

2. Rheumatism, Rochelle Salts for.--"One teaspoonful rochelle salts in one-half glass water every other morning." This acts on the bowels and cleanses the system.

3. Rheumatism, Flowers of Sulphur Will Relieve Pain of.-- Sciatica is sometimes very much improved by wrapping the limb for one night with flowers of sulphur."

4. Rheumatism, Three Simple Ingredient Liniment for.--"One pint pure cider vinegar, one pint of turpentine, four fresh eggs, put the egg shells and all in the vinegar, let stand until the vinegar eats the eggs all up, then add the turpentine." This makes a fine liniment.

5. Rheumatism, Sulphur Good for.--"Cases of chronic rheumatism are often relieved by sulphur baths and sulphur tea. Dose:-- Powder sulphur and mix with molasses. A teaspoonful three times a day," Sulphur is a good blood purifier and laxative.

6. Rheumatism, Horse-Radish for.--"An excellent and well-known remedy for rheumatism is to make a syrup of horse-radish by boiling the root and add sufficient sugar to make it palatable. Dose:-- Two or three teaspoonfuls two or three times a day,"

7. Rheumatism, Simple Remedy to Relieve Pain of.--

"Peppermint	1 ounce
Oil of Mustard	1/4 ounce
Vinegar	1 pint
White of one egg.	

Beat egg; stir all together."

8. Rheumatism, Liniment for Chronic.--

"Olive Oil	1 pint
Sassafras Oil	2 drams
Camphor Gum	2 ounces
Chloroform	1/2 ounce

Dissolve the camphor in the oil and when dissolved add the chloroform and four ounces of turpentine or rosemary. Rub the parts well night and morning. If the limbs are very sensitive to cold, add to the mixture two ounces of tincture of capsicum."

9. Rheumatism, Herb Remedy for.--

Tincture Colchicum Seed	4 ounces
Gum Guaiacum	4 ounces
Black Cohosh Root	4 ounces
Prickly Ash Berries	4 ounces
Iodide Potash	1 ounce

Dose for adult, one teaspoonful three times a day in wineglassful of water or milk."

10. Rheumatism, Three Things that Will Help.--

"Best Rye Whisky	2 pints
Ground Burdock Seed	1/2 pound
Poke Berry Juice	1/2 pint

Mix, shake well before using.

Dose for adults, one and one-half or two tablespoonfuls night and morning." In severe cases take three times a day. This is a thoroughly tried remedy and is a very successful one.

11. Rheumatism, Good Liniment for.--

"Alcohol	1 ounce
Oil of Wintergreen	1 dram Chloroform
	5 drams
Gum Camphor	1/2 ounce
Sulphuric Ether	3/4 ounce
Oil of Cloves	1/2 dram
Oil of Lavender	1 dram

Mix and apply externally for rheumatism and you will find it a very beneficial remedy."

12. Rheumatism, Camphor and Alcohol for.--"Soak cotton batting in alcohol and camphor and apply on part." Application to the affected parts will frequently give relief in some rheumatic patients, when in others no relief is obtained by this method, it being necessary to take something internally.

13. Rheumatism, Sweet Fern Tea Excellent for.--"Sweet fern tea taken three times a day. Dose, one cupful. Father has used this successfully himself."

14. Rheumatism, Well-known Celery Remedy for.--"Celery tea several times a day with plenty of celery cooked or raw as a regular table food. Cut the celery in pieces, boil until soft in water and let the patient drink the tea, then make a stew of the remaining bits. If fresh celery cannot be obtained, celery preparations can be found at the drug store.

15. Rheumatism, Flowers of Sulphur Relieves.--"Rheumatism is effectually removed by enveloping the limb one night with flowers of sulphur." The flowers of sulphur can be purchased at any drug store, and will give great relief, especially in severe cases.

16. Rheumatism, Poultice for.--"Apply belladonna ointment to seat of pain, poultices applied very hot. Sulphur applied to painful part is very effective, after which the parts should be enveloped in flannel." The belladonna ointment acts like a fly blister, but not quite so severe. The ointment can remain on for some time without blistering. This treatment relieves by removing the inflammation from the sore parts.

17. Rheumatism, Novel Relief for.--"The best remedy is electricity. It cured me; I used medical battery." Electricity has been known to help in a great many cases, but should be applied by a competent person.

18. Rheumatism, Snake Root and Lemons Good for.--"Make use of lemon juice freely. Use decoction of black snake root, one ounce to pint of boiling water; a tablespoonful four times a day. Wet compress renewed every two hours applied to painful joints."

The black snake root is a remedy that was used by the early settlers for this trouble. The wet compresses are very soothing, but care should be taken not to wet the bed clothing, as the patient would then take cold.

19. Rheumatism, Another Good Liniment for.--

Alcohol	5 ounces
Amber	30 drops
Tincture of Pinoum	30 drops
Hemlock Oil	30 drops
Tincture of Iron	30 drops
Aconite	30 drops

DIABETES MELLITUS.--A disorder of nutrition in which sugar accumulates in the blood and is excreted in the urine, the daily amount of which is greatly increased.

Causes.--Hereditary influences play an important role and cases are on record of its occurrence in many members of the same family. Men are more frequently affected than women, the ratio being about three to two. Persons of a nervous temperament are often affected. It is a disease of the higher classes. Hebrews seem especially prone to it.

The disease is comparatively rare in the colored race; women more than men in the negro,-nine to six. In a considerable proportion of the cases of diabetes the patients have been very fat at the beginning of or prior to the onset of the disease. It is more common in cities than in country districts. The combination of intense application to business, over-indulgence in food and drink, with a sedentary life, seem particularly prone to induce the disease. Injury to or disease of the spinal cord or brain has been followed by diabetes. It is much more frequent in European countries than here. Acute and chronic forms are recognized in the former.

Symptoms.--The only difference is that the patients are younger in acute forms, the course is more rapid and the wasting away is more marked. The onset of the disease is gradual and either frequent passing of urine (six to forty pints in twenty-four hours) or inordinate thirst attracts attention. When it is fully established, there is great thirst, the passage of large quantities of sugar urine, a terrible appetite, and, as a rule, progressive emaciation. The thirst is one of the most distressing symptoms. Large quantities of water are required to keep the sugar in solution and for its excretion in the urine. Some cases do not have the excessive thirst; but in such case the amount of urine passed is never large. The thirst is most intense an hour or two after meals. The digestion is generally good, but the appetite is inordinate. Pain in the back is common. The tongue is usually dry, red and glazed, and the saliva is scanty. The gums may become swollen. Constipation is the rule. The skin is dry and harsh and sweating rarely occurs. The temperature is under normal. In spite of the enormous amount of food eaten a patient may become rapidly emaciated. Patients past middle life may have the disease for years without much disturbance of the health; on the other hand I have seen them die after that age. Progress is more rapid the younger the person. Death usually occurs from coma of diabetes. This is most common in young patients.

1. There is a sudden onset after exertion of weakness, feeble pulse, stupor, coma, death in a few hours.

2. Sudden headache, coma, death in a few hours.

3. After nausea, vomiting or a lung complication, there are headache, delirium, abdominal pain, rapid labored breathing, sweetish odor of the breath, stupor, rapid feeble pulse, coma and death within a few days.

Recovery.--Instances of cure in true diabetes are rare.

Treatment. Preventive.--The use of starchy and sugary articles of diet should be restricted in families with a marked disposition to this disease. Sources of worry should be avoided and he should lead an even quiet life, if possible, in an equable climate. Flannel and silk should be worn next to the skin, and the greatest care should be taken to promote its action. A lukewarm and, if tolerably robust, a cold bath should be taken every day. An occasional Turkish bath is useful.

Diet.--Let the patients eat food of easy digestion, such as veal, mutton and the like, and abstain from all sorts of fruit and garden stuff. In Johns Hopkins' Hospital these patients are kept for three or four days on the ordinary ward diet, which contains a moderate amount of carbo-hydrates, in order to ascertain the amount of sugar excretions. For two days more the starches are gradually cut off. They are then placed on the following standard non-carbohydrate diet.

Breakfast: 7:30, six ounces of tea or coffee; four ounces of beefsteak, mutton chops without bone, or boiled ham; one or two eggs.

Lunch: 12:30, six ounces of cold roast beef; two ounces celery, fresh cucumbers or tomatoes with vinegar, olives, pepper and salt to taste, five drams of whisky with thirteen ounces of water, two ounces of coffee without milk or sugar.

Dinner: 6:00 P. M., six ounces of clear bouillon; seven and a half ounces of roast beef; one and one-half drams of butter; two ounces of green salad with two and a half drams of vinegar, five drams of olive oil, or three tablespoonfuls of some well-cooked green vegetable: three sardines; five drams of whisky with thirteen ounces of water.

Supper: 9:00 P. M., two eggs, raw or cooked, thirteen ounces of water .

The following is a list of articles which a diabetes patient may take as given by one of the best authorities in the world on diabetes:

Liquids: Soups.--Ox tail, turtle bouillon and other clear soups. Lemonade, coffee, tea, chocolate and cocoa; these to be taken without sugar, but they may be sweetened with saccharin. Potash or soda water and appollinaris, or the Saratoga-vichy and milk in moderation may be used.

Animal Food.--Fish of all sorts, including crabs, oysters, salt and fresh butcher's meat (with the exception of liver), poultry and game, eggs, buttermilk, curds and cream cheese.

Bread.--Gluten and bran bread, almond and cocoanut biscuits.

Vegetables.--Lettuce, tomatoes, spinach, chickory, sorrel, radishes, asparagus, water-cress, mustard and cress, cucumber, celery and endives; pickles of various sorts.

Fruits.--Lemons and oranges, currants, plums, cherries, pears, apples (tart), melons, raspberries and strawberries may be taken in moderation. Nuts, as a rule, allowable.

Must Not Take--

Thick Soups and Liver. Ordinary bread of all sorts (in quantity), rye, wheaten, brown or white. All farinaceous (starchy) preparations, such as hominy, rice, tapioca, arrowroot, sago and vermicelli.

Vegetables: Potatoes, turnips, parsnips, squashes, vegetable--marrows of all kinds, beets, common artichokes.

Liquids: Beer, sparkling wine of all sorts and the sweet aerated drinks.

Medicines. Codeine.--A patient may begin with one-half grain three times a day, which may be gradually increased to six or eight grains in the twenty-four hours (under the doctor's care); withdraw it gradually when sugar is absent or reduced as far as possible.

DIABETES INSIPIDUS.--A chronic affection characterized by the passage of large quantities of normal urine of low specific gravity.

Causes.--It is most often found in young males and is probably of nervous origin. It may follow excitement or brain injury.

Symptoms.--The onset is usually gradual. The urine is pale; ten to twenty quarts a day. Thirst, dryness of the mouth and skin. Appetite and general conditions are usually normal; sometimes there are feebleness and emaciation. Death usually occurs from some other disease.

Treatment.--There is no known cure. Keep the general health in good condition according to the advice of your family physician.

OBESITY.--An excessive development of fat; it may be hereditary. It occurs most frequently in women of middle age and in children. Its chief cause is excessive eating and drinking, especially of the starch and sugar foods and malt liquors, and lack of exercise. The increase of fat is in all the normal situations and the heart and liver are often large and fatty. The condition in general may be good or there may be inactivity of the mind and body. Disturbances of digestion and symptoms of a fatty heart. There is less power to resist disease. Death may occur from fatty infiltration of the heart, resulting in dilatation or rupture.

Treatment.--Must be in regulating the diet. The person must avoid all excess in food and drink, and avoid especially foods that contain starch and sugar. There must be regular and systematic exercise, hot baths and massages are helps. Medicines made from the poke berry are much used and are successful in some cases.

Diet.--The food of a fleshy person should be cut down gradually. Its bulk can be great, but its nourishing properties should be small. The diet for reduction of obesity should consist chiefly of bulky vegetables, but not too much of any one article or set of articles. The following list is recommended by Dr. Hare of Philadelphia:

For Breakfast.--One or two cups of coffee or tea, without milk or sugar, but sweetened with a fraction of a grain of saccharin. Three ounces of toasted or ordinary white bread or six ounces of brown bread; enough butter may be used to make the bread palatable, not more than one ounce. Sliced raw tomatoes with vinegar, or cooked tomatoes without any sugar or fats. This diet may be varied by the use of salted or fresh fish, either at breakfast or dinner. This fish must not be rich like salmon or sword-fish, but rather like perch or other small fish.

Noon Meal--Dinner.--One soup plate of bouillon, consomme julienne, or other thin soup, or Mosqueras beef-jelly, followed by one piece of the white meat of any form of fowl or a small bird. Sometimes a small piece, the size of one's hand, of rare beef, or mutton but no fat, may be allowed, and this should be accompanied by string beans, celery (stewed or raw), spinach, kale, cabbage, beans, asparagus, beets and young onions. Following this, lettuce with vinegar and a little olive oil (to make a French dressing), a cup of black coffee or one of tea, and a little acid fruit, such as sour grapes, tamarinds and sour oranges, or lemons may be taken, and followed by a cigar, if the patient has such a habit.

Supper.--This should consist of one or two soft boiled eggs, which may be poached, but not fried, a few ounces of brown bread, some salad and fruit and perhaps a glass or two of light, dry (not sweet) wine, if the patient is accustomed to its use.

Before Going to Bed.--To avoid discomfort from a sensation of hunger during the night, the patient may take a meal of panada, or he may soak graham or bran crackers or biscuits in water and flavor the mess with salt and pepper. The reduction of the diet is generally best accomplished slowly and should be accompanied by measures devoted to the utilization of the fat present for the support of the body. Thus, the patient should not be too heavily clad, either day or night, should resort to exercise, daily becoming more severe, and should not drink freely of water, unless sweating is established sufficiently to prevent the accumulation of liquid in vessels and tissues. Baths of the proper kind, cold or Turkish, should be used, if the patient stands them well. The bowels should be kept active by laxative fruit or purges. Salts are useful if drinks are thrown off rapidly. If proper exercise is impossible the rest cure with massage, electricity, passive exertion and absolute skimmed milk diet may be resorted to, particularly in those persons known as "fat anemics," who have not enough red corpuscles in their blood to carry sufficient oxygen to the tissues to complete oxidation.

CANCER.--(In the following article on cancer we quote in part from material issued by the Public Health Department of the State of Michigan).

Cancer is curable if it be operated upon in its early stages.--If it be left to grow and develop, cancer is always fatal. It may be partially removed when in an advanced stage, and relief may be had for some time after operation; but beyond the early stage, cancer cannot at present be permanently removed, nor permanently cured. Permanent cure of a cancer is possible if the afflicted person obtains an early diagnosis and receives early attention from a skilled surgeon. The only permanent cure for cancer known at the present time is early surgical operation.

Have Operations Failed to Cure?--Very few persons die from operations performed by skilled surgeons for the removal of cancer. Where cancer operation is done by experienced surgeons the fatality in America for the past fourteen years is less than one case out of a hundred, or in other words ninety-nine persons out of a hundred survive operation for cancer. Many persons have died from the return of the cancerous growth even after operation by a skilled surgeon, and this fact has led many persons to believe that operation for cancer is, therefore, unsuccessful, that it does not cure. This is not the fact. It is true that cancer often returns after operation, and that this method does not always effect a permanent cure; but it is not true that operations are, therefore, useless. The reason that operations do not remove cancers permanently in a great number of cases is that such cases do not submit to operation soon enough. The majority of persons suffering from cancer seek surgical aid too late. If a house is on fire and one refuses to turn in an alarm until the fire has spread from cellar to garret, neither blame nor disparagement must be placed upon the fire department if it failed to save the burning house. So with cancer; if the public refuses or neglects to operate for cancer at the time when it can be eradicated, the public cannot censure or belittle surgery. A cancer is like a green and ripe thistle. Pull up the green thistle and you have gotten rid of it. But if you wait until the thistle is ripe, and the winds have blown away the seeds, there is no use of pulling up that thistle. Early operations are successful. Late ones are not.

No reliable surgeon claims to save his patient or cure him of cancer if the disease be in an advanced stage. But experienced surgeons do recognize the fact that cancer in its early stage can be permanently removed and a permanent cure can be effected by surgical operation. No other means of permanent cure are known.

Caustic pastes applied to cancerous growths or sera, are sometimes successful in obliterating the cancer for a time; but they are not reliable for effecting enduring cures, and usually are merely palliative, The fact that a cancer does not return for three years after removal is not sure proof that it will not return; the return of a cancerous growth depends upon its state of development and other conditions at the time of removal from the cancer. In Johns Hopkins' Hospital forty-seven per cent of all patients with cancers of the breast operated upon remained well for three years or more, and seventy-five per cent of this forty-seven per cent were cured, being in the most favorable condition for cure at the time of the operation. But where conditions are not favorable at the time of the operation, many patients have a return of the cancer even after the three years of apparent cure have elapsed.

What is Cancer?--A cancer is a growth of cancerous cells in a network of connective tissue. The cause of cancer is not known. It has not been proved to be communicable and the majority of investigators of this subject believe that it is not caused by a germ. Nor is it thought to be inherited. Out of 8,000 cases of cancer at Middlesex Hospital, London, no evidence of heredity was found. Until the cause of cancer is known, it cannot be prevented. The only safeguard lies in an early diagnosis of the condition and an immediate operation. Eminent investigators are carrying on extensive research and thousands of dollars are being spent annually to ascertain, if possible, what is the cause of this dread disease, and it is confidently believed that final success will crown this labor.

When to Suspect Cancer and What to Do.--External or Exposed Cancer.--Cancer of the exposed or surface parts of the body, such as the skin of the lip, nose, cheek, forehead, temples, etc., is more readily recognized than internal cancer, and is therefore more liable to early operation and prompt cure. One rarely sees these forms of cancer in an advanced stage, because such cases are readily seen and recognized by physicians in the early stage of development, when operation can be sufficiently early to effect a lasting cure.

The least malignant of all cancers is that kind which first exhibits itself by a hardening of the skin, forming a nodule looking pimple or a mole and having a dark red color, due to tortuous blood vessels, upon the sides of the nose near the eyes, upon the cheek bones, forehead or temples. This form of epithelioma is called rodent ulcer, flat epithelioma or cancroid and sometimes does little harm for many years, but should receive the attention of a physician familiar with cancer and its eradication.

Deep or squamous cancer occurs on the lip, the tongue or the forehead or wherever the mucous membrane joins the skin, and is characterized by a hard, deep-seated sore formed upon any such part, growing down into the flesh and having a dark red or purplish-red color.

If such a cancer is suspected of being present, the patient should at once seek diagnosis from a competent physician. Cancer of the lip is more frequent in men than in women, occurring usually in the under lip and called "Smoker's Cancer." Any hard persistent nodule in the under lip should cause suspicion and should be taken to a skilled surgeon, as cancer of the under lip is easily removed when in its early stage of development.

CANCER OF THE STOMACH.--The beginning of cancer of the stomach is very difficult to recognize and it is far safer and wiser, upon the appearance of the first suspicious symptom, to seek the aid of some physician skilled in cancer diagnosis than to ignore and neglect these early warnings of the disease. Although cancer of the stomach may occur in younger persons, it is usually met with in persons after forty years of age. Therefore, any person at this age who suffers from continuous indigestion or characterized by retention and prolonged fermentation of food in the stomach, should at once consult a competent physician. In the early stages of the cancer of the stomach the patient loses weight, but in the later stages there is more or less pain.

Whenever a physician finds that a patient has a pappy, insipid taste with a furred, pale, rarely dry and red tongue, and is suffering from continuous, dull sensations or pain in the region of the stomach, periodically increasing to paroxysms, often induced by pressure or increased by it, together with a sensation of weight, drawing pains of varying character, and frequent pain in the shoulder, loss of appetite, frequent belching of fetid gas from the stomach, severe and frequent vomiting, often periodical, often occurring before partaking of a meal but more often afterwards with slight indigestion, but vomitus being more or less watery and containing mucus and blood, usually decomposed and recurring frequently, together with constipation of the bowels, the skin being sallow, yellowish, dry and flaccid, and losing weight and strength, he should suspect cancer of the stomach and where possible advise an immediate surgical operation for the removal of the cancer.

CANCER OF THE UTERUS.--What women should know regarding it. The menopause or change of life comes on gradually, rarely suddenly. It is not preceded by excessive flowing or discharge or pain in a healthy woman.

By cancer period is understood those years after forty, although rarely it may occur earlier. The first symptoms of uterine cancer are:

1. Profuse flowing, even if only a day more than usual. Flowing or spotting during the interval or after the use of a syringe or the movement of the bowels.

2. Whites or Leucorrhea, if not existing previously. If existing but getting more profuse, watery, irritating, or producing itching is a very suspicious symptom.

3. Loss of weight, if no other cause is apparent. Pain in the region of the womb, back or side.

If any of the above symptoms occur after the age of thirty-five or forty, a woman should seek relief and insist on thorough investigation of the cause and prompt treatment.

Cancer is always at first a local disease and can be removed if early recognized and an absolute, permanent cure brought about.

CANCER OF THE BREAST.--Eighty-one per cent of an tumors of the breast are cancer or become so. Whenever a woman feels a lump in her breast, particularly if she be at the cancerous age, she should consult a skilled physician at once and keep that breast under medical observation. If so advised by her physician or by a skilled surgeon, she should have an operation for the removal of the cancer, as it can be completely eradicated when operated upon in its early stages. If left to grow and develop it will get beyond the aid of even the most skillful surgeon. Early diagnosis plus surgery is the only hope for a cancerous person. Operation offers a most hopeful outlook for those afflicted with cancer. It is more important to make an early diagnosis in cancer of the breast than it is in appendicitis.

CANCER (CARCINOMA).--This is very malignant. This kind is divided into two classes, Scirrhus and Epithelial.

1. Scirrhus cancer. This is a hard, irregular growth of moderate size. Its special seat is the breast, the pyloric (smaller) end of the stomach and in few instances the glands of the skin.

Soft Medullary or Encephaloid cancer. This type resembles brain tissue both in appearance and consistence. It appears quite soft and may be mistaken for an abscess. In form, it differs according to the organ attacked. Special seats: The testicle, liver, bladder, kidney, ovary, the eye and more rarely the breast.

Colloid cancer; jelly-like substance.--The cancer cells have undergone a degeneration in one of the preceding varieties. The material it contains is a semi-translucent, glistening, jelly-like substance. Its special seats are the stomach, bowel, omentum, ovary and, occasionally, the breast.

Diagnosis.--This kind is very rare before thirty years of age and common after forty. They involve the gland early, contrary to what the sarcoma variety does. Innocent growths occur, as a rule, in younger patients, do not grow so rapidly, do not become adherent to neighboring parts and do not ulcerate.

2. The Epithelial Cancer (Carcinoma).--These always spring from free epithelium-clad surfaces, as the skin, and mucous membranes or from the glands of the same. These growths appear with great frequency at the points of junction of mucous membranes and skin surfaces, probably because these parts are subjected to more frequent and varied forms of mechanical and chemical irritation, Special seats: Skin surfaces, the nose, the lower lip, the penis and scrotum, the vulva, the anus (mucous surfaces), tongue, palate, gums, tonsils, larynx, pharynx, gullet, bladder, womb.

MOTHERS' REMEDIES.--l. Cancer, Simple Remedy for.--- "Give a teaspoonful of sarsaparilla tea four times daily, made with two ounces of sarsaparilla root and quart of water boiled to one pint and apply to cancer growth a poultice made of carrots scraped or mashed cranberries." These simple remedies will relieve and often cure growths taken for cancers, but if it is really a cancerous growth no medicine will help and a physician should be consulted at once.

2. Cancer, Nettles and Laudanum Will Help.--"Take the juice of common nettles inwardly and mix a little laudanum with the juice and rub the parts outwardly. Cancer has often yielded to this treatment." This remedy will no doubt help an ugly looking ulcer, repeatedly taken for cancer, by the patients themselves and frequently the doctor. It is always well to give this simple home remedy a trial, at least, for it is frequently admitted by the medical fraternity to-day that ugly ulcers are often treated in this way as cancers, sometimes to the lasting detriment of the sufferer. Then why not try some efficient home remedy like the above until you are certain that it is a cancer?

TUMORS.--A tumor is a new growth which produces a localized enlargement of a part, or an organ, has no tendency to a spontaneous cure, has no useful function, in most cases tends to grow during the whole of the individual's life. Clinically, tumors are divided into the benign and the malignant.

A benign tumor is usually composed of tissues, resembling those in which it originates.

A malignant tumor usually consists of tissues widely different from those in which it originates; its growth is rapid and therefore often painful; it infiltrates all the surrounding tissues, however resistant, even bone, because it is never encapsulated; it thus early becomes immovable; the overlying skin is apt to become adherent, especially when the breast is involved. Sooner or later it usually infects the group of lymphatic glands intervening between it and the venous circulation and from these new centres, or directly through the veins, gives rise to secondary deposits in the internal organs.

Some varieties. 1. Fibrous tumors; these consist of fibrous tissues. 2. Fatty tumors (or lipomata); these consist of normal fat tissue. 3. Cartilaginous tumors; consist of cartilage. 4. Osseous (bony) tumors. 5. Mucous tumors (myxomata). 6. Muscular tumors (myomata). 7. Vascular tumors (Angeiomata). 8. Nerve tumors (Neuromata).

Malignant Sarcoma (Sarcomata).--These are a variety of tumors. The result of these varies with the location of the tumor. If located in the jaw, an operation may cure it. If in the tonsil or lymphatic gland, it destroys life rapidly. If in the sub-cutaneous tissue, it may be repeatedly removed, the system remaining free, or the amputation of the limb involved will probably cure the disease.

TUMORS.--Diagnosis. It is uncommon under thirty, quite common after. Epithelioma of the lower lip is limited almost entirely to men. If, then, a man of from forty to seventy develops a small tumor in the lower lip which ulcerates early, it is likely to be the cancer. The same applies to some extent to the tongue. These growths and sores need attention early.

Treatment.--The best treatment is early free removal of the entire growth before the glands are involved.

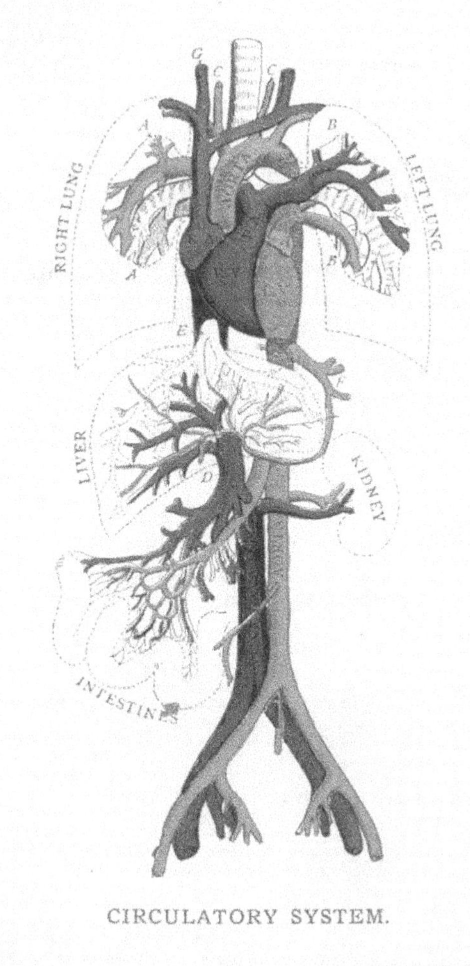

CIRCULATORY SYSTEM.

Circulatory system.

DISEASES OF THE CIRCULATORY SYSTEM

HEART DISEASE, Emergency Treatment.--For collapse or fainting, loosen clothing, lie down, rub camphor on forehead, and keep quiet.

To Revive When Fainting.--Smell of camphor or aromatic spirits of ammonia. Put one to two teaspoonfuls of whisky or brandy in eight teaspoonfuls of hot water, and give one or two teaspoonfuls at a time and repeat often. Some are not accustomed to stimulants and it may strangle them, so give it slowly. Pulse is weak in such cases, calling for stimulants.

2. Pearls of Amylnitrite. Break one in a handkerchief and put the handkerchief to the patient's nose so that he may inhale the fumes.

Stimulant.--A person with heart valvular trouble should always carry pearls of amylnitrite. Inhale slowly so as not to get too much of it at once.

HEART FAILURE.--The pulse may be slow and weak or fast and weak.

Digitalis.--Give five drops of the tincture in a little water. Another dose can be given in fifteen minutes. Then another in an hour, if necessary.

PALPITATION OF THE HEART.--Irregular or forcible heart beat action usually perceived by the person troubled.

Causes.--Hysteria, nervous exhaustion, violent emotions or sexual excesses; overdose of tea and coffee: alcohol or tobacco.

Symptoms.--There may be only a sensation of fluttering with that of distention or emptiness of the heart. There may be flushing of the skin, violent beating of the superficial arteries, with rapid pulse, difficult breathing and nervousness. Attack lasts from a few minutes to several hours.

22

MOTHERS' REMEDIES.-l. Palpitation of the Heart, Tea of Geranium Root for.--"Make an infusion of geranium root, half an ounce in pint of boiling water, strain, cool, and give wine glass full three or four times a day." The geranium root will be found to be an excellent remedy where female weakness has caused the palpitation of the heart.

2. Palpitation of the Heart, Hot Foot Bath and Camphor for.--"Place the feet in hot mustard water and give two grains camphor every two or three hours, or two drops aconite every hour. This remedy is very good and is sure to give relief."

3. Palpitation of the Heart, Valuable Herb Tea for.--"All excitement must be avoided. Where there is organic disease, all that can be done is to mitigate the severity of the symptoms. For this take the following herb tea: One ounce each of marigold flowers, mugwort, motherworth, century dandelion root, put in, two quarts of water and boil down to three pints; pour boiling hot upon one-half ounce of valerian, and one-half ounce of skullcap. Take a wineglassful three times a day. Let the bowels be kept moderately open and live principally upon vegetable diet, with plenty of outdoor exercise."

MOTHERS' REMEDIES.--1. Heartburn, Home Remedy for.--"A few grains of table salt allowed to dissolve in the mouth and frequently repeated will sometimes give relief." People who have too little acid in the stomach will be much benefited by this remedy.

2. Heartburn, Soda a Popular Remedy for.--"One-half teaspoonful soda in glass of water. Everybody uses this in the neighborhood."

3. Heartburn, Excellent Remedy for.--

"Powdered Rhubarb	1/2 ounce
Spirits of Peppermint.	2 drams
Water	4 ounces
Bicarbonate of Soda	1/2 ounce

Dose--One Tablespoonful after meals."

The bicarbonate of soda relieves the gas and swelling of the stomach, while the rhubarb has a tonic action and relieves the bowels. The spirits of peppermint stimulates the mucous membrane.

4. Poor Circulation, Remedy for Stout Person.--"Ten cents worth of salts, five cents worth of cream of tartar; mix and keep in a closed jar. Take one teaspoonful for three nights, then skip three nights." This is an old-time remedy known to be especially good, as the salts move the bowels and the cream of tartar acts on the kidneys, carrying off the impurities that should be thrown off from these organs.

PHYSICIAN'S TREATMENT FOR PALPITATION.--When caused by valvular trouble, digitalis can be given as above directed under heart failure.

When Caused by the Stomach.--From gas or too much food, take salts to move the bowels. Hot whisky is good when caused by gas; or soda, one teaspoonful in hot water is also good when gas causes palpitation.

Difficult Breathing.--If caused by gas, soda, hot whisky or brandy will relieve. If caused by too fast beating of the heart, give digitalis as above directed. If caused by dropsy, the regular remedies for dropsy. If the dropsy is due to scanty urine you can use infusion of digitalis, dose one to four drams; or cream of tartar and epsom salts, equal parts, to keep the bowels open freely.

PHYSICIAN'S CAUTIONS:--Quiet the patient's mind and assure him there is no actual danger; moderate exercise should be taken as a rule with advantage. Regular hours should be kept and at least ten hours out of twenty-four should be spent in lying down. A tepid bath may be taken in the morning, or if the patient is weakly and nervous, in the evening, followed by a thorough rubbing. No hot baths or Turkish bath. Tea, coffee and alcohol are prohibited. Diet should be light, and the patient should avoid overeating at any meals. Foods that cause gas should not be used. If a smoker the patient must give up tobacco. Sexual excitement is very pernicious, and the patient should be warned especially on this point. Absolute rest for the distressing attacks of palpitation which occur with nervous exhaustion. In these cases we find the most distressing throbbing in the abdomen, which is apt to come after meals, and is very much aggravated by the accumulation of gas.

Diet.--A person with heart disease should not bring on palpitation from over-eating or eating the wrong kind of food. Such a person dare not be a glutton. The diet must be simple, nutritious, but food that is easily digested. Any food that causes trouble must be avoided; starchy foods, spiced foods, rich greasy foods, are not healthy for such a person. The stomach must be carefully treated by such a patient. The bowels should move daily. The kidneys should always do good work and pass enough urine and of the right color and consistency. Stimulants like alcohol, tea and coffee are not to be used. Weak cocoa is all right in most cases. Hot water, if any drink must be taken, at meals. Such a patient in order to live and live comfortably, must take life easy. He cannot afford to run, to over lift, or over exert, to walk fast upstairs, hurry or to "catch the car." He must not get angry or excited. Games of all kinds that have a tendency to make him nervous must be avoided. The same caution applies to exciting literature. In short, a patient with organic heart disease must be a drone in the hum of this busy, fast-rushing life, if he would hope to keep the spark of life for many years. Sleep, rest and quiet is a better motto for you than the strenuous life.

The Heart.--The heart is the central organ of the entire system and consists of a hollow muscle; by its contraction the blood is pumped to all parts of the body through a complicated series of tubes, termed arteries. The arteries undergo enormous ramifications (branchings) in their course throughout the body and end in very minute vessels, called arterioles, which in their turn open into a close meshed network of microscopic (very minute) vessels, termed capillaries. After the blood has passed through the capillaries it is collected into a series of larger vessels called veins by which it is returned to the heart. The passage of the blood through the heart and blood vessels constitutes what is termed the circulation of the blood. The human heart is divided by a septum (partition) into two halves, right and left, each half being further constricted into, two cavities, the upper of the two being termed the auricle and the lower the ventricle. The heart consists of four chambers or cavities, two forming the right half, the right auricle and right ventricle, and two forming the left half, the left auricle and left ventricle. The right half of the heart contains the venous or impure blood; the left the arterial or pure blood. From the cavity of the left ventricle the pure blood is carried into a large artery, the aorta, through the numerous branches of which it is distributed to all parts of the body, with the exception of the lungs. In its passage through the capillaries of the body the blood gives up to the tissues the material necessary for their growth and nourishment and at the same time receives from the tissues the waste products resulting from their metabolism, that is, the building up and tearing down of the tissues, and in so doing becomes changed from arterial or pure blood into venous or impure blood, which is collected by the veins and through them returned to the right auricle of the heart.

From this cavity the impure blood passes into the right ventricle from which it is conveyed through the pulmonary (lung) arteries to the lungs. In the capillaries of the lungs it again becomes arterialized by the air that fills the lungs and is then carried to the left auricle by the pulmonary veins. From this cavity it passes into that of the left ventricle, from which the cycle once more begins. The heart, then, is a hollow muscular organ of a conical form, placed between the lungs and enclosed in the cavity of the pericardium. It is placed obliquely in the chest. The broad attached end or base is directed upwards, backwards and to the right and extends up to the right as high as the second rib and the center of the base lies near the surface underneath the breast bone. The apex (point) is directed downwards, forward and to the left and corresponds to the space between the cartilage of the fifth and sixth ribs, three-fourths of an inch to the inner side, and one and one-half inches below the nipple, or about three and one-half inches from the middle line of the breast bone. The heart is placed behind the lower two-thirds of the breast bone and extends from the median line three inches to the left half of the cavity of the chest and one and one-half inches to the right half of the cavity of the chest.

Size: In adults it is five inches long, three and one-half inches in breadth at its broadest part and two and one-half inches in thickness. Weight in the male ten to twelve ounces; in the female eight to ten. It increases up to an advanced period of life. The tricuspid valve (three segments) closes the opening between the right auricle and right ventricle. Pulmonary semilunar valves guard the orifice of the pulmonary artery, keeping the blood from flowing back into the right ventricle. The mitral valve guards the opening to the left ventricle from the left auricle. The semilunar valves surround the opening from the left ventricle into the aorta and keep the blood from flowing back. If any one of these valves becomes diseased it may not thoroughly close the opening it is placed to guard and then we have a train of important symptoms.

PERICARDITIS.--This is an inflammation of the pericardium, the sac containing the heart.

Primary or First Causes.--They refer in this disease to a peculiar constitution. Children that have a tuberculous constitution are more liable to this disease. Acute rheumatism or tonsilitis are the causes and this trouble follows or goes with them. Infectious diseases also cause it.

Symptoms.--Slight pain in the heart region, fever moderate. These subside or effusion may set in and this usually occurs with acute rheumatism, tuberculosis and septicemia. Sometimes these symptoms are absent.

Treatment of Pericarditis.--The patient must rest quietly in bed and a doctor should be in attendance. An ice bag placed over the heart frequently gives relief and quiets the distress and pain. There is apt to be liquid in the sac (pericardium) and to lessen the tendency to this there should not be much drink or liquid food taken. There should be what is called a dry diet. (See Nursing Department for this.)

ENDOCARDITIS.--Inflammation of the lining of the heart chiefly confined to the valves; it may be acute or chronic.

Simple Kind, Cause.--Occurs at all ages, but most often in children and young adults. It most frequently comes with acute rheumatism, chorea, tonsilitis, scarlet fever, and pneumonia. The valves in the left heart are most often affected, the mitral simply swollen or bearing small growths.

Symptoms.--If it is caused by acute rheumatism, there may be higher temperature, without increase of joint symptoms. Heart beats faster and is irregular. It may run into chronic valvular disease.

Treatment of Endocarditis.--Preventive.--Much can be done to prevent this disease by closely watching the patient having the disease that causes it. The heart should be closely watched. Acute inflammatory rheumatism is a frequent cause and the heart must be watched continually in this disease. When the patient has this disease he must be quiet and in bed. This is essential. A doctor must be called, for the disease is serious and dangerous.

Diet.--Should be liquid. Milk or preparations made with it is the usual diet. Care must be taken that the stomach and bowels be not disordered. Gas collecting in the stomach causes much distress to one who has endocarditis or valvular disease.

Caution.--Avoid early exertion after getting well.

CHRONIC ENDOCARDITIS.--Usually occurs in persons under middle age. Generally follows acute endocarditis. It may be caused by syphilis, alcoholism, gout, and prolonged over-exertion. The edges of the valve become thickened and then the thickened parts separate and cannot meet exactly and therefore fail to close the opening they are set to guard.

CHRONIC VALVULAR DISEASE.--Results of valve lesions. Narrowing of a valve causes increased difficulty in emptying the chamber of the heart behind it. Insufficiency of a valve allows the return of the blood through the valve during the dilation of a chamber, thus increasing the amount of blood entering the chamber beyond the normal. Either trouble causes dilation of the chamber and compensatory hypertrophy. Enlargement of its wall must take place in order to perform the extra work demanded constantly, for the normal reserve force of the heart muscles can accomplish the extra task only temporarily. This enlargement increases the working power of the heart to above normal, but the organ is relatively less efficient than the normal heart, as its reserve force is less and sudden or unusual exertion may cause disturbance or failure of the compensation acquired by the enlargement. If this loss of reserve force is temporary, compensation is restored by further enlargement and by diminution, by rest, of the work demanded of the heart. Any valvular lesion, whether a stenosis (narrowing) of the outlet or insufficiency from the moment of its origin, leads to certain alterations in the distribution of pressure upon each side of the affected valve. If the body of the heart itself did not possess a series of powerful compensatory aids, that is, the power of making good a defect or loss, or restoring a lost balance, to improve this relation of altered pressure, then every serious lesion at its very beginning would not only cause serious general disturbances of circulation, but very soon prove fatal. Without compensation of the power of making good the defect or loss, the blood in every valvular disease or lesion would be collected behind the diseased valve. The heart's reserve power prevents to a certain extent such a dangerous condition; the sections of the heart lying behind the diseased valve work harder, diminish the blood stoppage and furnish enough blood to the peripheral arteries. The reserve force is used in stenosis to overcome the obstacle, whereas in insufficiency it must force more blood forward during the succeeding phase through the diseased valve. To effect this increased work permanently, anatomic changes in the heart are bound to follow. The changes consist in hypertrophy (enlargement of the heart muscle) and dilatation of the different chambers. Under this head, compensation, is included the increased filling and increased work of certain heart chambers with their resulting dilatation and hypertrophy. But this compensation cannot last forever. It fails sometimes and certain symptoms follow as hereafter related. Therefore persons who have valvular disease and who have been informed that the heart has adapted itself to the condition by enlarging of its walls and chambers and thus forming the condition called compensation, should be very careful of their mode of living and not put any undue or sudden strain upon the heart that might destroy the conditions that make compensation continue. In the following pages symptoms are given showing what happens when compensation continues and when it fails.

AORTIC INSUFFICIENCY OR INCOMPETENCY.--The valves are not doing their work thoroughly.

Symptoms.--They are often long absent; headache, dizziness, faintness, flashes of light, difficult breathing, and palpitation on exertion, and pain in the heart region may occur early. The pain may be dull and localized, or sharp and radiating to the neck or left arm. When *compensation* fails, we have difficult breathing, which is worse at night, swelling of the eyes and feet, cough, anemia. Sudden death is more common in this than with any other valvular disease. You can hear a soft blowing sound by listening with your ear.

NARROWING (Aortic Stenosis).--Caused by chronic endocarditis, etc. Their valve segments are usually adherent to each other by their margins and are thickened and distorted.

Symptoms.--When compensation is gone, diminished blood in the brain causes dizziness and faintness.

MITRAL INSUFFICIENCY OR INCOMPETENCY.--This is the most common valvular disease. The segments of the valve may be shortened and deformed. There is often stenosis (narrowing) caused by this deformity. The effects are regurgitation, flowing back of blood from the left ventricle into the left auricle, which is also receiving blood from the lungs, causing dilatation of the auricle and its enlargement to expel the extra blood; dilatation and other enlargement of the left ventricle occurs on account of the large quantity of blood forced in by the auricle; obstruction to flow of blood from pulmonary veins due to extra blood in left auricle, hence dilatation and enlargement of right ventricle which forces blood through the lungs; dilatation and enlargement of right auricle.

Symptoms.--If compensation is slightly disturbed we have blueness (cyanosis), clubbing of the fingers, hard breathing on exertion, and attacks of bronchitis and bleeding from the lungs. If compensation is seriously disturbed we are likely to have the blueness (cyanosis) more marked, heart beat feeble and irregular, constant hard breathing, with cough and water or bloody sputum, dropsy in the feet first and going up and involving the abdomen and chest cavities.

MITRAL STENOSIS.--This is the narrowing of the valve opening. It is most common in young persons, chiefly females. The narrowing of the valve opening may be due to thickening or hardening of the valve segments, adhesion of their edges, thickening and contraction of the tendinous cords of the valve ring.

Symptoms.--Similar to mitral insufficiency, but they develop slower and those symptoms of venous congestion of the lungs, liver, etc., are more marked; bleeding from the lungs is more common.

TRICUSPID (VALVE) INSUFFICIENCY.--Cause.--Usually due to dilatation of the right ventricle in mitral disease or with lung emphysema or other obstruction to the lungs' circulation.

TRICUSPID STENOSIS (NARROWING).--Rare except in cases from the time of birth.

Recovery from the valvular disease, depends upon the degree of compensation maintained and is best when this is acquired spontaneously. This is to be judged by the heart action. The prognosis is poor in children. It is better in women than in men.

Treatment (a) While Compensated.--Medicine is not necessary at this period. The patient should lead a quiet, regulated, orderly life, free from excitement and worry; and the risk of certain death makes it necessary that those suffering from a disease of the aorta should be especially warned against over-exertion and hurry. An ordinary healthy diet in moderate quantities should be taken, tobacco and stimulants not allowed at all.

The feelings of the patient must control the amount of exercise; so long as no heart distress or palpitation follows, moderate exercise will be of great help. A daily bath is good. No hot baths should be taken and a Turkish bath absolutely prohibited. For the full-blooded, fleshy patient an occasional dose of salts should be taken. Patients with a valvular trouble should not go into any very high altitudes; over-exertion, mental worry and poor digestion are harmful.

(b) The stage of broken compensation. Rest. Disturbed compensation may be completely restored by rest of the body. In many cases with swelling of the ankles, moderate dilatation of the heart and irregularity of the pulse, the rest in bed, a few doses of the compound tincture of cardamon and a saline purge suffice within a week or ten days to restore the compensation. For medicine a doctor must be consulted as each individual case must be treated according to its peculiar symptoms.

FATTY HEART.--This occurs often in old age, prolonged, infectious, wasting disease, anemia, alcoholism, poisoning by phosphorus and arsenic.

ANGINA PECTORIS.--True angina, which is a rare disease, is characterized by paroxysms of agonizing pain in the region of the heart, extending into the arms and neck. In violent attacks there is the sensation of impending death. Usually during the exertion and excitement, sudden onset of agonizing pain in the region of the heart and a sense of constriction, as if the heart had been seized in a vise. The pains radiate up the neck and down the arm. The fingers may be numb. The patient remains motionless and silent, the face usually pale or ashy with profuse perspiration. Lasts for several seconds or a minute or two.

Treatment.--Live an absolutely quiet life, avoid excitement and sudden muscular exertion. During the attack, break a pearl of amyl-nitrite in a handkerchief and inhale the fumes. These should always be carried. If no relief is had in a minute or two chloroform should be given at once. It is dangerous and you must look to your physician for advice and treatment.

ARTERIOSCLEROSIS.--A localized or diffused thickness of the inner coat and then of the other coats of the arteries. Arteries look lumpy and are crooked, dilated with stiff, thin or calcified walls. All coats, especially the middle, show degeneration. It usually comes in later life.

Treatment.--Regulate the mode of life, avoid alcohol, excess of eating, drinking, exertion, excitement and worry. Keep the bowels and kidneys acting regularly. There is no medicine for it.

ANEURISM.--This is a local dilatation of an artery. A local tumor.

Treatment.--Absolute rest, restrict fluids. There is always danger from rupture.

MYOCARDITIS.--This is an inflammation of the muscle substance of the heart. It may be acute or chronic.

Causes.--Endocarditis and pericarditis in the course of rheumatism; acute fevers like typhoid, etc.; clots lodging in the heart arteries, coming from diseases such as septicemia and pyemia.

Symptoms.--The heart is weak. The pulse is rapid, small and irregular, palpitation and fainty sensations come on suddenly during the course of diseases mentioned. The outlook is serious and life may end suddenly.

Treatment.--The same as that given for endocarditis. Absolute rest is necessary. A good nourishing diet must be given and a doctor is always needed.

PHLEBITIS, INFLAMMATION OF THE VEINS.--Causes.--Some irritation of the vein, as a puncture or any other injury accompanied by infection.

Symptoms.--Pain and tenderness along the course of the vein with discolored skin and acute swelling (watery) below the obstruction. Pulse rapid, high temperature, chills, dry and brown tongue and pain.

Treatment.--Absolute quiet is necessary, with the affected limb elevated. Lead and laudanum wash should be applied, or hot antiseptic fomentations if an abscess is forming. An abscess should be opened, keep up the patient's strength.

VARICOSE VEINS (Varix).--This term means an enlarged, elongated, tortuous, knotty condition of the veins. The term "varicose veins" is restricted in general use to the veins of the extremities, and especially those belonging to the lower extremity. The disease begins with a slow dilation of the vein, which gradually becomes thickened and tortuous. The inner lining membrane or coat of the vein is altered, the valves are shortened and thus rendered insufficient to support the column of blood. The outer coat becomes thickened. The varicose conditions affect chiefly the superficial veins.

Predisposing Causes.--They are most frequent in the female sex. The tendency increases as the age advances. Obstruction. Anything that obstructs the full return of blood in the veins, as tight garters below the knee, etc. Standing work may bring it on.

Exciting Causes.--Tumors in the pelvis; diseases of the heart and lungs; pregnancy. These all obstruct the full return of blood in the veins.

PHYSICIANS' TREATMENT FOR VARICOSE VEINS.--**Palliative.**--Remove the cause if possible. Treat the heart and lung troubles. Remove the pelvic tumors. In pregnancy, the woman afflicted with this trouble should not be much on her feet, but should remain lying down in bed as much as possible. This position removes the weight of the pregnant womb from the veins and allows a free return of the venous blood. An elastic bandage, or a perfectly fitting elastic stocking, supports the veins, equalizes the circulation and turns the flow to the deeper veins, which do not, as a rule, become varicose. This silk stocking should be made to order. This treatment gives much comfort in chronic varicose veins.

DISEASES OF THE EYE AND EAR

The first thing we notice in looking at the eye may be the lids and at each edge are the eyelashes. When this edge becomes inflamed it is called Blenharitis Marginalis or inflammation of the margin of the eyelids. It is called thus from the name of the eyelid "Blepharon;" Itis always means inflammation.

If we turn down the lower lid and turn up the upper, we see a red membrane called the conjunctiva (connecting). This is the mucous membrane of the eye. It lines the inner surface of both lids and is reflected over the fore part of the Sclerotic and Cornea--two other coats of the eye, The palpebral or eyelid portion of the conjunctiva is thick, opaque, highly vascular (filled with blood vessels) and covered with numerous papillae. It turns back (reflects) over the Cornea, but it consists only of a very thin structure (epithelium) forming the anterior layer of the cornea and is, in health, perfectly transparent. Upon the sclerotic it is loosely attached to the globe. When the conjunctiva becomes inflamed it is called (Conjunctiv(a)itis) conjunctivitis. The sclerotic-cornea forms the external tunic (coat) of the eyeball, the sclerotic being opaque and forming the posterior five-sixths of the globe; the cornea, which forms the remaining sixth (the front white part that is plainly seen) being transparent. The sclerotic (means dense and hard) serves to maintain the form of the globe, the eyeball.

The cornea.--This is almost circular in shape. It is convex anteriorly and projects forward from the sclerotic in the same manner that a watch glass does from its case. This layer covers what we call the pupil.

The second tunic or coat (membrane) is formed from behind forward by the Choroid, the ciliary body and the Iris. The choroid is the vascular and dark coat covering the posterior five-sixths of the globe. The ciliary body connects the choroid to the circumference of the iris. The iris is the circular muscular septum (division) which hangs vertically behind the cornea, presenting in its center a large rounded opening, the pupil.

The choroid is a thin highly vascular membrane of a dark brown or chocolate color and is pierced behind by the optic nerve and in this situation is firmly adherent to the sclerotic.

The ciliary body comprises three muscles for its make-up and connects the choroid to the circumference of the iris.

The Iris (rainbow) has received its name from its various colors in different individuals. It is a thin, circular shaped, contractile curtain, suspended in the aqueous (watery) humor behind the cornea and in front of the lens, being perforated a little to the nasal (nose) side of its centre by a circular opening, the pupil, for the transmission of light. By its circumference it is continuous with the ciliary body, and its inner or free edge forms the margin of the pupil. The anterior surface of the iris is variously colored in different individuals and marked by lines which converge toward the pupil.

The Retina.--This is a delicate membrane, upon the surface of which the images of external objects are received. Its outer surface is in contact with the choroid; its inner, with the vitreous (glass) body. Behind it is continuous with the optic nerve; it gradually diminishes in thickness from behind forward. The retina is soft, semi-transparent and of a purple tint in the fresh state. Exactly in the centre of the posterior part of the retina corresponding to the axis of the eye, and at a point in which the sense of vision is most perfect, is an oval yellowish spot, called after its discoverer, the yellow spot or Macula lutea of Sommering.

Refracting Media.--The aqueous humor completely fills the anterior and posterior chambers of the eyeball. The anterior chamber is the space bounded in front by the cornea; behind by the front of the iris. The posterior chamber is a narrow chink between the peripheral part of the iris, the "suspensory ligament" of the lens and the "ciliary processes."

The vitreous body forms about four-fifths of the entire globe, It fills the concavity of the retina and is hollowed in front, forming a deep cavity, for the reception of the lens. It is perfectly transparent and of the consistency of thin jelly. The fluid from the vitreous body resembles nearly pure water. The crystalline lens enclosed in its capsule is situated immediately behind the pupil, in front of the vitreous body. The lens is a transparent, double-convex body. It is more convex on the posterior than on the anterior surface. The rays of light go through this body and converge to a point at the back of the retina.

BLEPHARITIS MARGINALIS.--This means a chronic inflammation of the margin or edge of the eyelids accompanied by congestion, thickening and ulceration of the parts and the formation of scales and crusts.

Causes.--The underlying cause is often an inflammation of the conjunctiva where the proper care is not taken in cleansing the roots of the lashes when the discharge collects.

Other causes are keeping late hours, smoke and dust.

Symptoms.--The red swelling along the roots of the lashes is often the only symptom. This comes and goes at the least excuse, such as eye strain, late hours, dust and wind. Scales and dust form in the severe forms, of the disease. It is most common in children, extends over many years and may finally result in the loss of the lashes, with the edge of the lid, thickened, reddened and turned out.

Treatment.--This is tedious. Fit glasses if there is eye strain, reform the mode of life and attend to any constitutional disease that may tend to make it worse.

Local treatment.--Keep the parts thoroughly clean. The edges of the lids should be washed carefully with soap and warm water or mild solution of borax or soda until the crusts are all cleaned off and then use at night an ointment composed of the following ingredients:

Yellow oxide of Mercury 2-1/2 grains

Petrolatum 2-1/2 drams

Mix and make an ointment and rub on the edge of the lids every night, first cleaning them. The conjunctivitis must be cured.

STYE (HORDEOLUM).--This is a swelling beginning in a gland or glands at the edge of the lid and pus forms finally.

Causes.--Inflammation of the edge of the lid, stomach trouble, run down condition, poorly fitted glasses, when glasses should be worn to relieve the eye strain.

Symptoms.--Itching and burning feeling followed by a red swollen area (lump) at the edge of the lid. Later it comes to a point and discharges.

Cause.--Styes usually run their course in a few days or a week; another frequently follows. When it does not reach the pus stage, it often leaves a hard swelling (blind stye).

MOTHER'S REMEDY. 1. Stye.--Home Method to Kill.--"To hasten the pointing of a stye apply hot compresses for fifteen minutes every two hours. As ill health may be the cause, a tonic may be needed; glasses properly fitted should be worn and a boric acid eyewash used until long after the stye has disappeared." Applying hot compresses will relieve the congestion and gives much relief. Ill health produces a poor circulation of the blood and a good tonic will be found beneficial. Styes are frequently produced by need of glasses.

Treatment.--Treat the stomach and system if necessary. Ice or cold cloths against the stye may abort it. If it goes on, hot fomentations will hasten it. It should then be opened up and scraped out. It will soon heal then and will not leave a lump.

ACUTE CATARRHAL CONJUNCTIVITIS (Pink Eye).--Definition.--This is an acute inflammation of the mucous membranes under the eyelids, and there is congestion (too much blood), swelling and a discharge of mucus and pus.

Causes.--Exposure to wind, dust, smoke, or irritating foreign substance, cinder, sand, etc. It may occur in epidemic form and then is contagious and is called "pink eye."

Symptoms.--The lids appear stiff to the patient, the light causes discomfort and the patient fears it. Burning feeling as if there was some dirt, etc., under the lid, not much pain, but discomfort especially in the evening.

The lids look swollen and red. The conjunctiva on the cornea is reddened and that on the lid is thickened, reddened and rough. The discharge collects at the roots of the lashes or lies on the conjunctiva. The lids are stuck together in the morning. The sight is slightly affected by the discharge on the cornea, which is otherwise clear. Sometimes little (minute) ulcerations are seen.

Course.--It may run into a chronic conjunctivitis. One eye is usually attacked a few days before the other. The first stage lasts a few hours or a day and then the discharge follows which may last a few days or a week or more.

Treatment.--First: Use gauze or cotton and dip in ice or cold water and apply to the eyelids. A wash of hot water can be used to cleanse the eye or ten to sixty grains (one teaspoonful) of boric acid to an ounce of water can be used as a wash also.

The following remedies are good in combination as follows:

Alum	3 grains
Sulphate of Zinc	2 grains
Distilled Water	1 ounce

Mix and drop one drop into the eye two or three times daily.

A weak solution of tea can be used also as a wash. Anoint the lids at night with white (tube) vaselin.

INFLAMMATION OF THE EYE OF NEWLY BORN (OPHTHALMIA NEONATORUM).--This is a severe inflammation of the conjunctiva in the new born infant, usually due to a discharge from the mother and it is characterized by a discharge of pus.

Causes.--Mild cases may come from a less violent form of infection from the mother's discharge from the vagina, or from outside causes. The majority of the severe cases is due to a poison (the gonococcus infection).

Symptoms.--The first symptoms are swelling and redness, usually of both eyes, usually occurring a few days after birth. Soon the discharge appears and shortly becomes creamy pus, which runs from the eyes when the swollen lids are partly opened. As the disease continues to advance, the membrane of the lid is thickened, red and velvety looking and the conjunctiva (membrane) in the eye is swollen, puffy and watery.

The disease may last from two to six weeks or longer.

If the pus is not cleaned from the eye, the cornea may look dim and ulcers may appear. If the ulcer eats through the cornea the iris is apt to be caught in the opening and in the scar resulting from the ulcer. The cornea may later bulge and protrude or the disease may involve the whole eye in an inflammation which may destroy it.

The result generally depends upon how soon treatment is begun. If attended to early the great majority of cases recover. It is serious to neglect early treatment for this disease. It causes a great many cases of blindness and generally the cases are neglected too long. Treatment must begin before the disease begins. Immediately at the birth of the child, when if there is any poison in the eye due to a discharge in the mother's vagina, it can be immediately cleansed.

TREATMENT PREVENTIVE. What to do first.--As soon as the child is born and before its eyes are opened the discharges should be carefully wiped away from the lids with small squares of cotton or gauze, pieces wrung out of a weak solution, three per cent (three parts to one hundred of warm, boiled, water) of boric acid. The eyes should not be exposed to the light. At the first both the eyes should be bathed and the same piece of linen should not be used for both eyes.

As soon as any redness appears the eye should be frequently bathed with this warm, weak solution of boric acid and sometimes cold compresses should be used by taking squares of folded gauze or masses of absorbent cotton. Take them cold from a block of ice and lay them over the eyes, and keep constantly changing to keep them cold. This relieves the congestion and prevents a great amount of blood from flowing and settling (congestion) there. When pus appears in the eye it should be cleansed every half hour at least. You can do this by letting the solution run over it from a medicine dropper. After being allowed to trickle from the outer to the inner angle (corner) of the eye, it will then run down beside the nose and can be caught in a piece of absorbent cotton or sponge. If there is a great amount of pus in the eye, the eye may have to be washed out in this manner, every fifteen minutes, day and night, so that the cornea will be kept clean. If this must be done a small fountain syringe with a glass tube (eye-dropper) attached will cause a steady flow of the solution. The boric acid can be increased to five or ten grains to the ounce of water. If only one eye is diseased the other eye may be covered.

All cloths, etc., should be burned at once and the basin which has held them, filled with carbolic acid solution of the strength of one part acid to twenty parts water. The nurse's hands should be thoroughly scrubbed in hot water and soap and disinfected in the same strength of carbolic acid solution, as the disease is very contagious and dangerous to adults. An attendant should not touch her face or hair with her hands unless they have been washed quite clean. The conjunctiva should be brushed with a solution of nitrate of silver of two per cent strength (two parts to one hundred of distilled water) and then neutralized with a salt solution, not strong enough to burn.

When the cornea is diseased one per cent solution of atropine may be necessary once or twice a day.

Caution.--In the cities this disease is disastrous in its results to the sight of babies. This is due to the want of necessary care. Persons who must be with the patient should be very careful not to get any of the discharge upon their clothes or person, as it is very contagious.

ULCER OF THE CORNEA.--Causes.--Poor general health is

an underlying cause or the cornea itself may be poorly nourished. Ulcers are common among the poor classes. They often begin through a rubbing of the cornea by a foreign body. They also come from diseases of the conjunctiva. Weakly babies are easily affected.

Symptoms.--The light hurts the patient; there is a feeling of something in the eye. When the ulcer is over the pupil the sight is impaired. The eyeball shows a ring of pink congestion about the cornea, with congestion of the conjunctiva. The form of the ulcer may be irregular, circular, etc.

Course.--The simple ulcers heal in a week or two. Infected ulcers may spread, or they may sink deeply into the substance of the cornea and eat through. The danger to the sight depends upon the kind and severity of the ulcer. There is apt to be more or less film over the eye for some time and if the ulcer eats through it may destroy the sight.

Treatment. Preventive.--When the cornea has been injured and there has been some rubbing off of its tissue (abrasion) mild antiseptic solution in the form of eye drops should be used. Boric acid, as much as will dissolve in warm, distilled water and some dropped in the eye three or four times a day. If there is a foreign body in the cornea, clean instruments should be used to remove it. The cocaine used to render the eye painless must be pure.

General Treatment.--If the patient is "run down" the general system should be built up.

Local Treatment.--One to two per cent solution of Atropine should be put into the eye three to six times a day to keep the pupil dilated and prevent it from adhering to the cornea. Hot fomentations repeated according to the severity of the case and the amount of "easing" they give. A three per cent solution of boric acid should be used for cleansing purposes. The bowels should be regular. The patient should remain in one room.

FILM ON THE EYE PTERYGIUM.--This is a growth beginning near the inner or outer corner and extending with its point towards the center of the cornea.

Symptoms.--The patient only complains when it has advanced toward the center of the cornea and the vision is lessened or cut off. It occurs more often from the inner corner. It keeps growing for many years and may cease advancing at any time.

Treatment.--Surgical treatment is often necessary. Dr. Alling says: "Dissect off the growth from the cornea and sclera coats, leaving the base attached (toward the corner of the eye) and bury its point under the undermined conjunctiva below. If the growth is dissected off the cornea, which may readily be done, and then cut off (towards its base) it would recur."

IRITIS. (Inflammation of the Iris.)--This is an inflammation of the iris, characterized by congestion, small pupil and posterior synechia.

Causes.--It occurs in the second stage of syphilis, second to eighteenth month, from rheumatism, diabetes, gout, injury, and without any known cause (idiopathic).

Symptoms.--More or less severe pain in the eye, forehead and temple, worse in the night and early morning especially. There is fear of the light and the eyes water very much. The sight is affected and there may be some fever. On examination the lids are found swollen and red, the eyeball shows congestion in the cornea and ciliary body, with some congestion of the conjunctiva. The cornea looks hazy. The anterior surface of the iris looks muddy and does not look so fine and delicate. The pupil is small and the light does not make it contract readily. If atropine is put in the eye (one per cent solution) the pupil will not dilate regularly, because at different points the pupillary edge of the iris is held to the lens by an exudate that lightly holds it.

Course and Recovery.--The disease may occur at any age, but it is most common in children. It may last from one to six weeks.

Chances of recovery are good if treatment is begun early. There is a tendency to recurrence.

MOTHER'S REMEDY.--1. Iritis.--Sensible Remedy for.-- "Doctor the blood with sulphur and lard, a teaspoonful three times a day. Refrain from using the eyes. This disease is said to be brought on by rheumatic fever, and rheumatism is a disease of the blood." This is a very serious disease and a physician should be called.

Treatment. What to do first.--Confine the patient in a darkened room and if the attack is severe in bed.

Local Treatment.--Dry or moist heat should be applied, according to the ease they give. Leeches are good in severe cases placed near the outer corner of the eye. Atropine usually made of about the strength of two to four grains Atropine to an ounce of water; or one per cent (1 to 100) may be used, and it should be dropped into the eye from three to six times a day. The pupil must be dilated and kept so from the beginning to keep the adhesions from forming between the iris and lens. If too much is used the throat and tongue will feel dry, face will flush, and there will be dizziness and a rapid pulse. Stop it until that effect is gone and then cautiously use it again. The bowels should be kept open.

The diet should consist of milk to a great extent. Water of course can be taken freely. Soups, broths, gruels, etc., can be used if desired; but meats should be withheld for a time unless the patient runs down.

Caution.--If a person has any of the special symptoms above mentioned it would be prudent to begin treatment at once. The great danger is permanent adhesion of the iris to other parts, especially the lens, and the dilating and contracting power may be lost.

INJURIES OF THE IRIS.--Concussion of the eyeball may produce an irregular dilation of the pupil. This is due to paralysis of the sphincter muscle of the pupil, but it generally disappears. The edge of the pupil may be torn in the form of one or more rents, or the iris may be separated from its root at its circumference, leaving a clear space, or it may be entirely torn from its attachment.

Perforating wounds are accompanied by injury to the lens and other structures; when the cornea is wounded it is often complicated by falling of the lens. When a small foreign body passes through the cornea and iris a small opening may be seen. The greatest danger from wounds is due to infection and if it reaches the iris, it may produce violent iritis. If the lens is displaced or absent the iris being without support, will tremble with every movement of the eye. In some cataract operations, if there is a loss of the "Vitreous" body a part of the iris may be folded upon itself, thus enlarging the pupil in that point.

CATARACT.--This is an opacity of the crystalline lens or its capsule. The lens is not clear and bright and keeps the light from going through it. Then it is called opaque.

23

SENILE CATARACT.--The vast majority of these cataracts are found after the age of fifty. They simply come without any known cause. Of course, injury can cause a cataract and it is then called traumatic cataract.

Symptoms of Senile (Old Age) Cataract.--Blurred vision, flashes and streaks of light, dark spots, double vision. There is no pain. Eye strain due to imperfect sight. Sometimes the first symptom is ability to read without glasses (second sight). This is due to the increased refractive power of the lens from swelling. The lens looks a little whitish through the pupil opening and looks more so as time goes on.

Course.--The progress is slow. It usually takes a number of years before it is "ripe" for operation. They may remain in the same condition sometimes. In this kind of cataract both eyes are affected sooner or later, although one eye may be fully matured before the other is much changed.

The result of an operation depends upon the condition of the eye. The eye should be free from evidence of disease. "The anterior chamber should be of normal depth. The pupil should react to light. There should be a homogeneous (all alike) white or gray opacity immediately back of the pupil, with no shadow from the edge of the pupil (except in cases of sclerosis, already mentioned). A candle carried on all sides of the patient while the eye is fixed, should be properly located by him. The tension of the eyeball should be normal."

The operation is very frequently done and it is very successful. The patient should be ready and willing to place himself in the charge of the operator and do as he says.

SYMPATHETIC INFLAMMATION OF THE EYE.--(Sympathetic Ophthalmia.)--A condition in which the healthy eye becomes the seat of a destructive inflammation transferred from the other eye which has been the subject of a similar inflammation usually following a perforating injury of the eyeball. The injured eye is called the exciting eye; the other, the sympathetic eye.

This is a rare disease, but it may occur when one eye is injured or diseased and on the first indication of trouble in the injured eye the other eye should be closely watched for symptoms of sympathetic trouble so that if can be removed.

Symptoms in the Exciting Eye.--This is more or less congested and painful; when pressure is made upon the upper lid, it shows tenderness. The tension is not as strong; the pupil may be blocked with an exudate.

In the Sympathizing Eye.--There is an inflammation involving the choroid, ciliary body and iris. There is pain, tenderness, small blocked pupil and sight is poor.

Course.--It usually appears between the third week and the sixth month after the original injury. "The extreme limits are two weeks and twenty years." The sound eye is likely to be attacked when the exciting eye is in a state of active inflammation.

Treatment.--The "exciting eye" should be enucleated (taken out) before any signs of sympathetic inflammation appears in the healthy eye. If it has appeared, enucleation will be of no value; at all events if there is vision in the exciting eye, the operation should not be done then.

INFLAMMATION OF THE RETINA FROM BRIGHT'S DISEASE (Albuminuric Retinitis).--The retina is a very delicate structure and we are often able to diagnose Bright's disease from the peculiar effect it produces upon the retina.

Causes.--The cause is usually Bright's disease, (nephritis) and usually the chronic Interstitial variety. Pregnancy causes it sometimes. Interference of the vision, sight, is what the patient complains of. This may be very slight, when you consider the great changes occurring in the retina. Such patients are subject to attacks of temporary blindness of uremic origin. The vessels of the retina are swollen and tortuous. Bleeding and shining white patches are scattered through the back part of the eye and a peculiar arrangement of glistening white dots around the yellow spot. This disease shows itself late in Bright's disease and the patient is not likely to live more than two years after the appearance of this eye lesion.

Treatment.--It sometimes occurs during pregnancy. Then the question of inducing premature labor arises. There is no local treatment that can be of any use when it is caused by Bright's disease.

FITTING GLASSES.--This is done by lenses and prisms, etc.

Lens.--A lens is made of glass and prisms graded in strength, one surface curved, and has the power of refracting or changing the direction of the rays of light. A prism is wedge-shaped and bends rays of light towards its base. A great many people are troubled with their eyes, much more than years ago. We even see little children wearing glasses. It is unfortunate, but true, that even more children and grown people should wear them. Fitting glasses is an art in itself. It takes more ability to fit glasses well than it does to operate well. Poorly-fitted glasses are not only annoying to the wearer, but dangerous. Glasses rest the eyes, not tire them. When the eyes water and feel tired or strained, even after using them but little, glasses are needed. Headaches are frequently caused by the eye strain. When glasses are needed it does not pay to put off getting them and the person needing them should go to one competent to properly fit them. A great many eyes are hard to fit, and they need not only ability to fit them well, but time and attention must be given to fitting them properly.

SQUINT OR STRABISMUS.--Both lines of sight are not directed towards the same object of fixation.

Internal or Convergent Squint.--Where one eye is turned inward toward the nose.

External or Divergent Squint.--One eye turns outward toward the temple. Squinting upward and downward are uncommon.

Causes of Convergent (Internal) Squint.--It generally appears between two and five years; at first periodically, later constantly. The patient is generally far-sighted.

Treatment.--Internal squint in very young children may be treated by covering the well eye and forcing the child to use the other. When the child is old enough, proper glasses should be worn. Operation can be done when needed and is generally successful.

External (Divergent) Squint.--This may appear at any age and is often associated with near-sightedness. An operation is necessary and the tendons on both sides must generally be cut and properly placed. Parents should always attend to a child who has this trouble. The operation is not difficult to perform and it will not only, as a rule, give the child good sight, but better looks. Parents who are able to have an operation or glasses fitted when needed, and who neglect their children, should be punished; they are guilty not only of neglect, but cruelty.

MOTHERS' REMEDIES. Inflammation of the Eye. 1. Chickweed a Relief for.--"The juice of chickweed is good for inflammation of the eyes, when dropped into them."

2. Inflammation of Eyes, Sassafras, Excellent Remedy for.--"Take sassafras bark and make into a tea. Apply this externally to the eyes, and it will be found very beneficial for this trouble." This is a very good remedy, on account of its oily soothing nature.

3. Inflammation of Eyes, Tried Remedy for.--

Boric Acid	10 grams
Camphor Water (not spirits)	1/2 ounce
Water	1/2 ounce

Apply this with a soft cloth.

This trouble usually results from or is associated with constitutional disease and requires treatment for same, but the above wash is good for local applications. This prescription was given me by an oculist."

4. Inflammation of Eyes, Common Potato Will Cure.--"Scrape raw potato and apply to the temple until relieved." This helps to draw the blood away and relieves the inflammation.

5. Inflammation of Eyes, Milk Curd Relieves.--"Make a curd of sweet milk; that is, set it on the stove till it forms a curd; then add quite a little alum and wash eyes." The milk is very soothing and the alum acts as an astringent. Care should be taken in using this remedy that none of the mixture gets into the eyes.

6. Inflammation of Eyes, Wild Hairs Cause.--"A few years ago, I had trouble with my eyes. They felt as though there was something in them scratching the eye-ball. I went to an eye specialist, and he gave me two little vials of medicine to drop into my eyes six times a day. I doctored with him several months, and while the medicine reduced the inflammation largely, it did not relieve the scratching sensation in the eyes. Then I was away from home for about ten days and did not use the medicine, and when I returned my eyes were very much inflamed, and very painful. I visited the doctor again, and he said I had a little ulcer on the eyeball, and he pulled out several hairs or winkers from the eyelid. I asked him if wild hairs were the cause of the ulcer and he admitted they were. After a few days' more treatment by the doctor I learned of a neighbor who understood a little about wild hairs in the eyelid and had him examine my eyes. He pulled out more wild hairs, and my eyes got well. Ever since then, when my eyes begin to hurt me as though there was some foreign substance in them, I go to my neighbor and he pulls out the wild hairs, and that was the trouble with my eyes. My experience in obtaining this knowledge cost me twenty dollars in fees to the eye specialist, which I could have saved by going to my neighbor at first,"

MOTHERS' REMEDIES.--Sore Eyes. 1. Rose Leaves Rest.-- "Steep rose leaves and apply often." Apply the leaves as a fomentation and relief will soon follow. This is very soothing and very easily applied.

2. Sore Eyes, Soothing Remedy for.--"Use a wash of borax and water. One-half teaspoonful to a cupful of water." This is very good.

3. Sore Eyes. Slippery Elm Excellent for.--"This is a very soothing dressing far the eyes. You can buy a small package of the slippery elm at any drug store, and prepare it by making a tea and using externally.

4. Sore Eyes, Common Remedy for.--"Use a wash night and morning of common table salt and water." This is often sold by druggists for 10 or 15 cents an ounce under a medical name.

5. Sore Eyes, Elder Berry Flowers Relieve.--"In a severe case of inflammation of the eyes apply a poultice of elderberry flowers; bathe the eyes with warm water and witch-hazel." This remedy was given by a mother who tried it a great many times and always had success.

6. Sore Eyes. Borax and Camphor Good Wash for.--"Borax one teaspoonful, spirits of camphor fifteen drops, distilled water one-half cupful. This makes a fine wash for sore eyes, and is perfectly harmless."

7. Sore Eyes, Tested Eye Wash for.--

"Hydrastis (Golden Seal Root)	1/2 ounce
Best Green Tea	1/2 ounce
Sulphate of Zinc, Pulverized	1 dram

Steep the root and tea for a few minutes in a pint of boiling water; while cooling add the sulphate of zinc; when cold strain well and bottle. Use as an eye wash three times a day. In severe cases a poultice is useful, made of pulverized slippery elm and warm milk and water. All eye washes should be used with caution and especially those containing belladonna or caustic solutions,"

8. Sore Eyes, Borate of Soda and Camphor Water Relieves.--

"Borate of Soda	2 grains
Camphor Water (not spirits)	1 ounce

Mix, drop one or two drops in the eye four times a day.

Camphor water is made by allowing the gum to dissolve in water instead of alcohol, also saturate lint in this mixture and apply on the eyes."

EAR AND ITS DISEASES.

The external ear is called auricle or pinna. It is an oval funnel--shaped organ. The canal leading in to the membrane (drum) is called the external auditory meatus. It extends inward about one and one--quarter inches and terminates in a membrane.

Membrane Tympani (drum) which separates the external ear from the tympanic cavity. To examine the drum, you must pull the ear backward and outward to make the canal straight.

Membrane Tympani (the drum) Membrane.--This is situated at the inner end of the canal and separates it from the tympanum or middle ear. It is placed like the membrane in the telephone. It is pearly gray in color. This membrane not only serves as a protection to the delicate structures within the tympanum, but also receives the sound vibrations from without and transmits them to the ossicular (bony) chain of the middle ear.

The Tympanum or Middle Ear.--This cavity just beyond the drum, which forms the greater part of its outer wall, is an irregular cavity, compressed from without inward and situated in the petrous bone. The mastoid cells lie behind. It is filled with air and communicates with the nose-pharynx (naso-pharynx) by the eustachian tube. The upper portion of this cavity, the attic, lies immediately below the middle lobe of the brain, separated from it by a thin layer of bone, which forms the roof of the cavity. This cavity is separated from the internal ear.

The Eustachian tube.--This is the channel through which the middle ear communicates with the pharynx. With an opening in the anterior of the middle ear, a bony canal passes from this point, inward, forward, and downward through the petrous bone, when it merges into a cartilaginous canal, which terminates in a funnel-shaped protuberance, with a slit-like orifice, located in the nose pharynx. This is the eustachian tube. It is lined with mucous membrane like the throat. The air goes up from the throat, through this canal to the middle ear. The mucous membrane of the middle ear is continuous with that of the nose-pharynx through the eustachian tube. So you can readily understand how easy it is for an inflammation of the throat to extend to the middle ear through the eustachian tube.

The posterior wall which has the greatest height, reveals in its upper portion a passage (antrum) through which the vault of the tympanum (attic) communicates with the cells of the mastoid process, situated posteriorly. From this description you see how near to each other these parts are placed and when one becomes diseased the disease can extend to the other part or parts. The brain is separated from some of these cavities by a very thin shell of bone, and the disease can soon affect the brain through infection or breaking through the thin structures that separates the parts.

Diseases of the middle ear and the mastoid are always to be considered serious, and should be very closely watched. A child with a running ear is in danger, for it may at any time become closed up and serious.

ECZEMA OF THE EXTERNAL EAR (Auricle).--This is an inflammatory disease of the skin, and in the poorer classes it is very frequent. It is quite a common disease in old age. It develops in other parts of the body at the same time in a certain percentage of cases.

Causes.--Soaps, alkalies, foreign bodies in the ear, removing ear wax and a chronic discharge from the middle ear. There is a tendency to it in some families; stomach trouble, improper food are also causes.

Symptoms.--Itching,--and this is very pronounced,--burning feeling. The part is somewhat reddened, fluid oozes out, crusts form, the skin thickens, and scales. Sometimes it swells very much.

Treatment.--Regulate the bowels, give a simple easily digested and proper food for children and adults. Cleanse the inflamed skin gently with castile soap and tepid water once a day. Cloths dipped in some cooling lotion, such as the lead and opium wash, or in plain water to which has been added a little alcohol or eau de cologne, should be wrapped around the inflamed ear during the acute stage and they should be kept wet. Clean vaselin, etc., is good to put on the scabs. The ear should be covered as before directed to keep dirt, dust, etc., out.

HARDENED WAX OR IMPACTED CERUMEN.--This mass may be mixed with foreign bodies or be made up of "wax" alone.

Symptoms.--A large mass of wax may remain in the ear for many years without causing any special loss of hearing so long as the plug does not rest against the drum and there remains a passage between the mass so that the sound-waves can strike the drum. Generally the hearing gradually grows less. Loss of hearing may take place suddenly, as after washing the head, or after a general bath, or after an attempt to clean the ear with the end of a towel. Patients will often say the dullness of hearing appeared suddenly. This no doubt was due to the fact that the mass of wax was displaced against the drum suddenly by an unusual movement of the head or the jaws, or the mass became swollen through fluids getting into the canal. If the canal is filled there will be more or less deafness, ringing in the ear, and there may be piercing pain produced by the hardened mass, especially if the jaws are moved from side to side. If the mass is thoroughly and carefully removed, the hearing may entirely return if it was caused by this wax.

Treatment.--The mass is best removed by syringing the hardened plug and softening it gradually. Removing it with a currette and forceps without softening it may do injury to the parts. The syringe and hot sterilized, boiled water should be used for some time, and the patient asked occasionally if there is any faintness or dizziness caused by it. It often comes, in a lump after the water has been used for some time. A strong solution of bicarbonate of sodium is also good to use.

FOREIGN BODIES IN THE EAR.--These are not of frequent occurrence. In the case of children these bodies may comprise such objects as pebbles, beads, beans, pieces of rolled paper, fly, bed-bug; insect of any kind may get into ear of adults. If they reach the drum a very unpleasant sensation is produced by the attempt to escape. Sometimes a layer of wax may gather around the dead object. These bodies should be removed, for their presence may produce a swelling or soreness in the canal. If the object is a dried pea or bean the syringe should not be used. The object must be carefully removed. Sometimes an operation is necessary to remove the object.

DISEASE OF THE MIDDLE EAR.--The ordinary cold in the head rarely runs its course without one of the eustachian tubes at least is involved to some extent.

SIMPLE INFLAMMATION OF THE EUSTACHIAN TUBE.--Causes.--Acute colds, inflammation of the nose and pharynx, tonsilitis.

Symptoms.--The ear may feel full and numb, roaring in the ear may occur. There may be pain on swallowing, shooting up through the tube.

Treatment.--Remove the cause. Treat the nose and pharynx. Spray and gargle with solutions advised for throat trouble. If it continues the throat should be examined for adenoids, enlarged turbinate bones and so on.

ACUTE CATARRHAL INFLAMMATION OF THE MIDDLE EAR. Causes.--Acute coryza, acute pharyngitis, influenza, scarlet fever, inflammation of the eustachian tube, gargling, bathing, employing the nasal douche or violently blowing the nose.

Inflammation of the eustachian tube is, in many cases, simply the first stage or onset of this disease. The congestion extends beyond the tube and involves to a greater or less degree this cavity. If it continues for a few hours or an entire day, the watery elements of the blood will begin to escape from the distended vessels into the tissues of the mucous membrane and ooze out upon its free surface. If this is copious enough pressure may be developed within the cavity, middle-ear, to cause pain. These cases vary much in severity. In the mildest ones there may be a few twinges of pain in the affected ear, but nothing more; and even in the most severe cases the pain does not last longer than a few hours, although it may return on several successive days.

Very many of the earaches of young children, from two to ten years of age, are due to this disease. The pain is very likely to come on late in the afternoon or during the night, while earlier in the day the child may be free from pain. In the milder forms the condition of the drum is similar to that existing in inflammation of the eustachian tube. It is not then much changed from normal. There may be more congestion than in this condition. In a fairly severe case the membrane (drum) a few hours after the onset presents a most striking change. It is a picture of obstructed venous (dark blood) circulation of a high degree. In some cases one or more of these distended veins may rupture and form a blood tumor in the external ear canal. The drum is red and more or less swollen.

Treatment.--Very little is needed for this kind, except care and watching. Use the simple hot water in the ear carefully or poulticing when there is pain with onions, bread and milk, and puncture of the drum if it bulges or is too tense. Hot water for gargle, steaming of the pharynx. Keep the patient in a room with an even temperature. The patient must not take cold as it might extend farther.

Recovery.--The outcome is usually good in this disease if proper care is taken; Generally in a few weeks the inflammation is gone and the hearing is restored.

SEROUS MUCOUS EXUDATION INTO THE MIDDLE EAR.--The disease just described is often associated with an (exudation) watery oozing of fluid into the middle ear, but the following condition is different. Sometimes a comparatively normal middle ear is found to contain a variable amount of either fluid or mucus, or a fluid which represents a combination of both. The failure of the fluid to absorb is due first to the fact that the drainage through the eustachian tube is still obstructed; second, that the absorbing process in the cavity is not acting normally.

Symptom.--Sudden change from somewhat poor to good hearing and the reverse. It is due to the changing in the position of the fluid. The hearing may be normal when the head is thrown far backward, for the fluid then escapes into the antrum, or when the chin is resting upon the chest.

Another symptom that is peculiar is a feeling of something moving in the ear. This is only felt when the head is moved suddenly. Sometimes the patient says: "I went in bathing and got some water into my ear, and I am unable to get it out." He thinks the water went into the ear by the way of the external ear canal. It was due to the chilling of the surface of the body, or the water accidentally entered into the ear through the mouth, or nose, throat, and eustachian tube, and this caused an exudation of fluid to take place in the middle ear. Hearing gurgling sounds in the ear during coughing, sneezing and swallowing is an important symptom. The drum on being examined varies greatly. The simplest case is seen when fluid contained in the cavity is small in quantity and consists of a thin serum. The upper level of this fluid can then be seen like a hair crossing the drum in a more or less horizontal direction. It retains its horizontal position when the patient moves his head backward and forward.

Treatment.--The fluid can be evacuated by an opening made into the drum, but it usually accumulates again. The proper treatment is to treat the diseased condition of the nose and throat, as described in other parts of this book.

CHRONIC CATARRHAL INFLAMMATION OF THE MIDDLE EAR.--The expression, acute inflammation of the middle ear, is rightly employed when it is applied to a case in which the underlying cause is of a temporary nature, as for example, a cold in the head, and mild attack of influenza, perhaps also in an attack of hay fever. But when the causes are of a more permanent character and the middle ear continues for an indefinite period to be the seat of all sorts of disturbances the combination of these different diseased phenomena receives the name of chronic catarrhal inflammation of the middle ear.

Causes.--Troubles (lesions) located in the upper pharynx, the naso-pharyngeal (nose-pharynx) vault and the nasal passages. Adenoids may cause it.

The course of this disease has of recent years been growing more favorable, because the causes are being removed more and more.

Symptoms.--Symptoms of the acute inflammation would be present, and impairment of hearing which sometimes comes so gradually as not to be noticed by the patient. It will be better and then worse. A harassing, hissing, blowing, ringing, usually accompanies it. Pains soon or later add to the discomfort. One side is usually affected first.

Treatment.--It must be devoted to removing the causes just mentioned. Restore the general health. Abstain from alcohol, tobacco and excess of all kinds. Active outdoor exercise, horseback riding, mountain climbing, rowing, walking, etc., are great health producers.

ACUTE SUPPURATIVE INFLAMMATION OF THE MIDDLE EAR.--This inflammation of the middle ear is one in which, at an early stage of the disease, the free liquid poured out assumes a pus-like character. At the onset the mucous membrane of the eustachian tube and middle ear becomes first congested and afterward oedematous (watery swelling). Then a serous or a bloody-serous fluid is poured out into the middle ear; and finally this assumes all the outward characteristics of pus. In a few exceptional cases this pus fluid will find a sufficient passage through the eustachian tube; but in the great majority of cases this passageway becomes closed almost at the very beginning of the attack, and then the free exudation; under an ever increasing pressure and on account of the softening and breaking down of the tissues of the drum forces an opening for itself directly through the drum membrane.

Causes.--The same causes that produce the acute variety will produce this variety of the disease. It occurs more frequently during the spring and fall months as the result of changes in the climate. Acute and chronic catarrh of the nose and pharynx are causes. It frequently occurs in connection with scarlet fever and measles. It complicates nose and pharyngeal diphtheria.

Symptoms.--Pain in the ear is the most striking symptom noticed by the patient. In infants and young children of two or three years of age it may appear and not be recognized until a slight discharge appears at the opening of the external ear. The child is feverish, fretful and peevish, seemingly suffering great pain, and the parents think it is, not very sick or has only an earache. Sometimes physicians fail to recognize the trouble until the discharge appears in the external ear. The symptoms are more severe at night. Any physical or mental exertion increases the plain. The pain is sometimes very severe, and a spontaneous or artificial rupture of the drum eases the suffering very quickly in some cases, and a bloody, serous, pus-like discharge escapes into the external ear canal. Often a patient will say: "I felt something give away in the ear, a watery discharge appeared, and the pain soon subsided." In many cases the rupture of the drum gives little or no relief from suffering. This is due in some cases to the small and insufficient size of the opening in the drum. If the pain persists, after a free opening has been made, it may indicate that pressure exists in some cavity or cavities other than the middle ear proper. A sensation of fullness and sometimes of throbbing or pulsation in the affected ear; roaring, singing, whistling, etc.; impairment of hearing; increased pain, when the jaws are opened and shut, are symptoms of minor importance. If there are no complications after free discharge sets in the pain disappears, the fever gradually returns to the normal point, and the patient drops to sleep. In the course of a week or two the discharge subsides and if the rupture is not too extensive the wound will close and the patient will soon be well. Frequently, however, on account of disease of one or more of the bony parts, the wall of the middle ear or the mastoid cells, the discharge continues for weeks and may become chronic in its character.

Treatment.--Apply heat or cold first. Open the bowels.

How to apply heat.--With the patient lying on his side with the affected ear turned upward, fill the external ear canal with hot water (about 105 degrees F.), then place immediately over the affected ear a hot flaxseed meal poultice, five or six inches square and one-half inch thick, and spread a folded blanket or shawl over the whole to keep it warm as long as possible. Bread and milk with catnip, or onions will do if flaxseed is not at hand. The flaxseed holds the heat longer. Water is a good conductor of heat, and that which fills the external auditory (ear) canal may rightly be considered as an arm of the poultice which extends down to the drum itself.

Leeches also can be applied in front and below the tragus (front of the opening). If the symptoms do not improve under this treatment and especially if the drum is bulging, an opening should be made at the bulging point of the drum. The canal is now syringed with a warm antiseptic solution--like one part listerine, etc., to twenty parts of warm boiled water, with a clean syringe, or warm boiled water can be used alone. If there is any odor carbolic acid one part, to fifty or sixty of water can be used. A strip of sterile gauze is put into the canal for drainage and protection. This syringing can be done from two to four to five times a day, and gradually decrease the number of times as the discharge lessens. It must be syringed and dressed often enough to allow a free discharge and produce cleanliness.

Recovery.--The result of this disease cannot be told at the outset. The majority of such attacks end favorably, with care and treatment; this in persons of good constitution and health. It may run ten days to three to six weeks. In tuberculous patients the result is not so favorable. Recovery follows as a rule in this disease following scarlet fever and measles, but not so quickly, and there may be a discharge for some time, due to chronic disease of the ears, etc.

Complications and results.--In the majority of cases, in ordinarily healthy persons, this disease runs its course without doing any great amount of damage to the organ of hearing, and without involving any structure lying outside of the middle ear proper. In scarlet fever, measles, la grippe, or nasal diphtheria, actual destruction of tissue often takes place in some part of the middle ear before it is recognized. Sometimes it results the same way even when it is discovered in time.

Caution.--A person who has had this disease should be very careful not to take cold. The patient should take plenty of time to get well and strong. The diet should be liquid mostly.

CHRONIC SUPPURATIVE INFLAMMATION OF THE MIDDLE EAR.--An inflammation that forms pus; hence called suppurative. This is an inflammation that has become chronic (continued) and has one characteristic at least that is very noticeable, and that is the discharge. This may last for an indefinite period. The acute suppurative (pus-forming) inflammation just described in the foregoing pages, may have inflicted various kinds and degrees of damage upon the mucous membrane which lines the cavities, and as a result of the conditions thus established there will be a discharge which may last an indefinite time.

Causes.--Improper or lack of treatment for the acute suppurative inflammatory attack. This is the chief cause. The first attack may have been caused by scarlet fever, measles, etc. They are prone to become chronic, especially if not recognized early and treated properly.

Symptoms.--The main symptom is the discharge from the ear. This may be abundant or scanty. It may stop for a time and begin again. The hearing may be slightly or seriously impaired. Such patients are not accepted by life insurance companies.

Treatment.--Cleanliness of the parts and perfect drainage must be secured. Syringing with one to fifty carbolic acid solution (acid one part, warm water fifty parts) is good treatment. The opening in the drum should be made large enough to give free discharge to the pus in the middle ear.

The patient's strength must be built up if necessary.

INFLAMMATION OF THE MASTOID' CELLS. (Acute or Chronic Mastoiditis).--This disease represents one of the most serious terminations of an acute or a chronic suppurative inflammation of the middle ear. This is fortunately a comparatively rare event. There are, however, quite a good many cases of this terrible disease.

Causes.--It occurs as a primary or secondary disease. The first condition is rare and the result from injury, exposure to cold and dampness, or from syphilis or tuberculosis. *Secondary disease* is catarrhal or pus-like in form. This results from an extension of middle ear disease through the antrum, as a rule. The disease may develop at any time and endanger the life of the sufferer.

Symptoms.--Dull constant pain behind the ear and tenderness on pressure, more severe at night, the tenderness is very apt to be followed in a short time by redness and swelling of the skin in the same region. The pus may drain from the mastoid into the middle ear cavity. If this does not happen it may swell behind the ear and break through some other place. It may involve the structures within the brain. If meningitis develops, the patient has headache and later it becomes very severe. Lights hurts the eyes, The patient is restless, sleepless, may have nausea and vomiting and a constant high temperature. The neck is stiff and rigid. If there is more brain involvement (phlebitis) there will be sudden rise of temperature, followed by a rapid fall of temperature and attended by profuse sweating and chills,--a dangerous condition. There can be abscess of the brain also.

In abscess of the brain symptoms are less severe and localized; the rigid neck and fear of light and vomiting are absent.

Treatment.--If seen early it may be aborted. If an examination of the drum shows bulging, an incision of the drum head should be made. If an opening is there it should be enlarged, if necessary. Cold applications are valuable and should be applied directly over the mastoid behind the ear. Sometimes hot applications are better, hot poultices, cloths, etc., syringing the canal with hot water. These applications, etc., should be constantly used for a day or, so, unless unfavorable symptoms set in, when if a marked improvement, especially in the local tenderness and pain, has not occurred, an operation should be done and the mastoid opened.

The diet should be liquid (milk), nourishing and sustaining. Bowels should be kept open.

This disease must be carefully watched. It is not only dangerous to life, and very quickly, but it is full of disagreeable and dangerous possibilities, lifelong discharge from the ear, an external fistulous opening, a permanent paralysis of the facial nerve, abscess in the brain. Brain symptoms, paralysis and pus symptoms do not now preclude an operation on the mastoid for mastoid disease. The patient should be closely watched and an operation performed as soon as called for.

I have given a longer description of the diseases of the ear than I intended when I began this part of the work. Diseases of the ear are becoming quite frequent, and the subject is important. I did not give much general medical treatment because I consider the local treatment is of more importance in a work of this kind. In treating the baby, I shall give more medical treatment. I shall treat the disease also, especially in relation to the baby. There can be more local applications used than those given. If the hot treatment is thought best, not only hot water and poultices of many kinds can be used, but fomentations of hops, etc., and hot water cloths alone. The intent of such treatment is to keep hot moist applications to the part continually. The use of laudanum in poultices used for ear trouble is not recommended because its soothing power may obscure symptoms that might appear and be dangerous in themselves and need quick and thorough treatment. The syringing of hot water into the external canal is often of great help. Five to ten grains of boric acid can be used in an ounce of water. If there is much odor to the discharge, you can use one part of carbolic acid to fifty parts of boiled water. The water should not be used too hot. One teaspoonful of the acid to fifty teaspoonfuls of water, or that proportion. After using the hot water, the canal should be filled with gauze for protection and drainage. For the fever, the first twenty-four hours, one-tenth to one drop of aconite can be used every one to three hours. By putting one drop in ten teaspoonfuls of water you get one-tenth of a drop at a dose.

DEAFNESS.--This is usually the result of a disease and is merely a symptom. Diseases of the middle ear, rupture of the drum membrane, and large ulceration of this membrane cause it. Ear wax causes temporary deafness. Diseases of the throat and nose cause it very often, and deafness frequently accompanies catarrh of the nose. Adenoids cause it sometimes, especially in children.

Treatment.--The only way to prevent this trouble is to treat the disease that causes it. Discharge from the ear, due to ear disease should be treated from the first or it may cause permanent deafness in that ear. Many cases of scarlet fever leave deafness behind in one ear at least. This trouble should be closely watched during an attack of scarlet fever, and in other infectious diseases and proper treatment given.

Chronic deafness is hard to cure; so often some of the deeper parts of the ear are diseased. When a person recognizes that his hearing is growing less acute he should have his ear examined. People often let the trouble go too long before beginning treatment.

MOTHERS' REMEDIES. Deafness. 1. Quick and Effective Remedy for.--"Five or ten drops of onion juice put in the ear several times a day is very good. If there is any pain in the ear, add a drop or two of laudanum, or you may just use two or three drops of glycerin with the other ingredients. In about an hour after treating the ear in this manner, syringe it well with warm castile soap suds or warm milk."

2. Deafness. Often Tried Remedy for.--"Take one dram each of tincture of lobelia, tincture of gum myrrh, oil of sassafras, tincture of opium and olive oil, mix and apply lint wet with the liniment in the ear, night, and morning, then syringe out with warm water and castile soap."

3. Deafness, My Mother, in Galt, Found Mullein Good for.--"Small blossoms of mullein, fill bottles and cork, hang in sun till oil forms, drop three drops every third day in the ear for three or four weeks. We tried this successfully in our family."

EARACHE.--The general belief exists that earache is something which is quite harmless and entirely different from a genuine inflammation of the ear. This belief is strengthened by the fact that the great majority of earaches subside without inflicting any harm upon the ear. As soon as a discharge appears, in many cases, there is relief. If a discharge appears, the earache was the result of an inflammation in the ear. So-called earache lasts but a short time, and can be relieved by either hot or cold applications; but when the earache continues for a day or more it is an indication of more than pain in the ear and if a thorough examination is made there will, no doubt, be found disease of the ear that is causing the earache. Then the disease proper should be treated.

Treatment.--Hot or cold applications are of benefit. With the patient lying upon the well ear, fill the canal with hot water (105° F.).

Then place over the ear a flaxseed poultice or a roasted onion poultice, four to five inches square and one-half inch thick and spread over all a folded shawl. Bread and milk makes a good poultice also. A hot bran bag or a hot salt bag is good. The heat must be continuous.

MOTHERS' REMEDIES. 1. Earache, Hot Raisin for.--"Hot raisins sometimes relieve earache. Soak them in hot milk and change frequently." This is an excellent remedy. The raisins should be placed in the ear canal, and they are sure to give relief.

2. Earache, Flax and Cornmeal for.--"Flaxseed and cornmeal in oil." Take equal parts of flaxseed and cornmeal and mix together, then add enough sweet oil to moisten this mixture. This should be applied hot and kept so by repeating as each poultice is cold. This will be found very beneficial.

3. Earache, Soothing Home Remedy for.--"Glycerin and laudanum heated and dropped in the ear. Hot poultice of hops inclosed in cotton bag and applied to the ear is very soothing." The glycerin and laudanum will give temporary relief and the hops poultice retains the heat, which is one of the essential things in earache.

4. Earache, Horse-radish Leaves for.--"Steaming the face and ear with crushed horseradish leaves will give relief and soothes one to sleep." When through steaming the face the horseradish leaves should be applied to the face and ear as a poultice. This is very soothing.

5. Earache, Onion Sure Cure for.--"The heart of an onion." Roast the heart of an onion and put in the canal of the ear. Then apply heat to the outside of the ear and relief will soon be obtained.

6. Earache; Temporary Relief for.--

"Gum Camphor	1/2 dram
Olive Oil	1/2 ounce
Glycerin	1/2 ounce

Mix and drop in ear."

This is good to relieve, but should not be continued, as this oily substance lodges in the ear and may cause trouble.

7. Earache, Sweet Oil and Pepper for.--"Take a piece of cotton batting, cover with sweet oil, then cover that with black pepper, inserting into ear." This is a good remedy.

8. Earache, Steaming With Hot Water for.--"Steam the ear and side of the head with cloths wrung out of hot water; put feet in hot mustard water; do not put anything in the ear but keep steaming it and you will find relief in a few hours, even if it is a gathering."

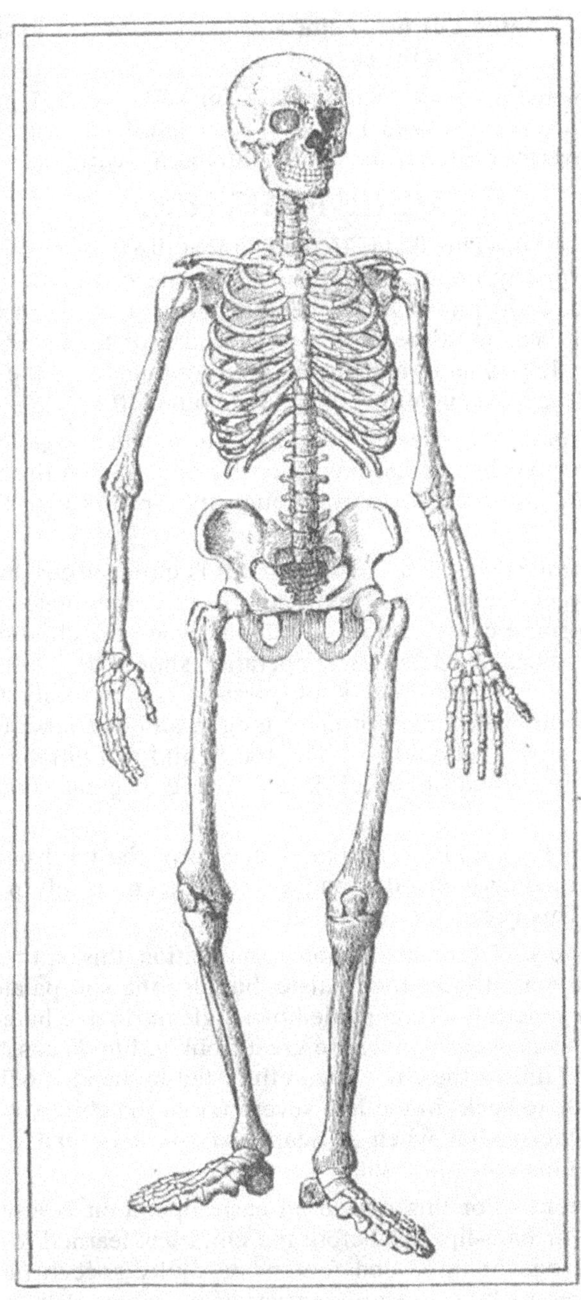

SKELETON.

SKELETON

9. Earache, Castor Oil for.--"Put a drop of castor oil in the ear. Fill hot water bag and warm the ear that aches."

10. Earache, Fresh Warm Milk for.--"The warm milk from a cow will cure earache and has also been known to cure deafness." While still warm from the cow drop a little in the ear.

DEFORMITIES.

HARE-LIP.--This is due to the fact that the flesh or bony parts do not quite properly unite. It may form a single or double hare-lip, or complicated, or it may involve the soft parts, or the hard (bony) and soft parts at the same time. It is always to one or the other side of the middle line. It is double hair-lip in about one-tenth of the cases, and when double it is frequently complicated with cleft palate.

Symptoms.--Upon examination you notice that there is a split in the lip, either partly through the lip or entirely, so that the bone is exposed; or the slit goes not only through the lip, but also through the bone.

Operation.--This is necessary, and it is quite successful. The best time is between the third and sixth month, especially when it is a simple case. In some cases of double hair-lip, when the child cannot take the breast and has to be fed, early operation should be done if the child is strong. The operation for a simple hare-lip is very easily and quickly done. For complicated cases it takes longer, and of course is not without some danger. It should be done, for a child is a pitiable sight with this deformity. When grown up it is a source of great annoyance and shame.

CLEFT PALATE.--The bones that form the hard palate do not unite in the median line and a longitudinal opening is left in the roof of the mouth. This is called Cleft Palate.

Symptoms.--Of course, upon examination this split is seen. It may involve not only the hard palate, but also the soft palate and uvula. It is then generally accompanied by single or double hare-lip. When the severe forms occur they cause great trouble. Fluids pass freely into the nose, and unless the child is carefully fed by hand it will soon die, as it is unable to suck. In the less severe forms the child soon learns to swallow properly, but when he learns to speak he cannot articulate properly and his voice is nasal.

Treatment.--For this reason an early operation is advisable, not so early as for hare-lip, but before the child has learned to speak, say between the age of three and four when faulty speech (articulation) may be overcome by successful closure of the palate. When the operation

is done late, the patient will not be able to overcome the bad habits of articulation acquired in his childhood.

Operation.--The anaesthetic is necessary. The end of one-half of the cleft palate is seized with an instrument and the edge freely pared with a thin bladed sharp knife; same with the other half. Then the stitches are put in of silk worm, gut or wire. The patient is fed on liquid food for three or four days, and afterwards on soft food until the stitches are removed. They are removed about the sixth or eighth day, and the wound should be completely healed.

CROOKED FEET. Talipes.--There are many varieties. The treatment should be begun, under the instructions of a physician, and continued from infancy and many a good foot can be obtained.

KNOCK KNEE. (Genu Valgum).--This is due to an overgrowth of the internal knuckle (condyle) on the knee joint, and curving inward of the shaft of the thigh-bone (femur) in its lower parts, with relaxation and lengthening of the ligaments of the knee joint.

It usually shows itself soon after the child begins to walk, but may not do so until puberty,--rarely later. It is due in the child to rickets; in the latter form, it is caused by an occupation that requires continued standing, by a person of feeble development of the muscles and ligaments. "Flat-foot" is often associated with it and, at times, may be the real cause. It may affect one or both knees, may be so slight as to escape detection, except upon a very careful examination, or so severe as to separate the feet very widely and render walking difficult and wobbling. In children other symptoms of rickets can generally be found. If not severe it may often get better spontaneously as the rickets condition improves and the general strength increases. This result is common in the cases occurring later, from standing if the general condition improves.

Treatment.--Should be begun early and both general and local treatment should be given. The quicker the treatment is begun, the quicker will be the recovery and the deformity will be less. The ordinary medical and hygienic treatment should be given for rickets.

Local Treatment.--This is mechanical, supplemented by baths, rubbing, friction, electricity and preceded, if necessary, by attending to the bones. If the rickets is still active, and the bones are soft and yielding, standing and walking should be forbidden, the limb should be straightened by manipulation and the correct position secured and maintained by an outside splint and bandage. Sometimes operative measures are needed.

BOW LEGS. (Genu Varum).--This is the opposite of knock knees, and the deformity usually affects both limbs, the knees being widely separated. The disease begins in early childhood; the cause is rickets, and the deformity is the direct result of the weight of the body and muscular action.

Treatment.--Spontaneous recovery occurs; but if the case is at all severe, and the child is young enough that the bones have not become firmly set in the abnormal curves, mechanical treatment should be employed to bring the limbs to a better position. This may be done by plaster of paris or braces. This must be used intelligently and continuously. Children should not be allowed to walk so early, especially those of slow development.

CLUB FOOT (Talipes).--Varieties:

1. The heel may be drawn up and the foot extended (Talipes Equinus).

2. The foot may be flexed, bent up, (Talipes Calcaneus).

3. The foot may be drawn inward, adducted, (Talipes Varus).

4. The foot may be drawn outward, abducted, (Talipes Valgus); or, two may be combined, extended, and drawn inward (Equino Varus).

In the congenital (born with it) variety the displacement is almost always one of adduction, that is, drawn inward, with commonly some elevation of the heel. It generally affects both feet, but it may be confined to one and if only one is affected, the right is oftener affected than the left. The deformity varies. At the time of birth and for some months afterwards the deformity can usually be corrected by proper manipulation, but later, if left to itself, it becomes in greater or less measure fixed, because of the muscular contraction, and developed changes in the shape of the bones.

Cause--It is not known.

Treatment is successful if it is begun early. Each case should be treated as it needs. The treatment should be varied to suit each case. Bandaging or adhesive straps properly applied has been used with success. Sometimes the leg must be kept motionless by plaster of Paris or gutta-percha bandages. They must be frequently removed and reapplied. In older cases the tendons must be cut and braces applied. Parents are careless who neglect such a case for even one month.

INTOXICANTS AND SUN STROKES

ALCOHOLISM. Acute Symptoms.--The face is flushed, the breath has the odor of liquor, the pulse is full and bounding with deep respiration. Reason, memory, judgment and will are first stimulated and then blunted. The drinker's peculiarities are exaggerated, the person becoming affectionate or quarrelsome. There is a loss of coordination as shown by the staggering, swinging, the relaxation of the muscles, and finally deep sleep, with snoring breathing. The person is unconscious, but can be partly aroused and will mutter when questioned or disturbed. The pupils are contracted or dilated, and they will dilate when the face is slapped. The urine is increased, but it is often retained.

CHRONIC ALCOHOLISM.--This results from protracted or periodic "sprees."

Symptoms.--The face is red, the capillaries are dilated, eyes are watery, conjunctiva is congested. There is chronic inflammation of the stomach, which is characterized by morning vomiting; there is often hardening of the liver, trembling of the hands and tongue; the memory is weakened and judgment and will as well, especially until a stimulant has been taken; often the person is irritable, careless, with loss of moral sense and in extreme cases dementia. Peripheral neuritis is more common in men than in women. It begins with sharp pain and tingling in the feet and hands; paralysis affects the lower extremities, then the upper, and is most marked in the further muscles of the limbs. The pain may be very severe, with great tenderness. There is Arteriosclerosis (hardening of walls of the arteries); often heart dilation.

DELIRIUM TREMENS.--This is a brain manifestation of chronic alcoholism occurring in steady drinkers after excessive drinking or sudden withdrawal of alcohol, or after sudden excitement or accident, pneumonia or other illness, or lack of food.

Symptoms.--There are restlessness, insomnia (sleeplessness), mental depression, then active delirium with great restlessness, talking, muttering, hallucination of sight and hearing. He thinks he sees objects in the room such as rats, mice, or snakes, and fancies that they are crawling over his body, has them in his boots, etc. The terror inspired by these imaginary objects is great, and has given the popular name of "horrors" or "snakes" to the disease. You must watch the patient constantly, or he may try to jump out of the window or escape. The patient may think he hears sounds and voices, threats of imaginary enemies. There is much muscular "shakings," the tongue is coated with a thick white fur and, when protruded, trembles. The pulse is rapid and soft, sleeplessness is a constant feature. Favorable cases improve in the third or fourth day, the restlessness abates, the patient sleeps and the improvement sets in. The shakings persist for some days, the hallucinations disappear gradually, and the appetite returns. In the more serious cases, the sleeplessness (insomnia) persists, the delirium is incessant, the pulse becomes more frequent and feeble, the tongue dry, the prostration is extreme and death takes place from gradual heart failure.

Treatment.--In acute alcoholic cases special measures are seldom required, as the patient sleeps off the effect of his "spree." If there is deep profound alcoholic coma, it may be proper to wash out the stomach and if symptoms of collapse occur, the limbs should be rubbed, and hot applications made to the body.

Chronic Alcoholism.--This is different; withdraw the alcohol and substitute strychnine, one-thirtieth of a grain three or four times a day, nourishing food, confinement in a sanitarium if necessary. Give the bromides for the restlessness and sleeplessness. Drugging of the liquor with apo morphine or tartar emetic.

MOTHER'S REMEDY. Drunkenness. 1. Effective as Cure for.--

"Arsenious Acid	19 grains
Bromine Water	sufficient
Tribromide of Gold	14 grains
Distilled Water	sufficient

Ten drops of this solution for injection, which equals one thirty-second grain of gold tribromide." This is an active tonic, powerful sedative and destroys the appetite or cravings for alcoholic stimulants; the medicine is to be taken regularly four or five times a day for several weeks until the alcohol is out of the system even though he may appear cured. This is a good remedy, but should be given under the supervision of a doctor.

Treatment.--The patient must be put into a bed and carefully watched; withdraw alcohol at once unless the pulse is too feeble. Procure rest and sleep for the patient. How? In mild cases, thirty grains (one-half dram) of bromide of potassium, combined with tincture of capsicum five to ten drops, may be given every three hours. Call a doctor for the rest. One hundredth grain hyoscine hypodermically is sometimes good; one-fourth grain morphine hypodermically is sometimes given. For heart weakness: Aromatic spirits of ammonia.

MORPHINE HABIT. (Morphinomania--Morphinism).--This is usually acquired by the repeated use of the hypodermic syringe for pain. It is also used by the mouth or opium smoking.

Symptoms.--At first it causes a sense of well-being and exhilaration, but it must be gradually increased to produce the result; when the effect wears off, the person feels weary, mentally and physically; has nausea, slight distress in the stomach region or pain like intestinal colic. Another dose relieves these feelings, eventually the person becomes thin, his face is sallow, the pupils are dilated or unequal, except when he is under the influence of the drug. His appetite is poor with indigestion. Sometimes itching of the skin, restlessness; irritable, disturbed sleep, and a tendency to lie about everything.

Treatment.--The patient must be taken from home and friends and be constantly watched. The drug should be withdrawn gradually and nourishing food given at stated intervals.

COCAINE HABIT.--The drug is taken as a snuff, hypodermically, or in sprays and often the habit is formed when given as sprays, etc., in disease.

Symptoms.--Large doses cause great excitement, sometimes convulsions, followed by weak heart and respiratory weakness, general prostration, convulsions and coma.

The cocaine habit causes emaciation, anemia, disturbances of the stomach, etc., disordered heart action, weakness of the body and mind, nervous and great depravity.

Treatment.--Same as for the morphine habit.

CHLORAL HABIT. Symptoms.--After a slight primary exhilaration there is depression of the mind and body; skin eruptions, bad breath, spongy gums, poor appetite, indigestion, bad nutrition, permanent dilation of the cutaneous (skin) blood vessels, intermittent pulse, blunting of the higher mental faculties, restlessness, sleeplessness, irritability, sometimes dementia.

Treatment.--Same as for morphine.

LEAD POISONING. (Plumbism-Saturnism). Causes.--It is common in lead smelters and grinders, painters, glaziers, and plumbers, whose hands are not washed before eating. The lead is absorbed by the mouth, skin and lungs. It may be taken into the system by drinking water, cider, etc., in new lead pipes, or from hair-dyes or cosmetics containing lead.

Symptoms of Acute Case.--These develop rapidly from continued exposure. There is rapidly progressing anemia, with acute neuritis, epilepsy, convulsions or delirium or with severe stomach and bowel symptoms.

Chronic Cases. Symptoms. 1.--Anemia, lead line on the gums, paralysis, colic, and brain symptoms.

2. Blue-black line of lead in the gums near the teeth.

3. This is preceded by an obstinate constipation. It resembles severe intestinal colic. There may be vomiting.

4. Paralysis. This is the result of peripheral neuritis, localized or generalized.

Wrist drop and many other symptoms of local and general paralysis.

TREATMENT. Prevention.--The hands and finger nails of the lead workers should always be thoroughly cleaned before eating. Use respirators if lead is present in the form of dust.

For chronic poisoning remove the cause. Potassium iodide, five to ten grains three times a day. Not to be given in acute cases or when the symptoms are very severe, until what is in the bowels is removed.

Constipation.--For this give a half ounce of epsom salts before breakfast when needed, or repeat in small doses.

For pain.--Heat over the abdomen and give morphine, if necessary.

FOOD POISONING. (Bromototoxismus).--Food may contain the specific organisms of disease, as of tuberculosis or trichinosis; milk and other foods may become infected with typhoid bacilli, and so convey the disease.

Animals (or insects or bees) may feed on substances that cause their flesh or products to be poisonous to man. Meat poisoning. Eating sausage or pork pie or headcheese has caused poisoning. Poisoning from impure milk, shell fish, pellagra, from using altered maize, etc.

Symptoms.--Acute inflammation of stomach and bowels, with great prostration, ending in collapse. In shell fish poisoning, there are numbness, weakness, dilated pupils, rapid and feeble pulse, temperature under the normal and collapse.

Treatment.--In all cases empty the stomach by emetics or stomach tube and the bowels by cathartics. Stimulate if necessary.

HEAT STROKE.--Called also heat exhaustion; thermic fever, coup de Soleil. A condition produced by exposure to excessive heat.

Heat Exhaustion.--This is caused by continued exposure to high temperatures, especially while working hard.

Symptoms.--Prostration with cool skin, temperature often below normal, 95-96, pulse is small and frequent, sometimes restlessness and delirium. The person need not necessarily be exposed to the direct rays of the sun, but the condition may come on at night, or while at work in close, confined rooms.

Treatment of indoor heat exhaustion.--Aromatic spirits of ammonia one to two drams and strychnine; avoid alcohol. If the temperature is below normal, (98.6) a warm bath can be given. Rest in bed in a well ventilated room.

SUNSTROKE. Heat Stroke, Thermic (heat) Fever.--This occurs in persons chiefly who, while working very hard are exposed to the sun. Soldiers who are marching with their heavy accoutrements are very liable to be attacked. In large cities the most of the cases are confined to workmen who are much exposed and at the same time, have been drinking beer and whisky.

Symptoms.--The patient may be struck down and die very soon with symptoms of failure of the heart, difficult breathing and coma. This kind is most frequent in soldiers. In ordinary cases there may be failure to perspire, premonitory headache, dizziness, sometimes nausea and vomiting, colored or poor sight (vision); insensibility follows, which may be temporary or increased deep coma. The face is flushed, the skin is dry and hot, the pupils are temporarily dilated, then usually greatly contracted, the pulse is rapid and full, and the temperature ranges from 107 to 110 degrees or higher. The breathing is deep, labored and snoring (stortorous). Usually there is complete muscular relaxation, with twitchings, jerkings, or very rarely convulsions may occur. In fatal cases, coma (deep sleep) deepens, the pulse becomes more frequent and feeble, the breathing becomes more hurried, shallow and irregular and death may occur within twenty-four to thirty-six hours. In others, the consciousness returns, the temperature falls, the pulse and breathing become normal and recovery may be complete or leave bad results. The patient may be predisposed to future attacks or suffer from weakness or headache, and disturbance of the mind when ever the weather is warm.

Prognosis.--The death rate is higher when treatment is delayed, and when alcohol has been used as a beverage.

MOTHER'S REMEDY. Sunstroke, Quick Method to Relieve.--"Apply alternately hot and cold applications to forehead and base of the brain or back of the neck, place the feet in warm mustard water, and apply mustard to the stomach and calves of legs. This remedy was tried by my brother's wife, who is a trained nurse. She says it is very effective," The hot and cold applications help to draw the blood from the brain. Placing feet in warm mustard water will help to give relief.

Treatment.--Avoid exposure and alcohol. For a mild case--Rest in a cool place, cool sponging, aromatic spirits ammonia or strychnine if needed for the prostration.

For severe cases.--The temperature must be reduced as rapidly as possible. Pack the patient in a bath of ice. Rubbing the body with ice is an excellent procedure to lower the temperature rapidly. Ice water enemata (injections in bowel) may also be employed. If ice cannot be obtained strip the patient and sprinkle him with water until the temperature is reduced. Use a thermometer to see it does not go too low. Ice cap or cold water to the head. Keep working for hours.

Medicine.--Glonoin, 1/100 to 1/200 grain is of help in severe cases.

ACCIDENTS, EMERGENCIES AND POISONS

COLLAPSE.--1. Place the patient flat on his back.

2. Raise the feet and lower his head, unless blueness of the face occurs.

3. Make the patient warm by applying warm coverings and hot water bottles, bricks or wood.

4. Enema of strong coffee.

5. If necessary the legs and arms can be bandaged beginning at the feet and hands and then bandage up. Use above in order given.

FAINTING.--Place the patient on her back, with the head low and feet raised unless the face is flushed. The face is generally pale.

Loosen the clothing about the waist, throat, etc.

Plenty of air and no crowding around the patient.

Cold water on the face with cloths. It is not necessary to wet her all over. Ammonia or camphor near the nostrils to inhale. Lie still for some time and do not attempt to rise while still feeling dizzy or faint.

MOTHERS' REMEDIES.--1. Sea Sickness, Red Pepper and Molasses Relieves.--"A teaspoonful of red pepper mixed with molasses and taken in one dose is considered one of the best remedies for this trouble."

2. Sea Sickness, Peppermint an Excellent Relief for.--"A teaspoonful of essence of peppermint put in a tumbler of hot water, sipped occasionally, is both a preventive and cure for sea-sickness."

Sea Sickness.--Dr. Hare, of Philadelphia, says: "The bromides should be used in the dose of five to ten grains three times a day for several days before the patient sails to quiet the vomiting center." After sea sickness begins the following combination is good:

(a)	Citric Acid	2 drams
	Distilled Water	4 ounces
	Make a solution.	
(b)	Bromide of Potash	1 dram
	Bicarbonate of Potash	1 dram
	Distilled Water	4 ounces
	Make a solution.	

Then a tablespoonful of each of these solutions should be added to one another and taken during effervescence. Lemon juice can be used in place of citric acid in the first combination.

DOG BITES (Not Rabid).--Treat the same as for any torn wound, wash out thoroughly with hot water and an ounce of salt in a pint of water. There is no danger of hydrophobia from the bite of a dog, cat or any animal unless that animal has hydrophobia. No one can take hydrophobia from an animal that does not have it. (See Hydrophobia).

POISONED WOUNDS. Mosquito Bite.--Remove the sting in the wound. Diluted vinegar applied to the bites is sometimes of help. Camphor is also good.

Snake Bite.--Naturalists have discovered twenty-seven species of poisonous serpents and one poisonous lizard; eighteen species of these are true rattlesnakes; the remaining nine are divided between varieties of the moccasin, copperhead or the viper. The poisonous lizard is the Texan reptile known as the "Gila Monster." In all these serpents the poison fluid is secreted in a gland which lies against the side of the skull below and behind the eye, from which a duct leads to the base of a hollow tooth or fang, one on each side of the upper jaw; which fang, except in the case of vipers, is movable and susceptible of erection and depression. When not in use the fang hugs the upper jaw and is ensheathed in a fold of mucous membrane. In the vipers the fang is permanently erect. In the case of biting the contents of the poison sac are forcibly ejected through the hollow fang.

Symptoms of a Snake Bite.--The symptoms are similar in bites of poisonous snakes. Pain in the wound, slight at first, but becoming more severe, with rapid swelling and spotted discoloration in the vicinity of the wound. Symptoms of heart and lung depression soon show themselves by feeble and fluttering pulse, faintness, cold sweating, mental distress, nausea and vomiting and labored breathing. Death may occur very soon in intense poisoned cases, but more frequently the struggle extends over a number of hours.

Treatment.--First thing to do.--When the bite is on a limb, tie the limb above the bite toward the body and twist the ligature so tight that the circulation is cut off, or checked. Then cut the wound open very freely. When the bite is on the body, make a free cut, and when this cannot be done suck the wound vigorously, which can done without danger, if there are no cracks or abrasions of the lips or mouth, as the poison is harmless when taken into a well mouth. If a hot iron is at hand apply it freely within the wound and this may take the place of the knife or suction. Salt put in the cut wound will be of help, or fill the wound with permanganate of potash and inject a solution of the same, diluted three-quarters with water, around the wound. Strychnine one-fifteenth of a grain every two hours until the symptoms are better. This is not given until the symptoms of snake poisoning have shown themselves.

If such agents are not at hand, brandy or whisky should be given freely. The pulse will show when the patient has had enough.

MOTHERS' REMEDIES. INSECT AND OTHER BITES.--1. Simply Use Pepper for Dog Bite.--"My son had his hand bitten by a dog and it was over a week before it was brought to my notice. The sore was then filled with green pus and the pain went up to his jaw, so we were afraid of lockjaw. I had him cleanse it thoroughly in a basin of warm saleratus water, then filled and thickly covered it with black pepper. The pain stopped almost instantly. It seems as though pepper would smart a cut terribly, but it does not." This is a good remedy and worth trying. The black pepper did not smart the wound because the flesh was dead.

2. Bites, Tobacco Good for Dog.--"Immediately wash the parts with clear water; then take leaf or cut tobacco and bind over the part bitten, changing it two or three times a day for a week. This effectually absorbs the poison. It is a good prevention of any future trouble."

3. Bites, Ammonia Good for Insect.--"Rub the affected parts with ammonia, which will draw out the poison. For mosquito bites have often used baking soda. This always gives relief and is very cooling."

4. Bites, Baking Soda for Insect.--"Cover the affected parts with baking soda and keep moist." A mud poultice is an old tried remedy.

5. Bites, Hartshorn Old Time Remedy for.--"Apply hartshorn or spirits of ammonia to part which neutralizes the formic acid, the active principle of the poison." This is an old-time remedy and will always give relief if applied immediately.

6. Bites, Carbolic Acid Draws Poison from.--"Bathe frequently in a weak solution of carbolic acid." The carbolic acid is a very good remedy and seldom fails to cure, but if you do not happen to have the acid, use vinegar, and it will have practically the same effect.

7. Bites, Alum and Vinegar Good Remedy for.--"Alum and vinegar. Purchase five cents' worth of powdered alum and dissolve in a pint of vinegar and apply freely. This is a very good remedy."

8. Bites, Salt Water for Mosquito.--"Take salt and water in a little dish and keep wetting the bite for a few moments. This will soon destroy the poison," This will be found a very simple but effective remedy, especially in children or small babies, as we mothers all know how very annoying a mosquito bite is to children. The salt water will remove all the poison and at the same time relieve the itching and swelling. Care should be taken not to make it too strong for a small baby.

9. Bites, Spirits of Ammonia for Snake.--"Strong spirits of ammonia applied to the wounds of snake bites or rabid animals is better than caustic. It neutralizes the poison." Enough of the ammonia should be used to irritate the parts. It is harmless treatment and should be used freely.

STINGS, MOTHERS' REMEDIES.--1. Leaves of Geranium Good for Bee or Wasp.--"Bruise the leaves of geranium and bind on the affected part. This has proved an excellent, though simple remedy."

2. Stings, Simple Remedy for.--"Take a dresser key or any with a good sized hole and press over the sting. If used very soon this will remove the stinger, then cover with wet salt."

DISLOCATIONS.--A dislocation is the putting out of joint some bone, such as the elbow or shoulder bone or bones. The bone has slipped out of its socket. They are called after the joints involved.

General Causes.--Blows, sudden contraction of the muscles; also due to some diseases of the joints.

General Symptoms.--There is a deformity at the joint, pain and sometimes it is not possible to make all the joint movements.

General Treatment.--Of course it is to replace the bone, as soon as possible, before there is much swelling, inflammation and consequent adhesions.

DISLOCATION OF THE JAW.--It is not possible to close the mouth. The chin is too far forward. The jaw may turn toward the other side in one-sided dislocation.

Treatment.--Hold something hard between the teeth in front so that when the jaw snaps in place your thumbs will not be bitten. A piece of wood as thick as your fingers will do. Stand in front of the patient, who should be sitting in a high chair. Put your thumbs in the mouth upon the lower jaw two-thirds of the length backwards, and your forefingers directly underneath the jaw; with the thumbs press down and with the fingers pull forward.

Oblique Bandage of Jaw.

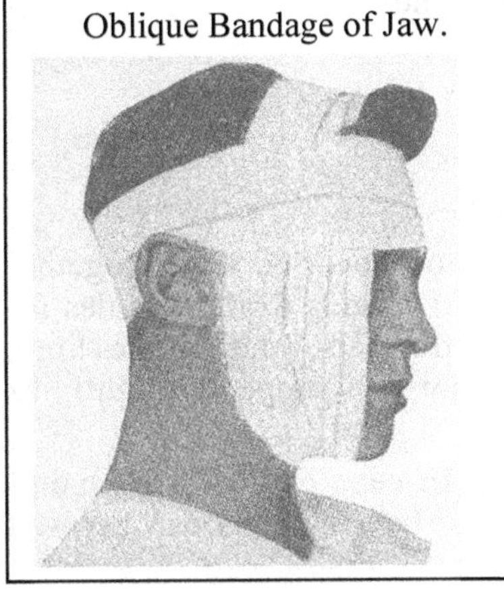

Medicated Cotton can readily be applied with this style of Bandage.

Bandaging and Photograph by

DR. W. E. ZIEGENFUSS, of Detroit.

Done expressly for this book.

Sometimes it is necessary to hold the jaw in place for some days. For that purpose the bandage for a broken jaw can be used.

SHOULDER JOINT DISLOCATION.--There is a depression of the skin over the cavity. The shoulder is flattened. The bone of the arm points to where the head of the bone is.

Treatment.--Carry the elbow to the side with the forearm at right angles to the arm: turn the arm around until the forearm points away from the body. Then carry the arm up from the body until it is level with the shoulder. In this position gradually rotate the arm again and then bring the arm to the side, with the forearm across the chest, hand pointing to the other shoulder when it should be bandaged by pieces of bandages three inches wide passing around the arm, elbow and body.

A pad should be placed under the hand to keep it from making the flesh sore.

FINGER OR THUMB DISLOCATION.--If the joint is dislocated forward pull the front part forward and backward. If it is dislocated backwards, pull the front part of the finger forward and upward. If reduced immediately this needs no bandaging.

FRACTURES.--They are simply broken bones or cartilage, usually applied popularly to a broken bone.

Varieties.--Simple fracture means a break of the bone only.

Compound fracture is where the broken bone sticks out through the skin.

Comminuted is where the bone is broken into small parts.

Impacted is where one part of the broken bone is driven into the other part.

Green stick break. This is not really a break, but only a bending of the bone, seen mostly in children.

Bandages for fractures can be made of muslin. They should be six to eight to twelve yards long for large bones.

Width. For a finger one inch.

For arm or head two and one-half inches.

For the leg three to four inches.

For the body six to eight inches.

An old sheet can be used and the ends of the strips sewed together and then wrapped tight in a roll, with the ravelings from the sides removed. The bandage should be started from the end of the limb, wrapped towards the body. They should not be wrapped so tightly as to shut off circulation,

Padding.--This should be of cotton. In case of necessity, handkerchiefs, towels, pieces of muslin, cloths; hay or grass can be used temporarily.

Splints.--In emergencies splints can be made from shingles, pasteboards or even bark.

How to Take Hold of a Broken Leg or Arm.--Never take hold of it from above, but slip the hands underneath, and then take a firm but gentle hold at two points a short distance from the break on each side, and all the while making slight extension with the hand on the end part (distal part) so as to keep the ends from rubbing together, and lift with both hands at the same time slowly and evenly until the limb is in the required position. Then apply the emergency treatment. This is to help keep the broken parts in place until proper care can be given, or to assist in safely and comfortably moving the patient to the place desired. Support the broken limb with something smooth and stiff, such as a thin narrow shingle, three inches wide perhaps, or thin board, stout pasteboard, or the bark of trees, and padded with something soft, such as cotton, wool, hay, straw, leaves, which can be held by bandages of required width, or handkerchiefs folded in triangular shape, or by strips of linen, muslin, ribbon or anything with which the splint can be temporarily held fast.

For the Forearm.--Two padded splints three to four inches wide and long enough to take in the hand also should be applied, one to the thumb, and the other to the back of the forearm, slight extension being made by pulling on the patient's hand. This pulls the broken end in place. Tie on the splints over the hand, wrist and just below the elbow. Two or three wraps of adhesive plaster or five or six wraps of a bandage or handkerchief or towel folded and pinned will temporarily hold the limb in place. Put on a sling reaching from the finger tips to beyond the elbow.

For the Arm.--Put on two padded splints from the shoulder to the elbow, one in front and the one behind, and bind on at the bottom and top. Then place the forearm on the chest pointing to the well or sound shoulder and bind the arm with bandages or a long towel to the body.

For a Broken Leg.--Pull on the foot gently to make slight extension, and lift the leg on a pillow or some sort of pad, and tie this firmly about the leg; or broad strips of wood may be padded and placed on either side of the broken leg and securely tied.

For a Broken Thigh, Upper Leg.--The splint should extend from under the arm to the ankle, padded and bound to the body and to the leg by means of long towels or pieces of sheeting applied six inches apart. If the patient is in a wagon and no splint can be had, bags of dirt or sand applied around the thigh will hold some. But there is always something at hand to use as a splint and to bind the splint to the leg.

For a Broken Collar Bone.--Place the patient on his back if he is to be moved and put a firm pad in the arm pit and bind the arm to the side with the forearm across the chest; or if you have a roll of adhesive plaster two or three inches wide, after putting a pad in the arm pit (sometimes this is not necessary) put the adhesive strip around the arm midway to the shoulder. The arm should be lifted up and a little back. Run the strip of adhesive plaster around the body and fasten to the first part. Then put another strip fast to the band around the arm and run this down around the bent elbow and over the forearm placed on the chest, the fingers pointing to the sound shoulder. This strip can pass over the sound collar bone and fasten to the strip about the body. If it is put on properly, the injured part will feel comfortable.

Broken Ribs.--Put on a towel, about eight to twelve inches wide. This should go around the body and be pinned tightly; or, if you have a roll of adhesive plaster, two and one-half to three inches wide, use this. Start at the backbone, at the lowest point necessary, about two ribs below the broken one, and carry it straight across the chest to the breast bone; put on about eight of such strips, lapping each about one-half inch. Fasten the ends with a strip running up and down one-half on the flesh and the other half on the strip. This is to keep the strips from slipping any. The arms should be held up while the strips are being applied.

A Broken Jaw.--Take a strong piece of muslin, long enough to reach around the neck and eight inches longer. Split this through the center to within about seven inches of the center of the band. Put this unsplit part above, over and under the chin. Tie the upper tails around the neck and run the under tail pieces up in front of the ear to the crown of the head. Tie each end on the back part of the head to the pieces left over after tying back of the neck.

Broken Nose.--Put the parts in place by pressure and moulding. It is easily done. Do not hurry. Put a strip of adhesive plaster across the bridge of the nose over the break reaching to the cheek.

If the injury causes bleeding, the wound should be washed with clean linen and boiled water and covered with clean linen. To wash the wound, one teaspoonful of salt to one pint of boiled water. Salt is usually at hand.

If an artery is cut, this bleeding must be stopped. The blood spurts out. Press your hands hard on the back of the thigh towards the body of the wound. Another should tie some cloth around the thigh above the wound tightly. It can be made tighter by putting a stick under the band and twisting it around as much as possible. Raise the leg high up and put the head low. If the cut is below the knee or on the foot, bend the leg back. First put a pad or your fist in under the knee joint and bend leg over the pad or your fist. Sometimes the spurting artery can be caught or pressed upon with your finger. If the arm is injured, bandage as for the thigh. If the forearm, the same as for the leg.

If a finger is cut clean off, pick the piece up and wash it and the stump clean and then place the cut off part against the stump and tie on, or stick on with adhesive plaster. It sometimes grows fast.

SPRAINS.--Sprains or wrenches of the joints are caused by a twist or a blow. The injury consists in the tear or rupture of a number of the fibres of the ligaments.

Symptoms.--Severe pain, the joint is practically useless for a time; swelling, heat and later the joint discolored from effusion of the blood into the tissues.

MOTHERS' REMEDIES.--1. Sprains, Ointment for.--"The

bark of bittersweet with chamomile and wormwood simmered in fresh lard make an excellent ointment for sprains and swellings."

2. Sprains, Vinegar and Bran Poultice for.--"Make a poultice with vinegar and bran only, or with the addition of oatmeal, or bread crumbs. As the poultice becomes dry it should be moistened with vinegar."

3. Sprains, Turpentine Most Common Remedy for.--"Rub the injured part with turpentine and keep warm and you will find this remedy to be one of the best to keep proud flesh out that has ever been used. I always have turpentine in my home and find that I have to use it often, and it always does as I said above, if once used you will never be without it."

4. Sprains, Quick Relief for.--"Bathe the parts with hot water as hot as one can bear it and relief comes at once." This is an old tried remedy, but if hot water does not give relief use cold water.

5. Sprains, Relieves Pain of.--"Put warm woolen cloth over sprain, drip hot water as hot as can be borne on cloth for half hour. Bathe with spirits of camphor."

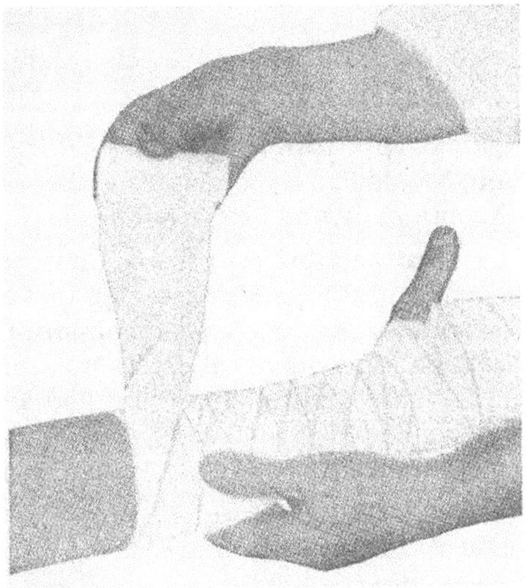

Method of applying Bandage to the Arm.

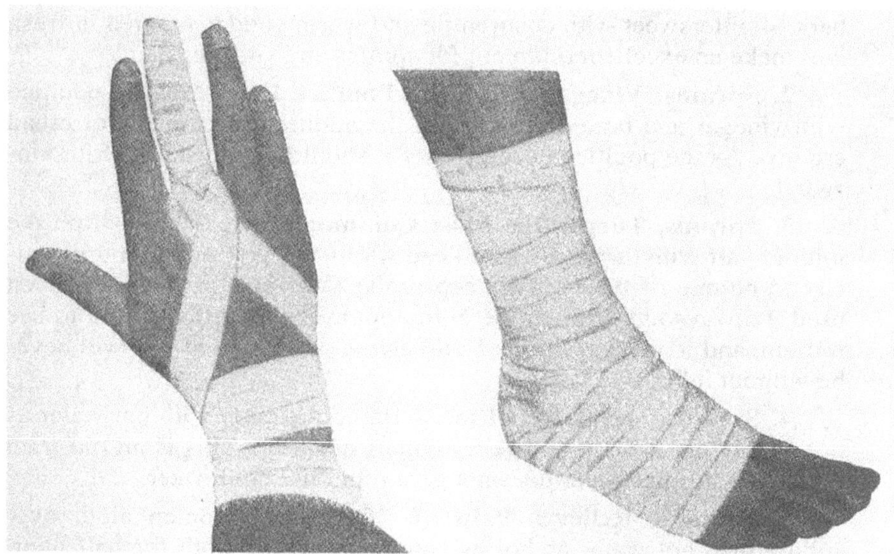

Spiral Bandage of the Finger

Simple Method of applying Bandage for Sprained Ankle.

Bandaging and Photographs by DR. W. E. ZIEGENFUSS, of Detroit. Done expressly for this book.

6. Sprains, Quick Application for.--"A poultice of stiff clay and vinegar." Add enough vinegar to the clay to make a nice moist poultice. The clay is exceptionally good for swellings and sprains.

7. Sprains, Turpentine Liniment for.--"Equal parts of spirits of turpentine and vinegar and the yolk of one egg make a valuable liniment in cases of sprains, bruises and rheumatism poultice. Take common salt, roast it on a hot stove till dry as possible. Take one teaspoonful each of dry salt, venice turpentine and pulverized castile soap. Excellent for felon, apply twice daily until open." This is a very good liniment and if applied often will draw, which is one of the essential things for a felon.

8. Sprains, Old English White Oil.--

"Alcohol	1/4 pint.
Turpentine	1/4 pint.
Hartshorn	1/2 ounce.
Oil Origanum	1 ounce.

For sprains and rubbing around sores."

9. Sprains, Arnica Much Used for.--"Tincture of arnica." This should be diluted with water about one and one-half for adults and one and three-fourths for a child. This is one of the best known remedies for sprains that can be obtained. Apply freely to the bruise or sprain.

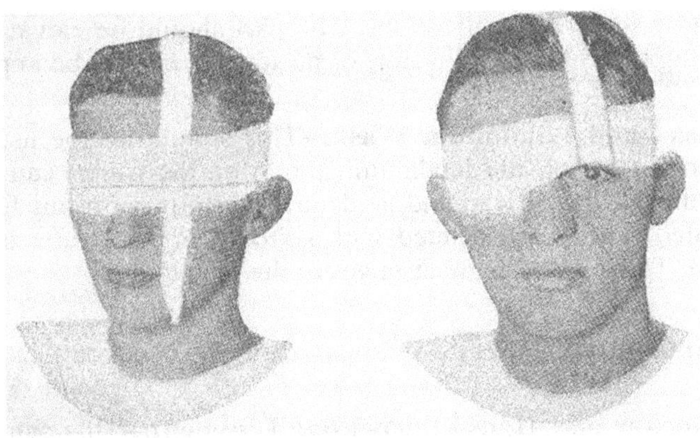

Most efficient way of Bandaging Eyes showing how Bandage may be lifted from one eye.

Usual Spiral Reverse Bandage of the Arm.

PHYSICIANS' TREATMENT for Sprains.--Rest for a time (for some weeks). The parts should be raised to lessen the blood supply. Hot applications, through fomentations, or cold evaporations, lotions, massage later, and support with a pad and a firm bandage, in some cases. When there is not much swelling, a plaster of Paris bandage is sometimes applied at once in order that absolute rest can be secured.

1. Tincture of Arnica.--This is an excellent remedy for sprains When the part is much swollen and looks bluish is when it is especially beneficial. It can be used full strength by saturating cloths and applying either hot or cold, or diluted to half strength.

2. Hot Water.--Applied with soaked cloths on the part is very grateful in some cases. It should be kept hot and plenty of water on the part all the time. This should be applied for hours. Between the soakings, the parts should be dressed with the lead and laudanum wash, and rubbed with ichthyol ointment or camphor and laudanum liniment.

3. Cold Applications.--Cold water.--Some patients are more benefited by the cold applications. The part should be elevated and a cloth wrung out of ice cold water, or an ice bag should be kept on the part.

4. Lead and Laudanum Wash.--This should not be used if the skin is broken. Then the laudanum, three-fourths water, can be used alone. Composition of lead and laudanum wash, proportions four parts of undiluted lead water, diluted with sixteen parts of water to one of laudanum. This can be made stronger in the laudanum.

25

5. Fomentations of hops, or smartweed or wormwood, etc., are also good.

6. Vinegar and Hops--Turpentine Liniment.--This can be used later, for stimulating purposes.

Bandaging and Photographs by DR. W. E. ZIEGENFUSS, of Detroit. Done expressly for this book.

The following is a liniment made by an old gentleman I used to know. I was well acquainted with him while he was living, and I know he was a good, competent man. Following is the recipe:

"Oil of Amber	1 ounce.
Oil of Wormwood	1 ounce.
Oil of Tansy	1 ounce.
Camphor Gum	2 ounces.
Ammonia	2 ounces.
Oil of Spike	1 ounce.
Small piece castile soap.	
Spirits of Wine	1 pint.

Rub in thoroughly. In some cases it should be diluted one-fourth to one-half strength. Full strength for much pain.

BURNS. SCALDS.--

A Burn is caused by dry heat.

A Scald is caused by moist heat.

A superficial burn, upon a young child, that involves the third of the body will almost certainly prove fatal, while a very deep burn, provided it is localized, may not be so serious, unless important nerves and blood vessels have been destroyed.

Burns may be divided into three degrees:

First degree are those burns that only affect the outer or superficial layer of the skin, producing a redness with some small vesicles.

Second degree burns: These extend through the true skin and blisters result.

Third degree burns: This goes down underneath and involves the deeper tissues. Charring and destruction of tissue takes place.

MOTHERS' REMEDIES. 1. Burns, Linseed Oil for.--"Quick application of linseed oil." The oil forms a coating and is very soothing.

2. Burns, Common Soda for.--"There is nothing better than common baking soda for burns and scalds; apply a thick coating of dry soda. Bind a cloth over it, and keep on until the pain ceases, after which any good healing salve will do."

3. "Apply crushed onion poultice; cover to keep out the air. This will soon extract the heat and pain." Onions seem to possess many medicinal properties. They are very soothing, and in a case of scalds keep out the air and relieve the pain.

4. Burns, Molasses Takes Pain from.--"Apply New Orleans molasses to the burn and cover with flour. This forms a coating over the affected parts, keeping the air from it, thereby relieving the burning. This is an excellent remedy and one easily prepared."

5. Burns, Butter a Relief for.--"Spread butter on the affected parts and bandage well. This is one of the remedies our grandmothers used to use and is a good one."

6. Burns, Oil of Peppermint Draws Fire Out of.--"Apply oil of peppermint; it will take the fire out almost immediately."

7. Burns, Sweet Oil and Cotton Batting Relieves.--"Saturate cotton batting in sweet oil and cover the burns and keep covered until the fire is out. I had my hand burned with steam until the skin peeled off, and this remedy relieved the smarting."

8. Burns, Vinegar Prevents Blistering from.--"Vinegar applied every few minutes will keep it from blistering." This is a remedy always at hand, and will do just what it says.

MOTHERS' REMEDIES. 1. Scalds, Elder Berries Soothing for.--"The flowers of the black elder berries and the bark all possess valuable medicinal properties. An ointment made by stirring the fresh flowers into melted lard or vaselin and occasionally stirring it, will be found an excellent remedy for scalds or burns." It is not only soothing, but forms a coating thereby keeping the air out.

2. Scalds, Alum for Slight.--"Put a teaspoonful of alum in a pint of water, and bathe the parts frequently. Keep the parts well wet with this solution which extracts the heat in a remarkable manner and soothes the patient into a calm and refreshing sleep." This remedy is most always at hand and will relieve if the case is not too severe.

3. Scalds, Scraped Potatoes will Relieve.--" A few raw potatoes scraped or grated and beaten in a bowl, then add a dram of laudanum; apply to the affected parts as you would a poultice."

4. Scalds, Crackers and Slippery Elm as Poultice for.--"Apply a poultice of cracker and slippery elm, made of raspberry leaf tea. Guard against taking cold." Use enough of the raspberry tea to make a soft mixture. This is very soothing, and keeps the air from the scald which is one of the essential things in order to get relief.

5. Scalds, Raisins' and Lard with Tobacco Helps.

"One pound Raisins, chopped.

One pound Lard.

Five cent package of Chewing Tobacco.

Mix all together and let this simmer about three hours slowly, strain it and put in a jar."

6. Scalds, Sweet Oil Soothing for.--"I know of nothing better than equal parts of sweet oil and lime water." This is very good and should be applied freely.

PHYSICIANS' TREATMENT for Superficial Bums.--Exclude the air; protect and treat the parts is the theory of treatment.

Superficial Burn.--When the skin is not broken, bicarbonate of soda may be sprinkled thick over the burn, then wrap the part in moist gauze, lint or linen, and over this a layer of common cotton, and hold in place with a bandage. Flour can be used in place of the soda. Oatmeal flour, rice flour, etc., will do also. The objection to all powders is that the moist gauze, etc., will make the flour form cakes and make removal painful and difficult. Applications in liquid form are therefore better.

Liquid Forms.--If the blisters are large, open them with a clean (sterile-boiled) instrument (scissors or knife) and absorb the fluid with a clean gauze. Then dissolve bicarbonate of soda in water--a saturated solution. This term means as much soda as the water will dissolve. Then gauze, lint or linen pads may be wrung out of this solution or the same strength of boric acid solution and applied. Put over this a layer of clean cotton and hold in place by a bandage or strip of adhesive plaster. (Keep parts always moist). Baking soda will do about as well as bicarbonate of soda.

Oil and ointments are also very beneficial. Spread the ointments or oil over the burn thick and cover with lint or soft linen, and change frequently to keep from smelling badly.

1. Carron oil made of equal parts of lime-water and linseed oil is good.

2. Carbolized oil or simple pure sweet oil is good.

3. Cosmoline, Vaselin, Pineoline (salves) are all good; they cover and protect.

4. Cold cream is very good.

5. Thick lather from any good pure soap spread over the part thick and then covered with the cloth dressing. This is very good and is always at hand.

6. Dr. Douglas, of Detroit, very strongly recommends the following simple remedy: One teaspoonful of common salt to one pint of boiled water, used comfortably warm. Old clean muslin or gauze cloths of several thicknesses should be dipped in this solution and spread evenly over the sores in several layers and over this oiled paper or paraffine paper should be applied to prevent evaporation or drying and bind all with a bandage. The covering should not be too thick or it might make the part too warm. This should be avoided in all dressings.

This salt water dressing can be moistened and changed when necessary.

7. Beeswax ointment. (Dr. Douglas).-

"Benzoinated Lard	6 ounces.
Yellow Beeswax	1 ounce.
Salicylic Acid	20 grains."

Mix the wax in a tin cup, then add the lard, when all is melted remove from the fire and stir till cool, then add the salicylic acid and continue stirring until cold. This makes an excellent covering, excludes the air.

8. Ointment of Oxide of Zinc is very good. The following are the ingredients:

"Oxide of Zinc	2 drams.
Lanoline	5 drams.
Alboline	1 dram.
Salicylic Acid	10 grains.

Mix, and make ointment and apply."

The following is not very pleasant to think about, but farmers have frequently used it: Cow manure as a poultice.

Another: The inner bark of elder boiled in cream. Use the salve resulting. This is good for burns and sores.

Another: Slippery elm bark tea boiled down so it will be thick and oily, is very good.

Some claim that immersing the part in milk and keeping it so is a very good remedy. We know that cream is, but it will soon become rancid.

Remedies must be of an oily covering nature to do good, or else do it by their antiseptic qualities like salt, boric acid, etc.

Another:

"Picric Acid	75 grains.
Alcohol	20 ounces.
Distilled Water	2 pints.

Mix and apply."

Cleanse the burns of dirt and charred clothing and then soak strips of clean gauze in this solution and apply to the part. Place over this a pad of dry absorbent cotton which can be fastened by a light bandage or adhesive straps. The dressing dries rapidly, and may be left in place for several days. Then moisten it with the same solution so as to soften the dressing and remove it. Then apply a fresh dressing of the same kind and leave on a week. This dressing soon relieves the pain, prevents the formation of matter (pus), hastens healing and, leaves a smooth surface. The dressing stains the hands so it is best applied with rubber gloves. This is good for all degree burns.

For Severe Case.--There may be and is shock and great weakness after some burns. The patient should be put to bed and given strong black coffee, or if you have it one teaspoonful of aromatic spirits of ammonia in a glass of water. Hot water bags and jars should be applied to the feet and one teaspoonful of paregoric may be given to an adult for the pain. Give the patient ice to hold in his mouth, as he is very thirsty. Cold water and milk to drink also. If the burn is severe put oil cloth or rubber on the bed to protect the bed from the wet dressing. Do not put a night-shirt or pajamas on him, as it pains to remove and renew the dressings, if such are used as need frequent removal and renewal. Cover warmly, but keep covers lifted so that their weight will not give unnecessary pain. The bowels can be kept open with soapsuds enemas. Watch carefully, especially a man, if urine is passed and enough in quantity. It must be drawn if it is not passed within twelve hours.

For Third Degree Burns.--In this kind there is a great shock. Stimulate the patient with whisky, etc. Put one ounce in a glass one-half full of water, and give two teaspoonfuls frequently, dependent upon how much stimulant the patient has ever used; or an enema of one ounce of hot coffee can be given.

The first dressings may be the same, but when the patient is stronger others should be used.

Warm Baths are now used when the deep tissues are burned, and the sloughs and charred material are removed.

When convenient, begin with a warm tub bath, with boric acid added to the water--handful to the tub. This is good for stimulating purposes, and also to relieve pain and for cleansing the surfaces before the applications of the dressings, these can be of those recommended.

When the air passages have been scalded by hot steam or hot liquids, the steam of lime-water, not too hot, may soothe.

Burns from Acid.--Soda, chalk, whiting, sprinkled over the surface of the skin and covered with moist coverings of gauze. Egg albumen is also good applied, on the part.

Bums from Alkali (like potash or strong ammonia).--Vinegar poured over the part, or dress with a mild solution of boric acid. One teaspoonful to four ounces of water.

MOTHERS' REMEDIES. 1. Bruises, Cold Water Prevents Coloring.--"Bathe the parts in cold water, prevents turning black and blue."

2. Bruises, Kerosene Relieves the Pain of.--"Bathe freely with kerosene."

3. Bruises, Turpentine to Keep Proud Flesh from.--"Rub the injured part with turpentine and keep warm, and you will find this remedy to be one of the best to keep proud flesh out and gangrene that has ever been used. I always have turpentine in my home, and find that I have use for it often. If once used you will never be without it."

4. Bruises, Bread and Vinegar Quick Remedy for.--"Apply a poultice made of hot vinegar and bread. A girl bruised her fingers with some iron rings in a gymnasium. She applied this poultice at night, and they were well in the morning. Since then I always use it for a bruise."

5. Bruises, Good Liniment for.--"Where inflammation is under the thin covering of the bone, dissolve chloral and camphor gum together. They dissolve each other by putting together, and looks like glycerin. Apply very little with tip of finger, put absorbent cotton on and bind up with pure gum rubber band to keep it from evaporating as it is very volatile. Rubber band must not be too tight, as it will cut off the circulation."

6. Bruises, Liniment Used in Ohio for.--"Five cents' worth spirits ammonia, five cents' worth spirits turpentine, whites of two eggs beaten, one cup cider vinegar, two cups rain water." This gentleman from Ohio says he has used the liniment for many years, and his neighbors have used it with the utmost success. He recommends it as the best he ever used.

PHYSICIANS' TREATMENT. Bruises.--1. Tincture of Arnica applied from one-half to full strength is very good.

2. Alcohol about two-thirds strength is also very good, gently rubbed in the parts.

3. Cold or hot water applied with cloths.

4. Raw beefsteak (lean) is excellent. Place it on the bruise.

5. Lead and laudanum wash if the skin is not broken.

Of course bruises usually disappear in time. The above remedies will help.

Heat applied at some distance from the parts relaxes the surrounding vessels and promotes absorption of the blood in the bruise.

CUTS. WOUNDS.--They are named cut (incised); contused, such as made by a blunt instrument.

Lacerated or torn, when the tissues are torn or ragged.

Punctured, stab-wounds, when made by a pointed instrument.

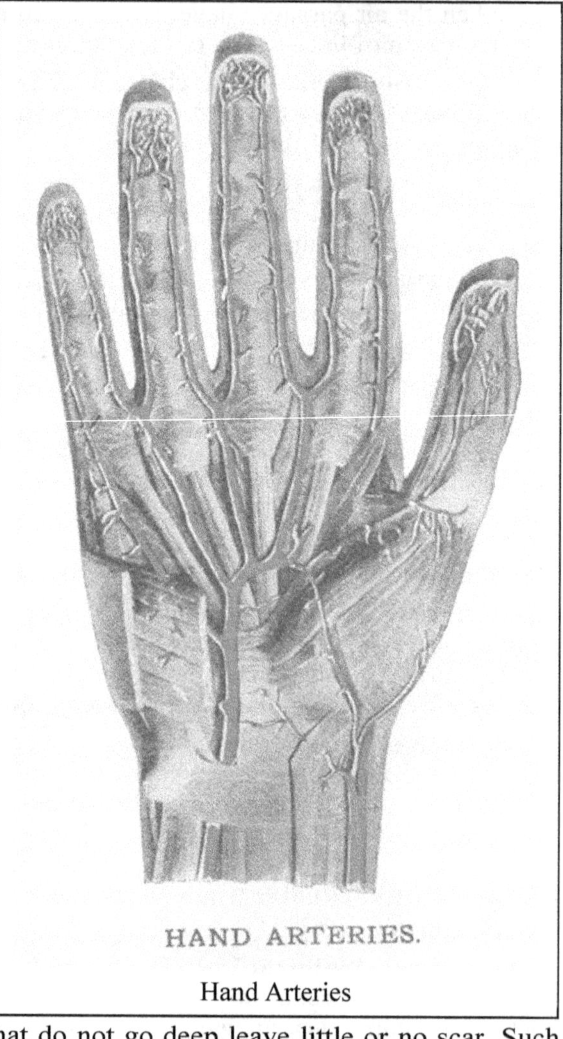

Hand Arteries

Treatment.--There may be pain, gaping (opening) of the edges and bleeding. In order to gape, the cut must pass through the deep skin. Cuts or wounds that do not go deep leave little or no scar. Such require only a little antiseptic dressing like this remedy:

"Boric Acid	1/2 ounce.
Boiled Water	1 pint."

Wash the cut thoroughly and cover with gauze or clean linen. Cuts or wounds should always be washed first with boiled water, cooled enough to use. Do this with absolutely clean muslin, absorbent cotton or gauze and boiled water. After being thoroughly cleansed and washed with hot water and cloths, a thick pad of muslin, absorbent cotton or gauze thoroughly soaked with the boric acid solution, (strength one-half ounce of boric acid to a pint of boiled water) should be applied on the wound, and for an inch or two around it. Over this lay a thick layer of absorbent cotton or muslin, bandage all securely with a bandage or adhesive strap, so the dressing cannot slip.

Gaping Wounds generally need stitches. These should be put in deep enough to draw the deep edges together. If that is not done, a pocket will be left where the parts are not together and "matter" may form there. Plaster will not draw the deeper parts of wounds together. They should then be covered the same way as superficial wounds; of course the wound should be thoroughly cleansed in the same way before the stitches are put in. Such wounds unless they are large, need not be dressed for a day or two, unless there is soreness or pain. If the wound is sore and throbs it should be redressed immediately. Some discharge will no doubt he found penned in, and needs a drain through which to escape. This does not usually happen, and if it does, the wound was infected (poisoned) and then needs dressing once or twice a day, and full vent given to any discharge that may be present. The dressing immediately over the wound should then be thick and soft so as to absorb the discharge that may be present. The stitches are usually removed in small wounds the third or fourth day. This is easily done, with a sharp pointed scissors or knife; put one point underneath the stitch next to the knot, cut it off and with the forceps take hold of the knot and pull it out gently. It comes away easily as a rule.

Torn Wounds should be trimmed. That is, cut away the torn pieces and then stitch together as for other wounds. Of course all the tissue possible should be saved and only ragged flesh should be cut away. This would die anyway, and prove a foreign body, and would be very apt to cause pus. These wounds should be dressed the same way as previously directed.

Sometimes bleeding may cause trouble. Usually, hot water constantly applied will stop it. Pressing above the part will often stop bleeding. If an artery is cut it will spurt red blood. The artery should be tied and pressure made upon the limb above the cut toward the body; or tying the limb tight. If a finger or toe is cut and bleeds much, press on each side. The arteries are there. Put the limb high and the head low. Bandaging a limb tight, beginning at the end, often stops bleeding. Stimulants' are sometimes necessary for a time.

Punctured Wounds.--From a sharp pointed instrument, nail, etc. The first thing to do is to cleanse the wound thoroughly with hot water and about one-half ounce of salt to a pint of water. Keep this up constantly for one-half hour. Then if it is from a nail, put on a bread and milk poultice hot, and keep changing it every ten minutes to keep it good and hot. Keep this going for at least an hour. Salt pork can then be put on and kept on; or a cloth dipped in hot salt water can be applied, and kept on for a few hours when it can be dressed as other wounds are. There should be no throbbing pain the next day. A wound of this kind should be dressed every day, with great care in the matter of cleanliness. It is lack of cleanliness that usually causes trouble, either the poison that gets into the wound at the time of injury or that is allowed to get in and infect the wound afterwards. Clean hands, tools, basins, dressings and boiled water are essential to a quick healing.

Rusty Nail Wound, Simple Guard Against Serious Results from.--"Every little while we read of someone who has run a rusty nail in his foot or some other part of his person, and lockjaw has resulted therefrom. All such wounds can be healed without any fatal consequences following them. It is only necessary to smoke such wounds or any wound or bruise that is inflamed, with burning wood or woolen cloth. Twenty minutes in the smoke will take the pain out of the worst case of inflammation arising from any wound I ever saw." Put on a poultice of bread and milk, changing every five or ten minutes. After this bind on salt pork and keep on for several days.

MOTHERS' REMEDIES. 1. Cuts, Iodoform and Vaselin Salve for Barb Wire.--

"Iodoform	1 teaspoonful.
Vaselin	1 ounce."

Before applying the above salve it is very necessary to cleanse the affected parts with a solution made of one teaspoonful of salt to a pint of water. If the iodoform is offensive to some people, you may use the vaselin alone, although the iodoform is known to be one of the best healing remedies that can be obtained.

2. Cuts, Turpentine Good in Small Quantities for.--"For cuts and any open wound pour turpentine in and put a piece of absorbent cotton on and soak well with the liniment, tie up, and leave it so until dry, then pour on some more." Care should be taken in using turpentine, not to put too much on the wound, as it may cause proud flesh in some people; a little of it is very healing and effective.

3. Cuts, Tincture of Myrrh for Fresh.--"Use freely of the tincture of myrrh by saturating a cloth and applying to the parts affected." This tincture of myrrh may be purchased at, any drug store, and is a very effectual remedy for fresh wounds of any description. It is slightly contracting, and has great healing qualities.

MOTHERS' REMEDIES. 1. Bleeding, Unusual Way to Stop.--"If fresh, sprinkle full of black pepper. It will not smart, and is soon healed. If not fresh, clean with a weak solution saleratus and cover while wet with pepper. This has been tried many times in our home and has never failed."

2. Bleeding, Cobwebs to Stop.--"Make a pad of cobwebs and apply to cut. I have never found anything to equal this remedy." This simple remedy has been known to save many lives, and can always be obtained. As most housekeepers know; cobwebs are easily found in every home, and perhaps after reading this remedy they will not seem such a pest as heretofore, if we stop to think that at some future date our baby's life might be saved by using them.

3. Bleeding, Powdered Alum and Hot Water Stops.--"A heaping teaspoonful of powdered alum, placed in a teacup of water will stop the flow of blood in ordinary wounds, where no large artery has been cut. This will be found very beneficial for children, when their finger has been cut and bleeding badly." Alum is something that should always be kept in the home, using it in a case of emergency when there is no time to run to the drug store.

4. Bleeding, Salt and Flour Successful Remedy for.--"Equal parts of fine salt and flour placed on cut. I have seen this tried and it proved successful." The salt will stop the bleeding by its astringent action and mixed with flour forms a coating over the cut.

5. Bleeding, Boracic Acid Excellent for.--"Bind up in boracic acid powder." The boracic acid is very healing and a good antiseptic, which is one of the important things to be attended to in a bad cut or wound.

6.--Bleeding, Tobacco Will Stop.--"Bind in tobacco." Very few people know that the nicotine in tobacco is very healing, and by applying it to a cut, not only stops the flow of blood, but heals.

THINGS IN THE EAR; Buttons, Beads, etc.--The bent hairpin is good to use for removing these objects, unless it is too far in. Sometimes the object can be washed out with a stream of water. This will kill and destroy insects. A small stream from a pitcher will do, if there is no fountain syringe handy. Water should not be used for corn, peas or beans, for if they are not removed the water will cause them to swell up and enlarge. A competent person should then be called, but no injury will be done for a few hours.

GAS from wells, cisterns, mines, illuminating gas and coal gas.

Treatment.--Fresh pure air. Open all windows in the house and remove patient from a house filled with coal gas. Artificial respiration: Inject salt enemas; teaspoonful of salt to one pint of warm water.

FITS. (Convulsions).--Loosen all clothing. Put something hard between the teeth to keep the patient from biting his tongue. Allow plenty of sleep afterward.

IN-GROWING TOE-NAILS. Causes.--Pressure from improperly fitting shoes, or a wrong way of cutting the nails. The flesh along the nails becomes inflamed. Toe-nails should be cut straight across, and not trimmed too closely at the corners.

Treatment.--Wear broad-toed shoes with low heels. The high heels push the toes against the shoe and besides are unhealthy and dangerous in walking.

Hot poultices will relieve the inflammation and pain. Soak the toe in hot water and push the flesh back from the nail. Cotton under the edge and corner of the nail helps to keep it away. Dust a boric acid powder, mixed with an equal quantity of starch flour, on the parts. Mennen's borated talcum powder is good.

MOTHER'S REMEDY. 1. In-growing Toe-Nail, Popular Remedy for.--"Shave a little common laundry soap and mix with a little cream and pulverized sugar, work to the consistency of salve and apply to the affected part night and morning. It will take off the proud flesh in about ten days and then heal. This is a good salve for bed-sores or cuts, that, have dirt in them, and will also draw out a splinter. To prevent in-growing toe-nails, scrape the center of the nail very thin and cut a V in the top. This will allow the nail to bend and the corners will have a chance to grow up and out. Avoid short shoes and stockings." Anyone suffering from this dreaded thing will be willing to try anything that will give relief. The above treatment is always at hand, and has been known to cure in severe cases.

FALLS.--If one has had a severe fall and is wholly or partially conscious, move as little as possible, in case of broken bones. Remain in a comfortable position until proper aid can be given. If unconscious stimulation may be necessary.

FIRE in Clothing.--Keep quiet, and away from a draught. Wrap anything handy around him and roll him. Leave only the head and face uncovered. Keep mouth closed.

CHOKING. (Foreign bodies in the larynx).--Produce vomiting. Give an emetic, warm water, melted lard, vaselin or one teaspoonful of mustard in one-half glass of warm water and drink. Tickle the throat with your finger or a feather. For a child, sometimes by taking hold of the feet with the head down and give a few slight jerks frequently expels the foreign body. Slap patient's back. The last resort is an operation,--tracheotomy.

MOTHERS' REMEDIES. 1. Choking, Fish Bone to Stop.--"A fish bone stuck in the throat can often be dislodged by swallowing a raw egg or raw oyster."

2. Choking, Simple Remedy to Stop.--"Hold both hands high above the head. If necessary tap gently between the shoulders."

3. Choking, Pennyroyal Tea and Lard Relieves.--"Pennyroyal tea and hog's lard; drink hot." The pennyroyal may be purchased at any drug store for ten cents. Make a tea of this, then add the hog's lard. As we all know, that this will produce vomiting and relax the tissues so that any foreign matter will come out.

4. Choking, Grease and Meat Common Remedy for.--"Warm lard, or any kind of grease, and give the patient. Have seen it used with success." The warm grease will usually cause vomiting, and in that way remove the foreign matter.

In the Gullet.--An emetic is good to give if the body cannot be reached with the hand. Doctors use forceps or another instrument called a probang. Pennies will go down into the stomach and pass out through the bowels and usually cause no trouble. Fish bones can generally be reached with the finger or crochet hook. This is also good for foreign bodies in the nose, such as beans.

THINGS IN THE NOSE. Corn, Peas, Beans, Buttons, etc.--Children frequently get such things in their nose and also ears. They should be removed soon and then there will be no harm done. They have been known to remain for years, and they have been the cause of catarrh. A small curved hair-pin makes a good instrument to use and is always handy. Also a crochet hook, though not so good, for it will not bend as well as the hair-pin. The mother should sit facing a window or open door. The child should be placed on its back with its head resting between the mother's limbs and an assistant holds the child's hands. Its legs will be hanging down. The light now shines into the nostril and the bent hair-pin can be slipped over the foreign body and easily hooked out. The head must be held quiet by the mother. The mother can do this herself, with one hand holding the head quiet and with the other can introduce the hair-pin and remove the object. But the position of the child must be reversed with the head between her knees and the light shining in the nose; or place the child on a bench or cradle or buggy, head on a pillow, and to the light. Hold the head and legs quiet; by kneeling by the child's side, you can easily see the object and remove it. If they are too far back, they can be pushed over into the throat, but parents should never attempt to remove an object in the nose they cannot see. Sometimes causing sneezing with a feather or pepper will expel the object.

TREATMENT OF THE DROWNED, SUFFOCATED OR ELECTRICALLY SHOCKED. Accidents, etc.--The one action of first importance in the treatment of the drowned, the suffocated or the electrically shocked is to restore breathing. This must be done by expelling from the lungs the poison or water which has caused the trouble, and by establishing artificial respiration. Avoid delay. One moment may lose or save a life.

Schaefer Method of Effecting Artificial Respiration In Case of Drowning.--After an investigation and comparison of the different methods of artificial respiration, Schaefer suggests one which is by far the simplest and easiest and at the same time one of the most effective and least injurious to the patient. In describing it he says: "It consists in laying the subject in the prone posture, preferably on the ground, with a thick folded garment underneath the chest and epigastrium, (region above the stomach). The operator puts himself athwart or at the side of the subject, facing his head (see plate) and places his hands on each side over the lower part of the back (lowest ribs). He then slowly throws the weight of his body forward to bear upon his own arms and this presses upon the thorax of the subject and forces air out of the lungs. This being effected, he gradually relaxes the pressure by bringing his own body up again to a more erect position, but without moving his hands." These movements should be repeated regularly at a rate of twelve to fifteen times per minute, until normal respiration begins or until hope of its restoration is abandoned. Some claim there is no hope of restoring respiration after half an hour of artificial respiration. Others claim there is a chance of saving the patient even then, and say that artificial respiration should be kept up for two or three hours.

TO RESUSCITATE THE DROWNED.--First: Lose no time in recovering the body from the water. Always try to restore life; for while ten minutes under the water is usually the limit, still persons have been resuscitated after being under water for thirty or forty minutes. Do not lose time by taking the body to a place of shelter--*operate immediately.*

Second: Quickly lay the person prone, face downward with stomach resting on a barrel or roll of clothing, so the head will be lower than rest of the body and the water will run out from the throat and lungs. Wipe dry mouth and nostrils. Wrap the corner of a handkerchief about the forefinger and clear the mouth of all mucus and

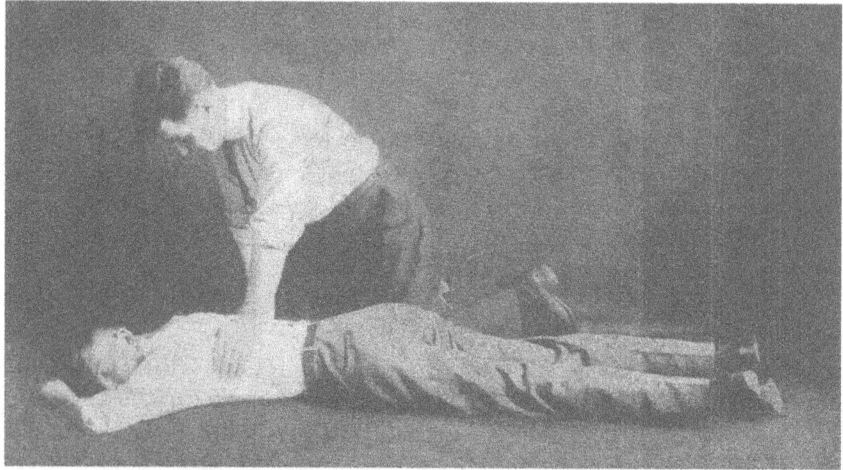

The Schaefer Position to be Adopted for Effecting

Artificial Respiration in Case of Drowning.slimy substance back as far as the top of the throat. Rip open the clothing on chest and back and keep the face exposed to the air. Separate the jaws and keep them apart with a cork, stone, or knot in a handkerchief.

Third: Remove the roll of clothing from underneath the stomach of the patient. Kneel by the side of or across the patient. Place your hands over the lowest ribs. Lean forward and put your weight straight over the lowest ribs. Exert this pressure for three seconds. To count three seconds, say: "One thousand and one, one thousand and two; one thousand and three,"

Fourth: Do not remove the hands from the ribs; but release the pressure from the ribs for two seconds, by squatting backward. To count two seconds, say: "One thousand and one, one thousand and two,"

Fifth: Again exert pressure straight over the lowest ribs for three seconds. Alternate thus (three seconds pressure and two seconds release), about twelve times a minute, until breathing is restored. This method of resuscitation at once expels water and produces the identical results of normal breathing.

Sixth: If another person is at hand to assist, let him do everything possible to keep the body warm, by sheltering it from the wind, rubbing hands and soles of feet, making hot applications. Warm the head nearly as fast as the other parts of the body to avoid congestion. Camphor or ammonia may be applied to nostrils to excite breathing.

Seventh: Do not give up too soon. Any time within two hours you may be on the point of reviving the patient without there being any sign of it. Send for a physician as soon as possible after the accident. Prevent friends from crowding around the patient and excluding fresh air.

AFTER-TREATMENT.--After breathing is restored, remove the patient to a warm bed where there is free circulation of fresh air. Administer in small doses stimulants (hot coffee, ginger tea, hot sling) being careful not to let the patient choke or strangle. There is danger that the patient may suffer congestion of the lungs and have great difficulty in breathing. When this occurs, a large mustard plaster should be placed over the lungs.

HOW TO KEEP FROM DROWNING.--To keep from drowning it is advisable, but not necessary, to know how to swim. The human body in the water weighs little more than a pound; so that one finger placed upon a piece of board, an oar or a paddle, will easily keep the head above water, and the feet and the other hand can be used to propel the body toward the shore. It is all important for the person in the water to breathe and keep a cool head, and the mouth closed.

HOW TO FIND DROWNED PERSONS.--Make a board raft, ten or twelve feet square. Cut a round hole in the center, eight or ten inches in diameter. Lie down on the raft with the face over the hole, covering the head with a coat or shawl, to exclude the light. By this contrivance the rays of the light are concentrated directly under the raft, and objects of any size can be seen a considerable distance below the surface. Tow the raft over the place where the drowned person is supposed to be. If the body has just gone under and no raft can be provided at once, dive or drag the bottom with line and hooks. The important object is to rescue the body at the earliest possible moment. If the body is not rescued, it will rise to the surface within a week or ten days.

Three hundred lives are lost in Michigan every year from drowning. If by studying and learning how to carry out the directions in this article, you can be a life saver at some critical moment, the few moments spent in careful reading will be well repaid. Master the directions so that you will be able to do everything possible in case of accident.

ELECTRIC SHOCK, ETC.--In suffocation by smoke or any poisonous gas, as also by hanging if the neck is not broken, and in suspended breathing from effects of chloroform, hydrate of chloral, or electric shock, remove all obstructions to breathing, instantly loosen or cut apart all neck and waist bands, taking special pains to keep the head very low, and placing the body face downward, to prevent closure of the windpipe by the tongue falling back. Then proceed to induce artificial respiration the same as in drowning, described above.

BATHING IN SEWAGE POLLUTED WATERS IS DANGEROUS.--Cases have been reported where typhoid fever has been contracted by bathing in streams below cities and villages. Probably this occurred through accidentally or carelessly taking the infected water into the mouth. No person should bathe in an ordinary stream just below any city or village, or other source of sewage or privy drainage, or in any harbor or lake near the entrance into it of a sewer or the drainage of a privy.

POISONS

An antidote is something given that counteracts poison, such as soda, chalk, magnesia, soap, whiting, milk mixed with magnesia, soda diluted, etc., followed by whites of eggs and bland drinks such as flaxseed tea, slippery elm tea, quince seed tea, and sweet or castor oil given after regular antidote.

For Shock, inject hot black coffee into the rectum.

Emetic is some medicine given to produce vomiting. The simplest emetic is mustard and warm water. If one does not know what poison has been taken, the best thing to do is to give an emetic first.

Mustard.--One-half ounce or four teaspoonfuls for an adult, one to two teaspoonfuls for a child, of mustard to a cup of warm water may be given and repeated every ten or fifteen minutes until free vomiting is produced.

Salt and warm water may be used in the same way. Tickling the throat with a finger or a feather produces vomiting.

Goose grease, lard, lard drippings, vaselin, all in large amounts.

Other medicines: Sulphate of zinc, ten to twenty grains at a dose, in a cup of warm water; or fluid extract of ipecac fifteen to thirty drops, or syrup of ipecac one teaspoonful.

Poisons may be divided into corrosive and irritant.

Corrosive poison: This is a poison that is likely to eat or burn through organic tissue immediately.

Irritant poison acts more slowly and produces inflammation which later may result in suppuration and perforation.

An emetic or stomach pump cannot be used in some poisons, such as suphuric acid, because the tissues are quickly injured by the acid and the emetic and pump would only injure farther.

ACONITE. Symptoms.--Sudden collapse; slow, feeble, irregular pulse, and breathing; tickling in the mouth and the extremities, giddiness, great muscular weakness; pupils generally dilated, may be contracted; mind is clear.

Antidotes: Solution of tannic acid, twenty drops to a glass of water, to wash out the stomach.

Treatment.--Stimulants, whisky or brandy; digitalis, artificial respiration, warmth and friction of the body. Lie in recumbent position.

ALCOHOL. Symptoms.--Stupid, confused, giddy, staggers, drowsy, but can be aroused; full pulse, deep snoring, respiration, injected eyes, dilated pupils, low temperature.

Emetics.--Strong hot coffee, inhale amyl nitrite; hot and cold douches.

AMMONIA. Symptoms.--Intense inflammation of the stomach and bowels, often with bloody vomiting and purging; lips and tongue swollen; violent difficulty in breathing; characteristic odor.

Antidotes.--Lemon juice and water, vinegar and water half and half.

Treatment.--Milk, soothing drinks; sweet oil or castor oil, bland drinks like flaxseed tea, slippery elm, albumen (white of egg) water. The oil should be used last.

ANTIMONY. Symptoms.--Metallic taste, violent vomiting, becoming bloody, feeble pulse; pain and burning in the stomach. Violent watery purging, becoming bloody; cramps in the extremities, thirst, great weakness; sometimes prostration, collapse, unconsciousness.

Antidotes.--Tannic acid, twenty drops to a glass of water.

Treatment.--Soothing drinks, milk, white of egg and water, flaxseed tea, etc.; external heat.

ARSENIC, Symptoms.--Violent burning in the stomach, nausea and vomiting, retching, thirst, purging of blood and mucus, suppressed urine, cramps in the legs, intense thirst, collapse.

Antidotes.--Jeaunel's antidote.

Treatment.--Emetics freely, mustard water, salt and warm water, goose grease, etc. White of egg and milk, and then sweet oil or castor oil.

ARSENICAL POISONING, Chronic Cases, Causes.--Inhaling arsenic from dyes, in wall-paper, carpet, etc, Taking it in by the mouth in handling dyed paper, artificial flowers, etc., and in many fabrics employed as clothing. The glazed green and red papers used in the kindergartens also contain arsenic. The drug given in repeated and excessive doses causes poisoning sometimes.

Symptoms.--Dry throat, watery swelling of the eyelids, sometimes coryza, nausea, burning vomiting, and burning watery diarrhea; skin eruptions, falling off of the hair, paralysis of the arms and legs, with wasting and numbness, but little pain, The legs are most affected, causing steppage gait.

Treatment.--Remove the cause in these chronic cases and treat the symptoms. It may be best for a physician to prescribe treatment.

ATROPINE. Symptoms.--Flushed face, red eyes, throbbing head, pulse fast, dizzy, staggering, hot and dry throat, dilated pupils, scarlet rash on the skin. Patient may be delirious and wildly so.

Antidotes.--Tannic acid, twenty drops in glass of water. Emetics to produce vomiting, such as mustard water, salt and warm water, goose grease, vaselin, etc.

Stimulants.--Coffee to drink or by enema, artificial respiration.

BELLADONNA, Symptoms.--Flushed face, red eyes, throbbing head, pulse fast, dizzy, staggering, hot and dry throat, dilated pupils, scarlet rash on the skin. Patient may be delirious and wildly so.

Antidotes.--Tannic acid, twenty drops in glass of water,

Treatment.--Emetics to produce vomiting, such as mustard water, warm salt water, goose grease, vaselin, etc.

Stimulants.--Coffee to drink or by enema, artificial respiration,

BLUE STONE. Symptoms.--Vomiting and purging, taste of metal, severe pains, dizziness and headache and sometimes insensibility.

Treatment.--Emetics such as mustard water, warm salt water, goose grease, vaselin, etc. Then white of eggs, followed by milk and soothing drinks, flaxseed tea, etc.

BLUE VITRIOL. Symptoms.--Vomiting and purging, taste of metal, severe pains, dizziness and headache and sometimes insensibility.

Antidote.--Jeaunel's antidote.

Treatment.--Emetics such as mustard water, warm salt water, goose grease, vaselin, etc., then white of eggs, followed by milk and soothing drinks, flaxseed tea, etc.

CARBOLIC ACID. Symptoms.--Immediately burning pain from mouth to stomach; giddiness, loss of consciousness, collapse, partial suppression of the urine; characteristic odor and white color of lips, etc.

Antidotes. Epsom salts or glaubers salts, and water very freely to drink; drink a pint of flaxseed tea. Later strong coffee or whisky and water as stimulants.

External.--If burned externally by carbolic acid, apply immediately some oil-sweet oil, olive oil or any good oil at hand-or wash freely with baking soda water. Should the acid get into the eye continue application of oil or soda water and send for a physician. Hold lower lid down to prevent acid getting into pupil until you are sure all the acid is off of the lids.

CHLORAL. Symptoms.--Deep sleep, livid look, pulse weak, breathing slow, pupils contracted during sleep, but dilated when awake, temperature low.

Antidotes.--Permanganate of potash, four to five grains every half hour.

Treatment.--Emetics at first, if seen early, such as mustard water, and warm salt water, vaselin, goose grease, etc. Keep person awake by walking, slapping and cold applications; give strong coffee enemas.

COPPER. Symptoms.--Intense corrosion of the mouth and stomach, bleeding and cramps in the bowels.

Treatment. Emetics.--Mustard water, warm salt water, lard, vaselin, etc. Then milk and eggs, black coffee enema.

CORROSIVE SUBLIMATE. Symptoms.--Burning heat in stomach and bowels, vomiting, diarrhea, with bloody stools, tongue white, shriveled: suppressed urine, gums sore, salivation.

Antidote.--Milk or white of eggs; one egg for four grains of drug; milk, flour paste.

Treatment.--Cause vomiting after the antidote has been given, and follow with soothing drinks, castor oil.

CHEESE, Spoiled. Symptoms.--Vomiting, cramps, diarrhea, weakness, cold hands and feet.

Treatment.--Emetics, such as warm water and salt until patient vomits freely; or mustard water, lard, vaselin, tickle throat with feather, etc. Enema to empty lower bowel; stimulants, such as strong coffee or whisky.

DEADLY NIGHT-SHADE. Symptoms.--Flushed face, red eyes, throbbing head, pulse fast, dizzy, staggering, hot and dry throat, dilated pupils, scarlet rash on the skin. Patient may be delirious and wildly so.

Antidotes.--Tannic acid, twenty drops in glass of water. Emetics to produce vomiting, such as mustard water, salt and warm water, goose grease, vaselin, etc.

Stimulants.--Coffee to drink or by enema, artificial respiration.

FOWLER'S SOLUTION. Symptoms.--Violent burning in the stomach, nausea and vomiting, retching, thirst, purging of blood and mucus, suppressed urine, cramps in the legs, intense thirst, collapse.

Antidote.--Jeaunel's antidote.

Treatment.--Emetics freely, mustard water, salt and warm water, goose grease, etc., then white of egg and milk and follow with sweet oil or castor oil.

HYDROCHLORIC ACID, Symptoms.--The stomach and bowels are irritated and inflamed, the mouth may burn and bleed; swallowing is difficult; "coffee grounds" vomiting.; pulse feeble, clammy skin.

Treatment.--Usually the first thing to do is to give an emetic. Send for a doctor and give an emetic. Then give chalk or, if necessary, take plaster from the wall, mix it with a glass of water. Also three or four eggs (raw) in a glass of milk can be taken.

HELLEBORE, WHITE AND GREEN. Symptoms.--Pain and burning in the bowels, vomiting and diarrhea, slow weak pulse, pupils dilated usually.

Treatment.--Emetics, such as mustard water, warm salt water, goose grease, vaselin, etc.; stimulants, strong coffee, brandy, whisky. Keep patient quiet and warm.

IODINE. Symptoms.--Pain in throat and stomach, vomiting is yellow from the iodine, or blue if starch is in the stomach; color and odor of iodine on lips and in mouth.

Antidote.--Starch or flour mixed into a paste with water, should be given and followed by emetics.

Treatment.--Emetics, something to cause vomiting, warm salt water, mustard water, etc. Then sweating drinks, such as hot flaxseed or hop tea, etc.

LYE. Symptoms.--Intense inflammation of the stomach and bowels, often with bloody vomiting and purging; lips and tongue swollen; violent difficulty in breathing; characteristic odor.

Antidotes.--Lemon juice and water; vinegar and water, half and half.

Treatment.--Milk, soothing drinks; sweet oil or castor oil, bland drinks like flaxseed tea, slippery elm, albumen (white of egg) water. The oil should be used last.

LAUDANUM. Symptoms.--Excitement at first, soon weariness weighty limbs, sleepiness, pin-point pupils, pulse and breathing slow and strong, patient roused with difficulty and later it is impossible, snoring breathing.

Treatment.--This is a dangerous poison. A stomach pump should be used. Emetics, such as mustard and warm water or warm salt water or vaselin, etc. Keep patient awake, stimulants, coffee enemas, artificial respiration, etc.

MERCURIC CHLORIDE. Symptoms.--Burning heat in stomach and bowels, vomiting, diarrhea, with bloody stools, tongue white, shriveled, suppressed urine, gums sore, salivation.

Antidote.--Milk or white of eggs; one egg for four grains of drug, flour paste.

Treatment.--Cause vomiting after the antidote has been given, then give soothing drinks and dose of castor oil.

MORPHINE. Symptoms.--Excitement at first, soon weariness, weighty limbs, sleepiness, pin-point pupils, pulse and breathing slow and strong; patient roused with difficulty and later it is impossible; snoring breathing.

Treatment.--This is a dangerous poison. A stomach pump should be used. Emetics, such as mustard and warm water or warm salt water, or vaselin, etc. Keep patient awake; stimulants, coffee enemas, artificial respiration, etc.

NUX VOMICA. Symptoms.--Appear quickly. Terrible convulsions, in paroxysms, devilish grin, the body is curved backward, jaw set.

Treatment.--Cause vomiting with warm salt water, warm mustard water, lard, vaselin, etc.; sixty grains of bromide of potash and thirty grains of chloral hydrate by the rectum. Dark quiet room.

NITRIC ACID. Symptoms.--The stomach and bowels are irritated and inflamed, the mouth may burn and bleed; swallowing is difficult. "Coffee grounds" vomiting. Pulse feeble, clammy skin.

OXALIC ACID. Symptoms.--Hot acrid taste; burning, vomiting, collapse, numb and stupid.

Antidotes.--Lime or chalk.

Treatment.--Medicines, soothing drinks, flaxseed tea, etc.

OPIUM. Symptoms.--Excitement at first, soon weariness, weighty limbs, sleepiness, pin-point pupils, pulse and breathing slow and strong, patient roused with difficulty and later it is impossible, snoring breathing.

Treatment.--This is a dangerous poison. A stomach pump should be used. Emetics, such as mustard water, or warm salt water or vaselin, etc. Keep patient awake, stimulants, coffee enemas, artificial respiration, etc.

PARIS GREEN. Symptoms.--Violent burning in the stomach, nausea, and vomiting, retching, thirst, purging of blood and mucus, suppressed urine, cramps in the legs, intense thirst, collapse.

Antidotes.--Jeaunel's antidote.

Treatment.--Emetics freely, mustard water, warm salt water, goose grease, etc. White of egg and milk first, and then sweet oil or castor oil.

PAREGORIC. Symptoms.--Excitement at first, soon weariness, weighty limbs, sleepiness, pin-point pupils, pulse and breathing slow and strong, patient roused with difficulty and later it is impossible, snoring breathing.

Treatment.--This is a dangerous poison. A stomach pump should be used. Emetics such as mustard and warm water or warm salt water, or vaselin, etc. Keep patient awake, stimulants, coffee enemas, artificial respiration, etc.

PHOSPHORUS MATCHES. Symptoms.--Vomiting and pain, the vomit may be luminous in the dark, characteristic odor, after several days deep jaundice, blood in vomited matter and bloody stools, pulse is rapid and weak.

Treatment.--Emetics to cause vomiting such as warm salt water, warm mustard water, etc., followed by epsom salts in large doses; five to ten drops of turpentine.

POTASH, CAUSTIC. Symptoms.--Intense inflammation of the stomach and bowels, often with bloody vomiting and purging; lips and tongue swollen; violent difficulty in breathing; characteristic odor.

Antidotes.--Lemon juice and water, vinegar and water half and half.

Treatment.--Milk, soothing drinks; sweet oil or castor oil, bland drinks like flaxseed tea, slippery elm, albumen water, white of egg water. The oil should be used last.

POISONOUS PLANTS. Symptoms.--Vomiting, terrible weakness.

Treatment.--Emetics such as warm mustard water, warm salt water, goose grease, vaselin, lard, etc.; strong coffee, brandy; heat to extremities, artificial respiration.

ROUGH ON RATS. Symptoms.--Violent burning in stomach, nausea, and vomiting, retching, thirst, purging of blood and mucus, Suppressed urine, cramps in legs, intense thirst, collapse.

Antidote.--Jeannel's antidote.

Treatment.--Emetics freely such as warm mustard water, warm salt water, goose grease, etc. White of egg and milk first, and then sweet oil or castor oil.

SALTPETRE. Symptoms.--Intense inflammation of the stomach and bowels, often with bloody vomiting and purging; lips and tongue swollen; violent difficulty in breathing; characteristic odor.

Antidotes.--Lemon juice and water, vinegar and water half and half.

Treatment.--Milk, soothing drinks; sweet oil or castor oil, bland drinks like flaxseed tea, slippery elm, albumen (white of egg) water. The oil should be used last.

SANTONIN. Symptoms.--Object looks blue, then yellow, ringing ears, dizziness.

Treatment.--Emetics such as warm mustard water, warm salt water, goose grease, lard, etc.; stimulants, brandy, strong coffee.

STRYCHNINE. Symptoms.--Appear quickly. Terrible convulsions, in paroxysms, devilish grin, the body is curved backward, jaw set.

Treatment.--Cause vomiting, with warm salt water, warm mustard water, lard, vaselin, etc.; sixty grains of bromide of potash and thirty grains of chloral hydrate by the rectum. Dark, quiet room.

SPOILED FOODS. Symptoms.--Vomiting, cramps, diarrhea, weakness, cold hands and feet.

Treatment.--Emetics such as warm salt water until patient vomits freely; or mustard water, lard, goose grease, vaselin, tickle throat with feather, etc.

SULPHURIC ACID. Symptoms.--The stomach and bowels are irritated and inflamed, the mouth may burn and bleed; swallowing is difficult. "Coffee grounds" vomiting. Pulse feeble, clammy skin.

Treatment.--Usually the first thing to do is to give an emetic. Send for a doctor and give an emetic. Then give chalk or, if necessary, take plaster from wall, mix it with a glass of water. Also three or four eggs (raw) in a glass of milk can be taken.

TARTAR EMETIC. Symptoms.--Metallic taste, violent vomiting, becoming bloody, feeble pulse; pain and burning in the stomach. Violent watery purging, becoming bloody; cramps in the extremities, thirst, great weakness; sometimes prostration, collapse, unconsciousness.

Antidotes.--Tannic acid, twenty drops to glass of water.

Treatment.--Soothing drinks, milk, white of egg and water, flax-seed tea, etc., external heat.

TOBACCO. Symptoms.--Vomiting, terrible weakness.

Treatment.--Emetics, such as warm salt water, warm mustard water, goose grease, lard, vaselin, etc.; then stimulants such as strong, coffee, brandy; heat to extremities, artificial respiration.

WINE OF ANTIMONY. Symptoms.--Metallic taste, violent vomiting, becoming bloody, feeble pulse; pain and burning in the stomach. Violent watery purging, becoming bloody; cramps in the extremities, thirst, great weakness; sometimes prostration, collapse, unconsciousness.

Antidotes.--Tannic acid, twenty drops to glass of water.

Treatment.--Soothing drinks, milk, white of egg and water, flax seed tea, etc.; external heat.

HERB DEPARTMENT

OVER ONE HUNDRED (100) MEDICAL HERBS

Partially Illustrated, with Full and Detailed Explanation as to Their Internal and External Uses, Part to Be Used, When to Gather, Time of Flowering, Where Found, Preparation for Medicine,

Teas, Etc., and Full Directions for Using.

In preparing this department we have been governed by two essential observations. First, that the tendency in American and Canadian homes is to the return to the good old home remedies that mother and grandmother used so successfully. We have, therefore, tried to choose in this list of over one hundred herbs, the most common ones, ones that could be prepared at home easily and quickly and which would be perfectly safe for the average person to administer as medicine.

Second, upon a close examination of the herb departments of practically all of the medical works or receipt books sold for family use today we discovered that only *general* information and directions were given. In this connection, we have endeavored, and we believe successfully, to supply what other books have neglected,--*definite directions for the preparation, dose, etc.* Should a physician leave a bottle of medicine at your home without directions you would not think of using it, and it is just as useless and indiscreet for a young mother to attempt to use herbs from the field without explicit directions for their preparation and administration.

We give below a few important directions for gathering, keeping and preparation of herbs, etc., for reference when using herbs not in this list. Those in the list are explained under their respective headings.

Drying and Preserving Roots, Herbs, Barks, etc.--Gather herbs when the weather is fine, when there is no dew upon them, when the flowers are in full bloom or the seeds are ripening. By gathering the herbs yourself you are assured of their being fresh although, if living in the city, you can purchase them ready prepared in ounce packages for about five cents at any drug store. Should you gather them yourself dry them in the shade, after which they should be kept from exposure to the air by wrapping up in paper or keeping in paper bags, tied and hung up in the attic or other dry place. If hanging exposed in your home for a long time watch them that moths do not gather in them and make their nests.

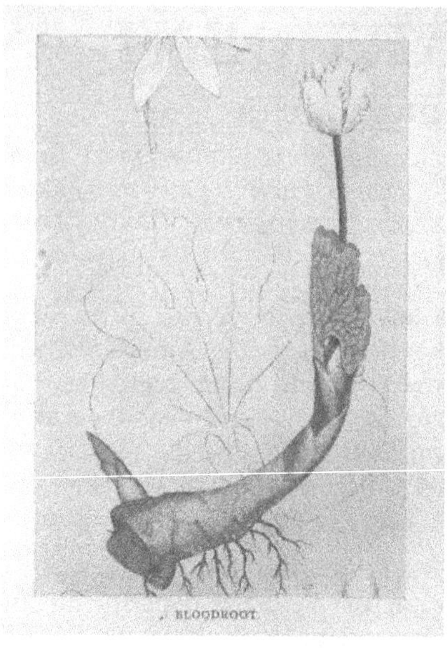

BLOODROOT.

ELDER FLOWERS.

Bloodroot

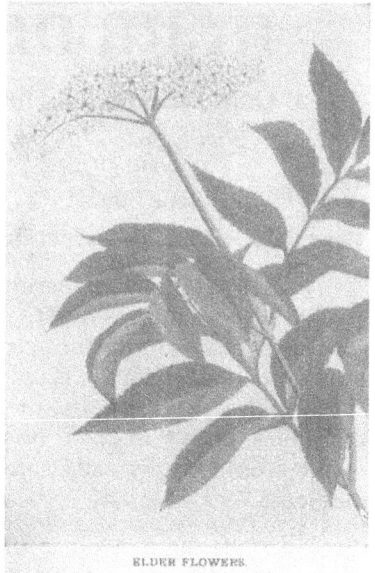

Elder Flowers

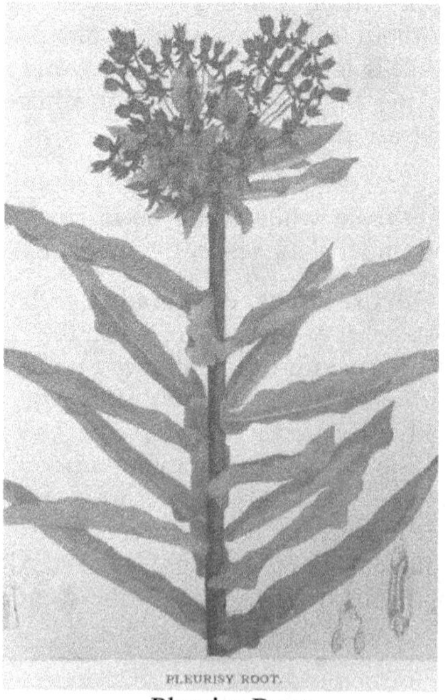

PLEURISY ROOT.

Pleurisy Root

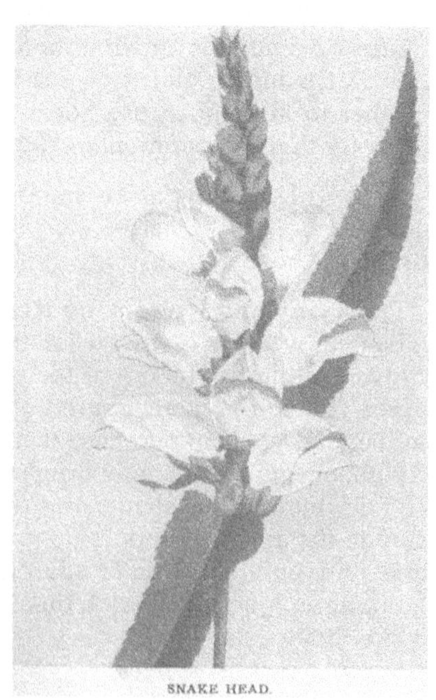

SNAKE HEAD.

Snake Head

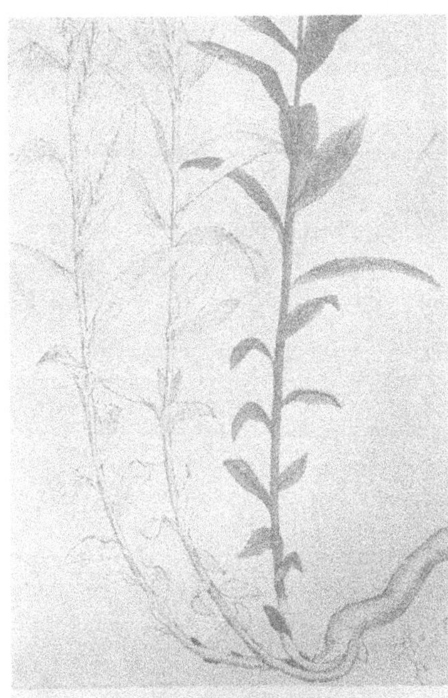

SENECA SNAKE ROOT.

Seneca Snake Root

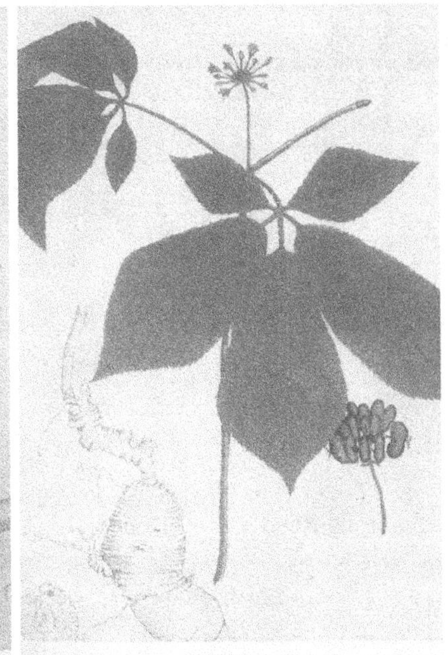

GINSENG.

Ginseng

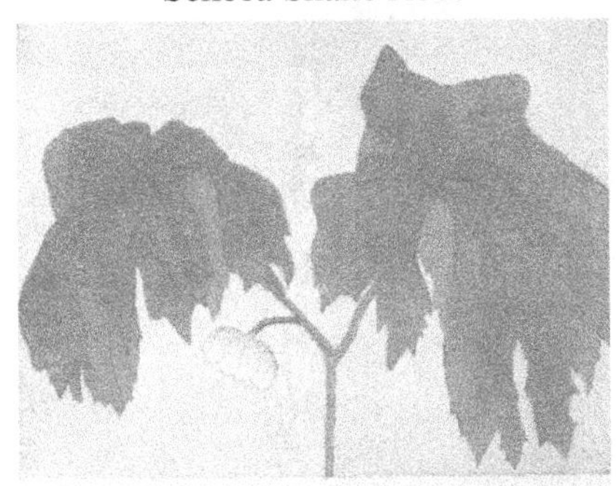

MANDRAKE OR MAY-APPLE.

Mandrake Or May-Apple

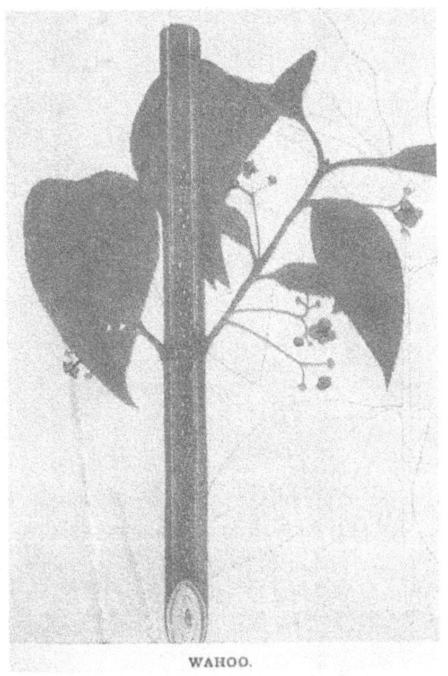

WAHOO.

Wahoo

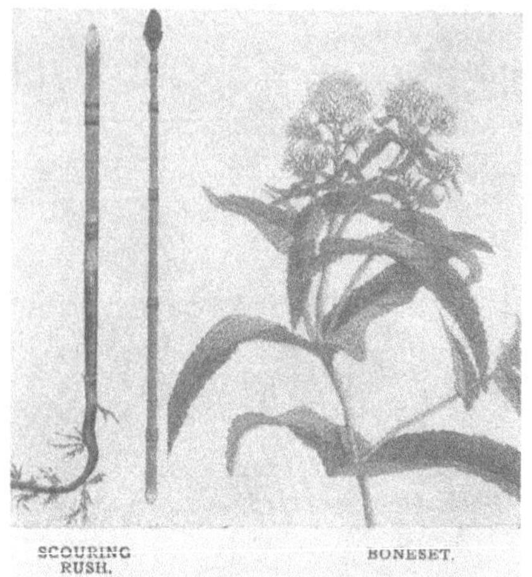

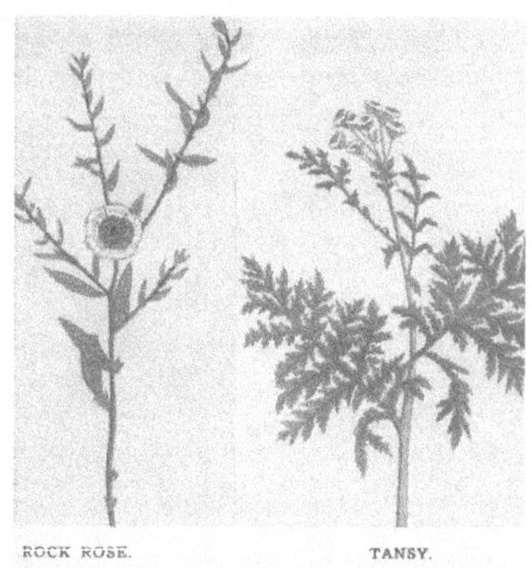

Scouring Rush Boneset Rock Rose Tansy

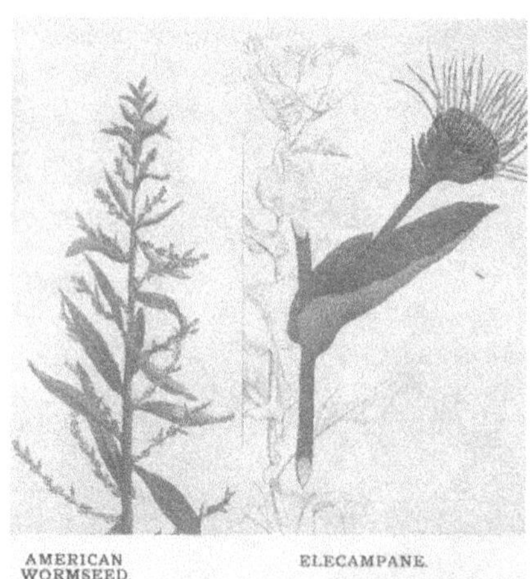

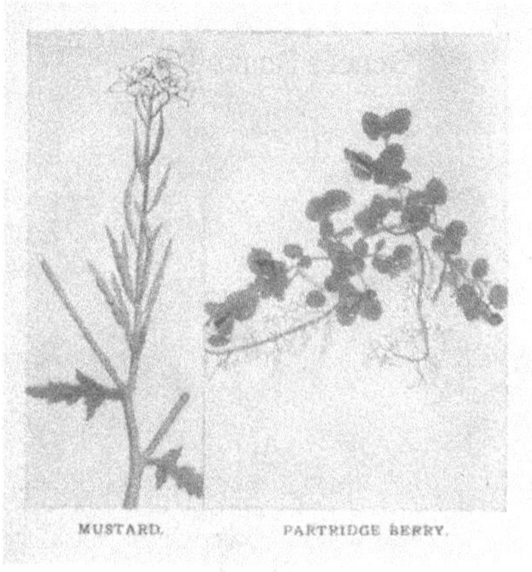

American Wormseed Elecampane Mustard Partridge Berry

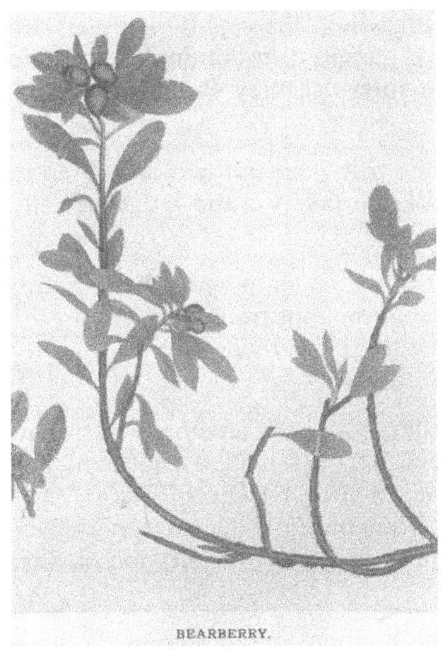

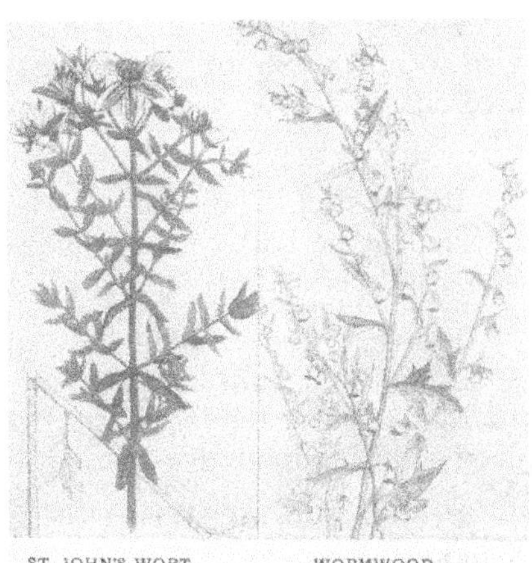

St. John's Wort Wormwood

Bearberry

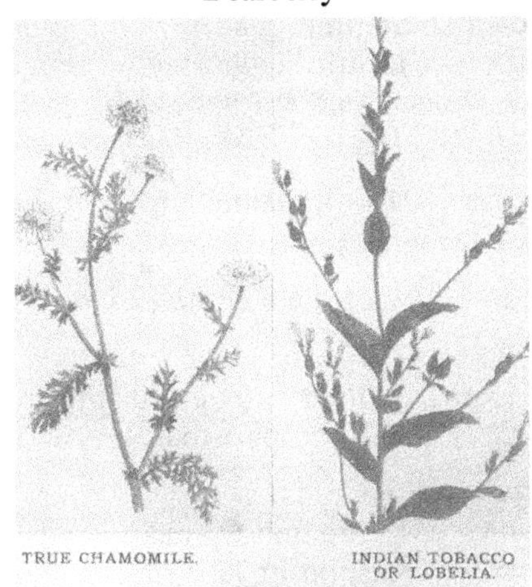

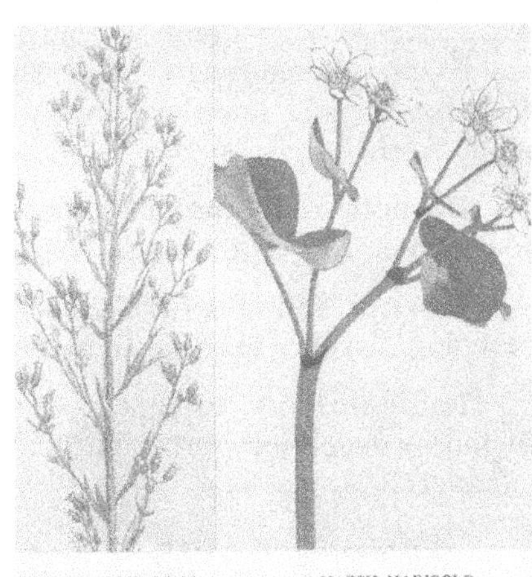

True Chamomile Indian Tobacco Or Lobelia Canada Fleabane Marsh Marigold

Roots should be dug in the spring when the sap is rising if you wish to make extract; or they may be gathered in autumn when they have ceased to vegetate. To dry for winter use they should be sliced, dried and kept from the air.

Barks should be stripped when the tree is in full leaf and dried in the shade. The bark of the roots should be taken in the fall, when the sap has descended.

Flowers and Seeds.--Flowers should be gathered when in full bloom and free from the dew and should be kept from exposure to the air. Be sure that seeds have fully matured; dry them also in a shady place and keep ready for use.

Preparation of Herbs for Medicine.--There are many different methods of preparing herbs for medicine,--Infusion, Decoction, Fomentation, Ointment, Plaster, Poultice, Powder, Essence, Tincture, etc. Only five of these, Plaster, Poultice, Fomentations, Decoction and Infusion are commonly used. An infusion is more commonly called "tea."

Infusion or Tea, to make.--Usually about one ounce of the herb to a pint of water is used for an infusion. Sometimes cold water is poured over the herb, but the most common method is to pour boiling water over the herb and let stand for a short time, just as you would make common tea for the table. Sometimes a little sugar may be added to make the tea more palatable. An infusion or tea should be used while fresh.

Decoction, to make.--Make same as for infusion and boil for some time, just as you would make coffee.

Essence, to make.--Take about an ounce of the essential oil of the herb and dissolve in a pint of alcohol.

Fomentations, to make.--Dip cloths or heavy towels in the infusion or decoction, wring out and apply locally to part that you wish to cover.

Ointments or Salve, to make.--An easy method to make a salve or ointment is to take about eight parts of vaselin or lard or any like substance and add two parts of the remedy you wish to use. Thus, if you were to make a sulphur salve you would use eight ounces of vaselin and two ounces of sulphur; stir and mix well while hot and when cool you would have a regular sulphur salve or ointment.

Plasters, to make.--Bruise the leaves, root, or other part of the plant and place between two pieces of cloth, just as you would a mustard plaster, and apply to the surface you wish to cover.

Poultices, to make.--Poultices are used to apply heat (moist heat), to soothe or to draw. Usually a soft substance is used, such as soap and sugar, bread and milk, mustard, etc. Some cause a counter-irritation, some draw the blood from a congested part and thus relieve pain. In the chapter on nursing many different poultices are given with methods of preparing them.

Powder, to make.--The part to be used is crushed, pounded, or ground until it is made very fine. It is best to have substance dry if to be prepared for powder.

Syrups, to make.--After preparing the substance for a tea boil for some time, then add considerable sugar and stir until all is nicely dissolved. To each pint of this syrup add one ounce of glycerin and seal up in bottles or cans as you would fruit.

Tincture, to make.--Take one ounce of the powdered herb and add 4 ounces of water and 12 ounces of alcohol, let stand for two weeks. A dram of glycerin may be added. After standing for two weeks pour off liquid and bottle for use. If it is necessary for you to use a tincture we would advise that you buy it at a drug store, as it is not often made properly at home. The above is a safe method for making a tincture and would not be especially strong. Should the herb used have a very weak medicinal power one to four ounces of the herb may be used for the above amount of water and alcohol.

ALDER, SPOTTED.--Snapping Hazelnut. Winterbloom. Witch Hazel. *Hamamelis.*

Internally used for.--Falling of the womb, sore mouth, falling of the bowel, piles, bleeding diarrhea.

Externally used for.--Sore eyes, ulcers, sores, enlarged veins, sprains, bruises and ivy poisoning.

Part used.--Leaves and fresh bark.

Gather.--In the fall.

Flowers (when).--From September to November.

Grows (where).--In all sections of the United States, especially in damp woods.

Prepared (how).--As a poultice, ointment, decoction. Make a decoction by using one and one-half ounces of the fresh bark or leaves, boiled in a pint of water. The medicine can be bought at any drug store.

Diseases, Dose, etc.--For sore mouth, throat, leucorrhea, falling of the womb and bowel, use the decoction strong locally. It should not cause any pain. For falling bowel, use a full strength injection and apply locally with cloths on the sore bowels. Used locally for bleeding from the nose or from pulling teeth. For piles, an ointment can be made by using strong decoction and cosmaline mixed. Apply decoction locally on varicose veins or varicose ulcers. It is often used in the form of "Pond's Extract." For diarrhea one to three ounces every three hours. Good also applied locally for burns, old sores, eczema, ivy poisoning, bruises.

BALMONY. Snakehead. Fish Mouth. Turtlebloom. Bitter Herb. Salt Rheum Weed. *Chelone Glabra.*

Internally used for.--Dyspepsia, weak digestive organs, jaundice.

Part used.--Leaves are best for medical use.

Gather.--In the fall.

Flowers (when).--From July to late Autumn.

Grows (where).--Found in the United States in wet grounds.

Prepared (how).--Leaves made into a powder or tea. One ounce of the leaves to a pint of boiling water to make the tea. Let steep.

Diseases, Dose, etc.--Dose of the powder, for above-named diseases, one-half to one even teaspoonful, four times a day. Dose of the tea for the above diseases, one to two ounces three or four times a day. The tea is the best to use. Gentian can be added to this remedy, if desired, when a more active bitter tonic is wanted. Use same amount of each and make into a tea. Dose of combination, one to two ounces before meals.

BAYBERRY.--Wax Myrtle. Waxberry. Candleberry. *Myrica Cerifera.*

Gather.--Collect it late in the fall, dry without exposure to moisture, pound with a hammer to separate the bark, powder and keep in dark, sealed vessels.

Grows (where).--In damp places in United States, especially in New Jersey.

Prepared (how).--As a powder, poultice, decoction. To make decoction use one ounce of the bark to a pint of water and boil.

Diseases, Dose, etc.--For jaundice, use the decoction, one to three ounces, every two to five hours. For diarrhea and dysentery one-half ounce every two hours. For blood diseases and scrofula, take two ounces four times daily. Poultice for scrofulous tumors and ulcers, alone, or with elm. For sore throat, mouth and gums gargle freely with the decoction. A plaster can be made and used on ulcers. Dose of powder: twenty to thirty grains, three times a day.

BEARBERRY. Upland or Wild Cranberry. Mountain Box. Red

Berry. *Arbutus Uva Ursi.*

Internally, used for.--Its special use is in kidney and bladder troubles. It may be used in diarrhea, dysentery, leucorrhea, but as stated it is better for cystitis, urinary trouble, etc., gonorrhea.

Part used.--The leaves.

Gather.--In autumn, and use only the green leaves.

Grows (where).--On mountains and dry land in United States, Europe and Asia.

Prepared (how).--As a powder or decoction. For decoction use one ounce of the leaves and boil in one and one-half pints of distilled water. Boil down to a pint.

Diseases, Dose, etc.--One to three ounces every two to four hours for gonorrhea, with bloody and mucous discharges and pain in the bladder. For cystitis one ounce every two hours. For kidney troubles one ounce four times a day. If taken long or in too large doses it irritates the kidneys.

BEECHDROPS. Cancer Root. *Epipegus Virginiana.*

Internally, used for.--An astringent for bleeding from the bowels and womb, and for diarrhea.

Externally, used for.--Erysipelas and skin eruptions, ulcers, and also good as an injection in leucorrhea.

Part used.--Roots and tops.

Flowers (when).--In August and September.

Grows (where).--All parts of North America.

Prepared (how).--As a powder, decoction, and poultice. To make a decoction take one ounce of the root to a pint of water and boil. Keep adding water to make a full pint.

Diseases, Doses, etc.--The decoction has been used in erysipelas, one-half to one ounce every two hours. Same dose for bleeding and diarrhea. Dose of powder ten to fifteen grains, four times a day. Decoction can be used locally in erysipelas. This is also good for ulcers and wounds, and for skin affections applied locally; or a poultice can be used. A poultice of this remedy, poke and white oak, equal parts, is very good for old sores. Useful locally also for sore mouth and throat, and as an injection for leucorrhea.

BETHROOT. Birth Root. Ground Lily. Lambs Quarter. Wake Robin. Indian Balm. Three-Leaved Night-Shade. *Trillium Purpureum.*

Internally used for.--Astringent, tonic, antiseptic. For bleeding from lungs, kidneys and womb, for leucorrhea and for confinement. Also for diarrhea, nose-bleed.

Externally.--The root is used as a poultice for tumors, lazy ulcers, buboes, carbuncles, stings of insects.

Part used.--The root. This contains volatile oil, tannic acid, etc.

Gather.--In autumn.

Flowers (when).--In May and June.

Grows (where).--In middle western and southern states.

Prepared (how).--As a poultice, powder and infusion. Use one to one and one-half ounce of root to a pint of boiling water for infusion.

Diseases, Dose, etc.--For female weakness, bleeding, leucorrhea, and bearing down particularly, bloody urine, two to four ounces, of the strong tea, four times daily, and also used as an injection in leucorrhea, once daily. For bleeding from the lungs, one ounce every hour for a few doses. For dysentery and diarrhea boil one ounce in a pint of milk and use two ounces every two to four hours. Powdered root, given in hot water, may be used in doses of one-half to one teaspoonful three times a day, instead of infusion. Taken after confinement, use the infusion four times a day, smell of the red bethroots.

BLACKBERRY. Dewberry or low blackberry. Red Raspberry.

Internally, used for.--Tonic and astringent, diarrhea, bleeding from the bowels and womb, injection for leucorrhea.

Externally, used for.--Gonorrhea, gleet.

Part used.--Leaves of the raspberry and the bark of the other two.

Flowers (when).--Spring.

Grows (where).--Almost everywhere.

Prepared (how).--Use one ounce of the leaves of raspberry or bark of either of the others, to a pint of water and boil to make a decoction.

Diseases, Dose, etc.--For diseases mentioned, such as diarrhea, take one tablespoonful every four hours. For injection use the decoction. This is used once daily for leucorrhea, gleet, gonorrhea, falling of the womb and bowel. Internally it is also used as a diuretic.

BLACK HAW. *Viburnum Prunifolium.*

Internally, used for.--Tonic, astringent, diuretic and alterative. Tonic for the womb, for threatened abortion and prevention of miscarriage. Good for severe after-pains, and for bleeding from the womb.

Part used.--Bark of the root.

Flowers (when).--From March to July.

Grows (where).--Most abundant in the middle states and southern.

Prepared (how).--As an infusion and tincture (or fluid extract).

Prepare infusion by adding one ounce of bark of the root to a pint of boiling water.

Diseases, Dose, etc.--For threatened abortion or miscarriage use infusion three or four times daily, in two teaspoonfuls doses, a week or two before, it usually has occurred; or the tincture in ten to twenty drop doses five times daily. For bleeding from the womb take ten to twenty drops, four times daily, a few days before the time for the flow.

BLOOD ROOT. Red Puceoon. Red Root. *Sanguinaria Canadensis.*

Internally, used for.--Tonic, emetic, and for sick headache.

Externally, used for.--Ulcers, ringworms and warts.

Part used.--Root and should be kept dry.

Flowers (when).--Appears early in March and April.

Grows (where).--Most parts of United States in woods, groves, in shaded banks, in rich light soil.

Prepared (how).--An Infusion and powder. For an infusion one ounce to one pint of vinegar.

Diseases, Dose, etc.--Dose of powder as an emetic, ten to twenty grains. Dose of infusion as an emetic one to four teaspoonfuls: For ringworm, tetter and warts, it is applied locally, freely. Applied to ulcers and growths, it often cures, and removes the growths. As a tonic for the stomach, the dose should be small, one to one and one-half teaspoonful of the infusion four times daily, and for sick headache it should be half as much and not repeated oftener than twice, a half hour apart.

BLUE FLAG. Flower de Luce. Flag Lily. Snake Lily. Liver Lily. *Iris Versicolor.*

Internally, used for.--Chronic liver troubles, sick or bilious headache, cathartic, catarrh of the upper bowel, jaundice, round worms, indigestion, chronic rheumatism.

Part used.--The root. Make a tincture immediately or dry it quickly before the fire, clean, powder, and bottle tight for use.

Gather.--In the fall. It must be kept fresh.

Flowers (when).--May or June.

Grows (where).--Found in all parts of the United States, growing in wet places, in meadows and borders of swamps.

Prepared (how).--In powder, tincture or fluid extract. They can all be bought.

Diseases, Dose, etc.--As a cathartic, five to twenty grains of powder. If it nauseates, mix with it a few grains of capsicum or ginger. Dose of saturated tincture, ten to sixty drops. Fluid extract, twenty to sixty drops. For sick headache one drop doses every hour. For chronic liver troubles, five to ten drops of tincture, four times daily. Same dose for all chronic diseases. For round worms, large doses must be used, enough to move the bowels. Following is good for indigestion and biliousness: Fluid extract of blue flag and golden seal each; one-half ounce, simple elixir, one ounce. Take a dessertspoonful in hot water, before meals.

BONESET.--Thoroughwort. Fever Wort. Sweating Plant. Cross Wort. Indian Sage. Ague Weed. Vegetable Antimony. *Eupatorium Perfoliatum.*

Internally, used for.--Ague, malarial fevers, influenza, colds, tonic, cathartic.

Externally, used for.--A fomentation.

Part used.--The top and leaves.

Gather.--When at its best in early autumn.

Flowers (when).--In August and September.

Grows (where).--All over the United States.

Prepared (how).--Powder. Infusion, one and one-half ounces to a pint of water.

Diseases, Dose, etc.--For malarial fever, a hot strong infusion taken freely as hot as possible. Teacupful at a time often enough to produce sweating. Same way for colds and influenza. Use the cold infusion as a tonic and laxative. As a tonic it is useful after fevers, etc. Dose of powder ten to twenty grains. Dose of infusion two to four ounces. It can be combined with tansy and hops and makes splendid fomentation.

BROOKLIME. *Veronica Beccabunga.*

Internally, used for.--Scurvy and for the menses, obstructed menstruation.

Part used.--Leaves and top.

Gather.--Early autumn.

Flowers (when).--From April to August.

Grows (where).--Eastern and northern states, and grows in small streams and near watercourses.

Prepared (how).--As a decoction, and it may be used freely.

Diseases, Dose, etc.--For scurvy used to purify the blood. It is used in decoction to regulate menstruation, and should be taken freely and warm and begun a day before the menstrual period.

BUCHU. A South African plant of the genus Barosma.

Internally, used for.--Bladder troubles. In irritable bladder and urethra, due to increased sand in the urine, inflammation.

Part used.--Leaves.

Gather.--Buy in drug store.

Grows (where).--In Africa.

Prepared (how).--Infusion; make it by putting one ounce of the leaves to a pint of boiling water and let it steep.

Diseases, Dose, etc.--Dose is two to four ounces, three or four times a day in chronic cases of bladder trouble, or one ounce every two or three hours in acute cases. It is very good when the urine is not free or is painful to pass. In acute and chronic inflammation, but more especially in the acute form. If it injures the stomach it can be used in alternation with pumpkin seed tea.

BURDOCK. *Arctium Lappa.*

Internally, used for.--Kidney troubles, rheumatism, syphilis, skin diseases. Must be used a long time.

Externally, used for.--Can be used as an ointment.

Part used.--Roots and seeds.

Gather.--In the spring.

Grows (where).--Almost everywhere.

Prepared (how).--As a decoction, two ounces to a pint of water or fluid extract can be bought.

Diseases, Dose, etc.--Dose of decoction: This should be used freely as it is not strong, one pint can be taken in twenty-four hours. Used as an ointment for skin diseases; the juice, of the leaves, is mixed with lard, cream or vaselin. This remedy is used frequently in combination with other blood remedies, for the above named diseases and is very beneficial.

CARROT. Wild Carrot. Bird's Nest. Bee's Nest. *Daucus Carota.*

Internally, used for.--Dropsy, chronic kidney troubles and gravel.

Externally, used for.--Ulcers: as a poultice.

Part used.--Roots and seeds. Garden carrot, only the root is used.

Flowers (when).--June to September.

Grows (where).--In neglected fields and by roadsides.

Prepared (how).--In infusion (tea) by using one ounce to a pint of boiling water and allow it to steep, but not to boil.

Diseases, Dose, etc.--Dose, two to four ounces of the infusion, three or four times a day, for diseases mentioned. When the infusion is made from the seeds the dose is only about one-third of a teaspoonful four times daily. For external use for troublesome ulcers, scrape or grate the root and apply to the ulcers.

CATNIP. Catmint. Catwort. *Nepeta Cataria.*

Internally, used for.--Sweating, nervous troubles, colic and tonic.

Externally, used for.--Poultices and fomentations.

Part used.--Leaves and top.

Gather.--Early autumn.

Flowers (when).--June to September.

Grows (where).--Grows in dry neglected places, about old buildings and fences.

Prepared (how).--The infusion should be prepared by adding one ounce of the plant to a pint of boiling water, Do not let it boil, but only steep; stand only a few minutes; when wanted as a tonic, use it cold. When used for sweating purposes, etc., it must be used hot.

Diseases, Dose, etc.--Drink as freely as the stomach will permit. It is frequently used for colic in babies in doses of half to one teaspoonful, warm. To produce sweating it should be used hot and freely taken. A combination of catnip, lady's slipper and skullcap, equal parts, either in the infusion or fluid extract, one dram doses, is good for nervous headache, hysteria, chorea. Leaves are used as a fomentation. The expressed juice of the plant is good for amenorrhea in one to two teaspoonful doses five times daily.

CELANDINE.--Tetter Wort. *Chelidonium Majus.*

Internally, used for.--Liver and skin troubles.

Externally, used for.--Warts, corns, salt rheum.

Part used.--Herb and root. Latter is the best.

Flowers (when).--Throughout the summer.

Grows (where).--In the United States in waste places.

Prepared (how).--It is best used internally in the tincture, powdered root, or fresh juice.

Diseases, Dose, etc.--For liver disease, it is especially good where the pain is under the right shoulder blade. Use the tincture in ten-drop doses three times a day. Externally rub the juice on the corn or wart. Make an ointment from the root and rub this on the skin for salt rheum. It is said to be good for piles also. Dose:--Powdered root ten to twenty to thirty grains. Tincture, ten to twenty drops, and of the juice ten to twenty drops.

CHAMOMILE. Roman Chamomile. *Anthemis Nobilis.*

Internally, used for.--Tonic in small doses, dyspepsia, colic, cramp, diarrhea, dysmenorrhea.

Externally, used for.--Fomentation, boiled in vinegar and applied to painful swellings.

Part used.--Leaves and herb.

Gather.--When in bloom.

Flowers (when).--Summer.

Grows (where).--Native of Europe. It grows wild in the United States.

Prepared (how).--As an infusion use a half ounce to a pint of boiling water, steep and take freely.

Diseases, Dose, etc.--Use cold infusion in dyspepsia; warm infusion for colic and cramps, and for diarrhea in children, especially of the green kind of stools. Dose:--One teaspoonful every two or three hours. Good for nervousness in teething children. An oil also is used, two to five drops on sugar. This is given for colic, cramps, and in painful dysmenorrhea.

CLEAVERS. Goose Grass. Catch Weed. Clivers. Bed Straw. *Galium Aparine.*

Internally, used for.--Suppression of the urine, gravel, inflammation of the kidneys and bladder, and for scalding urine in gonorrhea.

Externally, used for.--Freckles.

Part used.--The plant.

Gather.--Early autumn.

Flowers (when).--From June to September.

Grows (where).--Common in the United States, growing on cultivated grounds, moist thickets, and along fences and hedges.

Prepared (how).--Infusion. Use one and one-half ounces of the herb in a pint of warm water and allow it to steep for two hours.

Diseases, Dose, etc.--Take two to four ounces of the infusion three

27

or four times a day, when it is cold. The dose can be lessened and taken oftener. It may be sweetened with sugar when taken for the diseases named above. Also equal parts of cleavers, maidenhair, and elder blows, steeped in warm water for two or three hours and drank freely when cold forms an excellent drink in erysipelas, scarlet fever and measles. An infusion made with cold water is good to remove freckles; wash the parts several times daily for two or three months.

CLOVES. *Caryophyllus.*

Internally, used for.--Flatulent colic, diarrhea, cholera morbus, toothache, (oil of cloves).

Gather.--Collect flowers in October and November, before they are fully developed and dry quickly.

Grows (where).--In tropical climate.

Prepared (how).--Boil two or three teaspoonfuls of the ground cloves in a half pint of milk.

Diseases, Dose, etc.--Two to four teaspoonfuls every twenty to thirty minutes for gas colic, or diarrhea where the bowels need tone. The oil can be used in three to five-drop doses. Also good to place in hollow teeth. Put a little of the oil on cotton and insert into the tooth. It is also good to add to other medicines to stop griping and nausea.

BLUE COHOSH. Squaw Root. Papoose Root. Blue Berry. *Caulophyllum Thalictroides.*

Internally, used for.--Nervous affection, rheumatism, womb troubles, such as amenorrhea, leucorrhea; used previous to labor it is beneficial and also good for afterpains.

Externally, used for.--Sore throat. **Part used.**--Root.

Gather.--Latter part of summer or in autumn.

Grows (where).--All over the United States in low moist rich grounds, near running streams, in swamps, etc.

Prepared (how).--As an infusion or decoction. It can be bought in the fluid extract form. Make a tea by adding one ounce of the root to a pint of boiling water. Decoction is made by allowing it to boil some length of time.

Diseases, Dose, etc.--Dose of fluid extract fifteen to thirty drops. Dose of tea, two to four ounces, three or four times daily. Dose of decoction, one-half the amount. When used in acute disease, the dose should not be more than one-fourth as much and given every one or two hours. For rheumatism it is especially valuable, when small joints like the fingers and toes are involved. It is very good in the chronic womb diseases named above. It should be used in small doses several weeks prior to labor. It is said to assist in making labor easier.

BLACK COHOSH. Rattle Root. Black Snake Root. Squaw Root. Rich Weed. *Cimicifuga Racemosa.*

Internally, used for.--Chorea, dependent upon rheumatism; rheumatism, amenorrhea, dysmenorrhea, leucorrhea, afterpains.

Part used.--Root.

Gather.--Early in the autumn and dry in the shade.

Flowers (when).--In June and July.

Grows (where).--Native of United States. Grows in shady and rocky woods, rich grounds and on sides of hills.

Prepared (how).--Powder; decoction, one ounce to a pint of water; and tincture.

Diseases, Dose, etc.--Dose of decoction half to one ounce; of powder ten to twenty grains. For chorea, use powder, twenty grains, three times a day. Use tincture or fluid extract or the decoction for womb affections. Dose of tincture, thirty to sixty drops three times daily. Fluid extract, ten to thirty drops three times daily; for afterpains give half as much about every three hours. In making the decoction you can make it stronger by boiling longer. The dose must then be less, according to the strength. This is a very useful remedy. For rheumatism, especially the chronic kind, it is often beneficial.

COMFREY. Healing Herb. Gum Plant.

Internally, used for.--An astringent and soothing agent in diarrhea, dysentery, coughs, lung affections, female weakness, leucorrhea, and urinary diseases.

Externally, used for.--Bruises, ruptures, fresh wounds, sore breasts, ulcers and swellings.

Part used.--Root.

Flowers (when).--May or June.

Prepared (how).--It is boiled in water or wine or it can be made into syrup. For external use bruise the root and apply it to the diseased part.

Diseases, Dose, etc.--Dose of the syrup one to four ounces, two or three times a day. For the diseases named it is best to take it in smaller doses and oftener, say four teaspoonfuls every hour or two; children in proportion.

CORN SILK. *Zea Mays.*

Internally, used for.--Diuretic, quieting to the urinary passages. Congested kidney, dropsy from heart disease, chronic nephritis, suppression of the urine, renal colic, haematuria, cystitis.

Prepared (how).--Make a tea and drink freely. Fluid extract can be bought.

Diseases., Dose, etc.--Dose: One to two teaspoonfuls of fluid extract three or four times a day, or drink freely of tea for above diseases.

CRANBERRY (High). Cramp Bark. *Viburnum Opulus.*

Internally, used for.--Cramps and spasms of all kinds, asthma, hysteria; cramps in the legs, especially during pregnancy, or at labor.

Part used.--Bark.

Gather.--Early autumn.

Flowers (when).--In June.

Grows (where).--In Canada and northern United States, in low rich lands, woods, borders of fields.

Prepared (how).--Use an ounce of the bark, powdered, to a quart of wine.

Diseases, Dose, etc.--Take half a wineglassful four times a day for continued use. For hysteria attacks, asthma spasms, less should be used and taken oftener for a few doses. The following combination is effective for the spasmodic attacks, above named: Cramp bark two ounces, scull cap and skunk cabbage one ounce each, cloves one-half ounce, capsicum two even teaspoonfuls. Powder all, and bruise and add to them two quarts of good native wine. Dose: one or two ounces two or three times a day; oftener and smaller doses for hysteria, etc. It should be taken for two or three months during pregnancy.

CRAWLEY. Dragon's Claw. Coral Teeth. Fever Root. Chicken Toes. Albany Beechdrops. *Corallorhiza Odontorhiza.*

Internally, used for.--Sweating purposes in fevers and inflammatory diseases, acute erysipelas, pleurisy, low stages of fevers, amenorrhea and dysmenorrhea, in afterpains, and suppressed lochia.

Part used.--The root.

Gather.--In the fall.

Flowers (When).--In July. No leaves.

Grows (where).--Found on barren hills and shady uplands in northern states and Canada.

Prepared (how) .--Powder and keep it in well closed bottles.

Diseases, Dose, etc.--Dose of powder, from ten to twenty grains in hot water and repeated every hour or two as needed. Combined with blue cohosh, it is very beneficial in amenorrhea, etc., as above stated. In fevers, Culver's root can be added to it, if the bowels need regulating. It is also good for flatulent colic in twenty-grain doses. Some combine pleurisy root with it in pleurisy. It should be given in acute diseases every one to two hours as needed.

CRANESBILL (spotted). Crowfoot. Tormentil. Storkbill. Alum Root. *Geranium Maculalum.*

Internally, used for.--Second stage of dysentery, diarrhea in an infusion of milk; in bleedings, sore mouth, leucorrhea, gleet, menorrhagia and excessive mucous discharges, nose-bleed, bleeding from extracted teeth, piles, bleeding after labor, sore throat.

Part used.--The root.

Gather.--Collected in late autumn.

Flowers (when).--From April to June.

Grows (where).--In United States in open woods, thickets and hedges.

Prepared (how).--Powder. Use one and one-half ounces of the root and boil it in a pint of water or milk.

Diseases, Dose, etc.--Dose: one to two tablespoonfuls. Use the watery decoction as a gargle for sore mouth and throat. For piles:--

Inject a strong decoction and retain as long as possible; or apply an ointment of two ounces of the root to tobacco ointment seven ounces, and apply three or four times a day. Nose-bleed and bleeding from teeth extraction:--Apply the powder or strong decoction to the part. Bleeding from the womb:--Inject strong decoction or apply on gauze or cotton to inner womb. Decoction, two parts to one part blood root, forms a good injection for leucorrhea and gonorrhea. Good in latter stages of diarrhea and dysentery of children, boiled in milk, given in teaspoonful doses, every one to three hours.

CULVER'S ROOT. Veronica. Black Root. Culver's Physic. Tall Speedwell. *Leptandra Virginica.*

Internally, used for.--A laxative, bilious fever, dyspepsia due to inactive liver and bowels.

Part used.--Root. Age impairs its virtues. The dried root is safest to use, if not too old.

Gather.--In the autumn.

Flowers (when).--In July and August.

Grows (where).--In limestone lands and in rich moist places, woods, thickets, and barrens.

Prepared (how).--As a powder, extract and infusion. Fluid extract can be bought. To make decoction, use one ounce of the powdered root to one pint of water and let boil. If you use the green root put one ounce in cold water, and let it remain there for one hour.

Diseases, Dose, etc.--Dose of the powder of dry root, one small teaspoonful as a cathartic. This will bring away a black tarry discharge. Then it is better to use the decoction; one to two teaspoonfuls every two hours. Dose of extract is one-fourth of a grain. This is a good form to give, when the liver is acting badly. Good also for indigestion, in this form when due to inactive liver and costive bowels.

DANDELION. *Leontodon Taraxacum.*

Internally, used for.--Liver when it is torpid and engorged. It is also laxative and tonic.

Part used.--Root. The green plant is good to use in the form of greens. Milky juice is also good when fresh.

Gather.--July, August and September.

Flowers (when).--During spring and summer.

Grows (where).--Everywhere, it seems.

Prepared (how).--Juice is used, also infusion, extract and fluid extract. Infusion, two ounces of root to the pint of water.

Diseases, Dose, etc.--Dose of infusion one to two ounces. Juice, ten drops to one-half teaspoonful. Extract, ten grains. Fluid extract, one to two teaspoonfuls. It should be taken often enough, when the liver is torpid, to move the bowels once or twice a day. If the infusion is used, begin with a half ounce and take every three hours; increase or decrease as necessary. The extract is pleasanter and less bulky and best to use in winter. Take two or three grains every three hours more or less.

DEVIL'S BIT. False Unicorn Root. Drooping Starwort. Blazing Star. *Helonias Divica.* Somewhat similar to true unicorn root.

Internally, used for.--Used mainly in womb troubles, strengthens the womb and prevents miscarriages. Good also for leucorrhea, amenorrhea and dysmenorrhea.

Part used.--Root. Root is two to two and a half inches in length.

Gather.--In autumn.

Flowers (when).--June and July.

Grows (where).--In low grounds in United States and Canada.

Prepared (how).--Powdered root and decoction.

Diseases, Dose, etc.--It is a tonic to the womb and should be used for two months before the time the miscarriage usually occurs. For the other womb troubles, it should be taken four times a day. The fluid extract can be bought at any drug store, and can be used. Dose: Fifteen drops, four times daily. Dose of powder, ten to twenty grains. Decoction, one to two ounces.

ELDER (Sweet). Black-berried Elder. *Sambucus Canadensis.*

Internally, used for.--Erysipelas, kidneys, for sweating purposes, blood diseases and scarlet fever.

Externally, used for.--Burns, scalds, ulcers, skin diseases and weak eyes.

Part used.--Flowers and berries. Bark of the root also is used.

Gather.--Gather when in flower and when berries are ripe.

Flowers (when).--In summer.

Grows (where).--Grows in all parts of United States and Canada.

Prepared (how).--Infusion, one ounce of the flowers or root to a pint of boiling water.

Diseases, Dose, etc.--Use warm infusion for sweating and for erysipelas, half teaspoonful every three hours. Too much taken will move the bowels and also cause vomiting. Same for scarlet fever in adults. Infusion of the bark of the root may be taken in doses of half ounce twice daily, to act as a cathartic. Local, use inner bark of the limbs and steep with cream and apply freely and often for burns, sores, etc. For weak eyes make a tea from the flowers and use as an eye wash for children.

ELECAMPANE. *Inula Helenium.*

Internally, used for.--For sweating, expectorant, bronchitis, dyspepsia and dysmenorrhea.

Part used.--Root of the second year.

Gather.--Autumn.

Flowers (when).--In July and August.

Grows (where).--In Europe and Japan. Cultivated in United States and grows in moist places and about houses.

Prepared (how).--Use half ounce of the powdered root to a pint of boiling water and boil to make a decoction.

Diseases, Dose, etc.--For bronchitis, dyspepsia and dysmenorrhea, take half ounce doses four times daily. For sweating and painful menses take two teaspoonfuls of the hot decoction every two hours until relieved.

FLEABANE. Pridewood. Blood Staunch. Mare's Tail. Colt's Tail. Fireweeds. *Erigeron Canadensis.*

Internally, used for.--Diarrhea, dysentery, gravel, painful urination, piles, bleeding from the womb and bowels.

Part used.--The whole plant.

Gather.--Collect while in flower.

Flowers (when).--July and August.

Grows (where).--In United States and Canada. In fields and meadows, by roadsides, etc.

Prepared (how).--Powder, oil and infusion. To make infusion, use one ounce to pint of boiling water.

Diseases, Dose, etc.--The infusion, one to two ounces, should be used three or four times daily; powder, ten to twenty grains, the same. The oil is more effective in bleeding and dysentery and bleeding piles. Oil is very good, in doses of one to five drops every three hours for acute diseases, or three times a day for chronic cases. Put on sugar.

GARLIC. *Allium Sativum.*

Internally, used for.--Nervous children, coughs, colds, hoarseness, worms, croup, nervous vomiting.

Externally, used for.--Poultice.

Part used.--The bulb.

Gather.--When ripe.

Grows (where).--Native of Asia and Egypt; now cultivated.

Prepared (how).--Juice, syrup, powder, or may be taken whole. Juice or syrup is the best form.

Diseases, Dose, etc.--For coughs, bronchitis and worms, should be taken five times daily; croup, every half hour for a few doses. Nervous cough and vomiting only a few doses. Local.--Bruise bulbs and apply warm as a poultice in bronchitis, croup and tumors. For retention of urine, place a poultice in the perineum or over bladder on the abdomen. Dose of juice, twenty to thirty drops. Dose of syrup, ten drops to one teaspoon; this is very destructive to round worm.

GENTIAN. *Gentiana Lutea.*

Internally, used for.--Tonic appetizer, dyspepsia, ammenorrhea.

Part used.--Root used and imported. **Grows (where).**--In the Alps.

Prepared (how).--Powder, tincture and infusion. To make infusion, use one ounce of the root to a pint of boiling water.

Diseases, Dose, etc.--Dose of powder, ten to twenty grains. Tincture, one teaspoonful. Infusion, one to two ounces. Taken before meals for dyspepsia and loss of appetite. It should not be taken when the stomach is irritable. It is a good bitter tonic.

GINSENG.--Red Berry. Five Fingers. *Panax Quinquefolium.*

Internally, used for.--Gravel, general weakness, poor appetite.

Part used.--Root.

Flowers (when).--In May.

Grows (where).--In United States, in rich soil and in shady places.

Prepared (how).--Powder. Infusion is made by adding one ounce to a pint of boiling water.

Diseases, Dose, etc.--It should be taken three or four times a day for gravel or general weakness. As an appetizer it should be taken before meals. Dose of powder, ten to sixty grains. Dose of infusion, one to three ounces.

GINGER. *Zingiber Officinale.*

Internally, used for.--To increase gastric juice secretions, stimulating tonic, diarrhea, dysentery, flatulency, cramps and nausea.

Externally, used for.--Ulcers.

Grows (where).--Native of Asia.

Prepared (how).--Powder. Infusion made by adding half ounce of the powdered or bruised root to a pint of boiling water.

Diseases, Dose, etc.--For diarrhea, dysentery and cholera infantum, mix it with rhubarb, equal parts, or take alone. If with rhubarb it should be stopped if it becomes too laxative. Used alone for want of tone of stomach, flatulency, cramps and colic. It tones up the stomach and bowels temporarily, but should not be used long or frequently. Dose of powder, ten to twenty grains. Dose of infusion, one to two ounces.

GOLDEN SEAL. Orange Root. Yellow Puccoon. Ground Raspberry. Turmeric Root. *Hydrastis Canadensis.*

Internally, used for.--Tonic in dyspepsia, chronic stomach and bowel trouble. Torpid liver, sore mouth; gonorrhea (injection), leucorrhea, gleet.

Part used.--The root.

Gather.--In autumn.

Flowers (when).--In May or June.

Grows (where).--United States and Canada.

Prepared (how).--Powder, infusion, tincture, fluid extract. Use half ounce of root to a pint of boiling water for infusion.

Diseases, Dose, etc.--Of the powder, five to ten grains; of infusion, one ounce; of tincture, half to one teaspoonful and of fluid extract, five to twenty drops. When it is called for, the tongue is generally coated whitish; it will soon clear that. Diarrhea, etc., due to stomach and bowel troubles are benefited by it. Two parts of the decoction of golden seal and one of cranesbill used as an injection is good for gonorrhea, gleet, and leucorrhea. Same is good for chronic cystitis. If too strong, weaken it. Good in this form, mixed with cranesbill, for diarrhea and dysentery; taken in two teaspoonful doses every three hours.

GRAVEL PLANT. Gravel-Weed. Mountain Pink. Ground Laurel. May Flower. Trailing Arbutus. *Epigea Repens.*

Internally, used for.--Gravel and irritable bladder, causes more urine to flow, just as buchu does.

Part used.--The leaves.

Gather.--In summer.

Flowers (when).--Appear in April and May.

Grows (where).--Canada and United States, on sides of hills with northern exposure.

Prepared (how).--Infusion, and fluid extract which can be bought. Use one ounce of the leaves to one pint of boiling water and let it steep to make an infusion.

Diseases, Dose, etc.--Dose: One to two teaspoonfuls. For gravel, take one teaspoonful every three hours. For irritable bladder take half teaspoonful every three hours.

HOPS. *Humulus Lupulus.*

Internally, used for.--Nervousness, sleeplessness, hysteria, in afterpains, to prevent chordee.

Externally, used for.--Used as a fomentation in many inflammatory diseases.

Part used.--Cones.

Gather.--In the fall or when fully ripe.

Grows (where).--Native of North America and Europe.

Prepared (how).--Infusion, tincture and fluid extract lupulin.

Diseases, Dose, etc.--Dose of infusion, two to four ounces; tincture one to four drams. Fluid extract, five to twenty drops. For nervous troubles, take one ounce of the infusion, or one dram tincture, every hour or two until quiet; same for sleeplessness. In delirium tremens, infusion drank with some red pepper in it settles the stomach and quiets the craving for drink. Following is good for chordee, etc.:

Lupulin	1 dram.
Camphor monobromate	1 dram.
Cocoa Butter, sufficient.	

Make twelve suppositories and insert one in rectum every three or four hours. Take at the same time, the infusion or tincture every two or three hours. Fomentations are good in pleurisy and many other inflammations. Inhale steam in throat and chest troubles.

HORSE CHESTNUT. *Aesculus Hippocastanum.*

Internally, used for.--Rheumatism. Used especially for piles.

Part used.--Bark and fruit which contains tannin.

Gather.--Late autumn.

Flowers (when).--In May and June, and fruit ripens late in autumn.

Grows (where).--Native of Asia. Naturalized here.

Prepared (how).--Powder of the rind of the root or powdered fruit. Decoction made of the bark by using one and one-half ounces to a pint of water and boiling.

Diseases, Dose, etc.--Dose: For rheumatism two ounces, three times a day. For piles, make an ointment of the powdered nut and apply. This is very good.

HOARHOUND. White Hoarhound. *Marrubium Vulgare.*

Internally, used for.--Coughs, colds, bronchitis, chronic asthma, sweating, hoarseness.

Part used.--Whole herb.

Gather.--When fresh.

Grows (where).--Naturalized in United. States. Grows in dry sandy fields, waste grounds, roadsides; etc.

Prepared (how).--Infusion hot and cold by adding one ounce to pint of water; fluid extract.

Diseases, Dose, etc.--Dose of infusion, two to four ounces; fluid extract, one to two teaspoonfuls. A syrup is also made; dose, two ounces. Infusion used hot for sweating, freely and often; cold and chest troubles about every two to four hours; or use fluid extract. The hot infusion should be used in asthma, amenorrhea, and hoarseness.

JUNIPER. *Juniper Communis.*

Internally, used for.--Dropsy, and to increase flow of urine in kidney troubles.

Part used.--Berries.

Gather.--August.

Flowers (when).--In May and June and ripe in August.

Grows (where).--Grows in United States and Canada, in dry woods and hills.

Prepared (how).--In infusion or oil. For infusion, use one ounce of the berries to a pint of boiling water. It can be made more effective by adding half ounce of cream of tartar to the infusion.

Diseases, Dose, etc.--It should be used within the twenty-four hours for above troubles, dropsy, etc. The oil can be bought and used in doses of five to twenty drops, three or four times a day.

LADY'S SLIPPER. American Valerian. Yellow Umbel. Nerve Root. Yellow Moccasin Flower. Noah's Ark. *Cypripedium Pubescens.*

Internally, used for.--Hysteria, chorea, nervous headache, nervousness, delirium, hypochondria.

Part used.--The root.

Gather.--In autumn, cleanse from dirt and dry in the shade. Virtue impaired by boiling.

Flowers (when).--In May and June.

Grows (where).--Most parts of United States in rich woods and meadows.

Prepared (how).--In infusion, powder and tincture.

Diseases, Dose, etc.--Dose of powder, thirty to sixty grains in hot water. Tincture, one to two teaspoonfuls. Infusion, one to four ounces. For chronic cases large doses three or four times daily. For acute cases half as much every two or three hours. For nervous headache two doses, half hour apart. Following is a good preparation for nervous or sick headache: catnip, scullcap and lady's slipper, in powder, of each one-half ounce. Pour on a pint of boiling water and steep for fifteen minutes, and take half ounce every half hour, for three or four hours.

LIFE ROOT. Rag Wort. Squaw Weed. Female Regulator. *Senecio Gracilis.*

Internally, used for.--Mainly for menstrual disorders, when suppressed or too profuse, dysmenorrhea.

Part used.--Root and herb.

Gather.--In autumn.

Flowers (when).--May or June.

Grows (where).--Northern and western United States on banks of creeks and in low marshy grounds.

Prepared (how).--In infusion, by adding half ounce to a pint of boiling water and let steep and take throughout twenty-four hours. Take four or five days before menstruation is expected.

Diseases, Dose, etc.--For amenorrhea and dysmenorrhea it may be combined in equal parts with savin and wild ginger, and take one to two ounces four times a day some days before menstruation. In menorrhagia--too much flow--cinnamon and raspberry leaves can be combined with it. Dose, two to four ounces four times a day.

LOBELIA. Wild or Indian Tobacco. Emetic Herb. Puke Weed. Asthma Weed. *Lobelia Inflata.*

Internally, used for.--Asthma, emetic for croup (but very weakening), and lung diseases.

Part used.--Leaves and seeds. Dry carefully in the shade. Keep whole or powdered.

Gather.--August or September.

Flowers (when).--July to September.

Grows (where).--Very common, growing in fields and roadsides.

Prepared (how).--As an infusion, one ounce to pint of water, steeped; also tincture.

Diseases, Dose, etc.--Dose of the tincture, five to ten drops. Infusion, one to two teaspoonfuls. It should not be used strong enough to produce vomiting, as it is too weakening. In small doses and given often in infusion it produces sweating and relaxation of the tissues, thus helping in asthma and lung diseases; For asthma, dose:-- Ten drops of tincture every ten minutes at the onset until better or until there is a little nausea, and then lengthen the interval.

MAIDENHAIR. *Adiantum Pedatum.*

Internally, used for.--Expectorant, tonic and cooling uses; in fevers, erysipelas, and pleurisy, coughs, hoarseness, influenza.

Part used.--Part above the ground.

Gather.--In autumn.

Grows (where).--In United States in deep woods, on moist rich soil.

Prepared (how).--As a decoction or syrup. Take an ounce of the herb to a pint of boiling water and boil to make a decoction.

Diseases, Dose, etc.--Use freely. For feverish conditions use one to two ounces every two hours. In coughs and hoarseness, take four to five times daily. For influenza and pleurisy enough to produce perspiration.

MANDRAKE. May Apple. Wild Lemon. Indian Apple. Raccoon Berry. *Podophyllum Peltatum.*

Internally, used for.--A cathartic, alterative action in liver troubles in chronic hepatitis; in blood diseases as syphilis, rheumatism; clears liver; for constipation.

Part used.--Root.

Gather.--In autumn soon after fruit has ripened.

Flowers (when).--May and June and fruit ripens in September.

Grows (where).--In all parts of the United States, in damp and shady woods and sometimes in dry and exposed places.

Prepared (how).--In powder and tincture. To make tincture: Gather the fresh root before the fruit is ripe, chop and pound to a pulp, and weigh. Then take two parts of alcohol by weight, mix the pulp thoroughly with one-sixth of the alcohol and then add the rest of the alcohol. Stir all, pour into a well stoppered bottle, let stand eight days, in a cool place. Pour off, strain, filter.

Diseases, Dose, etc.--The resin, called podophyllin, can be obtained, and is used in one-fourth to one-eighth grain as a laxative; one-sixteenth of a grain can be taken four times a day for chronic liver trouble. Take ten drops of tincture four times a day for chronic diseases. Some can take more. For blood diseases., rheumatism, etc.

MARSHMALLOW. Mortification Root. *Altheae Officinalis.*

Internally, used for.--Hoarseness, gonorrhea, irritated bladder, acute dysentery, and diarrhea, blood in urine and gravel.

Externally, used for.--Poultice for painful swellings, bruises, scalds, burns, poisons.

Part used.--Root.

Gather.--Autumn.

Flowers (when).--July to September.

Grows (where).--Europe and this country.

Prepared (how).--Poultice; cut up finely and apply hot. Decoction half ounce to two pints of boiling water and boil down to one pint.

Diseases, Dose, etc.--Take one to three ounces four times a day for chronic diseases, and one ounce every two hours for acute troubles mentioned above. It is a mild soothing drink and medicine.

MARIGOLD. *Calendula Officinalis.*

Externally, used.--As a local remedy for cuts and wounds, applied constantly, it is the best remedy I know.

Part used.--Leaves and flowers.

Gather.--When in full bloom.

Grows (where).--Well-known garden plant.

Prepared (how).--Make a tincture of the flowers and leaves, or buy it. To make tincture: Take the fresh leaves at the top of the plant with the blossoms and buds, chop and pound to a pulp, enclose in a piece of new linen and press. Shake the expressed juice, with an equal part of alcohol by weight, allow it to stand eight days in a well stoppered bottle, in a dark cool place and then filter.

Diseases, Dose, etc.--Use freely on clean linen or gauze on wounds, cuts, etc.

MILKWEED. Also called Silkweed. *Asclepias Syriaca.*

Internally, used for.--Dropsy, retention of urine, scrofulous and rheumatic troubles.

Part used.--Root. Plant gives out a milky juice when wounded.

Gather.--In autumn.

Flowers (when).--July and August.

Grows (where).--Common in United States and grows in sandy fields, on the roadsides and on bank of streams.

Prepared (how).--Powder, decoction and tincture. Decoction is made by using three ounces of the root to one quart of water, and boil.

Diseases, Dose, etc.--Take as directed four times a day. Dose of tincture, ten to thirty drops four times a day. Can be bought. Dose, of the powder, ten to twenty grains. Decoction, two to four ounces.

MOTHERWORT. *Leonurus Cardiaca.*

Internally, used for.--Menstrual disorders, nervousness, cramps, amenorrhea from colds, suppressed lochia, hysteria, pains peculiar to women, disturbed sleep.

Externally, used for.--Used as a fomentation over womb in dysmenorrhea.

Part used.--Tops and leaves.

Gather.--Early autumn.

Flowers (when).--May and September.

Grows (where).--In fields and pastures.

Prepared (how).--Decoctions, use two ounces of dried herb to a quart of water and boil down to a pint.

Diseases, Dose, etc.--One to two tablespoonfuls every two hours. Smaller doses can be used for nervous women every hour, and when there are painful menstruations, suppressed lochia, hysteria, sleeplessness, etc.

MUSTARD. *Sinapis Alba.*

Internally, used for.--As an emetic, condiment, hiccough.

Externally, used for.--Counter-irritation.

Part used.--The seeds or leaves.

Gather.--While fresh, so the leaves can also be used. Seeds when used should be ripe.

Grows (where).--Almost everywhere.

Prepared (how).--In many ways, poultices, plasters, etc.

Diseases, Dose, etc.--Mustard leaves dampened with cold water are good for pleurodynia, lumbago, neuritis, cramps in legs, inflammations, croup, etc., applied locally. For apoplexy and convulsions, mustard poultices of the seeds to feet, and mustard foot baths, handful of ground mustard to hot water. Same is good in colds, sleeplessness, dysmenorrhea, headache. Mustard water is good for poisoning as an emetic. Hiccough: Teaspoonful of mustard in four ounces of boiling water, steep for twenty minutes, and take in four doses.

OAK BARK. (Red and White). *Quercus Alba.*

Internally, used for.--Leucorrhea, piles, diarrhea, sore throat and mouth.

Externally, used for.--Sores on man or beast.

Part used.--The bark; white oak is more astringent.

Prepared (how).--Decoction.

Diseases, Dose, etc.--This decoction is used as an injection in leucorrhea, piles and as a gargle in sore mouth, etc. Its astringent property is due to the tannic and gallic acid it contains.

ONION. *Allium Cepa.*

Internally, used for.--Coughs, catarrh, croup, laxative.

Externally, used for.--Poultice for boil, inflammation, earache, etc., raw and roasted and used locally.

Part used.--Bulb. It contains many constituents, such as citrate of lime, allyl sulphide, volatile oils, sulphur.

Gather.--In autumn.

Grows (where).--Native.

Prepared (how).--As a poultice, raw; when boiled volatile oil is cast off.

Diseases, Dose, etc.--Juice mixed with sugar is good for colds, coughs, catarrh, croup, chronic bronchitis. Roasted Spanish onion is good, eaten at bedtime, as a laxative; fried in lard and applied locally it makes a splendid poultice. Roasted in coals it makes a good poultice for earache, toothache, sore throat and sore chest.

PARSLEY. Rock Parsley. *Petroselinum Sativum.*

Internally, used for.--Dropsy, especially following scarlet fever, retained urine, painful urination, gonorrhea.

Externally, used for.--Seeds and leaves sprinkled on the hair, in powder, destroy vermin. Bruised leaves applied as a fomentation, cure the bites or stings of insects.

Part used.--Root, seeds and leaves.

Gather.--In autumn.

Grows (where).--Cultivated.

Prepared (how).--Infuse the whole plant, or a decoction can be made of the root and seeds.

Diseases, Dose, etc.--Drink freely of the infusion or decoction. Dose, two to four ounces three times a day, or less dose and oftener. The oil can be bought and used, two to three drops three or four times, daily.

PARTRIDGE BERRY. Squaw Vine. Checker Berry. One Berry. Winter Clover. Deerberry. *Mitchella Repens,*

Internally, used for.--Dropsy, suppressed urine, tonic and alterative action on womb.

Externally, used for--Cure for sore nipples.

Part used.--The vine.

Gather.--During the season.

Flowers (when).--June and July.

Grows (where).--In United States and Canada; in dry woods, among hemlock timber and in swampy places.

Prepared (how).--Infusion, tincture, fluid extract, decoction. Infusion, one ounce to pint of boiling water. Tincture: chop fresh plant and pound to a pulp and weigh. Then take two parts, by weight, of alcohol; mix pulp with one-sixth part of it thoroughly and rest of alcohol added, stir all well, pour into a well stoppered bottle and let stand eight days in a dark cool place; pour off, strain and filter.

Diseases, Dose, etc.--Dose of tincture, one-half to one teaspoonful. For chronic diseases take one to two ounces of infusion four times a day. For suppressed urine take half ounce every two hours. Dose of infusion, from one to two ounces every three hours. To tone the womb and make labor easier, the Indians used to take it several weeks before confinement. For sore nipple: two ounces (fresh, if possible) and make a strong decoction in a pint of boiling water. Boil down thick and apply on nipple after each nursing.

PEACH TREE. *Amygdalus Persica.*

Internally, used for.--Constipation, tonic to the stomach and bowels, leucorrhea, worms, inflammation of stomach and bowels, irritable bladder. haematuria, dysentery.

Part used.--Leaves and kernels.

Gather.--When ripe.

Grows (where).--Cultivated.

Prepared (how).--By infusion; put ounce of leaves in one pint of cold water and let it steep.

Diseases, Dose, etc.--For inflammations take one tablespoonful of the cold infusion every hour or two. For bladder and urinary troubles and leucorrhea, put four ounces of the kernels in a quart of brandy; dose,--teaspoonful three or four times a day. For bowel troubles use half ounce of the flowers and half ounce of the kernels to a pint of water; boil to make a decoction and sweeten; dose,--teaspoonful occasionally, until relieved; for teething children and for worms use about five doses.

PENNYROYAL. Squaw Mint. Tickweed. *Hedeoma Pulegoides.*

Internally, used for.--Stimulant, sweating, menstrual troubles, suppressed lochia, suppressed menses, flatulent colic in children.

Part used.--The herb. **Gather.**--In fall. **Flowers (when).**--June to October.

Grows (where).--In dry sterile places in calcareous soils. In all parts of the United States, etc.

Prepared (how).--An infusion, one ounce to a pint of boiling water and only steep, not boil.

Diseases, Dose, etc.--Use infusion freely. Dose of oil two to five drops. For menstrual troubles, checked lochia and perspiration, take a hot foot bath in bed and drink freely of the tea until sweating occurs. It is frequently taken at bedtime for painful menstruation, etc.

PEPPERMINT. *Mentha Piperita.*

Internally, used for.--Tone stomach, colic, spasms, or cramps in stomach, to check nausea and vomiting.

Externally, used for.--Fresh herb bruised and laid over the abdomen, to allay sick stomach and diarrhea of children.

Part used.--The whole herb.

Gather.--Early autumn.

Flowers (when).--July to September.

Grows (where).--Native of England, cultivated here and grows wild in wet places.

Prepared (how).--Essence, oil; infusion made by adding one ounce of herb to a quart of boiling water and steep.

Disease, Dose, etc.--One to two ounces of infusion at a dose. The best form is the essence or oil. Dose of the essence five to ten drops; of oil one to five drops. It should be used carefully.

28

PLANTAIN. *Plantago Major.*

Externally, used for.--It is better used externally; the bruised leaves are good for poisonous wounds, bites of snakes, spiders and insects, ulcers, sore eyelids, salt rheum, erysipelas, poisoning from ivy and other skin affections.

Part used.--Roots and tops.

Flowers (when).--From May to October.

Grows (where).--Well known and grows in rich moist places.

Prepared (how).--Tincture, infusion, bruised leaves for external use.

Diseases, Dose, etc.--Some claim the infusion is good for snake bites or the expressed juice can be used. This, to my mind, is doubtful and I would advise the usual remedies first. The tincture is good for some kinds of toothache, in one to two drop doses. The bruised leaves or the tea may be used for other diseases mentioned as poultice or wash.

PLEURISY ROOT. Butterfly Weed. Wind Root. Tuber Root. Orange Swallow Wort. *Asclepias Tuberosa.*

Internally, used for.--Pleurisy, pneumonia, catarrh, acute rheumatism, diarrhea, dysentery, sweating and expectorant, falling womb.

Part used.--Root.

Gather.--Autumn.

Flowers (when).--July and August.

Grows (where).--In gravelly and sandy soils.

Prepared (how).--Infusion, one ounce to a pint of boiling water and let steep. Tincture; buy powder.

Diseases, Dose, etc.--Dose of powder, ten to thirty grains three times a day in womb diseases. For falling womb use one ounce pleurisy root and one-half ounce unicorn root (true), mix powder and give in twenty to thirty grain doses three times daily; and an injection of the same, in infusion, may be given once a day. For pleurisy, etc., in first stage give the warm infusion to promote sweating. Dose,--Four teaspoonfuls every half hour, until sweating is produced. Following is good for diarrhea and dysentery: Tincture pleurisy root two ounces, brandy one ounce, syrup of raspberry three ounces. Half to one teaspoonful everyone or two hours.

POKE. Garget. Coakum. Pingeon Berry. Scoke. *Phytolacca Decandra.*

Internally, used for.--Chronic rheumatism, syphilis, sore throat, sore, inflamed breasts, scrofula.

Externally, used for--For fat people. Caked breasts, felons and tumors.

Part used.--Root, leaves and berries.

Gather.--Root late in November, cut in thin transverse slices and dry with moderate heat. Berries, when ripe.

Flowers (when).--July to September.

Grows (where).--Native of United States along fences in newly cleared spots, in cultivated fields, roadsides, etc.

Prepared (how).--Juice of plant. Powdered root, poultice, fomentation.

Diseases, Dose, etc.--One to five grains of powdered root as an alterative in chronic blood diseases, syphilis, etc. Juice of plant, half teaspoonful three times a day, for same diseases can be used. For caked breasts one to three drops of the tincture every one to three hours, at same time applying the root (roasted in ashes until soft) mashed and applied as a poultice; good also for a felon or can apply a hot fomentation of the leaves instead.

PRICKLY ASH. Toothache Tree. *Xanthoxylum Fraxineum.*

Internally, used for.--Chronic rheumatism, syphilis, skin affections, dysmenorrhea.

Externally, used for.--Decoction used as a wash or gargle in sore throat.

Part used.--Bark and berries.

Gather.--Autumn or earlier in some climates.

Flowers (when).--April and May.

Grows (where).--United States in woods, thickets and moist shady places.

Prepared (how).--Tincture. Powder. Decoction of root one ounce to a pint of water and boil.

Diseases, Dose, etc.--Dose,--half ounce every four to five hours. Tincture of the berries is also used for nervous diseases, dysmenorrhea, etc., in ten to thirty drops every two to four hours. Good also in blood diseases, four times a day. Powder for same troubles in doses of five to ten grains four times a day.

PRINCE'S PINE. Wintergreen. Ground Holly. Pipsissewa. Rheumatism Weed. *Chimaphila Umbellata.*

Internally, used for.--Kidney and bladder troubles, chronic rheumatism, syphilis, scrofula, gout, gleet.

Part used.--Whole plant.

Gather.--In autumn or late summer.

Flowers (when).--June and July.

Grows (where).--United States, etc., under the shade of woods and prefers a loose sandy soil enriched by decaying leaves.

Prepared (how).--Decoction and tincture; put a pound of the dried herb into a quart of water and three quarts of spirits; let stand for twelve days, and then turn off the liquid. This makes a tincture. To make decoction use one ounce of plant to a pint of boiling water and boil.

Diseases, Dose, etc.--Take one to two ounces of the decoction three or four times a day; fluid extract can be bought, dose fifteen drops four times daily. Dose of tincture, one-half to one teaspoonful.

PUMPKIN. *Cucurbita Pepo.*

Internally, used for.--For tape worm and for urinary troubles, suppressed or retained urine.

Gather.--When ripe.

Grows (where).--Common.

Prepared (how).--A tea can be made of the seeds, or an oil gathered from them.

Diseases, Dose, etc.--A tea strong or weak as the age and case demand, may be given freely and is very effective. Do not bruise the seeds, as the virtue resides in the covering. An oil can be gathered from the seeds and is good for same purpose. Dose.--Six to twelve drops several times daily or three drops every two hours. For Tape worm, see article on another page. If it is best to take it as an emulsion get druggist to make it. Taken at night with fasting. In the morning take dose of salts. Watermelon seed tea is also good for kidney trouble.

QUEEN OF THE MEADOW. Purple Boneset. Gravel Root. Trumpet Weed.

Joe-Pye Weed. *Eupatorium Purpureum.*

Internally, used for.--Gravel stone in the bladder, kidney or stone colic, or other urinary troubles.

Part used.--The herb.

Gather.--Autumn.

Flowers (when).--August to November.

Grows (where).--In wet places in United States.

Prepared (how).--Fluid extract; or an infusion, one ounce of the dried leaves or plant in a quart of boiling water and steep.

Diseases, Dose, etc.--Half teacupful of the infusion may be taken every hour or two as hot as possible. This is a splendid remedy. Drug stores keep the fluid extract, which can be bought and given in doses of fifteen to thirty drops every three or four hours. Some claim it relieves the pain in the kidney stone colic; the Indians used it for that purpose.

QUEEN'S ROOT. Queen's Delight. Yaw Root. Cock-up-Hat. *Stillingia Sylvatica.*

Internally, used for.--Secondary syphilis, scrofula, chronic skin diseases.

Part used.--The root. **Gather.**--Autumn.

Flowers (when).--April to July.

Grows (where).--In United States, etc.

Prepared (how).--An infusion of the fresh root, or use the tincture or fluid extract. One ounce of root to pint of water for infusion.

Diseases, Dose, etc.--Dose of infusion one to two ounces. Tincture; dose, twenty to sixty drops. Extract; dose, ten to thirty drops; smaller doses given every two or three hours; larger dose three or four times daily. This is a good remedy. It can be given with other remedies like poke root, sarsaparilla, etc.

RED CLOVER. *Trifolium Pratense.*

Internally, used for.--Blood diseases and is often used with other remedies; good drank warm in whooping cough.

Externally, used for.--Ulcers. **Part used.**--Blossoms.

Gather.--When fresh. **Flowers (when).**--Throughout summer.

Grows (where).--Common.

Prepared (how).--In infusion and salve.

Diseases, Dose, etc.--Use blossoms to make tea and drink freely; tea boiled down thick makes a good salve for ill-conditioned looking sores.

ROCK ROSE. Frost wort. Frost Plant. *Cistus Canadensis.*

Internally, used for.--Scrofula and blood diseases.

Part used.--The herb. **Gather.**--In autumn early.

Flowers (when).--From May to July.

Grows (where).--In United States in dry sandy soil.

Prepared (how).--Infusion. Fluid extract. Decoction, use four ounces of the dried leaves to one quart of boiling water and boil.

Diseases, Dose, etc.--Dose of infusion or decoction, one ounce three times a day. Fluid extract is the best form, can be bought and given in doses of half to one teaspoonful three or four times a day. The following combination is good one for secondary syphilis: Rock rose, turkey corn, Queen's root, equal parts; either the infusion, decoction or fluid extract.

SAGE. Garden sage. *Salvia Officinalis.*

Internally, used for.--To stop sweating in consumption, used cold; and used warm to sweat. Gargle in sore throat, colds, coughs, etc., alone or combined with sumach berries or vinegar, or honey or alum.

Part used.--The leaves.

Gather.--In early autumn;

Flowers (when).--In June.

Grows (where).--Cultivated.

Prepared (how).--As an infusion cold or hot; half ounce of leaves to a pint of boiling water.

Diseases, Dose, etc.--Dose, an ounce or two. To produce perspiration give warm. To check perspiration give cold, in smaller doses and oftener. For sore mouth, sore throat, tonsilitis and quinsy, use hot infusion strong as a gargle.

SCOURING RUSH. Horse Tail. Shave Grass. *Equisetum Hyemale.*

Internally, used for.--Dropsy, suppression of the urine, blood in the urine, gravel, gonorrhea and gleet.

Part used.--The stalk.

Gather.--Matures in June and July,

Grows (where).--In wet grounds in river banks, hillsides, and borders of woods in United States.

Prepared (how).--Infusion, one ounce to the pint of water.

Diseases, Dose, etc.--For above diseases drink in half ounce doses every two hours.

SASSAFRAS. *Laurus Sassafras.*

Internally, used for.--Syphilis, scrofula, skin eruptions, bland drink after poisoning,

Part used.--The bark of the root. **Gather.**--In autumn.

Flowers (when).--April and May. **Grows (where).**--Common.

Prepared (how).--Infusion of the bark, one ounce to a pint of water; as a mucilage made by using two parts of the pith to one hundred of water. Do not boil.

Diseases, Dose, etc.--Dose of infusion, one to two ounces. Oil, five to ten drops on sugar for menstrual pain, and in painful urination. The mucilage is good for chest disorders, bowels, kidneys and for inflammation after poisoning, as a bland demulcent drink.

SENECA SNAKE ROOT. Mountain Flag. Milk Wort. Seneka or Senega. *Polyagla Senega.*

Internally, used for.--Second stage of bronchitis in aged people, bronchial asthma, coughs.

Part used.--The root.

Gather.--In autumn.

Flowers (when).--June to August.

Grows (where).--In United States in woods and on hillsides.

Prepared (how).--Powdered root. For decoction use one ounce of the dried root to a pint of boiling water and let boil. You can buy the syrup and fluid extract.

Diseases, Dose, etc.--Dose of the decoction, half to one ounce three or four times a day. Dose of the syrup, one to two teaspoonfuls. Dose of the extract, ten to twenty drops. This remedy is frequently used with other remedies for bronchitis and cough.

SHEEP SORREL. *Rumex Acetosa.*

Internally, used for.--Scurvy.

Externally, used for.--Good for wens, boils, tumor, ulcers.

Part used.--Plant. **Gather.**--Autumn. **Grows (where).**--Well - known plant.

Prepared (how).--Decoction; poultice made of roasted leaves.

Diseases, Dose, etc.--Decoction, freely drank for scurvy. Poultices should be applied to above troubles.

SKUNK CABBAGE. Swamp Cabbage. Meadow Cabbage. Polecat Weed. Fetid Hellebore. Dracontium. *Ictodes Foetida.*

Internally, used for.--Asthma, whooping cough, nervousness, hysteria, convulsions of pregnancy.

Part used.--Root. **Gather.**--In autumn or early spring and dried carefully.

Flowers (when).--March and April.

Grows (where).--Various parts of United States in moist places.

Prepared (how).--Powder. Tincture.

Diseases, Dose, etc.--Dose: Five to ten grains of powder three times a day. A saturated tincture of the fresh root is much better, of which half a teaspoonful can be given everyone to four hours for above diseases.

SKULL CAP. Madweed. Hoodwort. Blue Pimpernel. *Scutellaria Lateriflora.*

Internally, used for.--Chorea, delirium, convulsions, neuralgia, restlessness, insomnia.

Part used.--The whole herb.

Gather.--Late summer while in flower.

Flowers (when).--July and August.

Grows (where).--In moist places.

Prepared (how).--Infusion, one ounce to the pint.

Diseases, Dose, etc.--The infusion may be drank freely, Fluid extract, dose, half to one teaspoonful, every two or three hours.

SLIPPERY ELM. Red Elm. *Ulmus Fulva.*

Internally, used for.--As a mucilage for stomach and bowel and urinary troubles when a mild, soothing demulcent drink is needed; in diarrhea, dysentery, coughs, painful urination, constipation.

Externally, used for.--As a poultice.

Part used.--Inner bark.

Gather.--Early fall. **Flowers (when).**--In April.

Grows (where).--In United States, in open elevated situations in rich firm soil.

Prepared (how).--Infusion of two ounces to pint of water. Mucilage made by using six parts of the dried bark to one hundred of water and allow to steep.

Diseases, Dose, etc.--The infusion and mucilage may be taken freely. The infusion can be injected for dysentery, diarrhea, gonorrhea, gleet and leucorrhea. Mucilage is taken after poisoning to allay inflammation of the membranes, etc. Eat bark or take prepared tablets for constipation.

SPEARMINT. *Mentha Viridis.*

Internally, used for.--Nausea and vomiting, internal and external scalding urine. For fever is superior to peppermint.

Externally, used for.--For piles. **Part used.**--The herb.

Gather.--Just as the flowers appear in dry weather, and dry in the shade.

Flowers (when).--July and August.

Grows (where).--United States in moist places.

Prepared (how).--Warm or cold infusion.

Diseases, Dose, etc.--Warm infusion, a handful of the herb to a quart of water and used freely to allay fever in inflammations, colds, etc. Cold infusion is good in highly colored or scalding urine. Local, saturate cotton with the strong infusion or diluted tincture, and apply to piles; use it hot.

SPIKENARD. Spignet. Pettymorrel. Pigeon-weed. *Aralia Racemosa.*

Internally, used for.--Coughs, colds, chronic rheumatism, syphilis.

Part used.--Root.

Gather.--In autumn.

Grows (where).--In dry rocky woods in United States.

Prepared (how).--Decoction. Syrup.

Diseases, Dose, etc.--Decoction, used freely in above diseases. It is an old home remedy. A syrup can also be made of it.

SMARTWEED. Water Pepper. *Polygonum Punctatum.*

Internally, used for.--Suppressed menstruation, to wash out the bladder, good for gravel, colds and coughs.

Externally, used for.--Fomentations.

Part used.--The whole herb.

Gather.--Autumn. **Flowers (when).**--August and September.

Grows (where).--About brooks and streams.

Prepared (how).--An infusion or a tincture made from the fresh plant. Use cold water to make infusion. Fomentations, simmer in water and vinegar.

Diseases, Dose, etc.--Dose of infusion, one to three ounces. Tincture, one to two teaspoonfuls. Apply fomentations for colic, bloating of abdomen; used often with other plants externally. For menstruation give half teaspoonful of the tincture four times a day a week before menstruation. Use small doses for other troubles.

SNAKE ROOT, VIRGINIA. *Aristolochia Serpentaria.*

Internally, used for.--Sweating for feverish conditions where eruptions are tardy in coming out.

Externally, used for.--For snake bites.

Part used.--Root.

Gather (when).--May and June.

Grows (where).--Hill-sides, in rich shady woods.

Prepared (how).--Powdered root. Infusion made by using four teaspoonfuls of the powdered root to a pint of water and let steep.

Diseases, Dose, etc.--Take two to three tablespoonfuls of the hot infusion every three to four hours. Dose of powdered root, ten to twenty grains in hot water.

SOLOMON'S SEAL. *Convallaria Multiflora.*

Internally, used for.--Female weakness, leucorrhea, menorrhagia.

Externally, used for.--Poultice for piles.

Part used.--Root.

Gather.--Autumn.

Flowers (when).--May and August.

Grows (where).--In United States and Canada, sides of meadows, high banks, woods, and mountain.

Prepared (how).--Decoction, use one ounce of the root to pint of water and boil. Poultice, bruise the root.

Diseases, Dose, etc.--Dose of the decoction, one to two ounces. Take less when it is taken oftener, as much as the stomach will bear. Make a poultice of the bruised root for piles and local inflammation.

STONE ROOT. Horse Balm. Rich Weed. Knob Root. Hard Hack. *Collinsonia Canadensis.*

Internally, used for.--Cramps, colic, dropsy, bladder troubles, gravel, leucorrhea.

Externally, used for.--Poultice for bruises, blows, wounds, strains.

Part used.--The plant.

Gather.--Autumn.

Grows (where).--United States and in Canada.

Prepared (how).--In infusion and poultice, steep the root in a covered dish.

Diseases, Dose, etc.--Dose of the infusion half to one ounce, three or four times a day.

STRAWBERRY. *Fragaria Vesca.*

Internally, used for.--Gravel, gout, irritable bladder, nettle rash, eruption.

Part used.--Fruit, roots, and leaves.

Gather.--When ripe.

Flowers (when).--Spring; April, May and June.

Prepared (how).--As an infusion.

Diseases, Dose, etc.--Leaves are astringent and good in infusion for sore mouth, diarrhea, and dysentery. Infusion of the root is a good diuretic and is effective in difficult urination and gonorrhea. Drink freely.

STRAMONIUM. Thorn-Apple. Stink Weed. Jimson Weed. Apple Pern. *Datura Stramonium.*

Internally, used for.--Used mainly for asthma.

Externally, used for.--Piles.

Part used.--Leaves.

Gather.--When leaves are green and when flowers are in bloom.

Flowers (when).--July to September.

Grows (where).--Along roads, etc.

Prepared (how).--Ointment. The leaves should be dried for smoking. It is rather dangerous.

Diseases, Dose, etc.--For asthma, the leaves are mixed with tobacco leaves and smoked. It must be done carefully as it is poisonous. The leaves are good to cure piles when rubbed on them, or made into an ointment and used locally.

SUMACH. *Rhus Glabra.*

Internally, used for.--Sore mouth and throat, quinsy, diarrhea, leucorrhea, gonorrhea, suppressed urine.

Part used.--Bark and fruit.

Gather.--Autumn. Berries earlier.

Flowers (when).--June and July.

Prepared (how).--Make an infusion as usual. Use either bark or berries.

Diseases, Dose, etc.--Fluid extract can be used and is safer; in doses of ten drops three times a day. The infusion will do as a gargle and a wash.

SWEET FLAG. Calamus. Flag Root. Sweet Rush. *Acorus Calamus.*

Internally, used for.--Disorders of the stomach, flatulency, dysentery, colic.

Part used.--Root.

Gather.--Late autumn or early spring, wash clean and dry with moderate heat.

Grows (where).--Borders of small streams, ponds, wet meadows, swamp.

Prepared (how).--Infusion made by scalding one ounce of the root in a pint of water.

Diseases, Dose, etc.--Dose: One to three ounces, warm, for general troubles; give hot for colic. One-third to a teaspoonful of the root can be taken.

ST. JOHN'S WORT. *Hypericum Perfoliatum.*

Internally, used for.--Suppressed urine, chronic urinary affections, diarrhea, menorrhagia, hysteria, etc.

Externally, used for.--Fomentations for caked breasts, hard tumors, bruises, swellings, stings and wounds.

Part used.--Tops and flowers.

Gather.--When fresh.

Flowers (when).--From June to August.

Grows (where).--In this country.

Prepared (how).--Ointment. Infusion of powder or blossoms. Infusion one ounce to one pint of boiling water.

Diseases, Dose, etc.--Dose of infusion, one to two ounces, three or four times daily or less. Powder; dose, thirty to sixty grains can be put in hot water and drank. Children's dose: Half to one teaspoonful. It should be taken three or four times daily in regular full doses for chronic diseases, and in half doses every two or three hours for acute diseases. Local.--Make an ointment of the tops and flowers, or boil down the infusion until thick, and make an ointment. First way is the best.

TANSY. *Tanacetum.* (Sometimes called double tansy).

Internally, used for.--Womb troubles and sweating, amenorrhea, dysmenorrhea, hysteria.

Part used.--The whole herb.

Gather.--In the summer.

Flowers (when).--July to September.

Grows (where).--Cultivated and also grows wild.

Prepared (how).--As an infusion and fomentation. The oil can be bought. To make infusion use one ounce of the plant to one pint of boiling water and let steep.

Diseases, Dose, etc.--Dose of the infusion one to two ounces. Oil, half to one drop. This oil is dangerous, so it must be taken carefully. For dysmenorrhea, take half ounce of infusion every hour or two.

Same for hysteria. For amenorrhea, two ounces three times daily. For sweating, it should be taken in one to two-ounce doses and hot. Fomentations should be used hot and are good placed on the abdomen, over the womb, in painful menstruation.

TURKEY CORN. Wild Turkey Pea. Stagger-Weed. *Corydalis Formosa.*

Internally, used for.--Tonic, diuretic and alterative, for syphilis and scrofula. (Eclectics esteem this a great remedy).

Part used.--Root, small round ball.

Gather.--While the plant is in flower.

Flowers (when).--In March.

Grows (where).--In rich soils, on hills and mountains, etc.

Prepared (how).--Tincture. Infusion, four teaspoonfuls of the powdered bulb to one pint of boiling water and let steep.

Diseases, Dose, etc.--Dose of the infusion, one to three ounces three or four times daily. Tincture, half to one teaspoonful. Tincture can be bought at a drug store.

TURNIP, INDIAN. Jack-in-the pulpit. Wild Turnip. Dragon Root. *Arum Triphyllum.*

Internally, used for.--Expectorant and sweating purposes in chest troubles. Also good for sore mouth and sore throat if given in honey or syrup.

Part used.--Root.

Gather.--In autumn.

Flowers (when).--From May to July.

Grows (where).--Common in South America in all moist and damp places.

Prepared (how).--Dry the root and powder it and give in honey or make into a syrup or given in powder.

Diseases, Dose, etc.--For sweating use powder in hot water, ten grains three times a day or smaller dose oftener. For bronchitis, etc., use in syrup or in honey, three or four times a day, five to ten grains at a dose. Same way for sore mouth and throat.

TRUE UNICORN ROOT. Star Grass. Colic Root. Ague Root. Crow Corn. *Aletris Farinosa.*

Internally, used for.--Its tonic influence upon the womb to prevent a tendency to miscarriage, for amenorrhea, dysmenorrhea, falling, also for chlorosis.

Part used.--The root.

Gather.--In autumn.

Flowers (when).--June and July.

Grows (where).--Most parts of United States, usually in dry sandy soils and barrens.

Prepared (how).--Powdered root. Tincture. Fluid extract.

Diseases, Dose, etc.--Powdered root, five to ten grains three times a day. Saturated tincture, two to five drops, three times a day. Fluid extract, five to ten drops. Tincture and fluid extract can be bought at any drug store. For the above diseases it should be taken regularly four times a day. The fluid extract is the best form in which to take it and is often given by doctors.

WAHOO. Indian Arrow Wood. Burning-Bush. Spindle Tree. *Enonymus Atropurpureus.*

Internally, used for.--Dyspepsia, torpid liver, laxative, tonic.

Part used.--The bark of the root.

Gather.--Autumn.

Flowers (when).--In June.

Grows (where).--In woods and thickets.

Prepared (how).--Powder. Tincture.

Diseases, Dose, etc.--Dose of powder, ten to twenty grains; saturated tincture, one to two teaspoonfuls; extract, one to five grains. This is a good remedy; smaller doses can be given every two hours for dyspepsia and liver complaint. It is often combined with remedies, like dandelion, yellow dock, burdock.

WILD CHERRY. *Prunus Virginianus.*

Internally, used for.--Tonic, dyspepsia, scrofula.

Part used.--The bark of the root.

Gather.--In autumn.

Flowers (when).--In May.

Prepared (how).--Powdered bark or infusion. One ounce of bark to one pint of cold water to make infusion, allow it to stand for a few hours.

Diseases, Dose, etc.--Take of infusion one to three ounces four or five times a day. Dose of powdered bark, one to two teaspoonfuls in hot water. For tonic action and for dyspepsia it should be taken oftener and in half the given doses.

WILD YAM. Colic Root. *Dioscorea Villosa.*

Internally, used for.--Bilious colic.

Part used.--Root.

Gather.--In autumn.

Flowers (when).--June and July.

Grows (where).--United States and in Canada, twining over bushes and fences, thickets and hedges.

Prepared (how).--Decoction of the root. Pour a pint of boiling water on two ounces of the bruised root, let steep slowly for half hour, strain.

Diseases, Dose, etc.--Give half cupful of decoction every twenty minutes for bilious colic. Some have given half a pint at once in a severe case.

WORMWOOD. *Artemisia Absinthium.*

Internally, used for.--Worms, jaundice, dyspepsia, amenorrhea and leucorrhea.

Externally, used for.--Bruises, local inflammations.

Part used.--Tops and leaves.

Flowers (when).--In July and August.

Grows (where).--United States.

Prepared (how).--Fomentations. An infusion is made by adding thirteen of the herbs to a pint of cold water.

Diseases, Dose, etc.--Dose of infusion one to four teaspoonfuls. Use fomentations for bruises and local inflammation.

WORMSEED. Goose Foot. Stinking Weed. *Chenopodium Anthelminticum.*

Internally, used for.--Worms, round worms.

Part used.--Seeds and herb.

Gather.--In late autumn.

Flowers (when).--July to September.

Grows (where).--United States, in waste places.

Prepared (how).--Oil.

Diseases, Dose, etc.--Four to eight drops of oil to be given night and morning, for four or five days, and then followed by a purgative. Combination: Oil of wormseed one ounce, oil of tansy one ounce, spirits of turpentine one and one-half ounce, castor oil one pint. Dose for a child, a teaspoonful every hour until it operates; for an adult one tablespoonful. Powdered herb: Dose, half to one teaspoonful.

YARROW. Milfoil. Thousand Leaf. *Achillea Millefolium.*

Internally, used for.--Bleeding from the lungs, kidneys, piles, dysentery, menorrhagia.

Part used.--The herb.

Flowers (when).--Nearly whole summer.

Grows (where).--Europe and America in fields, woods, pastures.

Prepared (how).--Decoction, half ounce of plant to six ounces of water and boil down to three ounces. Juice of the herb is also used.

Diseases, Dose, etc.--In menorrhagia either can be used, as well as in other diseases. Tablespoonful of decoction every hour. The expressed juice in two or three tablespoonful doses may be taken three times a day.

YELLOW DOCK. *Rumex Crispus.*

Internally, used for.--Skin disease, scrofula, syphilis, scurvy.

Externally, used for.--Fresh root bruised in cream is good applied to ulcers, tumors and itch.

Part used.--The root.

Gather.--Early autumn.

Flowers (when).--June and July.

Grows (where).--In pastures, dry fields, etc.

Prepared (how).--One ounce root to a pint of boiling water. Let steep.

Diseases, Dose, etc.--One or two ounces, three times a day; or half ounce every three hours. This is a good remedy. Some people should commence with smaller doses.

T. J. Ritter

HOMEOPATHY

The Treatment Of About One Hundred Twenty Diseases According To Homeopathy

In cities and in most towns Homeopathic medicine will be found in drug stores in their special preparations. Some drug stores handle Homeopathic medicines exclusively.

MEDICINES.--Homeopathic medicines should be kept in a dry cool place. Do not leave them standing open among odors or exposed to bright lights. The following are among those common for home use:

List of Remedies.

Aconitum
Antimonium crudum
Antimonium tartaricum
Apis
Arnica radix
Arsenicum
Belladonna
Bryonia
Chamomilla
China
Cina
Cinchona (see China)
Colocynthis
Cuprum metallicum
Gelsemium
Hepar Sulphuricum
Hyoscyamus
Ipecacuanha
Lycopodium
Mercurius
Natrum muriaticum
Nux Vomica
Opium
Phosphoric acid
Phosphorus
Pulsatilla
Rhus toxicodendron
Sanguinaria
Sepia
Silicea
Spigelia
Spongia
Sulphur
Veratrum album

Fluid for External Use.

Arnica.
Calendula.

Care of Medicine in the Sick Room.--Use a *clean* tumbler and when not using cover the tumbler with a small saucer or piece of cardboard. Set it in a cool place and where it is free from odors, as liquid medicines exposed are likely to take up such impurities.

DIRECTIONS FOR USING HOMEOPATHIC MEDICINES.

They are prepared in two forms, Dilutions and Triturations (powdered form). From the triturations tablets are made. When we write "3X dil." that means 3X dilution; when we write "3X trit." that means 3X trituration. The 3X means or indicates the strength of the medicine. We have different dilutions and triturations, as IX, 2X, 3X, 4X, etc., according to the strength of the medicine used and we say dil. or trit., for dilution or trituration, depending upon the form to be used. Tablets are handier to use than the triturations or powder. In this book when I write trituration I shall always expect you to use it in the form of tablets. Instead of giving directions in every disease how to prepare the medicine, I will give it here.

When you use the medicine in the dilution (liquid) form, you put ten to fifteen drops of the dilution (say the 2X or any one) in a glass half full of water and give one to two teaspoonsful everyone-half to one to two or three hours, as the case may be, according to the age of the patient, etc. This is for acute cases.

For chronic cases.--You give medicine three or four times a day, one to two teaspoonfuls at a time. When you use it in trituration (tablet) form, you give one to two tablets at a dose every one-half to one, two or three hours, etc. In chronic cases three or four times a day, one or two tablets.

For the beginning of a common cold.--Aconite 2X dil. Put ten drops in a glass half full of water and take two teaspoonsful every one-half hour for three doses, then every three hours for twelve hours. Tincture of camphor in drop doses is also good.

If throat feels raw and sore.--I give three tablets of Mercurius bin. 2X trit. (tablet form) in alternation with the Aconite for three doses. Then stop it.

LA GRIPPE.--Gelsemium IX dil. Put ten drops in a glass half full of water and give one to two teaspoonfuls everyone-half to two hours. Feels sick, achy and bad all over; generally good at the beginning.

Belladonna 3X dil. if throat is raw and sore, throbbing, beating arteries, tickling annoying hard cough.

Mercurius 3X trit. (tablet form). When throat is sore with much saliva, sticky sweat which does not relieve.

Bryonia 2X dil. Grip with cold on chest, hurts to cough.

Phosphorus 3X dil. In bronchial tubes under breast bones.

Arsenicum 3X trit. (tablet form) stopped nose, watery burning discharge; feverish, thirsty and restless; chills and fever.

STOMATITIS.--Meaning a simple inflammation of the mouth.

Mercurius sol. 3X trit. (tablet form). Give one to two every one to three hours, according to the case.

APHTHAE (Thrush) in Children.--1 Mercurius sol. 3X trit. (tablet form). Indicated when it extends downward and produces diarrhea. Give one tablet every four hours for a few days.

29

2. Arsenicum 3X trit. (tablet form). Give one tablet every two to four hours, when the parts look bluish and livid, with great weakness, much thirst and restlessness, with burning watery diarrhea.

In Adults.--Arsenicum 3X trit. (tablet form). Give about two tablets every three hours when the edge of the tongue is ulcerated and whitish with violent burning pains.

Mercurius 3X trit. (tablet form). Give two tablets every three hours, when the ulcerated gums discharge a fetid matter; loose teeth or teeth feel long, much sticky saliva in mouth.

GLOSSITIS. Inflammation of the tongue.

Aconite 2X dil. if there is much fever, fast pulse, dry skin. Prepare:--Put ten drops in a glass half full of water and give one to two teaspoonfuls everyone to three hours.

Mercurius 3X trit. (tablet form) indicated in most cases. Take two tablets every two to four hours.

DISEASES OF THE TEETH.--Chamomilla 1X dil. Put ten drops in one-half glass full of water and give one to two teaspoonfuls everyone to three hours. This is especially good in cross, nervous, teething babies.

Aconite 2X dil. Prepared and given as above stated. When there is much fever, dullness and stupor.

Mercurius sol. 3X trit. (tablet form). When the teeth are sore and feel too long; one to two tablets everyone to three hours.

DISEASES OF THE GUMS.--Hepar sulph. 3X trit. (tablet form) is good when teeth are ulcerated and decayed. Take one to two tablets every three hours. Or use,

Mercurius sol. 3X trit. (tablet form) if there is much saliva in the mouth and teeth feel too long.

UVULA, INFLAMMATION OF.--Aconite 2X dil. Ten drops of this in a glass half full of water and give one to two teaspoonfuls everyone to three hours, when there is fever, furred tongue, dry and hot skin.

Belladonna 3X dil., prepared and given same as Aconite, instead of Aconite when the parts are red, congested and painful.

Mercurius 3X trit. (tablet form). Good when the parts are much swollen, sore and very sensitive, darkish, with much sticky saliva in the mouth.

THROAT, INFLAMMATION OF.--Aconite 2X dil. Ten drops in a glass one-half full of water and give two teaspoonfuls everyone to three hours, in the first stage attended by fever, hot and dry skin.

Belladonna 3X dil. Is better in second stage, when there is some sweating, parts are red and swollen that interfere with swallowing.

Mercurius 3X trit. (tablet form). Given when there is much saliva with pain, soreness and difficulty in swallowing.

PHARYNGITIS, Inflammation of the Pharynx.--

Aconite 2X dil., Belladonna 3X dil., and Mercurius 3X trit. (tablet form) according to symptoms given above.

TONSILS, TONSILITIS AND QUINSY.--Aconite 2X dil. In the first twenty-four hours when there is fever, full pulse and dry skin.

Belladonna 3X dil. instead, when there is much redness and swelling of the parts with much trouble in swallowing, great pain. Prepared as above directed and given.

Hepar Sulph. 3X trit. (tablet form). One to two tablets every one to two to three hours when suppuration is threatened and where there is constant throbbing and pain in the tonsil.

Mercurius 3X trit. (tablet form). One to two tablets everyone to three hours, when the trouble continues after suppuration, parts are dark red and much thick sticky saliva and foul breath.

ENLARGED TONSIL (Chronic).--Baryta Carb. 3X trit. (tablet form). Take one to two tablets daily for some time.

DIPHTHERIA.--Antitoxin is the best remedy.

Belladonna 3X dil. Ten to fifteen drops in one-half glass of water and give two teaspoonfuls every one to two hours when there is fever, marked inflammation of the tonsils, no spots as yet, red face and throbbing arteries.

Kali bichrom 2X trit. (tablet form). Put ten to fifteen tablets in a glass half full of water and give one to two teaspoonfuls every one to two hours, when the discharge is thick and stringy.

Mercurius protoid 2X trit. (tablet form). Prepare and give same way as Kali bichrom when membrane is dark, foul odor, tongue thick and pasty.

ESOPHAGUS, INFLAMMATION OF.--Aconite 2X dil. if there is much fever.

Belladonna 3X dil. If there is much local pain.

GASTRITIS, ACUTE INFLAMMATION.--Aconite 2X dil. Put ten drops or fifteen drops in a half-glass of water and give when there is active and violent inflammation with full and rapid pulse, shivering and bilious vomiting.

Arsenicum 3X trit. (tablet form). Give one to two tablets every one to three hours. Where there is great soreness and burning, much thirst, vomiting, dry, red and cracked tongue.

Nux Vomica 3X trit. (tablet form). One to two tablets every one to three hours. When there is a dull pain and nausea, but no active vomiting; especially good in cases from drinking.

CHRONIC GASTRITIS.--Arsenicum alb. 3X trit. (tablet form), one to two tablets four times a day when there is much emaciation and when there is much desire to vomit.

Nux Vomica 3X trit. (tablet form). One to two tablets after meals when it is caused by intemperance, eating too highly seasoned food, too much tea and coffee. Bowels are generally constipated.

Pulsatilla 3X trit. (tablet form). One to two tablets after meals, when it is caused by rich, greasy foods, such as cakes, pies, puddings, pork and greasy gravies.

Carbo veg. 3X trit. (tablet form). Two tablets after meals when there is much wind (gas) in the stomach.

Bryonia alb. 2X dilution, ten drops put in a glass half full of water and take two teaspoonfuls after every meal and before retiring, when the stomach is sore to touch, food feels like a load in the stomach, with sour water coming up.

HEART-BURN.--Nux vomica 3X trit. (tablet form), Mercurius vivus 3X trit. (tablet form), Bryonia alb. 2X dil. are main remedies.

GASTRALGIA (Cardialgia).--Pains in the stomach.

Nux vomica 3X trit. (tablet form) with pressure and cramps in the stomach, more particularly if the patient uses coffee, tea and liquors, or is troubled with piles, constipation, with indoor life and headaches, two tablets every half hour until better.

Ignatia 3X trit. (tablet form) especially for morose, nervous females, same dose as Nux Vomica, and same way.

Pulsatilla 3X trit. (tablet form). Two tablets every half hour until better. When brought on by rich food, as pork, pies, cakes. It is especially good in blonde women with scanty and painful menstruation. Sepia 6X trit. (tablet form). One tablet everyone to three hours. It is especially good in brunette type with irregular and painful menstruation.

VOMITING.--Nux Vomica 3X trit. (tablet form). For acid vomiting, one tablet dry on the tongue every fifteen minutes.

Ipecac 3X trit. (tablet form) for bilious vomiting.

Cocculus 2X dil. for vomiting from riding. Ten drops in a half glass full of water; take one teaspoonful every ten minutes until better.

Arsenicum alb. 3X trit. (tablet form). One tablet every ten minutes until better when the vomit is watery, burning liquid, patient is very restless and thirsty. Generally found in disease.

ENTERITIS.--Acute inflammation of the small intestines.

Aconite 2X dil. Put ten drops in a glass half full of water and give one to two teaspoonfuls everyone to three hours. When it is at the commencement, caused by cold, with dry skin, dry tongue and fever.

Arsenicum alb. 3X trit. (tablet form). One to two tablets every one to two hours, when the pains are burning, tearing, cutting in the bowels, restless and anxious, vomiting and thirsty.

Belladonna 3X dil. Prepare and give as usual. When the ordinary symptoms are accompanied by delirium or spasms with throbbing head.

Chamomilla 1X dil. For children during teething, with foul green diarrhea.

Mercurius 3X trit. (tablet form). One to two tablets everyone to three hours with usual pains, pasty, coated tongue, foul breath, painful diarrhea with it.

Nux Vomica 3X trit. (tablet form). One to two tablets every one to three hours. Caused by sudden suppression of piles, especially in drinkers and high livers, with lazy habits.

LARGE INTESTINE, INFLAMMATION.--Aconite 2X dil. at the beginning. Chilly, fever, hot dry skin, usual symptoms and dose.

Arsenicum alb. 3X trit. (tablet form). One to two tablets every one to three hours, with retching, vomiting, intense thirst, great prostration.

Mercurius viv. 3X trit. (tablet form) same dose as Arsenicum. Stools are green and watery, with much pain before and after stools.

Nux Vomica 3X trit. (tablet form) constipated bowels, nausea and vomiting.

DYSENTERY AND DIARRHEA.--Nux Vomica 3X trit. (tablet form). One to two tablets every one to two hours when there is pain before stool and relieved by the passage.

Mercurius 3X trit. (tablet form) same dose, etc. When there is pain and it is not relieved by the passage, stool is sometimes slimy, bloody and very little in quantity.

Arsenicum alb. 3X trit. (tablet form). One to two tablets every one to three hours. The person is very restless, thirsty, anxious, vomiting, and burning watery stool.

Podophyllum 3X dil. Put ten drops in a glass half full of water; take two teaspoonfuls every hour or two; especially good in children with large watery mealy stools of so large quantity of mealy liquid that the mother wonders where it all comes from.

Mercurius corr. 3X trit. (tablet form) instead of Mercurius 3X trit. (tablet form) when the bladder also is affected.

CHOLERA INFANTUM:--Chamomilla 1X dil. in teething children, with sour mucous vomiting, frequent greenish stools.

Mercurius vivus 3X trit. (tablet form). For mucous, painful slimy stools, child strains at every stool, sometimes mixed with blood. Pain is not relieved by a stool.

Arsenicum alb. 3X trit. (tablet form). One tablet every one to three hours, for watery burning vomiting and same kind of stools, very restless, thirsty and drawn looking.

CHOLERA MORBUS.--Arsenicum alb. 3X trit. (tablet form). One to two tablets on tongue every fifteen minutes until better, when there is watery burning vomiting, with terrible thirst, great prostration.

Veratrum alb. 2X dil. in water, etc. When there is vomiting with great prostration, cold hands and feet, cold sweat.

APPENDICITIS.--Aconite 2X dil. at the beginning.

Belladonna 3X dil. after the first twenty-four hours.

Bryonia alb. 2X dil. Pains are sharp, shooting, better quiet. Can alternate with Aconite or Belladonna.

Mercurius Viv. 3X trit. (tablet form) given later.

CONSTIPATION.--Correct diet and habits.

Bryonia 2X dil.

Nux Vomica 3X trit. (tablet form).

Sulphur 6X trit. (tablet form).

Opium 6X dilution. Taken 4 times daily.

COLIC.--Colocynthis 1X dil. Put ten drops in a glass half full of water and give two teaspoonfuls every fifteen minutes until better. When the pains are cutting, pinching, cramping, as if the bowels were pierced with knives in the region of the navel and when the patient bends forward.

Nux Vomica 3X trit. (tablet form). One to two tablets every half hour until better. When there is constipation, acid vomiting, distended abdomen.

Chamomilla 1X dil. Colic in stomach region and is caused by bad food. Face flushed, in teething children.

Mercurius 3X trit. (tablet form). One tablet every hour, when the pain is in the liver, patient vomits much bile and has a diarrhea, both bilious and fecal, with straining.

Podophyllum 3X dil. Ten drops in a half glass of water, two teaspoonfuls every hour when the liver is too active, too much bile, colic is aggravated by the bilious vomiting--jaundiced skin, bitter taste in the mouth.

PAINTER'S COLIC.--Opium 6X dil. As usual, prepared, and given every one to two hours, when the constipation is obstinate, hard abdomen, with intense pain, griping and pinching.

Belladonna 3X dil. same way. When bowels feel constricted or seem as if grasped by the finger nails.

PILES.--Nux Vomica 3X trit. (tablet form). One tablet after each meal and before retiring. Constipation with pain in the lower back and in the lower part of the rectum; piles may protrude and be sore.

Sulphur 6X trit. (tablet form) Tablet at night in connection with Nux Vomica in the morning.

Aloes 3X dil. One drop of it four times a day when the piles are very painful, and in the lower part of the bowels, and lots of them.

BOWEL FALLING (Prolapsus ani).--Tincture Cina is good when caused by worms, one-tenth to one drop of the tincture every two hours.

Mercurius 3X trit. (tablet form) when caused by dysentery or loose bowels.

Mercurius Corr. 3X trit. (tablet form) when caused by dysentery. Last two use 3X; one to two tablets every two hours.

WORMS.--Tincture of Cina from one-tenth drop to two drops four times a day for pin (seat) (thread worms) and round worms.

Symptoms.--Boring of the nose, livid, semi-circle under the eyes, restless sleep, cross, etc.

CHOLERA ASIATIC.--Aconite first stage.

Tincture Camphor in drop doses second stage every fifteen minutes.--Follow with Arsenicum, Veratrum alb.

Carbo veg. 3X trit. (tablet form) third stage.

PERITONITIS.--Aconite 2X dil. at first.

Arsenicum 3X trit. (tablet from) when patient is thirsty, very restless. Dose every hour.

Bryonia alb. 2X dil. Prepare. Pains worse from motion,--cutting shooting; constipated.

Mercurius 3X trit. (tablet form) Later, skin yellow, coated pasty tongue.

DROPSY.--After scarlet fever. Apis Mel. 3X trit. (tablet form). One tablet every two hours.

In feet, ankles, and abdomen.--Arsenicum alb. 3X trit. (tablet form). One tablet every three hours.

LIVER, INFLAMMATION (Hepatitis) Bryonia 2X dil. Prepare as usual and give, etc. When some fever; lies on affected side. Severe pains when moved.

Mercurius 3X trit. (tablet form). One tablet every two to four hours, after first remedy, when heavy odor from the breath, dry mouth, bitter taste, yellow (pasty) coated tongue, yellow color of skin.

Nux Vomica 3X trit. (tablet form), etc. When severe pains in region of liver extending to the back; nausea, vomiting and constipation.

LIVER, ENLARGED.--Phosphorus 3X dil. Prepare and give two teaspoonfuls every four hours.

BILIOUSNESS, LIVER.--With vomiting of bile and mucus use Nux Vomica 3X trit. (tablet form) one every three hours, also from stimulants and over feeding.

Sulphur 6X trit. (tablet form) when associated with piles. One tablet night and morning.

Mercurius 3X trit. (tablet form). Two tablets four times a day, when associated with white costive stools and depression of spirits.

BILIOUS DIARRHEA.--Give Podophyllum 3X dil. one drop every three hours.

BILIOUS ATTACKS.--In children brought on by teething, cold or anger give one drop of Chamomilla 1X dil. every three hours.

Chelidonium 3X dil. Is good for chronic liver disease, when there is a thick yellow coating on the tongue, pains, aching under right shoulder blade, also constipation. Give two drops four times a day of 3X dil.

Nux Vomica 3X trit. (tablet form). Liver troubles of drinkers. Use two tablets every three hours.

JAUNDICE.--Aconite 2X dil. Beginning from taking cold. Nux Vomica 3X trit. (tablet form). Constipation prominent. Chamomilla IX dil. From fright, anger, teething.

DISEASE OF THE RESPIRATORY ORGANS.--Coryza, cold in the head.

Aconite 2X dil. Prepare as usual. Use first twenty-four hours.

Arsenicum 3X trit. (tablet form). One tablet every hour for burning watery discharge from the nose; nose stopped up, discharge makes nose sore.

Mercurius 3X trit. (tablet form). One to two tablets everyone to three hours, for thick mucous discharge.

CATARRH, CHRONIC.--Sulphur 6X trit. (tablet form). Use tablets; take about four times a day.

Kali Bich 3X trit. (tablet form) thick crusts from ulcers in the nostrils, one tablet four times a day.

LARYNGITIS, (Inflammation of the Larynx).-Aconite 2X dil. In first twenty-four hours; give one to two drops every hour.

Belladonna 2X dil. (second day) after aconite; give same way.

Kali Bich 3X trit. (tablet form). One to two tablets everyone to three hours when hoarseness is present.

CHRONIC LARYNGITIS.--Belladonna 3X dil.

Hepar sulph. 3X trit. (tablet form).

Phosphorus 3X dil.

CROUP.--Aconite 2X dil. Put ten drops in a glass half full of water, and give two teaspoonfuls every fifteen minutes in alteration with Spongia 3X trit. (tablet form) one at a dose. If there is no fever the Spongia can be used alone. Cough is hard, rasping, barking, sawing.

Hepar sulph, 3X trit. (tablet form), This can be used in place of Spongia in light haired children. Cough may be a little looser than the spongia cough.

BRONCHITIS, ACUTE AND CHRONIC.--Aconite 2X dil. Ten drops, etc. One to two teaspoonfuls everyone to three hours in first stage for the fever, etc.

Belladonna 2X or 3X dil., etc., same. Chilly, dry throat and dry cough, soreness, and rawness beneath the breast bone, pain in the head.

Phosphorus 3X dil. etc, Constant cough, pressing feeling under breast bone, a little mucus expectorated.

Tartar Emetic 3X trit. (tablet form), One tablet every four hours. Better for old people and chronic cases, when the cough is loose and much rattling from mucus. Also good in children for capillary bronchitis.

INFLUENZA.--Gelsemium 1X dil. generally at the beginning twenty-four hours one drop every hour.

Belladonna 3X dil. for sore throat.

Phosphorus 3X dil. for bronchitis.

Bryonia 2X for the lungs.

WHOOPING-COUGH. (Pertussis).--Belladonna 2X or 3X dil. Ten drops in a glass half full of water and two teaspoonfuls given every one to three hours for sudden tight, violent cough, with sore throat, headache and nose bleed.

Cuprum Met. 3X trit. (tablet form). One to two tablets every hour, for the violent forms causing convulsions.

Hyoscyamus 1X dil. Ten drops in a half glass of water; a dessertspoonful after each paroxysm until they get better. This is indicated when the paroxysms are frequent but not so violent, and when they are worse at night; no fever, mucus of a thick greenish color; and when the cough produces a sparkle or spots before the eyes.

PNEUMONIA, Inflammation of the Lungs.--Aconite 2X dil., etc. every hour for first twenty-four hours.

Bryonia 2X dil., etc. Given same way, when the patient lies quietly, hurts to move, stitching pain in chest when coughing and attended by a pain in the head. Goes well after Aconite. Aconite and Bryonia are frequently alternated every hour.

Phosphorus, 3X trit. (tablet form). One tablet everyone to three hours. Tight cough, with little mucus.

PLEURISY, Inflammation of the Pleura.--Aconite 2X dil., etc., one to two teaspoonfuls every hour, for the chill and fever, dry hot skin, full bounding pulse, shortness of breath. First stage.

Byronia 2X dil. One to two teaspoonfuls every hour. Head aches as if it would split open, sharp stitching pain in the affected side. Constipation.

PLEURODYNIA, (Intercostal Neuralgia).--Belladonna 3X dil. Bryonia 2X dil.

ENDOCARDITIS.--Inflammation of inner lining of the heart.

Aconite 2X dil.

Spigelia 3X dil.

Cactus 3X dil.

ANGINA PECTORIS.--Cactus 2X dilution.

Spigelia 3X dil.

Arsenicum 3X trit. (tablet form).

PALPITATION.--Aconite 2X dil. One drop. Arising from excitement.

Chamomilla 1X dil. and Nux Vomica 3X dil. (tablet form) caused from anger.

Nux Vomica 3X trit. (tablet form) for palpitation from indigestion.

Pulsatilla 3X dil. (light haired people).

PULSE INTERMITTENT.--Give digitalis, spigelia 2X dil. Gelsemium 2X dil.

VEINS VARICOSE.--Hamamelis locally is good.

Sulphur 6X trit. (tablet form) for varicose ulcers.

SPLEEN, ENLARGEMENT.--Arsenicum 3X trit. (tablet form) two tablets three times a day.

China 3X di!. Two drops four times a day.

Bryonia 2X dil. One drop four times a day. Worse on motion and on touch.

KIDNEY (NEPHRITIS). (Inflammation of the Kidneys).--Aconite 2X dil. Ten drops in a glass half full of water and two teaspoonfuls everyone to two hours, when there is much fever.

Belladonna 3X dil. can follow.

BRIGHT'S DISEASE.--Arsenicum 3X trit. (tablet form). One tablet four times a day.

DIABETES MELLITUS.--Phosphoric acid 3X dil. Two drops four times a day.

Uranium nitrate 3X trit. (tablet form). One tablet three times a day.

CYSTITIS (Inflammation of the Bladder).--Acute and chronic. Aconite 2X dil. One drop everyone to two hours first twenty-four hours.

Cantharis 3X dil. For painful urination, and small amount; one to two drops every two hours.

RENAL CALCULI.--Sand in the urine. Lycopodium 30X trit. (tablet form). One tablet three times a day, for red sand.

Sarsaparilla 2X dil. Two drops three times a day for white sand.

Berberis Vulgaris (tincture). One drop four times a day for thick urine, pain in the back running down to the bladder.

HEMATURIA.--(Blood in the urine). Aconite 2X dil., etc., beginning, when there is fever.

Cantharis 3X dil. Ten drops every two hours. Urine pains in passing little at a time.

Terebinth 3X dil. When the urine has a good deal of blood in it.

RHEUMATISM.--Acute inflammatory. Aconite 2X dil. At first, and when new joints are attacked.

Belladonna 2X or 3X dil. When the parts throb and beat, and are swollen a bright red.

Bryonia 2x dil. Pains are cutting, lancinating. Worse on least motion and touch; better by rest.

Rhus tax 6X dil. Parts sore and stiff, but better, for a time, when moved a little. Opposite to Bryonia.

GOUT.--Aconite 2X dil. At first for the fever.

Colchicum 3X dil. every two hours.

For chronic and muscular Rheumatism; above remedies are good but given four times a day.

ERYSIPELAS.--Belladonna 3X dil. Bright red color, pain in head and eyes; full throbbing, bounding pulse.

Rhus tax 6X dil. When swelling is dark and in the form of vesicles.

Apis Mel 2X trit. (tablet form) for puffy swollen kind. Urine is generally light yellow color and lessened. Give a tablet generally every hour.

ACNE.--Sepia 6X trit. (tablet form). When caused by menstruation in dark haired women.

Pulsatilla 3X dil. For blondes, and when caused by rich foods.

HIVES.--Apis Mel. 2X trit. (tablet form). One to two tablets every two hours.

ITCH.--Sulphur 6X trit. (tablet form). One tablet four times daily and sulphur ointment.

ECZEMA.--Graphites 6X trit. (tablet form).

Hepar sulph. 3X trit. (tablet form).

Rhus tox 6X trit. (tablet form).

Arsenicum 3X trit. (tablet form).

PEMPHIGUS.--Cantharis 3X dil. Dose every two hours.

PSORIASIS.--Arsenicum 3X trit. (tablet form). Rhus tox 6X tablet.

IMPETIGO.--Arsenicum 3X trit. (tablet form). Rhus tox 6X, Graphites 6X.

BOILS.--Belladonna 2X dil. Hepar sulph 3X tablets.

CARBUNCLE.--Arsenicum 3X trit. (tablet form).

SCURVY.--Carbo Veg. 3X trit. (tablet form). Mercurius 3X tablet.

SCARLET FEVER.--Belladonna 3X dil. Put ten drops in a glass half full of water and give two teaspoonfuls every two hours for usual kind.

Apis Mel. 2X trit. (tablet form). One to two every three hours when the kidneys secrete less and there is some dropsy.

MEASLES.--Aconite 2X dil. in the beginning.

Belladonna 3X dil. for sore throat, dry spasmodic cough, headache delirium.

Bryonia 2X dil. When lungs are sore and hurts much to cough.

CHICKEN POX.--Aconite 2X dil. for fever stage. Rhus tox 6X trit. (tablet form). Tablet every three hours.

SMALL POX.--Aconite 2X dil. for fever. Tartar Emetic 3X trit. (tablet form). 2 Tablets every two hours after fever is low.

FEVER, INTERMITTENT, AGUE, ETC.--Arsenicum 3X trit. (tablet form).

Natrum Mur. 30X trit. (tablet form) especially after Quinine has failed.

INFANTILE REMITTENT FEVER.--Aconite 2X dil.

Belladonna 3X dil.

Mercurius 3X tablet.

INFLAMMATORY CONTINUED FEVER.--Aconite 2X dil. for the fever.

Nux Vomica 3X trit. (tablet form). One every two to three hours for the stomach.

TYPHOID FEVER.--Gelsemium 1X dil. Ten drops in a half glass, etc., 2 teaspoonfuls every hour, generally good in beginning stage.

Arsenicum 3X. trit. (tablet form). One to two everyone to three hours, later when there is sunken countenance and eyes; dry, cracked, tongue, burning thirst, restless, burning and involuntary diarrhea.

Rhus tox 3X dil. Delirium, nose bleed, sordes on teeth, brown dry tongue, wants to change position often, muttering, drowsy sleep, picking at things.

YELLOW FEVER.--Tincture Camphor drop doses every hour followed by Belladonna and Arsenicum.

CONGESTION OF BRAIN.--Aconite 2X dil. Prepare, and give one to two teaspoonfuls everyone to two hours.

Belladonna 3X dil. Prepare and give one to two teaspoonfuls everyone to two hours. When head bounds and throbs much.

Bryonia 2X dil. Aggravated by motion; more fullness in the forehead; bilious temperament.

BRAIN, INFLAMMATION OF.--Aconite 2X dil. at beginning.

Belladonna 3X dil. This follows well after Aconite.

Chamomilla 2X. Good in teething children.

CORD, INFLAMMATION OF (Myelitis).--Aconite 2X dil. At beginning.

Belladonna 3X dil. and Bryonia 2X dil. following.

SPOTTED FEVER (Cerebro-Spinal Meningitis).--Aconite 2X dil.

Belladonna 3X dil.

Bryonia 2X dil.

Arsenicum 3X trit. (tablet form).

APOPLEXY.--Belladonna 3X dil. When arteries beat violently at first.

WATER ON THE BRAIN (Acute Hydrocephalus).--Helleborus nig. 3X dil.

HEADACHE (Cephalalgia).--Belladonna 3X dil. One to two drops every half hour until better. Pounding throbbing headache, eyes red, and pain.

Bryonia, 2X dil. same way. Stomach trouble, headache, worse on motion, in forehead, full forehead, bilious feeling.

Nux Vomica 3X trit. (tablet form). One to two every one-half to two hours. Begins in morning after eating, nausea, especially when from too much coffee, liquor, etc.

Gelsemium 2X dil. For nervous headache.

SICK HEADACHE.--Bryonia 2X dil. Vomiting (bilious) worse from motion.

Pulsatilla 3X dil. Blondes with menstrual troubles.

Iris vers. 2X dil. Ten drops in water. Bilious sick headache, frequent nausea and vomiting.

Sanguinaria 2X dil. Ten drops, etc. Dose every fifteen minutes to an hour. Stomach sick headache. Nausea and vomiting of stomach material, sick waves from stomach to head.

Sepia 6X trit. (tablet form) for brunettes; bilious jaundiced appearance.

Spigelia 2X dil. Neuralgic headache, one sided, in one eye, heart palpitates.

CONVULSIONS, IN CHILDREN.--Belladonna 3X dil. Ten drops in a half glass of water, one teaspoonful every half hour to one hour. Flushed face with wandering look, half open, staring eyes.

Chamomilla 2X dil. Spasms during teething, screaming, tossing, restless sleep, irritable cross children.

Cina 1X dil. Two drops every half hour. When caused by worms.

Nux Vomica 3X trit. (tablet form). When caused by indigestion from a hearty meal; constipated bowels.

ST. VITUS' DANCE (Chorea).--Arsenicum 3X trit. (tablet form) emaciated, tired girls, weak.

Belladonna 3X dil. suited to rugged looking girls, with rush of blood to the head.

Nux Vomica 3X trit. (tablet form) constipated, stomach bad.

Pulsatilla 3X dil. For blonde girls, menstrual troubles.

Sepia 6X trit. (tablet form). For brunettes, menstrual troubles.

NEURITIS (Inflammation of the Nerves).--Aconite 2X dil. when caused from cold or congestion.

Belladonna 3X dil. sore to touch and movement.

Arnica 2X dil. when caused by injury,

Rhus tox ex trit. (tablet form) when caused by strain.

NEURALGIA or pain in the nerves, Tic douloreux infraorbital. Facial, intercostal, sciatic, etc.

Aconite 3X dil. when caused by cold, fever, hot dry skin.

Belladonna 3X dil. Beating throbbing pain, red parts, faceache, pain in the eyeballs, bright eyes.

Arsenicum 3X trit. tablet form. Periodical in character, burning pain, relieved temporarily by heat, aggravated by cold.

TOOTHACHE.--Aconite 2X dil. Fever, heat, and from cold or wet.

Arsenicum 3X trit. (tablet form) when cold brings on a paroxysm or aggravates the pain.

Belladonna 3X dil. Throbbing pain, great in extent, aggravated by heat.

Mercurius 3X trit. (tablet form). Hollow teeth, ulcerated, feel too long.

Pulsatilla 3X dil. Persons of blonde type, menstrual troubles.

SCIATICA.--Rhus tox 6X trit. (tablet form). Pains better on motion, must move.

Bryonia 2X dil. must keep quiet.

Arsenicum 3X trit. (tablet form) restless, burning, shooting pains.

LUMBAGO.--Rhus tox 6X trit. (tablet form).

Bryonia 2X dil.

PALPITATION OF THE HEART.--Nux Vomica 3X trit. (tablet form) from over eating, drinking, sedentary life.

Pulsatilla 3X dil. Blondes who have menstrual troubles also when caused by fat greasy foods.

Sepia 6X trit. (tablet form). Brunette type, womb troubles.

EYES, Simple Inflammation of.--Aconite 2X dil. First stage.

Belladonna 3X dil. Second stage.

Mercurius 3X trit. (tablet form) when there is a thick discharge.

EYES, weak and watery.--Ruta 3X dil. (may need glasses).

EYES, stye on lids. Pulsatilla 3X dil. Four times daily.

EARS, boils in the canal.--Belladonna 3X dil. hourly doses.

Hepar sulph. 3X trit. (tablet form) when suppuration (pus formation) appears.

EAR, inflammation or.--Aconite 2X dil. First stage, followed by Belladonna 3X tablet; then Hepar sulph. 3X trit. (tablet form) or Mercurius 3X trit. (tablet form).

DISEASES OF WOMEN.

METRITIS, (inflammation of the womb)--Aconite 2X dil. followed by

Belladonna 3X dil. when the skin is moist.

Mercurius 3X trit. (tablet form) when there is a thick discharge.

MENSES, suppression of.--Aconite 3X dil. when caused by cold.

Caulophyllum 3X dil. can alternate this with aconite every hour.

OVARY, inflammation of.--Aconite 2X dil.

Apis Mel 2X trit. (tablet form). These can be alternated.

DYSMENORRHEA, Painful Menstruation.--Cocculus 2X dil. Put ten drops in a glass half full of water and give two teaspoonfuls every fifteen minutes.

Caulophyllum 3X dil. can be used if Cocculus fails.

Pulsatilla 3X dil. used in blondes.

Sepia 6X trit. (tablet form) used in brunettes.

MENORRHAGIA (too much flow).--Sabina 3X dil. pains between sacrum and pubic bones most, bright red blood.

Ipecac 3X dil. especially when there is much nausea.

China 3X dil. especially when it is a chronic case.

WHITES, Leucorrhea. Pulsatilla 3X dil. In blondes.

Sepia 6X trit. (tablet form). In brunettes.

China 3X dil. When it follows loss of blood, long sickness, malaria, etc.

MUMPS.--Mercurius 3X trit. (tablet form). Tablet everyone to three hours.

Pulsatilla 3X dil. When it goes down. Give every hour.

NIGHT SWEATS.--China 2X dil. and Phosphoric acid 3X dil. These can be used alternately, giving each one three times a day.

PATENT MEDICINES AND SECRET FORMULAE

About One Hundred and Twenty Medicines in Common Use, How to Prepare Them and Their Approximate Cost.

In giving the following recipes and formulae to the public, we wish to offer a word of explanation. Many, in fact, *most* of the above are the exact formulae. Others were secured from analysis by reliable institutions and you need entertain no doubt whatever as to their reliability as far as chemical analysis could determine their ingredients. Some of the patent medicines are changed a trifle from time to time to conform with the Pure Food Laws, etc. We can supply many others not in this list and will be pleased to do so to our subscribers at any time upon request.

ALLEN'S WORLD'S HAIR RESTORER.

Sulphur	1-1/2 drams
Plumbi Acetatis	2 drams
Glycerin	3 ounces
Water, flavored to make	6-1/4 ounces

Dissolve the plumbi acetatis in the water then add the glycerin and sulphur. Any aromatic water may be used for making the restorer.

The above amount would cost about 20 cents.

RELIEF FOR ASTHMA.

Powdered Lobelia	1 ounce
Powdered Stramonium Leaves	1 ounce
Powdered Saltpeter	1 ounce
Powdered Black Tea	1 ounce

Mix and sift. Burn and inhale the fumes.

The above amount would cost about 25 cents.

ANTI-CONSTIPATION PAD.

Podophyllum	3 ounces
Aloes, powdered	1/2 ounce
Extract Colocynth compound, powdered	1/2 ounce
Croton Oil	1 dram
Oil of Sassafras	1 dram
Black Root	1/2 ounce
Lady's Slipper	1/2 ounce

Mix. Wear pad directly below pit of stomach.

The above amount would cost about 50 cents.

BLOOD AND LIVER REGULATOR.

Potassii Iodidi	1/2 ounce
Fluid Extract Senna	1/2 ounce
Fluid Extract Cascara Sagrada	1/2 ounce
Fluid Extract Sarsaparilla	1/2 ounce
Fluid Extract Stillingia	1/2 ounce
Simple syrup to make	8 ounces

Dose: One teaspoonful three times daily.

This is conceded by all to be one of the finest combinations for regulating blood and liver known.

The above amount would cost about 75 cents.

AYER'S CHERRY PECTORAL.

Acetate of Morphia	3 grains
Tincture Sanguinaria	2 drams
Wine Antimony	3 drams
Wine Ipecac	3 drams
Syrup Wild Cherry	3 ounces

Mix.

The above amount would cost about 35 cents.

SALVE FOR BOILS AND OLD SORES.

Rosin	1 ounce
Beeswax	1 ounce
Mutton Tallow	4 ounces
Copper Acetate	1 dram

Melt the rosin, tallow and wax together, then add the copper acetate, stir until cool.

The above amount would cost about 50 cents.

AYER'S HAIR VIGOR.

Plumbi Acetate	3 drams
Flowers of Sulphur	2 drams
Glycerin	14 drams
Water enough to make	1 quart

The above amount would cost about 25 cents.

BURNS AND SCALDS.

Raw Linseed Oil	3 ounces
Lime Water	3 ounces
Acidi Carbolici	15 drops

This preparation for burns is used in all hospitals and is prescribed every day by the best physicians in the United States.

The above amount would cost about 20 cents.

AYER'S SARSAPARILLA.

Fluid Extract Sarsaparilla	3 ounces
Fluid Extract Queen's Root.	3 ounces
Fluid Extract Rumex Crispus	2 ounces
Fluid Extract Mandrake	2 ounces
Sugar	1 ounce
Iodide Potassium	90 grains
Iodide Iron	10 grains

The above would cost about $1.00.

FOR AGUE, CHILLS AND FEVER.

Quinine	2 drams
Tincture Chloride Iron	6 drams
Simple Syrup	2 ounces
Fowler's Solution Arsenic	128 drops
Glycerin to make	8 ounces

Mix. Dose: Teaspoonful three times a day in chronic ague.

The above amount would cost about 60 cents.

ROYAL CATARRH CURE.

Muriate of Berberine	0.65 parts
Acidi Carbolici	1.35 parts
Common Salt	98.00 parts
Total (parts by weight)	100.00 parts

The above amount would cost about 15 cents.

FOR CATARRH OF LONG STANDING.

Menthol	10 grains
Gum Camphor	10 grains
Chloroform	10 drops
Oil Petrolatum	8 ounces

This prescription is used by the most successful specialists and physicians. You can have this filled for about 25 cents and the aboline atomizer, which is used in administering the medicine, can be bought cheaply.

BARKER'S BONE AND NERVE LINIMENT FOR MAN OR BEAST.

Cures rheumatism, sprains, bruises, chilblains, etc. We have made an examination of the foregoing liniment and find it to be essentially a liquid petroleum product, containing large quantities of camphor and turpentine, and with smaller quantities of oil of tar and probably oil of thyme. The bottle is square and deeply paneled and holds two fluid ounces of a dark colored fluorescent liquid. The following formula, according to H. W. Snow, makes a preparation not to be easily distinguished from the original:

Camphor	70 grains
Oil of Tar	1/2 fluid dram
Oil of Thyme	1 fluid dram
Oil Terebenthene	2 fluid drams

Franklin Oil (Black oil, lubricating oil) sufficient to make 2 fluid ounces

The above amount would cost about 25 cents.

CATARRH OINTMENT.

Eucalyptol	4 drops
Terebene	8 drops
Menthol	4 grains
Cosmaline to make.	1 ounce

Mix. Good.

This ointment will cure any ordinary catarrhal trouble of the nasal cavities unless too far advanced.

The above amount would cost about 25 cents.

LAXATIVE BROMO-QUININE TABLETS.

Aloin	1/9 grain
Podophyllin	1/9 grain
Sodii Bicarbonatis	1 grain
Quinine Sulphate	1 grain
Acetanilid	2 grains

Mix. The above makes one capsule.

Would cost about 25 cents for 25 capsules.

CATHARTIC AND SURE CURE FOR CONSTIPATION.

Fluid Extract Rhamnus Purshiana	1 ounce
Syrup Rhubarb	1 ounce
Simple Syrup	2 ounces

Mix.

Dose: Teaspoonful four times a day. Is a sure cure for constipation and the very best cathartic and laxative.

The above amount would cost about 35 cents.

BRINKERHOFF SYSTEM OF TREATING PILES AND OTHER DISEASES OF THE RECTUM.

There have been so many inquiries of late concerning the above treatment that we deem it a duty to tell our readers, as nearly as possible, of what the alleged specific treatment consists. The following is the Brinkerhoff secret pile remedy or injection:

Carbolic Acid	1 ounce
Olive Oil	5 ounces
Zinci Chloridi	8 grains

Mix.

The above amount would cost about 40 cents. Inject into the largest piles, eight drops; into the medium sized piles from four to six drops; into small piles from two to three drops; into club-shaped piles near the anal orifice two drops. He directs hot sitz baths for cases where violent pains follow an injection. He recommends an interval of from two to four weeks between each injection.

COUGHS.

Hydrochlorate Ammonia	1 dram
Syrup Pruni Virginani	1 ounce
Syrup Squills	1 ounce
Tincture Opii Camphor	1/2 ounce
Syrup Tolu	1/2 ounce
Syrup Rock Candy to make	4 ounces

Mix. Dose: Teaspoonful every three to four hours.

This cough remedy is simple, but very effective remedy for coughs, such as are generally experienced after catching a severe cold. Keep bowels open with good cathartic.

The above amount would cost about 45 cents.

COLIC, CHOLERA AND DIARRHEA.

Laudanum	2 drams
Oil Cloves	15 drops
Oil Cassia	15 drops
Compound Tincture Catechu	4 drams
Alcohol to make	4 ounces

Mix. Dose: Teaspoonful every ten minutes to produce vomiting.

This prescription is said to be one hundred years old, and has cured thousands of dysentery and diarrhea, as well as other bowel troubles.

The above amount would cost about 35 cents.

LYDIA PINKHAM'S COMPOUND.

High Cranberry Bark	1/2 pound
Partridge Berry Vine	1/2 pound
Poplar Bark	1/4 pound
Unicorn Root	1/4 pound
Cassia	1/4 pound
Beth Root	3 ounces
Sugar	3 pounds
Alcohol	1 pint
Water, sufficient quantity.	

Reduce the six first named ingredients to Number Forty powder, add boiling water enough to cover, let stand till cold, and then percolate with water until two and one-half gallons of liquid are obtained. To this add the sugar, bring to a boil, remove from the fire, strain, and when cold add the alcohol.

The above amount would cost about $2.70 or about 40 cents per pint.

CROUP.

Powdered Alum	2 drams
Honey Strained	1/2 ounce
Syrup Simple	1 ounce
Mucilage Acacia to make	2 ounces

Mix. Dose: Take one teaspoonful as required.

The above amount would cost about 30 cents.

SMITH'S ELECTRIC OIL.

Chloroform	1 ounce
Sassafras Oil	2 ounces
Linseed Oil	8 ounces
Cotton Seed Oil	1 pint

Mix. The above, nearly two pints, would cost about 60 cents.

EARACHE.

Tincture Opium	1 dram
Olive Oil	1/2 ounce
Glycerin	1/2 ounce

Mix.

This is another prescription you should have made up and keep on hand, as children are very subject to earache, especially in the winter.

The above amount would cost about 15 cents.

BULL'S BLOOD SYRUP.

Potas. Iodid	12 drams
Red Iodide of Mercury	2 grains
Tincture of Poke Root	3 drams
Compound Syrup of Stillingia	6 ounces
Simple Syrup to make	1 pint

Mix.

The above, about three 8-ounce bottles, would cost about $1.25.

SORE EYES.

Acetate Lead	2 grains
Sulphate Zinc	2 grains
Glycerin	1 dram
Pure Water	1 ounce

Mix. Good.

Drop a few drops in the eye, once or twice daily. For inflamed or granulated sore eyes there is no better remedy. The above would cost about 25 cents.

CALIFORNIA LINIMENT.

Tincture Myrrh	1 ounce
Tincture Capsici	1 ounce
Sweet Spirits Nitre	1 ounce
Sulph. Ether	1 ounce
Chloroform	1/2 ounce
Tincture Arnica	1 ounce
Oil Spearmint	2 drams
Oil of Wintergreen	2 drams
Oil Lobelia	1 dram
Aqua Ammonia	1/2 ounce
Alcohol to make	1 quart

Mix.

The above, about four 8-ounce bottles, would cost about $1.50.

CONSTIPATION.

Fluid Extract Cascara Sagrada	1 ounce
Fluid Extract Wahoo	1 ounce
Neutralizing Cordial	2 ounces

Mix. Dose: One-half teaspoonful three times a day (more or less).

This prescription is one of Dr. John Pitzer's of St. Louis, dean of the faculty of the Missouri Medical College. The above amount would cost about 50 cents.

CANCER PASTE.

I will tell you how I made it for the last twenty-three years. Take equal parts (by weight) of chloride of zinc, pulverized bloodroot, and wheat flour; mix well, add enough water to form a paste; spread the paste, just the size of the sore, on a rag and apply, put olive oil around the ulcer before applying, in order to protect the sound tissues. Leave the paste on as long as the patient can bear it. Then remove and if convenient apply a mild poultice or salve. In six or eight days the cancer will come out; if it leaves a smooth and healthy surface, all is well; if not, repeat the application until all diseased tissue is removed. This has never failed me, but remember that many so-called cancers are not cancers at all; then again, some are so malignant that this paste and all others will not cure, but all the cases I have had for twenty-three years were healed. One that I have on hand now, on the lower lip of a man thirty-four years old, is stubborn, but I hope it will finally yield. I will be pleased to furnish any further information in my power.--Jer. Hess, M. D., in Med. World.

Arsenic	2 ounces
Sulphur	2 ounces
Zinc Sulphate	2 ounces
Rochelle Salts	2 ounces

Of each equal parts; add yolk of one egg, till of the consistence of paste; bake with slow heat, until dry, and then pulverize. When desired for use mix again with egg, and apply as paste or on cloth.

The above amount would cost about 35 cents.

COLIC IN INFANTS.

Dewee's Carminative	1 ounce

Dose: One week old, three to five drops; one month old, five to ten drops; three months old, ten to twenty drops. One ounce would cost about 15 cents.

LOMBARD SECRET CANCER REMEDIES.

Dr. J. L. Horr says in Boston Medical and Surgical Journal: "Having without solicitation on my part, become possessed of the knowledge of the 'secret remedies' employed by the late Doctor Lombard, the 'famous cancer doctor' of Maine, I feel it my privilege, as a member of a scientific profession that has only for its object the advancement of knowledge and the relief of suffering to make a simple statement of the remedies and methods which were employed in the so-called 'treatment of cancer.'

The remedy employed, if the cancer was small, was the inspissated juice of leaves of the phytolacca decandra (garget) which was applied in the form of a plaster until sloughing took place. The after treatment was some dressing like simple cerate. If the tumor had attained considerable size, Dr. Lombard first used a paste composed of chloride of zinc and pulverized sanguinaria until an eschar was produced and then the same plaster as before was applied until the mass sloughed away. The knowledge of these remedies was given to me by Dr. Lombard himself, while I was attending him during his last illness and a few days before his death."

CORNS.

Salicylic Acid	1 dram
Muriate Ammonia	1 dram
Acetic Acid	1/2 dram
Lanoline	1 dram
White Wax	1 dram
Lard to make	1 ounce

Mix. Excellent remedy. The above amount would cost about 25 cents.

CARTER'S LITTLE LIVER PILLS.

For headache, torpid liver, constipation, and the complexion take one pill every night. As a purgative take four to eight. Weight of twelve pills about seven and one-half grains of which probably two to two and one-half grains is sugar coating. They contain Podophyllin and aloes made into a pill and coated with sugar. On the above we deduce the following formula as closely resembling the original:

Podoph (resin)	1-1/2 grains
Aloes (Socotrine)	3-1/2 grains
Mucilage of Acacia	sufficient

Mix; divide into twelve pills and coat with sugar.

The above amount would cost about 25 cents.

FOR DIARRHEA, FLUX AND DYSENTERY.

To one teaspoonful of Epsom Salts add eight drops of laudanum in one-fourth glass of water. An excellent medicine. The above amount would cost about 5 cents.

CASTORIA.

Senna	4 drams
Manna	1 ounce
Rochelle Salts	1 ounce
Fennel Seed	1-1/2 drams
Sugar	8 ounces
Oil of Wintergreen	sufficient

Boiling Water, enough to make 8 fluid ounces or a half-pint.

Pour the water over the ingredients, then cover and macerate until cool, after which strain, add the 8 ounces of sugar and dissolve by agitation; add enough oil of wintergreen for suitable flavoring.

The above amount would cost about 25 cents.

DYSPEPSIA TONIC.

Tincture Gentian Compound	2 ounces
Tincture Rhubarb	2 ounces
Tincture Ginger	1/2 ounce
Essence Peppermint	2 drams
Sodium Bicarbonate	1/2 ounce
Water to make	8 ounces

Mix. Dose: Teaspoonful after meals.

For acute cases of indigestion where the stomach and bowels are full and distended, or sour stomach and spitting up of food, this will relieve at once; and with continued use relieve entirely. The above amount would cost about 50 cents.

MADAME RUPERT'S FACE BLEACH.

Analysis assigns the following composition to this cosmetic:

Corrosive Sublimate	1 grain
Tincture of Benzoin	7 grains
Water	10 ounces

Mix. The above amount would cost about 15 cents.

TO REMOVE BLOTCHES AND PIMPLES FROM THE FACE.

Acidi Carbolici	20 drops
Powdered Borax	1 dram
Listerine	1 ounce
Alcohol	1 ounce
Aqua Rose to make	8 ounces

Mix.

For young ladies, this will prove more beneficial than any face preparation on the market. It is very refreshing and will remove black heads, tan and blemishes, leaving the skin clear and smooth. The above amount would cost about 50 cents.

CHAMBERLAIN'S COLIC, CHOLERA, AND DIARRHEA REMEDY.

Tincture Capsici	2-1/2 ounces
Tincture Camphor	2 ounces
Tincture Guaicum	1-1/2 ounces

Mix. The above amount would cost about 50 cents.

FEMALE REGULATOR.

Carbonate Iron	1 Ounce
Tincture Gentian Compound	2 ounces
Powdered Rhubarb	1/2 ounce
Powdered Cinchona	1 ounce

Mix. Add to one pint Sherry Wine. Dose: Teaspoonful three to four times a day.

We warrant this to be one of the best tonics that can be procured for general female weaknesses.

The above amount exclusive of pint of sherry wine, would cost about 50 cents.

CUTICURA OINTMENT.

The much advertised "Cuticura Ointment" has been found to consist .of a base of petroleum jelly, colored green, perfumed with oil of bergamot and containing two per cent of carbolic acid. Four ounces would cost about 25 cents.

FLUX.

Prepared Chalk	2 drams
Tincture Catechu	1/2 ounce
Tincture Opii	1/2 ounce
Aqua Cinnamon to make	8 ounces

Mix. Dose: One-half to one teaspoonful every three hours. For adults, only.

The above amount would cost about 40 cents.

CUTICURA RESOLVENT.

This preparation is said to be:

Aloes, Socot	1 dram
Rhubarb Powdered	1 dram
Potas. Iodidi	36 grains
Spirits Frumenti	1 pint

Macerate over night and filter.

The above amount exclusive of whisky would cost about 15 cents.

FOR FEVER.

Quinia Sulp	50 grains
Capsicum	6 grains

It will make twenty-five capsules. Mix. Dose: One every three hours.

This has been used for years. You should keep the bowels open to remove the cause.

The above amount would cost about 25 cents.

ELY'S CREAM BALM.

This is a proprietary article, largely advertised in the Eastern states, and meets with rapid sales and is used for catarrh. The directions are to dip the little finger into the balm and insert up the nostrils giving two or three inhalations. It is as follows:

Thymol	3 grains
Bismuth Carbonatis	15 grains
Oil of Wintergreen	2 minims
Vaselin to make	1 ounce

The above amount would cost about 25 cents.

FOR SORE THROAT.

Listerine	2 ounces
Glycerin	1/2 ounce
Pure Water to make	4 ounces

Mix. Use as a gargle.

This will cure any ordinary case, but do not mistake sore throat for diphtheria.

The above amount would cost about 25 cents.

FELLOW'S HYPOPHOSPHITES.

Glucose	1 lb.
Simple Syrup	1 pint
Hypophosphite Calcium	128 grains
Hypophosphite Potassium	48 grains
Ferri Sulp	48 grains
Sulphate Manganese	32 grains
Sulphate Quinine	14 grains
Sulphate Strychnine	2 grains
Water	sufficient

Dissolve the calcium and potassium hypophosphites in two fluid ounces of warm water. Add to one ounce of water, three fluid ounces of the syrup and dissolve in the mixture, by the aid of heat, the remainder of the salts. Mix the solutions and set by a few hours, covered, to deposit the sulphate of calcium which is formed. Filter into bottle containing the remainder of the syrup, wash the residue with an ounce of boiling water, mix filtrate and washings with the syrup; dissolve the glucose in the mixture, and add through the filter enough water to make two pints. The formula would be improved by substituting for the glucose, a refined extract of malt like that prepared by Gebe, in Germany. The proportion of the medicinal ingredients in the syrup it is true is small; I shall not warrant it to perform miracles of cure. It is simply offered as a substitute for Fellow's Hypophosphites; whatever therapeutic efficiency that nostrum has, we may count upon obtaining equally from this syrup.

The above, about four pints, would cost about $1.00.

GENERAL TONIC.

Citrate of Iron and Quinine	2 drams
Simple Syrup	2 ounces
Pure Water	2 ounces

Mix. Dose: Teaspoonful four times a day.

This tonic is good to build up the system and to make rich, new blood. People who feel tired and do not rest well at night cannot use a better remedy.

The above amount would cost about 25 cents.

GENUINE WHITE OIL LINIMENT.

Carbonate of Ammonium	19 drams
Camphor	20 drams
Oil of Turpentine	21 drams
Oil of Origanum	20 drams
Castile Soap	19 drams
Water to make	1-1/2 pints

Mix. The above amount would cost about 60 cent.

HEADACHE.

Acetanilid	160 grains
Citrate Caffein	1 dram
Sodae Bicarbonatis	15 grains
Tartaric Acid	5 grains
Simple Elixir to make	4 ounces

Mix. Dose: One-half to one teaspoonful half hour apart for two doses.

Two doses of this remedy will generally relieve any headache. Be careful of this. It is good but all these are sometimes dangerous. The above amount would cost about 35 cents.

GOOD SAMARITAN LINIMENT.

Oil of Sassafras	2 drams
Oil of Hemlock	2 drams
Spirits of Turpentine	2 drams
Tincture of Capsicum	2 drams
Tincture of Myrrh	1 ounce
Laundanum	2 drams
Oil of Origanum	2 drams
Oil of Wintergreen	1 dram
Gum Camphor	1/2 troy ounce
Chloroform	3 drams
Alcohol, to make	1 pint

Mix. The above amount, about twenty ounces, would cost about 90 cents.

HEARTBURN.

Tincture Nucis Vomicae	1 ounce

Dose: Take five drops three times a day before meals. This is good.

The above amount would cost about 15 cents.

GRANDMOTHER'S OWN COUGH REMEDY.

One green paneled bottle contains seven and one-half fluid ounces of a brownish-yellow, semi-clear, very sweet, thickish liquid, of a tarry odor, and pronounced taste and smell of chloroform. From a close examination we have ascertained that an exactly similar preparation is easily made In the following way:

Rub well together:--

Liquid Tar	5 grains
Fluid Extract Hemlock	1 fluid dram
Powdered White Sugar	2 ounces av.
and add	
Alcohol	1/2 fluid ounce
Aquae	1-1/2 fluid ounces
Molasses	3 ounces av.
Fluid Extract Ipecac	8 minims
Mix well and add finally	
Chloroform	1 fluid dram

Mix. The above amount would cost about 25 cents.

HEART DISEASES, FLUTTERING, PALPITATION, ETC.

Tincture Digitalis	2 drams
Elixir Valerian	1 ounce
Simple Syrup to make	4 ounces

Mix. Dose: Teaspoonful at once. In ten minutes another, and afterward every four hours for twenty-four hours or less.

When there is fluttering or palpitation of the heart, do not get excited but use the above, it is the best thing you can use in this trouble.

The above amount would cost about 30 cents.

GREEN MOUNTAIN SALVE.

Resin	1 pound
Burgundy Pitch	1 ounce
Beeswax	1 ounce
Mutton Tallow	1 ounce
Oil of Hemlock	2 drams
Balsam Fir	2 drams
Oil Origanum	2 drams
Oil of Red Cedar	2 drams
Venice Turpentine,	2 drams
Oil Wormwood	1/2 dram
Copper Acetate	2 drams

Melt the first articles together, and add the oils; having rubbed up the copper acetate with a little oil, put it in with the other articles, stirring well; then put into cold water and work until cold enough to roll.

The above amount, over thirty-six ounces, would cost about 50 cents.

IRON TONIC BITTERS.

Elixir Calisay and Iron	4 ounces
Alcohol	1 ounce
Pure Water	2 ounces
Syrup Simple	1 ounce

Mix. Dose: One teaspoonful four times a day.

The above amount would cost about 35 cents.

GUNN'S RHEUMATIC LINIMENT.

Oleum Olivi	1 ounce
Oil Cedar	1 ounce
Oil Amber	1 ounce

Take camphor gum one-half ounce; rub in a mortar with alcohol or sulphuric ether till pulverized, and while damp add

Oleum Olivi	1/2 ounce
Turpentine	1/2 ounce
Laudanum	1/2 ounce

After which add the first three articles. The above amount would cost about 40 cents.

ITCH OINTMENT.

Lac. Sulphur	160 grains
Naphthaline	10 grains
Oil Bergamot	4 drops
Cosmoline	1 ounce

This is good.

Rub Lac. Sulphur into fine powder, sift it into the melted cosmoline and stir until nearly cool, then add napthaline and oil bergamot. Stir until cool.

The above amount would cost about 25 cents.

HAINES'S GOLDEN SPECIFIC FOR OPIUM HABIT.

Myrica Cerif	8 ounces
Ginger Powdered	3 ounces
Capsicum, powdered	1/2 ounce

Mix. The above amount would cost about 40 cents.

KIDNEY AND LIVER CURE.

Fluid Extract Cascara Sagrada	1 ounce
Fluid Extract Uva Ursi	1 ounce
Fluid Extract Buchu	1 ounce
Tincture Gentian Compound	1/2 ounce
Syrup Simplicis to make	16 ounces

Mix. Dose: Teaspoonful four times daily or less dose if bowels move too freely.

The above amount would cost about 80 cents.

DR. B. W. HAIR'S ASTHMA CURE:

Potassii Iodidi	1 ounce
Tar Water	16 fluid ounces
Carmel sufficient to color light brown or about	30 grains

The above amount would cost about 60 cents.

LINIMENT.

Chloroform	3 drams
Oil Cloves	1 dram
Tincture Opii	1 ounce
Oil Sassafras	2 drams
Aromatic Spirits Ammonia	2 drams
Alcohol to make	6 ounces

Mix. This is excellent.

This liniment is for household use; in sprains, bruises, cuts, and bites from insects it cannot be excelled. It is a very fine liniment to keep on hand.

The above amount would cost about 50 cents.

HALL'S HAIR RENEWER.

Sulphur Precipitated	1/2 dram
Lead Acetate	1/2 dram
Sodium Chloride	1 dram
Glycerin	4 ounces
Bay rum	1 ounce
Jamaica rum	2 ounces
Water enough to make	8 ounces

The above amount, nearly pint, would cost about 35 cents.

LINIMENT.

Camphor Gum	1/2 ounce
Tincture of Capsid	1/2 ounce
Oil of Turpentine	1/4 ounce
Water Ammonia, U. S. P	5 ounces
Alcohol enough to make	12 ounces

Dissolve camphor gum and turpentine in alcohol and add balance of ingredients. Do not use internally. The above amount would cost about 35 cents.

HAMBURG DROPS.

Powdered Socotrine Aloes	1-1/2 ounces
American Saffron	1/2 ounce
Tincture Myrrh	16 ounces

Macerate for fourteen days and filter through paper.

The above amount would cost about $1.00.

LIVER PILLS.

Aloin	5 grains
Podophyllin	10 grains
Capsicum Powder	5 grains
Extract Nux Vomica	10 grains
Henbane	1 grain

Mix. Make fifty pills. Dose: Take one or two at night.

This little pill is one which you can always depend on and in old chronic cases, torpid liver and constipated bowels, these pills if kept up will make a permanent cure.

The above amount would cost about 40 cents.

HAMLIN'S WIZARD OIL.

Alcohol	1 pint
Gum Camphor	1 ounce
Oil Sassafras	1/2 ounce
Tincture Myrrh	1/2 ounce
Tincture Capsicum	1/2 ounce
Chloroform	1/2 ounce

Mix.

I consider this recipe as harmless (and useful too) as Hamlin's famous Wizard Oil, and I believe it is as perfect an analysis as we can get.

The above amount would cost about 60 cents.

NEW YORK SUN CHOLERA CURE.

Essence Peppermint	1 ounce
Laudanum	1 ounce
Tincture Rhei	1 ounce
Tincture Camphor	1 ounce
Tincture Capsicum	1 ounce

Mix. Dose: Teaspoonful every ten minutes for three doses if necessary.

This preparation has a national reputation, and is certainly the very best preparation you could keep on hand for immediate relief from cramps, colic, and diarrhea, and no family should be without it. This preparation alone is worth the price of the book.

The above amount would cost about 50 cents.

HINKLEY'S BONE LINIMENT.

Oil of Wormwood	40 minims
Oil of Hemlock	2 drams
Oil of Thyme	2 drams
Oil of Turpentine	4 drams
Fluid Extract Capsicum	1 dram
Alcohol to make	4 ounces

Mix. The above amount would cost about 25 cents.

NERVOUSNESS.

Tincture Chloride of Iron	1 ounce
Aromatic Spirits Ammonia	1 ounce
Compound Spirits Lavender	1 ounce

Mix. Good when run down. Dose: Fifteen drops four times a day.

People suffering from nervousness, fainting spells or shortness of breath, can obtain relief from a few doses of this medicine. The above amount would cost about 30 cents.

HOLLOWAY'S OINTMENT.

The formula for this preparation is said to be:

Yellow Wax	2-1/2 drams
White Wax	2-1/2 drams
Terebinth	6 drams
Lard	13 drams
Sweet Oil	19 drams

Mix. The above amount would cost about 40 cents.

NEURALGIA.

Acetanilid	160 grains
Sodium Bicarbonate	15 grains
Tartaric Acid	5 grains
Simple Elixir	4 ounces

Mix. Dose: Teaspoonful at a dose. Should not take more than two doses. Shake bottle. The above amount would cost about 30 cents.

KELLOG'S RED DROPS.

Spirits of Camphor	1 ounce
Spirits of Origanum	1 dram
Oil of Sassafras	1 dram
Oleum Terebinth	2 drams
Color Tincture (about)	2 ounces

Mix. The above amount would cost about 25 cents.

PAIN KILLER-EXTERNAL.

Chloroform	3 drams
Tincture Opii	3 drams
Tincture Camphor	3 drams
Aromatic Spirits Ammonia	3 drams
Spirits Vini Gallici	4 ounces

Mix. Do not use internally. Good liniment.

The above amount would cost about 35 cents.

KICKAPOO INDIAN OIL.

Camphor Gum	1/2 ounce troy
Oil Turpentine	1 fluid dram
Oil Peppermint	1/2 fluid dram
Oil of Wintergreen	1/2 fluid dram
Tincture Capsicum	1/2 fluid ounce
Alcohol sufficient to make	1 pint

The above amount would cost about 60 cents.

POISON OAK AND IVY.

Zinci Oxide	1 dram
Bismuth Sub. Nit.	1 dram
Carbolic Acid	10 drops
Glycerin	2 ounces

Mix. This is excellent. There are a number of remedies, but this is the best known for poison oak. The above amount would cost about 20 cents.

RHEUMATISM, INTERNAL USE.

Iodide Potash	1/2 ounce
Fluid Extract Phytolacca Decandra	1 ounce
Compound Syrup Sarsaparilla to make	8 ounces

Mix. For Chronic Rheumatism.

This is the oldest rheumatism remedy known. Rheumatism being a blood disease, requires constitutional treatment. The above amount would cost about 80 cents.

MITCHELL'S EYE SALVE.

Saxoline Snow White	175 grains
White Wax	65 grains
Zinc Oxide	22-1/2 grains
Oxide of Mercury	2-1/2 grains
Oil of Lavender	5 drops

Melt the white wax and saxoline together, and stir constantly while cooling. As soon as the mass begins to solidify incorporate the oxides and oil of lavender. The above amount would cost about 25 cents.

SCROFULA.

Iodide Potash	192 grains
Fluid Extract Queen's Root	1 ounce
Fluid Extract Prickly Ash Bark	1/2 ounce
Fluid Extract Yellow Dock	1 ounce
Compound Syrup Sarsaparilla	8 ounces

Mix. Dose: Teaspoonful four times a day.

We do not claim this remedy will cure every case of scrofula, but will give relief, and if continued for several weeks will generally produce a cure.

The above amount would cost about 75 cents.

MOTHER SIEGEL'S SYRUP.

Conc. Decoction of Aloes (1 to 4)	60.0 m.
Borax	1.3 gm.
Capsicum, Powdered	0.13 gm.
Gentian, Powdered	2.3 gm.
Sassafras Oil	0.3 gm.
Wintergreen Oil	0.12 gm.
Rectified Spirits	7.5 gm.
Fluid Extract Taraxici	7.5 gm.
Syrup	125. gm.

The above amount would cost about 40 cents.

SCALD HEAD.

Acidi Boracici	2 drams
Salol	2 drams
Balsam Peru	1 dram
Carbolic Acid	20 drops
Vaselin	1 ounce
Lanoline	2 ounces

Mix. This is excellent. First wash the head thoroughly with castile soap and apply morning and night. The above amount would cost about 25 cents.

PATTERSON'S EMULSION OF PUMPKIN SEEDS.

Patterson's Emulsion of Pumpkin Seeds is said to be a good emulsion for expelling tapeworms. Take two ounces of pumpkin seeds, peel and pound to a paste with sugar, then add by degrees eight fluid ounces of water, the whole to be taken in two or three draughts at short intervals. The above amount would cost about 25 cents or less.

TAPE WORM.

Powdered Kamalia	3 drams
Syrup Simple	3 ounces

Mix. This is very good. Two doses of this mixture hardly ever fails to bring the worm.

Give oil and turpentine two hours after the last dose.

The above amount would cost about 25 cents.

SOUTHERN CHOLERA CURE.

Tincture Laudanum or Opii	1 ounce
Tincture Capsicum	1 ounce
Spirits Camphor	1 ounce
Chloroform	180 minims
Alcohol to make	5 ounces

Mix. Dose: One-half to one teaspoonful fifteen minutes apart for two doses or one-half to one teaspoonful every four hours. The above would cost about 40 cents.

PARRY'S COMPOUND SARSAPARILLA BLOOD PURIFIER.

Turkey Corn Root	1/4 lb.
Stillingia Root	1/4 lb.
Sarsaparilla Root	1/4 lb.
Yellow Dock Root.	1/4 lb.
Sassafras Bark	2 ounces
Simple Syrup	1 qt.
Diluted Alcohol	4 ounces.
Iodide of Potassa	1/4 lb.
Water	sufficient

Percolate roots and bark with diluted alcohol, add syrup, then iodide of potassa. Dissolve in water to make 6 gallons. The above amount, six gallons, would cost about $2.00.

TOOTHACHE.

Gum Camphor	1 grain
Chloral Hydrate	1 grain
Oil of Cloves	2 drams
Chloroform to make	1 ounce

Mix. Put on some cotton and put around the tooth. No physician can give a better prescription for toothache than this.
The above amount would cost about 25 cents.

PERRY DAVIS'S PAIN KILLER.

Gum Myrrh	7-1/5 ounces
Cayenne Pepper	2 ounces
Gum Opium	1-3/5 ounces
Gum Benzoin	1-1/5 ounces
Gum Guaiac	3/5 ounce
Gum Camphor	2 ounces
Alcohol enough to make	1 gallon

The above amount would cost about $3.50 or 45 cents per pint.

WHOOPING COUGH.

Extract Belladonna	1 grain
Powdered Alum	1/2 dram
Mucilage Acacia	1 ounce
Syrup Scillae	1/2 ounce
Syrup Simple to make	4 ounces

Mix. Dose: Ten drops to use for whooping cough. It has been in use for years and some of our best doctors employ it in their practice. The above amount would cost about 30 cents.

BRODIE'S LINIMENT FOR ASTHMA.

Oil of Queen's Root	4 drams
Oil of Cajeput	2 drams
Oil of Lobelia	1 dram
Alcohol	1 ounce

Mix. Bathe the chest and throat three times a day. The above amount would cost about 35 cents.

JOHNSON'S LINIMENT.

Chloroform	4 drams
Sulph. Ether	4 drams
Oil Spearmint	2-1/2 drams
Oil of Wintergreen	2-1/2 drams
Tincture Myrrh	1 ounce
Tincture Capsicum	1 ounce
Tincture Arnica	1 ounce
Water of Ammonia	2 ounces
Alcohol enough to make	32 ounces

Mix. The above amount would cost about $1.10.

SAGE'S CATARRH REMEDY.

Powdered Hydrastis Canadensis	1 ounce
Powdered Borax	10 grains
Sodium Chloride	10 grains
Ferro-cyanuret of Iron	sufficient to color

Mix. The above is the formula of Dr. Sage, and sold by him to Dr. Pierce, of New York, for $500.00. The above amount would cost about 35 cents.

SAUL'S CATARRH REMEDY.

Tincture of Benzoin Compound	1 ounce
Tincture of Tolu	1 ounce
Chloroform	1/2 dram
Sulphuric Ether	1/2 dram
Aromatic Spirits of Ammonia	4 drams
Oil of Tar	1/2 dram
Rectified Spirits	2-1/2 ounces

Mix. Use with Cutler's Inhaler. The above amount would cost about 40 cents.

SEVEN SUTHERLAND SISTERS' HAIR GROWER.

Stearns' Bay Rum	7 fluid ounces
Dist. Extract of Witch-Hazel	9 fluid ounces
Sodium Chloride	1 dram
Hydrochloric Acid (5 per cent)	1 drop
Magnesia	sufficient

Mix the bay rum and distilled extract of witch-hazel, and shake with a little magnesia; filter, and in the filtrate dissolve the salt and add the hydrochloric acid. The agitation with magnesia causes the preparation to assume a yellow color; but by rendering it very slightly acid, with one drop of five per-cent hydrochloric acid, this color all disappears. The above amount would cost about 50 cents.

SKINNER'S DANDRUFF MIXTURE.

Hydrate of Chloral	1 dram
Glycerin	4 drams
Bay Rum	16 drams

The above amount would cost about 25 cents.

ST. JACOB'S OIL.

Gum Camphor	1 ounce
Chloral Hydrate	1 ounce
Chloroform	1 ounce
Sulp. Ether	1 ounce
Laudanum	1/2 ounce
Oil Origanum	1/2 ounce
Oil Sassafras	1/2 ounce
Alcohol enough to make	1 gallon

Mix. The above amount, eight pints, would cost about $2.25.

SYRUP OF FIGS.

Senna Leaves	7 ounces
Coriander Seed	3 ounces
Figs	12 ounces
Tamarind	9 ounces
Cassia Pulp	9 ounces
Prunes	6 ounces
Glycyrrhizae	3/4 ounce
Essence Peppermint	3/4 ounce

Syrup Simple, to make 1/2 gallon The formula omits directions; but probably a water extract should be made of the drugs, so as to measure about four pints, and in this dissolve eight pounds of sugar to make the syrup. The above amount, four pints, would cost about $1.00.

THOMAS'S ELECTRIC OIL.

Gum Camphor	1 dram
Oil Wintergreen	1 dram
Oil Origanum	1 dram
Chloroform	2 drams
Tincture Opium	2 drams
Oil Sassafras	2 drams
Oil Hemlock	2 drams
Oil Turpentine	2 drams
Balsam fir	2 drams
Tincture Guaiacum	2 drams
Tincture Catechu	2 drams
Alcohol, to make	1 pint
Alkanet	sufficient to color

Mix. The above amount would cost about 40 cents.

KELLY'S TONIC.

Tincture Nux Vomica	2 drams
Dilute Nitro-hydrochloric Acid	3 drams
Compound Tincture Cinchona	1-1/2 ounces
Compound Tincture Gentian	3 ounces

Mix. Dose: Two drams in water three times a day.

The above amount would cost about 35 cents.

VAN BUSKIRK'S FRAGRANT SOZODONT.

The following formula may be regarded as making an article identical with the original in all essential features:

Alcohol	1 fluidounce
Water	1-1/4 fluidounces
Soap	120 grains
Oil of Gaultheria	2 minims
Red Sanders	sufficient

Dissolve the soap in the mixture of alcohol and water; add the color, perfume with oil of wintergreen, add enough water to make the fluid measure three ounces. The above amount would cost about 15 cents.

The following is suggested as a similar article to the Fragrant Sozodont powder, which accompanies the liquid.

Infusorial Earth	40 grains
Orris Root	125 grains
Precipitated Chalk	200 grains
To make	365 grains

Perfume very tightly with Oil of Cloves. The above amount would cost about 10 cents.

WATT'S ANTI-RHEUMATIC PILLS.

Powdered Aloes	4 drams
Powdered Gamboge	4 drams
Powdered Hellebore	2 drams
Powdered Guaiac	1/2 dram
Hydrargyrum Chlorid Mite	1/2 dram
Precip. Sulphide of Antimony	15 grains
Oil of Cloves	1/2 fluid dram
Soap	1 dram
Spirits of Camphor.	sufficient

Mix. Make into five-grain pills. The above amount would cost about 50 cents.

WHITE'S COUGH SYRUP.

Syrup Tolutani	4 drams
Glycerini	8 drams
Hive Syrup	12 drams
Syrup Ipecacuanhae	12 drams
Tincture Lobelia	12 drams
Tincture Opii Camphor	12 drams
Extract Pilocarpi Fluid	4 drams
Ammonia Chloridi	2 drams

Mix. Dose: Take a teaspoonful three times during the day, and every hour or two before going to bed. The above amount would cost about 60 cents.

EDWARD'S ALTERATIVE AND TONIC BITTERS.

Fluid Extract of Hops	2 ounces
Fluid Extract of Red Cinchona	2 ounces
Fluid Extract Sarsaparilla	6 drams
Fluid Extract Golden Seal	6 drams
Fluid Extract of Podophyllum	4 drams
Oil of Wintergreen	6 drams
Oil Sassafras	3 drams
Oil of Peppermint	2 drams
Oil of Lemon	2 drams
Sugar	12 ounces
Alcohol	1 quart
Water enough to make	6 quarts

The above amount would cost about $1.75.

HARTER'S WILD CHERRY BITTERS.

Wild Cherry Bark	1 ounce
Yellow Cinchona Bark	1 dram
Orange Peel	2 drams
Cardamon Seed	1 dram
Wild Ginger	1/2 dram
Alcohol Dilute	12 ounces
Honey	2 ounces
Syrup	2 ounces

Percolate the drugs in moderately fine powder, with the dilute alcohol and when six pints are obtained add the honey and syrup.

The above amount would cost about 40 cents.

HAMBURG BREAST TEA.

Marshmallow Flowers	2 ounces
Glycrrhiza Root	6 drams
Iris Florentina	2 drams
Coltsfoot	1 ounce
Mullein Flowers	1/2 ounce
Anise Seed	1/2 ounce

Mix. The above amount would cost about 25 cents.

PAINE'S CELERY COMPOUND.

Celery Seed	2 ounces
Red Cinchona Officinalis	1 ounce
Orange Peel	1/4 ounce
Coriander Seed	1/4 ounce
Lemon Peel	1/4 ounce
Hydrochloric Acid	15 min.
Alcohol	5 fluid ounces
Glycerin	3 fluid ounces
Water	4 fluid ounces
Syrup	4 fluid ounces

Grind the solids to No 40 power, mix the acid and the water, add the glycerin and alcohol, and in the menstruum so prepared macerate the powder for twenty-four hours; then percolate, adding enough alcohol and water in the proportion given to make twelve fluid ounces. Finally add the syrup, and, if necessary, filter.

The above amount would cost about 60 cents.

RADWAY'S PILLS.

Aloes	4 parts
Jalap	2 parts
Zingiber	2 parts
Myrrh	2 parts

Make into a mass with mucilage and divide into two grain pills, of which about four dozen are put into each box. The above amount would cost about 35 cents.

BRITISH OIL.

Petroleum	1 ounce

Oil Juniper	1 dram
Oil of Terebinth	1 ounce
Oil Amber	4 ounces
Linseed Oil	12 ounces

Mix. The above amount would cost about 50 cents.

PIERCE'S COMPOUND EXTRACT OF SMARTWEED.

Smartweed	10 drams
Alcohol	6 ounces
Water	2 ounces
Camphor	22-1/2 grains
Oil of Hemlock	30 drops
Oil of Sassafras	30 drops

Extract the smartweed with the alcohol and water and to the liquid obtained add the camphor and oils. The above amount would cost about 30 cents.

WOMAN'S DEPARTMENT.

I

CAUSES, SYMPTOMS AND TREATMENT OF DISEASES OF WOMEN,

With Advice regarding the Health of YOUNG WOMEN AND GIRLS

II

OBSTETRICS OR MIDWIFERY INCLUDING NURSING THROUGH PREGNANCY AND CONFINEMENT; PREPARATION, DIET, CARE OF CHILD, ETC., ETC.

"Sickness is the vengeance of nature for the violation of her laws,"--C. Simmons.

Our busy life, our manner of dress, with all its attending demands are causing havoc with the health of women who are under its terrible strain. The number of women undergoing operations in our public and private hospitals from day to day bears witness to the ravages of the strenuous social life and mute testimony of the neglect of the laws of nature. Good health is the fruition of eternal vigilance and a blessing that money cannot buy. The conduct and health of our women represents the life of our nation; individually, in a measure at least, health governs the happiness of the home. Steele says: "All a woman has to do in this world is contained within the duties of a daughter, a sister, a wife, and a mother." But how many girls grow to womanhood untaught; enter wifehood in ignorance, and assume motherhood wholly unprepared for the duties that are thrust upon her. It would be out of place in a work of this nature, a family table book, to take up all the questions involved in such a subject; we can only leave with you a word of warning. Before puberty the girl should be taught to lead a life that will make her strong and healthy to prepare her for the coming strain upon her system. Once she has reached puberty parents should remember, above all things, that HEALTH is far more important than high grades in school. Do not offer prizes for high marks and otherwise add to the pressure of the present school system. Relieve her of worry, do not add to it. A cheerful mind, plenty of fresh air and sunshine is more important at this period than school work. We have paid special attention to "Causes" in this department; may we ask you, Mother and Daughter, to read "CAUSES" of disease and thus render unnecessary in later life, drugs, medicines, headache tablets and, perhaps, operations.

The Pelvis. It is so called from its resemblance to a basin, is stronger and, more massively constructed than either the skull or chest cavity; it is a bony ring, interposed between the lower end of the spine, which it supports, and the lower extremities, upon which it rests. It is composed of four bones, the two innominated, (nameless), which bound it on either side and in front, and the Sacrum and Coccyx, which complete it behind. Further description will be given in the department of Obstetrics.

The cavity of the pelvis contains the bladder, the rectum, and some of the generative organs peculiar to each sex and some windings of the small intestine; they are partially covered by the peritoneum (lining membrane of the abdominal cavity).

Anatomy of the Female Genital Organs.--The external genital organs, to which the term vulva is usually given, consist of the mons veneris, labia majora, labia minora, clitoris, vestibule, meatus urinarius, hymen, fossa navicularis, fourchette and perineum.

Mons Veneris.--This is a rounded eminence surmounting the pubic bones, and is composed of fatty tissue, covered by skin and hair.

The Labia Majora.--There are two more or less prominent longitudinal folds of cutaneous (pertaining to the skin) tissue, covered by hair and mucous membrane, which is continuous with the mucous membrane of the genital organs and urinary tract. They join at each extremity, forming the anterior and posterior commissures (uniting together). Between the posterior commissure (union) and the margin of the bowel is a space of about an inch in extent, the Perineum. It is important to remember this part, for it is often torn in labor, to a greater or less extent.

The labia are the analogue of the scrotum in the male.

The Labia Minora.--These are two smaller folds situated within the labia majora, extending from the clitoris, downward and outward for about one and one-half inches on each side of the vaginal opening. At their convergence at the clitoris each lip (labium) divides into two folds and these surround the glans (clitoris) forming its covering (prepuce) above and the bridle (frenum) below. These lips (labia) are composed of mucous membrane covered by a thin epithelial layer. They contain a network of vessels and numerous large mucous crypts (small sacs or follicles) which secrete a quantity of (fatty) matter.

The Clitoris.--This is an erectile structure, the analogue anatomically of the cavernous body of the penis, and is an elongated organ partially covered by the anterior extremities of the labia minora and connected on each side with the rami (slender process of the bone) of the pubic bones and the ischia (two bones) by a band. The clitoris is surmounted by a small tubercle (a small nodule) of spongy erectile tissue, the "glans clitoris," Two cavernous bodies of erectile tissue enclosed in dense fibrous tissue compose the body of the organ.

The Vestibule.--This is the smooth surface of triangular form situated between the clitoris and the entrance to the vagina. The labia minora bound it on either side. It contains the opening of the urethra.

The Hymen is a thin fold of mucous membrane of half moon in shape (semi-lunar) and is spread across the lower opening of the vagina.

The Glands of Bartholin are small oblong bodies, two in number, situated on each side of the commencement of the vagina above the deep fascia band like tissue. Each gland has a single duct and by this duct opens the inner surface of the adjacent labia minoris just external to the hymen. They are made up of mucous glands and a colorless tenacious fluid is secreted by them, which lubricates the vagina. These glands sometimes become diseased. Hence the description.

The Vagina.--This is a membranous canal and extends from the vulva to the uterus (womb) and connects the external and internal organs of generation. It is four to six inches in length, the anterior wall being from one to two inches shorter than the posterior. It lies in the cavity of the pelvis in front of the rectum, behind the bladder and follows first the line of axis of the cavity of the pelvis, and afterwards the axis of the outlet.

The vagina consists of an internal mucous lining (membrane) continuous above with the mucous membrane lining the womb and below with the covering of the labia majora. The next covering (inward) is a muscular coat consisting of two layers--an external longitudinal and an internal circular. There is a layer of erectile tissue between the muscular coat and mucous lining. The lower end of the vagina is surrounded by a band of striped muscular fibers comprising the sphincter muscle of the vagina (sphincter vagina).

The internal organs of generation, more commonly called the pelvic organs. These comprise the womb, fallopian tubes and ovaries.

The womb is the organ of pregnancy, and receives the fruitful egg (ovum), supports it during its development and expels it at the time of labor (parturition). In form it is pear-shaped, weighs from 12 drams to 3 ounces and is situated in the pelvic cavity, between the bladder and the rectum, with its base upwards and its apex, smaller end downward.

Its upper broad extremity is called the fundus--base of the organ, and the lower, constricted, narrowed portion is called the Cervix (neck or constricted portion). The body of the womb gradually becomes narrower from the fundus to the Cervix.

Its anterior surface is covered on its upper three-quarters by the peritoneum, while the lower fourth is connected with the bladder. The peritoneum covers the whole of the posterior surface. The womb is held up (suspended) in the pelvis by ligaments; two anterior, womb and bladder (utero-vesical), two posterior, womb-sacral (utero-sacral), two lateral broad ligaments, and two round ligaments. The womb sacral (utero-sacral) which holds the womb well up in the hollow of the sacrum and the round ligaments which keep the womb well forward enter most actively into the support of the womb. The round ligaments are strong muscular fibrous cords and serve to hold the womb forward. When pregnancy exists they increase in size with the womb, and keep the fundus forward in its excursion upwards into the abdominal cavity, and after confinement, become smaller with the womb, guiding the womb back again to its regular position. The broad ligaments are little more than reflection of the peritoneum serving to support the vessels that nourish, as they go to and from the womb.

The womb has three coats, enclosing a central cavity. This cavity of the womb is small by comparison with the size of the organ and it communicates with the Fallopian tubes by two minute openings at each side of the body, and with the vagina below, through the mouth or opening of the womb.

The external coat of the womb is called servos, derived from the peritoneum; the middle or muscular coat, which forms the chief substance of the womb, consists of bundles of unstripped muscular fibers intermixed, with loose connective tissue, blood vessels, lymphatics and nerves; the internal or mucous coat is continuous through the fringed extremity of the fallopian tubes, with the peritoneum, and through the mouth of the womb (os uteri) with the mucous membrane of the vagina. This mucous membrane is lined in the body of the womb by epithelium arrayed in columns (Columnar Epithelium) which loses its ciliated (eye-lash) movement character during pregnancy. In the lower half of the Cervix, the epithelium (this kind of cell lines all canals having communication with the external air) is of the stratified (arranged in layers) variety. The appendages of the womb are the fallopian tubes, the ovaries and their ligaments and the round ligaments. The fallopian tubes convey the ova (eggs) from the ovaries to the cavity of the womb. They are two in number, one on each side, situated in the free border of the broad ligaments and extend from each horn, an excrescence of the womb that looks like a horn, of the womb outward to the sides of the pelvis; each is about five inches in length, and has a small canal beginning at the womb in a very small opening called the internal mouth (ostium internum). This canal gradually widens to its ending, the abdominal mouth (ostium abdominal) by which it communicates with the peritoneal cavity, the timbrae. A series of fringe-like processes surround this mouth or opening and this farther end is known as the fimbriated extremity. The tube has three coats, serous or external or peritoneal; the middle or muscular, continuous with that of the womb, and an internal or mucous coat continuous also with the lining of the womb and peritoneum (covered with ciliated Columnar Epithelium).

The Ovaries.--They are analogues, anatomically, of the testes in the male. They are two egg-shaped bodies situated one on each side of the womb on the posterior aspect of the broad ligament, below and behind the fallopian tubes; each is connected by its anterior margin to the broad ligament; internally to the womb by the ovarian ligament, externally to the fringe-like extremity of the fallopian tubes by a short cord-like ligament. They are white in color; about one and one-half inches long, three-quarters of an inch wide and one-third of an inch thick and weigh about two drams each.

The ovarian ligament extends from the inner side of the ovary to the superior angle of the (Uterus) womb. The round ligaments, two in number, are about five inches long and are situated between the layers of the broad ligament, one on each side of the womb in front and below the fallopian tube. They pass forward and outward from the womb through the internal abdominal ring, along the groin canal and out at the external abdominal ring.

I have given a lengthy description of these organs; I think it will repay a careful reading. To understand a disease one should understand the organs that are subject to the disease.

CAUSES OF DISEASES OF WOMEN.

Dr. Child says among primitive people, woman is notoriously free from many of the diseases to which her sister in our present-day civilization is especially prone. As we ascend the scale of civilization, departing from a natural and adopting an artificial mode of life we find nature enacts due penalties for the transgression of her laws. The female among savage tribes has every advantage and opportunity to develop physical perfection, and her endurance suffers little, if any, by comparison with the male. How different is our modern system when the young girls are sent early to school and subjected daily to long hours of study, often in badly ventilated class-rooms, for nine months in the year, and this at the time of puberty, one of the most important periods of their life when they need plenty of out-door exercise. Surely, as Goodell says, "If woman is to be thus stunted and deformed to meet the ambitious intellectual demands of the day, if her health must be sacrificed upon the altar of her education, the time may come when to renew the worn out stock of the Republic it will be necessary for our young men to make matrimonial excursions into lands where educational theories are unknown."

Menstruation.--Many of the disorders of menstruation are due to carelessness and neglect of this function. There should be rest of both body and mind at this time, and especially at puberty. Rest is seldom allowed, but the daily routine is gone through, regardless of what may happen.

Dress.--The way the abdomen is now constricted, and this is now a prominent feature of women's mode of dress, is without doubt an important predisposing cause in female diseases. This contraction of the normal size of the cavity of the abdomen, with the subsequent compression and displacement of its organs, must of necessity produce dynamic (powerful) changes in the pelvis that cannot be otherwise than injurious to the pelvic organs. Tight lacing or any lacing, aside from the remote effects so unnatural a practice must produce, causes marked atrophy (dwindling) of the abdominal muscles. These are often so weakened that during labor they cannot properly assist the uterus (womb) in effecting delivery, and as a result instrumental interference, with its attendant dangers becomes necessary.

Prevention of Conception.--This is a very common practice among civilized women, and it has a most destructive effect upon the pelvic organs, as well as upon the general system.

Criminal abortion.--The chief danger from the criminal interruption of pregnancy is sepsis (absorption of poisons) into the system. This may be acute in character and have a fatal termination, or chronic in nature, leading to permanent injury of the womb and fallopian tubes, sterility and chronic invalidism.

Child birth.--Pelvic diseases frequently come from injuries received during labor.

Venereal diseases.--Dr. Child says, "Syphilis exerts its usual baneful influence, but gonorrhoea is responsible for more pathological (diseased) lesions (conditions) in the female pelvis than any other one factor. Its attack, if not resulting in ultimate loss of life, always leaves the tissue in an impaired condition, from which resolution (returning to natural condition) is rare. It is doubtful if a woman once infected with gonorrhoea ever recovers from its ravages. As a cause of sterility its power is beyond estimation."

INFLAMMATION OF THE VULVA.--(Vulvitis).--An acute or chronic inflammation of the vulva (external genitals) either from a specific, like gonorrhoea, or non-specific cause.

Causes.--Veit says, "Seventy-five per cent of the cases are caused by gonorrhoea."

Other Causes.--Accumulation and decomposition of discharges from the womb and vagina, inflammation of the inner lining of the womb and of the vagina. Foul, putrid discharges from neglected supports (pessaries) and tampons in the vagina; sloughings from cancer may act as exciting causes. Contact with ammoniacal and sugar urines has a similar effect.

In Infants.--It is usually due to want of cleanliness in failing to remove decomposing urine and feces. Mothers often allow soiled, foul smelling diapers to remain for a long time on the baby.

Symptoms and Condition of the Parts.--In the acute stage the mucous membrane around the opening of the vagina is red, swollen, painful and bathed in pus. The glands in the groin and glands of Bartholin are usually enlarged and tender. The glands of Bartholin and those around the urethra may become infected and fill with pus. The fatty glands of the labia majora are also sometimes affected and then appears the disease called Follicular Vulvitis (in the chronic stage secretion is abundant). The parts feel hot and there is more or less burning and itching. Walking makes the trouble worse, due to rubbing of the parts. Passing of urine increases the distress.

When the disease is caused by gonorrhoea it is more extensive and involves the vagina, urethra, the glands around the urethra and glands of Bartholin. This gland infection frequently results in an abscess.

Treatment.--In the acute form the patient should go to bed and remain there for some time. The parts should be kept constantly moist with a wet antiseptic dressing, listerine, hot water, etc., applied to the vulva and kept there.

1. If there is much pain the following solution may be used:

Acetate of lead	1 dram
Laudanum	1/2 ounce

Water enough for six ounces.

Mix and apply constantly with sterile cloths.

2. For chronic form Dr. Child says, "The vulva should be shaved, thoroughly cleansed and a mild ointment applied daily thereafter," such as:

Salicylic acid	20 grains
Oxide of zinc	2 drams
Petrolatum	enough for 1 ounce

Mix and make an ointment and apply daily.

If it is due to irritating discharges that cannot be checked, cleanse the parts thoroughly and use the Zinc ointment to protect.

ITCHING OF THE VULVA.--Vulvae or Pruritus.--This intense itching is the characteristic symptom. With the itching there is more or less swelling of the parts and extreme nervous irritability.

Causes.--This is doubtful; some think it is a purely nervous condition.

Parts irritable.--The upper angle of the labia majora and the mons veneris are the usual locations. The skin is inflamed thickened, raw, from the continual scratching."

Symptoms.--The itching and burning are almost unbearable at times, beginning most often around the clitoris, coming in paroxysms and made worse by warmth and motion.

In chronic cases the skin is a little thickened and looks dull and dry and is covered with small cracks and scratches, the result of the patient's efforts to stop the itching.

Treatment.--Systematic, general tonic treatment. Diabetes, gout, irritating discharges from the vagina and rectum should be removed. Pin worms and highly acid urine sometimes cause it in children. Internally the bromides to quiet the nerves and arsenic to build up the system should be given.

Local.--Strong solutions of corrosive sublimate (1 to 1000), nitrate of silver, tincture of iodine, and cocaine ointment give temporary relief.

Sometimes an operation is necessary.

CYSTS OF THE VULVA.--A cyst is a cavity containing fluid and surrounded by a covering (capsule). The duct (canal) of the gland of Bartholin, situated in the labia majora, sometimes closes and the secretions of the gland are not cast out, thus forming the cyst.

Cause.--The closing is nearly always the result of gonorrhea.

Condition.--The cyst is formed in the duct, the gland itself being affected rarely. It contains a thin sticky mucus. If the cyst arises in the gland, the swelling is more deeply situated. These cysts may be attacked with an acute inflammation and finally pus is formed in them, and a very painful abscess is the result,

Symptoms.--There are no symptoms except from the size of the swelling unless an abscess occurs. Then there is an acute local pain, quite tender on pressure, and often high fever.

Treatment.--If the cyst is large it should be removed, especially if it causes annoyance. If it becomes inflamed, rest in bed and cold applications are indicated. If it goes on to an abscess, a free cut should be made, the abscess scraped and good drainage given. Sometimes it is best to use pure carbolic acid in the walls of the cyst.

INFLAMMATION OF THE VAGINA, (Vaginitis).--Vaginitis

is an inflammation of the mucous membrane of the vagina.

Varieties.--1. Catarrhal or simple 2. granular; 3. gonorrheal; 4. diphtheritic, and 5. senile.

1. Catarrhal or simple form.--This is the most usual form. There is a general redness of the membrane with swelling and increased secretion.

2. Granular.--This is an advanced stage of the simple type, and is due to long continued or repeated attacks.

3. Gonorrheal form.--Is due to infection by the gonococcus of Neisser (due to gonorrhea). This form is hardest to cure and may continue for years or life, The infection may extend to the womb, fallopian tubes and peritoneal cavity and produce inflammation of the womb (endometritis) pus in the tubes, (pyosalpinx) and peritoneal cavity. This is more common than even some physicians realize.

4. Diphtheritic--Due to diphtheria, not frequent.

5. Senile type.--This comes only after the change of life.

Symptoms.--There is pain in the lower abdomen. Passing of urine is frequent and is attended with smarting and burning pain. There is a feeling of heat and burning in the vagina, and a copious discharge of mucus and pus. In the gonorrheal variety the urinary disturbances are most marked.

In gonorrheal variety the symptoms date from a distinct onset, last longer, do not yield so rapidly to treatment, and complications, such as enlarged glands in the groin and in the vulva and vagina, inflammation of the lining of the womb and fallopian tubes, inflammation of the bladder, often make their appearance early.

Treatment (in acute cases).--Rest in bed and prolonged vaginal injections of a solution of corrosive sublimate (1 to 4000 strength) three times a day. If the gonorrheal poison is present in the pus, the walls of the vagina, cervix and cervical canal should be dried and thoroughly painted with a twenty per cent solution of nitrate of silver. The patient should be in the knee-chest position for this treatment.

In chronic cases the gonorrhea poison (gonococcus) is found most frequently just behind the posterior lip of the cervix and here the silver solution should be applied very thoroughly.

VAGINISMUS.--This is a painful reflex muscular contraction of the vaginal orifice, and is most often observed in patients of a nervous and sensitive temperament.

Treatment.--Any local cause of irritation should be removed. If there is no local irritation, the opening should be dilated under an anesthetic. Tonics, exercise, and a complete change of scene are beneficial.

DISEASES OF THE CERVIX.

TEAR OF THE CERVIX (Laceration).--This is a tear in the lower part of the cervix. There may be one or more. The left one-sided tear is the usual form. Next comes the tear on both sides (bilateral). Tears on front and behind are not frequent. Tears are found in about thirty per cent of women who have had children.

Causes.--The majority of cases are caused by labor, and is due to a cervix that is not perfectly dilated. Very hurried, quick labors cause it sometimes, but the greatest injuries are due to the various operations for delivering the child through a cervix that is not fully dilated.

Symptoms. Immediate and remote.--On the immediate, when the tear is severe, there is bleeding; later, sub-involution, that is, the womb does not return to its normal size and weight.

Remote symptoms.--Leucorrhea, thick and mucus in character; profuse menstruation and inability to become pregnant. When the tear has extended through the internal opening the woman win not be able to carry the child to full term, even if she becomes pregnant.

32

Treatment.--Tampons of ichthyol (ten per cent), mixed with glycerin, introduced twice a week against the cervix and permitted to remain forty-eight hours will often afford relief.

The tear should be repaired after child-birth, if possible. If not then, and if it does not heal, it should be repaired later when the tear extends through the internal (opening) or in case of extensive raw surface on the cervix.

INFLAMMATION OF THE CERVIX.--This is an inflammation of the mucous membrane lining the canal of the cervix (cervical canal), known as Endocervicitis; it may be acute or chronic. The acute form is seen most often as a part of a general infection involving both womb and cervix, and will be described later. The chronic form is a very common condition and it is difficult to treat.

Cause.--Injury and tear of the cervix.

Symptoms.--Leucorrhea, profuse and frequent menstruation, pain in the back and loins. On examination a string of thick mucus is seen at the external opening (os) of the cervix; and of women who have borne children there are usually signs of tear and rawness of the cervix present; (Endometritis usually produces a thin watery discharge, while gonorrhea produces a thick, pus-like discharge).

Treatment.--Hot vaginal douches, containing one dram of sulphate of zinc to one pint of water, used every night for ten minutes. Hot water with witch-hazel, about four drams to the pint, is also good. Tincture of iodine applied locally twice each month. White oakbark tea used as an injection once a day for this trouble; also good for vaginitis.

INFLAMMATION OF THE LINING OF THE WOMB. Endometritis.--Endometritis is an inflammation of the lining membrane of the womb, with a tendency to extend to the lining membrane of the fallopian tubes and to the peritoneum. These are the acute and chronic varieties.

Causes.--It may occur during an acute skin disease eruption, like that of scarlet fever, and occasionally upon exposure to cold during menstruation. The most frequent exciting causes are the micro-organisms, like the gonorrhea poison, etc.

Acute Variety.--The whole mucous lining is inflamed. In severe cases the whole mucous lining is destroyed and the deeper muscular tissues of the womb are invaded.

Gonorrheal Variety. Symptoms.--There is general pain in the lower bowel region, in spells at first, later constant, with rapid rise of temperature and pulse. A purulent (pus) discharge appears early from the cervix, usually about the second day, and difficult and burning passing of urine are early symptoms. There is inflammation of the vagina accompanying it in about fifteen per cent of the cases, while inflammation of the fallopian tubes, pus in the tubes, and local peritonitis are common results.

MOTHER'S REMEDY. Inflammation of the Womb. 1. A Good Tonic for.--"For inflammation of the uterus or ovaries try a hot sitz bath every day for a week, and then every other day. In case of hemorrhage this bath is invaluable, and will relieve when all other means have failed. It can be taken during the hemorrhage, or at frequent intervals between times. Remember, one should always lie down after a sitz bath. If desired you may give aconitum tincture. Dose:--Two drops in a half glass of water, tablespoonful doses every ten to thirty minutes according to the severity of the case." If a woman has taken a severe cold, then the aconite should be given, but under no other condition.

PHYSICIANS' TREATMENT.--Dr. Child advises that the cervix be dilated, and the interior of the womb, cervical canal and vagina swabbed out with a ten per cent silver nitrate solution. Subsequently vaginal douches (1 to 5000) corrosive sublimate solution followed by a salt solution, one dram of salt to a pint of water, should be given for at least one week. Keep the bowels open.

SEPTIC PUERPERAL ENDOMETRITIS.--This is an inflammation of the inner lining of the womb that occurs after child-birth during the first few weeks, and is due to a poison.

Symptoms.--The attack usually begins with a chill, preceded by a regular increase of the temperature and pulse. The face looks flushed at first, but it soon becomes pale and the patient has an anxious look, as the disease goes on. There is very little pain, if any. The discharge that always follows labor is diminished or stops and has no odor, if there is any discharge.

The death rate is from five to twenty-five per cent.

Treatment.--Never scrape out (curette) the womb for this disease. The womb should be washed out with a hot salt solution, one teaspoonful of salt to one pint of water, and then packed with ten per cent iodoform gauze. This solution should also be injected hot into the rectum and frequently. The bowels should move freely, and if necessary injections may be given for that purpose.

The strength must be kept up by a liquid diet. Milk, brandy and strychnine, if necessary; 1/100 of a grain of strychnine can be given every four hours. Milk should be given every half hour, about two ounces at one time: or more if it agrees well.

The gauze should be removed gradually, beginning on the third day and ending on the ninth day.

In this disease the interior of the womb is smooth and contains no broken down or foreign tissue. In the next disease, Putrid Endometritis, it is far different, for this is caused by the presence of dead material, such as parts of the after-birth, left in after labor, or sloughing tumors. This material becomes putrid (rotten), and thus causes the disease called "Putrid Endometritis."

PUTRID ENDOMETRITIS.--An inflammation of the inner lining of the womb caused by putrid (rotten), decaying material.

Symptoms.--A chill is sometimes present at the beginning. The fever is high, pulse bounds and feels hard and strong, the face is flushed but there is little or no pain. The discharge from the womb, unless it is blocked by a clot, is foul smelling. The flow after childbirth is scanty, sometimes suppressed. The womb and ovaries are not very tender.

Treatment.--The first thing to do, of course, is to get the dead material, such as parts of an after-birth, clots, shreds, etc., out of the womb, and then scrape the rough surfaces. This must be done carefully and with perfectly clean tools and liquids of every kind. Then wash the womb thoroughly with the hot salt solution. One teaspoonful of salt to one pint of boiled water. After this pack the womb with ten per cent iodoform gauze, which may be bought in this strength. Remove this from the womb about the third to the ninth day. The bowels should be kept open.

Diet.--Should be of milk or at least of liquids only. The patient can be given whisky or brandy and 1/60 grain of strychnine every four hours if needed.

MALIGNANT DISEASES OF THE WOMB.--Cancer or carcinoma is a malignant disease of the neck (cervix) of the womb.

Causes.--The immediate cause is not yet known. Tears and erosions (scraping off and making raw) are supposed to act as direct causes.

Symptoms.--Bleeding is the early and very important symptom. After the change of life (menopause) is over if bleeding occurs and continues it is a very bad sign and the womb should be examined immediately. Later, a watery bloody discharge appears, with pain, loss of weight and general weakness. Pain is not an early symptom. It appears when the disease has spread to the nearby tissue.

Treatment.--The only thing to do is to operate and the earlier the better. The womb and all its belongings should be removed. If this is done early it is very successful. If the case is too far advanced, the only thing to do is to make the patient as comfortable as possible.

For the pain, morphine or opium should be given.

For the discharge, hot water and corrosive sublimate (1 to 2000) is the strength to be used. This should be used daily as an injection into the vagina.

Cancer of the Body of the Womb is found in only about two per cent of womb cancers.

Treatment.--An early operation is then necessary. The chances of obtaining a cure if operation is done is better even than in cancer of the neck of the womb. There is less chance for the adjoining structures to be affected so early and readily.

FIBROID TUMORS OF THE WOMB or Fibromata, Frequency.--Some observers state that twenty to forty per cent of all women over thirty-five years have one or more of these tumors. They are not malignant. They are more common in women who are sterile, unable to become pregnant. They appear early in life and attack all classes. They appear oftener in the body of the womb than in the neck. When in the body of the womb the back wall is the common site. A covering of loose fibrous tissue surrounds the growth. Few blood vessels appear in the tumor, nourishment being received from the surrounding tissues. Their growth is slow, except during pregnancy, when they grow rapidly. There are three varieties named according to their location and the structure covering: or surrounding them. 1. Interstitial; 2. sub-mucus; 3. sub-peritoneal or sub-serous.

1. Interstitial.--They are in the substance of the womb wall. They are usually many and vary in size.

2. Sub-mucus (under the mucous membrane).--They project into the cavity of the womb, are covered by mucous membrane and are attached to the womb by a broad base or pedicle. This is sometimes cut off spontaneously, and then the tumor is expelled from the womb.

3. Sub-peritoneal.--They are under the peritoneum, which forms its outer cover.

Causes.--Are not known. They are more frequent between thirty and forty.

Symptoms.--Difficult monthly sickness, too much blood flowing from the womb, unable to become pregnant, sometimes, and abortion. Bleeding comes more from the sub-mucus variety generally. Pain is caused by the size and weight and by pressure upon the bladder, rectum and the nerves. Death rarely results except from the complications.

MOTHER'S REMEDY. 1. Ulcers of the Womb, Common Wood Cactus for.--"Common wood cactus tea. Take wineglassful three times a. day." Should remove all thorns, chop fine and boil in sufficient water; add gin to make dose more pleasant.

Treatment.--Operation is needed when the symptoms are pressing. The sub-mucus variety may make an early operation necessary on account of their location.

Symptoms Calling for an Operation.--Size of the tumor; from the pressure symptoms; persistent bleeding from the womb. Sometimes it is necessary to remove the entire womb, especially in the interstitial variety, for the walls of the womb may be filled with the tumors.

SUBINVOLUTION OF THE WOMB.--This simply means that the womb, after miscarriage or child-birth, fails to return to its normal size and weight.

Causes.--This is frequently due to getting up too soon after labor.

Symptoms.--Menstruation or too much flow of blood (menorrhagia), dull, heavy feeling in the pelvis, backache or leucorrhea.

Results.--The womb frequently becomes misplaced.

Treatment.--Proper supports should be put in after the womb has been placed in its proper position.

If seen early enough some cases can be cured by tampons of ichthyol used three times a week and prolonged hot water injections at bed time. Cotton soaked in ichthyol and glycerin are frequently of benefit three times a week used as a tampon. The patient should not be on her feet much, or be active. Witch-hazel water can be added to the hot water injection if so desired.

DISEASES OF THE FALLOPIAN TUBES.--These are named after their discoverer, Fallopian, an Italian anatomist. These tubes begin at the part of the body of the womb that extends out like a horn. This is on the sides near the top of the body of the womb. They are two in number and extend outward on each side for about four inches; each end forms a fringe or finger shape to catch the egg, as it emerges from the ovary. Through the center there is a tube or canal, and the inner lining of the womb continues on and lines this canal, the mucous membrane of the Fallopian tubes. When this lining or membrane becomes inflamed it is called Salpingitis or Inflammation of the Fallopian tubes. Salpingitis is derived from two words: Salping, meaning tube; ltis, meaning inflammation; Fallopian was the discoverer. Thus we have Salping(x)itis, or Inflammation of the Fallopian tubes. Unfortunately in medical description it is generally called Salpingitis.

SALPINGITIS. Inflammation of the Fallopian Tubes.--It may be either acute or chronic in character.

Condition.--The tissues of the tubes become swollen when the inflammation runs into the pus stage; the finger-shaped end (outer end) is usually closed by adhesions, the pus accumulates in the tube and we have pus in the tube, or what is technically called [pyo. (pus) Salpinx (tube)] Pyosalpinx. In long standing cases the pus is absorbed or degenerates into a thin watery fluid, forming watery fluid in the tube or [hydro (water) Salpinx (tube)]--hydrosalpinx.

The tube may become attached to neighboring organs. The pus or fluid may drain occasionally into the womb and vagina. It may go into the bladder or bowels.

Causes.--It is usually caused by invading germs from the womb. Gonorrhea is the cause of the most cases.

Symptom.--This disease follows the same kind of an infection in the womb and vagina; the patient complains of pain in the region of the tube, a little to the side or sides of the womb, and the pain is made worse by motion, exercise or long standing. If it is the acute variety, the temperature rises, the pulse grows faster, and sometimes there is nausea and vomiting.

The Symptoms of the Chronic Variety are due to congestion and adhesions. There is a constant pain in the region of the tube and the patient protects herself when she walks, rides or sits down. There are difficult, painful monthly periods and too much flow. The history shows gonorrhea or septic infection, that is, disease caused by the absorption of products of putrefaction.

Treatment of the Acute Kind.--First thing is absolute rest and quiet in bed. Then prolonged hot injections in the vagina of hot water, and if you wish, one teaspoonful of listerine, etc., in each injection. Put a hot-water bag to the sore side, or fomentations of different remedies, like hops, catnip, pennyroyal, smart-weed. The applications should not be of great weight. The bowels should be kept open.

For Chronic Variety.--This frequently calls for an operation. When the symptoms are due to inflammation in the tube alone, ten per cent strength of ichthyol and glycerin tampons placed behind the lower part of the womb three times a week do much to improve the condition.

This is an unfortunate disease, and it must be closely watched for symptoms that may arise from a pus condition. There are many cases of this kind in our public hospitals, and when they are due to gonorrhea they may have been caused by the husband who had an acute or latent gonorrhea--an attack he thought cured.

DISEASES OF THE OVARY.

Inflammation of the Ovary or Ovaritis.--This is an inflammation of the ovary and it may be either acute or chronic.

In the acute form the ovary is slightly enlarged and the follicles on the circumference are distended and filled with thick fluid or pus.

In the chronic variety the ovary may be small and contain cysts; there is a destruction of the follicles and a hardened condition develops. The function of the ovary is then impaired.

Causes.--Gonorrhea, septic infection from adjacent tissues, acute fever diseases, mumps, and peritonitis. Falling (prolapse) often gives rise to chronic inflammation.

Symptoms.--Pain in the lower abdomen (pelvis), difficult and painful menstruation, too much monthly flow (menorrhagia), and painful intercourse.

Treatment.--Ichthyol (ten percent) and glycerin tampons placed behind the lower back part of the womb three times a week. The bowels should be kept open with salts. The diet should be milk or liquid. Sometimes an operation is necessary. In the department on operations this subject will be touched upon in regard to operations.

PHYSICIANS' TREATMENT.--Change of the mode of life, and proper hygienic measures will generally be all that is needed.

TUMORS OF THE OVARY.--Cystoma is the most common tumor of the ovary. The word "cystoma" means a cyst tumor, or cystic tumor. A cyst means a cavity containing fluid and surrounded by a covering (capsule). Ovarian cyst or tumors is often seen in print these days. Ovarian tumor takes in the cystic variety, cancer and sarcoma, two malignant tumors.

Symptoms.--These depend upon the size of the tumors. The large tumors are generally cystic. Examination of the vagina shows the pelvis filled by a tense, watery, fluctuating mass. Examining the abdomen, the abdomen is seen more or less distended by a regular swelling, and sometimes this is enormous. The abdomen is rounded and there is no bulging at the sides like there is in ascites (dropsy). The navel is not prominent. The tumor can be outlined. It cannot be in ascites.

Treatment.--In bygone years tapping was done for these tumors. If it gets large or the health fails, an operation should be performed. This is very successful in uncomplicated cases. Inside of two months the patient is about well. I know I have saved many lives of women by recommending an operation for such tumors.

For the congested ovary, treatment by tampons and medicine often helps. I have frequently given a medicine called Apis-Mel for this condition and with success. I give it in tablets of 1/100 of a grain regularly four times a day.

MENSTRUATION AND ITS DISORDERS.--Normal menstruation occurs monthly in the female. There is a flow of blood from the cavity of the womb. The time for its beginning is different in different countries, it being earlier in warm climates, ten to twelve years, and later in cold ones (fifteen to seventeen years); the average is fourteen years.

Pregnancy suspends menstruation and often nursing the child does, also. Menstruation continues longer in robust, healthy women. Change of life (Menopause) occurs usually between forty and fifty years. The healthy girl and woman comes around every twenty-eight to thirty days. This is the usual time. The flow lasts from two to eight days and the quantity is about one ounce each day. A slight feeling of weight and fullness in the lower abdomen (pelvis) should be the only symptom present in a healthy female. The blood lost should not cause any special degree of weakness.

PREMATURE MENSTRUATION. Too early menstruation.--Premature or precocious menstruation is when it occurs before puberty. This is in part hereditary, but bad associations may be a cause of this early menstruation.

Treatment.--The cause, if possible, should be removed. The nerves should be kept quiet by rest and, if needed, general tonics like iron, arsenic, and nux vomica prescribed and given.

DELAYED MENSTRUATION.--This is often caused by slow development of the generative organs. The girl may not come around until seventeenth to nineteenth year.

Causes.--It may be due to heredity. Lack of proper nourishment and proper exercise are the most important causative factors.

MOTHERS' REMEDIES.--l. Obstruction of Monthly Flow.-- An herb combination for.

Poplar Bark	2 ounces
Ginger	1/2 ounces
Bayberry	1 ounce
Cinnamon	1/2 ounce
Anise Seed	1/2 ounce
Golden Seal	1/4 ounce

Mix well and give a teaspoonful in a cup of boiling water sweetened with sugar two or three times a day. Excellent in obstructions of the monthly periods, debility, loss of appetite, etc. This combination is fine when used as a tonic. It is stimulating and has been known to cure many severe cases.

2. To Promote the Menses, Smartweed for.--"Smartweed is good to promote the menses. Always steep in cold water; never boil. Dose.--Two teaspoonsful every hour. Be sure to take warm."

VICARIOUS MENSTRUATION (In place of).--When menstruation is absent or suppressed, bleeding sometimes occurs periodically, from the ear, nose, any existing raw surface, leg, ulcer, and from the respiratory (breathing) tract, and also from the bowels.

AMENORRHEA.--This is absence of menstruation.

Causes.--Delayed puberty, anemia (want of proper blood) chlorosis (green sickness). diabetes, malaria, tuberculosis and acute illness may cause it. Sometimes change of climate causes it and nursing baby too long.

Symptoms.--If it is associated with atresia, that is, want of the normal outlet, of course no signs of flowing can show, but colicky, cramp-like, monthly pains appear in the lower abdomen. These increase in severity as the retained blood distends the womb.

Treatment.--If there is no opening for the vagina or cervix one must be made, by operation. If it is due to anemia or chlorosis, Blaud's pills will benefit. The following is the formula:

Dried Sulphate of Iron	2 drams
Carbonate of Potash	2 drams

Syrup--Sufficient quantity to make forty-eight pills.

Take one to three pills three times a day, after meals.

MENORRHAGIA.--Too much bleeding at the monthly periods.

If it occurs between the monthly periods it is called Metrorrhagia, womb-bleeding at any time, especially between the periods.

Causes.--These may be constitutional or local, the latter being the most important.

Local Causes.--These are inflammation of the womb, displacements of the womb, malignant disease of the womb, fibroid tumors and disease of the ovaries.

Symptoms.--Sudden or gradual increase in the amount of blood lost at the monthly periods. Then secondary anemia, weakness and run-down feeling.

PHYSICIANS' TREATMENT. 1. Profuse Menstruation, an Easily Prepared Herb Remedy for.--

"Cranesbill Root	1 ounce
White Poplar Bark	2 ounces
Bistort Root	1 ounce
Golden Seal	1 ounce
Geranium	1/2 ounce
Cloves	1/2 ounce
Ginger	1/2 ounce
Ground Sugar	1/2 pound

Mix. This compound is excellent for complaints of weak females, such as leucorrhea, bearing-down, or profuse menstruation, etc. Dose: One teaspoonful of the powder, in a half cup of boiling water three times a day. Drink the clear liquid only." Any woman suffering with, female trouble will find the above combination very beneficial.

2. In young girls and women who are not married, thirty drops of the fluid extract of Ergot three times a day. This medicine will cause the womb to contract. Hot douches can be given to married women. If the bleeding is severe it may be necessary to pack the vagina with sterile gauze. Ergotin ten to twenty drops, may be needed, given hypodermically. If it is due to constitutional causes, like anemia, a played-out feeling, paleness. weakness, etc., a tonic treatment is needed.

3. Blaud's pills will do well. This is the formula:

Dried sulphate of iron	2 drams
Carbonate of potash	2 drams
Syrup	enough to make a mass

Mix and make forty-eight pills. Take one to three, three times a day after meals.

4. If the appetite is poor, bitter tonics such as gentian, quassia, cinchona, or nux vomica are needed.

Compound Tincture Cinchona	2 ounces
Compound Tincture Gentian	2 ounces

Mix. Take one teaspoonful before meals, in a little water.

5. Tincture of nux vomica in doses of two to three drops after meals is a good stomach and bowel tonic.

6. Golden seal root made into a tea is good in some cases, especially if the tongue is much coated.

7. Oil of Erigeron or flea-bane is good for oozing bleeding. Dose: Three to five drops in a capsule every four hours.

8. Oil of cinnamon in one dose of one-half dram is good where flea-bane oil cannot be used or obtained; *usual dose,* one to five drops. An infusion can be made of the cinnamon bark and drank freely.

9. Cranesbill (Geranium maculata). The fluid extract is splendid when diluted three or four times with boiled water, used locally for bleeding from the womb, or as an injection for the same; or an infusion can be made of the plant and injected into the vagina. The local cause mentioned should be treated. The displacement should be corrected.

DYSMENORRHEA or Difficult Menstruation.--This term means difficult and painful monthly periods. The pain may occur before, during or after the periods.

Causes.--It may be caused by a narrow cervical canal, the canal from the inner womb to the vagina. This is often very narrow and almost closed. Again it is produced by the womb being turned back and bent on the canal, thus partially closing it. This causes the blood to be retained in the womb and then the womb contracts to expel the blood, pains being the natural result. Diseases of the womb and ovaries also cause it. Sometimes the membrane of the womb is cast off in the form of shreds or even a cast of the inner womb.

Symptoms.--The flow may be scanty, moderate or profuse, often clotted. The pain varies. It may be slight before the flow, or the first day or two, or it may be severe, agonizing and continuous for one or two days, or during the whole period and sometimes for some days after there may be pains.

MOTHERS' REMEDIES. 1. Painful Menstruation, a Good Tonic for.--"This may be relieved by sitting over the steam of a strong decoction of tansy, wormwood, and yarrow, and fomenting the abdomen with the same. Then take the following in wineglassful doses:--One ounce each of ground pine, southern wood, tansy, catnip and germander, simmering in two quarts of water down to three pints and pour boiling hot on one ounce of pennyroyal herb, strain when cold and take as per dose above."

2. Painful Menstruation, a Home Remedy for.--"Let the patient take an active cathartic; then when put to bed let a half cup of hop tea be given; and a douche of one quart of hot water into which ten drops of laudanum have been dropped, be injected." A cathartic is not necessary in all cases. If the bowels have been moving freely do not take one. The douche will give great relief providing the woman can take one while menstruating. Some women can and some cannot.

PHYSICIANS' TREATMENT.--If the womb is displaced it

should be corrected. Any disease of the womb or ovaries should be treated. If the canal is too much closed, gradual and careful dilation between the periods, will often remove this cause in time. The bowels should be kept regular at all times.

1. For the attack.--Never take opium or alcohol for it in any form; it is so easy to form the habit and a doctor who gives it is simply dodging effective general and local treatment between the periods. If it is due to taking cold, or from any local cause, the following

treatment is good: The patient should take a hot sitz bath, being well covered by a blanket, while in the tub and afterwards, and should immediately get into bed as soon as the buttocks are dried and remain there well covered. A turpentine stupe is now to be used, prepared as follows: Place a tin cup containing the turpentine in a vessel containing hot water. This will keep the turpentine warm. Dip a piece of flannel into very hot water and wring it out in a twisted towel, and after it is perfectly dry and no dripping, dip it into the hot turpentine and wring it out again to free it from too much of the drug. Apply the cloth while hot and allow it to remain until it causes discomfort. Then withdraw it or it will blister the skin if left on too long. Fomentations wrung out of teas like hop, pennyroyal, smart-weed, etc., applied and kept warm often do much good. At the same time pennyroyal tea can be drank freely. A five-cent package can be bought at any drug store. Hot lemonade will help also. The object is to produce relaxation of the tissues through the local applications and tea drinking. If there is constipation, the bowels should be moved freely with epsom salts, half ounce dose, in the morning before breakfast. If there is much pain a belladonna suppository, one-half grain of the extract, can be inserted into the rectum.

2. If the patient's nervous system is run down the "Rest Cure" will be of benefit, and medicines to strengthen the nerves. Exercise, outdoor life, horseback riding are of great benefit in toning the system.

3. Fluid extract of blue cohosh is a good medicine in this disease, especially if there is some rheumatism during the interval. One or two drops every hour will be enough.

4. Tincture of Pulsatilla in doses of three drops every hour is good for the pain, especially in blonde girls and women.

5. Tincture of Cocculus I have found to be of great benefit. Put five drops of a good pure tincture into a glass half full of water and give two teaspoonfuls every ten to fifteen minutes until relieved. This I give in cases I am called to and have not the time then to find out what the real cause may be.

DISPLACEMENTS.--Turning back or retro-displacements. This includes retro-version and retro-flexion. Retro-version means turning back, in plain terms. Retro-flexion means bending back, bending of the body of the womb, or the neck, backward. Retro-flexion is more common than retro-version.

Causes.--Some are congenital, that is, from birth, and a few are the result of some injury, falls or blows. It is more often found in child-bearing women, and this may be due to the fact that the womb has not returned to its normal size and weight, and therefore there is more weight for the ligaments to hold up. The ligaments often relax and do not support the womb as thoroughly as before.

Symptoms.--Backache, a sense of weight in the lower abdomen, difficult menstruation, leucorrhea, sterility, or repeated abortion and constipation. The constipation is often due to the womb lying on the rectum.

Treatment.--This is to replace the womb and keep it in position. Supports of various kinds are used to keep the womb in position after it has been replaced, They must fit thoroughly and give no pain or any discomfort whatever. They are called supports or pessaries. If they are fitted properly they do much good. They should be removed often (every month) and not allowed to grow fast or cause sores in the vagina. There are the ring support and the stem variety and others. The stem variety can be taken out and replaced by wearer at any time. They are made to buckle around the abdomen. They are bungling but effective. The ring kind should be introduced by a competent person who should see that it is of correct size and shape, and worn with comfort. Sometimes these supports fail to cure when adhesions and other diseases exist; it may be impossible to wear them.

Operations.--One operation is to break up the adhesions, the body of the womb brought forward and sewn (sutured) to the abdominal wall. Another operation is to shorten the round ligaments in the inguinal (groin) canal. These are the usual operations, and they are quite successful.

FALLING OR PROLAPSE OF THE WOMB.--The womb may come down and remain in the vagina (incomplete falling). When the womb escapes at the vulva it is called a complete falling (prolapse or procidentia).

For the Incomplete Kind.--Replace the womb and wear a support for months.

For the Complete Falling.--Replace the womb. The patient should remain in bed with daily, hot, prolonged vaginal injections of water for a few weeks. The injection daily of white oak bark tea, of the strength of one ounce of the bark to a pint of hot water, is often of great benefit.

If these measures fail to cure, an operation may be necessary.

MOTHERS' REMEDIES. 1. Falling of the Womb. Unicorn Root for.--"Make a strong tea of unicorn root, and take a half teaspoonful three times a day, This is an excellent remedy for falling of the womb," This is very easily prepared and not bad to take, and in addition to this use an injection of witch-hazel or golden seal.

2. Falling of the Womb, a Fine Herb Combination for.--"Peach leaves, mullein leaves and hops made into a tea, and a pint used twice a day as an injection often cures when other remedies fail." We all know that this combination of herbs is healing and especially in female trouble. The hops, especially, are very soothing to the affected parts.

3. Falling of the Womb, a Physician's. Treatment.--"Knee-chest position. Get down on the knees and put chest and chin to the floor.

Retain this position about three minutes several times a day." This is a splendid thing to do, and is recommended by all physicians.

4. Falling of the Womb, a Never Failing Remedy for.--"Ague root (Aletris Farinosa) is a valuable agent to prevent tendency to miscarriage and falling of the womb. It is especially useful for the purpose of restoring the activity of the generative organs giving them vigor and healthy action. Dose of the tincture is from six to ten drops three times a day and of the powdered root five to eight grains." This is an old tried remedy, and is frequently used by physicians alone or in combination with other remedies.

5. Falling of the Womb, White Oak Bark for.--"A mild infusion of white oak bark, or of alum or tannin, used in quantities of a pint, as a douche, will often give immediate relief."

LEUCORRHEA. (The Whites).--This is an over-secretion from the glands that pour out their contents into the vagina or the cervical canal of the womb.

Causes.--It is dependent upon many causes. Tear of the neck of the womb (cervix), displacements, inflammation of the womb and vagina, a run-down condition of the system from any cause. The character of the discharge varies.

From a Torn Cervix, the discharge is thick and mucus-like in character.

In Inflammation of the Canal of the Cervix.--A thick mucus discharge also comes from this trouble.

Inflammation of the Body of the Womb.--The discharge is thin and watery.

If the Inflammation is Caused by Gonorrhea the discharge would partake of the pus-like variety.

Symptoms.--Local: is of course mainly the discharge or the irritation often produced by it, especially if it is thin. It then irritates the parts. The patient will be run down. It will be hard to do anything, frequently the patient is very nervous and irritable.

MOTHERS' REMEDIES. 1. Leucorrhea, Slippery Elm for.---"The immediate cause of leucorrhea is either congestion or inflammation of the mucous membrane of the vagina or womb, or both. It is not a disease, but a symptom of some vaginal or uterine disorder; hence, general or specific tonics may be needed but appropriate injection as auxiliary treatment will very much assist in cure. The patient should bathe frequently and freely expose herself to the sunshine, and have good ventilation in the house. If the vaginal passage is very tender and irritable, an infusion, or tea, of slippery elm bark is very soothing and may be used freely with a vaginal syringe. Whatever injection is employed, should be preceded by the free use of castile soap and warm water to thoroughly cleanse the parts." Always lie down after an injection.

2. Leucorrhea, Glycerin for.--"One part glycerin to six parts water is a very soothing lotion when there is much tenderness, pain or heat in the vagina. A teaspoonful of tartaric acid in a pint of warm water is a specific, in some cases, acting like magic. Whatever lotion is employed, always use it warm. After cleansing with soap suds, the medicated lotion of not less than two ounces should be injected."

3. Leucorrhea, Common Tea for.--"A very simple remedy that every woman has in the home is a decoction of common tea; used as an injection twice daily is very beneficial." The tea has an astringent action and the tannin contained in the tea leaves is very effective. This remedy is a harmless one, and every woman suffering with this disagreeable disease should give this remedy a trial.

4. Leucorrhea, Witch-hazel for.--"Cleanse the parts well with clear warm water, then inject two quarts of warm water in which has been dropped a tablespoonful of witch-hazel." This is a very good remedy and sure to give relief.

5. Leucorrhea, White Oak Bark for.--"White oak bark one ounce, water one pint. This makes a very good injection and will be found very effective,"

6. Leucorrhea, a Good Herb Remedy for.--"Inject into the vagina with a female syringe, a tea of bistort or beth root, and cranesbill, night and morning and take the following night and morning in wineglassful doses.

White Pond Lily Root.	2 ounces
Unicorn Root	2 ounces
Wahoo Root	1 ounce
Golden Seal	1 ounce
Cinnamon	1 ounce

Add three pints of water, simmer to one quart, pour boiling hot upon one ounce of grated nutmeg, one-half ounce ginger, powdered, one - half pound of granulated sugar. Exercise in the open air and nourishing food are indispensable."

7. Leucorrhea, Common Vinegar for.--"Two tablespoonfuls vinegar in two quarts of water (warm or hot), used as a douche at bed-time, until cured," This will cure some mild cases and has an astringent action.

8. Leucorrhea, an Easily Prepared Remedy for.--"Red oak bark tea used with syringe; follow with hot water." Steep the red oak bark and make a tea of it, using about two or three teaspoonfuls of the bark to a pint of hot water. This acts as an astringent and the red oak bark contains a good deal of tannin which is very beneficial in cases of this kind.

9. Leucorrhea, Home-Made Suppositories for.--"Take a small piece of medicated cotton, and saturate in pure glycerin and insert in the vagina at night, after a warm salt injection has been taken to thoroughly cleanse the parts." So many women of today are careless about taking injections, at least once or twice a week. Many of these diseases could be avoided in the beginning by women being more cleanly. This saturated cotton acts as a suppository absorbing the mattery secretion and in that way relieves the congestion.

10. Leucorrhea, a Good Home Remedy for.--"Cleanse the parts affected with warm water with a little castile or ivory soap in it, by means of an injection. Then inject a full syringe of the mixture, made by dropping a tablespoonful of extract of witch-hazel (Pond's is best) into warm water; repeat each night until cured." The injection of soap and water is one of the essential things to do for leucorrhea, as it cleanses the parts thoroughly and the witch-hazel is very soothing and healing.

11. Leucorrhea, a New York Doctor's Remedy for.--"Fluid extract of Oregon grape root (sometimes called mild grape) mixed with a simple syrup and given in teaspoonful doses, three times a day, is recommended by Dr. W. W. Myers, as a curative for leucorrhea."

PHYSICIANS' TREATMENT.--First is to do away, if possible, with local disease, like inflammations, tear of the cervix, etc. The general system should be built up with tonics. The same treatment as for anemia and chlorosis will be usual for this trouble. Refer to those diseases.

Local.--The vagina should be kept as clean as possible with the hot water injections. To the hot water many simple remedies can be added with much benefit.

1. One ounce of white oak bark in a pint of boiling water makes a good injection for this trouble. Before any medicine is used the vagina should always be washed out by an injection of warm water. Then follow with the indicated injection and retain it as long as possible.

2. Tannic acid and glycerin, equal parts, one ounce to two quarts of warm water, is a good injection.

3. Lloyd's Golden Seal is splendid, used in the proportion of four teaspoonsful to a pint of warm water.

4. This combination gives good service:--

Sulphate of Zinc	1 dram
Sulphate of Alum	1 dram
Glycerin	6 ounces

Put a tablespoonful to each quart of warm water and use as injection.

It is well to remember the injections must be given in large quantities, and used in a fountain syringe. A gallon can be used at one time.

5. Witch-hazel in warm water makes an excellent injection in many cases. It can be used in the proportion of one-fifth water of witch-hazel to four-fifths of warm water.

6. Many other simple remedies may be named, Cranesbill is one. Vaginal cones are now made for leucorrhea. These are used about every third night and a thorough injection taken the next day. There are many varieties, most of them are good and can be bought at any drug store.

MENOPAUSE. (Change of Life). The active menstrual life lasts on an average for thirty years and ends between forty and fifty years of age. The courts have recognized the age of fifty-three years as the limit that a woman can become pregnant.

The onset of the change of life, may be sudden or gradual. The organs shrink and waste. The womb shrinks and part of its muscular tissue disappears and its walls become thin, soft and relaxed. The ovaries become small and harder. The vagina shortens and also becomes narrower. Sudden mental shock, wasting disease or change of climate, may cause a sudden appearance of the change of life.

Symptoms.--Many women hardly notice any change, as it comes on gradually. Other women have all kinds of bodily and mental symptoms, and some are afraid of becoming insane. The heart palpitates readily, feelings of heat and cold, flushes of heat of the face, followed by sudden sweating. Rush of blood to the head so quickly sometimes as to make the patient lose temporary consciousness. The spirits are very much depressed, sleeplessness is common in some women.

MOTHERS' REMEDIES. 1. Change of Life, a Useful Herb Remedy for.--"Motherwort is one of the most useful herbs to relieve obstructed menstrual flow. There is no better herb for cleansing the womb and removing obstructions in the female at change of life. Dose: A wineglassful of the decoction three times a day."

2. Change of Life, excessive Flowing. An Old Tried Remedy for.--"One ounce of nutmeg, grated, one pint Jamaica rum. Mix well and shake before taking. Dose :--One teaspoonful three times a day as long as necessary." I tried this remedy upon the advice of a physician at the time of "change of life" and was very soon relieved, so I heartily recommend it.

3. Change of Life. Good Advice From an Experienced Mother.--"The first and most important point to consider is the general health of the patient. If the general health can be sustained there will be no danger attending this critical period of life. Therefore whatever form of disease may manifest itself the one object should be to seek a remedy in time. Take special pains to preserve general good health and take care not to overwork, take plenty of outdoor exercise and keep up a regular action of the bowels. Purify the blood with tonics if necessary."

PHYSICIANS' TREATMENT.--Exercise, fresh air, with freedom from worry, anxiety and care. Many women at this time of life need much encouragement, and cheerful company is a good tonic. Prominent annoying symptoms should be met with the proper medicine.

33

Irregular bleeding of the womb at this time or after should lead to an examination as to its origin.

CYSTOCELE--Cystocele is simply a tumor formed by the bladder pressing into the walls of the vagina. The bladder descends into the pelvis on account of relaxation or destruction of its normal support. The anterior wall of the vagina yields.

Causes.--Tear of the perineum allows the bottom of the pelvis to relax. Undue relaxation of the ligaments of the bladder and of the floor of the pelvis, with over distention of the bladder, are responsible for the majority of the cases.

Symptoms.--Weight and dragging feeling. A tumor can be felt in the vagina. It decreases when the bladder is emptied.

Treatment.--Supports are suitable in some cases (Skene's pessary). An operation is necessary in many cases.

RECTOCELE.--The muscle that holds up the lower end of the rectum is relaxed or torn and this deprives the lower end of the rectum of its support so that during expulsion of the feces forward distention of the anterior wall of the rectum into the vagina results. The posterior wall of the vagina is carried before the advancing anterior rectal wall, and appears at the entrance of the vagina as a bulging tumor which is increased in size with every effort of the rectum to cast out the feces.

Causes.--Hard child-birth (labor) and the long time the head of the child was resting on the perineum. This resulted in an over-stretching or tear of the muscle that holds up the lower end of the bowel and the parts were necessarily weakened.

Symptoms.--It is hard to entirely empty the rectum because of the presence of the tumor. This is soft, rounded, increasing and decreasing in size and disappears upon pressure.

Treatment.--Keep, if possible, the tumor from getting larger, regulate the bowels.

An operation may be necessary to restore the parts to their normal condition. A physician must be consulted.

OBSTETRICS OR MIDWIFERY

Small bodies are contained in the ovaries. These are called eggs or ova. The human egg is about 1/125 of an inch in diameter. This egg enlarges and one or more escape from the ovaries, usually about the time of the monthly sickness, and are caught by the ends of the Fallopian tube, enter its canal and are carried into the womb. After they have arrived in the womb they are, as a rule, cast off with the secretion and leave the body. If in the course of its travel from the ovaries, through the tube to the womb, the female ovum or egg meets with the male elements, fertilization or impregnation may take place. If then it is not cast off it generally lodges in the womb and pregnancy has begun. The male and female elements are usually supposed to meet in the outer portion of the Fallopian tubes, fertilization then taking place; but this can occur any place from the ovary to the womb. When the fertilized egg enters the womb it is usually arrested in the folds of the womb membrane nearest the opening of the tube and at once attaches itself to the womb wall. The folds by which it is surrounded then grow forward and their edges unite over the egg or ovum forming a sac--the decidua reflexa. Then follows the development of this ovum and with it the development of the womb, and this growth or development constitutes the process which is called pregnancy.

The Embryo or impregnated egg is nourished in the womb by measures preparing for it. The placenta or after-birth forms during the third month of pregnancy. Its function is to furnish nourishment breathing (respiration) and excreting power to the embryo or impregnated egg. The fully developed after-birth is a roundish spongy mass with a diameter of about eight inches and weighs about one pound. It is usually thickest at the center, the edges thinning out to the membranes. The inner surface is smooth and glistening and is covered by a membrane (amnion) and beneath this two arteries and a vein branch in all directions.

The cord is attached to the inner surface of the after-birth and is of a glistening white color, varying in thickness, and is about twenty-two inches long, but it may be longer or shorter. It contains two arteries and a vein, which run in a somewhat spinal course.

DEVELOPMENT AT DIFFERENT MONTHS.--

First month.--There are indications of the eyes, mouth and anus. The extremities are rudimentary. The heart is 4/10 of an inch long.

Second month.--It is now about one inch long. The eyes, nose and ears can be distinguished. External genitals. There are suggestions of the hands and feet.

Third month.--The ovum is now the size of a goose-egg. Fingers and toes separate, nails look like fine membranes. The neck separates the head from the body. The sex can now be told. Length is five inches. Weight about 460 grains.

Fourth month.--Six inches long and now weighs 850 grains. Short hairs are present. Head equal to about one-fourth entire body. May perceive quickening.

Fifth month.--Ten inches long; weighs eight ounces. Eyelids begin to separate. Heart sounds can he heard. Quickening takes place.

Sixth month.--Twelve inches long; weighs 23-1/2 ounces. There is hair on the head, eyebrows and eyelashes are present. Testicles show near the abdominal rings (openings).

Seventh month.--Fifteen inches long; weight 41-1/2 ounces. Pupillary membrane disappears.

Eighth month.--Sixteen inches long; weight 3-1/2 pounds. Left testicle has descended into the scrotum. Nails protrude to end of finger tips.

Ninth month.--Eighteen inches long; weighs 4-1/2 to 7 pounds. Features are complete.

While this growth goes on in the embryo the womb itself shows changes. The virgin womb averages 2-3/4 inches in length, 1-3/4 inches in width and 1 inch in thickness and weighs about 12 drams. At term (confinement) the womb is about 14 inches long, 10 inches wide, and 9-1/2 inches thick. This increase in size is necessary for its growing contents and is due to both an enlargement of its tissues (hypertrophy) and to an increase in the number of its cells (hyperplasia). The muscular fibres are elongated to about 11 inches, and they are five times thicker than they are in a womb that is not pregnant. The cervix or neck of the womb participates but little in these changes, and remains practically the same until a few weeks before confinement. It becomes softened as the result of congestion, and the glands are more active, secreting a thick glairy mucus. The canal also is more or less dilated.

While this process is going on in the womb, various other conditions show themselves, sometimes in the parts of the body so distant that it may not be easy to discover the connection with the womb. Almost any part of the body is liable to show changes from its normal condition; and yet some of these changes are so constant and regular as to be regarded as signs of pregnancy. It must not be forgotten, however, that sure signs of pregnancy, such as cannot be induced by other causes, are very limited, especially in the early months.

Changes occur in the genital organs that may lead a physician to suspect that pregnancy may exist; but the first symptom that attracts the attention of the woman, is the passing of the monthly period. This is not an absolute sign of pregnancy, since other things or conditions may cause it. The effect of the mind upon the body may cause it, and it also occurs sometimes in early married life without any appreciable cause, unless it may be then due to the effect upon the nervous system of the marital relation. Again, the monthly sickness sometimes continues in a greater or less degree, during a part or even the whole of pregnancy. Usually this discharge is due to some diseased condition of the cervix. The fear of impregnation in unmarried women after illicit intercourse will occasionally suspend menstruation for one or two months.

Nausea and Vomiting.--Another symptom upon which considerable dependence is placed is the morning sickness (nausea and vomiting). While this symptom is common, yet its absence does not prove that the woman is not pregnant. Some women go through the whole pregnancy without any sign of this symptom.

Nausea accompanied or not by vomiting may appear at the very time of conception, but it usually appears about the fourth or fifth week of pregnancy and continues until the sixteenth week or longer. In some cases it may last but a short time, in others it may continue until confinement. It may be light or severe; It generally manifests itself upon arising in the morning and subsides in a short time, but it may occur at any time of the day and continue during the entire waking hours. It may be absent entirely and, in rare instances, manifest itself in the husband alone. I have known of one such case. This nausea may be excited only by various odors or sights or may be caused by constipation. An increased secretion from the salivary glands usually accompanies the stomach disturbances and in some cases it may amount to salivation. An irresistible desire for certain articles of food or drink, generally of a sour or acid nature, is often developed. Indigestion, gas in the bowels and belching of gas are frequently present. The appetite is often capricious or it may be entirely lost (anorexia).

Breasts.--Changes in the breasts also constitute a sign of pregnancy. As an early symptom, there may be a feeling of fullness, sometimes pain. They become larger and firmer from the development of the individual lobules, which have an irregular knotty feel. A fat deposit takes place between the lobules and in the other parts of the breast. The nipples increase in size, are harder to the touch, become more prominent. A few drops of a turbid fluid, colostrum, may be pressed from the nipple as early as the third month. The veins under the skin become larger and more conspicuous. The rose-colored circles (rings) around the nipples are broadened and are slightly elevated above the surrounding skin and there is a marked increase in their pigmentation, the color varying with the complexion of the individual from reddish pink to brown and black. These changes usually occur at the beginning of the third month, and if the woman has already had a child the question of pregnancy has been decided by inspection of these breast changes.

Bladder.--This is sometimes irritable in the later months, causing a frequent desire to pass urine. It sometimes occurs in the second or third week and is sometimes followed, later, by an inability to retain the urine which escapes at any time. This, however, is not frequent.

Abdominal changes.--There is a slight flattening of the lower abdomen at the second month, due to the sinking of the womb. There is also a slight retraction (drawing back) of the navel. After the third month, when the womb begins to ascend out of the pelvis, a progressive enlargement of the abdomen begins and continues until near the end of pregnancy, when the womb again sinks and the so-called lightening occurs. The protrusion of the abdomen is more marked usually on the right side. There is often an increased deposit of fat in the lower portion of the abdomen, as well as on the hips and thighs. The navel may protrude after the sixth month,

Pigmentation.--Pigmentation or darkening of the middle line of the abdomen begins by the eighth or twelfth week, and a dark band about 1/8 of an inch wide extends from the pubis (bone) to and around the navel or even higher. This shows plainer in brunettes, where it is quite conspicuous. Discolorations also appear on other parts of the body, especially on the face, "moth patches."

Quickening.--This is caused by the movement of the child (foetus) in the womb. The impact of the enlarging womb, through the child (foetal) movements, against the abdominal wall about the sixteenth week of pregnancy gives rise to this sensation called quickening. Some women claim to have experienced this sensation at a much earlier date, and by some it is not felt at all. Gas in the bowels and contraction of the muscles of the abdomen may give a chance for mistakes. In the later months of pregnancy, the movements sometimes become so violent as to produce perceptible movements of the womb and the abdominal muscles, and sometimes they are the cause of the pain.

The Blood.--The blood is increased in quantity and slightly altered in its composition. The water, fibrin and white corpuscles are increased; the red cells are at first relatively diminished, but later return to normal.

Nervous System.--The nervous system is over sensitive and the disposition of the woman may undergo a radical change, mental exaltation and depression are often exhibited.

Constipation is the Rule.--Neuralgias in different parts of the body, especially in the face and teeth, are common. Palpitation of the heart and difficulty in breathing may be experienced. A discharge from the vagina is almost always present, due to the increased circulation in the cervix and vagina.

The Foetal Heart-beat.--This is the one positive sign of pregnancy and it may be heard as early as the sixteenth to the twentieth week. It has been compared to the ticking of a watch under a pillow. It ranges in frequency from one hundred and ten to one hundred and fifty to a minute.

Pelvic Signs.--As early as the first month of pregnancy a faint violet color of the anterior wall of the vagina just below the opening of the urethra may be distinguished. In the third month this color has become purplish and pronounced. This sign is present in eighty per cent of cases. There is also a more or less marked lividity of the vaginal portion of the cervix from the first month of pregnancy. Also there is softening of the cervix as early as the sixth week, and as pregnancy advances the whole of the cervix is softened.

Duration of Pregnancy.--This is for all practical purposes two hundred and eighty days.

How to Determine Date of Confinement.--The best rule is to count backward three months from the first day of the last menstrual period and add seven days to it. To be more accurate, in April and September only six days should be added; in December and January, five days; and in February, four days.

Position of the Womb.--At four months the top of the womb has risen above the pelvic brim bone in front; at five months, it is midway between the bone (pubic) and the navel; at six months, it is at the navel; at seven months, it is four fingers breadths above the navel; at eight months, it is midway between the navel and the bottom of the breast bone; at nine months, it is to the breast bone; from the middle to the end of the ninth month, the top of the womb sinks to about the position occupied at the eighth month.

Twins occur about once in ninety to one hundred and twenty, triplets once in one thousand eight hundred and seventy-five, and quadruplets once in three hundred and seventy-one thousand one hundred and twenty-six pregnancies. The causes are unknown. Twin conception is more common in women who have borne children, and more so in the elderly than in the young, first bearing women (primiparae).

Sex.--Children from the same ovum (egg) are always of the same sex. Of twins in general, more than one-third are males, less than one-third are females, and in the remaining one-third both sexes occur. The after-birth is always, at least at first, double.

Diagnosis.--In twin pregnancy the symptoms and disorders of pregnancy are apt to be exaggerated, and watery swelling above the pubic bone is almost always present in the latter months. The abdomen is larger and broader and there may be a depression dividing the abdominal wall in two spaces. The womb is much distended and the walls are thin.

Hygiene of pregnancy.--In pregnancy the dividing line between health and disease is often so shadowy that every care should be given the pregnant woman, not only that she shall escape dangers that may come, but that the future health of the coming baby may be safeguarded.

The care taken in pregnancy therefore should include attention to clothing, food, exercise, rest, sleep, functions of all excreting organs, the breasts, nervous system and the mind.

Clothing.--This should be worn loose. The heavier garments should not be held by the waist but suspended from the shoulders. Flannels, if possible, should be worn next the skin excepting, possibly, during the warmest weather. Every precaution should be taken not to take cold or to chill the surface of the body, as this might bring on an acute trouble of the kidneys. As soon as the womb has risen out of the pelvis during the fourth month, the corset should be absolutely abandoned, since pressure upon the enlarging womb tends to cause acute Bright's disease and uraemia, and these troubles are always to be guarded against. During the later months of pregnancy, when the abdominal enlargement is great, a linen or elastic bandage may be worn with great comfort, but it must be so put on as to support and not press upon the womb.

Food.--The food of the pregnant woman should be simple, wholesome, nutritious, of the kind that is easily digested and enough to satisfy the demands of her system; excessive eating should be avoided. A mixed diet is to be preferred, but the diet should be of such kind as to help to overcome the constipation, usual in pregnancy. Meat should not be eaten in as great quantities. It not only tends to produce more constipation but also has injurious effect upon the kidneys, and anything that in any way puts a greater burden upon the kidneys in pregnancy should be avoided. All foods that are likely to produce indigestion, heart burn, or irritation of the stomach and liver, such as sweets, fried. greasy, highly spiced foods; greasy rich gravies, or pastry should not be eaten.

The heartiest meal should be taken near midday and the stomach, especially at night, should never be overloaded. Water should, be drank freely, as it tends to overcome the constipation and wash out the kidneys. Some women do better with lighter meals and taken more frequently. Some do better by taking their breakfast before rising.

Bathing.--Extremes in hot and cold bathing should be avoided. The skin should be kept active by daily comfortable baths, followed by a brisk rubbing with a rough towel.

The Bowels and Bladder.--The bowels, as before stated, are usually constipated and should be kept open by coarse foods, fruit and, when necessary, mild laxatives; mineral waters and enemas especially should not be given. It should not be forgotten that in some women injections into the bowel are liable to bring on contractions of the womb.

No woman, and especially no pregnant woman, should ever neglect the bowels, as much discomfort and ill health are caused by improper eliminations of the bowel contents. The bladder should also have proper care. This is apt to be irritable during the early and later months of pregnancy, owing to being pressed upon by the womb. A mild inflammation arises in some cases. The woman should take plenty of water, either pure or effervescing, to induce sufficient secretion in the kidneys, and also to flush them. This is also very good for an irritable bladder. In order that the physician may keep himself informed regarding the condition of the kidneys, the urine of every pregnant woman should be examined, both chemically and microscopically, every two weeks from the beginning of pregnancy; during the late months of pregnancy the urine analysis should be made weekly. Catherized specimens should be used because leucorrheal discharges, so common in pregnancy, may give the albumin reaction. If the above advice of Dr. Manton, of Detroit, was followed in every case there would be fewer cases of trouble during the confinement. I remember one case; the lady was seven months along when I was called. She was feeling badly and complained much of her eyes; an analysis of the urine showed thick with albumin. The failure of her sight was due to thc condition of her kidneys. If the urine had been examined early and often, her condition might have been prevented. Watch the kidneys, have the urine examined frequently and carefully.

Exercise, Rest and Sleep.--Plenty of exercise in the open air should be taken daily, without this health cannot be maintained. It should not be violent or so great as to fatigue and overtire. Slow riding in a carriage and walking will give the best results. Horseback riding and riding in an automobile should be avoided. The woman should sit out of doors as much as possible. Plenty of sleep is also necessary. Eight hours are not too much at night, and lying down an hour or two during the forenoon and afternoon is very restful and desirable.

The Vagina.--When there is a profuse discharge of leucorrhea, a daily vaginal douche is necessary. This should consist of a quart of warm solution (as much as the water will dissolve) of boric acid, or an equal amount of mild carbolic acid (one to eighty). The temperature of the solution should be about 100 degrees F., and it should be injected slowly, and without any force to the stream.

It is also best to remain in the recumbent position for some time after the injection, to rest.

The Breast and Nipples.--These should be bathed once or twice daily in cool or tepid water until the last month or two of pregnancy. Astringent application should not be applied to the nipples to harden them. If the nipples are small, undeveloped or retracted they should be pulled out several times daily by the fingers and gently rubbed, and this will usually stimulate their growth. Cocoa butter or castor oil may be applied during the last month.

Nervous System and the Mind.--The pregnant woman is very susceptible to annoying conditions of the social and domestic surroundings; such should be removed, if possible, and excitement of every kind should be avoided. Everything should be made bright and comfortable around her, cheerfulness should be the rule in the home and she should be treated with every care and consideration. Surroundings will influence the coming baby's future.

Disorders of Pregnancy.--Nausea and vomiting.--The simple nausea

and vomiting of pregnancy needs no treatment. This kind generally disappears by the third or fourth month, but it may persist in a mild form during the greater part of pregnancy. Generally the regulation of the diet and attention to the bowels are all that is necessary to be done for this trouble. Foods should be chosen carefully and only such foods taken that agree with the stomach and lessen the constipation. Sometimes taking a light breakfast in bed saves the usual morning sickness. It is best then to remain lying for some time after eating. When the condition is annoying the following powder will give much relief: powder Ingluvin, oxalate of cerium, of each five grains. Mix thoroughly and take one, every one or two hours as needed. A physician should be consulted if this trouble is very severe.

MOTHERS' REMEDIES.--1. Pregnancy, A Great Aid for.--- "Soothing syrup or Mother's friend, while pregnant. Two ounces each of cramp bark, blue cohosh, slippery elm, raspberry leaves, squaw vine, orange peel and bitter root. Simmer gently in sufficient water to keep herbs covered for two hours, strain and steep gently down to one quart. Let it stand to cool, then add one cup granulated sugar, and four ounces alcohol. Dose.--One tablespoonful two or three times a day for several weeks before the birth of the child. This has been thoroughly tried and causes an easy birth where difficulty has been expected."

2. Nausea of Pregnancy, Menthol and Sweet Oil for.--"Vomiting and nausea of pregnancy; a twenty per cent solution of menthol in sweet oil; use ten drops on sugar when nausea appears." The menthol acts on the stomach and quiets it. This will be found very beneficial.

3. Pregnancy, Bouillon or Broth for.--"Was weak and generally run down. Family physician warned me I would never survive the birth of another child. I bought each day several beef bones and boiled them for three hours. I also bought chicken feet, scalded them and scraped them until the outside skin peeled off, then boiled the chicken feet with the bones. Skim surface from time to time. I would then heat up a raw egg in a glass and fill glass with this broth and drink it warm." This lady would take a glass whenever thirsty or six or seven times a day. She increased in strength immediately, within a year was the mother of a healthy baby girl now nineteen years old and believes her life was saved by the above. Anyone will find this worth trying.

Indigestion and Heart-burn.--This should be treated the same as under other conditions. Diet, habits, should be regulated. The bowels and kidneys should be regulated and do their eliminating work. For heartburn the popular remedy, magnesia may be taken or dilute hydrochloric acid with nux vomica. One teaspoonful or effervescing citrate of magnesia dissolved in water and drank, is a convenient remedy. Also, five drops of diluted hydrochloric acid in water, taken after meals, through a tube, and one or two drops of nux vomica before meals is beneficial. The following is an excellent combination from Dr. Hare, of Philadelphia:.

Dilute Hydrochloric Acid	2 drams
Essence of Pepsin	1 ounce
Compound Tincture of Gentian enough to make	4 ounces

Mix. Take one or two teaspoonfuls in a little water with meals.

In cases where it is impossible to eat anything the patient must be fed by the rectum. In such cases a doctor must be called. Fortunately such severe cases are very rare. The following for rectal feeding is given by Dr. Manton, of Detroit, and is a good combination. Give every four hours:

Liquid Beef Peptonoids	3 drams
White of an Egg	
Whisky	3 drams
Beef Tea or Warm Water enough to make	3 ounces

The rectum should be washed out once or twice daily in the interval between the feeding.

Teeth.--The teeth are often affected during pregnancy, softening and decaying rapidly, causing severe neuralgia. The teeth should be cleaned frequently during the day to get rid of the secretions of the mouth, and at night before retiring. Milk of magnesia should be held in the mouth for a few minutes; cavities in the teeth should be stopped with a temporary filling. Teaspoonful of lacto phosphate of lime can be taken three times a day with benefit.

Constipation.--The enlarging womb pressing upon the rectum and also irregularity in diet causes constipation at this time. Daily free bowel movements are necessary to prevent the kidneys from overworking. As stated before, the diet should be strictly regulated. Cascara sagrada cordial is a good mild laxative to take, if necessary.

Difficult Breathing.--This usually comes late in pregnancy and is due to the pressure of the womb upon the diaphragm; the patient should avoid excitement and sleep with the shoulders well elevated. In the ninth month the womb drops lower and the breathing is better.

Varicose Veins and Piles.--Varicose veins: These are due to the pressure on the veins so that the return flow of blood is impeded and occur as a rule late in pregnancy. They are seen oftenest on the inner side of the thighs, the lower extremities, the vulva, and in the region of the anus. As a rule, they do not give much trouble. When they become painful or inflamed the patient should lie down, with the legs elevated and use water of witch-hazel applied with cloths. Elastic stockings, properly fitted, give much relief when the trouble is on the thigh and leg.

Piles.--When these are troublesome the rectum should be emptied by a small dose of salts, and the parts thoroughly washed with warm water, the piles pushed back and local lotions applied (see treatment of piles). Hot fomentations of witch-hazel frequently give great relief to the piles as well as to the varicose veins. Regular movements of the bowels usually will prevent piles. Piles will not usually give rise to much trouble unless constipation exists.

Albumin in the urine. (Albuminuria).--While the urine of about six to ten per cent of all pregnant women contains albumin, the appearance of this symptom should always be regarded with apprehension. Women who are in their first pregnancy are most frequently affected. If the woman has had disease of the kidneys before her pregnancy began this symptom will likely appear in the early months; if it is caused by pressure, etc., it may not appear until after the sixth month, but both acute and chronic. inflammation of the kidneys may develop at any period of pregnancy. Dr. Manton, of Detroit, states, "In the majority of cases, the albuminuria is due to the so-called kidney of pregnancy, in which there is no inflammation, but a fatty infiltration of the epithelial cells associated with anemia of the organ." The urine may also contain casts. Whatever the cause it indicates a condition of insufficiency of the kidney which may lead to serious consequences to the mother and it is also injurious to the (foetus) child. If this symptom develops suddenly the danger to both is greatly increased. For this reason physicians should urge pregnant women to have their urine examined frequently, especially during the later months of pregnancy.

Treatment.--Regulation of the diet; in pronounced cases the diet should consist entirely of milk and the patient should take three or four quarts in twenty-four hours. Meats, pastry and sweets must be prohibited, but vegetables such as squash, spinach, salads may be added to the dietary in ordinary cases. Vichy water may be taken alone or with the milk, and may be taken freely. The bowels should be kept open with citrate of magnesia (one to two teaspoonfuls in water) or epsom salts in peppermint water. Exercise in the open air can be taken in moderation. Warm clothing should be worn and flannel next the skin; exposure to cold and draughts should be carefully avoided. If the more special symptoms appear, such as persistent headache, vertigo, ringing in the ears, black or bright spots floating before the eyes, dimness of vision, an abortion of miscarriage should be induced without delay. Fortunately such cases are rare and with care from the beginning seldom occur. Pregnant women should inform their family physician at the beginning of pregnancy of their condition, and in the great majority of cases serious troubles can be prevented. Physicians expect this information and receive it as a matter of course, and no woman should hesitate to inform her physician either personally or through her husband.

Abortion, Miscarriage, Premature Labor. (Accidents of pregnancy).--These three terms indicate a premature expulsion of the products of conception. Let us medically define these terms as follows; Abortion implies expulsion of the foetus before the sixteenth week. Miscarriage, the expulsion between the sixteenth and twenty-eighth weeks. Premature labor designates the time of expulsion as between the twenty-eighth week to within a few weeks before the normal termination of pregnancy. Miscarriage is the term popularly used for the accidental loss of the products of conception.

Abortion, in the popular mind, expresses the intentional loss of the products of conception. Abortion in the medical sense, takes place about once in every four or five pregnancies. It occurs more frequently in those who have borne children, occurring generally in the third or fourth pregnancy, or toward the end of the child-bearing period, and it takes place more frequently between the ninth and sixteenth week, when the after-birth is in process of formation; and it is more liable to occur at the time of the month when the normal menstruation would be due. It should be borne in mind also that abortion occurring at this period is quite dangerous to the mother's future health, and also dangerous to life; so that at the first indication of abortion a physician should be called for this trouble, because it needs care, both to prevent it and to assist the woman to a successful ending when it is impossible to prevent it. This is more dangerous to life than confinement at full term, and is apt to leave behind a tendency to recurrence at the same time in the future pregnancies, and also makes the woman liable to inflammatory conditions of the womb.

Causes.--Abortion may be induced by many causes due to the mother, father, and child. Among maternal causes may be mentioned any serious disease, especially fevers, when accompanied by a rash on the skin, such as smallpox, measles, scarlet fever. It is hard for a pregnant woman to go through one of these diseases, without having an abortion. Syphilis, tuberculosis, malaria, organic heart and kidney disease, diabetes, anemia, and systemic poisoning also are causes; nervous disturbances as shock, fright, sorrow, convulsions, chorea; mechanical causes, violent exercise, lifting, blows, falls, coughing, vomiting; local causes, as wrong position of the womb, inflammation of the womb, etc.; all are causes.

Causes. Due to the Father. Paternal.--Syphilis, alcoholism, lead poisoning, excessive venery, extremes of youth or old age.

Foetal Causes.--Disease of the after-birth, other parts, of cord, death of the foetus, placenta pravia, and yet many women are subjected to falls, blows, etc., who carry their child to full term.

Symptoms.--These vary with the period of pregnancy where they occur. In the earlier months the symptoms are those of profuse menstruation, sometimes accompanied by more pain perhaps than usual. The ovum is then so small that it escapes notice. In the profuse flow there may be unaccustomed clots of blood; when this trouble occurs later in pregnancy there are two constant symptoms which, together with the history of the case, render the diagnosis easy. These prominent and constant symptoms are pain and bleeding. The symptoms may be preceded by a bearing down feeling in the lower abdomen, with backache, frequent calls to pass urine, and a discharge from the vagina, that is a mixture of mucus and water. After these symptoms last for a shorter or longer time, labor pains set in, the bleeding increases and the contents of the womb are discharged. The ovum may be expelled whole when it looks like a huge blood clot, or it may be expelled partly and the membranes left behind; or the embryo (child) alone, surrounded by the transparent membrane, escapes.

If the after-birth has formed it may be cast off entire or piecemeal. The embryo (child) alone may escape, the neck of the womb contracts and shuts; bleeding persists for an indefinite period, for weeks and weeks, until the health of the poor woman is seriously affected. Persistent bleeding of this kind is almost always due to the retention of portions of the after-birth or membranes, and should prove to the woman that there is a serious condition existing which should be speedily corrected. A physician should be called who should make a thorough examination; and if such a condition as above described is found, should free the womb from its retained products, which are not only sapping the woman's life, but also rendering the future health of the womb very uncertain.

Threatened Abortion.--If a bleeding takes place in the woman who is pregnant, abortion may be assumed to threaten; a careful examination will usually settle this matter.

Inevitable Abortion.--The abortion is probably inevitable if the bleeding becomes persistent and free, the cervix softens, the womb dilates and the labor pains set in. Still in spite of all these conditions, the bleeding and pain may cease, and the pregnancy go on to full term, The result of these cases, if carefully and properly treated, is favorable as far as the mother is concerned.

Treatment. Preventive. In women where repeated abortions have occurred, the cause should be diligently sought for. If syphilis exists the treatment should be begun at the beginning of pregnancy. But when no special cause can be found, and an irritable condition of the womb is suspected to be present, the patient must be kept quiet in bed, especially at the time when menstruation would normally occur. She should also be guarded against lifting, fright, worry, over-exertion; and medicines like bromide of potash, five to fifteen grains at a dose, given to quiet and allay the nervous irritability.

Treatment of Threatened Abortion.--The patient should go to bed, lie down and remain there, and if possible be not only quiet physically, but also quiet mentally. The main remedy is opium, and if necessary to obtain a quick action it can be given hypodermically in the form of morphine. Otherwise, laudanum may be given by the mouth, twenty drops, repeated cautiously, every three or four hours as required, or it can be given in thirty-drop doses combined with a couple of ounces of starch water by the rectum. Extract of opium in pill form, one grain three times a day by the month; or a suppository of opium, one grain, may be inserted into the rectum every four to six hours. After the bleeding and pain have ceased, the emergency is probably passed; but rest in bed and quiet should be the routine for one or more weeks, and the patient should always rest in bed at the usual time of the menstrual period, during the remainder of the pregnancy.

Treatment of the Inevitable Abortion.--If the cervix is hard and the canal is not dilated, especially if the bleeding is free, the vagina should be packed full at once, if possible, with iodoform gauze. Rolls five yards long and two inches wide can be bought perfectly adapted to this purpose. A speculum should be used (Sims' or Graves') and the gauze should first be packed tightly into corners (fornices) around the cervix, then over the cervix and well down to the outlet. This should be held in place by a proper (T) bandage. The gauze can be removed in from twelve to twenty-four hours, and the ovum will generally be found lying upon the upper part of the packing, or in the canal that is now dilated, from which it can easily be removed. Sometimes it is necessary to repack and allow it to remain for another twelve hours as the canal has not been sufficiently dilated by the first packing. This packing not only causes the canal to dilate but usually stops the bleeding. After the ovum has been expelled an antiseptic vaginal douche should be given twice a day for a week or longer.

If at the first examination the cervix is found softened and the mouth of the womb is open, but the womb has not yet expelled its contents, the sterile (clean) finger may be introduced into the womb and the ovum and membranes loosened and taken away, while this is being done counter pressure should be made over the abdomen. After the womb has been cleared of all its contents an antiseptic solution should be used, carefully, in the womb to wash it out, and this followed by washing out of the vagina. The after treatment is the same as that for labor at full term. The woman should remain in bed at least ten days.

Placenta Praevia.--The after-birth is placed in the lower part of the womb; (after-birth before the child). This is a dangerous condition and terrible bleeding may occur. It occurs about one time out of every one thousand. The main symptom is bleeding and this may occur at any period of pregnancy. It usually appears from the seventh to the ninth month. The outset is without any appreciable reason and without pain. The amount of blood lost at the first attack may be so slight as to escape notice or copious enough to endanger the life of the mother. This flow may occur at any time during these months, and it may be small or great. If during the course of pregnancy the bleeding occurs at intervals in the increasing amount, the greater will be the loss of blood during the labor.

Treatment.--There is little danger of dangerous bleeding before the seventh month, and a waiting treatment may be adopted, but the woman should be closely watched and told what the trouble is, so she will be willing to remain quiet. Rest in bed, the avoidance of all muscular exercise and quieting medicines may enable the mother to carry the child until it can live, when pregnancy must be quickly terminated. If the child is dead the womb must be emptied at once. After the seventh month an expectant treatment is no longer allowable, and authorities declare the pregnancy should be terminated without delay. The mother is in great danger from sudden free flow. This treatment must be given by an experienced hand and only a physician can do it. If the pregnancy is allowed to continue to full term the danger to the woman is very great, as the mortality runs from thirty to sixty-five per cent; but under modern treatment it has been brought down to five to ten per cent. The death rate of the child is between fifty and seventy-five per cent.

Labor.--Labor may be defined as the physiological termination of pregnancy whereby the mature foetus (child) and its appendages (after-birth, etc.), are separated from the maternal organism.

Premonitory Signs of Labor.--Premonitory signs of labor, usually observed from one to two weeks before the onset of the labor pains, is a sinking down of the womb in the abdomen, whereby some of the unpleasant features of pregnancy are relieved, and the so-called "lightening" takes place. The waist line becomes small, the breathing is easier and the general well-being of the woman is better, so that her friends are attracted by her feeling of relief. But as a result of the womb descent and the consequent pressure, irritation of the bladder and rectum may occur, and she may have frequent calls to empty these organs. The vagina secretes more actively, the veins enlarge, some dropsy may appear in the extremities, and the womb contractions of pregnancy, which have been painless, begin to cause more and more discomfort.

These false pains recur at regular intervals of hours or even days, and generally at night, last for a varying period and usually disappear in the morning. They often deceive the woman and lead her to the belief that the labor has already begun; but examination of the cervix will reveal that this is not so. It is well to bear in mind that the true labor pains usually begin in the back, extend down to the thighs and often around to the front and they recur at regular intervals, and with increasing intensity.

The beginning of labor is characterized by recurring pains at regular intervals and of increasing severity. There is also a discharge from the vagina of mucus, and this is sometimes tinged with blood, "the show." If an examination is now made, it will be found that the cervix (neck of the womb) is shortened, and that the mouth of the womb is beginning to dilate. At the beginning, the pains are usually in the back and spread to the abdomen and down the thighs; but they may be felt first in the abdomen. They return every half hour or twenty minutes, but as labor goes on the interval is shortened, so that toward the end of the second stage when the child is being born, they appear to be continuous, and the patient feels as if she is encircled by a belt of pain; however, with all this, she will bear the suffering easier and better for she knows that progress is being made, and that she will soon be over the pains and the child born. A pain rarely lasts more than one minute.

STAGES OF LABOR.--First stage extends from the beginning of labor until the mouth of the womb is dilated. Second stage, from the complete dilation until the complete birth of the child. Third stage, from the birth of the child until the expulsions of the after-birth--Placenta.

The First Stage.--The first stage varies greatly in different women. The average duration of this stage is from ten to fourteen hours in the woman with the first child, and six to eight hours in the woman who has borne children. During this stage the woman prefers to remain on her feet, sit, stand or walk about. The amount of pain experienced varies greatly, according to the temperament of the patient; in nervous women it may be excessive. The pains now have nothing of that bearing down character which they afterward acquire; they are described as "grinding," are usually felt in the front. The genitals become bathed with secretions, which are sometimes tinged with blood. This is an especially trying period to a young wife, for she cannot see that the pains are doing any good, only making her restless, tired and nervous. Little can be done by the physician in this stage except to encourage and explain what is really being accomplished by these seemingly futile pains and by tact and proper encouragement, a physician tides this stage over and gives great comfort to the needy patient. This stage ends with the opening and dilation of the mouth of the womb and the second or expulsive stage sets in, with pains altered in character.

Second Stage.--The pains now become more frequent and severe and last longer, and the patient now manifests a strong desire to expel the contents of the womb. The woman now feels better in bed and when the pains come she involuntarily bears down, with each contraction she sets her teeth, takes a deep breath, fixes the diaphragm, contracts the muscles of the abdomen and bears down hard if you allow her to do so. The knowledge that she is working to overcome an obstacle gives her some satisfaction and she feels that she is accomplishing something by the efforts she is making. The physician can aid greatly by suggesting to the patient how to use the pains and how much bearing down to do. He can tell her when not to bear down, and so save her strength for the next real pain when bearing down will do good. Although the pains are really harder in this stage, nervous women suffer no more, for their mind is now concentrated upon the work at hand. Sometimes at the beginning of this stage the patient feels chilly or has a severe chill; a hot drink and more covering counteract this.

Another phenomena is the escape of the waters and a lull in the pains for a little time, when they come on more effectively than before as the womb contracts down upon the child and is not hindered by the "bag of water." The pains keep on at intervals until the child is born and the physician can now be of help by guiding, directing and assisting the birth of the head. This stage averages about two hours.

34

Third Stage.--The birth of the head is very soon followed by the shoulders and the rest of the body, and the woman is now at comparative rest. The cord is now tied and cut and the child laid away, if all right, in a warm place until it can be washed and dressed. Following the birth of the child there is a short resting period, the contractions of the womb cease and it becomes smaller through retraction. After a few minutes the pains begin again, the after-birth separates from its attachment in the womb, and together with the membranes is extruded into the vaginal canal and vulvar opening; whence it can be easily delivered by pressing upon the abdomen over the lump (womb) and by guiding the after-birth with the cord. This should be done slowly so that the membranes will all come away with the after-birth.

This should always be examined to be certain that everything has come away. A greater or less amount of clots of blood come with the after-birth. The contraction of the womb stops the bleeding, one hand should be kept on the abdomen over the womb, to see that it remains hard and retracted. The womb moves under the hand. If it softens, gentle rubbing should be kept up and the womb will soon remain contracted. This stage averages about fifteen minutes.

MANAGEMENT OF LABOR.--Preparation of the Bed.--The bed should be high, springs not soft, with a firm and smooth mattress. It should be placed so that both sides are accessible. The bed should be made up on the right side as a rule, as the woman usually lies on her left side when delivered. Place a rubber, or an oil cloth sheet, over the mattress, and over this an ordinary muslin sheet and secure this with safety pins to the corners of the mattress. This is the permanent bed; on top of this is the second rubber sheet and this is covered with another muslin sheet and both held by safety pins. This is the temporary bed. Plenty of hot and cold boiled water should also be at hand. Frequently only a temporary bed is made with rubber or oil cloth underneath, blanket and sheet above this. They should be fastened so that the movements of the woman will not disorder them. These can be removed after the confinement and new, clean warm clothes put in their place. The objection to this is the woman may be too tired to be moved, while, with the permanent and temporary bed arrangement she need not be moved at all, only lifted, while the temporary bed is being removed and she is then let down easily upon clean bedding.

Preparation of the Patient.--The patient, if she desires, can take a full bath. The bowels should be moved thoroughly with a soap and water injection so that the rectum will be fully emptied. This makes labor not only easier, but pleasanter, as no feces will be discharged during labor. The bladder should also be emptied. The external organs should be scrupulously cleansed and bathed with some antiseptic solution, like glycothymoline, listerine, borolyptol, etc. A fresh suit of underwear may then be put on and over this a loose wrapper.

Examination of the Patient.--The physician needs to satisfy himself as to the position of the child, etc. This can be done by an examination of the abdomen and also of the vagina. He must determine whether the child is alive, its position, the condition of the cervix and mouth of the womb. In making such examination a routine plan should be adopted. The coat must be removed, the shirt sleeves turned up and the hands and arms washed with soap and water. The abdomen should be thoroughly palpated (felt) and listened to with the ear or stethoscope to determine the character of the child's heart beat, whether it be very slow, one hundred and twenty or less, or a very rapid one, one hundred and fifty or more. It may indicate danger to the child and necessitate a hurried delivery. After these things have been done, the hands and arms must again be thoroughly washed and sterilized, the fingers anointed with carbolated vaselin and the examination of the vagina made.

This cleanliness is necessary, and if this plan were carried out by everyone connected with the patient during the whole confinement, there would be fewer cases of "child-bed" fever, with its resultant diseases. The patient should lie on her back with the knees drawn up. There is no need for any exposure now, for the covering can be held up by an attendant so that it will not touch the physician's hands. The soft parts are now separated by the fingers of one hand while the examining fingers are introduced into the vagina. These fingers should never touch any external part and especially the parts near the anus. If the cervix is found to be long and the canal still undilated, or only slightly so, and especially if it is the first child (primipara), the physician's presence is not needed and he may safely leave for an hour or two. But if the mouth (os) of the womb is dilated to the size of a silver dollar he should on no account leave the house.

Frequent examination of the vagina should not be made. In ordinary cases during the first stage, the woman should be up and encouraged to walk about the room, to sit or assume any comfortable position. During a pain she may stand beside the bed resting her hands upon something or kneel in front of the bed or chair. The standing position assists in the birth. The bladder should be emptied frequently, as a distended bladder retards labor and may even stop the womb contractions. The pains become more frequent and severe as the end of this stage approaches and each contraction is now accompanied by straining or a bearing down effort on the part of the woman, and as a rule the membranes rupture spontaneously about this time. An examination of the vagina should now be made with the woman in bed, and if the membranes have not broken and the womb is completely dilated as shown during the pain, they may be ruptured by pressing against them with a finger-nail during a pain. Sometimes we use every means to retain the membranes intact, but that is when protection for the child is needed for sometime longer. If the suffering is very severe, during this stage, fifteen grains of chloral hydrate, well diluted with water, may be given every fifteen or thirty minutes until sixty grains have been given. (This medicine should never be given to a person with heart trouble). I find one drop doses of the tincture of Gelsemium every fifteen to thirty minutes of benefit, especially if the womb does not dilate well, or the patient is very nervous. The patient may receive and can receive light nourishment during this stage.

Management of the Second Stage.--After the rupture of the membranes the labor proceeds faster and a termination may be expected within a reasonable time. There is a short lull in the pains, usually, after the waters have escaped and during this time the patient should remove her clothing and put on a night dress, and to prevent its being soiled roll it well up under the arms and retain it there. After labor it can be very easily pulled down and made comfortable for the patient. A folded, clean, sterile sheet is now placed about the body and extremities and held in place by a cord around the waist. The opening in the sheet should be in the right side, as this will allow the assistance being given as needed. The powerful force of the abdominal muscles is now brought into action; the force is best utilized with the woman lying on her back.

She should now be encouraged to bear down during the pains and she will be greatly assisted by pulling on a sheet or long towel tied to the foot of the bed, or by holding the hand of the nurse. A support for her feet frequently aids the woman. Pressing low on her back relieves her to some extent. In the intervals between the pains she should rest, do nothing, and be perfectly passive. It is now that an anesthetic may be used to relieve the suffering. She should not be put completely under its influence for that is not only unnecessary, but injurious. Chloroform when used should be given on a handkerchief opened and loosely held over the woman's face, and administered drop by drop on the handkerchief. The handkerchief should be placed over the face at the beginning of the pain and be taken away as soon as the pain is stopped. The woman inhales the chloroform during the pains and their sharpness is blunted. Given in that way it is not considered dangerous. It should only be pushed to unconsciousness during a forceps delivery, and even then it is not always necessary to render the woman unconscious. I have used the forceps without giving an anesthetic. They should be placed without causing any special pain, and assist in delivery without causing any more pain when the head is down low. Of course if the forceps must be used when the head is high up a greater amount of anesthetic is needed.

Dr. Manton, of Detroit, says:--"The dangers of anesthetics are the same when employed for obstetric purposes as in surgery, and then use should be governed by the same rules in each instance." As soon as the head begins to dilate the vulvar opening, the patient should be turned on her left side with her knees drawn up and her body lying diagonally across the bed, with the buttocks close to and parallel with the edge. This position allows the physician to give better assistance and is no harder for the patient.

The physician with his hands thoroughly sterilized and with a clean sterilized gown, seats himself on the edge of the bed and watches the progress of the labor, ready to assist the woman at any moment. And at this time he can do much by words of encouragement and proper directions to the laboring woman how to use her pains so as to get the most from them; and also by manipulation of the soft parts and the head. The head advances more and more with each succeeding pain, and the perineum is put on the stretch, each contraction is followed by a resting pause during which the head slips back a little and relieves the perineum. Tear of the perineum is liable to take place when the head is about to escape through the vulvar opening, especially if the contractions are strong, the woman bears down forcibly and the interval between the pains is short, so that the head is forced out before the parts have time to completely dilate and soften. Here is where the physician's work comes in, by holding the head back and fully flexed (bent), chin upon the breast, and keeping the back of the head (occiput) well up towards the bone in front (pubic arch) until thc perineum is completely dilated.

The effect of the pains can be lessened, if necessary, also, by telling the woman to open her mouth and not to bear down during the pain for a few times. In this way the perineum will dilate properly and be torn little, if at all, and perhaps much future trouble for the woman saved. I always tell my patient why I ask her to do certain things in labor and I have never found any woman who, when able, was not willing to do as I asked. A torn perineum is not desirable, because even when sewn up immediately after labor, it may not unite thoroughly, and thus cause displacements of the womb in the future. A little time and care at the time of labor will save the perineum and every woman is willing to do her share when the conditions are plainly explained to her. It takes only a few minutes longer, and only a few more pains to bear. When the head begins to stretch the opening, the left hand of the physician should be carried over the woman's abdomen and between the thighs, her right leg being supported by a pillow placed between her knees, and this left hand presses the back of the head (occiput) forward and against the "pubic arch." The right hand may also press the head upward by being placed against the posterior portion of the dilated perineum. The edge of the perineum should now be closely watched. A small towel wrung out of a bowl of hot water placed handy on a chair, should be held constantly against the perineum to hasten the softening and dilatation of these tissues. Plenty of hot water and small towels should be at hand. The head advances with each pain and again recedes until the parts are properly dilated, and the perineum slips backward over the child's face.

If torn, it should be sewed before the physician leaves, as it can be done easily and without pain to the mother. As the head of the child emerges, the anesthetic should he pushed, or the woman told to open her mouth and cry out. This lessens the pain and the child's head emerges slower, and the perineum is saved. The child's head should be received in the hand. After the head is born, there is a lull

for a few moments. Then the shoulders rotate into the proper position and are easily born. There may then be a flow of watery fluid for a few seconds. Before this time the physician has examined to see whether the cord is around the child's neck, released it if it has been, and also cleaned out the child's mouth. The child usually cries a little about this time and it is soon seen whether it needs quick attention. The perineum should be guarded also while the shoulders are being born as it can be torn by them. The shoulders are generally born without any help. The child's head is held in the physician's hand. As soon as the body is born, the child should be laid upon the bed behind the mother's thighs, and the cord pulled down to prevent it pulling upon the after-birth. After the beating in the cord has ceased, generally from five to ten minutes have elapsed, the cord is then tied, tight enough so it will not bleed afterward, about one or one and one half inches (some say more) from the body and tied a second time an inch or so from the first ligature, and the cord cut between the two ligatures. Care should be taken so as not to cut a finger or toe of the baby. If the cord is very thick it is best to pinch it at the point of tying and the contents stripped away before the first ligature is applied. After the cord is cut it should be wiped off to determine that bleeding from the vessels has been permanently cut off, and if not it should be tied again. The child is now taken up by placing the back of its neck in the hollow between the thumb and forefinger, and the other hand over the backbone. It should then be placed in a warm receiving blanket, and put in a safe place.

Management of the Third Stage,--The contractions of the womb are renewed and with the second or third the after-birth may be expressed. The top (fundus) of the womb is grasped by the hand through the relaxed abdominal walls, and squeezed, and at the same time make a downward pressure. The after-birth is loosened from the womb and slides through the vagina and outlet, and it may be caught in a tray which has been placed between the patient's legs, or by the hand and given a few twists in order to roll the membranes together; while this is being done, gentle rubbing should be applied to the womb, when the membranes will slip out without tearing; no drawing on the cord should be done in delivering the after-birth.

From the time of the birth of the head to the delivery of the after-birth the womb must be controlled by the firm pressure of the hand on the abdomen. It is well for the nurse, when the after-birth is separating from the womb to follow the womb, throughout this whole stage, by keeping her hand upon it and if, while the physician is attending to the child, the womb softens and enlarges she should at once notify him. There may be bleeding within the womb. After the womb is empty, friction should be made over the womb whenever it softens at all in order to stimulate the womb to perfect contraction, and it should be kept up at intervals for one hour after the after-birth and membranes have been delivered.

THE CHILD.

The eyes should be washed soon and normal respiration established. If the child does not breathe well, cold water may be sprinkled in the face and chest and if this fails, immersions in hot water at 106 degrees F., and sprinkling with cold water must be resorted to. If necessary, artificial respiration must be given. Slap the child on the back and move the arms up and down by the side a few times, or breathing into the child's mouth.

Another method.--Face the child's back, put an index finger in each arm-pit and the thumbs over the shoulders, so that their ends over-lap the collar-bone and rest on the front of the chest, the rest of the fingers going obliquely over the back of the chest. The child is suspended perpendicularly between the operator's knees. Its whole weight now hangs on the first fingers in the arm-pit; by these means the ribs are lifted, the chest is expanded and inspiration is mechanically produced. The infant is now swung upward till the operative's hands are just above the horizontal line, when the motion is abruptly, but carefully, arrested. The momentum causes the lower limbs and pelvis of the infant to topple over toward the operator. The greater part of the weight now rests on the thumbs, which press on the front of the chest, while the abdominal organs press upon the diaphragm. By these two factors, the chest is compressed and we get expiration, mechanically. After five seconds the first position is resumed again, and the lungs expand and fill with air. This process may be repeated several times until the breathing seems to be going naturally, and with delicate infants it should be the last resort.

After the breathing has been established the child should be wrapped in a warm flannel with hot water bags or cans near it, and left until the mother has been cared for. Infants at birth are covered with a white greasy substance, vernix caseosa, or cheesy varnish; it is removed by applying olive oil, vaselin or fresh lard, and afterward rubbing the skin gently with a soft cloth. The eyes and mouth should be washed out with pure warm water--or a saturated solution of boric acid, used. Separate squares of soft linen being used for this purpose. If the baby is born too soon or is very small, weak and undeveloped, it should be given an oil bath, only, and then wrapped in cotton wool and kept at a temperature of not less than 80 degrees F., for ten days or two weeks.

To a fully developed child the first bath may be given at once. Have everything ready before beginning, a foot tub, warm soft towels, warm water, castile soap, olive oil or vaselin, small squares of muslin or linen, dusting powder, a dressing for the navel and clothing, the latter consisting of a diaper, a flannel band, a shirt, long woolen stockings, a loose long sleeved flannel petticoat and a simple soft white outside garment, the two last, long enough to more than cover the feet. The infant should be wrapped in flannel and only the part which is being bathed at the moment should be exposed. The eyes are first bathed separately and with different cloths, and afterward the face, no soap being used; the head is then washed with warm water; very little soap should be used with infants as it is more or less irritating, and it is likely to injure the fine texture of the skin. Next, one should carefully clean the parts behind the ears and the crevices of the neck, arm-pits and joints and those between the buttocks and the thighs, and it is well to notice if all the natural openings are perfect; finally the baby is put down into the tub of warm water at about 96 degrees F., and washed off, with the head and back firmly supported with the left arm and hand during the bath. The baby is lifted out in a minute of two, held face downward for a moment and rinsed off with clean warm water. It is then wrapped in a warm towel and flannel and dried by patting, not rubbing. It is best to do all this on a table, instead of on the lap, and it should be large enough to hold a bath tub, every thing necessary for the bath and a pillow upon which to place the baby. Everything then can be done without stooping and with greater comfort to the child. Powder should not he used except where there are signs of chafing, when stearate of zinc is the best to use.

The navel is then dressed. A hole is cut in the center of a square of sterilized lint or linen which is slipped over the cord and folded about it; the cord is then laid toward the left side, and over it is put a small sterilized cotton pad which is held in place by the flannel bandage and just tight enough to hold. The binder may be kept on by sewing it smoothly with half a dozen large stitches, thus doing away with any danger of being injured from the pins. A binder should only be tight enough to hold the dressing for the navel. After the cord drops off the looser knitted band should be used. The infant is not bathed in the tub again until after the cord has been dried up and ready to drop off, which usually occurs on the fifth or sixth day, although it may not drop off for nine days. The cord should not be redressed in the meantime. (See Baby Department for further directions).

THE MOTHER.

The first duty of the physician, following the third stage of labor, is to see that the womb is well contracted and control of this organ should be continued for at least one hour after delivery. This generally prevents excessive loss of blood. If necessary to promote womb contraction one teaspoonful of ergot can be given. After the womb has been kept in a state of contraction, the room should be rid of all evidences of labor and the woman made comfortable. The buttocks and thighs which have been soiled during the labor should be bathed with warm water and soap and the external genitals sprayed with an antiseptic solution, then dried with sterile gauze or cotton, the dressing applied to the vulva and the temporary bed removed, her night dress pulled down and the patient thus lying in a clean, comfortable bedding. The woman may then have a cup of weak tea, hot milk or broth and be left to rest; but during the first sleep the womb should be carefully watched lest it relax and serious, if not fatal, bleeding occur. In a normal confinement the dressings need not be changed, as a rule, oftener than six times in twenty-four hours, for the first few days. As soon as convenient after the first toilet is finished the physician sterilizes his hands and with the patient on her left side introduces one finger into the rectum and the thumb into the vagina to discover the condition of the perineum. Washing out of the vagina is not necessary as a rule.

The binder is considered indispensable, and should be made of unbleached muslin and wide enough to extend from the pubic (bone) to the breast-bone, and long enough to go around the patient's body and slightly lap. The binder should be pinned or sewed tightest in the middle, but it should not be so tight as to press upon the womb and crowd it backward or to either side. It acts as a splint to the muscles and assists in resting them to their natural condition.

Rest.--Complete rest of the body and mind is essential to the well being of the lying-in woman. She is better off without any company, and should see no one except her family for the first week or two. Outside visitors should be prohibited. The lying-in room should be kept free from noise and confusion, and the patient should be protected from annoyances of every kind. She should remain lying on her back for a few days and immediately following delivery she should not have a pillow for her head. Sleep is very necessary and desirable, and mild medicines should be given to produce it, if necessary. It is best not to sit up in the bed until the womb shall have had time to become smaller, and has resumed its natural position behind the pubis. Among the upper classes, when it takes the womb longer to regain its normal size, three weeks is a good rule to go by before sitting up in the room, and she should remain in her room until the end of the fourth week. Among healthy women of the laboring class, whose muscular system has not been injured by "culture" and social excesses, the womb and appendages regain their normal proportions more rapidly; but even they should remain in bed two weeks.

AFTER-PAINS.--Women who have borne children frequently suffer from the after-pains, occurring at irregular intervals, for two or three days and they may give rise to much distress. A few drops of spirits of camphor on a lump of sugar will often give relief when they are not severe. Also a drop of tincture of blue cohosh taken every two or three hours is valuable.

THE BLADDER.--If the patient is not able to pass urine it should be drawn once in eight or twelve hours or oftener if required. A No.7 rubber catheter is best. After it has been used, it should be sterilized by boiling and then kept in a bichloride solution (1-2000). It should be washed off with boiled water again before being used to remove the bichloride solution and greased with sterile oil. The parts should be exposed to pass the catheter, the labia separated by the finger and thumb, and the opening of the urethra and surrounding parts bathed clean with an antiseptic solution; unless you are clean decomposing discharges from the vagina may be introduced into the bladder and a cystitis set up. The care of the bladder is very important. It is not so sensitive after the labor and the woman may have urine when she does not think so. Sometimes she passes a little after trying and then thinks there is no more in the bladder. Even the attendants are deceived sometimes. I once had a case where the mother was the nurse. At each visit I inquired as to the amount of urine passed. I was told each time it was sufficient. She suffered severely the second day in the evening. I went to see her and against the protests of the mother I used the catheter and took away an enormous quantity of urine. In such cases the bladder should be emptied slowly to save the woman from shock.

A physician cannot always depend upon the patient's knowledge of her condition even in such matters and sometimes even the nurse is at fault.

THE BOWELS.--There should be a movement of the bowels the second or third day, and a soap and water enema containing a small teaspoonful of spirits of turpentine and one-half ounce of glycerin, will usually be sufficient. Later cascara cordial, castor oil, etc., may be used. Should the breasts be much swollen and painful and fever arise, saline laxatives are needed for two or three days, such as citrate of magnesia, rochelle salts, hunyadi water or seidlitz powder may be given.

Care of the Breasts.--Careful attention should be given them from the first. The nipples should be bathed after labor, with an antiseptic lotion (bichloride, 1-2000), dried and then covered with castor oil, a small square of clean sterile gauze being laid over each to protect the clothing. Bathe the nipples before and after each nursing with a warm saturated solution of boric acid and dry them carefully. The breasts may be supported by a binder, made of a strip of muslin sufficiently wide to extend from above to well below the breasts. If they are heavy and sagging place a layer of cotton at the outer border of each breast and they should be raised toward the middle line, the binder being pinned only tight enough to hold without pressing upon them. The breasts should not be pressed upon by anything. Shoulder straps can be pinned or sewed on the binder if it has a tendency to slip down. Should the breasts be much swollen relief can be obtained by massage with warm olive oil and by the use of a breast pump. The tips of the fingers only should be used in giving massage and the stroke should be light, from the circumference to the center. Roughness and pressure must be avoided.

INFLAMMATION OF THE BREAST, Abscess; Broken Breast.-- This usually results from germs. The breast inflames, the milk tubes are choked and distended, there may be fever. There is sometimes severe local pain, hard swelling and an abscess forms and if this breaks it is called broken breast.

Treatment, Preventive.--Support breast with a binder. The milk should not be allowed to accumulate and cake. The breasts and nipples should be kept clean and dry. Breast pump should be used if necessary to get out the surplus milk. If the lumps continue and are painful, put cold applications to the breast. Have child nurse at the other breast. If it continues and will suppurate, apply moist heat, such as fomentations or poultices, and then open thoroughly. Poke root makes a splendid poultice for caked breasts. I have great faith in it. At the same time I give of the tincture one drop doses every hour. It is a splendid remedy and the poultice and remedy frequently stop the trouble. Inflammation of the breasts sometimes occurs in babies, generally in the first weeks. The swelling can be reduced by mild rubbing with warm carbolized oil used every day. Do not rub hard enough to hurt the baby. After the rubbing, absorbent cotton with carbolized oil should be applied and cover all with a thick layer of cotton held on with adhesives. If the breasts form pus they must be opened.

MOTHERS' REMEDIES. 1. Sore Breasts, a Never-Failing Remedy for.--"Take a pint of raw linseed oil and four ounces tincture of camphor, mix and apply a cloth saturated in the liniment to the affected parts, taking care that the whole surface of the inflamed parts is covered with the liniment. When the breasts become swollen or painfully inflamed, apply the liniment often to prevent gathering." Even if they have gathered it is an excellent outward application. It allays pain, is extremely soothing and seldom fails to effect a cure.

2. Swollen Breasts, an Herb Treatment for.--"Chamomile flowers one ounce, marshmallow roots one ounce, bruise and boil in one quart of water down to a pint. Foment the breast with this liquor as hot as can be borne; and then place the flowers and roots in a cloth and apply as a poultice."

3. Sore Breasts, a Hot Poultice for.--"Apply hot pancakes made of sour milk, saleratus and wheat flour, large enough to cover affected parts. Keep them changed often enough, so they will not be cold. This is an excellent remedy to steam out the inflammation." This is an old tried remedy and one to be relied upon. The steaming relieves the swelling and inflammation and gives relief quickly.

4. Caked Breasts, Fresh Hops for.--"Fry one pint of fresh hops in a half cup of lard until the lard is a rich brown, then strain, set away to cool and use as a salve."

5. Sore Breasts, a Poultice of Peach Leaves for.--"Take enough peach tree leaves to mix well with meal and water to the consistency of a poultice." This poultice should be applied hot, but should only be used in cases where the breast has matter or pus in it.

MOTHERS' REMEDIES.--l. Sore Nipples, a Good Wash for.--"Brandy and water mixed together and put on the nipples will harden them but should be washed off before the child nurses. If they are cracked, apply glycerin with starch, or arnica ointment."

2. Sore Nipples, Good Family Ointment for.--"Four ounces of white wax, one ounce bayberry wax, three ounces of spermaceti, one pint olive oil. Mix briskly over a slow fire, taking care to stir it briskly until cool." This is an excellent ointment for mothers when troubled with sore nipples; it moistens the skin and forms a coating.

It is good for dry, scurvy, chapped hands, blotches on the face and all sores which require a mild ointment, but should be assisted with internal remedies when the case requires it.

The Lochia.--By this term is meant the discharges from the womb and soft parts after labor. They are mixed with blood at first and contain dark clots, mucus, shreds of the after-birth and pieces of the membrane. They become paler in color from the end of the third to the sixth day. After this the color is yellow, greenish and contains pus and fatty cells, with a little blood. This discharge varies in different women. In those who menstruate freely and do not nurse they are usually copious; when decomposed, they smell badly and the odor is penetrating. The flow may cease entirely between the second and sixth week. It is increased by exertions at about the time the patient begins to move about.

Diet.--This should consist at first of liquid, unstimulating food, given in small quantities and frequently. If the baby does not nurse, the liquids should be restricted. Some women on the first day can take milk, milk toast, or if desired, dry or buttered toast with coffee, tea, weak cocoa, according to the patient's taste. Water may be given if desired. On the second and third days, simple soups or any of the following may be added to the dietary: Meat broths, beef tea, soft boiled or poached eggs, raw or stewed oysters (no vinegar or spices) and some simple dessert, such as boiled custard or junket. During the next few days, chicken (white meat), scraped beef or mutton in small quantities, baked potato, rice and cereals may be given and by the end of the week a gradual return to the ordinary diet may be made. Should there be any tendency to constipation, the bowels should be opened by a simple enema (as before stated) or glycerin enema, etc.; or by one or more doses, 2 drams, of the compound licorice powder repeated in three or four hours, if necessary; or a half ounce of castor oil, or a half glass of hunyadi water. Cooked fruits for the constipation may also be given.

Bleeding After Delivery, Post-Partum Hemorrhage.--Bleeding from the womb occurring six hours after delivery is called post partum and after that time, is known as puerperal child-birth bleeding or hemorrhage.

Causes.--A relaxed condition of the womb, the retention of clots or parts of the membranes, etc., in the womb, a full rectum or bladder, fibroid tumors, deep tears of the cervix.

Symptoms.--If the bleeding is profuse, the pulse is fast, the woman looks pale, anxious and feels cold, restless, gaping, usually it comes from a relaxed, softened and enlarged womb.

Treatment.--In severe forms no time must be lost in securing contraction of the womb and the method employed for expelling the afterbirth should be employed to expel clots. Grasp the womb over the abdomen, employ firm but gentle kneading, pressing downward. The pillows should be removed, the foot of the bed elevated twelve to eighteen inches, a preparation of ergot given by the mouth or hypodermically in the thigh. If these measures fail the hand and arm should be sterilized and inserted in the womb, all clots, etc., removed and pressure made over the abdomen on the womb while the hand is still there. This pressure and presence of the hand close the bleeding vessels in the womb. The hand should remain, while the kneading goes on externally, on the womb.

This kneading should be kept up until the womb contracts. The hand can then be removed from the vagina, while gentle kneading is slowly kept up over the womb. The womb should be closely watched for hours after. Bleeding very seldom occurs again, but it might. If the bleeding is more of an oozing, an injection of very hot water, 120 degrees F., through a long douche nozzle, directly into the womb cavity may be given. This is very effective for any kind of bleeding. Lemon juice or boiled vinegar can be added to the injection. Everything used must be perfectly clean or child-bed fever may be caused by these measures. After the womb has thoroughly contracted, it is sometimes of benefit to place a rubber bag filled with cold water over the pubic bone to prevent subsequent relaxations of the womb. Weakness can be met by hypodermics of whisky or brandy and strychnine, one-thirtieth of grain, injected hypodermically to stimulate the heart.

Pulse and Temperature.--The temperature may rise one to one and one-half degrees without the case being abnormal. The pulse falls after labor, ranging between sixty and seventy. A rise of temperature, a rapid pulse, a flushed face, a chill, pain or tenderness of the abdomen, and abnormal increase or decrease of the discharge, bleeding, or offensive odor of the discharge should cause suspicion of child-bed (puerperal) fever. This is a grave condition and results from infection which has taken place during labor or afterward. The septic matter may be carried in on the fingers or instruments by the physician or attendants, etc. The most usual sources are unclean hands, instruments and clothing which come in contact with the woman's genitals. The attack is usually ushered in during the second to the fourth day by a chill, or chilly sensations, etc., rise of temperature, rapid pulse, accompanied by headache and a feeling of weariness. The discharge may be increased at first, but later diminished and may cease; or it may be abundant, frothy and of a very fetid odor. Secretion of milk may fail, the bowels are usually constipated, pain in the abdomen develops.

Treatment.--If the interior of the womb is smooth, a single antiseptic womb injection should be given; if it contains foreign material or is rough, it should be scraped and then a douche given. This must be done carefully and with absolute cleanness. Turpentine stupes should be placed hot on the abdomen for the pain, or where cold feels more grateful the ice bag or cloths wrung out of cold or ice water should be applied over the abdomen, and covered with several thicknesses of flannel and changed as soon as they become heated. Medicines to relieve the pain may be given. Hot and cold sponging may be given to reduce the temperature, a little alcohol can be added to the water or the cold or hot pack may be used.

Diet.--This should be nourishing and supporting, and at first, liquid and consist largely of milk; but concentrated broths, jellies, and liquid beef, peptonoids, are useful. Stimulants should be given in these septic conditions. From one to two ounces of whisky may be given every three to four hours in the form of milk punch and, if possible, as much red or port wine also. Women in this condition can stand this treatment. Salines (salts) should be given to keep open the bowels.

CONVULSIONS. (Eclampsia).--All forms of convulsions may occur during pregnancy. They may occur during pregnancy and during labor. These are usually the result of kidney trouble. The attacks occur most often during the last three months of pregnancy. Their frequency is one to three hundred to one to five hundred cases. It occurs oftener in the first pregnancy, three to one.

Treatment.--Inhalation of chloroform to control the convulsion. Morphine in one-half grain dose can be given if no chloroform is handy. Place the patient in a hot water or vapor bath, or wrap blankets wrung out of hot water around her, and pile the bedding on until a profuse sweat is started. The sweating aids in eliminating the poison. Change the hot wet blankets as often as necessary. If the convulsions do not cease the womb must be emptied of its contents. If the convulsions occur during labor they should be treated in the same manner. The mortality then is about seven per cent. Chloral hydrate in thirty to sixty grain doses in three ounces of water may be injected into the rectum if the other remedies fail.

MILK LEG.--This is due to infection. It usually arises from an extension of a blood clot (thrombosis) of the womb or pelvic veins, to the thigh (femoral) vein, resulting in a partial or complete obstruction of the vein. It may come in less frequent cases, from a lymphatic infection.

Symptoms.--They may develop at any time between the tenth and thirtieth days or even later. These are general feelings of weariness, stiffness and soreness of the leg, especially when it is moved. There may first be pain in the region of the groin; or pain from the ankle to the groin and followed by swelling. The skin of the leg becomes markedly swollen, white and shiny. Later there is pitting on pressure, but not at first, because the skin is extremely stretched. Fever may accompany the attack, but it will subside long before the swelling of the leg has disappeared.

The vein may be felt as a hard lash-like cord, a red line of inflammation marking its course along the inner and under side of the thigh. The disease may last weeks, depending upon the severity of the trouble.

The affected leg is disabled for a number of months after recovery. Recovery takes place as a rule. Absorption of the clot takes place, or the vessel remains closed, and another (compensatory) circulation is established.

Treatment.--The patient should lie in bed with the leg elevated and swathed in flannel or cotton wet with some quieting lotion. The following is a good lotion:--

Compound Soap Liniment	6 ounces
Laudanum	1-1/2 ounces
Tincture Aconite Root	1/2 ounce
Tincture Belladonna	1/2 ounce

Wet the flannel or cotton with this. After the acute symptoms have passed the following ointment may be put on the leg:--

Ichthyol	45 grains
Iodide of Lead	45 grains
Chloride of Ammonium	10 grains
Alboline	1 ounce

The parts should not be rubbed lest a clot be loosened and travel in the general circulation and thus endanger life.

Diet.--Should be supporting. Salts for the bowels.

ALL ABOUT BABY

QUESTIONS AND ANSWERS

Preparation, Outfit, Nursing, Formulas for Preparation of Milk for Bottle-Fed Infants; Weaning, Teething, Diet Through Childhood, All the Baby Diseases, etc., from the Best Medical Authority, Infant Hospitals and Nurses.

How long does pregnancy usually last? Two hundred and eighty days.

How can the time be reckoned? Count back three months from the first day of the last menstruation and add seven days to the date thus obtained. To be more accurate, you should add only six days in the months of April and September, five days in December and January, and in February four days.

What time of pregnancy does the form begin to change? It changes a little the first two months. It is flatter and lower down. After the third month there is a progressive enlargement.

What is quickening, and when first felt? It is a motion, of the foetus (child) in the womb, imparted to the abdominal walls, and is felt from the sixteenth to the twentieth week. It has been said to have occurred earlier in some cases.

Can you foretell twin pregnancy? Not to a certainty.

Can a mother influence her child as to character and temperament before birth? Authorities differ very much upon this point. The child inherits the physical characteristics of its parents. The frame of the mother's mind, some think, can be given in some degree to her offspring.

Will nervousness be inherited by the child? Not invariably; if the mother is fretful, irritable, cross, repining, etc., her child may be puny, cross and irritable, etc.

Do you believe in influences transmitted before birth (parental influences?) All must admit that there is a great deal in heredity, and the characteristics of parents are shown in their children.

Can a mother mark her baby? This is another disputed question.

When should the family physician be informed of the woman's condition? The first month.

Why? So that the woman will know how to live properly, and also that he will be given the urine twice each month to examine. This is for her protection and is necessary, because anything that may be wrong with the kidneys can be corrected much easier, and diet, etc. can be arranged to prevent future trouble.

What kind of diet should a pregnant woman have? She should eat only healthy articles of food. Stimulating, highly seasoned, rich, greasy foods should be avoided. Constipation is frequently present and the diet must be chosen with reference to that also. She should not restrict herself to one line of diet unless it is necessary.

Should she take a daily bath, if so, what kind and when? Yes, if it does her good. The pores of the skin should be kept open so that the kidneys will have less work to do. Spray and baths should be taken cold or lukewarm. Hot baths or Turkish baths are to be avoided. The time should be at the woman's convenience. Morning is preferable, if she does not feel the need of sleep.

Should she take a daily nap and when? Yes, one or two hours in the forenoon, and also in the afternoon.

Should she take exercise? Yes, exercise is necessary. This promotes the proper circulation of the blood, favors rest and sleep, relieves the "blues," tones the whole system, gives her good wholesome air and makes everything look better. It should not be violent. Slow walking and riding in an easy carriage. She should not ride a horse, run, jump, dance, or do any jerky or violent exercise; no heavy lifting or reaching up.

What about clothing? The clothing should be perfectly loose and comfortable. Garters and corsets are injurious, especially when the pregnancy has reached four or five months. The weight of the clothing should be borne by the shoulders instead of the hips. Special waists can be made for pregnant women. There should be no pressure on any part, especially on the womb and breasts.

What is the meaning of the word enciente? The Roman women were accustomed to wear a tight girdle about their waists which was called a cincture. This they removed when they were pregnant. They were then said to be *incincta,* or unbound. The term enciente is derived from this, and is frequently used to indicate pregnancy.

What are the main symptoms of miscarriage? Pain and bleeding.

35

Does it usually come on suddenly? Not as a rule. There are premonitory symptoms such as bearing down feeling in the pelvis, backache, frequent desire to pass water, a discharge from the vagina, and sometimes a little bloody flow.

At what period is it most common? Between the ninth and sixteenth weeks when the after-birth is forming.

What are the causes of miscarriage? Diseases of the womb, disease in the father, constipation, falls, over-exertion, violent emotions, such as shock, fright, anger, blows on the abdomen, over-lifting, reaching up, sewing on machine.

What is the first thing to do? Lie down, rest and send for a doctor.

Is it ever possible to stop it? Yes, and often.

Do the breasts need any special care? The nipple, if much drawn in and small, should be "pulled out" once or twice daily. It will do to rub sweet oil on the breasts every evening in order to relieve the tightness and discomfort, especially after the pregnancy has advanced some months.

Are there any diseases to which a pregnant woman is more subject? None. The kidneys need more watching.

Can any dentistry be done during pregnancy? Not if it makes her very nervous; but toothache can cause more harm from a diseased tooth than if it were treated carefully.

Why do pregnant women suffer from "varicose" veins? The enlarged womb presses upon the veins and thus obstructs the return flow of the blood. It is not so common during the first pregnancy.

Can anything be done for this trouble? The woman should lie down a good part of the time if possible, and also wear a perfectly fitting elastic stocking. They can be had of any size and length. The limb should be measured for them.

Does oiling and massaging the body do good? Some women claim it does; it certainly puts the muscles in better condition and strengthens the muscles of the abdomen which have so much part in the labor.

What is the morning sickness and are all women subject to it? Nausea and vomiting without any cause. No; many escape it entirely.

At what period of pregnancy does it usually occur? During the early months it is more frequent and troublesome.

How long does it usually last? Usually three or four months, but it may last during the whole pregnancy.

What can be done for it? In some cases arranging the diet to prevent and cure constipation relieves it. For fuller treatment see this heading under Obstetrics.

Does it ever endanger life? Not often, but a physician should be called if it is bad.

Can any strict rules be laid down for this trouble? No, but the food should be as concentrated as possible; egg-nog, ice cream, a bit of rare steak, etc., raw oysters, gruels, meat broths, etc., if liquids are well borne. It is surprising how little will keep up some women during pregnancy.

When and how often should the urine be examined? From the beginning and twice each month, and every week after the fifth month.

When should the nurse be called? Long enough before the expected time to get everything ready.

What is lightening? It is caused by the womb sinking down lower in the pelvis the last month, and this lightens the pressure upon the diaphragm and lungs.

What are false pains? They occur during the last few weeks of pregnancy at irregular intervals and are usually in the abdomen.

What is the bag of waters? It is a sac containing the fluid in which the child floats while in the womb. The amount of fluid varies from a pint to a gallon or more. When it ruptures there is a sudden flow of liquid, more or less continuous flow. It may occur at the very beginning of labor and is one of the signs of labor.

What are the other signs of approaching labor? A profuse discharge of mucus from the vagina, and this may be tinged with blood. The "show" pains begin generally in the back and are quite regular, one every twenty minutes or half hour. (Dilatation of the womb).

How should the baby be first washed? See Obstetrics.

What clothing should be put on? See Obstetrics chapter.

Care of the eyes.--Wipe the eyelids with clean gauze and water. If there has been much discharge from the vagina during pregnancy, the child's eyes should be washed cleanly and also one or two drops of the one per cent solution of silver nitrate should be put into each eye as a preventive. (See Obstetrics).

How often should the baby's bowels move? Two or three times daily for the first week, and then once or twice a day.

What is the appearance of the stool? It is soft, yellow and smooth and should not contain any lumps.

How about the urine? It should pass from six to ten times a day, and it should be colorless.

What is the average weight of a healthy baby? Seven to seven and one-half pounds.

Does it lose any weight during the first week? Yes, generally a few ounces, then it begins to gain at the rate of four to six ounces each week.

Should the newly-born babe have its eyes exposed to the light? The eyes are very sensitive, and the sun or artificial light should not be allowed to shine on them. The first day the baby is deaf, but his hearing develops and becomes very acute so that he is very much disturbed by sudden, sharp noises.

What is the "soft" spot on a baby's head? This is called the "fontanelle." Do not touch this spot. This closes in time. At six months of age the fontanelle is somewhat larger than it was at birth because the brain expands faster than the boney matter deposited around the edges in the skull bones. After this another deposit of bone goes on more rapidly than the growth of the brain substance, and by sixteen or eighteen months the opening should be entirely closed.

When should the baby be given the second tub bath? Not until the cord has dropped off.

How and when should this be given? The room should be warm. The head and face should be washed first and dried; then the body soaped and the infant placed in the tub with its head and body well supported by the hands. The bath should be given quickly with no special rubbing, drying with a soft towel. (An hour after feeding).

What should be the temperature of the bath? One hundred degrees F. for the first few weeks, later ninety-eight F. After six months ninety-five F.; during the second year from eighty-five to ninety degrees F.

What should you use in giving the bath? Soft, clean sponges or smooth cloths. There should be separate pieces for each eye, for the head, face and buttocks.

What are the objections to sponges? They are very apt to become dirty and are hard to keep clean.

When should the daily bath be omitted? In the case of infants who are delicate and feeble, when the bath seems to harm them; in all forms of acute sickness, unless the bath is directed. In eczema and many other forms of skin diseases a great deal of harm is often done by soap and water or water baths.

How should a genuine bath be given? If possible the bath should be given in front of an open fire, in a room where the temperature is from seventy to seventy-two F. and the draughts kept off by a large screen. Have everything at hand with which to give the bath. A folding rubber bath-tub is the best, next a papier-mache one; or if tin must be used, put a piece of flannel in the tub to protect the baby from the tin. If necessary place the tub on a low table, place another low table to the right of the one on which the tub sets, and on this table should be the baby's basket containing a soft brush, different sizes of pins in a pin-cushion, several threaded needles, a thimble, squares of soft linen, absorbent cotton, wooden tooth-picks, a powder-box and puff, or a powder-shaker containing pure talcum powder, a box of bismuth subnitrate, one of cold cream, a tube of white vaselin, a dish containing castile, ivory, or pure French soap should be placed by the basket on the table; also a cup containing a saturated solution of boric acid; two cheese-cloth washcloths, a soft towel, a thermometer to test the water, several toothpicks on which a little absorbent cotton is twisted, and the rolled flannel band. Then a basin containing warm water, 98 to 100 degrees F., also one with cold water. The baby-clothes should be hung on a rack close at hand.

How to take care of a sore navel.--If it looks red or has a thin discharge coming from it, wash it carefully twice a day with saturated solution of boric acid; or if pus is there use a 1-5000 solution of bichloride of mercury. Use for a dusting powder one part of salicylic acid and nineteen parts of starch on it. It needs a physician's attention if it does not soon heal.

Do any physicians advocate a daily bath before the cord drops off? Yes; but not a full tub bath.

When does the cord drop off? In from five to ten days.

Does soap hurt a baby's skin? Some doctors claim it does.

Is it necessary to use a powder after the bath? No, if all moisture is removed, there is no need of powder. The skin can be kept cleaner and healthier without it.

GENITAL ORGANS.

When is circumcision needed? Usually when the foreskin is very long and very tight, so that one must use force to push it back, and always if it produces local irritation.

How should you clean the genitals of a female child? Use good absorbent cotton and warm water, with a solution of boric acid if necessary, about two teaspoonfuls to a pint of warm water. This should be done once a day.

Is the hood of the clitoris ever too tight? Yes, and it needs to be loosened and kept so, or it will produce irritation and sometimes convulsions.

How should you wash the genitals of a male child? In infants and children, this should be attended to daily. The foreskin should be pushed back and the parts washed with absorbent cotton and water. Tight foreskin and unclean parts induce trouble and bad habits.

TREATMENT FOR SORE EYES.

How should a newly-born baby's eyes be treated? They should be kept clean with a soft cloth and warm water. Do not use the same piece of cloth for both eyes.

Should redness and pus appear in the eye or eyes a few days after birth, what should be done? Use a piece of soft linen or absorbent cotton and wet it in a solution of boric acid or salt (one-half teaspoonful to one pint of water, warm) and wash out the eye or eyes, and if pus appears, use a stronger solution of boric acid (ten grains to eight teaspoonfuls of water.) If the lids stick together grease them with vaselin from a tube and rub in at night. If the sore eyes are severe send for a physician as it may be the beginning of ophthalmia neonatorum.

MOTHERS' REMEDIES.--1. Sore Eyes, Mothers' Milk for.-- "There is nothing as good as mother's milk." This is very soothing and healing and seems to work better than medicines in small babies.

2. Sore Eyes. A Nurse from New York sends the following remedy for.--"Take a cup of water that has been boiled and cooled and dissolve in it one teaspoonful boracic acid powder. Bathe the eyes thoroughly and often." A nurse in New York state, gives this recipe, and says she has been a nurse for several years and has never had a case of sore eyes which did not heal with this treatment.

How is washing out the baby's mouth done? Use a swab made by twisting some absorbent cotton upon a toothpick. The folds between the gums and lips and cheeks may be gently and carefully cleaned twice a day unless the mouth is sore.

If a baby cries while nursing, what is the cause? It may have a sore mouth.

What is thrush or sprue? Patches looking like little white threads or flakes appear inside the cheeks.

What is the cause of sore mouth? It is usually due to uncleanness and carelessness. It may come in delicate babies without any special reason. Babies who suck a "pacifier" or a rag with sugar in it are very apt to have the disease. Bottle-fed babies get it because of uncleanness of the nipple and bottle.

Should the baby continue to nurse? Yes, but the mother should thoroughly cleanse her nipple with a solution of boric acid after each nursing.

What should be done for it? It should be washed before and after every feeding with a solution of baking soda or boric acid of the strength of one even teaspoonful to twenty-four teaspoonfuls of water, or listerine, one teaspoonful to twenty-four teaspoonfuls of warm water, can be used. (This will be treated more fully later under diseases). A solution of borax (twenty grains to eight teaspoonfuls of water) can be applied every two hours with a camel's hair brush. Borax, sage and honey are good old remedies.

Should the scalp have special care at birth? It should then and afterward be kept clean to keep scurf from accumulating. It should be wet before the body is immersed in the bath. The hair should always be dried carefully; brush first with a soft towel and then with a fine, smooth hair-brush. Never use a comb on an infant's head.

Should any dressing be put on the scalp? No, for if the hair is washed and brushed, the oil from the scalp will keep it soft, glossy and healthful.

QUESTIONS AND REMEDIES FOR SORE MOUTH. CANKER. THRUSH.

Explain more about thrush or sprue? It is an inflammation of the mouth where small particles looking like milk curds appear on the tongue, gums and cheek. This is really a more severe type of sore mouth, and is of a fungus origin.

Causes of sore mouth. Uncleanness, failing to keep the mouth---especially of bottle-fed infants--and the nipples and bottles, clean. Babies who are allowed to suck a "pacifier" or rag with sugar on it. Thrush is parasitic in origin and is always due to uncleanness in bottles, nipples and the mouth, and is commonly associated with the stomach trouble. Diarrhea frequently goes with it.

(See Mothers' Remedies for Sore Mouth, Canker, etc., in general department).

PHYSICIANS' TREATMENT for Thrush. Severe Sore Mouth. 1. Boric acid in a saturated solution (five teaspoonfuls to a pint of distilled water) is a specific for it.

Dr. Tuley, of Louisville, Ky., says:

2.	Powdered Borax	8 teaspoonfuls
	Strained Honey	3 teaspoonfuls
	Mix thoroughly.	
3.	Glycerin	1 ounce
	Distilled water	1 ounce
	Boric Acid	2 drams

4. Golden seal diluted one-half with boiled water makes an excellent mouth wash. Also a weak solution of alum. Use a piece of absorbent cotton or soft linen on your little finger or small round piece of wood and dip in solution and apply. Dr. Douglas, of Detroit, advises the use of a soft brush. This should be boiled after using.

5. In Mild Cases of Sore Mouth.--The medicines need not be as strong as for thrush. One teaspoonful of boric acid or baking soda to a pint of boiled water is usually sufficient; wash after each nursing or four or five times a day.

6.	Powdered Borax	1 teaspoonful
	Powdered Sugar	4 teaspoonfuls

Put a pinch on the tongue every two or three hours. The child's tongue will work it around. This avoids the pain from washing, etc.

7. Another Mouth' Wash.--

Borax	1/2 teaspoonful
Tincture of Myrrh	1/2 teaspoonful
Glycerin	1 teaspoonful
Boiled water	enough for one ounce.

Apply gently to the inside of the mouth several times a day in thrush or any form of sore mouth or gums. Use a camel's hair brush.

WHAT CARE SHOULD BE GIVEN THE DIAPERS?

A diaper should never be used more than once without washing. It should be removed as soon as it is wet and placed in a covered pail in the bathroom, etc., and washed at the first opportunity. Pure white soap only should be used, and the diapers should be thoroughly rinsed and boiled. Dry them in the sun and air and never before the nursery fire. They should be warmed before they are again used. Unclean, soiled diapers frequently cause chafing.

Should a baby cry while passing urine? No; it may be too acid, alkaline, too little of it or too concentrated, or have sand in it. Examine the diapers.

How about bands for the baby? Straight pieces of flannel, twenty-two by five inches or wider. They may be knitted.

How long should they be worn? The snug bands, flannel or knitted should be worn, not tight, three months; then if one is worn it should be loose. It may prevent rupture and bowel trouble.

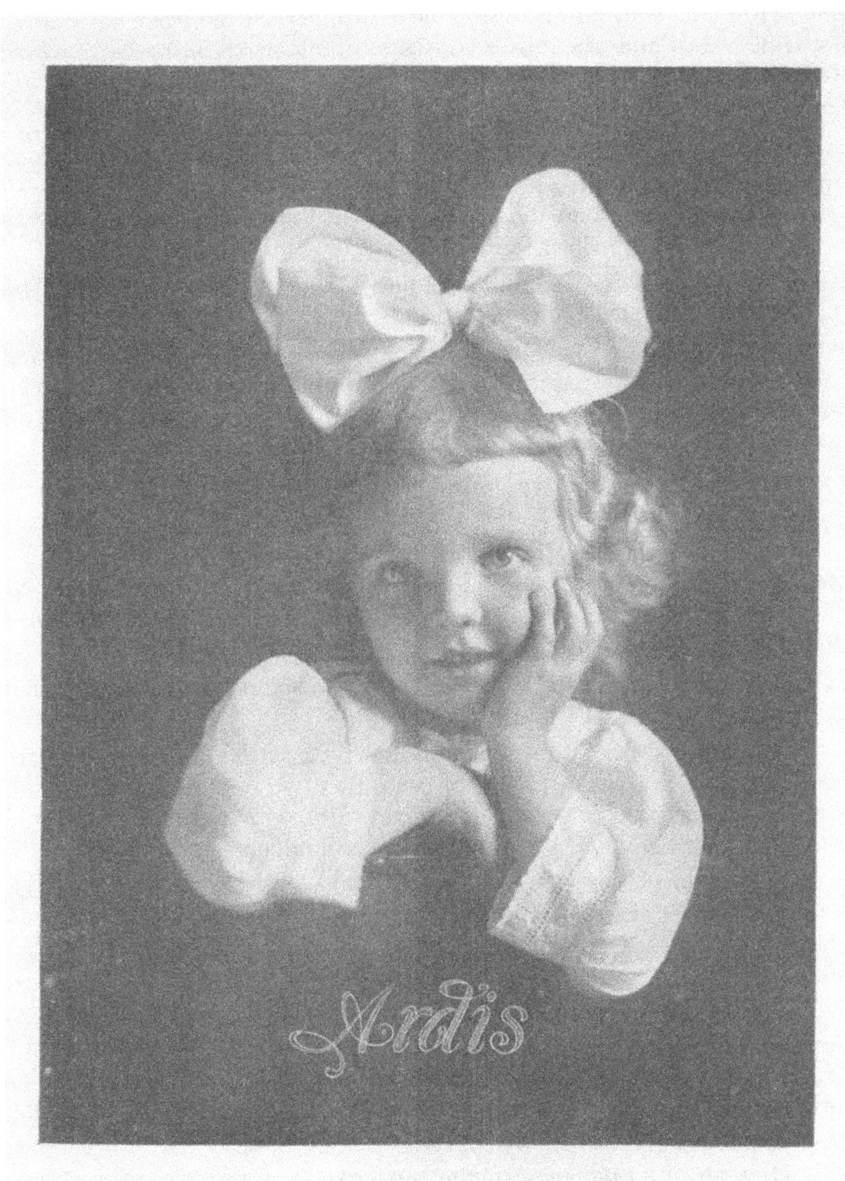

Ardis

Do you approve of rubber diapers as an outside covering? No, because they confine the dampness cause more sweating of the parts and may thus cause chafing, etc.

How large should a diaper be? A diaper should be twice as long as wide. They may be different sizes, eighteen by thirty-six inches, twenty-two by forty-four, or twenty-seven by fifty-four.

CHAFING.

Chafing is a very common trouble in infants. What causes chafing? A wet diaper left on too long; not drying the folds of the flesh properly; too much and too strong soap in the bath, or in the diapers when they are washed, or failure to wash the child clean.

Where are the places where baby is most likely to chafe? The buttocks, in the folds of the neck and in the groins.

How can you prevent chafing? Use very little soap; no strong soap; rinse the body carefully; dry thoroughly after rinsing; use clean diapers; use dusting powder in the folds of the flesh, especially in fat babies.

If the skin is very sensitive, what then? Do not use any soap, but use bran or salt baths.

How can you prepare a bran bath? Place one pint of wheat bran in coarse muslin or cheese-cloth bag and put this in the bath water. It should then be squeezed for five minutes until the water looks like porridge.

How is a salt bath prepared? One teaspoonful of common salt to each two gallons of water.

If the parts are chafed what should we do? Do not use any soap, and give only bran or salt baths or use pure olive oil and no water at all on the chafed parts. Dry the parts carefully with old, soft linen and dust them with a powder made of starch and talcum--equal parts

--with one-fourth as much boric acid, all carefully mixed together. Or use starch two parts and boric acid one part. Pure stearate of zinc powder is also good. Keep a little piece of soft linen between the folds of the flesh, so they will not be irritated by rubbing together.

MOTHERS' REMEDY.--1. Chafing in Infants, Mutton Tallow for.--"Five cents' worth of mutton tallow, melted. Apply at night." If there is a tendency to chafe during the day, use talcum powder, putting the mutton tallow on at night when the child will be quiet, giving it an opportunity to heal.

How shall I take care of the buttocks to prevent chafing? This is the most common place for chafing, as it is so frequently wet and soiled; hence all napkins should be renewed as soon as wet and soiled and the parts always kept perfectly clean.

What is prickly heat, and how caused? Fine, red pimples appear, caused by excessive sweating and from irritation of flannel underwear.

How should I treat it? Muslin or linen should be worn next to the skin. The entire body sponged frequently with vinegar and water (equal parts) and plenty of starch and boric acid powder used; starch, two parts; boric acid (one part) should be put on.

(See Mother's Remedies under "Prickly Heat," General Department.)

CLOTHING FOR THE BABY.

The chest should be well covered with soft flannel, the limbs protected, but not cramped, the abdomen supported by a band, not too tight. The clothing should be neither too tight nor too loose. No pins should be used, but all bands should be fastened to the body. The petticoats should be supported by shoulder straps.

How should a baby be held during dressing? It should lie on the lap until quite old enough to sit alone. Draw the clothes over the child's feet and do not slip them over the head.

Why use the band, and how long should it be worn? It protects the abdomen, but its main use is to support the abdominal walls in very young infants and thus prevents rupture. The snug flannel band should not be worn more than four months. Then in healthy infants a knitted band may be used and worn up to eighteen months. If the baby is thin and the abdominal organs are not protected by fat, they may be troubled with diarrhea and need protection. In such condition, the band may be worn until the third year.

BABY'S FIRST WARDROBE.

Four to six dozen diapers (bird's-eye cotton), two to three shirts (wool), four flannel skirts, two white skirts (nainsook), two to four night dresses (outing flannel), six day dresses, two wrappers, six pairs of socks, four to six flannel bands, two flannel sacks, two shawls or afghans. The dresses to be worn after the first four or six weeks. Of course this can be less or more elaborate, according to the conditions and circumstances of the parents, etc.

What changes should be made in the clothing in summer? The thinnest gauze flannel undershirts should be worn, the outside garments to be changed for the changing weather. They should not be kept too hot in the middle of the day, while in the morning and evening extra wraps should be used.

Should older children go with bare legs? There is no objection, if they are strong and well, to doing this in warm weather.

What kind of underwear should be worn in cold weather? Next to the heaviest is thick enough.

Do children require heavy flannels? Not as a rule, as they usually live in the nursery and they sweat readily while playing. When they go out-of-doors, coats and leggings render thick flannels unnecessary.

Are many children too thinly clad in the house? Very few. The usual mistake is excessive clothing and too warm rooms. These cause them to take cold so easily.

GENERAL DRESSING FOR DIFFERENT SEASONS.

At night baby may have a warm sponge bath, a fresh band, shirt and skirt put on. In the winter he should sleep in a flannel nightdress and this can be made with a drawing string or button on the bottom so that he cannot expose his feet. In the summer he can wear a cotton night-dress and after the third month the skirt may be left off in very warm weather. By the time baby has entered his second month he may wear simple little "Bishop" dresses instead of his plain slips. At the end of the third month, the flannel band may be discarded, usually, and a ribbed knitted one used. The band should be of wool in the winter, and of silk and wool in the summer. It should be put over the child's feet when he is being dressed each morning, and be changed for a fresh one at night, if possible. If the baby is healthy he may begin going out in March, if the days are mild and there are no stormy cold winds. Begin by letting him stay out one-half hour during the warmest part of the day, then one hour, etc. When there is much melting snow he should not be taken out. In cold weather the baby's cap and cloak should be lined with flannel or lamb's wool. Woolen mittens should cover his hands. A veil is not necessary.

Cap for Baby's Ears.--If baby's ears stand out from his head a considerable distance, it can be corrected best when he is young. A skeleton cap is made for this purpose. This can be bought or the mother can make one out of thin lawn or pieces of broad tape. It should fit snugly in order to do any good and be worn for some time.

Drooling.--If the baby drools much he is apt to wet any little bib he may wear and take cold by having damp clothing next to his throat and chest. Cut a piece of material now made (Linite, by Johnson & Johnson) in the shape of a bib, and bind with tape. This can be worn underneath the bib.

Short Clothes About the Fifth Month.--Short clothes should be prepared for the baby's wear at the beginning of the fifth month, and may consist of a shirt, knitted band with shoulder straps, flannel skirt made on a cotton waist, in summer or a flannel one for cold weather, and having a row of small flat buttons, on to which the white petticoat may be buttoned; a diaper, and a simple white dress. For summer, white cotton stockings should always be worn, woolen ones in the winter; and they should be long enough so that they may be pinned to the diaper. Moccasins or soft kid shoes should be the first kind worn. At night a baby (in short clothes) should sleep in a shirt, band, diaper and a night-dress of cotton in summer, and flannel in winter. The change to short dresses should not be made in very cold weather; and if the baby is born at such a time as to make it necessary, he may be put into short clothes as early as the end of his third or fourth month, rather than to wait until later and make the change in mid-winter.

Clothing in Summer.--Even in summer, the baby should have clothing which contains some wool. A mixture of silk and wool or cotton and wool may be used for the shirt, band and skirt. The band should never be left off; the shirt may be left off in the hottest weather and the long ribbed band with shoulder-straps may take its place, but the abdomen must be covered by means of the band. The nightdress should now be of cotton and the skirt left off at night, but the band and the thin skirt should be worn. Long, white cotton stockings reaching to the napkin should be worn all summer, and not short socks.

The head should be kept cool, therefore do not use a sunbonnet which shuts out all of the air. Muslin caps and light pique hats provide enough shade, if the baby-carriage has a parasol.

Creeping aprons can be used for babies. They are made of fine gingham and may be put over the dress or worn without one in very warm weather. Make them so as to button all the way down the back, and they sometimes have an elastic or draw-string run into the hem at the bottom of the apron so that the white skirts may be kept clean.

For early fall, two or three little jackets of light flannel or cashmere can be made; and the baby can wear one of these either over or under his white dress in the morning or evening when it is cool. The baby should be in the house by six o'clock unless the weather is exceptionally warm. In the fall, if he has been accustomed to having his nap on the piazza, in his carriage, a screen should-be placed around the carriage to protect him from any possible draught. After the first of October, in chilly days, he should have his nap in the house.

Winter.--A year-old baby in winter should wear a medium weight wool shirt, knit band with shoulder-straps, a flannel skirt on a flannel waist, white skirt buttoned on to the waist of the flannel skirt, woolen stockings pinned to the diaper, laced shoes, a white dress of some cotton

material and for very cold days, a little flannel, or cashmere sack. At night should be worn a band, shirt, diaper and flannel night-dress long enough to keep his feet warm. For an outing in the winter he should have on a light, but warmly lined coat; a wadded lamb's wool lining is best, but it is expensive, and flannel may be used. His bonnet should be lined with flannel; and leggings and mittens should be of wool.

First Half of Second Year.--A baby of this age may wear a thin gauze shirt with short sleeves, but he should wear under it the ribbed silk and wool band and also his flannel petticoat during the summer.

Summer complaint is often kept off by such clothing.

Second Half of Second Year.--A baby of this age is too young to walk in the streets in the winter, and his feet cannot be protected from the damp and cold sidewalks by the usual roomy shoes. When in the go-cart instead of his carriage, his legs should be well covered, so that dampness and wind will not chill and give him a cold. A large bag having a draw-string at the top is an excellent thing to use for the lower part of baby's body while in the go-cart, and the strings should be drawn up and tied under his arms. This bag may be made of any material (warm) from eiderdown, cloth, flannel to felting; or it may simply be made of an old crib blanket and a small carriage robe placed over it. Baby's ears should be covered at this age on very cold days, when out. The baby girl should wear a lined bonnet, well covering her eyes. Tam O'Shanter caps of angora wool can be made and pulled down over the eyes for both girls and boys alike; or a soft felt hat with rosettes of ribbon lined with flannel sewed onto the elastic can be made for the boy to protect the head and ears.

By the time baby is two years old, diapers should be given up and little drawers used instead. It may be frequently necessary to use diapers at night for several months longer, although if the baby be taken up at ten or eleven o'clock p. m. he will frequently go all night without urinating.

First Half of Third Year.--Children of this age should be put into night-drawers, cotton ones in summer and flannel ones either with or without feet, in winter. Tiny overalls or "rompers" are now used a good deal for both boys and girls while at play.

Second Half of Third Year.--Now he can walk in the street for a little while each day, even in winter, having his legs protected by warm leggings and with small rubbers for his shoes when the walks are at all damp. Woolen leggings should be used.

Children should not be allowed to race about in their night-drawers and bare feet. They should also have little wrappers and bedroom slippers.

What About the Nursery? The furnishings should be very simple. No unnecessary hangings or upholstered furniture. A large room, well ventilated and one in which the sun shines at some part of the day. The shades should be dark, but no extra hangings or curtains.

Nothing should be allowed about the baby's crib but what can be washed. The air should be kept pure. There should be no plumbing, no drying of napkins or clothes, no cooking of food, and no gas burning at night. A small wax candle will do for all usual purposes.

What kind of heat is best? An open grate fire is best; next, heat from a Franklin stove. Steam heat is bad in a nursery. Never use a gas stove unless for a few minutes during the morning bath.

What should the temperature be during the day? From 66 to 68 degrees with the thermometer hung three feet above the floor. It should never be allowed above 70 F. At night, not below 65 F. during the first three months. After that it may go to 55 F., and after the first year it may go to 50 and even to 45 F.

Does the fireplace furnish enough ventilation? No, the principal ventilation must be from the windows.

How soon can you leave the windows open at night? Usually after the third month, except when the outside temperature is below the freezing point.

How often should the nursery be aired? At least twice a day, after the baby has had his bath in the morning and also before putting him to bed for the night. This ventilation should be done thoroughly and the baby should be moved to another room. In the meantime, any time the child is out of the room it should be aired.

How can you ventilate the room at night? During the winter, while the baby is young, the sleeping room may be ventilated at night by opening a window in an adjoining room; or if the weather is not very severe, a window board may be used, or a frame on which has been tacked heavy muslin; this may be from one to two feet high and put into the window like an ordinary mosquito screen. In summer, a screen around baby's crib will furnish all needed protection from the open windows.

How does a room that is kept too warm affect the baby? He becomes pale, loses his appetite, has some indigestion, gains no weight, perspires very much and takes cold easily.

How early in baby's life may airing indoors be commenced, and how long continued? When the baby is one month old. For fifteen minutes at a time at first and may be lengthened ten to fifteen minutes daily. This airing may be continued in all kinds of weather.

Will the baby take cold? Not if the period is at first short and the baby becomes accustomed to it gradually. It is a cold preventive.

How should such an airing be given? The baby should be dressed with bonnet and tight coat and placed in a crib or carriage which should stand a few feet from the window; all the windows should be thrown open for baby's airing. Doors should be closed to prevent draughts.

How soon can baby be taken out of doors? In summer when one week old, with eyes thoroughly shaded. In spring and fall usually in about one month; in winter, when about three months old, on pleasant days, and kept in the sun and out of the wind.

What time of day is best? A baby may go out almost any time in the early summer and early autumn between 6 A. M. and 7 P. M. In winter and early spring a young child only between ten or eleven and three.

Can this be done in all kinds of weather? When the winds are sharp and the ground covered with melting snow, and when it is very cold, the baby should not go out. If the thermometer is below 32° F., a child under four month's should not go out. If below 20° F., a baby under eight month's should not go out.

What care should be taken? The wind should never blow in the baby's face, its feet and legs should be properly covered and warm and the sun should never be allowed to shine directly upon its eyes either sleeping or waking.

Does this outing do the baby any good? The fresh air renews and purifies the blood, and this is just as necessary for its health and growth as proper food.

How does it show in the baby? The appetite is good, also the digestion. The child sleeps better and all signs of health are seen.

Is it better for the baby to be carried by the nurse in this airing? No, for it can be made more comfortable in its carriage and as well protected from exposure.

Is there any objection to a baby sleeping out of doors in the daytime? No, it needs only to be kept warm and out of draughts. A covered inclosed porch is a good place.

What can be done for a child that takes cold easily? The room should be kept cool when it sleeps, the clothing should be light so that he will not perspire so freely. Every morning the chest and back should be sponged with cold water, 50 to 60 degrees°F.

How should such a sponge bath be given? The child should stand in a tub containing a little warm water, and a large bath sponge filled with cold water should be squeezed over the body two or three times. Follow this with vigorous rubbing with a towel until the skin shows quite red. This may be given at least at three years old. For infants the temperature should be 65 to 70 degrees F.

WEIGHING BABY FREQUENTLY.

Why is it necessary to weigh the baby regularly? To be able to tell how it is doing. This is especially necessary during the first year.

How frequently should this be done? During the first six months every week, and during the last six months at least once in two weeks; once a month during the second year.

How rapidly should the baby' gain weight during the first year? During the first week it loses a few ounces, after this it shows a gain of four to eight ounces a week up to the sixth month, then two to four ounces a week, up to the twelfth month.

Do bottle-fed infants gain so rapidly? Very seldom during the first month, but after that with favorable air and circumstances, the gain is quite regular, and they may gain faster during the latter part of the first year, because the nursing baby loses weight at weaning time.

Why do they not gain so rapidly at first? Because it takes a few weeks for the stomach to become accustomed to cow's milk and until this is accomplished it is necessary that the milk be made very weak or indigestion will result.

What is a baby's average weight at birth? Seven to seven and one-half pounds.

How much should it be at different months at this average birth? At three months it should be twelve to thirteen pounds; at six months fifteen to sixteen pounds; at nine months seventeen to eighteen pounds; at one year twenty to twenty-two pounds. A healthy baby will usually double its weight at five months and at twelve months it will nearly triple its weight.

Should a healthy baby gain steadily in weight during the first year? He usually does, but not regularly in every week during the year. There are periods when most infants do not gain any weight. This is most often seen from the seventh to the tenth month and frequently occurs when the child is teething and sometimes in the very hot weather.

Is gaining regularly in weight a sure sign that the child is thriving normally? Not always, some infants' foods produce weight, but not strength nor development in other respects.

Can the regular gaining in weight guide us as much in the second year? The gain after the first year is not so continuous; interruptions occur during change of seasons, sometimes without any apparent cause.

How soon should a child hold its head up? During the fourth, and sometimes in the third month, as a rule. If the body is supported the head can be held erect.

How early does a baby notice things? During the second month he shows pleasure by smiling and will turn his head in the direction of a sound. They should be kept quiet, or their sleep will be broken.

What will it do at three months? It will recognize its nurse or mother, and will smile and "coo" when she approaches, and now for the first time the tear glands become active and the baby cries with tears. At this age when taken out he should lie out straight in a heavy folded blanket, or hair pillow, having a small thin pillow under his head; a hot water bag should be near his feet; a light woolen blanket or afghan should be put into the carriage and the baby placed upon it, then it should be carefully wrapped around him and the outer carriage robe tucked in. These wraps should be modified according to the weather. Babies should not perspire much for they will take cold readily; so the covering should not be too heavy.

When does the baby laugh aloud? From the third to the fifth month.

When does it first notice toys, etc.? From the fifth to the seventh month. At four months he is able to hold his head without support. He begins to use his hands better. He will often grasp an attractive object; he will throw it on the floor and expect it to be picked up for him. And also frequently shows signs of fear at the end of the fourth month, and strangers will scare him. He can now be played with for a little time every day, but never before bedtime. The best time is after the morning nap. Do not toss him about, but be gentle with him or you will make him nervous and sleepless at night.

What is baby's condition at the fifth month? He is now a bright lively fellow, and may sit in a half upright position in his carriage or in his chair for a short time each day. When in his chair he should be tied in, a soft pad or pillow should be at his back to support him. He now enjoys exercise on a bed or in a large clothes basket, and may even have one toy at a time to play with. Do not shake rattles at him. It tires him. His naps now grow shorter gradually, but he should take two daily; a long one of two or three hours in the morning and about one hour in the afternoon. He should not sleep late in the afternoon, or he will not sleep as well at night. He now "drools." This is a sign of teeth coming, and baby will bite his fingers and put everything he can hold in his mouth. He may form the sucking habit now, and if he does, put a small toy in his hand, or dip his thumb in a solution of quinine or aloes. The habit of thumb sucking is an ugly one. Another way to stop it is to bind a piece of cardboard on the arm and long enough to reach a little above or below the elbow. Then the arm cannot be bent.

Should the baby use an ivory or rubber ring to bite on when teething? A special cracker is now made in the form of a ring; it is quite hard and composed mostly of malt sugar and is intended for teething babies to bite on.

MOTHERS' REMEDIES.-1. Teething, What One Quebec Mother did for.--"Rub paregoric on the gums. This always eased my children."

2. Teething, Novel Canadian Method to Aid in.--"Put a thimble on your finger and when holding the baby rub his gums gently with it, and let him chew on it. This cuts the gums and starts bleeding when the baby doesn't think of it."

How early should a baby be able to sit and stand alone? At seven to eight months he is usually able to sit erect and support his body.

He first attempts to bear the weight upon his feet at nine to ten months, and at eleven to twelve months babies can stand without assistance.

When should a child walk without help? At twelve to thirteen months he attempts to walk. At fifteen to sixteen months the average child is able to run alone.

What conditions postpone this? Premature birth, a delicate constitution, or prolonged illness and especially chronic or digestive disturbances. Rickets is a common sign of late sitting, standing or walking.

Should you urge a child to walk? No; his muscles and bones may not be ready. He will walk soon enough if able.

How early does a child begin to talk? Generally a child can say papa and mamma at one year. The end of the second year the average child is able to put words together in short sentences.

If a child does not attempt to talk in two years, what should be suspected? Child may be a deaf-mute or mentally deficient. It is sometimes seen in children who are very backward.

SPECIAL CARE OF THE BABY.

Baby will be sensitive to light, even the first day. Do not allow the sun to shine in his eyes, or gas or electric light if that must be used. The baby's skin may change to yellow for a few days, but this soon passes away and frequently there is scaling. The fine soft hair usually comes out and is replaced later by a second growth. The open spot on the head should not be touched. When the head is out of shape or is swollen, this need not cause worry for it will soon disappear. Mold it a little. Do not allow the baby to lie in one position, as the soft skull may become flattened or all the hair rubbed off in one place. The baby sleeps about nine-tenths of the time, but he should be wakened regularly for his food and kept awake while taking it. This will soon become a regular habit to him, and he will wake of his own accord in a short time. Do not allow the baby to fall asleep nursing at the breast or while taking food in his bottle. He will not get enough nourishment and will want to nurse too often. Also if he is bottle-fed the milk is apt to grow cold and cause colic. He should be taught to nurse slowly and if he tries to nurse too fast the breast or nipple should be taken away for a minute, and then given again. The baby should nurse from fifteen to twenty minutes. A certain amount of crying is necessary for a baby if he is to be strong and healthy. It exercises his lungs. "Soothing syrup" should never be given to quiet him.

THE CRY-HOW TO DISTINGUISH IT.

The cry of pain is strong, sharp, but not continuous, often accom-

panied by contractions of the features and drawing up of the legs.
36

The cry of hunger is a continuous, fretful sound, after feeding or sometime before the next feeding. The cry of temper is loud and strong, accompanied by kicking or stiffening of the body, and, this should never be given away to from the first. The cry of a sick child is feeble and whining. Baby should not be rocked to sleep, nor carried about the room.

Baby's First Meal.--He should be placed to the breast as soon as the mother can have him. He will not get much milk for the first few days, but he should be given the breast four or five times daily. He needs what is then secreted and it is also good for the mother to try to nurse as soon as possible. The baby may be given a few teaspoonfuls of boiled water between nursing, but no teas. At the third day the milk is usually established, and the baby should nurse regularly every two hours up to 10 p. m., and twice at night. He should not sleep in his mother's bed, but have his own crib and be taken to her at nursing time. There is danger of baby being smothered sleeping with its mother, and it will not sleep so well. As a rule it is best to wash baby's mouth out before nursing, and the mother's nipple should also be wiped off with a little boric acid solution.

Baby's Bed.--As before stated, baby should sleep in his own crib, an iron or brass crib without rockers is best. A screen or plain white curtain of some wash material may be used to protect him against draughts. If this cannot be had, he may sleep while very young in a large clothes basket placed on two chairs. The crib should have a good woven wire mattress and a pair of heavy airing blankets should be placed on top of the crib, folded so as to fit the mattress; a square of rubber or any waterproof material should come next, then a cotton sheet, a quilted pad, a second sheet, a pair of wool crib blankets and a light counterpane. This should be removed at night and a comfortable afghan be used in its place. The pillow should be of hair, never of feathers or down, about one inch thick. The bed clothes should be aired thoroughly and the heavy airing blanket be washed occasionally and thoroughly dried and aired before it is again used. The blanket can hang on a line out of doors on a bright sunny day for an hour or two; in this way the blanket will be kept cleaner and will last comfortably until baby is three years old. The baby should never be put in a cold bed; warm the sheets before the fire just before putting baby in his bed (or crib) or place a hot water bag between them until they are warm. Now (second month) the baby is old enough to use his chair, not to soil his napkin. Place a small chamber on the mother's lap and hold the child on it, supporting his head and back. Do this exactly the same hours every day, morning and afternoon, directly after a meal. This training should be continued, as the position alone often goes a great way in helping to over-come constipation or any tendency to irregularity of the bowels that may exist. They cannot be taught not to wet the napkin until they are some months older.

The baby needs water as much as any adult person. Boil a fresh supply daily and cool and keep it in a covered dish or bottle. A little,--four to eight teaspoonfuls,--should be offered to the baby between each meal. It can be given from a spoon, a medicine dropper, or taken from a nursing bottle, and either hot or cold. This aids in overcoming constipation and teaches a breast-fed baby to use a nursing bottle, which will be of much benefit should sudden weaning be necessary.

During the second month his meals should be given every two and one-half hours during the day, having eight meals in twenty-four hours of three to four ounces at each meal. At night he should be fed at ten and two.

Meals for the Third Month.--Baby should be regularly nursed or fed every three hours up to ten p. m. Then have one meal at two or three a. m., and nothing more until seven a. m. If bottle fed he should be given three and one-half to four ounces at each feeding.

Fourth Month.--If the mother is nursing her baby, it is a good plan now to teach him how to use the bottle. Some doctors advise one bottle feeding each day from the start, for, should the mother's milk suddenly fail, or should she be obliged to stop nursing for any reason, there will be no struggle, which would be very hard for the baby if it happened in hot weather. Also the gradual accustoming of the digestive organs to the cow's milk before weaning must be commenced and does away in some degree, at least, with the danger from indigestion from the cow's milk given regularly.

Fifth Month.--Night feeding should now be discontinued; he should be taught to sleep from ten p. m. to seven a. m. There may be a few nights of crying and a struggle when the night feeding is first stopped, but he will soon learn to sleep without waking for his meal. He should be fed every three hours until ten p. m., and if bottle fed he should be given five to six and one-half ounces at each meal, making six meals in twenty-four hours.

Sixth Month.--The baby sleeps about two-thirds of the time. He shows signs of increasing intelligence. The baby should now accustom itself to taking either condensed milk or only the best prepared foods once or twice daily. The mother may become ill or unable to nurse for some reason, or wish to take a journey, etc., and baby is then prepared for emergencies.

When the baby is seven months old he will need more exercise than a clothes basket will afford. An exercise pen should be made.

Teeth.--As soon as the teeth come they should be kept clean, otherwise they will decay, milk is likely to remain in the mouth, turn sour and gradually destroy the enamel of the teeth.

With a soft linen cloth or a piece of absorbent cotton dipped in a solution of boric acid wash out the mouth and teeth, twice a day at least, carefully. A soft brush may be used later when baby has eight or ten teeth, and a little finely prepared chalk may be put on the brush, if there are any specks on the teeth. The baby should have three meals in twenty-four hours of six or seven ounces at each meal, if bottle-fed.

Eighth Month.--Baby should be allowed to creep on the floor a little or in his pen. It is good exercise and it will benefit him, but he should not be urged to do it. Many mothers give baby potato, etc., at this period; this is bad, as potato is hard to digest on account of having so much starch. Bread and cakes are also prohibited; convulsions are often caused by such food. Milk gruel and broths are enough for the baby and he will thrive using them. Baby should feed every three hours up to ten p. m., six and one-half to seven and one-half ounces at each meal.

Mosquito Bites.--If baby is bitten by mosquitoes wash the spot off with a little camphor water, soda water, or a wet compress of witch-hazel should be kept on the bite or boracic acid or soda solution. Keep the baby from scratching the part by fixing his hands; scratching will further poison the part.

Flies.--They often carry germs of disease on their legs and wings, and they frequently light on baby's mouth or on the nipple of the nursing bottle. Diseases can be contracted in this way. The windows should be screened. Everything that the fly has touched should be washed with some light antiseptic solution.

Ninth Month.--His long morning nap should be *encouraged* and he should sleep in the early afternoon. If the baby is heavy his little moccasin or kid shoes will not now support his ankles and he should have a shoe with a piece of stiffening at the side. The shoe should have no heels; laced shoes fit better and should be preferred. The baby (bottle-fed) can take seven to eight ounces of the proper food every three hours until ten p. m.

Tenth Month.--He can now take a little beef juice, beginning with one teaspoonful once a day and soon twice a day; then increase to two teaspoonfuls at a time and keep on until he is taking eight teaspoonfuls daily.

This should be given between his regular meals. Some babies cannot take beef juice; orange juice may then be tried, strained through cheesecloth or fine muslin and be given at first in doses of one teaspoonful and increased until baby gets the juice of one-half an orange.

If the mother is nursing baby and he has been given one bottle of milk daily, as advised for a four-months-old babe, he can now have two bottle feedings daily. Every healthy baby should be weaned when one year old, and it is better to do it gradually in this way. The baby's food should now be given him every three and one-half hours up to ten p. m., thus making five meals in twenty-four hours of seven to eight ounces at each meal.

Eleventh Month.--Baby can now have added to his diet another cereal like farina well cooked,--twice as long as the directions advise and it should be half solid when finished. Begin with one teaspoonful and then try two. This should be given in addition to his beef juice or orange juice. It should come between his regular meals, which should now be given at four-hour intervals. He should take eight or nine ounces to a meal.

Twelfth Month.--Baby should go to bed at six p. m., and take long morning nap. He should have five meals a day of such food as directed later.

INFANTS' FEEDING.

What is the best food for an infant? Mothers' milk.

What is the composition of mothers' milk? About thirteen parts solids and eighty-seven parts water.

Name the solids? Fat, sugar, proteids and salts.

What is sugar? Milk sugar or "lactose."

What are the proteids? The curd of the milk, which is very similar to the white of an egg, and is the muscle making element in the milk.

Is it necessary to have all these elements? Yes.

What benefit is the fat? It is needed for the growth of the bones, nerves, fat of the body and also for producing heat.

Give the use of sugar? It is needed to produce heat and make fat in the body.

Use of the proteids? They are needed for the growth of the cells of the body, such as those of the blood, the various organs of the muscles.

What do the salts do? Help in the growth of bone.

What is the use of water? Water keeps the food minutely subdivided or in solution, so that the infant's delicate organs can digest it. It also enables the body to get rid of the waste material.

NURSING.

Should all mothers make an attempt at nursing their babies? Yes, as a rule.

What are the most important conditions that may prevent nursing? Tuberculosis now or in the past or, in fact, any other serious chronic diseases; very delicate health herself. Some acute disease like typhoid fever or cancer.

How soon after labor should the baby be put to the breast? As soon as the mother is able to have it.

What is the food called that it then obtains? Colostrum.

What does this do? It aids in cleaning the baby's system.

Should the mother nurse the baby inclining or lying? Yes.

Does nursing drain the mother? Not if she is reasonably well. It is a natural process.

If the mother cannot nurse immediately after labor, what should you feed baby? The baby will not starve in a few days. Give it warm water regularly every few hours, or a little cream and warm water.

Are there any impediments to nursing? Sometimes the baby is tongue-tied.

Is the baby ever too weak to nurse? Yes.

What should be done in that case? Draw the milk from the breast and feed it through a free flowing nursing bottle. Such babies are generally born prematurely.

Are the mother's nipples ever at fault? Yes, they are; poorly developed, retracted, that the baby's tongue cannot surround it to draw upon it.

What can be done for them? They should be drawn out, and sometimes a breast pump is needed for this.

Should the nipples be treated after nursing? They should be dried and clean clothing put against them. Some recommend washing them with a mild solution of boric acid.

Are they ever so tender that nursing is painful? Yes.

What can be done for this? The nipples should be drawn out before confinement; if neglected use the following: Compound tincture of benzoin one-half ounce. After each nursing wash them clean with warm water or water and a little alcohol and after drying them, put on the tincture of benzoin with a camel's hair brush. It will not hurt the baby.

What can be done with cracked nipples? Apply benzoin as before directed, and use a glass or rubber nipple shield until it gets well.

How can caked breasts be prevented? The breasts should be kept emptied and well protected, both while nursing and during the intervals. Empty with a breast pump if necessary.

If mother's clothes are wet by the excess milk, what can she do? Use a breast-pump and drink and eat less fluid; eat more solid.

Should a baby nurse at both breasts? It is better.

If the breast contains pus, what can be done? Nurse at the other breast, but if both breasts are affected it must stop breast nursing.

Should an infant nurse from a mother who is taking medicine? Not as a rule.

When will the mother be able to nurse again? It is hard to tell. If the child is six months old the child should be weaned if the mother is seriously ill, and children with delicate stomachs should always be weaned, when the mother is sick.

If the mother has not enough nurse, what can be done?-- Nurse partly and feed it the rest.

Can the milk secretion be increased? Yes, by regulating the mother's diet. She should drink freely of good cow's milk and have an occasional bowl of gruel, soup, etc.

How long can you wait to see if the mother can have milk? It is well to wait several days, nurse all there is and supply the deficiency by bottle feeding.

How often should the baby nurse at first, and how long? Every four or five hours for the first few days--usually nurses fifteen to twenty minutes; one night nursing.

When is there a full secretion of milk? Usually on the third day.

How often should the baby be nursed afterward? After the third day every two hours and twice at night.

How often during the rest of the year? For two to three months every two to two and one-half hours during the day, two times at night; three to five months about every three hours up to ten p. m.; and one time at night; five to twelve months every three to three and one-half or four hours and not at night.

Is it necessary as a rule to give additional food the first few days? No; give plenty of water.

What important things should be attended to in nursing? First, a regular time night and day. Second, nipples should be kept clean.

What should a nursing mother eat? Her diet should be simple and plentiful, and lots of fluids; she should have three regular meals a day, and gruel, cocoa, or milk at bedtime and sometimes between meals. She can use cereals, most soups, most vegetables; *avoid* sour tart fruits, salads, pastry, and desserts. She may eat egg, meats once or twice daily, but in most cases but once. Tea and coffee if taken should be very weak, and ordinarily no wine or beer.

Are fruits eaten by the mother likely to injure baby? Sour fruits do in some cases, but sweet fruits and most fruits that are cooked do not, and are useful for the bowels.

Should the mother take special care of herself? Yes, she should lead a simple, natural, happy life, with outdoor exercise, as soon as possible after the confinement. She should make her bowels move daily by food and habit; she should not worry, should sleep plenty and should nap for an hour during the middle of the day.

Will the milk of the mother be affected by nervousness? Yes, more so than by her diet; worry, anxiety, fatigue, loss of sleep, household duties, society functions, have an injurious effect upon the child. Mother's grief, excitement, anger, passion, act upon the child through the milk.

How does the return of the menstruation affect the milk? The quantity is lessened, the infant is not satisfied. Sometimes the quality is affected and the child may suffer from restlessness, colic, and acute indigestion.

Should regular menstruation prohibit nursing? Not always; as a rule both functions do not go together. If the child thrives, it can keep on nursing, although it might be well to feed the infant, at least partly, during the period.

How can you determine that the baby is well nourished? Good color, sleep for two hours after nursing, is quiet, good-natured and comfortable when awake; has normal bowel movements, three stools daily and gains gradually in weight.

How can you tell when a baby is poorly nourished? It neither gains nor loses weight; it is listless, tired, indifferent, cross, fretful, irritable and sleeps poorly. It looks pale, anemic, and it becomes soft and flabby. If the milk is scanty, it nurses long; at other times it tries the breast and turns away seemingly disgusted.

What should be done? This depends upon the conditions; should the child gain nothing for three or four weeks or lose weight, immediate weaning may be necessary; at least other food must be given in addition to the breast food. Feeding may be alternated with the breast nursing.

How do the symptoms show when the mother's milk disagrees? The child, is in constant discomfort; it sleeps little, is restless, cries much, gulps up gas, passes it by the bowels, or it accumulates in the bowels causing colic. There may be vomiting, but more often bowel trouble. The bowels may be constipated but usually there is diarrhea--frequent, loose, green, with mucus and gas.

What should you do in such a case? If the child does not gain or loses weight and there is little chance of improvement in the mother's milk, the child should be weaned immediately. If the child gains in weight, try a little longer to improve the mother's milk.

Why do some babies nurse so often? The milk does not satisfy.

When the baby has thrush, should the mother take special care of the breasts? Yes, they should be cleaned after every nursing.

How much does the baby's stomach hold at birth? Six to seven teaspoonfuls.

Is vomiting a healthy sign in infants? Frequent vomiting is not natural; see if his bands are too tight; find out if he has been danced or handled after nursing.

When is it harmful? When it is frequent. If it comes up directly after a meal looking just as it was when taken, the child may be overfed.

What can be done? Reduce the quantity, or do not let it nurse so long or so often. If vomiting takes place a half hour after feeding, in sour swelling masses, it may be getting food too rich in cream, and then the time between nursings should be lengthened; or dilute the breast milk by giving one to two teaspoonfuls of plain boiled water, barley water, five or ten minutes before nursing; the mother should eat less hearty food, especially of meat.

If baby has frequent colic, what is the cause? The milk has too much proteids.

What should be done? Eat less meat, keep quiet, and happy, do not worry, etc.

How many stools does a healthy baby have daily? About two.

What color? Yellow color and pasty consistence.

If a nursing baby has too many stools, what change should be made in the mother's diet? She should eat food that would cause costive bowels in her.

LOOSE STOOLS IN NURSING BABIES.

They are caused by the mother eating improper food. If the stools are very yellow, foul, greasy or ropy the mother is eating food that produces too much fat (cream) in her milk. If curds appear there is not enough fat, and too much of the proteids (skim milk). When the stools are very green with much mucus in them, the food should be reduced.

If a nursing baby is constipated, what can be done? More boiled water should be given between nursing. The mother should take exercise at least two hours each day out of doors; her bowels should move every day, even if she must take a laxative. She should take plenty of pure, rich milk, cocoa, oatmeal and cornmeal gruels, and some kind of tonic if she is weak. Tea and coffee should not be used. Ripe fruit (not tart), some green vegetables and a little meat can be eaten. Starchy foods should be avoided. Sometimes baby does not get enough nurse. Then she should be fed and given plenty of pure water between meals.

If a nursing baby has frequent colic attacks, what should be done? The food is probably too strong. The mother should eat food that will produce less fat (cream) in her milk. The baby can be nursed at longer periods for a time; or give an ounce of hot water just before nursing. The mother should take plenty of exercise, enough sleep and have a free movement of her bowels, so as to keep well and free from nervousness.

WEANING.

When and how should this be done? This may usually be begun at nine or ten months by substituting one feeding a day for one nursing. Later two feedings, etc., until weaning is gradually accomplished. Some advise one bottle feeding regularly each day much earlier, as before stated.

Give reasons for weaning earlier? Some serious illness of the mother, pregnancy, but the main reasons usually are that the child is not thriving.

When should the weaning be completed? Generally at one year, It may be advisable to wait longer in warm, damp weather.

Is there any danger in nursing longer? Yes, as the milk is scanty; the child may get rickets or anemia.

Is gradual weaning the best method? Yes.

Should a wet nurse be preferred to bottle feeding? Yes, if you are sure you can get a good and perfectly healthy wet nurse. Her habits, etc., must be unobjectionable--she should be chosen by a physician.

When should a "weaned" child use the bottle, and when the cup? If the weaning is done at the eighth or ninth month the bottle should be used; if weaning is done from the tenth to the eleventh month, the baby should be taught to drink or be fed with a spoon.

How can you overcome some of the difficulties of weaning? As before recommended, by feeding every nursing infant once a day or by giving water regularly from out a feeding bottle, as this accustoms the baby to the bottle. This is very good, for the mother is sometimes away at nursing time, for a few hours and the baby can be fed, and when weaning comes, it is much easier.

How soon should a child stop nursing from a bottle? If the child is well this should be begun at the end of the first year, and after it is fourteen months old, it should not have the bottle except at the night feeding.

What is the objection to longer bottle nursing? They become attached to the bottle and refuse solid food when it is proper to give it. They get the bottle habit; also, it is troublesome and unnecessary. Then they will not take milk in the future, when the bottle is finally taken from them; an exclusive milk diet for children of two to three years old often results in poor nutrition and anemia.

Give the process of training a child to give up the bottle? There is little trouble if it is begun at the right time; pour the milk in a small cup or glass and the child will drink little by little. Give only a small portion of the food in this way, at first, and the balance from the bottle. The child will in a few weeks time learn to drink out of the cup without difficulty. If the child is two or three years old, take the bottle away entirely and let the child get hungry, and give it only milk in the cup and nothing else. Some children may go for a day without food, but hunger will master them finally. As soon as he has learned to drink milk from his cup, cereals and other solid foods are gradually added to his dietary and the child has not only been taught to give up his bottle, but he has also a training which is often necessary.

Can you give a baby just weaned as strong cows' milk as one of the same age who has been fed upon cows' milk from birth? Not generally; it would be almost certain to cause indigestion. You must remember that the change in food is a great one, and the feeding should be begun with a weak milk and increased gradually in strength as the baby becomes accustomed to the cows' milk.

What are the proper proportions for an infant weaned at four or five months? About the same as that given to a healthy bottle-fed baby of two months, except the quantity should be larger. The food can be gradually increased, in most cases, so that by the end of two or three weeks the usual strength can be given.

What strength is given to a bottle-fed baby of two months? From the top of a quart bottle of pure milk, that has stood from three to six hours, skim carefully off the top six ounces and then pour off three ounces of milk and mix them with the top milk (first skimmed off) making nine ounces in all; add to this nine ounces twenty-four ounces of boiled water in which you should have dissolved four teaspoonfuls of granulated sugar, or six or seven teaspoonfuls of milk sugar; add a pinch of salt and a pinch of bicarbonate of soda, or else two ounces of lime water.

Give the proper proportion for a baby who is weaned at nine or ten months? About the same as for a bottle-fed baby of four or five months. The increase to be as above given.

What is the formula for a bottle-fed baby of four months? For a healthy baby, six ounces of top milk skimmed from the top of a quart bottle of milk, six ounces of milk, then poured off, twenty-four ounces of barley or oatmeal gruel, six teaspoonfuls of milk sugar or three of granulated sugar, a pinch of salt and a pinch of bicarbonate of soda or if lime-water is used instead take one ounce of lime-water to each twenty of the milk or gruel. He should have four ounces of this mixture every three hours up to ten p. m., and then one meal at about two a. m.; none until six or seven a. m.

Will a child lose weight when placed upon this diet? It will often do so for a week or more, but he will soon gain gradually and regularly.

SPECIAL MONTHLY RULES FOR A BOTTLE-FED BABY.

Formula of food.--For the first month: skim off carefully the top six ounces from a quart bottle of pure milk, add to this twenty-four ounces of boiled water, in which water three teaspoonfuls of granulated or six teaspoonfuls of milk sugar have been dissolved, and then add a pinch of soda, or else one and one-half ounces of lime-water. Mix all these ingredients thoroughly, and then pour the correct quantity into each of ten clean nursing bottles. Tightly cork these bottles with clean cotton, and they can all be pasteurized or heated to a temperature of 155 degrees F. (Some say higher).

What strength is given to a bottle-fed baby of two months? From the top of a quart bottle of pure milk that has stood from three to six to eight hours, skim carefully off the top six ounces and then pour off three ounces of milk and mix them with the top milk (first skimmed off) making nine ounces in all; add to the nine ounces, twenty-four ounces of boiled water in which you should have dissolved four teaspoonfuls of granulated sugar, or six or seven teaspoonfuls of milk sugar; add a pinch of salt and a pinch of bicarbonate of soda, or two ounces of lime-water.

Formula for the third month.--(This is often used), Carefully skim off the top six ounces from a quart bottle of pure milk, then pour off six ounces of milk, twelve ounces in all, and now add twelve ounces of boiled water in which three teaspoonfuls of granulated or six of milk sugar have been dissolved, with a pinch of soda or else two ounces of lime-water; add then twelve ounces of barley or oatmeal gruel, divide into eight bottles, pasteurize, etc.; cool quickly and place where the temperature is 50 degrees F., until meal time, when one of the bottles should be warmed by placing it in warm water. Pour a little out in a spoon to test the warmth, etc.; when the milk is lukewarm remove the cotton cork and attach the rubber nipple. He should be fed regularly and equally every three hours up to ten p. m., then have one at two or three a. m., and nothing until seven a. m. He should get three and one-half to four ounces at each meal, so that much should be put in each bottle.

What is the formula for a bottle-fed baby of four months? For a healthy baby, six ounces of top milk skimmed from the top of a quart bottle of milk, six ounces of milk then poured off, twenty-four ounces of barley or oatmeal gruel, six teaspoonfuls of milk sugar or three of granulated sugar, a pinch of salt and a pinch of bicarbonate of soda; or if lime-water is used instead, take one ounce of lime-water to each twenty of the milk and gruel. He should have four or five ounces of this mixture every three hours up to 10 p. m., then one meal at about 2 a. m. None until 6 or 7 a. m.

Will a child lose weight when placed upon this diet? It will often do so for a week or more, but he will soon gain gradually and regularly.

Formula for the fifth month.--Skim off the top six ounces as before, then pour off nine ounces of milk and mix it with the top-milk, add twenty-four ounces of barley or oatmeal gruel, a pinch of salt, four teaspoonfuls of granulated or seven of milk sugar, a pinch of bicarbonate of soda and proceed as before. He should be fed every three hours during the day until 10 p. m. Give five to six and one-half ounces at each meal, making six meals in the whole twenty-four hours.

Formula for sixth month.--Six ounces of the top-milk skimmed off from a quart of pure milk, ten ounces of milk then poured off. Twenty-four ounces of barley or oatmeal gruel, in which has been thoroughly dissolved four teaspoonfuls of granulated or seven of milk sugar, a pinch of bicarbonate of soda, and a pinch of salt. Pasteurized as before, etc. Give baby from four to six ounces at each meal every three hours up to 9 or 10 p. m. If the day is exceedingly warm, pour out one or even two ounces from each bottle of the regular mixture and substitute boiled water for it. If the baby is inclined to vomit, it will be better during the hot weather to use less of the top milk, four, or five ounces instead of six or eight, and add so much more gruel. Barley gruel is better than oatmeal gruel unless baby is constipated. Again if the baby has delicate digestive organs, one meal each day during the very hot weather, can be made of mutton broth prepared as follows: Cut up one pound of neck of mutton, one pint of cold water and a pinch of salt; this is cooked very slowly for three hours until half a pint is left, adding a little water from time to time as it boils away; strain through muslin and allow to cool, and when cool take off all of the fat. Add this to an equal quantity of barley water and feed lukewarm to the baby from the nursing bottle. These measures may ward off summer complaint and assist in teething.

Formula for the seventh month.--From a quart of pure milk carefully skim off the top six ounces, pour off fifteen ounces of the milk and add twenty-one ounces of barley or oatmeal gruel to which has been added dissolved four teaspoonfuls of granulated or seven of milk sugar, a pinch of bicarbonate of soda. Give six or seven ounces at each meal and six meals in twenty-four hours.

Formula for the eighth month.--Skim six ounces of top-milk as before directed, pour off seventeen ounces of milk, add twenty-one ounces of barley or oatmeal gruel, four of granulated or seven teaspoonfuls of milk sugar, a pinch of salt and bicarbonate of soda. Give six and one-half to seven ounces every three hours up to 10 p. m.

Formula for the ninth month.--Use six ounces of top-milk skimmed off as before, twenty ounces of milk poured off, twenty-two ounces of either barley or oatmeal gruel, a pinch of bicarbonate of soda and salt added to the gruel, and five teaspoonfuls of granulated or eight of milk sugar dissolved in boiled water and put in the gruel. Give seven or eight ounces of this every three hours up to 10 p. m.

Formula for tenth month.--The milk in a quart bottle is stirred and thirty ounces of this is taken and twenty ounces of either barley or oatmeal gruel is added to it, to which three teaspoonfuls of granulated or seven of milk sugar, a pinch of salt and a pinch of bicarbonate of soda have been added. Feed the child every three and a half hours up to 10 p. m., making five meals in twenty-four hours, and seven to eight ounces at each meal.

Formula for eleventh month.--Stir up the entire quart of milk, add thirteen ounces barley or oatmeal gruel and to this add one tablespoonful of granulated or two of milk sugar dissolved in boiled water, a pinch of salt and a pinch of bicarbonate of soda. Treat as used; eight or nine ounces are given at each feeding, and five feedings given during the twenty-four hours.

Formula for twelfth month.--Stir up the entire quart of milk; add eleven ounces of gruel, one tablespoonful of granulated or two of milk sugar, a pinch of salt and bicarbonate of soda. The child should now have five regular meals daily, arranged about as follows: Six a. m., nine ounces of this modified milk; 8 a. m., teaspoonful of prune jelly or strained juice of an orange; 10 a. m., seven ounces of the modified milk and two tablespoonfuls of a well cooked cereal; 2 p. m., five ounces of beef juice or six ounces of mutton or chicken broth, or else a coddled egg (alternate on different days), five or six ounces of modified milk and a small piece of zwieback; 6 p. m., nine ounces of modified milk; 10 p. m., ten ounces of modified milk.

BARLEY AND OATMEAL GRUELS.

How is barley gruel made? Rub up one teaspoonful of the flour with a little cold water, and then stir this into a pint of boiling water, add a pinch of salt and boil it fifteen minutes, strain if it is at all lumpy.

How is oatmeal gruel made? In the same way, but use two teaspoonfuls of the flour.

SPECIAL RULES OF FEEDING AND NURSING FOR EACH MONTH IN CONNECTION WITH THE FORMULA GIVEN.

How can milk be pasteurized? A regular pasteurizer can be bought for three dollars; or the bottles, ten or less, can be placed in a pot partly filled with water which is rapidly brought to the boiling point about 155 degrees F. These bottles are filled with each regular feeding before being put in the water. The milk should not boil. Then remove the pot from the fire and allow the bottles to stand in it for one-half hour, then take them out and cool them as quickly as possible by allowing first warm and then cold water to run over the outside of the bottles; when they are cold, place them on ice or where the temperature is about 50 degrees F., and keep them until meal-time. Then one of the bottles is placed in warm water until the milk is lukewarm, the cork can then be removed and the nipple applied. These ten bottles were equally filled with the modified milk as prepared under the formula for the first month.

How much modified milk should be placed in each bottle? For the first week of life one to two and one-half ounces are placed in each of the ten bottles, and two or three and one-half ounces for the last two weeks of the first month.

What should be done if the baby vomits or has curds in his stools? Use a little less cream and a little more water. Remember, two tablespoonfuls equal one ounce.

What kind of bottles should be used? Round cylindrical bottles with the ounces marked on them.

What color of nipples? Black rubber nipples.

How should the bottle be treated when emptied? Rinse it out with cold water and then allow it to stand full of cold water with a pinch of soda or borax in it.

How should the bottles be prepared before the food for the whole day is put in them and pasteurized, etc.? They should be thoroughly rinsed in hot soap suds, and then rinsed and boiled in clear water for ten minutes.

What about the nipples? Rinse them first in cold then in hot water and allow them to stand in a covered cup of boric acid solution or borax water solution one teaspoonful to a pint of water. Once or twice each day they should be turned inside out and scrubbed with a brush and water. The hole in the nipple should be only large enough for a rather coarse needle to go through. The hole in the nipple can be made by such a needle heated red hot and then run through the nipple.

When can you begin to add barley and oatmeal gruel to the baby's milk? In the third month. The gruel should be made daily. If the child is not constipated use barley gruel; if constipated use the oatmeal gruel.

If you cannot get the flour, how can you prepare the gruel from the grain? Take two teaspoonfuls of barley or three of oatmeal and allow it to soak over night in cold water; add one quart of cold water the next morning and boil steadily down to a pint, (for about four hours), then strain through muslin.

Do some physicians advise feeding nursing babies one or two meals daily, beginning the fourth month? Yes.

What strength should it be? Use the formula for bottle-fed babies of the first month and the same amounts.

How can you calculate the amount necessary? Take one-eighth or one-fourth either for one or two meals daily of the separate ingredients mentioned in the formula for the first month.

Following order may be as follows: First give baby three ounces of the formula, and if all goes well in a day or two give him three and one-half ounces and miss one meal at the breast. After one week if the baby is well suited, give him three ounces of the formula for the two-months-old baby; wait a few days, then give him four ounces of this formula at the one meal. Then in a week's time if all goes well, give him four ounces of the formula for the three month's baby. Use this for one week, and then give him four and one-half ounces of the same formula. If after another week is past, there are no signs of indigestion, give him four ounces of the four-month formula, and if he enjoys this very much wait for a day or two and then increase the amount to four and one-half ounces of the same formula, and then to five ounces; as he grows older give him of the same formula as the bottle-fed infant of the same age, and the same amount at the one feeding; if he vomits or has curds in his stools or colic keep him on a weak formula longer than formerly advised.

If you have fed a breast-fed baby one meal a day from the bottle when can he be given two feedings from the bottle? During the tenth month.

COWS' MILK.--Does cows' milk contain all the elements present in the mother's milk? Yes, but in different proportions.

Why not use prepared foods? They are not thought so good, and are more likely to produce poor nutrition.

What is, the difference between cows' milk and mothers' milk? Cows' milk contains nearly three times as much casein (curd) or cheesy matter, and only about one-half as much sugar.

What kind of cows should be selected? They should be healthy and the milk should be clear and fresh.

Is it best to select Jersey cows? The milk from Jersey and Alderney cows is generally too rich; common grade cows are best.

Should the milk be from one cow? It should be from the mixed or herd milk since that varies little from day to day.

How fresh should the milk be? In winter it should not be used after it is forty-eight hours old; in summer not after it is twenty-four hours old, and sometimes it is unsafe in a shorter time.

How should the milk be cared for at the dairies? It must be kept clean and free from being contaminated. Cows, milkers and stables must all be kept clean, and the milk must be carried in sealed bottles; those that handle the milk must not be near a contagious disease; all milk pails, bottles, cans, etc., used for the milk must be steamed and boiled before being used.

Should it be immediately cooled after leaving the cows? Yes, and kept at a temperature of about 50 degrees F.

How should the family care for it after it is delivered fresh from the cows? Strain it for infants through a thick layer of absorbent cotton or through several thicknesses of cheese-cloth into quart jars or milk bottles, covered and cooled immediately. This is best done by placing the bottles in ice water or cool spring water that comes up to their necks and allow them to remain there at least one-half hour. What you wish to use for the children who drink plain milk you may pour into one-half pint bottles, and these should be placed in an ice chest or in the coolest possible place. The first rapid cooling is very important and adds greatly to the keeping qualities of the milk, for the milk loses its heat quickly when cooled in water, but very slowly when it is simply placed in a cold room. After standing for four or five hours or longer, the top milk can be strained off; the cream may be removed after waiting twelve to sixteen hours.

How should it be cared for when received in bottles? The temperature of the milk is always raised during the delivery, so it should be cooled as before described. If it was bottled at a dairy the cream or top milk can be removed in an hour or two.

How should milk and cream be cared for by the family when purchased in bulk? This milk should never be used for infants, as it is liable to be contaminated. Both cream and milk should at once be poured into vessels, covered and kept in a cool place. There will not be much cream or top milk upon such milk.

How should refrigerators be treated? The inner portion should be of metal. An ordinary metal refrigerator, as sold, if encased in a wooden box makes the best kind. A covering of felt and heavy quilting can be made for the refrigerator which can be removed easily when wet or soiled--it must be kept absolutely clean. The compartments for the milk should be so arranged that the milk bottles be either in contact with the ice or near it. The supply of ice should always be abundant, or the temperature of the milk will not be low enough. The temperature should not be higher than 50 degrees F.; it is oftener 60 to 65 degrees F. To tell the temperature, use a nursery thermometer and this should be used from time to time to know what temperature the milk is in. Milk is often spoiled in too warm temperatures in refrigerators, and also in unclean refrigerators. Many cases of sickness are caused by it. The refrigerator should carry a temperature of near 50 degrees F., and be absolutely clean, and the compartment for the milk should be absolutely separated from other food compartments.

MODIFIED COWS' MILK.

Can cows' milk be fed to infants without being modified? No; because, although the elements are similar to those in mothers' milk, they are not identical, and are present in different proportions.

Is this a matter of great moment? Yes, for very few infants can digest cows' milk unmodified.

What does modifying cows' milk mean? It is changing cows' milk so as to make it more nearly like mothers' milk.

What is this changed milk called? Modified milk; and the original milk is known as "plain milk," "whole milk," "straight milk" or "milk."

State the principal differences between cows' milk and mothers' milk? Cows' milk contains a little more than half as much sugar. It contains nearly three times as much proteids (curds) and salts, and the proteids are different and much harder to digest. The reaction is decidedly acid, while the mother's milk is faintly acid or neutral.

Any other things of importance to consider? Yes; mothers' milk is always fed fresh and sterile, while cows' milk is always more or less contaminated by dust or germs which increase rapidly with the age of the milk in proportion to the amount of dirt in it and with any increase of temperature at which the milk is kept. So pasteurization and sterilization are done to destroy the effect of germs.

How can the acidity of cows' milk be overcome? By adding lime-water or bicarbonate of soda.

How much lime-water should be used? About one ounce to twenty ounces of food.

How much bicarbonate of soda? About twenty grains to twenty ounces of food.

Suppose there is a tendency to constipation in the infant? You can then use Phillip's milk of magnesia, or some other good preparation, adding one-half to one teaspoonful to each twenty ounces of food.

How can the sugar be increased? By adding milk or granulated sugar to the cows' milk.

37

How much milk sugar is added to twenty ounces of food? About one ounce will do for the first three or four months. This makes it between six and seven per cent sugar.

How should you prepare the sugar? Dissolve it in boiled water and strain if there is a deposit after standing, by pouring it through a layer of absorbent cotton one-half inch thick placed in an ordinary funnel.

Is not granulated (cane) sugar recommended also? Yes; but all infants cannot use it. It is cheaper, but a good article of milk sugar should be bought. It costs from twenty to sixty cents per pound. The cheap variety contains many impurities.

But if cane sugar is used, how much is needed? Usually about one-half or a little over one-half as much as milk sugar, or about one - half ounce to twenty ounces of food.

What occurs if too much is used? The sugar is likely to ferment in baby's stomach and cause colic. The milk is made too sweet.

If you continue to overfeed granulated sugar, what happens? Gas, colic, restlessness, uneasiness, lining of the bowels becomes reddened and irritated; the redness shows externally around the rectum, and in severe cases around the hips.

Unless the amount of sugar is now reduced, what occurs? There follow frequently watery, splashy stools with much gas and foul odors.

Is cane or granulated sugar safe to use after six months? It does not usually produce so much trouble later on.

Suppose milk sugar produces irritation? The quantity used should be reduced to one ounce to twenty-five ounces of food or even less for a short time.

As a rule should milk sugar be preferred the first six months? Yes.

What are the best grades of milk sugar? Merck's, Mallinkrotz's, or Squibb's.

Is sugar added to sweeten and make the milk palatable? No; although it does that, its use is to furnish one of the needed elements for the growth of the baby, and it is required by young infants in the largest quantity.

How do we know that this is true? Because in good mothers' milk the amount of sugar is greater than that of the fat, proteids, and salts combined.

As cows' milk has nearly three times as much proteids (curds) and salts as mothers' milk, how can these be diminished? By diluting the cows' milk.

How much should cow's milk be diluted for a very young infant? Diluted twice will give almost the same proportion of proteids present as in mothers' milk, but as the proteids of cows' milk are so much harder for the infant to digest, the milk should, in the beginning, be diluted five or six times for most infants.

Does the diluted cows' milk with lime-water and sugar added resemble mothers' milk? No; for this mixture does not contain enough fat.

How can this be remedied? By increasing the fat in the milk before it is diluted.

How is this done? By adding top milk or milk and cream.

What is the top-milk? It is the upper layer of milk, one-third or one-half of milk removed after it has stood a certain number of hours,--six to eight hours.

How is the strength of the top-milk measured? By the fat it contains. A ten per cent milk contains a ten per cent of fat; a seven per cent milk contains a seven per cent of fat.

Are these strengths used for infant feeding? Yes, they are most used.

What increases the percentage of fat in the top-milk? 1. The longer time it stands. 2. Manner of its removal. 3. Number of ounces removed. 4. Thickness of the milk used.

When is top-milk removed? If milk is fresh from the cow or before the cream has risen, is bottled and rapidly cooled, it may be removed in four hours. It does not make much difference in bottled milk, and it may stand much longer.

How should top-milk be removed? Skim carefully off with a spoon, or cream-dipper (specially prepared) holding one ounce. It may be taken off with a glass or rubber syphon, never pour it off.

How can ten per cent top-milk be obtained from the different kinds of cow's milk? From rather poor milk (three to three and one-half per cent fat) remove the upper eight ounces from a quart.

How can it be obtained from good average milk (four per cent fat?) Remove the upper eleven ounces or one-third.

From rich Jersey milk (five and five one-half per cent fat)? By removing sixteen ounces or upper one-half from the quart.

How is seven per cent top-milk obtained? 1. By removing the upper eleven ounces or one-third of a quart from poor milk. 2. By removing the upper half from average milk. 3. By removing two-thirds or about twenty-two ounces from rich Jersey milk. As stated before the seven per cent and ten per cent are the two kinds generally used.

If top-milk is treated in this way, is it like the human milk? The proportion of the fluids and solids are about the same, but the elements are different. The curd (albuminous element) is still different in structure and action from the same element in human milk. The curd of human milk when it is met by the gastric juice in the stomach coagulates in minute particles, and the pepsin acts upon this very readily, but the curd of cows' milk being much coarser and firmer coagulates under these conditions, into large hard clots or masses, and these are quite indigestible if the child's stomach is sour from an under amount of acid being present.

How can we prevent this? By adding some bland and non-irritating substance to the milk which will mingle with the particles of curd and separate them until the gastric juice can act upon each separate particle and digest it.

What can we use for this purpose? Barley or oatmeal water or gruel is best.

What is cream? It is the part of the milk containing the most fat.

How is cream now obtained? By skimming after it has stood for twenty-four hours, "gravity cream"; by a separator, and it is then known as "centrifugal cream"; (most of the cream now sold in cities is "centrifugal cream").

How much fat has the usual "gravity cream?" Sixteen to twenty per cent.

How much fat is contained in cream removed from the upper one fifth of a bottle of milk? About sixteen per cent.

How much does the usual centrifugal cream contain? Eighteen to twenty per cent fat.

How much does the heavy centrifugal cream contain? Thirty--five to forty per cent fat.

Should the milk be boiled for babies in the summer time? No, not usually.

FOOD FOR HEALTHY INFANTS.--FOR EARLY MONTHS.

These directions, etc., are for healthy infants. Directions for such as are suffering from digestive disturbances will be given later. I have in preceding pages given formulas for feeding children. I give these additional, because not all children can be fed the same way and it may be well to have the two sets of formulas.

What important parts are to be remembered when we are modifying cow's milk for the early month's feeding? That sugar is the most easily digested, fat comes next, while the proteids (curd) are the most difficult.

What relation should the fat and proteids bear to each other during the earlier periods? Usually in healthy infants the fat (cream) should be three times the proteids (curds). Some healthy infants do not digest fat so well and they should have only twice as much fat as proteids (curds--skim-milk).

What per cent milk must be used to obtain three times as much fat as proteids? Ten per cent milk.

How can we obtain ten per cent milk? As top milk, described on another page, or by using plain milk and ordinary cream (sixteen per cent), in equal parts mixed; or it may be obtained directly from the milk laboratories.

Which is better to do, use the top-milk or mix plain milk and ordinary cream?

If the milk is fresh from the cows, it is best then to use the top-milk, because the food can then be made up after it is only a few hours old.

If one uses bottled milk, in cities, the upper third may be used, but if milk and cream are bought separately it is usually more convenient to mix these, as cream will not rise uniformly upon the milk a second time.

What per cent milk must be used to obtain twice as much fat as proteids? Use for dilution a seven per cent milk, that is, milk containing seven per cent fat, as in this milk the fat is just twice the proteids.

How is this obtained? Same as top-milk, described on another page; or by mixing three parts of plain milk and one part of ordinary cream (sixteen per cent), or by obtaining it directly from the milk laboratories.

How should we prepare the food for the early months? Granted you make up twenty ounces at a time, first obtain the ten per cent, or seven per cent, milk to be used, then take the number of ounces of this called for in the formula desired. One must remember that to make twenty ounces of food one ounce of milk sugar (or three even tablespoonfuls) and one ounce of lime-water must be used. The rest of the food is boiled water and the per cent milk.

FIRST SERIES--Five formulas for early months for ten per cent milk:

Formulas.	1	2	3	4	5
10 per cent milk	2 oz.	3 oz.	4 oz.	5 oz.	6 oz.
*Milk Sugar	1 oz.	1 oz.	1 oz.	1 oz.	1 oz.
Lime-water	1 oz.	1 oz.	1 oz.	1 oz.	1 oz.
Boiled water	17 oz.	16 oz.	15 oz.	14 oz.	13 oz.
	-----	-----	-----	-----	-----
	20 oz.	20 oz.	20 oz.	20 oz.	20 oz.

*The milk sugar takes no space as it is always dissolved in the boiled water.

How can we strengthen this food? By gradually increasing the milk (top milk) and decreasing the amount of water.

SECOND SERIES--Of five formulas for the early months from the seven per cent milk. This is weaker in fat (cream), etc., about one-third:

Formulas	1	2	3	4	5	
7 per cent, milk		2 oz.	3 oz.	4 oz.	5 oz.	6 oz.
Milk Sugar	1 oz.	1 oz.	1 oz.	1 oz.	1 oz.	
Lime-water	1 oz.	1 oz.	1 oz.	1 oz.	1 oz.	
Boiled water	17 oz.	16 oz.	15 oz.	14 oz.	13 oz.	
	-----	-----	-----	-----	-----	
Food	20 oz.	20 oz.	20 oz.	20 oz.	20 oz.	

How can I decide which series of formulas to use? A strong child with good digestion can be given from the first series, ten per cent milk.

A smaller, weaker child, and whose digestion is not so good, or with one who has tried the first series and did not do well, should use the second series of formulas.

What is the reason the food is made so weak at first? The infant's stomach is made to digest mother's milk, not cows' milk, so we must begin with weak cows' milk, and the infant's stomach can thus be trained to digest it. Strong milk would be very liable to seriously upset the child's digestion.

How rapidly can I increase the food in strength, that is, go from formula 1 to 2, 3, 4, and 5, of either series? This can not be told, absolutely. It depends upon the infant, how it bears the food. Usually you can begin on formula one on the second day, formula two on the fourth day; three, after seven or ten days, but after that make the increase slower. If the infant is large, strong and of good digestion, he may be able to take of formula five by the time he is three or four weeks old. A weak child, or one with feeble digestion must go much slower, and such an one may not reach formula five until it is three or four months old. Mothers should remember it is safer to increase the strength of the food very gradually; some infants should have an increase of only one-half ounce instead of one ounce; thus: three to three and one-half ounces, etc. Two or three days should be allowed at least between each increase of food.

May I not go by a general rule in increasing the food? Yes, increase the food when the infant is not satisfied, but is digesting well.

How does an infant show this? He drains the bottle hungrily and cries when it is taken away. He may begin to fret a half hour or so before the time for the next feeding. He often sucks his fingers immediately after feeding.

If I wish to prepare more than 20 ounces of food, what proportions shall I use? To make 25 ounces, add one-fourth more of each ingredient. To make 30 ounces, add one-half more of each ingredient. To make 35 ounces, add three-fourths more of each ingredient. To make 40 ounces, double each ingredient.

For example, 25 ounces of food would call for--2-1/2 ounces of milk; 1-1/4 ounces of milk sugar; 1-1/4 ounces of lime-water; 21-1/4 ounces of boiled water.

For 30 ounces of food, proportions would be--Milk, 3 ounces; milk sugar, 1-1/2 ounces; lime-water, 1-1/2 ounces; boiled water, 25-1/2 ounces.

How much more should be made at one time? Five ounces may be made, but the first few days only two or three ounces of the additional should be given; four ounces the next two days, and after two days more may give the five ounces additional that has been made; that is, twenty-five ounces in all.

How much increase can be given at each feeding? Not more than one-quarter of an ounce.

FOOD FOR HEALTHY INFANTS DURING THE LATER MONTHS.

How long shall I continue this proportion, that is, the fat three times the proteids (curd)--skim-milk? Usually for three or four months.

What changes shall I then make in the food? After you are using formula five of the first series; that is, six ounces of the ten per cent milk in twenty ounces of milk, increase the fat slowly, for the proportion of fat (three per cent), is near the limit for healthy children.

How then shall I strengthen the milk? By raising the percentage of proteids (curds, skim-milk).

How can I do this? Use the formulas derived from the seven per cent milk and discontinue the ten per cent milk.

THIRD SERIES.--Five formulas for seven per cent milk for the later months--

Formulas.	1	2	3	4	5
7 per cent milk	7 oz.	8 oz.	9 oz.	10 oz.	11 oz.
*Milk Sugar	1 oz.	1 oz.	1 oz.	3/4 oz.	1/2 oz.
Lime-water	1 oz.	1 oz.	1 oz.	1 oz.	1 oz.
Boiled water	12 oz.	11 oz.	10 oz.	4 oz.	3 oz.
Barley Gruel	0 oz.	0 oz.	0 oz.	5 oz.	5 oz.
	-----	-----	-----	-----	-----
	20 oz.	20 oz.	20 oz.	20 oz.	20 Oz.

*(As the milk sugar is dissolved in the boiled water the quantity is twenty ounces instead of twenty-one.) Oatmeal gruel can be substituted for barley gruel if there is constipation. To increase the food to twenty-five, thirty, or thirty-five ounces increase the milk ingredients by 1/4, 1/2, 3/4 and for forty ounces using two times as much.

How shall I increase the food during this period? Beginning with formula one of this series, which should usually follow five of the first or second series, you can usually make the increase in ten days to No. 2; in two weeks you can use No. 3; but proceed more slowly to four or five when you have reached them. The same formula may be continued sometimes for three or four months with no other change, except an increase in the quantity of the food, that is from twenty ounces to twenty-five, etc.

Is it necessary or important to reduce the proportion of fat as it is at first, reduced in passing from formula five of the first series to formula one of the third series? It is not necessary.

How much is this reduction? From 3 to 2.50 per cent.

How much increase of fat is there from the fifth formula of the second series to the first formula of the third series? From 2.00 to 2.50 per cent.

Can the first decrease be avoided? Yes, by taking off at first the upper thirteen ounces as top-milk, and using in a twenty-ounce mixture seven ounces of this in place of formula No. 1, and also by using for the next increase the upper fifteen ounces as top-milk--taking of this eight ounces in a twenty-ounce mixture in place of formula No. 2. Then follow three of this third series. This is only done when you think the formulas two and three of the third series do not give enough fat.

Can I add any other food about the sixth or seventh months? Yes, foods in the form of gruel, and have this take the place of part of the boiled water and part of the sugar. Oatmeal and barley gruels can be added.

Can I make further changes at ten or eleven months? The proteids (skim-milk) may be further increased, sugar and lime-water reduced until plain milk is given.

How can I do this? Give at first one feeding of plain milk and barley gruel daily; later two feedings, then three feedings, etc. For example, suppose one infant was being fed with modified milk as formula 4 or 5, series 3, six feedings daily. The plain milk diluted with boiling water would take the place of one such feeding at first, then two, three, four, etc., feedings. Such changes to be made at intervals of two weeks. Proportions of milk and barley gruel should be, at first, about five and one-half ounces milk, two and one-half ounces barley gruel; later six ounces milk, three ounces barley gruel and then seven ounces milk, two ounces barley gruel until plain milk is alone used, and this can usually be reached at twelve to thirteen months. For five months' infants a pinch of soda may be added to each feeding when the lime-water is omitted. It is not generally necessary, however.

Do some infants dislike the milk after the milk sugar has been omitted? Yes; for such 1/4 to 1/2 teaspoonful of granulated sugar may be added for a time to each feeding and gradually reduced.

RULES FOR USING THESE FORMULAS.

They are only for healthy infants. Begin always with a weak formula, especially with an infant previously nursed at the breast, with one just weaned and with infants who have poor digestive powers, or whose digestive powers are unknown. Should the first formula tried be too weak the food can be strengthened every three or four days until the right formula is found. If the food is made too strong at first an attack of indigestion is liable to follow.

How shall I increase the strength of the food? This should be done very gradually. Do not advance more than one formula in the given series. It is frequently better to make the increase in half steps. Say when it is from three to four, give three and one-half, and then four.

How rapidly can I increase the quantity of food? This should not be more than one-fourth ounce in each feeding, one to one and one-half to two ounces daily.

When should the amount of food be increased? An increase may be necessary every few days in the early weeks, but the same formula is often continued for two or three months during the later months.

What signs in the infant demand an increase? The infant is not satisfied, does not gain in weight, but it has good digestion--that is, it does not vomit and has good stools.

When should I not increase the food? So long as the child is satisfied, gains four to six ounces weekly, even when the quantity and strength of the food is considerably below the average.

Should you then increase the food if the child seems somewhat hungry, but still gains from eight to ten ounces weekly? It is not always a safe rule to be guided by the appetite.

How can I know whether to increase the strength or the quantity of the food? In the early weeks it is well first to increase the strength, the next time the quantity of the food, then the strength, then the quantity, etc. The quantity chiefly should be increased after the fourth or fifth month.

Should a slight stomach discomfort or disturbance follow after the food has been strengthened, what shall I do? If the disturbance is marked and continues and the infant does not seem able to accustom itself to the new food, you should go back to the weaker one and the next increase should be smaller.

Should I be worried if the gain in weight for the first few weeks of artificial feeding is slight, or even no gain? Not as a rule; if the infant loses no weight, sleeps well, is comfortable, does not suffer from vomiting, nausea, colic, you can feel sure the baby is doing well and is becoming used to his new food. As his appetite improves and his digestion is stronger the food may be increased every few days. Then the weight will soon increase.

Is constipation likely to occur from such a weak food? This is very often seen owing to the fact of their being little residue in the bowels, so if he has a daily stool, even if it is small and dry, it need not cause worry as it soon passes away with the using of stronger food.

What circumstances indicate that the food should be reduced? When the child becomes ill from any causes, or when there are any marked symptoms of indigestion.

How can I reduce the food? If there is but a slight disturbance and the daily food has been prepared, pour off one-third from each bottle just before each feeding and replace this quantity of food with boiled water; if the disturbance is more severe, immediately dilute the food at least one-half and also reduce, at the same time the quantity given; for a severe attack of indigestion, omit the regular food altogether and give only boiled water until a doctor has been called.

How shall I return to the original formula after it has been reduced for a disturbance of digestion? The increase must be very gradual after the immediate reduction. After a severe attack of indigestion, the milk should not be made more than one-fifth the original strength, and ten days or two weeks should elapse before the original strength food is given and, as stated, there should be a gradual slow increase.

ABOUT ADDING OTHER FOODS TO MILK.

How long shall I continue the modified milk? Usually for about six months; but if the infant is doing well you can continue it for ten or eleven months. If the infant has trouble in digesting cows' milk other foods can be added at three or four months or even at the beginning.

What food can I first use? Barley, oatmeal, arrowroot, and farina.

Is it better to make them from the flour? Yes, they are more simple to prepare from the flour.

How shall I cook them? Cook them separately, and when used they take the place of some of the boiled water.

(For another way, see former pages.)

How shall I prepare barley gruel water? Take one teaspoonful of the flour and rub it up with a little cold water, and then stir this into a pint of boiling water; add a pinch of salt and boil it fifteen minutes; strain if it is lumpy. Oatmeal gruel is made the same way, only using two teaspoonfuls instead of one.

Barley Jelly.--One rounded tablespoonful of the flour, mixed with a little cold water, is added to one pint of boiling water containing a pinch of salt; cook twenty minutes in a double boiler and strain. A thinner gruel (barley water) is made by using half of the quantity of flour.

How much of the gruel can I use? If prepared by the last method one-sixth to one-half the total quantity of food; if the barley water is used it can be used in greater quantity if desired, as it is weaker by half.

Which one shall I use? Barley and oatmeal are generally used; oatmeal is more laxative.

What is their value as infant foods? Their chief value is to prevent the curd from coagulating in the stomach in hard masses, thus rendering it more digestible.

Would you advise this addition for all infants? No, for it does not agree with them all, and so it cannot be recommended for all infants.

Can I give anything more during the first year? Beef juice, white of an egg, and orange juice.

How and when may I use the beef juice? It may be begun at ten or eleven months in infants who are strong and thriving well. Two teaspoonfuls may be given daily, diluted with same amount of water, fifteen minutes before the midday feeding; in two weeks it may be doubled; and six teaspoonfuls can be given, in four weeks. Two or three tablespoonfuls is all that can be given a child of one year.

Is beef juice of value in delicate pale infants? Yes, of much value, and it is more important for them, and it may sometimes be given them at five or six months in one-half the quantity mentioned.

When shall I give the white of egg (albumen) or albumin water? When the conditions are similar to those requiring beef juice especially in infants who digest the proteids (curd) with difficulty. You can give the one-half of the white of one egg at six months, and soon the entire white of one egg can be given.

What is the best way of preparing this? By coddling the egg.

Describe the way of preparation? Place a fresh egg with the shell on in boiling water and immediately remove all from the fire. The egg cooks slowly in the water for seven or eight minutes as the water gradually cools, and the white part becomes like jelly. Give the white with only a pinch of salt--it can be easily separated from the yolk.

When can I give orange juice? Usually about the eleventh or twelfth month, and it should be given about one hour before the feeding. You can begin with two teaspoonfuls at first, then one tablespoonful at a time, and later three or four tablespoonfuls. Orange juice is very good when constipation exists--strain it always, and it must be always fresh and sweet.

OVER NURSING.

Mothers who have a very large supply of milk are very likely to overfeed their babies if the milk is of good quality. This will drain the mother's strength. Some mothers allow their babies to nurse to relieve the uncomfortable feeling. If the infant vomits the surplus immediately they are not injured. Where the baby does not vomit, the surplus food passes into the bowels and causes colic and green and yellow gassy stools. If the mother's milk is too rich, only, and not too much and the baby vomits, this can be corrected by giving the baby some boiled water before each meal. The baby will not nurse so much then.

OVER-FEEDING.

What do you mean by this term? The infant gets too much food, and this is chiefly done at night.

Can I depend upon the infant's natural desire for food as to the quantity to be given? Not always, the habit of over-eating is frequently acquired, and is frequently seen in infants with a good digestion.

What harm results from over-feeding an infant? The food lies in the stomach or bowels, undigested, ferments, and causes gas and colic, and if the over-feeding is long continued, serious trouble arises.

The baby becomes restless, fretful, irritable, sleeps badly, stops gaining weight and may lose weight.

LOSS OF APPETITE.

What may cause this? Over-feeding or the use of milk too rich in fat.

What can I do for this trouble? If the child is well, offer food to him at regular hours only. Do not coax or force him to eat even though he takes only one-half or one-third of his usual quantity. Lengthen the intervals between the feedings. It may be necessary with a child under a year old to reduce the number of feedings to three or four in twenty-four hours. Give water at more frequent intervals, weaken instead of strengthening the food.

FOODS FOR SPECIAL CONDITIONS.

Some infants with weak digestive powers, and those suffering from various forms of indigestion, have often much trouble in digesting the fat of milk. To meet such troubles a series of formulas are given obtained from plain milk.

FOURTH SERIES-Formulas containing four per cent fat:

1	2	3	4	5	6	7
Plain Milk	5 oz.	6 oz.	7 oz.	8 oz.	9 oz.	10 oz.
*Milk Sugar	1 oz	1 oz.	1 oz.	1 oz	3/4 oz.	3/4 oz.
Lime-water	1 oz.	1 oz.	1 oz.	1 oz.	1 oz.	1 oz.
Boiled water	14 oz.	13 oz.	12 oz.	7 oz.	6 oz.	5 oz.
Barley Gruel.	0 oz.	0 oz.	0 oz.	4 oz.	4 oz.	4 oz.
-----	-----	-----	-----	-----	-----	-----
20 oz.	20 oz.	20 oz.	20 oz.	20 oz.	20 oz.	20 oz.

*(Milk sugar is not counted in totals.) If more than twenty ounces are needed get the proportions by adding one-fourth, one-half, three-quarters, or double each ingredient.

Why does an infant so often vomit some of its food soon after feeding? The quantity may be too large or too rich food, the baby may feed too fast, the hole in the nipple may be too large, the clothing too tight, or you may press upon its stomach in moving the baby.

What are the causes of and changes needed for stomach troubles? It is usually a symptom of indigestion and is frequently caused by too much fat or sugar.

How can I remedy this? Reduce the fat or sugar, and increase the lime-water. Avoid the formulas made from the top-milk, or cream and milk. Those made from the seven per cent milk are not so likely to cause trouble; but you had better, if the symptoms are severe, use formulas of the fourth series.

What symptoms indicate that the baby is getting too much fat

(cream)? Vomiting and yellow, foul, greasy, or ropy stools.

How much shall I reduce the milk sugar? Use only one-half ounce to twenty ounces of food or leave it out altogether.

How shall I know when to reduce the sugar, etc.? When there is excessive formation of gas in the stomach, causing distention and pain, or belchings of gas, and often a sour stomach. Reduce the amount of sugar and increase the lime-water one and one-half to two ounces in twenty ounces of food, increase intervals between the meats one-half hour and give less quantity.

What food usually causes habitual colic? This is due to gas accumulating in the bowels, and is usually caused by the want of digestion of the proteids (curd).

How shall I overcome this? Use a weaker formula. Use formula 4 or 3 of first series; or use partially pasteurized milk, or use barley water instead of plain water.

If curds regularly or frequently appear in the stools, what changes shall I make? This usually accompanies colic, so use means just described--reduce the proteids (skim milk).

How shall I modify the milk for chronic constipation? This is difficult to overcome, and it is more frequent when infants are fed upon a plain milk diet, variously diluted, than when seven or ten per cent milk is used and diluted to a greater degree. But you cannot use food containing more than four per cent fat, that is, eight ounces of ten per cent milk or twelve ounces of seven per cent milk in twenty ounces of food. In some cases ordinary brown sugar in one-half the quantity can take the place of milk sugar, or Mellin's food, malted milk or cereal milk can be used in the place of the milk sugar. Milk of magnesia can be used for lime-water as before directed. Orange juice can be given to infants over nine months old.

What modifications should I make in very hot weather? The proportion of fat (top-milk or milk and cream mixed) should be less and when it is very hot, for a short period, it should be much less. Use seven per cent milk in place of ten per cent, that is, formulas from the second series, or plain milk, in place of the seven per cent milk, fourth series.

If a child has good digestion, but gains very little or no weight, what changes in the food should I make? Increase the quantity of the food if the child seems hungry; or increase the strength of the food, if the child will not take a greater quantity; do not coax or force the baby to eat, give him more sleep; fresh air, etc.

If there is no modified milk that will agree with the baby, what shall I do? If the infant is under four or five months old, a wet nurse would likely succeed. If a wet nurse cannot be obtained or if the child is older use some of the substitutes for cows' milk, like Borden's Eagle Brand, canned or condensed milk. This is better to use when the trouble is in the bowels and shows colic, gas, curds in the stools, constipation, or diarrhea. If it is due to indigestion it shows in vomiting, etc.

How shall I use condensed milk? The directions are on the bottle. But if the baby is three or four months old, and has symptoms of indigestion, dilute its food with sixteen parts of boiled water, or sometimes barley water if there is no constipation. As the symptoms improve it can be made stronger, one to fourteen, one to twelve one to ten, one to eight, such changes to be made gradually.

How long can I use the condensed milk? Generally for a few weeks only as the sole food, then give one feeding a day of modified milk, for instance, No. 3 or 4 of the series; later two feedings and gradually increase until the milk feeding is entirely used.

Why can I not continue to use condensed milk? It is very low in fat and proteids and has much sugar in it; children who take this food for sometime often gain rapidly in strength and weight, yet have not much resistance, and they are very prone to develop rickets and scurvy.

Suppose baby is teething, has a cold, sore throat, etc., what change shall I make? Dilute the food for two or three feedings by using boiled water in place of an ounce or two of food; this much to be removed from the bottle before being given; if it is necessary to continue for several days, use a weaker formula.

What changes shall I make in this for serious acute sickness? For, diseases with fever like measles, bronchitis, pneumonia, etc., dilute the food and reduce the fat (cream from top-milk). Give the food at regular intervals, but not so often. Do not force food in the early part of acute sickness.

Suppose baby has acute gastritis, what changes shall I make? Stop all food and give boiled water, only, for ten or more hours, then try barley water or whey, but do not give any milk for at least twenty-four hours after all vomiting has ceased. When you again begin the modified milk use a small quantity with a low proportion of fat, and you can secure this by using a formula from the fourth series. You may also double the proportion of lime-water.

If baby is attacked with intestinal indigestion accompanied by loose bowels, what food shall I give? If it has but two or three passages daily, lower the proportion of fat (cream, etc.), in the manner above directed, and boil the milk for five minutes. Dilute it still more if curds are present in the stools.

But suppose the attack is more severe? If there is fever and the passages smell badly and are more frequent, stop all milk and use the diet given for acute gastritis. (Acute indigestion).

Do other conditions besides the food influence digestion? Yes, use proper clothing, keep warm feet, regular habits, fresh air. Clean bottles and food, given at proper intervals and temperature, quiet surroundings and absence of excitement are needed.

What common mistakes are often made in modifying milk and feeding infants? Never fail to follow the directions given for removing the top-milk. Remove *all* the top-milk of any given strength in making a formula, and not only the number of ounces needed for the formula. By using rich Jersey milk as if it were more common milk. The formulas given are based upon about four per cent fat. Food is very often increased too rapidly, particularly after stomach and bowel indigestion. The food in an infant of three or four months old attacked by acute indigestion should seldom be given in full strength for two weeks afterwards, only half steps should be taken like two to two and one-half, etc. Another mistake, when indigestion symptoms show the food is not reduced quickly enough; reduce the food immediately by at least one-half.

How to prepare cows' milk at home; what is needed? Feeding bottles, rubber nipples, an eight-ounce graduated measuring glass, a glass funnel, a brush for bottles, cotton, alcohol lamp, a tall quart cup for warming bottles of milk, a pitcher for mixing food, a wide mouthed bottle of boric acid and one of bicarbonate of soda, a pasteurizer, and later a double boiler for cooking cereals will be needed.

What kind of bottles shall I buy? A cylindrical graduated bottle with a wide neck holding about 8 ounces. This makes washing them easier. You should have as many bottles for use as the baby takes meals a day (ten at first).

How shall I care for the bottles? Rinse them, as soon as the child is through nursing, with cold water, and let stand filled with cold water and a little bicarbonate of soda in the water. Before using them again wash them thoroughly with the bottle brush and hot soap suds and place them for twenty minutes in boiling water.

What kind of nipples are best? Straight ones which slip over the neck of the bottle, of black rubber, and the hole should only be large enough for the milk to drop rapidly when the bottle is held upside down.

How shall I care for the nipples? Boil new ones for five minutes at first. After using rinse them carefully in cold water and keep them covered in a glass containing a solution of borax or boric acid. Turn them inside out once a day and wash thoroughly with soap and water.

(There is a slight difference in the directions given by different authorities as to cleaning bottles and nipples, but the general way is the same.)

What kind of cotton shall I use for corking the bottles? Refined non-absorbent cotton is best, but the ordinary absorbent cotton will do.

Which is the best--an alcohol lamp, or the Bunsen burner? The Bunsen burner is the best, cheaper and simpler if there is gas in the house. Should you use the lamp, put it upon a table covered with a plate of zinc or tin, or upon a large tin tray. The French pattern is the best.

Give special directions now for preparing the food according to any of the given formulas? The hands must be clean, as well as everything else--food and utensils. First dissolve the milk sugar in boiling water, filtering, if necessary, then add to the boiled water and sugar the milk, cream, and lime-water, mixing all in the pitcher; a sufficient quantity for twenty-four hours is always prepared at one time. Divide this in equal quantities into the number of feedings for the twenty-four hours and cork the bottles with the cotton cork and cool the bottles rapidly, after having been pasteurized by standing first in tepid and then in cold water, and then place in an ice chest at 50 degrees F.

FEEDING DIRECTIONS.

How shall I prepare the bottle at feeding time? Take one from the ice chest, warm it by placing it in warm water deep enough to cover the milk in the bottle. Then thoroughly shake it, remove the cotton cork, and adjust the nipple.

How shall I know that the temperature of the milk is correct? Pour a teaspoonful from the bottle before adjusting the nipple, and taste it, or pour a few drops through the nipple upon the inner surface of the wrist. It should feel quite warm, but not quite hot; or a baby thermometer may be placed in the water where the milk stands, and the temperature should be between 98 and 100 degrees F.

How can I keep the milk warm while the baby is feeding? Slip over the bottle a warm flannel bag with a draw-string.

What position should a child be in when feeding? During the first few months, except at night, it had better be held in the arms; later it can lie on its side in the crib, but the bottle must then be held by the nurse until it is emptied, or the baby will nurse and sleep, and nurse and sleep, etc.

How much time shall I give the baby for one feeding? Not longer than twenty minutes. Take the bottle away then and do not give it until the next feeding. Keep a sleepy baby awake, when well, until the food is taken, or remove the bottle.

Can I play with the baby after feeding? Never. It may cause vomiting and indigestion. Baby should lie quietly and sleep if possible, or at least not be disturbed.

FEEDING INTERVALS.

How often shall I nurse or feed baby during the first month? Ten times in twenty-four hours at intervals of two hours during the day and two times at night.

Why can I not feed baby oftener? Because it takes nearly two hours to digest a meal at two months, about two and one-half hours at five or six months, and if another meal is given before the former meal is digested, vomiting and indigestion will result. The following schedule is given by one authority on children for healthy infants for the first year:

	Night Interval between meals by day.	No. feedings 10 P. M. to 7 A. M.	Quantity of feedings in 24 hours.	Quantity for one feeding, ounces.
2d to 7th day	2 hrs.	2	10	1 to 1-1/2
2d to 3rd week	2 hrs.	2	10	1-1/2 to 3
4th to 5th week	2 hrs.	1	10	2-1/2 to 3-1/2
6th to 8th week	2-1/2 hrs.	1	8	3 to 5
3d to 5th Month	3 hrs.	1	7	4 to 6
5th to 9th month	3 hrs.	0	6	5 to 7-1/2
9th to 12th month	4 hrs.	0	5	7 to 9

This schedule is for healthy children. The smaller amounts are required by smaller children with weak digestion; the larger amounts are required by large children with strong digestion. The interval is from the beginning of one feeding to the beginning of the next feeding.

How soon can I make the intervals at two and one-half hours? Generally at five or six weeks.

When may I increase it to three hours? Usually at eight weeks or two months.

When should I lengthen the interval between feedings? When there is poor stomach digestion.

How is this shown? By habitual vomiting or regurgitation of food long after nursing is finished; also when the baby has a very poor appetite so that it always leaves some of its food.

When can I shorten the intervals? It is not generally advisable to feed any baby oftener than given by this schedule.

REGULAR FEEDING.

How can I teach baby to take regular meals? By commencing at birth to feed at exactly regular hours every day.

Shall I awaken baby to feed it? Yes, for a few days. In a short time he will waken at the same hours himself.

Should this regularity extend through the night? Only up to nine or ten o'clock. After ten let him sleep as long as he will.

How soon can baby go without food from 10 p. m. to 7 a. m.? At four months usually and always at five or six months; night feeding causes restlessness and poor sleep.

STERILIZED MILK.

What do you mean by sterilizing milk? It means to heat milk so as to destroy the germs.

Does cows' milk contain germs? Yes, even if it is handled faultlessly; but when carelessly handled the number of germs is enormous.

Are all of the germs injurious? Most are harmless or cause only the souring of the milk.

What other germs are occasionally present? Typhoid fever, diphtheria, scarlet fever, cholera, tuberculosis and many forms of diarrhea germs.

Do I need to sterilize milk under all circumstances? When you cannot obtain it fresh in warm weather. Hence during warm weather in cities and towns; when you do not know that the cows are healthy or that the milk has been cleanly handled; when milk is kept over twenty-four hours, especially if there is no ice at hand. When there are epidemics of typhoid fever, scarlet fever, diphtheria, or any form of bowel disease accompanied by diarrhea.

How many methods of heating milk are there? First, sterilizing, in which the milk is heated to 212 degrees F., for one hour or one and one-half hours. Second, pasteurizing, when you heat the milk to 155 degrees or 170 degrees F. for thirty minutes.

Will the temperature of 155 degrees F. for one-half hour be sufficient to kill the germs of the diseases mentioned above? Generally.

How long will milk so treated keep on ice? Heated to 212 degrees F. for an hour will keep for two or three weeks; that heated (pasteurized) to 155 degrees F. will keep for two or three days.

Is cows' milk as digestible when sterilized? No, and it should be modified for infant feeding the same as milk not heated.

When milk is heated for an hour to 212 degrees F. (sterilization), is it injured in any way? It is rendered harder to digest, and is more constipating; scurvy may be caused if it is used as the sole food for a long time. It is so objectionable that the method is not recommended for general use.

When should I heat it 212 degrees F.? For use on long journeys of days traveling. Then you should heat for one hour upon two successive days, leaving the cotton stoppers in the bottles.

Does heating milk to 155 degrees F. for one-half hour injure it in any way? It does not affect the taste or make it more constipating. The unfavorable effects, if any, are slight. Get clean and fresh milk and the effects will be really of no account.

What pasteurizer would you recommend. Freeman's or Walker-Gordon.

What shall I do with the milk after it has been pasteurized? Cool it quickly by placing the bottles in cold water--never leave them in the room where pasteurized, and never place them, when warm, in an ice chest.

Why this caution? Because it requires from two to four hours to cool them in the air, or in the ice box, and during that time a good many undeveloped germs may mature and injure the keeping properties of the milk. You can cool the bottles of milk in cool water in from ten to twenty minutes if you change the water frequently, or if ice is put into the water.

What is modified milk of the laboratories? It is milk containing fat, sugar, proteids, etc., in definite proportions put up, usually, according to a physician's directions.

PEPTONIZED MILK.

What is peptonized milk? Milk that has been partially digested.

What part of the milk has been digested? The proteids (curd).

Does this alter its taste? No, if it is peptonized for only ten minutes, but if it is fully peptonized the milk has a bitter taste.

How can the bitter taste be avoided in partly peptonized milk? At the end of ten or fifteen minutes place the milk in a sauce-pan and raise it quickly to the boiling point; this kills the ferment so that the milk will not become bitter when it is warmed for feeding; or the milk can be cooled rapidly by placing the bottles first in cool and then in ice water; but in this way the ferment is not destroyed, and the milk may become bitter when warmed for feeding.

How is milk peptonized? By the action of a peptonizing powder composed of a digestive agent known as the extractum pancreatis and bicarbonate of soda. This is added to the plain or diluted milk. This agent can be bought in tubes or tablets, and is the active ingredient of the peptogenic powder.

Will you describe the process? Place the plain or modified milk in a clean glass jar or bottle, and then rub up the peptonizing powder or tablet with a tablespoonful of milk, and add it to the milk and shake the bottle. Place the bottle in a large pitcher or basin of water of about 110 degrees F., or as warm as the hand can bear comfortably, and allow it to remain for ten to twenty minutes if you wish to peptonize the milk but partially; or if you wish it completely peptonized let it remain for two hours.

Is it better to peptonize the whole day's supply, or each bottle separately just before feeding? If you peptonize the whole day's supply at once raise the milk to the boiling point after it has been peptonized; if only the one feeding do not peptonize it more than ten minutes before feeding for the ferment will work while the child is feeding. It can be done either way.

Is not the completely peptonized milk distasteful? Not so in the case of young infants; older infants will take a few feedings without objection, but it cannot be used for children much older than five months.

How much of the agent should be used? For a single feeding of four ounces one may use one-eighth of a tube with a weak formula of milk or one-sixth with a stronger formula. For one pint of plain milk five grains of the extract and fifteen grains of bicarbonate of soda will be needed. This amount is usually put up in one tube or tablet. Less will be required in weaker formulas of modified milk.

What advantages has peptonized milk? Partially peptonized milk assists greatly in digesting the curd of milk. Young infants sometimes have trouble in digesting the curd. When completely peptonized it is good in attacks of acute indigestion.

How long may I give it? It may be used for a few days when completely peptonized; when partially peptonized it can be used for two or three months, and when you wish to give other food, leave off its use gradually by shortening the time of peptonizing and lessening the quantity of the powder used.

FEEDING DURING THE SECOND YEAR

How many meals should a child have during the second year? Five.

Shall I prepare the milk for all day at one time? It is better to prepare the milk for all day during the second and third years. If you wish to modify it by adding cream, water, etc., prepare as done during the first year, and later when only plain milk is used, the quantities needed for the different feedings should be put into one or two bottles, pasteurized or not as necessary. In this way the different feedings are kept separate. Prepare the food as soon as possible in the morning alter the milk has been received.

FOR A HEALTHY CHILD OF TWELVE MONTHS.

6:30 a. m. or 7:00 a. m.--Milk, six to seven ounces, diluted with two or three ounces of barley or oatmeal gruel, and taken from a cup after thirteen months.

9:00 a. m.--One to two ounces of orange juice.

10:00 a. m.--Milk two parts, oatmeal or barley gruel one part, and from ten to twelve ounces in all may be given in a cup.

2 :00 p. m.--One or two ounces of beef juice, or the white of one egg, slightly cooked, and later an entire egg or mutton or chicken broth, four to six ounces.

6:00 p. m.--Same as 10 a. m.

10:00 p. m.--Same as at 6:30 a. m., except the milk can be taken from the bottle.

How long can this schedule be given? Until the fourteenth or fifteenth month, and then you can give the cereals thicker and with a spoon.

Can I give other fruit juices at fourteen or fifteen months? Orange juice is the best, but the juice of ripe peaches, red raspberries or strawberries in the order given, is good. Strain all carefully through muslin, for the pulp or seeds might cause serious trouble. You may now give one to four tablespoonfuls of the orange or peach juice, and about one-half the quantity of the others.

When shall I give the fruit juices? One hour before the second meal.

What diet shall I give between fourteenth and eighteenth months?

6:00 to 6:30 a. m.--Eight to ten ounces of plain milk from a cup.

8:00 to 9:00 a. m.--Juice of one-half orange strained.

10:00 a. m.--One, or later two or three tablespoonfuls of oatmeal or barley jelly, hominy cooked at least three hours, and on which you may put a little top-milk; a pinch of salt; no sugar and cup--about six ounces--of milk to drink; crisp dry toast, one piece.

2:00 p. m.--Beef juice one to two ounces, a soft boiled; coddled or poached egg, and a tablespoonful of boiled rice, or mutton or chicken broth, four ounces; one or two pieces of stale bread or zwieback; and if most of the teeth are present, one scant teaspoonful of scraped rare beef, slowly increased to one tablespoonful, alternating with two ounces of beef juice and a salt-boiled or coddled egg. (Some advise a little prune jelly, apple sauce, a baked apple or junket as a dessert). No milk, but little water can be taken.

6:00 p. m.--Two tablespoonfuls of thoroughly cooked farina, or cream of wheat or granum, or arrow-root, on which is a little top-milk; salt, but no sugar, and eight ounces of warm milk which may be taken from the bottle.

10:00 p. m.--Warmed milk and eight to twelve ounces if necessary, by bottle.

How shall I prepare the beef? Take round or sirloin steak and scrape it with a large spoon on both sides, so that you obtain the pulp only, salt it a little, and place it with a very tiny piece of butter in a saucer, cover it with another saucer, remove the cover from the boiling teakettle, and place the saucer in its place; let it steam until it is just heated through, as it must look rare when done, Give at first one teaspoonful and gradually work up to one tablespoonful, but do not begin this diet in midsummer. Give baby plenty of water to drink between meals, boil and cool.

A diet for the eighteenth month to end of twenty-fourth month? Follow the same order. For most children milk at 10 p. m. is desirable; but if a child sleeps during the whole night it is not necessary to wake it at 10 p. m. for the feeding.

6:00 or 6:30 a. m.--Warmed milk ten to twelve ounces.

9:00 a. m.--Two or three ounces of fruit juices.

10:00 a. m.--Cereals similar to the last schedule; they need not be strained, but well cooked; crisp, dry bread, zwieback, warmed milk one cup.

2 :00 p. m.--Beef juice and one egg or broth and meat; beefsteak, mutton chop or roast beef scraped, very stale bread or two pieces of zwieback; one or two tablespoonfuls of prune pulp, or baked apple and water, but no milk.

6:00 p. m.--Farina, cream of wheat, or arrow-root well cooked with milk, salt, but no sugar; or milk or stale bread and milk.

10:00 p. m.--If required, ten to twelve ounces of pure milk.

What fruits may I give during this period? If the child has a weak stomach, only the fruit juices mentioned, but strong children may have in addition, baked apple, apple-sauce and prune pulp. Stew the dried prunes without sugar until they are very soft, and put all the fruit through a strainer thus removing all the skin; you may give one to two tablespoonfuls of this at one time. No cream should be given with the baked apple, and very little sugar with the apple-sauce These are very good for constipation, Remember to give water freely between the feedings, especially in warm weather. From one to three ounces may be given at one time either with a spoon, glass or bottle. Boil the water daily and cool. Do not allow it to stand in the room, but give fresh water to the child each time.

SCHEDULE FOR THREE-YEAR-OLD CHILD.

7:30 a. m.--Cereal well cooked (over night) or at least for three hours, A larger variety of food can now be given and given as before with thin cream, salt, but little sugar. One glass of warm milk, a soft boiled, coddled or poached egg; bread very stale or dry, one slice with butter.

10:00 a. m.--One cup of warm milk, with a cracker or a piece of stale bread and butter.

2:00 p. m.--Soup, four ounces, or two ounces of beef juice. Meat: chop, steak, roast beef, lamb or chicken; white potato, baked or boiled rice. Green vegetables: Tips of asparagus, string beans, peas, spinach, all cooked until they are very soft, mashed or preferably put through a sieve, and only one to two teaspoonfuls at first. Desserts: Cooked fruit, baked or stewed apple, stewed prunes, water, but no milk.

6:00 p. m.--Cereal: Farina, cream of wheat, or arrow-root, cooked for at least one-half hour with plenty of salt, but no sugar; or milk toast; or old bread and milk or stale or dry bread and butter and a glass of milk.

BABY'S SECOND SUMMER.

Nearly all mothers dread baby's second summer. If the baby is born at such a time that he cuts his double teeth during the hot weather, and if it is attended by indigestion and fever, there is really some cause for worry, because the digestive organs during the hot weather are more difficult to manage than during the colder months; otherwise, if you feed your baby carefully and properly, and with the regularity that you did in the early months, there is no reason to dread the second summer, Mistakes are made by mothers and grandparents especially. They permit the child to come to the table and eat of the food prepared for adults. Sometimes it is only a little, but that little will gradually grow larger; and even that little may be enough to upset baby for weeks and then the illness that follows is in reality due to the parents' own foolishness when it is laid to the credit of the second summer, or regarded as "a mysterious dispensation of Providence." Do not give anything to baby between its regular meals but water; crackers, zwieback, and bread are prohibited between.

DIET OF OLDER CHILDREN-FOURTH TO TENTH YEAR.

Give the largest meal at midday and a light supper at night, very much like that recommended for the third year. For a few years you can give milk once between breakfast and dinner, or dinner and supper, and permit no other food between meals, but give water freely.

MILK AND CREAM.

What part of the diet should milk form now? Nothing can take its place, and it should be an important part of the diet. Most children can take and digest milk.

Why is this of so much advantage? Because it possesses a higher nutritive value than any other food, for the amount of work required of the digestive organs, and it is very especially adapted to a child's diet.

It must be clean and fresh and not too rich.

What essential point should I consider in its use? The Jersey cow gives too rich milk, and it must be greatly diluted. Children who digest milk with difficulty should take it diluted about four parts milk, one part water, a little salt or bicarbonate of soda should be added. Do not give milk at meals when fruits, especially if they are sour, are allowed.

How much milk can I allow to advantage? For an average child with good digestion, you can allow one and one-half pints to one quart daily, including what is also used upon cereals and in other ways. Two quarts are too much, for a mixed diet will do better.

How much cream can I allow? Older children do not need so much fat as do infants, and cream, especially when very rich, often produces indigestion. It is a common cause of the coated tongue, foul breath, and pale greasy stools, or biliousness so-called.

Will not cream overcome constipation? It does so in some degree in infants, but not so much so in older children; and if it produces the above given symptoms it should not be given.

EGGS.

What is the value of eggs in the diet of this period? They form a very valuable food. They must be fresh and only slightly cooked, being either soft-boiled, poached or coddled. Fried eggs and omelets are prohibited.

Is the white or yolk more digestible? Generally the white in most children. This is a very digestible proteid and can be used to great advantage even in the latter part of the first year.

Do eggs often cause biliousness? Very seldom if they are carefully prepared and fed.

How often may I give eggs to the child? Most children at this period will be able to take one egg for breakfast and one for supper, with relish and advantage; however, some few children cannot eat them at all.

MEAT AND FISH.

What kinds of meat can I give to my child? Beefsteak, mutton-chop, roast beef, lamb, boiled chicken and fish, such as shad or bass.

What points should I consider in feeding meat? Most meats should be rare, scraped or finely divided, as a child will not chew it properly. Boiled or roast beef is best; fried meats should not be given to a child.

How often can I give meats? Only at the midday meal, at this period.

Do you think it causes nervousness in children? Not unless too much is given and too often.

What meats should be forbidden? Ham, bacon, sausage, pork, liver, kidney, and all dried and salt meats; also mackerel, cod and shell fish. A child should not eat any of these until after the tenth year.

Are gravies healthy and nutritious? Beef juice or so-called "platter gravy" from a roast is very nourishing and desirable, but many of the gravies that are thickened are harder to digest and too much is given. Only a small quantity should be allowed.

What about vegetables? Baked, boiled or mashed potatoes may be given first, but never fried. After the sixth or seventh year baked sweet potato, turnips, boiled onions and cauliflower, all well cooked, may be given moderately. They must be thoroughly cooked and mashed. This is the great trouble.

Can I give canned vegetables? Peas, and asparagus of the best brands can be used. They are often better than stale green vegetables.

What vegetables should be prohibited? Any that are eaten raw such as celery, radishes, onions, cucumbers, tomatoes or lettuce; corn, lima beans, cabbage, egg plant, even when well cooked; none of these should be given to a child under ten years old.

Can I give vegetable salads? As a rule none should be allowed at this period. They are difficult to digest and create great disturbances in children of all ages.

CEREALS.

What points should I consider in selecting and preparing these? They must be properly cooked and not used in excess. He should not make a meal of them because he is fond of them, and eat two or three saucerfuls at once. Proper cooking is essential. Oatmeal, hominy, rice, wheaten grits need two hours' cooking at least, in a double boiler; cornstarch, arrow-root, and barley should be cooked twenty minutes or more. All the market preparations need cooking.

How should they be eaten? Usually with milk or milk and cream; plenty of salt, no sugar or very little--one-half teaspoonful to a saucer--syrups or butter and sugar are prohibited.

What broths and soup do you recommend? Meat broths are generally to be preferred to vegetable broths, mutton and chicken usually being the best liked. Almost all plain broths can be given. Those thickened with rice, barley or cornstarch make a good variety, especially with milk added. Tomato soup should not be given to young children.

BREAD, CRACKERS, AND CHEESE.

What forms of bread can I give? Stale bread cut thin and freshly dried in the oven until it is crisp is very useful, also the unsweetened zwieback. Fresh bread should not be eaten. Gluten, oatmeal, or graham crackers, or the Huntley and Palmer breakfast biscuits, stale rolls or corn bread which has been cut in two or toasted or dried to a crisp form a sufficient variety.

What kinds of breadstuffs should be prohibited? All hot breads, all fresh rolls, buckwheat and other griddle cakes, all fresh sweet cakes, especially when covered with icing and those containing any dried fruits. Lady finger (stale) or a piece of sponge cake is all that can be allowed to children up to seven or eight years old.

DESSERTS.

Can I give any desserts to young children? Mistakes are very often made here. Junket, plain rice pudding without raisins, plain custard, and not more than once a week, a small amount of ice cream are all that can be allowed up to six or seven years.

What are prohibited? Pies, tarts, and pastry of every kind and jams, syrups, and preserved fruits; nut candy and dried fruits.

Can I give a little? No, for it develops a taste for this sort of food, and then the plainer food is taken with less relish. The little is soon likely to become a great deal.

A child has an instinctive desire for sweets, why not satisfy it? A child's fondness for sweets is not a normal instinct. A free indulgence in desserts and sweets by young children produces more digestive disorders than any other causes. It is a growing tendency and hard to control as the child grows older. The only safe rule is to give none in early childhood.

FRUITS.

Are fruits an important or essential part of children's diet? Very important, and they should be begun young. They have a splendid effect upon the bowels. They should be carefully selected, especially in large cities. A greater latitude can be all owed in the country where fruit is fresh.

What fruit can I safely give to children up to five years? Generally only cooked fruits and fresh fruit juices.

What kind of fruit juices can I use? That from fresh, sweet oranges is best. The fresh juice of grape fruit, peaches, strawberries, and raspberries may also be used.

What stewed fruits may I use? Stewed and baked apples, prunes, pears, peaches and apricots.

What raw fruits should be avoided? The pulp of oranges or grape fruit, also cherries, berries, bananas and pineapple.

What care should be exercised in regard to the use of fruits? In hot weather they should be used with greater care, and in children who are easily attacked with intestinal indigestion.

What symptoms suggest that I should avoid fruits? Looseness of the bowels or a tendency thereto, with discharge of mucus, or frequent attacks of colic (abdominal pain) or stomach-ache.

At what meals should fruits be used? If the fruit juice is given upon an empty stomach early in the morning, it works more actively upon the bowels, than when given later.

Is it wise to give cream or milk with sour fruits? No, it is not wise, it is best to give it at midday when no milk is taken as a dessert. The quantity should always be moderate.

Can I give anything besides water and milk to drink? Cocoa, if made very weak, almost all milk is often useful as a hot drink. Tea, coffee, wine, beer and cider are all prohibited under puberty. Lemonade and soda water should not be given until the tenth year at least.

INDIGESTION IN OLDER CHILDREN.

Different ways in which indigestion shows itself in children? First as an acute attack which lasts for a few days only; second, as chronic disturbances which may last for weeks and months.

Which is the most serious? Chronic indigestion, for it often goes on for months and even years unchecked, because it is not recognized.

The symptoms of acute indigestion? Vomiting, pain, diarrhea of undigested food, often fever and prostration.

What are the common causes? Over eating or indulging in improper food or too hearty eating when very tired.

Is it sometimes the forerunner of some acute general sickness? Yes.

How shall I treat acute indigestion? Give castor oil to clean out all undigested food from the bowels. Vomiting usually frees the stomach of food; stop food for from twelve to thirty-six hours, only boiled water being allowed. Let the stomach rest.

Can I then begin with the former diet? No, give at first only broth gruel, very much diluted milk or whey. Increase the diet slowly as the appetite and digestion improve, but this should consume a week or ten days in most cases before the full diet is resumed.

Give the symptoms of chronic indigestion (dyspepsia) in children? Disturbed sleep, tired, grinding teeth, fretfulness, loss of weight and flesh, gas in the stomach and bowels, pain in the bowels, bloated bowels, constipation or loose bowels with mucus in the stools, foul breath, coated tongue, poor appetite, capricious appetite. Some may think worms are present.

Common causes of chronic constipation? Bad system of feeding, prolonged use of improper food or improper methods of feeding, such as coaxing the child to eat, rapid eating, eating between meals, child selects his own food and lives largely upon one article of diet; indulgence in sweets, desserts, pies, etc. Improperly cooked foods especially oatmeal, and vegetables and eating sour or stale fruits. Exclude articles of diet which are known to be hard for children to digest.

How shall chronic indigestion be treated? Remove all causes such as bad foods, habits, etc.

Is it curable? In most cases, but the rules for feeding must be carefully followed for a long period. Medicine will not cure such cases unless the proper food is given in a proper way. That is better than medicine.

How long must this proper feeding continue? For months, and with many children for two or three years.

Is medicine of any use? It will relieve the symptoms, but the main thing is proper feeding.

SLEEP.

Should a baby sleep with anyone? No, young infants have been smothered by their mothers. It is also a frequent temptation to nursing at night, and this is injurious to both mother and child.

How long does baby usually sleep at first? About nine-tenths of the time.

How should his bed be prepared? The mattress should be firm and soft, the pillow, of hair and very thin; you should change his position so as not to sleep always in the same position.

How many hours should baby sleep at six months? About two-thirds of the time.

How long should the daily nap be continued? Until about four years old.

How shall I put baby to sleep? Darken the room and have quiet. The child's hunger should be satisfied and make him generally comfortable and lay him in the crib while still awake.

Can I rock him to sleep? No. It is a bad habit and, he will readily acquire it. It will be hard to break, and besides it is useless and some times an injurious one. The same may be said of sucking a rubber nipple or pacifier, and all other devices to put baby to sleep.

What principal things disturb baby's sleep? Quiet, peaceful sleep is a sign of perfect health, and disorders of sleep may be produced by almost anything that is wrong with the child. Food and feeding cause disturbed sleep. It may come from chronic indigestion due to improper food. In bottle-fed babies it is often due to over-feeding. In those who nurse it may be due to poor food and hunger. Feeding three or four times during the night makes a restless baby. It may also be due to nervous causes such as bad habits due to faulty training, as when the nursery is light and the baby is taken from its crib whenever it cries or wakes, or when contrivances for producing sleep have been used. Any excitement in a nursing mother or child before sleeping time will cause wakefulness. Romping play just before bedtime and fears aroused by stories and pictures are causes, and children who inherit a nervous constitution are special sufferers from this cause. Cold feet, insufficient or too much clothing, want of pure fresh air in the sleeping room. Tonsils or adenoids may interfere with breathing in older children. Rousing a sleeping child from a good sound sleep, is a frequent cause of poor sleep. If a pregnant woman keeps herself in as good condition as possible, not only physically, but also mentally, she will not be likely to have a nervous baby; and if a baby is not born nervous there is no reason, at all, why it should not sleep well, for sleep is then its most normal condition, nine-tenths of the time. It will then depend upon the food and training it is given. The training many babies receive is enough to make them poor sleepers.

Unnecessary handling.--Babies are wakened from sleep to show to friends who wish to see them at almost any and all hours. They are handled, petted, and made restless. Sleep is their normal condition and they ought to be given the opportunity nature demands. They are only to be aroused from sleep for nurse, bathing and clothing, and immediately placed in their crib, covered comfortably and warmly with all light shut away from their eyes and quiet about them. They will soon wake of their own accord for meals.

Rocking baby.--Rocking and shaking cause an increased flow of blood to the brain, and this should be avoided, for it of itself will cause sleeplessness. The brain during sleep is comparatively empty of blood; warm feet and cool head tend to produce sleep. Rocking, etc., is unnatural, and baby is made to receive and enjoy the natural. If the baby is sick the mother may take it in her arms and sing to it and coddle it carefully, but it is then sick. If it is trained properly from the beginning, rocking to sleep will be unnecessary; walking with the baby is of the same nature. See that your baby has warm feet and legs and body and a cool head, with comfortable clothes and good careful feeding, and it will sleep. Singing lullabies are soothing, but they do no good at first as the baby is deaf. Such lullabies are good when baby is sick and nervous, and then the mother is allowed and expected to hold and quiet baby. Sleep perhaps as much or more than any other item of nursery regime, depends on habit and mild but decided purpose. A lack of firmness in the early months of the baby's life may not only render its early years a burden to itself, but an annoyance, if not a nuisance to the entire household. Baby's habits are quickly and easily formed, but hard to correct. Dr. Tooker says: "An infant is as plastic as moist clay, you can mold it to your will. But you must have a will and a purpose and a plan, and make your judgment and your duty law."

But suppose baby will not sleep, but continues cross and wakeful and peevish; can I not give medicines to produce sleep? Never. If baby is wakeful and refuses to sleep, there is something wrong with your training, his clothing, covering, or his food, or he may be sick, he may not get enough food, etc., or he may have worms. If everything is all right and you have trained your baby right from his birth, he will sleep. Find out the cause and remove it. All soothing syrups, cordials, and quieting medicines contain opium in some form, and all experienced physicians realize the danger of giving these mixtures to babies. Babies have been killed by medicines which were declared to contain neither opium nor anything else injurious. They are often used. Remember that opium, laudanum and paregoric are dangerous for babies and old people. Careful proper training, allowing plenty of sleeping time, no waking at wrong hours, warm feet, legs and body, cool head, proper modified food, and especially mother nursing, with mother careful with herself, will give a good baby in nine out of ten cases.

Will children ever sleep too much? Not if they are healthy; you must remember a newly-born baby sleeps nine-tenths of the time; excessive sleeping may indicate disease of the brain.

EXERCISE.

Is exercise necessary for infants? Yes.

How can it be obtained? A young baby usually gets its exercise by screaming, waving its arms, kicking, etc. It is a good plan to let baby lie in the center of a large bed, and with his long skirts drawn up, allow him to kick his little legs about for twenty or twenty-five minutes twice each day or one-half hour once a day. His clothing ought to be loose for this exercise. If the room is all right you can remove all clothing except his shirt, stockings and napkin; change his position sometimes and let him lie on his stomach for awhile. Of course this exercise cannot be taken after a meal and before the fourth month. Take a large clothes basket, put a blanket and some large pillows in it and prop baby up in a half sitting position for a little while each day, beginning with fifteen minutes, then one-half hour, and you can also at this time (fourth month) play with baby for a short time every day, but never just before bedtime, and the best time is just after his morning nap. Do not toss him in the air to make him laugh or crow; he is too tender and delicate for that. When baby is older and in short clothes, place a thick quilt upon the floor and allow him to tumble as he will; a fence two feet high which surrounds a mattress, makes an excellent place, or a box for this young animal to exercise his arms and legs without danger of injury. Before you put baby to sleep at night give him a warm sponge bath with a fresh band and shirt and he will sleep.

When, if ever, is crying useful in a baby? The cry expands the lungs of a new-born baby, and he should use his lungs a few minutes daily in order to keep them well expanded.

How much crying daily is necessary? Twenty to thirty minutes is not too much.

What kind of a cry is it? Loud and strong and infants get red in the face with it. Some call it a scream. It is exercise for baby and necessary for its health.

When is the cry abnormal? When it is very long and too frequent. It is not strong, but rather of a moaning or worrying nature or only a whine.

What causes such crying? Habit, temper, pain, hunger, illness.

What is the indulgence or habit cry? This is the cry of infants who cry to be rocked, or carried about, for a bottle to suck, etc.

Temper cry? This is loud and strong and is usually accompanied by kicking, stiffening of the body, bending backward and is usually quite violent.

Pain cry? This is generally strong, sharp and quick, but not usually continuous, the features contract, legs draw up and the baby plainly shows symptoms of distress,

Hunger cry? This is a continuous fretful, pitiful cry, not strong and lusty,--baby looks hungry.

The cry of illness? This is moaning, fretful, easily aroused to crying. This can be distinguished even from a little distance before seeing baby, if you have heard it once. A baby who cries to get things stops when he gets them.

If baby cries at night what shall I do? See that he is comfortable, clothing all smooth under and about him, with warm feet and hands, and clean unsoiled napkin. If he is all right, let him cry. If it is habitual, find out the cause.

If baby cries from temper or habit what shall I do? Let him cry it out, you must conquer him or he will make of your life a burden. Be sure first it is habit or temper and then conquer him. I have seen many babies who cried from cause and I have also seen those who needed conquering.

But will not crying cause rupture? Not in young infants if the band is properly applied and not under any conditions after one year.

HOW TO LIFT A CHILD.

Grasp the clothing below the feet with the right hand and slip the left hand and, arm beneath the infant's body to its head. It is then raised upon the left arm and its head is upon your arm or chest. This supports the entire spine and there is no undue pressure upon the chest or abdomen, as is often the case when baby is grasped around the body or under the arms.

How shall I lift a child who is old enough to run about? Place your hands under the child's arms, at the arm-pits and never by the wrists.

Can I injure the child lifting it by its hands or wrists? Yes, it often injures the elbows or shoulder joints.

TEMPERATURE.

Normal temperature of an infant? This varies more than it does in adults. In the rectum it varies from 98 degrees F. to 99.5 degrees F., and a temperature in the rectum of 98 degrees F. or of 100 degrees F. is not of much importance unless it continues.

Where should I take the temperature of infants and young children? First the rectum, next the groin, the first is from one-half a degree to a degree higher than that of the groin.

How long should the thermometer be left in place? Two minutes in the rectum and five minutes in the groin.

What meaning has the different temperature in a young child? 100 degrees F. to 102 degrees F. means a mild illness.

One hundred four degrees F. or over means a serious illness. The duration of the fever is more important. Slight causes often produce a high temperature in all young children which lasts for a few hours. There is then not much cause for alarm unless the temperature continues high or is accompanied by important symptoms of illness.

Is high temperature a more serious symptom in a young child than in an adult? No, for young children are very sensitive to conditions which produce fever and the thermometer often gives an unduly high idea of the severity of the symptoms. The same cause which would produce a temperature in an adult of 102 degrees F. or 103 degrees F. would likely produce a temperature of 104 degrees or 105 degrees F. in a child.

NERVOUSNESS.

What are the principal causes of nervousness in young infants and in children? The brain is a delicate structure at this time, and it grows rapidly, and during the first year of life grows as much as during all the rest of life. This needs quiet and peaceful surroundings and infants who are naturally nervous should be left almost alone, and few people should see them. Such babies should not play much. The poor little baby is often so tried by the attentions given him by older people that he does not know what to do, and as one author, a lady, says: "If he could speak he would beg for a quiet hour, and be perfectly happy if left alone with his own little hands and toes for his sole amusement." Babies of the very poor are less nervous than those of the wealthy and this is generally due to the fact that their mothers are too busy to constantly entertain and bother them. Children are better companions for babies than adults. Such little attentions given by the parents and relatives make sleepless and nervous babies very often. Playing with them before time and out of season, makes them not only nervous and irritable, but causes indigestion and allied diseases.

TOYS.

It is instinct for baby to put everything in its mouth. However, toys should be chosen that are smooth, easily washed and which cannot be swallowed. Avoid toys with sharp points like corners, or loose parts, small objects that can be pushed into the nose or ear or swallowed, such as coins, marbles, buttons, safety pins, beads, painted toys and those covered with hair or wool. Infants frequently swallow such wool or hair.

KISSING.

What objections are there to kissing babies? They are many and serious. No one, at least, outside of the immediate family has any right to kiss baby. Tuberculosis, diphtheria, syphilis and many other diseases are given by kissing. If infants are kissed at all, they should be kissed upon the cheek or forehead.

FOREIGN BODIES.

If in the throat, examine and remove with the finger. If it has gone into the stomach, give plenty of dry food, such as bread, potatoes, but do not give an emetic or cathartic. An infant should have its usual food. A cathartic would hurry the foreign body too rapidly through the intestines, and in this way do harm. In the usual way it becomes coated with fecal matter and usually passes the intestines without causing any injury.

What shall I do if it is in the ears? If you can easily remove it with your fingers or small hair pin or crochet hook, do it. If not, take the baby to a physician. If it is a corn, bean or pea, do not wet it, or it will swell and become larger.

What if it is in the nostril? Place baby upon the table with its face toward a good light and use a hair pin bent right and pass this slowly and carefully behind the object, and pull slowly forward; or compress the empty nostril and have the child blow the nose strongly. If not removed easily, see a physician.

COLIC.

This is a very common disturbance in children, and is always due to disturbed digestion. It occurs in both nursed and bottle-fed babies, and may appear in the healthiest baby from error in the last meal, or error of diet or habit in the mother. Some mothers cannot under any circumstances secrete good nourishing milk, suitable for their children, and continued stomach and bowel disturbances with colic and emaciation follow its use. Such mothers should not nurse their baby.

What are the causes of colic? As before stated, it is due to indigestion

What causes indigestion? In nursing babies this may be due to some irregularity in the health or habits of the mother, or change in her dieting, and if the colic is not persistent the cause is not hard to find. Worry, trouble, sorrow, anger, overwork, and errors of diet in the mother often cause this trouble or the child may nurse too fast, too long, too much, or too often, or the milk may be too rich. If so, give baby an ounce of hot water before nursing. Hand-fed children are too often over-fed, and this produces indigestion.

What are the symptoms of colic? The child screams sharply; the cry comes suddenly and returns every few minutes; he draws up his legs and feet; the muscles of his face contract and he has other signs of pain. The belly is usually hard and tense.

What can I do for colic? First warm his feet and hands by placing them against a hot-water bag, or holding them before the open fire, turn him on his stomach, letting him lie on a hot-water bag or hot piece of flannel; pat his back gently to help up the wind and give him a little hot water with a medicine dropper and a few drops of essence of peppermint may be added to the water. If the colic continues, put ten drops of turpentine into a half teacupful of warm water, and inject this slowly into the rectum, and at the same time gently rub the abdomen so as to start the wind. If the wind is in the stomach, give him one-half a soda mint tablet dissolved in a tablespoonful of very warm water, or a little soda. If the attacks are frequent, the foods are too strong; use less cream or milk and more water. Regulate the mother's diet carefully if the baby nurses, and she should take some exercise out of doors, if possible, and try not to be nervous. Cereals, cocoa, milk, eggs, gruels made of corn, oatmeal; most fruits, not tart, and vegetables, with some meat, make a good diet for a nursing mother. The bowels must move freely every day at least once.

MOTHERS' REMEDIES.--1. Wind Colic, Yarrow Tea for.--- "Steep the yarrow tea the same as for catnip tea or any ordinary herb, and give as often as necessary." This is a remedy that has been very much used, and will help in a great many cases. It is perfectly harmless, and no one need have any fear of trying it.

2. Colic, Camphor Cure for.--"One drop of camphor in a teaspoonful of water. This remedy worked like a charm with my little girl." This acts quickly, and is sure to give relief as it warms up the stomach.

3. Wind Colic, Castor Oil for.--"Give large doses of castor oil." Colic, as we all know, is frequently caused by fermentation of the food in the stomach and bowels, and castor oil is one of the best known cathartics in a case of this kind. This can be given to small babies, in small quantities of course.

4. Wind Colic.--A New York mother sends in the following relief for:--"Give enough essence of wintergreen in water to make it taste for a small babe, and more according to age. For mine I give 1/4 to 1/2, cup of warm sweetened water. I have always used this remedy, as it was recommended to me by my mother. It is better than peppermint as it is not so binding."

5. Wind Colic, a Good Herb Remedy for.--Add enough water to one ounce of snake root to make one-half pint." Give in doses according to the age of the child. This is a good remedy, and has been used by many mothers with good success.

6. Wind Colic.--A doctor in New York sends in the following remedy for.--"One-half teaspoonful sweet spirits of nitre in one-third glass of water, for baby. Increase the dose for older children or adults. This warms the stomach, and is highly recommended."

7. Wind Colic, Cloves for.--"Make an infusion of 1 or 2 ounces of cloves. Cloves are warming, cordial and strengthening; they expel wind, and are good for the colic." This treatment has been known to give many a fretful baby a good night's sleep, and will be found very useful in homes where babies have this disease.

PHYSICIANS' TREATMENT.--Temporary relief is obtained in attacks of colic by emptying the bowels of irritating materials, either

39

by an enema or medicine. Peppermint, anise seed, catnip are effective, but may be harmful if continued long. Gin and whisky, warm, are good when the gas is in the stomach and upper bowel. It is always best to mix them with a solution like the following:

Bicarbonate of soda	40 grains
Aromatic spirits of ammonia	30 drops
Enough peppermint water to make	2 ounces

Put one teaspoonful in a cup of hot water for a child one year old.

The following is good to move the bowels:

Bicarbonate of soda	40 grains
Aromatic syrup of rhubarb	4 drams
Syrup of senna	5 drams
Syrup of orange	1 ounce

One teaspoonful two or three times daily is needed in sour gassy stomach, with constipation or foul smelling stools. Fortunately such medicine is not often needed if the mother is careful, or baby is carefully bottle-fed. When there is vomiting with the colic and the stools contain curds the food is too strong. The nursing baby should be given one ounce of warm water before nursing, and the food for the bottle-fed baby should be made weaker by going back one formula. Sometimes peptonizing the food for a short time will do. This is very good when the proteids (curds) are hard for the baby to digest.

EARACHE.

Many young babies suffer from this trouble without the cause being even suspected. It may come after a cold, an attack of bronchitis or pneumonia, and sometimes during teething. It often accompanies scarlet fever and measles. The child screams, presses his head against his mother or nurse, pulls at his ear as if it hurt him. If you press in front of the ear the baby jumps as if in great pain and cries aloud. The pain is likely to be continuous and prolonged.

What can I do for it? Heat is the best remedy. Wash out the ear with a hot solution of boric acid fifteen to twenty grains to the ounce of water, and then apply heat in various ways. Have the child lie with the painful ear against a covered hot water bag or heat a flannel over a lamp and place it against the ear, changing it often to keep it hot. A bag of hot salt or bran is also very good. Laudanum and oil should not be used unless ordered by a physician. As soon as possible after the first attack of pain the baby should be examined by a doctor and unnecessary deafness is often avoided by such action. For a more extended account, see General Department. Fomentations applied are often beneficial, especially of hot water.

(See Earache, Mothers' Remedies, etc. under General Department).

CROUP.

This disease is treated fully in the general department; only a general outline is given here. This is a disease dreaded by most mothers. It is more distressing than dangerous. Its appearance is sudden and generally at night. The baby may have had a slight cold or have been exposed to a bad wind or it may have come on without any known cause.

Symptoms.--They are known to almost everyone. There is a hard, dry, barking, hoarse cough, generally with difficulty in breathing to a greater or less degree with a distressed look.

(For Mothers' Remedies, see General Department.)

Treatment.--If the child has eaten a big supper, it is well to give a simple emetic, such as warm mustard water, alum and molasses, or goose grease, or melted lard. Wring out pieces of flannel in hot water and put them on the child's throat as hot as he can bear them and change them often to keep them hot. Make a tent by spreading a sheet over an opened umbrella over the crib then place a croup kettle or teakettle close to the crib, directing the steam under the sheet into the tent so that baby may inhale the vapor, taking care not to burn him. This affords much relief. If necessary give ten drops of syrup of ipecac until vomiting occurs; a teaspoonful of castor oil should also be given and if the baby is constipated, give an enema of soapsuds and water. Keep the child indoors the next day.

CONSTIPATION IN BABIES.

MOTHERS' REMEDIES.--1. Constipation, Olive Oil Treatment for.--"Rub the abdomen with a firm yet gentle motion from left to right with pure olive oil. This is what the doctor told me to do for my babe of three years." This treatment will be found very beneficial as the olive oil is very strengthening and the rubbing will always give relief.

2. Constipation, A Pleasant Treatment for.--"One-half teaspoonful olive oil, one-half teaspoonful orange juice, three times a day after feeding."

3. Constipation, Prunes a Medicine for.--"Abate heat and gently open the bowels by the use of prunes. These should be fed to children more often. This would often prevent sickness. A very useful way of administering prunes as a medicine is to simmer for one-half hour, a few in water enough to cover, with 1/2 oz. senna leaves; remove the prunes, allow to dry and let the child eat them when needed. This is very good."

4. Constipation, Soothing Syrup Made by a Mother in New York for.--"One-half ounce spearmint, one-quarter ounce lady's slipper, one-half ounce rhubarb, one-quarter ounce cinnamon powder; pour one-half pint boiling water on the whole, mix and let stand to boil fifteen minutes, strain and sweeten well with syrup or honey. Give a teaspoonful every half hour, diminishing as the pain subsides." This will be found very beneficial in children, and may be used without any fear whatever, as it is perfectly harmless.

5. Constipation, Figs as a Medicine for.--"Grind up equal amounts of figs and senna leaves, put in closed jar and eat dry when needed." This will be found especially good for children, and most of them like it.

CONSTIPATION may be caused by many things, inheritance, malformation of the rectum and other parts, errors of food in the mother and in bottle-fed babies.

What is the treatment? If the baby is nursed and the mother is constipated, she should at once change her habits and diet. She should exercise in the open air at least two hours every day, and have a movement daily, even if she must take some mild laxative.

What should she drink and eat? She should drink plenty of water, and pure rich milk, cocoa, eat oatmeal and cornmeal gruels. She should not drink tea or coffee. She can eat fruit, most green vegetables and some meat, but not much starchy food. Baby may not get enough residue in his bowels. Give him one or two meals daily of modified milk made up of oatmeal gruel instead of barley, and give him plenty of water between his meals. One teaspoonful of cream in a little hot water given before nursing is often beneficial, or one or two teaspoonfuls of beef juice may be given night and morning, After six months a little orange or prune juice may be added.

BOTTLE-FED BABIES.

Add a little more top-milk or cream to each bottle than the formula gives; do not pasteurize the food unless it is necessary; do not use lime-water, but bicarbonate of soda in proper strength in its place, as lime-water is often very constipating. Malted food may be added to each bottle for some time. If necessary, stimulate the rectum mildly; this can be done by holding the baby over a small chamber at exactly the same time after a meal each day and insert into the bowel a small cone of oiled paper, or use a small castile soap suppository. This may form a habit in a few days. Suppositories of gluten are very beneficial if used in the morning. The child should not be allowed to go longer than twenty-four hours without a passage. A enema made up of one or two tablespoonfuls of sweet oil may be given with a bulb syringe, or an ounce of warm water to which has been added one-half teaspoonful of glycerin, or one-half pint of warm soap-suds. Do not give it every day; massage the baby's abdomen. Your hand should be warm. Begin at the right side groin and make a series of circular movements with your fingers, lightly at first, and then press down harder as the baby becomes accustomed to it; work your way up gradually to the ribs, then across to the ribs on the left side, and down to the left groin. This can be done twice daily for eight or ten minutes at a time, and always at the same time of day, but never soon after a meal. Olive oil may safely be given for constipation to a baby,--from twenty drops to one teaspoonful one or two times daily, but castor oil should *not* be given for constipation, as after a time it leaves the baby more constipated than ever. Sometimes inserting your finger, well oiled, into the rectum, will produce a passage. For older children, decrease the amount of white bread, toast, potatoes, and give green vegetables, oatmeal, and graham bread instead, with plenty of proper fruit twice daily; raw, scraped apples are sometimes the best fruit to use.

DIARRHEA. (For Older Children).

What shall I do for this trouble? Rid the system of the irritating matter by giving the baby one teaspoonful of castor oil. Then stop all solid food and give boiled water if there is only a moderate looseness. Keep the child perfectly quiet. If the attack is more severe and attended by fever and vomiting all food and milk should be stopped at once in children of all ages, and only broth, barley water or some thin gruel given. Castor oil is required for a severe attack. If the patient is an infant the milk should be diluted or stopped. In severe attacks with vomiting or frequent foul stools, stop all food for at least twelve hours and all milk for a longer time, and the bowels should be freely moved by a cathartic. Give plenty of water to drink.

Food.--Albumin water is often better than plain water or anything else. To make it stir the white of an egg into a pint of cold water. See that they are well mixed, add a pinch of salt and strain. Give baby one teaspoonful every one-half hour, and if he vomits all other food, give two ounces every two hours; barley gruel, wheat flour gruel, mutton broth may be given also.

MOTHERS' REMEDIES.--1. Inflammation of the Bowels, Poultice of Hot Mush for.--"Wrap the child in a poultice of hot mush. Place the poultice over the abdomen." A poultice of this kind retains the heat, and is very good for inflammation of the abdominal cavity, and would help to take away the soreness and bloating in the bowels that is always present in this disease.

2. Bowel Trouble, a Good Tonic for.--

Powdered rhubarb	1 heaping teaspoonful
Soda	1/4 teaspoonful
Sugar	1 teaspoonful
Peppermint essence	1/2 teaspoonful
Hot water	1/2 cup (scant)

Dose:--One-half teaspoonful every hour until bowels show signs of right color.

The soda and the peppermint will tone up the stomach and relieve any trouble present there, while the rhubarb will act on the bowels and carry off all impurities.

3. Bowel Trouble, Rhubarb and Licorice for.--"Compound tincture of rhubarb one ounce bicarbonate of soda 1 dram, fluid extract of licorice 1 dram, pure water 6 ounces. Give from one to two teaspoonfuls according to the age of the child." This will he found a very good treatment for this trouble, and one that has been thoroughly tried.

RICKETS.

You should always be suspicious if your baby has no teeth at the end of the first year. A hearty baby should have six or eight, and if the soft spot in the head just above the forehead is as much open as it was for months previously you should be doubly suspicious. This soft spot should be closed in a well-nourished infant between the fifteenth and twentieth months. If in addition to this the child sweats about the head whenever it sleeps, cries whenever it is handled (unless it has scurvy or rheumatism) and does not like to play, the indications of rickets are very nearly conclusive. Rickets is a constitutional disease showing itself in different ways.

At what age does it usually occur? Between six months and two and one-half years.

What are the causes of rickets? Improper food, or inability to absorb the food, unhygienic conditions. Nursing babies who have a healthy mother are not troubled with this disease unless she nurses too long into the second year. Starchy foods, too little milk or other animal food, taking the infant to the family table and allowing it to eat whatever it wants, these are the most common errors in baby feeding which very often result in rickets. Babies who are brought up on condensed milk, or other foods that contain little fat are likely to have rickets. Insufficient clothing, damp and badly ventilated buildings, a lack of out-door air and sunshine, and inherited constitutional weakness, are other causes.

When do the most marked symptoms usually occur? Between the sixth or fifteenth months.

What are the symptoms? Such children are likely to be nervous and irritable; child's head sweats profusely at night, so much so that the pillows are very wet. The chest is poorly shaped and frequently has depressions at the sides, and little nodules or "beads" in the ribs where the ribs and breast-bone join. The child's head is also peculiar. It is often very flat on the top and measures more around than a normal child at the same age. The forehead stands out and the sides and top are flattened. The soft spot in the skull is large and late in closing. He is late in cutting his teeth. His abdomen is generally large and prominent, pot belly; his muscles are soft and flabby, and his wrists and ankles are enlarged a little later. He takes cold easily. He is pale and anemic, although he may be plump and fat, and when he begins to walk his legs bend easily, and he will have bow-legs. When he sits, his back will look as if curved and this alarms his parents, who may think his spine is diseased.

Is such a disease curable? Yes, if taken in time; you can arrest its progress.

Do they ever die of rickets? Very seldom, but they do not stand other diseases very well.

When and what shall I do for it? If you recognize the condition, have the baby attended to immediately by a physician. The food should be changed--such children require fats; very little starchy or sweet foods allowed. A baby ten to twelve months old can suck a piece of boiled bacon for a few minutes every day. Fruit juices can be given early, raw meat juice once a day. Give him his tub bath daily, and if he is apt to take cold easily he should have a little cold water dashed over his chest and spine, followed by a gentle brisk rubbing to start up the circulation. Sun baths are beneficial. Place the baby directly in the sun with his back to it, for an hour every day. Give him plenty of air and sunshine, both indoors and outdoors.

Medicine.--Cod liver oil is an excellent remedy with the hypophosphites. Cod liver oil alone with calcarea phosphoricum 3X (homeopathic) is splendid treatment also. The whole treatment must be continued for months--calcarea phos. four times daily.

SCURVY.--This disease is sometimes seen in infants. It attacks infants who have been fed for a long time on a proprietary food or else on milk that has been over sterilized. Nursing children seldom have it, or those who have been properly fed on modified cows' milk. Babies who are delicate and poorly nourished are more subject to it. The first symptoms a mother notices is that it seems to hurt very much when his legs are touched; sometimes both hurt, and then again only one is painful; at other times the arms will be most painful and again both arms and legs seem to pain alike. So it goes on; the joints enlarge somewhat and sometimes little red spots appear just under the skin and very often the gums will become red and spongy; this is especially noticeable around the incisor teeth of the upper gums, if they have already appeared. Rheumatism is very rarely seen so early and with that, there is generally fever.

Treatment.--A cure is soon affected. Stop the patent food at once, or if the milk has been sterilized, it must be discontinued and the baby put on unsterilized milk diluted to the proper strength for his special age. Strained juice of an orange should be given him every day; if under six months he can have the juice of one-half an orange; over that the juice of one orange. This is given in intervals during the day. Beef juice is good, about two ounces in twenty-four hours. Smaller amount if necessary. Improvement is noticed twenty-four to forty-eight hours after treatment.

MALNUTRITION. (Marasmus).--Marasmus is a term applied to infants who grow thinner and thinner. No matter how much or little they eat there is a constant wasting or fading away of the body.

What are the causes? Syphilis, tuberculosis, chronic vomiting, persistent loose bowels, poor assimilation of the food. Marasmus is really a later and more severe form of malnutrition.

Symptoms.--He looks shriveled, the skin is dry, eyes are sunken, anemia is marked, the belly is much distended, while the other parts of the body seem to be all bones and no flesh; he is constantly whining and fretful, has a tired and anxious expression most of the time; under six months it is hard to cure.

Treatment.--A physician is needed to watch over and prescribe, no set rule can be given. Sometimes cod-liver oil or iron is needed. It needs constant care and watching to cure this trouble.

CONVULSIONS.--Young children are more subject to convulsions than older people. Convulsions may be due to brain trouble, but an overloaded stomach is the first thing a doctor thinks of, and so the mother should remember what was eaten that might be unusual.

First Thing for the Mother to do? Undress the baby and put him to bed in a quiet room, and place an ice bag on his head, or wring cloths out of ice water or very cold water and place them on baby's head, and change often to keep them cold. Warm the feet with a hot water bag. If the doctor can not be present soon, give baby a mustard foot bath in bed; use two tablespoonfuls to a gallon of water, some advise stronger. If the convulsions are severe wring towels out of mustard water and place a rubber sheet on the bed and wrap the child's body and feet in the hot wet towels until the parts are quite red, and afterward cover the body with warm flannels. Have plenty of hot water ready, so the doctor can give a full tub bath when he comes, if he thinks it necessary. If the child can swallow, give him a teaspoonful of castor oil; or if the convulsions continue, wash out the bowels or give an injection as soon as possible.

When is a hot bath needed and useful? If the convulsions have continued until the pulse is weak, the face is very pale, the nails and lips blue, the feet and hands cold: it will do good by bringing the blood to the surface and relieve the brain, heart and lungs.

How shall I give it? Use a thermometer to see that the temperature of the water is not over 106 degrees F.; if no thermometer is handy put your arm into the water to your elbow. It should feel warm, but not so hot as to be uncomfortable. Put one-half teacupful of powdered mustard in the tub. Place the baby in the tub, body all covered, and hold the head out of the water; keep him in the bath for five to ten minutes; wrap him in a blanket and put into bed without drying.

The following is given to prevent convulsions:--

Bromide of Potash	1/2 dram
Chloral Hydrate	15 grains
Simple Syrup	2 ounces

Mix thoroughly.

Give one teaspoonful every hour, while the baby is nervous or feverish. For one-year-old child.

MOTHERS' REMEDIES.--1. Convulsions, a Grandmother's Remedy for.--"Dip the feet and limbs in warm water; give dry salt in mouth." Care should be taken not to give too much salt as you may choke the child. Also apply cold cloths to the head, to draw the blood from the brain.

2. Convulsions, Hot Mustard Water for.--"Put patient in tub of hot mustard water, with cold cloths to the head," The hot mustard water draws the blood from the head to the feet and the cold cloths assist in doing good by keeping the blood away from the head. This is, an old, tried and effective remedy,

3. Convulsions, Old Tried Remedy for.--"Put patient in hot bath; give castor oil and rub vigorously." The castor oil does good in cases where the bowels are too loose or constipated, as the case may be, by carrying off the impurities, and the hot bath equalizes the circulation, relieving the convulsion.

4. Convulsions, A New York Mother's Remedy for.--"Chloroform one-half dram, tincture of cardamom, one-half ounce, spearmint water, two and one-half ounces. Shake well and give one-half teaspoonful in water to child one year old, smaller children a proportionate dose." The chloroform is very quieting, and the tincture of cardamom and spearmint act on the bowels. This combination will quiet the child, and in that way relieve the trouble.

(See "Convulsions" in General Department for Mothers' Remedies).

INFLAMMATION OF THE BRAIN.

What are the early symptoms of brain diseases? Temperature is usually very high, 104 degrees F. and over. There is stupor or delirium, and vomiting is common; light hurts the eyes; the child jumps and starts at the slightest noise, unless the hearing is affected. There is often a squint, the eyes may be turned upward, and the lids may be only half closed during sleep. The pupils are dilated or contracted, Sometimes one pupil is larger than natural, while the other is smaller.

What can I do for these symptoms? Cold to the head, either by ice bags or cold water cloths. The room should be dark and quiet. No food given unless ordered, and then bland and very little at a time. A doctor should always be called for such symptoms; castor oil to move the bowels should be given or an enema of soap-suds and water. This helps to draw the blood from the brain, also keep the feet warm and head cool.

SCALD HEAD (in Babies) Milk Crust.--This is often due to neglect in regularly removing the free secretion, or due sometimes to an inflammation of the little sebaceous follicles of the skin. It occurs on the scalp most. The hair should be cut short, and soften the crusts with warm olive oil, or vaselin may be left on the scalp over night, then wash off the crusts with warm water and castile soap. An ointment can be made of vaselin or cold cream, and two per cent resorcin, and applied after the crust is resumed. Spread on linen and hold it in place by a thin cap, wash this off every day with olive oil and apply the salve fresh. Water should not be used oftener than once a week--oxide of zinc ointment is also good.

MOTHERS' REMEDIES.--l. Cleaning Baby's Head, Common Lard for.--"Nothing is better than common lard. Grease the head good at night, using plenty of lard, especially if very heavily coated. Let stand over night, the lard softens the coating so you can take a fine comb and remove it. Comb from the forehead back. You need never have any scale on the baby's head." Care should be taken in using a fine comb, as it will very often make a child's head very sore.

2. Scald Head, An Experienced Mother's Remedy for.--

"Boracic acid	2 drams
Salol	2 drams
Balsam Peru	1 dram
Carbolic acid	20 drops
Vaselin	1 ounce
Lanoline	1 ounce
Mix."	

Then wash the head thoroughly with castile soap, and apply the above morning and night, and use internally the following:--

Iodide Potash	192 grains
Fluid Extract Stillingia	1 ounce
Fluid Ext. Prickly Ash Bark	1/2 ounce
Fluid Ext. Yellow Dock	1 ounce
Compound Syrup Sarsaparilla, q. s	8 ounces
Mix."	

Take about one-half teaspoonful from two to four times a day, according to the age of the child. If this treatment is kept up faithfully, you will be sure to obtain a cure.

TEETHING.--There are twenty teeth in the first set. There is sometimes slight fever, restlessness, sleepless nights, maybe loss of appetite and some indigestion. If signs of indigestion are seen, give less food, and replace same with boiled water. If he is a nursing baby give him an ounce of boiled water before nursing and nurse him only ten to fifteen minutes. If he is restless at night give him a warm sponge bath, and if there is any fever, add one teaspoonful of bicarbonate of soda to a basin of tepid water. If the gums are very much congested and swollen and the child suffers, they may need to be lanced. Sometimes the teeth come earlier, but generally between the fifth and ninth months. They appear usually as follows:--

2 lower central incisors 6 to 9 months (often earlier)	
4 upper incisors	7 to 10 months
2 lower lateral incisors	12 to 14 months
2 anterior upper molars	12 to 16 months

2 anterior lower molars	12 to 16 months
2 upper canines (eye teeth)	18 to 24 months
2 lower canines (stomach teeth)	18 to 24 months
2 lower and 2 upper posterior molars	24 to 30 months

During the first year the child should cut six teeth; next six months, six or more; at two years he should have sixteen; at two and one-half years twenty. About the sixth year the permanent teeth are cut and follow closely after the shedding of the milk teeth.

TEETHING.--PERMANENT TEETH, USUAL ORDER.

4 first molars	6 years
4 central incisors	7 years
4 lateral incisors	8 years
4 first bicuspids	8-1/2 to 9 years
4 second bicuspids	10 years
4 canines	11 or 12 to 14 years
4 second molars	12 to 13 years, (12 to 15)
4 wisdom teeth	18 to 25 years (17 to 25)

HICCOUGH.--Some infants are very liable to hiccoughs. It is generally a matter of little importance. It is a spasmodic contraction of the diaphragm, often caused by gas or wind or too much food in the baby's stomach. It is very annoying, and should not be allowed to go on indefinitely. Pat the baby gently, but suddenly, on the back, or give him a little hot water in which there are a few grains of sugar or a drop of essence of peppermint. See that he does not feed too fast or suck an empty bottle.

ENLARGED GLANDS.--Cutting teeth or sometimes a bad cold or other things cause the glands at the sides of the neck to swell and enlarge. This does not always give any discomfort to the baby, but it annoys and worries the mother. Frequently the enlargement will soon disappear of itself, but sometimes the gland grows larger, gets quite hard and often much inflamed--matter or pus will then form, and a discharge soon follows.

Treatment.--If the gland keeps on enlarging, a doctor should be seen, and if it needs lancing he can do so at the proper time, and save the neck from a bad scar. Medicine can also be given that will sometimes stop it. Syrup of iodide of iron three to ten drops, three times a day for a one-year-old child is good; cod-liver oil should be given to pale, thin children for a long time.

BED-WETTING.--If a child continues to wet the bed after he is three years old, something should be done for this annoying habit. The child should be examined by a doctor; circumcision will often effect a cure in boys; or pin worms may be the cause of the trouble; a stone in the bladder, or any trouble that makes him nervous, or it may be due to habit.

Treatment.--Scolding will not do any good. The child should not drink any fluids after four in the afternoon. He should not have any bread and milk or water for supper, but instead have bread and a dry cereal, with a little stewed fruit; sometimes a child needs a tonic. It is a tedious trouble to treat and it takes a long time to gain control of it. The mother must have a large stock of patience and co-operate with the doctor. The child should pass urine before retiring, have the foot of the bedstead elevated, not too warmly covered so as to become restless. His suppers should not be hearty, bowels should be regular. The following is a good remedy:--Tincture of belladonna; give five drops at bed-time and increase the dose, drop by drop, each night until it produces a fine scarlet rash upon the skin. This should be marked "poison" and only given under the care of a doctor. It is a good remedy, but it must be watched.

HIVES.--Hives, or urticaria, is often seen in young children, It is generally caused by indigestion. It is not a serious disease, but it is uncomfortable and makes a baby cross. The eruption is bright red in color, and appears in blotches or wheels.

Treatment.--Give the child a laxative like magnesia or citrate of magnesia, or epsom salts and cream of tartar, of each two ounces. Dose, one-half teaspoonful in water every three hours until the bowels move freely. (One-year-old).

To relieve the itching.--Sop the spots with warm water, and a little soda, or an entire bath can be given of this if the eruption is extensive.

RUPTURE in a Baby. (Navel).--Take a strip of oxide of zinc adhesive plaster about one and one-half inches wide and long enough to reach three-fourths around the baby's body. Fasten one end of this to one side of the abdomen and with the other hand gently push the rupture back; bring the skin on either side of the navel together so that it will meet and hold the rupture. Bring the plaster tightly across the abdomen, across the navel and attach it firmly to the other side; change this dressing every few days and continue treatment until healed.

COLDS in Babies.--Many babies seem to take cold without any cause. It is often due to the fact that the room is too warm, or they are clothed too warmly; they get easily overheated and feel the slightest draught of air. If it is in his nose and it is stopped up, twist a piece of cotton on a small wooden piece like a tooth-pick and dip it into olive oil and put it into the nostrils a short distance. If necessary, buy a nose syringe with a soft rubber tip, and use it twice daily. The following solution is good: one-half teaspoonful of boric acid powder, one ounce of glycerin, and eight ounces of warm water. Mix. Place the child on your lap, head against your chest, bend his head well forward and syringe one nostril and then the other. Camphor cream is a good remedy.

For a cough and much wheezing use a mustard plaster. Take one part mustard, six parts flour and mix it into a smooth paste with a little cold water, spread it between two layers of muslin, warm it and moisten with a little water if necessary, and put it on the upper part of the breastbone. Leave it on only long enough to redden the skin (five to six minutes). Put it on just before baby goes to bed. A drop of camphor every three hours is often good for a cold at the beginning. Aconite in small doses is also very good.

MOTHERS' REMEDIES. Colds, Catnip Tea for.--"Give a little sweetened catnip tea, then grease well with camphor and lard." This is a very simple and effective remedy, especially for small babies. (See "Colds" under General Department for more Mothers' Remedies,)

Early signs of sickness.--When a baby who persistently refuses his food is drowsy at unusual times, fretful, feverish, and is uncomfortable, the mother should look in baby's mouth, for sore throat or tonsils, or on his body for rashes. Undress the baby and put him to bed in a quiet room away from the rest of the family, and if he is hot and restless give him a sponge bath with one teaspoonful of bicarbonate of soda to a basin of luke-warm water. Give him also an enema to move his bowels, especially if they are not regular. Dilute his usual food with water or barley water to one-half the usual strength. If he is old enough to eat solid food, stop it. A dose of a teaspoonful of castor oil is safe to give until the doctor comes. Give him water to drink for he is thirsty. Take his temperature.

CARING FOR BURNS, BRUISES, CUTS, WOUNDS, ETC., IN BABY.

For Burns.--Keep away the air from the burn. Dust soda on the burn if the skin is not too much broken, and wrap it up in clean linen. Olive oil, linseed oil, is better, or cream should be put on if it is more severe. Then a layer of clean linen and then a thin layer of cotton wool. It must not be too warmly dressed. An ointment called pineoline is excellent for burns.

For a bruise or bump.--Apply cloths hot or cold,--you can do this with flannel wrung out of very cold or hot water. Ice may be wrapped up in cotton and put on the part.

Cuts.--Wash it with clean cold water, and bind it up with clean linen. If it bleeds much, let it bleed for a few seconds, and then stop it with a pad of clean linen pressed firmly on the part and held there until it stops.

SPLINTERS.--Remove them and dress as for any other wound.

POISONING.--Children will get hold of poison, and mother had better have antidotes, etc., to use in case of necessity. Rat poison, fly poison, matches, etc.

Treatment.--First use emetics; mustard and luke-warm water or one teaspoonful of alum in a glass of luke-warm water; a little salt and warm water; ten to fifteen drops syrup of ipecac, and then warm water. For fly poison, give one-half ounce of olive oil in same amount of lime-water, and repeat it every five or six minutes, for five or six doses, and then white of an egg, and keep child warm. Antidote for arsenic is freshly precipitated, sesquioxide of iron. Go to druggist and tell him to prepare it; tell him what it is wanted for, and give this in doses of an ounce at a time as the oil was given.

For poisoning from sucking matches.--Vomit the child freely, but do not give anything oily, as milk or egg, as this dissolves the phosphorus.

Oxalic acid is sometimes used for cleaning purposes, and mistaken for epsom salts. Give an emetic and lime-water.

For carbolic acid.--Give an emetic, and then white of an egg and epsom salts.

Overdose of soothing syrup.--Keep baby awake, slap with wet towel, etc.; or walk him about if he is old enough, inject strong black coffee in the rectum. Keep up the strength with stimulants.

PROPRIETARY FOODS.

These foods are sometimes of temporary use. As many of them contain very little fat, they may be used in cases of illness where fat cannot be borne. Some of these contain malt sugar, and when the baby is constipated this kind is useful when added to milk. Others can be made up of water only, and are useful and handy where it is impossible to obtain fresh milk. In cases of diarrhea the flour foods made up with water are very useful. Milk at that time acts as a poison. Some of the best foods on the market are the following--Condensed milk, Mellin's food, Horlick's Malted milk, Nestle's food, Imperial granum, Just's food, Carnrick's soluble food, Ridge's food, peptogenic milk powder, Lactated food, Eskay's, Albumenized food, cereal milk, Borden's food.

For constipation in a child.--One to two teaspoonfuls of Mellin's food, added to each bottle of his usual modified milk formula will often help a great deal. As soon as the bowels move naturally it should be gradually diminished until after four or six weeks, the child can do without it.

Condensed milk and Malted milk.--These can be prepared with water only, and so are best to use on a long journey. Give the baby one or two meals daily a week or two before the journey. Discontinue when at the end of the journey.

Imperial Granum.--This is often useful in acute diarrhea, when milk cannot be given. Mix the proportion as given on the box with water into a smooth paste, then add a pint of boiling water and boil for fifteen or twenty minutes.

Peptogenic Milk Powder.--This may be used for a short time during or after acute illness; you can add it to the formula used as directed on the package.

NURSING DEPARTMENT

Including

Care of the Sick and the Sick Room

FOODS, FORMULAE, DELICACIES FOR SICK ROOM, HOW TO PREPARE THEM; DIET IN FEVERS AND OTHER DISEASES, SECURED FROM TRAINED NURSES, PHYSICIANS AND HOSPITALS.

Every Phase of Nursing Given in Detail and in Plain Mothers' Language, including Latest Sanitary Care and Science.

VENTILATION.--The sick room should be ventilated without any draught hitting the patient. The patient's bed should be placed out of the line of air currents. If this is not possible he must be protected by means of screens, the head of the bed being especially guarded. That draughts are dangerous is founded on fact no less than is the modern idea that an abundance of fresh air is necessary and helpful. A nurse has been guilty of gross neglect of duty when the patient contracts pneumonia through exposure to too severe currents of air. A simple way to ventilate a private room is to raise the lower sash of window six inches and place a board across the opening below; the air will then enter between the two sashes and be directed upward, where it becomes diffused and no one in the room is subjected to a draught. In a room where there is only one window a pane of glass may be taken out and a piece of tin or pasteboard may be so placed that the current will be directed upwards; or a window can be opened in an adjoining room which fills with fresh air and the door of the sick room opened afterwards to admit the air; or, the patient may be covered up, head and all, for a few minutes two or three times a day, while all the windows are thrown open, The room should be thoroughly warmed before it is so thoroughly ventilated.

TEMPERATURE OF THE ROOM.--This should be regulated

by a thermometer suspended at a central point in the room. The temperature should be regulated according to the nature of the disease and the comfort of the patient. In fevers it should be lower, varying from 55 to 60 degrees F., but in bronchial troubles it should be kept about 70 degrees F. The mean temperature should be kept about 60 degrees to 70 degrees. It should be raised or lowered gradually, so that the patient will not be overheated or chilled.

LIGHT.--The patient should have plenty of light and sunshine, but do not let the sun or light shine directly upon the face.

CARE OF THE DISCHARGES (Excreta).--This is very important. Sputa, dirty vessels, soiled dressings and linen are prolific sources of impure air.

Sputum Cups.--These should be of glazed earthenware, without any corners or cracks and provided with a simple moveable cover when in use. They should be sterilized for one hour in every twenty-four hours.

Bed Pans and Urinals.--These should be washed out thoroughly. Allow boiling hot water to run on them for some time before they are put away after being cleansed.

Soiled Dressing and Linen.--These should be received in covered basins or in paper bags and at once carried away and destroyed or disinfected, or put in a metal dressing can and closely covered until the contents can be cared for at the earliest possible time. Vomited matter or the discharges from the bowels and the urine should always be covered in the vessel either with a lid, towel or rubber cloth. The rubber is better than the cloth as it keeps in the odor and can be scrubbed and disinfected.

If the patient is too sick to use a *sputum cup,* the expectoration can be received in a paper handkerchief or a piece of cheese cloth and placed in a small paper bag and burned at once.

SOILED AND STAINED LINEN.--These should be put away in a covered receptacle that contains enough disinfectant solution to keep them moist. They are removed as soon as possible to the wash room to be cleaned and sterilized.

Sterilization.--This term is usually employed when heat is used to sterilize.

Disinfection.--This is the term used when chemicals are relied upon to purify (sterilize).

Heat and Chemicals are much aided by sunshine, light and fresh air, especially that of high dry climates.

The germs (bacteria) are destroyed by dry or moist heat, the latter used in the form of steam. Dry heat is not so penetrating and requires a longer time and some goods are destroyed when exposed in it long enough to destroy the germs.

In order to destroy these organisms it is thought to be necessary to expose whatever is to be sterilized to the steam at 200 degrees F. for three successive days for thirty minutes or more each day, and during the interval to keep them in a room with a temperature of 60 degrees F.

A SIMPLE METHOD OF STERILIZING.--Put the articles (small articles) in an ordinary kitchen steamer; closely cover it and place it over a pot of boiling water. If you wish you can add two parts of carbonate of sodium to each ninety-eight parts of water.

Germicides are chemicals used to destroy germs.

Disinfectants are chemicals used to arrest and prevent their development. These disinfectants should always be fresh.

Carbolic acid is one of the most efficient and most frequently employed of the known chemical disinfectants. It comes to us in the form of white crystals and dissolves in water, glycerin, or alcohol.

Watery solutions cannot be made stronger than five per cent. Solutions weaker than this will not destroy all germs, but on account of its irritating qualities the weaker solutions are employed when used for the skin and mucous membranes. How to make a five per cent or one to twenty solution:

A bottle containing the crystals is placed in hot water until they are melted (or you can buy this dissolved product). Then take one part of the acid and add it to nineteen parts of boiling water and shake this vigorously until all has been thoroughly dissolved and mixed. To make a 1, 2, 3 or 4 per cent solution, you take 1/100 or 1/50 or 1/33 or 1/25 of acid.

Corrosive Sublimate or Bichloride of Mercury.--Tablets can be bought at any drug store containing the desired strength, and are better to use. This is a powerful irritant poison and must be used carefully. Tablets of the strength of 1-1000 and 1-2000 are most often employed for germicide action. The weaker solutions 1-5,000 or 1-10,000 were used to wash out the cavities. It is not now used much for that purpose; it stains clothing and corrodes instruments.

Milk of Lime is considered very valuable and safe to use in vessels to receive evacuations from the bowels. It should be freshly made or it is useless. Equal parts should be stirred up with the contents of the bed pan and this must be let stand at least one hour. This is the best way to disinfect stools.

To Prepare Milk of Lime.--The milk of lime is made by adding one part of slaked lime to four parts water.

Chloride of Lime (Chlorinated lime) is also a very good disin-

fectant. It has a bad odor and unless it is very fresh, is not reliable.
40

Boric acid disinfectant. This property is not very marked, but it is not irritating. The standard solution is five per cent. The weaker solutions are used to clean cavities, for superficial wounds, and to wash out the bladder.

The standard or saturated solution is made by using one part of the acid in crystal form to nineteen parts of water; or, this saturated solution can be easily made by putting a large quantity of the crystals in a filter and pouring the quantity of boiling water over them slowly until all are dissolved. Strain the solution to get rid of the excess of crystals or it can be allowed to cool when the liquid can be poured off.

Normal salt solution is made by using one teaspoonful of salt to a pint of water.

CARE AND DISINFECTION OF AN INFECTED ROOM.--- Carpets, upholstered furniture, hangings, bric-a-brac, or any personal clothing, the color of which may be destroyed by disinfection, should have been removed from the room at the beginning of the disease.

DAILY CARE OF THE ROOM BY THE NURSE.--The furniture should be wiped off with a damp cloth and the floor swept with a broom covered with a damp cloth wrung out of a 1-20 (five per cent) carbolic acid solution; besides this the floor must be rubbed thoroughly with a damp cloth every second or third day. If the disease is contagious a damp sheet kept moist should be hung in the line of the air currents. Cloths that are used daily should be washed in hot soap suds and when not in use left to soak in carbolic acid solution 1-20 (five per cent).

After the patient has recovered from an infectious disease he should receive a hot soap and water tub or sponge bath, thorough washing of the hair and irrigation of the ears included, followed by a thorough sponging with a one per cent carbolic acid or corrosive sublimate (1-10,000) solution. The finger-nails and toe-nails should be cut close and cleaned underneath.

A nasal douche is given, and the mouth should be washed with listerine or a saturated (five per cent) solution of boric acid. The patient is then wrapped in clean sheets or clothes and taken in another room. Then the bedding and clothing are made ready for sterilization.

DISINFECTION OF THE ROOM.--Brush off the mattress, wrap it in a damp sheet wrung out of a twenty per cent solution of carbolic acid, and send to the sterilizer. The clothes are steamed and sent to the wash room. When there is no sterilizer the bed must be soaked in a 1-20 (five per cent) carbolic solution, afterwards boiled and the mattress ripped apart and boiled or burned.

DISINFECTING THE ROOM.--Arrange all articles that are left in the room so as to expose them the best to the fumigating substance. To disinfect with formalin, close the room tightly, seal all cracks and openings with paste and paper. Place an alcohol lamp in a metal dish in the center of the room. Put in a receptacle over the lamp three fluid ounces of a forty per cent solution of formaldehyde; have a dish of water in the room for some time; moisten the air of the room, light the lamp and then close the room up tight for twenty-four hours, until the dust has settled; then enter gently so as not to disturb the dust and wipe off everything in the room with a cloth wrung out of a corrosive sublimate (1-1000) solution. Floors, woodwork, furniture, bedstead must be so washed or wiped, and use for crevices pure carbolic acid, applying it with a brush. The walls should be washed down with the 1-1000 corrosive sublimate solution. Then leave the windows wide open. Sulphur fumigation is not considered so certain in its results.

HOW TO TREAT SPUTUM FROM TUBERCULOUS PATIENTS.--Sputum is dangerous when it is dry. The sputum cups should be of china or paper, so that they may be either boiled or burned. There should be no crevices. The cup should be kept covered and the sputum moist so that none of the germs on the sputum becoming dry may escape into the air of the room. The china vessel should be frequently cleaned and, before the contents are thrown away, the germs must be destroyed by putting the sputum in a two per cent solution of carbonate of soda for one hour. The paper cups and contents must be burned before the contents have time enough to become dry. In infectious diseases, all discharges from the nose, mouth, bowels and bladder should be received in a china vessel containing carbolic acid or milk of lime.

In Diphtheria the expectoration, discharge from the nose and vomited matter should be received in paper napkins and burned at once in the room, or if this is impossible, boiled before being taken from the room.

Use the same treatment for the discharges in **Scarlet fever.** Two sets of cups should be kept and boiled in the soda solution before being used. All vessels, tubes or cups that are used for the mouth in diphtheria, syphilis, or cancer should be kept in a 1-40 solution of carbolic acid and boiled before being used by another patient.

Bed-pans used in cases of cancer, dysentery, typhoid fever and, in short, in all infectious diseases, are to be soaked in a 1-20 (five per cent) carbolic acid solution and boiled before again coming into general use.

Sheets and clothing stained with typhoid fever discharges must be washed out at once, or soaked in a disinfectant solution and steamed before being sent to the laundry. Also the bedding and clothing in any infectious or malignant disease should always be put to soak, at once, in a 1-20 (five per cent) carbolic acid solution, or else steamed or boiled before being brought again into general use.

The urine needs the same attention as the bowel discharges in typhoid fever.

Coughing in diphtheria, lung tuberculosis, scarlet fever, etc., sets free infectious germs. These may be received in the person of the attendant, or on the bedding and furniture. Care should be taken when attending such cases.

CARE OF THE MOUTH AND TEETH.--A weak solution of borax or listerine is very good. One-half ounce of listerine to a glass of water to be used by the patient as often as he desires to rinse his mouth. Lemon juice in solution is very good. For cracks in the mouth, vaselin or cold cream is good. A few drops of oil of peppermint can be added, or oil of wintergreen.

For spongy and sore gums.--A few drops of tincture of myrrh added to pure water may be used. Colorless golden seal in the same way is pleasant and successful.

Cloths for washing the teeth and mouth are made in small squares of gauze or old linen. They are best to use since they can be burned immediately after being used. Wrap one of the squares around the first finger, dip it into the mouth-wash and insert in the mouth. Go over the whole cavity, the cloth being passed along the gums and behind the wisdom teeth, thence over the roof of the mouth, inside the teeth and under the tongue. Use more than one piece for all this. This is very necessary in typhoid fever. If the tongue is badly coated, it can be soaked and gently scraped. A good mouth-wash for general use is the following:

Glycerin	1 dram
Soda	10 grains
5% solution of Boric Acid	1 ounce

BED SORES. Prevention and care of.--Very fat flabby people or thin emaciated patients are liable to suffer from bed sores. They result from constant friction or pressure on a certain spot or spots and when the body is poorly nourished. Moisture, creases in the under sheets, night gown, crumbs in the bed and want of proper care and cleanliness also are causes.

Bed-sores due to pressure occur most frequently upon the hips and lower back, the shoulders and heels; those from friction, in the ankles, inner parts of the knees, or the elbows and back of the head. In patients suffering from dropsy, paralysis or spinal injuries, or when there is a continuous discharge from any part of the body, the utmost care must be taken to prevent bed sores.

Treatment. Preventive.--Cleanliness and relief from pressure. Bathe the back and shoulders with warm water and soap night and morning and afterwards rub with alcohol and water equal parts. Dust the parts with oxide of zinc or stearate of zinc powder, or bismuth mixed with borax; all are good. If there is much moisture due to sweating or involuntary stools or urine, castor oil should be well rubbed in addition. The sheets must be kept smooth and dry under the patient.

Redness of the skin may be the first symptom of this trouble.

This may be followed by a dark color under the skin, and when the cuticle finally comes off the underlying tissues are found broken down and sloughing. Any skin scraped or worn off--abrasion--should be carefully washed and a small pad of cotton smeared with olive oil and stearate of zinc placed over it and kept there with collodion painted over it; or white of egg painted over the sore is sometimes very beneficial; also equal parts of castor oil and bismuth make an excellent dressing. Rubber rings or cotton rings over the part relieve the pressure. Changing the position is often beneficial.

Treatment of the Sore Proper.--Sponge with clean soft cloths, with a solution of boric acid or one per cent solution of carbolic acid and the cavity packed with iodoform gauze, or iodoform, or aristol ointment, over which apply a layer of borated cotton. Dress the sore daily. If it sloughs apply hot boric acid dressings every four hours and follow with an application of castor oil and balsam of Peru. When it is better treat as any other sore.

BATHS.

A hot bath temperature is from	100 to 112 degrees F. or higher.
A warm bath temperature is from	90 to 100 degrees F.
A tepid bath temperature is from	70 to 90 degrees F.
A cool bath temperature is from	65 to 70 degrees F.
A cold bath temperature is from	33 to 65 degrees F.

The entire bath should not last longer, when given in bed, than fifteen or twenty minutes. A few drops of water of ammonia or a little borax will help much in getting the patient clean and disguise the bad odor of the perspiration. A little alcohol or Eau de Cologne will be found refreshing. Cold damp towels should never be employed here. The water should be pleasantly warm and changed a few times during the bath. A glass of hot milk can be taken after the bath is given, if the patient feels exhausted, and if the feet are cool a hot fruit can is applied.

Foot Baths in Bed.--The patient should lie on her back, with the knees bent and place her feet in the tub, which is placed lengthwise in the bed on a rubber sheet spread across the lower part of the bed for protection. A mustard foot bath can be given the same way except that the knees and foot bath are enclosed in a blanket. These are often given for severe colds, with head symptoms (headaches), when it is desired to draw the blood from the head. Hot water alone will do this, but the mustard hastens the action. The mustard should be mixed with a small amount of water before being added to the bath. The amount will depend upon the sensitiveness of the patient. The feet may remain in the bath for fifteen to twenty minutes, the water kept at the same temperature or made warmer by adding more hot water from time to time. They are wiped gently afterward and tucked snugly in blankets.

Hot Bath, Hot Air, Vapor, and Steam Bath.--Given for sweating purposes. Fill the tub half full of water at 100 degrees F. and draw it to the bedside if necessary. Lift the patient into the tub and gradually increase the temperature by the thermometer to 110 degrees and 112 degrees F. Maintain it at this point for twelve or fifteen minutes. After this the patient is lifted out into a prepared bed on which a long rubber is spread with three or four hot blankets over it; these are wrapped all around the patient, tucked in closely about the neck and watched continually to see that no air enters. Give plenty of water to drink, as it promotes perspiration and helps in that way to cast off the impurities. Keep this up for an hour if possible, and then the patient is gradually uncovered, sponged under a blanket with alcohol and water and the wet blankets removed. Cloths wrung out of cold water are applied to the head during this bath. The pulse should be closely watched for any indication of faintness, when the patient should be put to bed, immediately. This bath should not be given during menstruation or pregnancy.

Warm Baths (90 degrees to 100 degrees F.) are frequently given to children for convulsions. They should be placed in the tub and cold applied to the head, while the body is washed and rubbed.

Local baths and packs.--For sprains, a foot bath. For menstrual pain, a sitz bath. The patient sits in the bath with only the thighs and part of the body immersed, while the upper part of the body and the feet are protected with blankets. Sitting on a cane-seated chair over a steaming pail with a blanket around the neck and body gives a good bath for pain during menstruation.

Salt-water bath. Tonic action.--Nine to fourteen pounds of sea salt to fifty gallons of water will redden the skin and give an exhilarating effect.

Dry Salt Bath sent us with Mothers' Remedies.--"To a basin of water put a big handful of salt, take a Turkish towel and soak it in the salt water, wring out and let dry. The salt will adhere to the towel. Use to rub the body. A tepid bath should be taken next day to remove the salt."

Starch bath.--Add eight ounces of laundry starch to each gallon of water. This allays skin irritation.

Bran bath.--Put the bran in a bag and allow this to soak in warm water for an hour before being used; or it may be boiled for an hour and then the fluid drained and added to the bath water.

Sponge bath.--Water and soap should be ready. Clothes to be put on, well aired and at hand. Then remove the patient's clothes and wrap him in an old blanket, expose only the part being washed at a time, wash and dry this part. Begin with the face and neck, then the chest, abdomen, arms and back, and lastly the lower extremities. Warm the water at least twice. Then put on his clean, well aired clothes and into a clean bed, and the patient will bless you.

Alcohol sponge bath.--This is given the same way, only sixty per cent alcohol is used and the parts are allowed to dry themselves.

Tub bath (common).--Prepare everything as to heat, etc. Then carry the patient or assist him to the tub. Soap him all over and pour water over him from a large pitcher. The temperature of the water depends upon the disease. One person should continually rub the patient in typhoid fever to keep up the circulation while the water is being poured over him. A hot drink is given before and after these baths and the patient is wrapped immediately in warm flannel.

Patients are frequently put into a tub with a water temperature of 85 to 90 degrees, and then the water temperature decreased by adding cold water. This bath must be carefully given.

The cold pack.--It is used to reduce fever, delirium and extreme nervousness and to induce sleep. Cover the bed with a rubber sheet or oilcloth, and over this a blanket. Wring a sheet out of cold water and place this over the blanket. Lay the patient on this sheet and wrap it around him so that every surface has the wet sheet next to it. Tuck the sheet in well at the neck and feet. Fold the outer blanket over the patient and tuck it in. Lay a wet towel over the head, or he can be enveloped loosely in blankets and allowed to remain twenty minutes to an hour, only ten to fifteen minutes by the tucked-in method and then dried and put to bed.

The hot pack.--This is given in the same manner except that the patient is wrapped first in a blanket wrung out of boiling water. More covering is put over the patient than in a cold pack, and something cold is applied to the head.

EXTERNAL APPLICATIONS.

General and Local.--For dry heat, for warmth alone, hot bags, bottles and cans are used. Hot flannels are sometimes used for inflamed joints. Make the flannel very hot, wrap in heated paper or cloth and apply quickly; cover all with a layer of cotton, wool and oiled muslin.

For neuralgia and earache, salt bags are used.

Fill flannel bags with salt, heat as hot as can be borne, and cover it so as to retain the heat after it is applied to the ear.

For moist heat.--This is more penetrating and has a more pronounced effect than dry heat. It also hastens suppuration when it cannot be prevented in acute inflammation like quinsy, etc.

For local pains, fomentations, stupes and poultices are used. Poultices are best for deep-seated pain or continuous inflammation.

Linseed meal poultice.--Stir the meal slowly and evenly in boiling water; boil this mixture for several minutes and stir briskly all the time, and when thick enough it is well beaten with a spoon to remove lumps. If this is properly done it will be a light smooth paste, just stiff enough to drop away from the spoon. Use a muslin or coarse cloth and spread the poultice on this to the depth of one-half inch, leaving one inch space to turn in. Put vaselin over the surface, thin, and cover with a thin layer of gauze or thin cloth. Turn the edges over and roll in a towel to keep it warm and carry to patient. Keep them warm,--one should never be removed until another is ready to be put on. The skin should always be wiped dry before another is applied. Oiling the poultice prevents irritation of the skin and pimples. Cover the poultice loosely if possible with a layer of cotton-wool and oiled muslin to retain the heat and moisture longer. It should be changed every three hours at least. Apply hot and never keep on when it is cold. It should never be used a second time.

Starch Poultice.--This is used in skin diseases for its soothing properties. Mix the starch first with a little cold water and then add enough boiling water to make a thick paste, which is then spread on muslin covered with a layer of gauze.

The Jacket Poultice. For lung affections.--Two layers of thin muslin are shaped so as to fit closely around the neck and under the arms and come over the chest and back, low enough to cover the lungs. Three sides are now closed, and the prepared linseed is poured into the bag and regularly distributed. Close the open end and then apply. Cover it with wool and oiled silk and keep in place with safety pins or tapes which are tied under the arms and over the shoulders. When changing the poultice be careful not to expose the patient. A cotton-wool jacket should be worn a few days after the poultice has been discontinued.

Cold is applied either by means of the cold bath or by compresses, pack, sponging, coils or ice.

Cold Compresses are made by using two or three thicknesses of lint or linen wrung out of cold water or ice water and applied over the inflamed part, and changed frequently. A little vaselin may be rubbed on to prevent the skin from becoming irritated. They are very useful where little weight can be borne. If iced compresses are used a small block of ice partially wrapped in flannel is placed in a basin; there should be two compresses, one of which is kept on ice while the other is on the patient.

Compresses are very good in the early stage of tonsilitis, quinsy, sore throat, laryngitis and croup.

Ice-bags (India Rubber).--With these, cold can be best applied and with less trouble. These are made in different shapes. For instance helmet-shaped to fit the head and long and narrow for the spine.

Crush the ice in small pieces and mix in it a little common salt,--never fill the rubber bags more than half full; expel the air as much as possible by pressing before screwing on the top. Always place a layer of lint, cotton or thin cloth between the skin and the bag. The extreme cold is not only painful but liable to irritate the skin, and may cause frost-bites. Its effect should be watched carefully. Sometimes the weight causes discomfort. In such cases suspend the bag. For the head, fasten a bandage to the neck of the bag and pin the two ends to the pillow just high enough to allow the cap (bag) to barely touch the head. Care should be taken to refill the ice-bags before the ice has melted. At times a piece of ice is wrapped in moist lint or old linen and passed gently over the head in order to cool the head.

For Appendicitis.--There should be quite a thickness of cloth between the ice bag and the skin. The latter must not become too cool. In this disease this bag is a great reliever of the pain and generally used.

Ice Poultices.--In some cases these are better than the ice bag for the reason that they fit the body better. They are usually made of two parts of crushed ice to one of linseed meal or bran, together with a small amount of salt. Make two bags of oiled silk,--one should be smaller than the other. Close all sides but one, with adhesive plaster. Fill the smaller bag two-thirds full of ice, close and slip it into the larger bag.

Ice Water Coils.--These can be bought. They can also be made from rubber tubing. Sew this upon a piece of rubber cloth in circles about one inch apart for five or six rounds; leave a yard or two of tubing at each end to be used as a siphon, A large pan of ice water is raised above the patient into which one weighted end of the tubing is placed, with a funnel inserted into it, covered with gauze to prevent clogging, while the other end is laid in a second basin on the floor which receives the water. The upper pan must be kept filled. This is very good for delirium in brain fever, etc., when applied to the head and also good for bleeding from the bowels in typhoid fever. The stream of water can be regulated if necessary by a stop-cock.

Lotions.--Lotions are medicated moist applications, and may be either hot or cold.

Counter--Irritants are agents applied externally to produce irritation or inflammation in order to relieve a diseased condition in an adjacent or deep-seated part of the body. Mustard foot-bath relieves pain in the head by drawing the surplus blood away from the head. The mildest mustard counter-irritant is the mustard poultice. It can be made with one part mustard to six of linseed meal. Never use boiling water with mustard.

Mustard Poultice.--Use of ground mustard, one-fourth to one-eighth of the amount of meal used. Make into a paste and stir this into the linseed, after it has been prepared for the poultices. The white of an egg is used in this poultice as it may keep the poultice from blistering.

Yeast Poultices.--These stimulate ulcers, gangrene and sloughing conditions. Mix eight ounces of soft yeast with as much water. Add enough flour to make a sponge, but not too stiff. It should be kept warm until fermentation begins; then apply every day. Finely powdered charcoal can also be added.

For Soothing Effect.--Hop bags or bran bags, dipped in hot water, may be applied, protected and kept in place with a bandage.

Spice Poultice.--This is very good for pain in abdomen in children especially. Equal parts of ground cinnamon, cloves, allspice and ginger, one-quarter part cayenne pepper, if needed very strong. Place all together in a flannel bag and spread equally. Wet with alcohol or brandy. When dry, re-wet. This is a mild warming dressing.

Spice Poultice from a Stanlyton, Va., Mother.--"Take one teaspoonful each of mustard, ginger, black pepper, cinnamon, cloves, nutmeg, or as many ground spices as one has in the kitchen; mix them well in a bowl while dry, adding boiling water slowly and stir constantly until it is of the consistency of soft putty; spread between soft thin cloths and apply to the affected parts as hot as the patient can bear it. When it is cool heat it again and apply."

Mother's Flour and Water Poultice.--"Make a thick poultice of flour and water; bake soft and apply hot. Have another ready for change, if necessary. This is good for any pain."

Poultice of Peach Tree Leaves from our Mother's List.--"Put a handful of peach leaves in a vessel and let boil well; add enough meal to thicken, spread between thin muslin cloth and apply to parts affected. This is a splendid poultice."

Mild Plaster for Children.--"Two teaspoonsful of flour, three teaspoonsful of mustard, a little fresh lard and a few drops of turpentine, Mix up with warm water."

Fomentations.--This is the best way to apply moist heat, but it is troublesome, as they should be changed very frequently, at least every ten minutes when heat is required. They should never be left on until they are cold and clammy. Sheets of lamb's wool make the best material. Cut these layers into sizes required and encase them in a gauze cover over which is put a layer of oiled silk. Coarse old flannel or an old blanket will do well. Take two layers of the flannels, dip in the boiling water and wring. Two should be at hand. Dry the skin first and then put on the flannel. It should be covered with enough material to keep in the heat and moisture. Hops, etc., can be put into the water.

Turpentine Stupes.--This is prepared the same way, except turpentine is added. After the flannel has been wrung out, add from ten to twenty drops of turpentine, or add two or three teaspoonfuls of turpentine to one pint of boiling water and put the flannel in it and wring out and apply. Put a towel over the stupe. This is especially for gas in the bowels.

Mustard Stupe.--Put a tablespoonful of mustard in one pint of hot water. Make a paste of the mustard before it is put into the hot water, to avoid forming lumps; never use boiling water. Wring the flannel out after it has been in this solution and apply to the part.

Mustard Plaster.--This is made of different strengths, depending upon the length of time it is desired to keep it on and the sensitiveness of the skin.

1. Equal parts of mustard and flour.
2. One of mustard and two of flour.
3. One of mustard and three or four of flour.

White of an egg added makes it better and not so blistering.

A paste is made with warm water and spread between the layers of muslin and left on no longer than ten minutes. When the skin is red remove the plaster. This is used when you wish a quick counter-irritation.

Mustard Plaster.--This is made stronger, 1 to 2 to 3 parts meal.

Mustard leaves or Sinapisms may be bought at a drug store. They are no better than you can make. Use plasters.

Capsicum and Belladonna Plasters.--May be bought. In applying, heat the back of the plaster slightly; the face of the gauze is pulled off and the plaster placed where wanted. To remove soak first with alcohol.

Spice plaster.--Mix two teaspoonfuls each of ginger and cloves with a teaspoonful of cayenne pepper, one tablespoonful of flour, enough brandy or water to make a paste. Spread this between two layers of muslin.

For Turpentine and Mustard Stupes see above.

Tincture of iodine, chloroform and liniments are also counter-irritants, also castor oil, and pure tartar emetic, and cartharides.

Cupping, Wet and Dry.--This is sometimes used to relieve inflammations of the eye, lung or kidney, or even muscular pains like lumbago. Wine-glasses will do as well as any you can buy.

Dry cupping.--Take a piece of wire, wrap a small piece of cotton about the end, dip this in alcohol, light it and swab the inside of the glass, remove and apply the glass. The heat causes the air to expand and it is driven off and the partial vacuum formed is filled by the skin and tissues over which the glass is placed. The edges of the cup must not be warm enough to burn the patient. Six or seven cups may be applied at one time and allowed to remain five minutes, after which they are removed by pressing the flesh around the edge and inserting the finger there so as to let in the air.

Linseed meal poultices can be applied afterwards to keep up the work begun.

Wet cupping.--Scrub the skin with hot water and soap, wash off with a five per cent (1-20) carbolic acid solution. Make a few cuts over the parts desired with a clean knife and apply the cup prepared in the way above directed. Remove the blood and check the bleeding, if necessary, by sponging. Place a pad on the part and hold this in place by a bandage or adhesive strap.

Blistered Skin. To dress.--Puncture the lower part with a clean instrument and catch the fluid on absorbent cotton. Dress it with oxide of zinc ointment or vaselin on lint or clean linen and strap on. It is best not to remove the skin from a blister at the first dressing.

HOW TO DETERMINE THE DOSE FOR CHILDREN.

We have endeavored to always give the dose throughout this book as we recognized the lack of accurate and detailed information regarding the administering of medicines as one of the weak features in practically all home medical books. If we have overlooked a few instances we wish to provide for such omissions by giving the table of doses generally used by nurses as a basis for determining the dose of any medicine she may be using for a particular age.

Rule usually followed.--For children under twelve years of age. Make a fraction. Use the age of the child for the upper number, numerator. The number below the line, denominator, is twelve, added to the age of the child. For example: If your child is two years old you would begin by placing two as numerator, thus 2/, then you add 2 + 12 = 14 and place 14 below the line and you have 2/14 or 1/7. You then take 1/7 of the adult dose for your two-year-old child. If the dose for an adult is 21 drops, a child of two years is given 3 drops, etc.

DOSE IN DROPS FOR DIFFERENT AGES.

If the dose is a spoonful or 60 drops for an adult, the other doses would be correct for the ages given below:

21 and over		60 drops	
15 years		33 drops	A few more or less if robust or weakly
12 "	"	30 drops	"
10 "	"	27 drops	"
8 "	"	24 drops	"
6 "	"	20 drops	"
5 "	"	17 drops	"
4 "	"	15 drops	"
3 "	"	12 drops	"
2 "	"	8 drops	"
1 "	"	4 drops	"

Exceptions to this rule are calomel and castor oil, when half an adult dose can be given between 12 and 18.

Opium is dangerous to children and old people and should be administered by a physician or trained nurse.

"Lest We Forget."

COMMON TABLES OF MEASURES.

APOTHECARIES' WEIGHT.

Apothecaries' Weight is used in prescribing and mixing medicines

Table.

20 grains	equal	1 scruple
3 scruples	"	1 dram
8 drams	"	1 ounce
12 ounces	"	1 pound

The pound is the same as the pound Troy. Medicines are bought and sold in quantities by Avoirdupois Weight.

1 grain	equals	1 drop or 1 minim
60 grains or drops	"	1 teaspoonful
1 teaspoonful	"	1 fluid dram
8 drams (or 8 teaspoonfuls) make		1 fluid ounce
2 tablespoonfuls make		1 fluid ounce
1/2 fluid ounce is a		tablespoonful
2 fluid ounces is a		wineglassful
4 fluid ounces is a		teacupful
6 fluid ounces is a		coffee cup
16 ounces (dry or solid) is a		pound
20 fluid ounces is a		pint

MEDICINE CHEST.--More important than the furnishing of the house is the medicine chest. If you are beginning housekeeping let this be your first consideration. Do not put it off because it is a little trouble and costs a few dollars. Yon would not think of leaving your front room or your "spare room" half furnished. Your health is of vastly more importance than the looks of your best rooms. There may come a time when you cannot secure the doctor for several hours or get into a drug store. Be prepared for this emergency and either fix up a home-made box with shelves, etc., or buy a regular medicine chest; in either case have a lock to it and the key where you can find it but where the children cannot reach it.

We give below a few of the necessaries and you will of course add to this list. One mother writes that she went to the store and bought several tiny little bells and tied one of these bells around the neck of each of the bottles in her medicine chest that contained poison. There was no danger of her getting the wrong bottle in the dark.

Contents of the Medicine Chest.

Ten cents worth of Alum.
A small bag of Burnt Alum.
A small bottle of Castor Oil.
A small vial of Bichloride of Mercury Tablets.
A box of Boric Acid Powder.
A $mall bottle of Glycerin:
A bottle of Extract of Witch-hazel
A small bottle of Syrup of Ipecac.
A bottle of Whisky and one of Brandy.
A box of English Mustard.
Medicine glass.
A small box of Cold Cream.
Soft rubber Ear Syringe.
A Clinical Thermometer.
An Eye Stone.
A pad, pencils, and labels.
A small bottle of Carbolic Acid.
A roll of Adhesive Plaster.
A small box of Pineoline Salve.
A bottle of Arnica.

Hung near the chest should be a fountain syringe with the rubber catheter for use in irrigating the bowels and a hot water bag.

HOW TO CARE FOR THE DEAD.

The limbs should be straightened before the body becomes stiff (rigor mortis). The eyes should be closed and the jaws held in position by means of a support placed firmly under the chin; for this a roller bandage or a small padded piece of wood is generally used. Of course if the person has worn false teeth, and they have been taken out during the last hours, they should be replaced immediately after death. The nostrils, mouth, rectum, and vagina should be packed with absorbent cotton to prevent the escape of discharges after death. After this bathe the body, if so desired by the relatives, with a two per cent watery solution of carbolic acid, and if there are any wounds they should be covered with fresh cotton and neatly fastened with a bandage. The hips may be enclosed in a large triangular binder; the knees are held together by a broad bandage; the hair should be brushed smoothly, and finally stockings and a simple nightgown should be put on. If the case be one of the infectious diseases, wrap the body in a sheet wrung out of a five per cent watery solution of carbolic acid and this sheet should be kept damp.

The room where death occurs should be tidied and regulated to make it look natural and comfortable. The undertaker can be sent for as soon as desired by the family. But if such care as directed has been given, the undertaker need not be hurried.

ENEMA.--Enemata (Injections).--There are various methods used for injecting fluids into the body. When they are introduced into the intestines, we speak of giving enemata (enema is the singular). They are named according to their purpose.

1. Simple laxative or purgative enemata.
2. Nutritive enemata for the purpose of nourishment.
3. Sedative enemata for local or systemic quieting effects.
4. Astringent enemata to check bleeding and diarrhea, like hot water, ice water, solution of alum or nitrate of silver.
5. Emollient (soothing) enemata for soothing irritated and painful mucous membrane; starch and drugs are also used.
6. Antispasmodic enemata to relieve flatulence such as the turpentine enemata.
7. Anthelmintic (against worms) for destroying worms; salt, turpentine and quassia are used.
8. Antiseptic or germicidal enemata used in dysentery.
9. Stimulating enemata, like hot water, hot strong coffee, hot whisky and water, salt water.
10. To relieve thirst, water one pint or normal salt solution (one dram to a pint of water) and injected high up.

ENEMATA are given either high or low.

A high enemas thrown high up into the bowel.

A low enema is injected into the rectum only, through a hard rubber tip to a syringe.

Directions.--There are many ways of giving a simple enema.

Position.--A good way is to place an adult patient on his left side, with the knees bent up close. Protect the bed with a rubber sheet and towel under the patient. The basin of water can be placed on the rubber sheet and the enema given under cover.

Amount.--An adult person will take one to four pints. A child one-half to one pint. For an infant about two ounces will do.

What material? A simple enema can be made with good castile soap or good brown soap and water, temperature about 95 degrees F. When ready for use make into a good suds.

Syringe.--Use a bulb syringe, see that the syringe is filled full to the nozzle before the nozzle is put into the bowel. Any air left in the syringe will pass into the bowel and cause pain. Oil the nozzle with vaselin or sweet oil and then gently put the nozzle into the rectum. It is better to introduce an oiled finger through the sphincter muscle and pass the nozzle along the finger and gently into the bowel. It should be in the bowel two or three inches. Do not attempt to force the nozzle through any obstruction. Introduce the water slowly in a gentle and steady stream. The main object is to distend the rectum by means of the water, thereby producing reflex stimulation. The worm-like movement of the bowels results, thus bringing about an evacuation. The patient should retain it for ten or fifteen minutes to get the best results. A folded towel placed against the anus will assist the patient in resisting the desire to expel the water. A large amount should be given in one-half hour if the first one does not produce the desired result.

Sometimes a laxative enema is necessary.--Olive oil or glycerin or castor oil may be used.

For olive oil, six ounces may be given in a hard rubber syringe; this is seldom successful unless followed by a soap suds enema in one-half hour.

Glycerin enema, one-half ounce with equal quantity of warm water 95 degrees F., and give with a hard rubber syringe. This generally proves successful, without an additional soap suds enema.

For infants and children the contents of a straight medicine dropper will be sufficient.

Glycerin irritates the mucous membrane, and it is best that we add an equal amount of olive oil.

If these enemata fail it will be necessary to use purgative enemata.

These are made by adding drugs, such as turpentine, rochelle or epsom salts or castor oil in certain proportions to the simple enema. In giving castor oil and water it is necessary first to mix the oil with the yolk of an egg and then add the warm soap suds.

1. Formula.--

Castor Oil	2 ounces
Turpentine	1/2 ounce

Mix thoroughly and inject with hard rubber syringe, followed in one-half hour by a quart of soap-suds.

2. Formula.--

Turpentine	1/2 ounce
Rochelle Salts	1 ounce

Mix with warm soap-suds, one pint.

The buttocks and anus should be washed off with warm water after turpentine has been used in the enema.

3. Molasses and Laxative Enema.--Mix from two to ten ounces, according to age, with one pint of soap suds and inject slowly.

Nutritive Enemata.--Food is given by the bowel when the stomach cannot retain it. It is then called **Nutritive Enemata**. They should be given only from four to six times in twenty-four hours and the quantity given at one time should not exceed four ounces. It must be introduced high up in the bowel, about ten inches, and therefore they should be given through a rectal tube made of heavy rubber one--quarter inch in diameter and at least eight inches of it should be inserted in the bowel. After it has been oiled the tube is gently inserted in a backward, upward, direction and a glass funnel is attached to the outer end. The enema has been already mixed in a small pitcher and gently poured (very slowly) into the funnel, which is then raised so that the contents will go slowly through the tube into the bowel. The patient is protected from drops by a folded towel underneath him. Then the tube is slowly withdrawn. The tube should then be cleansed by allowing warm water to run through it, and then kept in a one per cent solution of boric acid. Food given by enemata should be very nourishing and concentrated. The following are excellent formulas:

Formula 1.--

One whole Egg	
Table Salt	15 grains
Peptonized Milk	3 ounces or 3/8 of a cup
Brandy	1/2 ounce

Formula 2.--

White of two Eggs	
Peptonized Milk	2 ounces or 1/4 of a cup

The whole amount should never exceed four ounces. The addition of salt aids the absorption of the egg. Brandy, and whisky are very irritating and should be given only every other time.

The fresh raw milk can be used, if it is impossible to have it peptonized.

After a nutritive enemata the patient should lie quietly on his back for twenty or thirty minutes.

Turpentine enemata for distention may be given according to the following formula:

Mucilage of Acacia	1/2 ounce
Spirits of Turpentine	10 drops

This should be administered high up in the bowel.

Astringent Enemata. To check diarrhea.--They should be given slowly and injected high up, and they should be retained as long as possible.

Starch and Laudanum.--Boil the starch as if to be used in the laundry and dilute with luke-warm water, until it is thin enough to pass through a tube. Take of this three ounces. This can be given alone in mild cases; but if there is much pain and straining add ten to fifteen drops of laudanum to the starch water or thirty to forty drops of paregoric. This dose is for an adult.

Stimulating Enemata. 1. Black coffee.--One-half to one pint of strong coffee, injected as hot as possible. It should be strained before using. This is frequently given in poison cases.

2. Salt Enemata.--Two teaspoonfuls to one quart of hot water is mildly stimulating; one-half to one ounce of brandy or whisky may be added.

DOUCHES.--By this term is generally meant a jet of fluid directed with a certain amount of force upon a limited external or internal surface, for cleansing, stimulating purposes and to relieve inflammation. Three common douches are the ear (aural), the vaginal and the rectal.

The Vaginal Douche. For cleansing.--A one per cent solution of carbolic acid is often used in one to three quarts of water.

To allay inflammation.--A hot solution of the temperature of 105 degrees to 115 degrees is given, and three or six quarts may be used. Allow the stream to flow before the nozzle is inserted so as to have the warm temperature instead of cold at the start, and the nozzle should be introduced up towards the posterior vaginal wall. The fountain syringe bag should not be raised more than six to twelve inches above the patient who is lying down with her hips raised on pillows and her knees drawn up. Medicines can be used in all the douches.

Rectal douche.--This is to relieve piles and reduce inflammation. Hot or cold as needed. A rectal tube or fountain syringe is used.

Ear (aural) douche.--This is used for earache and inflammation. Salt or boric acid is generally used in the warm water. It should be allowed to flow in slowly and gently.

How to use a bed pan.--When you are placing the pan, you should slip one hand under the buttocks and then place the flat end of the pan under the buttocks. It should always be warm. Raise the patient in the same way before attempting to remove it. Do not pull it out.

TEMPERATURE (Fever).--A thermometer is necessary in taking the temperature. They can be bought for from fifty cents up. The temperature is taken by putting the thermometer under the tongue, in the arm-pit and in the rectum. For children it should be placed in the rectum or in the arm-pit or groin. Allow it to remain from two to five minutes. This depends upon the time limit of the thermometer. The normal temperature is 98-6/10 degrees F. This varies, some people are normal at times at 99 or 98 degrees. The temperature in the arm-pit is lower by 3/10 of a degree, but that in the rectum is 1/2 degree higher than that taken in the mouth. The normal point on the thermometer is marked by an arrow. The mercury in the tube must always be down to that at its highest point, before the thermometer is placed and the highest point the mercury goes indicates the height of the temperature (fever). If you take it in the rectum, that should be free from feces. Oil the thermometer and gently insert it into the bowel for one and one-half inches and hold the stem.

Under the Tongue.--Place the point under the tongue and instruct the patient to close his lips over the thermometer. He can also hold the stem with his fingers, It should never be taken here right after a cold drink. Unconscious patients may bite through the instrument, so care must be taken with them.

Arm-pit.--Wipe the part thoroughly dry and place the point directly in the arm-pit. Then place the elbow against the body and the hand on the chest pointing to the opposite shoulder. When ready to take it out move the arm away from the body and take the thermometer away gently for it sticks sometimes and you will cause pain if you draw it away quickly. The instrument should be cleansed in tepid mild salt solution.

PULSE.--Average in men, sixty to seventy. In women, sixty-five to eighty. Children ninety to one hundred to one hundred and twenty. Different authors vary. In men it is generally seventy to seventy-two. In women seventy-two to seventy-five.

It is better taken sitting. It is faster when walking, slower when lying down. I always take the pulse in the left arm unless there is a deformity there. I use my right hand with the third finger toward the elbow. By using the first three fingers you can find out different things about the pulse. Some people are very nervous and such an one will make your arm ache when feeling the pulse. The pulse should be regular, even beats, in health. Sometimes you can feel it best on the temple or on the neck.

RESPIRATION (Breathing).--In an adult the average is eighteen per minute. In a child the average is twenty to twenty-four. Respiration is the act of taking in (inspiration), and giving out (expiration) air by the lungs.

THE TONGUE.--This is coated in dyspepsia and fevers,--some healthy persons always have a coated tongue.

In **Ulcers** of the stomach there is no coating.

In **high fevers**, the tongue may also be red and cracked as well as coated in some parts.

A **dark brown or blackish** coating indicates a serious condition in acute diseases.

Strawberry tongue is seen in **Scarlet Fever**.

Cankered tongue and month may be due to local conditions, or to stomach, liver and bowel disorders.

In **Peritonitis** the tongue is generally dry and red (beefy).

Cholera Infantum.--At first coated, then dry and reddish.

Constipation.--Tongue is generally coated.

Biliousness.--Yellowish dirty coating.

DIET

FOODS AND DRINKS FOR THE SICK ROOM.

DIET.--The importance of diet and its relation to the needs of the system in disease can hardly be overrated. One should not only know what kind of food to give, but how much and how often it should be given to get the best result. Food should be given in small quantities in acute diseases and at regular intervals. It will digest better. The food should never be left in the sick room after a patient has finished with it. This applies to all kinds of food, but especially to milk, for it absorbs impurities from the air more readily than any other kind of food. How often do we see milk standing in a sick room and uncovered; how often is it placed in an ice box uncovered. I have often wondered how such people could eat some foods I have seen prepared for them in such a careless way and with no attempt to make it appear tempting to their poor appetite. Foods should be given just as regularly as medicines, when so ordered, especially in long wasting diseases like typhoid fever.

The kind of food.--Under each disease directions for the kind of food, time, and quantity have been given. In diseases like typhoid fever, special care must be given. It is better in that disease to give too little than too much food and the proper kind of food must be given. I shall never forget the death of a minister in my childhood days. I was about four years old. This minister was loved by everyone and when he died of typhoid fever, everyone was grieved and shocked and they could not understand why God should take such a useful man away. It made a great impression upon me. I found out more about the "why" afterwards. This minister was in the convalescent stage and very hungry.

He wanted a genuine boiled dinner. That is bad enough for a well man. The doctor forbade it, but the family gave him the dinner and the result, of course, was fatal. It could not be otherwise. We often blame God for our own sins. Many people are killed by kind friends. I have seen it more than once. Peanuts, popcorn, and candy have caused many convulsions in children and some deaths.

It is generally allowable to give a little liquid food every two hours in acute diseases. It should be given at regular intervals in the conscious or unconscious patients, especially in long continued diseases.

LIQUID DIET.

1. Cream soups; tomato, pea, corn, celery, rice, spinach, asparagus, potato.

2. Gruels; oatmeal, cornmeal, cream of wheat, flour gluten (for diabetes).

How to Albuminize Fruit Juices.--Into a cup of lemonade, orangeade, grape juice, etc., put white of an egg slightly beaten, mix thoroughly, strain and serve.

The following may or may not be albuminized.

3. Fruit juices; lemonade, orangeade, unfermented grape juice, currant, berry juice.

4. Milk; peptonized milk, albuminized, buttermilk, malted milk, and milk porridge.

5. Stimulating drinks; tea, coffee, cocoa.

6. Broths; beef broth, mutton broth, chicken broth, bouillon, consomme, oyster broth, clam broth, oyster soup, clam soup, beef tea, and beef juice.

7. Eggs; raw eggs and egg-nog.

8. Cooling and nourishing drinks; oatmeal water, rice water, barley water and toast water. Ices and ice cream may be included in the liquid diet list.

SOFT DIET.--This diet includes everything in the liquid diet list, and the following additional foods:

1. Bread: soft bread; dry toast; milk, water or cream toast, brown bread (after the first day on soft diet).

2. Eggs: poached, soft-boiled and shirred.

3. Cereals: all cooked for some hours; cornmeal, oatmeal rice, sago, wheaten grits and cream of wheat.

4. Desserts: junket, custards, milk puddings, rice, thoroughly cooked, tapioca, jellies, baked and stewed apples, prunes whipped and stewed, ices and ice cream.

CONVALESCENT DIET.--This includes everything in the liquid and soft diet lists and the following in addition:--

1. Breads: wheat, rye, Boston brown and graham bread and biscuits.

2. Meats: broiled steak, mutton, fish, game and fowl, or stewed fowl. Also calf's head, calf 's brains, shell fish and oysters.

3. Eggs, as in soft diet.

4. Drinks as in soft diet.

5. Vegetables: tomatoes, green peas, string beans, potatoes (Irish and sweet), lettuce, cresses, asparagus, onions, celery, spinach and mushrooms.

6. Desserts: custards, creams, jellies, ripe fruits and stewed fruits. No pastry or rich puddings.

FOODS FOR DIFFERENT MEALS FOR THOSE WHO CAN EAT,

BUT WHO DO NOT HAVE MUCH APPETITE.

Breakfast; drinks: tea, coffee, cocoa, milk or albuminized fruit juices; cereal with cream; eggs; omelet, scrambled or poached on a piece of round toast, or soft boiled in a hot cup; muffins or gems.

Dinner; broiled porterhouse or tenderloin steak; baked potatoes; bread or rolls; pretty salad, as apple salad in apple case; custard baked in souffle dish; tea, cocoa or milk.

Supper; broiled squab, raw oysters or meat balls, asparagus tips on toast, fresh or stewed fruit, bread cut in fancy shapes.

Foods that may be taken together.--Meat; eggs: soft boiled, poached, shirred or baked; potatoes, baked, boiled or mashed; fruit sauce and ices may go with the following: stewed tomatoes, salad, spinach, or cucumbers, acid drinks, etc., any foods prepared with vinegar.

Meats, vegetables cooked in milk, or served with cream sauce, cream soups and eggs prepared with milk may be given with fruits, vegetables, drinks, etc., containing no acids.

Foods that should not be taken together.--Any food prepared with milk should not be given with lemonade, tomatoes, salads containing much vinegar or any foods served with vinegar or lemon juice.

Diets in Fevers.--Furnished us by a Trained Nurse in a Hospital.

May Take--

Foods.--Soups, clear or thickened with some well-cooked farinaceous substance, mutton, clam or chicken broth, beef tea, peptonized milk, panopepton with crushed ice.

Drinks.--Pure cold water, toast water, lemon or orange juice in cold water, jelly water, cold whey; all in small quantities sipped slowly.

Must Not Take--

Any solid or vegetable food or fruit until so directed by the physician in charge, **Diet in Debility sent us from one of our Leading Hospitals.**

May Take--

Soups.--Any broth thickened with farinaceous material, chicken or beef soup containing chopped meat, rich vegetable soups, whole beef tea.

Fish.--All fresh fish, boiled or broiled, raw oysters.

Meats.--Beef, mutton, chicken, game, boiled ham, lamb chops or cutlet, broiled bacon, tender juicy steak, hamburger steak.

Eggs.--Soft boiled, poached, scrambled, raw with sherry wine.

Farinaceous.--Cracked wheat, rolled oats, mush, sago, tapioca, hominy, barley, macaroni, vermicelli, rolls, biscuits, cakes, whole wheat bread, corn bread, milk toast, dry toast, brown bread.

Vegetables.--Nearly all perfectly fresh and well cooked.

Desserts.--Custards, egg and milk, rice or apple pudding, baked apples, fruit jams, jellies, cocoa junket, marmalade, sweet fruits, calf 's foot jelly.

Drinks.--Cocoa, chocolate, milk hot, cold or peptonized, pure water, plain or aerated, wineglassful of panopepton.

Must Not Take-

Hashes, stews, cooked oysters or clams, pork, veal, thin soups, turkey, salt meats, except ham and bacon, cabbage, cucumbers, turnips, carrots, squash, spices, pickles, vinegar, pies, pastry, bananas, pineapples.

DISHES FOR THE SICK ROOM.

Oatmeal Gruel.--Boil one part oatmeal and two parts water in double boiler two hours; strain through gravy strainer, add one quart sweet cream, a little sugar, pinch of salt. Do not make it too sweet.

Raspberry Shrub.--Place red raspberries in a stone jar and cover them with good cider vinegar, let stand over night, next morning strain and to one pint of juice add one pint of sugar, boil ten minutes, bottle hot. When desiring to use place two tablespoonfuls full of the liquid in a glass of ice water; very nice.

Root Beer.--Take blackberry root, black cherry bark, spruce boughs, wintergreens, sarsaparilla roots; steep in a large vessel till all the goodness is out; strain, and when lukewarm put in a cup of yeast, let work, bottle up, sugar to sweeten.

Cream Toast.--Toast a piece of light bread and moisten it with hot water; butter and then put on a layer of sweet cream on top and place in oven a moment. This is easily digested.

Lemon Jelly.--On one box gelatine pour 1 pint cold water and let stand one or two hours. Then put on 4 cups of granulated sugar, squeeze juice of 4 lemons with the grated rind of one. When gelatine is dissolved, pour over it one quart boiling water and stir. Pour this over sugar and lemon juice and stir thoroughly until all is dissolved; strain. Put fruit in if desired--turn into molds, cool until firm.

Baked Custard.--One quart milk. 4 eggs beaten light (separately). 5 tablespoons sugar, mixed with the yolks; nutmeg and vanilla. Scald but do not boil the milk, add, gradually, yolks and sugar, then add whites and flavor. Pour into dish or cups, set in pan of hot water, grate nutmeg over top and bake until firm. Eat cold.

Mountain Dew.--Yolks of two eggs, 3 crackers (rolled),--four if small. 1 pint milk, pinch of salt, cook in double boiler. Beat whites of two eggs stiff, add 3/4 cup sugar, lemon extract for flavor. Set in oven and brown. This will serve four people.

Raspberry Vinegar.--Equal parts of red and black raspberries, wash them and cover with cider vinegar, let stand over night. Strain and to each pint of juice take 1 lb. white sugar and boil 15 minutes. Bottle ready for use. To drink use about 2 tablespoons in glass of ice water.

Milk Porridge.--l tablespoon each of cornmeal and wheat flour wet to a paste with cold water, cook in two cups boiling water twenty minutes, then add 2 cups milk and cook a few minutes, stirring often.

Lemon Velvet.--l qt. milk, 2 cups sugar, juice of 2 lemons. Chill the milk, then add the sugar and lemon mixed, and freeze like sherbet.

Ice Cream.--Mix 3 cups sugar and 2 tablespoons flour and stir into 2 qts. hot milk until flour is cooked. When cool add 1 qt. cream, whipped, and one tablespoonful vanilla. Freeze.

Sago Custard.--Soak 2 tablespoons sago in a tumbler of water an hour or more, then boil in same until clear. Add a tumbler of sweet milk; when it boils add sugar to taste, then a beaten egg and flavoring.

Crust Coffee.--Toast bread very brown, pour on boiling water, strain and add cream and sugar. Good for stomach and diarrhea.

Cream Soup.--One pint boiling water, one-half cup of cream, add pieces of toasted bread and a little salt.

Cinnamon Tea.--To 1/2 pint fresh milk add stick or ground cinnamon, enough to flavor, and white sugar to taste; bring to the boiling point and take either warm or cold. Excellent for diarrhea in children or adults.

Barley Water.--Add two ounces pearl barley to 1/2 pint of boiling water; simmer five minutes, drain and add 2 qts. boiling water, add two ounces of sliced figs, and two ounces of raisins; boil until reduced to one quart. Strain for drink.

Arrowroot Custard.--One tablespoonful of arrowroot, one pint milk, one egg, two tablespoons sugar. Mix the arrowroot with a little cold milk and beat in the egg and sugar, pour into the boiling milk and scald until thickened, flavor and pour into cups to cool.

Odors.--A few drops of oil of lavender poured into a glass of very hot water will purify the air of the room almost instantly from cooking odors; the effect is especially refreshing in a sick room.

Dainty Way to Serve Egg on Toast.--Pile the well-beaten white of an egg on a slice of buttered toast, which has been softened with hot water. Make a hollow in the white and drop the yolk therein. Set in the oven to cook the egg.

Oatmeal Gruel.--Pour boiling water over a cupful of rolled oats, stir and let stand a moment, then strain off the liquid. Season with sugar and a little cream if desired. Especially good for children.

Prepared Flour for Summer Complaint.--Take a double handful of flour, tie up in a cloth and cook from three to six hours in a kettle of boiling water. Take out and remove the cloth and you have a hard, round ball. Keep in a dry, cool place. Prepare by grating from this ball into boiling milk enough to make it as thick as you desire, stirring it just before removing from the fire with a stick of cinnamon to give it a pleasant flavor. Salt the milk a little. This is very good for children having summer complaint.

Chicken Broth.--Take the first and second joints of a chicken, boil in a quart of water until tender, season with a very little salt and pepper.

Fever Drinks--Pour cold water on wheat bran, let boil one-half hour, strain and add sugar and lemon juice. Pour boiling water on flaxseed and let stand until it is ropy, pour into hot lemonade and drink.

Egg Gruel.--Beat the yolk of an egg with one tablespoonful sugar, beating the white separately; add one cup boiling water to that yolk, then stir in the whites and add any seasoning. Good for a cold.

Diabetic Bread.--Take one quart of set milk or milk and water, one heaping teaspoonful of good butter, one-fifth of a cake of compressed yeast beaten up with a little water, and two well-beaten eggs. Stir in gluten flour until a soft dough is formed; knead as in making ordinary bread; place in pans to raise, and when light bake in hot oven.

Lime Water.--Into an earthen jar containing hot water stir a handful of fresh unslaked lime. Allow it to settle; then decant the clear fluid and bottle it. Water may again be added to the lime, and the mixture covered and allowed to stand to be decanted as needed.

Vanilla Snow.--Cook one-half cup of rice. When nearly done add one-half cup of cream, small pinch of salt, beaten white of one egg, one-half cup of sugar, flavor with vanilla. Pile in a dish and dot with jelly. Serve with sugar and cream.

Omelet.--One egg, white and yolk beaten separately; two tablespoons milk, one-third teaspoon each of flour and melted butter, a little salt. Add the beaten white last. Pour in small spider in which is a little melted butter (hot) and cook over moderate fire. When it thickens and looks from under the edges, fold it over and slip it on a hot dish.

Almond Milk.--Blanch one pound of sweet and two of bitter almonds that have been soaked in cold water for twenty-four hours. This is done by pouring boiling water over the almonds when, after a few minutes, they can easily be pressed out of their hulls. Grind the almonds in a mill or pound them in a mortar; mix with a half-pint of warm milk or water and allow the mixture to stand two hours after which strain through a cloth, pressing the juice out well.

Brandy and Egg Mixture.--Rub the yolks of two eggs with half an ounce of white sugar; add four ounces of cinnamon water; one coffee-spoonful of white sugar.

Cold Eggnog.--Beat up an egg; add to it two teaspoonfuls of sugar, a glassful of milk and a tablespoonful of brandy or good whisky; mix thoroughly.

Hot Eggnog.--Beat up the yolk of one egg; add a teaspoonful or two of sugar and a glassful of hot milk; strain and add a tablespoonful of brandy or old whisky, or flavor with nutmeg or wine.

Egg Broth.--Beat up an egg and add to it half a teaspoonful of sugar and a pinch of salt; over this pour a glass of hot milk and serve immediately. Hot water, broth, soup, or tea may be used in place of milk.

Egg Cordial.--Beat up the white of an egg until light; add a tablespoonful of cream and beat up together, then add two tablespoonfuls of sugar and a tablespoonful of brandy.

Caudle.--Beat up an egg to a froth; add a wineglassful of sherry wine, and sweeten with a teaspoonful of sugar; if desired flavor with lemon peel. Stir this mixture into a half-pint of gruel; over this grate a little nutmeg and serve with hot toast.

Albumin Water.--Beat the white of one egg until very light and strain through a clean napkin. Add six ounces of water. If intended for an infant a pinch of salt may be added. A teaspoonful or more of sugar and a teaspoonful or more of lemon juice, orange juice, or sherry wine may be added to enhance its palatableness. This drink may also conveniently be made by placing all the ingredients in a lemon-shaker, shaking until thoroughly mixed and then straining. Serve cold.

Apple Water.--Pour a cupful of boiling water over two mashed baked apples; cool, strain, and sweeten. Serve with shaved ice if desired.

Currant Juice.--Take an ounce of currant juice or a tablespoonful of currant jelly. Over this pour a cupful of boiling water (use cold water with the juice) and sweeten to taste.

Lemonade.--Take the juice of one lemon or three tablespoonfuls of lemon juice; add from one to three tablespoonfuls of sugar and a cupful (six ounces) of cold water. Serve with cracked or shaved ice if desired.

Syrup for Cough of Long Standing.--"Five cents worth of flax seed, a little rock candy, two tablespoons of best brandy and a lemon makes the finest cough syrup in the world. Steep flaxseed a short time, strain and add rock candy to sweeten, then juice of one lemon and the brandy. One physician says it is as good as anything he can put up."

Syrup of Lemons for Fever Cases and to Disguise the Taste of Bad Medicines.--"Boil for ten minutes a pint of lemon juice, strain, add two pounds of brown sugar and dissolve. When cold add two and one-half ounces of alcohol. A fine addition to drinks in fever cases and good to disguise the taste of medicines."

Lemonade.--Pare the rind from one lemon, cut the lemon into slices, and place both in a pitcher with an ounce of sugar. Over this pour a pint of boiling water and let it stand until cold. Strain and serve with cracked ice.

Albuminzed Lemonade.--Shake together a cupful of water, two teaspoonfuls of lemon juice, two teaspoonfuls of sugar, and the white of an egg. Serve at once.

Orangeade.--Cut the rind from one orange; over the rind pour a cupful of boiling water; then add the juice of the orange and a tablespoonful of sugar; cool, strain, and serve with shaved ice if desired. If this is too sweet, a tablespoonful of lemon juice may be added.

Imperial Drink.--Add a teaspoonful of cream of tartar to a pint of boiling water; into this squeeze the juice of half a lemon, or more if desired; sweeten to taste and serve cold. This drink is most useful in fevers and nephritis.

Flaxseed Tea.--Add six teaspoonfuls of flaxseed to a quart of water; boil for half an hour; cool, strain, sweeten, and if desired flavor with a little lemon juice.

Mulled Wine.--One-fourth of a cupful of hot water, one-half inch of stick cinnamon, two cloves, a tiny bit of nutmeg, one-half cupful of port (heated) two tablespoonfuls of sugar. Boil all the ingredients except the wine and sugar for ten minutes; then add the wine and sugar, strain, and serve very hot.

Grape Juice.--Pluck Concord grapes from the stem. Wash and heat them, stirring constantly. When the skins have been broken, pour the fruit into a jelly bag and press slightly. Measure the juice and add one-quarter the quantity of sugar. Boil the juice and sugar together and then pour into hot bottles; cork and seal with paraffin or equal parts of shoemaker's wax and resin melted together. Less sugar may be used.

Oatmeal, Barley or Rice Water. From the Grain: Use two tablespoonfuls of grain to a quart of water. The grain should have been previously soaked over night or at least for a few hours. When required for an emergency the soaking may be dispensed with and the grain boiled for five minutes instead. The water in which the grain was soaked should be poured off and fresh water added before cooking. The grain should be boiled for several hours, water being added from time to time to keep the quantity up to a quart. Strain. This makes a somewhat thin, watery gruel. From prepared flours: Various brands of prepared grain flours are on the market, such, for example, as Robinson's Barley flour. These are all somewhat similar in preparation. From two rounded teaspoonfuls to a tablespoonful of the prepared flour is added to a pint of boiling water and this is boiled from fifteen to thirty minutes and then strained. No previous soaking is required.

CEREALS AND CEREAL GRUELS.

Either the grain itself or the specially prepared flour may be used. When the grains are used they should be spread on a clean table and all foreign substances removed. If the whole grains be used, it is well to wash them, after picking them over, with two or three changes of cold water. Cereals are best cooked in a double boiler. The lower part should be filled about one-third full of water and, if more is added during the soaking, it should always be boiling hot. The cereal should be boiled over the fire for ten or fifteen minutes. The water should be boiled first and then salted. The cereal is added gradually and the whole stirred to prevent it from burning. It should then be placed in the double boiler and steamed until thoroughly cooked. Cereals, like other starchy foods, require thorough cooking. Most recipes allow too short a time. Oatmeal, especially, should be mentioned. It develops a better flavor if cooked for three hours or more, and is better when it is prepared the day before and reheated when used. It should be just thin enough to pour when taken out of boiler, and when cooled should form a jelly.

Any cereal mush may be thinned with water, milk or cream and made into a gruel, or the gruel may be made directly from the grain or flour. Gruels should be thin, not too sweet nor too highly flavored, and served very hot. Milk gruels should be made in a double boiler. Gruels can be made more nutritious by the addition of whipped egg, either the white or yolk or both, and the various concentrated food products.

When cereal flours are used, the flour should be rubbed to a smooth paste with a little cold water and added slowly to boiling water, stirring constantly until it is thoroughly mixed.

LENGTH OF TIME TO COOK CEREALS.

Cornmeal mush:	Boil 10 minutes, then steam for 3 hours or more.
Oatmeal:	Boil 10 mins, then steam for l-1/2 hours or more.
Irish oatmeal:	Boil 10 minutes, then steam for 8 hours or more.
Wheatena:	Boil 10 minutes, then steam for 10 hours or more.
Gluten mush:	Boil 30 minutes.
Steamed rice:	Steam for one hour.
Boiled rice:	Boil for twenty minutes or until soft.

Arrowroot Gruel.--Dissolve half a teaspoonful of sugar and a quarter of a teaspoonful of salt in a cupful of water and heat. Mix half a teaspoonful of arrowroot flour with a little water and add to the heated water. Boil for twenty minutes, stirring constantly; then add a cupful of milk, bring to a boil, strain, and serve hot.

Barley Gruel.--Proceed as above, using a tablespoonful of Robinson's Barley flour instead of arrowroot.

Oatmeal Gruel.--As above, but use oatmeal, and boil for half an hour or longer before adding the milk.

Farina Gruel.--Proceed as in making arrowroot gruel, using instead a tablespoonful of farina, and boil ten minutes before adding the milk.

Cracker Gruel.--Brown the crackers, and reduce to a powder by means of a rolling-pin. Add three tablespoonfuls of the powdered crackers to half a cupful of milk and half a cupful of boiling water; cook for ten minutes; then add one-fourth of a teaspoonful of salt and serve.

Cornmeal Gruel.--Take a tablespoonful of cornmeal and moisten with a little cold water. Stir this into a pint of boiling water to which a pinch of salt has been added. Cook for three hours in a double boiler, or for thirty minutes directly over the fire. In the latter case it must be stirred constantly.

Gluten Gruel.--Mix a tablespoonful of gluten flour with one-fourth of a cupful of cold water and stir this into one cupful of boiling salted water. Cook directly over the fire for fifteen minutes; then add one clove and cook over boiling water for a half hour.

Tapioca Jelly.--Soak a cupful of tapioca of the best quality in a pint of cold water for two hours; when soft, place in a saucepan with sugar, the rind and juice of one lemon, a pinch of salt, and another pint of water; stir the mixture until it boils; turn into a mold and set away to cool; if desired, a glassful of wine may be added.

Chestnut Puree.--One pound of chestnuts (not horse-chestnuts) are peeled, and boiled in water until the second (inside) skin comes off easily. The chestnuts are placed in a sieve until all the water drains off. They are then washed in a dish and afterwards passed through a sieve. Melt three ounces of butter in a stew-pan on the fire, add a little salt and sugar,--enough to cover the point of a knife, and then the chestnuts. Stew them for half an hour, stirring frequently; pour in enough bouillon so that the mush does not get too thick.

Brown Bread.--Take one-half cupful scalded milk, one-half cupful of water, one teaspoonful of salt, one-half teaspoonful of butter, one-half teaspoonful lard, two tablespoonfuls of molasses, one-half cupful of white flour, sufficient graham flour to knead, and three-quarters of a yeast cake dissolved in one-quarter of a cupful of lukewarm water. Prepare the same as white bread. Instead of graham flour, equal parts of graham flour and white flour may be used in kneading.

Whole Wheat Bread.--Dissolve a quarter of a yeast cake in a tablespoonful of lukewarm water. Pour half a cupful of hot water over half a cupful of milk and when lukewarm add the yeast and half a teaspoonful of salt. To this add a cupful of whole-wheat flour and beat for five minutes. Cover and allow this to stand in a warm place for two hours and a half. Then add whole-wheat flour gradually, mixing the mass until it can be kneaded. Knead until elastic; shake and place in baking pans. Cover and allow to stand in a warm place until it doubles in bulk. Prick the top with a fork and bake for one hour. The oven should not be as hot as for white bread.

Cream-of-Tomato Soup.--One can tomatoes, one-fourth teaspoonful soda, one-half cupful of butter, one-third cup of flour, 3-1/4 teaspoonfuls of salt, one-half teaspoonful of white pepper, one quart of milk. Stew the tomatoes slowly one-half to an hour, strain and add soda while hot; make a white sauce and add the tomato juice. Serve immediately.

Cream-of-Celery Soup.--One and one-half cupful of celery, one pint of water, one cupful of milk, one cupful cream, two tablespoonfuls of butter, one-half cupful of flour, one-half teaspoonful of salt, one-eighth teaspoonful of white pepper. Cook the celery in the boiling water until very soft; strain and add the hot liquid; make a white sauce and cook until it is thick cream.

Cream-of-Potato Soup.--Three potatoes, two cupfuls milk, one-half cupful of cream, yolks of two eggs, one teaspoonful of salt, pepper, one-half teaspoonful of onion juice. Cook the potatoes until soft, drain, mash, add the hot liquid, and strain; add the beaten yolks and seasoning. Cook in a double boiler until the egg thickens, stirring constantly. Serve immediately.

Oyster Stew.--One cupful of milk, one pint of oysters, one-fourth teaspoonful of salt, one tablespoonful of butter, pepper. Heat the milk. Cook and strain the oyster juice. Add the oysters, which have been rinsed, and cook until the edges curl. Add seasoning, butter and hot milk. Serve at once This soup may be thickened with a tablespoonful of flour cooked in butter as for white sauce.

Peptonized Milk.--Cold Process.--Mix milk, water and peptonizing agents, and immediately place the bottle on ice. Use when ordinary milk is required. This is particularly suited for dyspeptics and individuals with whom milk does not, as a rule, agree. The flavor of the milk remains unchanged.

Peptonized Milk.--Warm Process.--Put in a glass jar one pint of milk and four ounces of cold water; add five grains of extract of pancreas and fifteen grains of bicarbonate of soda. After mixing thoroughly, place the jar in water as hot as can be borne by the hand (about 115 degrees). This should be heated for from six to twenty minutes. At the end of this time it may be placed upon ice until required. The contents of one of Fairchild's peptonizing tubes may be used in place of the pancreas extract. If the milk is to be kept for any length of time, it should be brought to a boil, to prevent the formation of too much peptone, which renders the milk bitter.

Hot Peptonized Milk.--Mix together the usual peptonizing ingredients and add a pint of fresh cold milk; after thoroughly shaking the bottle, place it on ice. When needed pour out the required amount, heat it, and drink it as hot as it can agreeably be taken. If required for immediate use, the ingredients may be mixed together in a saucepan and slowly heated to the proper temperature.

Peptonized Milk Punch.--In the usual milk punch recipes the specially peptonized milk may be used in place of ordinary milk. Take a goblet one-third full of finely crushed ice; pour on it a tablespoonful of rum and a dash of curacao, or any other liquor agreeable to the taste. Fill the glass with peptonized milk; stir well, sweeten to taste and grate a little nutmeg on top.

Peptonized Milk Gruel.--Mix with a teaspoonful of wheat flour, arrowroot flour, or Robinson's barley flour with half a pint of cold water. Boil for five minutes stirring constantly. Add one pint of cold milk and strain into a jar; add the usual peptonizing ingredients, place in warm water (115 degrees) for twenty minutes, and then put upon ice.

Junket or Curds and Whey.--Take a half-pint of fresh milk; add one teaspoonful of Fairchild's Essence of Pepsin and stir just sufficiently to mix. Pour into custard cups and let it stand until firmly curdled. It may be served plain or with sugar and grated nutmeg. It may be flavored with wine which should be added before curdling takes place.

Junket with Eggs.--Beat one egg to a froth, and sweeten with two teaspoonfuls of white sugar; add this to a half-pint of warm milk; then add one teaspoonful of essence of pepsin and let it stand until curdled.

Milk Punch.--Shake together in a lemonade-shaker a glass of milk, a tablespoonful of rum, brandy, or good old whisky and two teaspoonfuls of sugar. After it has been poured into a glass a little nutmeg may be grated over the top.

Whey.--Take a half-pint of fresh milk heated luke-warm (115 degrees), add one tablespoonful of essence of pepsin and stir just enough to mix. When this is firmly coagulated, beat up with a fork until the curd is finely divided and then strain. For flavoring purposes lemon juice or sherry wine may be added.

Cream of Tartar Whey.--Add a heaping teaspoonful of cream of tartar to a pint of boiling water. Strain, sweeten to taste, and serve cold.

Wine Whey.--Cook together a cupful of milk and half a cupful of sherry wine. As soon as the curd separates, strain and sweeten. This may be eaten hot or cold.

Milk Mixture.--This is made of cream, two parts; milk, one part; lime water, two parts; sugar water, three parts (seventeen and three--fourths drams of milk sugar to a pint of water).

Milk-and-Cinnamon Drink.--Add a small amount of cinnamon to the desired quantity of milk and boil it. Sweeten with sugar and add brandy if desired.

Albuminized Milk.--Shake in a covered jar or lemonade-shaker, a cupful of milk, a tablespoonful of lime water and the white of an egg. Sweeten, flavor as desired and serve at once.

Milk-and-Cereal Waters.--A most valuable method of preparing milk for invalids with whom it disagrees is to mix equal parts of milk and thoroughly cooked barley, rice, oatmeal, or arrowroot water and boil them together for ten minutes. This may be served plain, or flavored by cooking with it a cut-up raisin, a sprig of mace, or a piece of stick cinnamon, which should be strained out before serving.

Irish Moss and Milk.--Soak about two tablespoonfuls of Irish moss for five minutes and wash thoroughly in cold water. Add to a cupful of milk and soak for a half an hour; then heat slowly, stirring constantly, and then boil for ten minutes, preferably in a double boiler; strain, pour into cups and cool. This may be served while hot and may be rendered more nutritious by the addition of the white of an egg stirred into it just before serving.

Eggs.--Eggs and all other albuminous food should be cooked at as low a temperature as possible in order to avoid rendering them tough.

Soft-Cooked Eggs.--Place in a pint of boiling water, remove from the fire, and allow to stand for eight or ten minutes. If the egg is very cold to start with it will take a little longer.

Hard-Cooked Eggs.--Place in water, bring to a boil and then set on the back part of the stove for twenty minutes.

Eggs should be served as soon as cooked and the dishes should be warm and ready.

Rules for Custards.--The eggs should be thoroughly mixed but not beaten light, the sugar and salt added to these, and the hot milk added slowly. Custards must be cooked over moderate heat; if a custard curdles, put it in a pan of cold water and beat until smooth. Custards should always be strained.

Soft Custard.--Take a pint of milk, the yolks of two eggs, two tablespoonfuls of sugar, and a pinch of salt. Mix all except the milk in a bowl. Heat the milk to the boiling-point and add, stirring constantly. As soon as mixed, pour into the saucepan in which the milk has been heated and cook from three to five minutes, stirring constantly until it thickens. Strain and pour into a cold bowl and flavor with from half to one teaspoonful of vanilla, a teaspoonful or more of sherry, or other flavoring material as desired. Custards may be cooked to advantage in a double boiler.

Soup Stock.--To make stock, use a chicken or several pounds of bones with some meat attached, or a pound of lean meat and one quart of water. Cut-up vegetables may be added as desired. For flavoring add a sprig of parsley and of celery, a peppercorn, a small onion, and a scant teaspoonful of salt. Any of the flavoring vegetables may be omitted as desired or others added. The meat should simmer for several hours, until but half the quantity of water remains. Then add the other ingredients, simmer half an hour longer, strain and cool. Remove the fat.

Chicken Broth.--Take one pound of chicken and a pint of cold water. Clean the fowl, cut it into pieces, and remove the skin. Separate the meat from the bone and chop the meat very fine. Place with the bones (if large they should be broken) in the water and soak for an hour. Cook over hot water for four or five hours at a temperature of 190 degrees. Strain and add salt. Water must be added from time to time to keep the quantity up to a pint. Remove the fat. If the broth is to be reheated use a double boiler.

Meat Broth: Beef, Veal, Mutton, or Chicken.--Cover one pound of chopped lean meat with one pint of water, and allow it to stand for from four to six hours. Then cook over a slow fire for an hour until reduced to half the quantity. Cool, skim, pour into a jar and strain.

Veal Broth.--Pour a pint of water on a half-pound of finely chopped lean veal and allow it to stand for three hours. Boil for a few minutes, strain and season with salt.

Clam or Oyster Juice.--Cut the clams or oysters into pieces and heat for a few minutes in their juice. Strain through muslin and serve while hot. In straining great care must be taken that sand does not pass through the muslin. The juices should be diluted and may be frozen.

Clam Broth.--Wash three large clams very thoroughly, using a brush for the purpose. Place in a kettle with a half a cupful of cold water. Heat over fire. As soon as the shells open, the broth is done. Strain through muslin, season and serve.

Mutton Broth with Vegetables.--Allow one pound of neck of mutton to each pint of water; add carrots, turnips, onions, and barley; let all simmer together for three hours.

Mutton Broth Without Meat.--Cook two "shank-ends" in a pint of cold water, and vegetables as directed in the foregoing recipe; simmer for three hours and strain.

Beef Tea.--Cut up a pound of lean beef into pieces the size of dice; put it into a covered jar with two pints of cold water and a pinch of salt. Let it warm gradually and simmer for two hours, care being taken that it does not at any time reach the boiling point.

Beef Tea with Oatmeal.--Mix thoroughly one tablespoonful of groats with two of cold water; add to this a pint of boiling beef tea. Boil for ten minutes, stirring constantly, and strain through a coarse sieve.

Beef Juice.--Broil quickly pieces of the round or sirloin of a size to fit the opening of a lemon squeezer. Both sides of the beef should be scorched quickly to prevent the escape of the juices, but the interior should not be fully cooked. As soon as they are ready pieces of meat should be squeezed in a lemon squeezer previously heated by being dipped in hot water. As it drips the juice should be received into a hot wine glass; it should be seasoned to the taste with salt and a little cayenne pepper, and taken while hot.

Cold Beef Juice.--Cover one pound of finely chopped lean beef with eight ounces of cold water and allow it to stand for eight or ten hours. Squeeze out the juice by means of a muslin bag; season with salt or sherry wine and drink cold or slightly warmed. It may be added to milk, care being taken that the milk be not too hot before the juice is added.

Raw Meat Juice.--Add to finely minced rump steak cold water, in the proportion of one part of water to four parts of meat. Stir well together and allow it to stand for half an hour. Forcibly express the juice through muslin, twisting it to get the best results.

Beef Essence.--Chop up very fine a pound of lean beef free from fat and skin; add a little salt, and put into an earthen jar with a lid; fasten up the edges with a thick paste, such as is used for roasting venison in, and place the jar in the oven for three or four hours. Strain through a coarse sieve, and give the patient two or three tablespoonfuls at a time.

American Bouillon (American Broth).--Place in a tin vessel that can be sealed hermetically alternate layers of finely minced meat and vegetables. Seal it and keep it heated in a water bath (bainmaire) for six or seven hours and then express the broth.

Bottle Bouillon.--Cut beef, free from fat, into squares. Place these in a stoppered bottle, put the bottle in a basin of warm water, heat slowly, and boil for twenty minutes. There will be about an ounce of yellowish or brownish fluid for each three-quarters of a pound of meat used. The flavor is that of concentrated bouillon.

Methods of preparing raw beef.--Meat given raw should always be

perfectly fresh and very finely divided. Scrape the meat with a sharp knife, which will separate the coarser fibers. If the resulting mass is stringy pass through a fine sieve. This may be seasoned with salt and pepper and served on toast, crackers or bread and butter. It may be rolled into small balls and swallowed. These may be flavored as desired. They may also be slightly browned by rolling about rapidly in a hot saucepan, care being taken not to change any but the outside of the ball, and that but slightly. Scraped beef may be served as a liquid or semi-solid food. Mix it with an equal quantity of cold water until it is quite smooth. Place in a double boiler and cook until thoroughly heated, stirring constantly. Add a little salt and pepper and serve at once. This may be made thicker by adding less water.

Raw-beef Soup.--This is made by chopping up one pound of raw beef and placing it in a bottle with one pint of water and five drops of strong hydrochloric acid. This mixture is allowed to stand on the ice over night and in the morning the bottle is placed in a pan of water at 110 degrees and kept at about this temperature for two hours. It is then placed in a stout cloth and strained until the mass that remains is almost dry. The filtrate is given in three portions daily. If the taste of the raw meat is objectionable, the meat may quickly be roasted on one side and the process completed in the manner previously described.

Barley Gruel with Beef Extract.--One-half teaspoonful of "Soluble Beef," two cupfuls of hot water, one tablespoonful of barley flour, one saltspoonful of salt. Dissolve the beef in the hot water, and mix the flour and salt together with a little cold water. Pour the boiling stock on the flour and cook for ten minutes. Strain, and serve very hot.

Beef Broth with Poached Eggs.--Prepare the broth in the proportion of half a teaspoonful of "Soluble Beef" to one cupful of hot water and add a poached egg.

A Nutritive Drink for Delicate Women and Children.--This is made by mixing one-fourth to one-half teaspoonful of "Soluble Beef," five ounces of boiling water and one-half ounce of cream; season with salt and pepper to suit the taste.

Beef Broth with Grain.--Take one teaspoonful of "Soluble Beef," one quart of water, one tablespoonful of rice, and salt to taste. Dissolve the "Soluble Beef" in the hot water and add the well-washed rice. Simmer slowly until dissolved and absorbed by the rice, adding more beef broth if too much boils away. If not entirely dissolved the broth should be strained before using.

Beef Tea Egg-Nog.--This requires one-eighth teaspoonful of "Soluble Beef," one-half cupful of hot water, one tablespoonful of brandy, and a pinch of salt. Beat the egg slightly and add the salt and sugar. Dissolve the "Soluble Beef" in the hot water, add to the egg and strain. Mix thoroughly, adding wine, and serve.

Chicken Jelly.--Half a grown chicken should be well pounded, and boiled in one quart of water for two hours until only a pint remains; season and strain. Serve hot or place on ice, where it will jelly.

Veal-bone Jelly.--Place ten pounds of veal bones and ten quarts of water or weak bouillon over the fire and bring to just a boil. Skim and add two pounds of barley and a little salt. Simmer for five or six hours and then strain. If too thick dilute, before serving, with bouillon. Stir in the yolk of an egg in a cup and serve.

Meat Jelly.--This is made by cooking good boneless, lean beef on a water bath with a little water for sixteen hours or until it becomes gelatinized. Of the artificial preparations on the market for making bouillon the most reliable is Leibig's Extract of Meat (10:250 gm.) or Cibil's Bouillon (one teaspoonfnl to 250 gm.), Inaglio's Bouillon Capsules are also very convenient. If it is desired to make a bouillon more nutritious one teaspoonful of meat peptone may be added.

Jelly for Dyspeptics.--Remove the skin and meat from one calf 's foot; wash the bone and place in cold water on the stove; when it begins to foam skim off the refuse which gathers on top. After rinsing off the scum with cold water put the bones into a pot with one-quarter kilo of beef or half an old hen, one-quarter liter of water, and little salt, and boil slowly for from four to five hours. Pour the jelly thus formed through a fine sieve and place overnight in a cellar. Next morning remove the fat and clarify the cold jelly by adding one egg with its shells mashed, beating and stirring steadily. Then, with the addition of a little cornstarch, subject the whole to a temperature not over 60 degrees F., or the white of the egg will curdle. Constantly beat and stir. If the jelly begins to get grainy, cover and let it cool until the white of the egg becomes flaky and separates. Then strain again several times until it becomes perfectly clear; add 5 gm. of extract of meat, pour the jelly into a mold, and let it cool again. The gravy from a roast may be utilized and is very palatable. It must be stirred in while the mass is still warm and liquid. This jelly is usually relished with cold fowl, but spoils easily in summer; it must therefore be kept on ice.

Gluten Bread.--Mix one pound of gluten flour with three-fourth of a pint or one pint of water at 85 degrees. (With some of the prepared flours--Bishop's, for example--no yeast is required). As soon as the dough is mixed put it into tins and place them immediately in the oven; should be made into small dinner rolls and baked on flat tins. The loaves take about one and one-half hours to bake, and the rolls three-fourths of an hour. Either are easily made. The addition of a little salt improves the bread. (When any special brand of flour is used, the directions that accompany it should be followed closely).

A GENERAL DESCRIPTION OF THE FOUR LEADING SCHOOLS OF MEDICINE:

ALLOPATHY, HOMEOPATHY, OSTEOPATHY AND ECLECTICISM.

ALLOPATHY.--Literally the word Allopathy means "other suffering," from the Greek "allos" meaning other, and "pathos" meaning suffering. A more liberal translation would be,--other methods of treating suffering. The term was first used during the latter part of the eighteenth century by Hahnemann, the founder of the Homeopathic School, to distinguish the ordinary or regular practice of medicine as opposed to Homeopathy.

Notwithstanding the comparatively recent origin of the term, however, the methods and theories of Allopathy are based empirically upon the results of the practice of medicine since the time of Galen, and logically upon the scientific facts disclosed by modern research and study. In its broad and popular sense, Allopathy is the preservation of health and the treatment of disease by the use of any means that will produce a condition incompatible with the disease.

The application of the theories and methods of this "old school" necessitates a thorough knowledge of anatomy, pharmocology, pathology, bacteriology, physiology and other sciences. At the present time much stress is also laid upon the means for the prevention and the eradication of diseases and their causes. The inefficiency of drugs is recognized and besides the articles of the Materia Medica the "regular" physician makes use of antitoxins, vaccines, surgery, electricity, baths, etc., in treating diseases. Everyday examples of their methods may be seen in the use of quinine in Malaria, antitoxins in Diphtheria and vaccines in Smallpox, etc.

HOMEOPATHY.--This school was founded by Hahnemann, who lived in Germany over a hundred years ago. Everyone now admits that he was a great scholar. In translating a materia medica he was very much struck with the article on cinchona, where it seemed to state that taken continuously in large doses it would produce all the indications of ague. He tested other remedies in the same way and finally announced his law "Similia Similibus Curantur."

Definition given by a Medical Dictionary of Homeopathy.--"A system of treatment of disease by the use of agents that, administered in health, would produce symptoms similar to those for the relief of which they are given." For instance, ipecac given in large doses, will produce certain kind of vomiting. If the same kind of vomiting, with the other symptoms agreeing, occurs in disease ipecac would be given for the trouble.

But if the vomiting was produced by ipecac, that same medicine would not be given to stop it, but treatment given for an over dose of the drug, ipecac. According to the principles of Homeopathy a medicine is selected which possesses the power (drug diseases) of extinguishing a natural disease by means of the similitude of its alterative qualities, (similia similibus curantur); such a medicine administered in simple form at long intervals, and in doses so fine as to be just sufficient without causing pain or debility, to obliterate the natural disease through the reaction of vital energy.

A great many medicines are used in this way by all schools, but the "regular" school claims it is not an universal law. Some homeopathic doctors claim that the antitoxin treatment for diphtheria, etc. is an application of the homeopathic law. The poison that produces the diphtheria is taken and from this by a thorough and precise process the serum is made and injected into the body of a person who has diphtheria.

Hydrophobia is successfully treated in the same way. A homeopathic doctor has a right to use any sized doses he wishes, but he claims experience has proven that large doses are not often necessary and that the medicine usually acts better attenuated.

ECLECTICISM.--An eclectic physician is a member of a school or system that claims to select "that which is good from all other schools."

This school uses very few mineral remedies, but uses many vegetable remedies. They have introduced a great many vegetable remedies into medical practice and very many of them are useful.

The homeopathic school has benefited very much by the experience of the eclectic system. This school uses remedies in large and small doses. Many of them use the homeopathic attenuated drugs.

OSTEOPATHY.--"The name 'Osteopathy' is made up of two Greek words: 'Osteon,' which means 'bone,' and 'pathos,' which means suffering (to suffer). 'Pathy,' our English equivalent for this word, by usage has come to mean "a system of treatment for suffering or disease. Hence, viewed strictly from its derivation, this term, Osteopathy, would carry only the meaning of bone suffering, 'bone disease' or 'bone treatment.'"

Definition.--"Osteopathy is that science of treating human ailments which regards most diseases as being either primarily produced or maintained by an obstruction to the free passage of nerve impulses or blood and lymph flow, and undertakes by manipulation to remove such obstruction so that nature may resume her perfect work."

Explanation.--"While it is a distinctive theory of osteopathy that disease conditions, not due to a specific poison, are traceable to mechanical disorder in the body, or some part of it, and that the correction of such disorder is not only the rational treatment, but is necessary to the restoration of a permanent condition of health, yet as a palliative treatment appropriate manipulations are occasionally employed to stimulate or inhibit functional activity as conditions may require. Osteopaths also employ such rational hygienic measures, common to all systems of healing, as has been proven of undoubted value, and take into account environmental influences, habits and modes of life, as affecting the body in maintaining or regaining health."

The "American School of Osteopathy" is located in Kirksville, Missouri.

The course of study required is of three years duration, of nine months each, and the degree of D. O. (Doctor of Osteopathy) is given to the graduates.

OPERATIONS.

There has been a great change in regard to operations among the laity of late years. There is much less opposition and prejudice. The people are being educated to the necessity for operating in many diseases. A great deal of the opposition was due to the doctors themselves. There have been doctors who would operate at every opportunity. Some doctors could not treat a woman for diseases of the womb and ovaries without suggesting that an operation was necessary. There have been a great many healthy organs removed, or at least organs that could have been saved by proper treatment. Fortunately such doctors are becoming less in number and there is more discrimination being used. On the other hand there has also been too much conservatism. Many persons have spent years in suffering who could have been relieved by an operation. Years ago a person suffering from terrific attacks of gall stone colic continued to suffer all their natural life. Now an operation is performed and relief is obtained at very little risk to life. The same is true of cancers, tumors, etc. These, if taken early, can be removed safely and successfully in very many cases and lives saved and suffering relieved.

If an operation is needed the family should go to their family physician, in whom they have confidence. He can do the operation or direct the family as to what surgeon to choose. Bad results of operations are, sometimes, due to the operator. It is the duty of the family to choose a competent and honest surgeon. There are plenty of them all over the world,--and very few competent surgeons operate simply for the money they receive. As a rule they earn all and more than they are paid. There are more surgeons today than ever and they are also more competent, for our medical schools prepare them in the hospitals for that kind of work.

The surgeons connected with our hospitals, public and private, are doing a great work in relieving the ills of humanity, others in private practice are doing great work. Here and there one is found who operates only for the money, but persons who employ such a doctor are usually entitled to the results they receive. Your family physician, even if he is not a surgeon, is the best person to consult when an operation may be necessary. He will send you to some honest and competent man. Operations usually should be performed as early as possible. In malignant disease the operation must be done early. This applies to cancers of the lip, face, tongue, breast, womb, ovaries, stomach and the abdominal cavity.

Then again, operations are far less dangerous now than before the days of aseptic and antiseptic surgery. Cleanliness on the part of the surgeon, nurses and patient is the first law of success in all operations. Any case that becomes infected through fault of the surgeon or attendants is no longer looked upon as a thoroughly successful operation, even though the patient recovers.

As in other branches of medicine, there are now many specialists in surgery. In the major operations it is best to employ a specialist, but in the minor cases the "family doctor" should be competent. If he does not care to perform the operation himself he can advise and direct you in selecting a competent surgeon. Always seek his advice early; do not wait until the patient is weak or dying before you decide to allow the operation, as then the chances are it cannot help. If you are in doubt as to the necessity of the operation consult more than one surgeon. There is a possibility of a wrong diagnosis in some cases.

SPECIAL OPERATIONS.

ADENOIDS.--Should be removed early when they obstruct the breathing. In another part of the book the reasons are given. The same advice is given for tumors and malformations in the nose passages. Such conditions should not be allowed to go on until the parts are permanently deformed or diseased. These operations are done very frequently and successfully now, and many people are saved years of worry and suffering. For more extended account see department of nose and throat.

APPENDICITIS.--There has been a great deal of discussion about this disease. It is no doubt true that many healthy appendices have been removed, but it is also true that many lives have been saved by operation. There is more discrimination now than formerly in this disease. Blood tests, etc., aid in telling when an operation is necessary in acute cases. There is very little danger in a chronic case if the operation is done during the interval of the attacks.

CATARACT.--The operation for this trouble is gloriously successful and the blind are daily recovering their sight through this operation.

MASTOID.--Operations on the Mastoid cells are frequently performed now and save many lives. When there is swelling behind the ear or there is much pain there a careful examination should be made. Chronic cases of Mastoid disease usually demand this operation.

OVARIES, TUMORS OF THE.--The operation for tumors is very successful. If the ovary is simply enlarged by congestion, medicine will frequently reduce it; but when the enlargement is due to a tumor, it should be removed if it continues to enlarge. Sometimes there is cancer of the ovary. If so, it should be operated upon early. Tumors of the womb, such as fibroids, are often observed. They sometimes require removal if they grow large. The symptoms will indicate when an operation is needed. These tumors often grow so large as to necessitate the removal of the womb.

PERINEUM AND CERVIX.--The perineum and cervix are sometimes torn during labor and should be immediately repaired. The perineum is the support for the organs of generation and if it is not solid the ovaries, tubes, womb and vagina will sag and fall. Neglect of this simple operation at the proper time results in backaches, headaches, etc. Many women have suffered for years and doctored for other complaints when proper attention to the real trouble would have saved all that expense and pain. Your physician should be requested, in advance, to attend before he leaves to any laceration that may occur during labor. At this time it causes little or no pain. If postponed until next day or later it would be painful and require an anesthetic. Many cases of cancer are caused by neglected lacerations.

PILES.--It is often necessary to operate both for external and internal piles. The result is usually complete relief and cure.

CANCERS.--Cancers should be operated on early. A sore on the womb, lip or tongue, or lump on the breast that continues for a little time without getting better, is dangerous. It may soon spread in the surrounding tissue and general system. Operations on the womb and breast, performed in time, are very successful. Such tumors or sores should not be neglected. A lump in the breast should be examined early. The womb should be examined if there is a discharge from the vagina that continues. In such a case the family doctor can determine what should be done. A sore on the lip, tongue, face, etc., that continues and refuses to heal should cause suspicion and be shown to a physician.

PLEURISY.--"Water in the chest" sometimes follows pleurisy. This, if not absorbed, must be drawn off and is quite easily done. After some cases of pneumonia the lung does not clear up properly and pus forms in it. An operation is sometimes necessary to evacuate it. This should be performed before the patient becomes very much exhausted. Some people allow it to continue too long and thus lessen the chances of recovery when an operation is at last performed.

SQUINT.--There is no need for any person being cross-eyed if attention is early given to the trouble. Sometimes properly fitted glasses will correct this trouble, but an operation is often necessary and is very successful and not serious or painful.

TRACHEOTOMY AND INTUBATION.--The operation of tracheotomy, opening of the wind-pipe, is performed where there is choking from a foreign body in the wind-pipe or when it has become suddenly closed in diseases such as croup and diphtheria. It is always an emergency operation and is only resorted to when it is evident that unless severe measures are taken the patient will choke to death. Intubation is more frequently practised in disease when the breathing has become difficult owing to the growth of membrane in the larynx. A tube of the proper size is placed in the wind-pipe and allowed to remain there until the disease has lost its force and the membrane no longer obstructs the air passage. This tube allows the patient to breathe freely as it furnishes an opening for the air and an attendant notices the change immediately. Intubation should be performed before the patient has become weak.

TONSILS.--A person who is subject to enlarged tonsils should watch them carefully. If they contain pus for any length of time they should be removed, for they not only obstruct the breathing, but are a menace to the health. Enucleation is usually the best method of removal. Enucleation means the operation of extracting a tumor in entirety after opening its sac, but without further cutting. Removal of the tonsils is a simple operation, usually not requiring the use of anesthetics and most physicians advise the removal of an enlarged or troublesome tonsil.

CALCULI OR STONES.--Calculi or stones are removed from the gall bladder, gall ducts, kidneys, ureter and bladder by operations, when it has been ascertained that the patient cannot "pass them." Many physicians prefer to locate the calculus by use of the X-rays before deciding to operate, and there can be no doubt as to the wisdom of this. In these, as in all operations, success depends largely upon the general condition of the patient. They are not considered dangerous operations, but the final decision as to their necessity should rest, in each case, with a competent physician or surgeon.

KIDNEYS, STOMACH, PROSTATE, ETC.--Little can be said in this brief paragraph concerning the many operations that are now performed upon the different organs. What applies to one applies, in general, to all. Operations are now performed, and successfully, for pus in the kidney, floating kidney, etc. Ulcers and cancers are removed from the stomach and reproductive organs. In some cases it has been necessary to remove the organs in their entirety. Pieces of the intestines have been removed with gratifying results in cases of ulcers and injuries. Enlarged prostate nearly always necessitates an operation before relief can be expected. It is impossible here to say much concerning the chances for recovery in each individual case, since they are decided by the strength and temperament of the patient, the care and skill of the surgeon and nurses, and whether the patient has submitted to the operation soon enough in the course of the disease. Let it suffice here to say that the majority of the above-mentioned operations are successful and result in the relief and often the complete recovery of the patient.

THE HOT SPRINGS OF ARKANSAS.

Government Ownership.--The ownership and control of the Hot Springs of Arkansas by the United States Government is absolute, and its endorsement of them for the treatment of certain ailments is unequivocal. After due investigation, congress took possession of the springs in the year 1832, and it retained around them a reservation ample to protect them from all encroachments, It was the first National park reservation of the country. They are set apart by this act as "A National Sanitarium for all time," and "dedicated to the people of the United States to be forever free from sale or alienation."

The Army and Navy Hospital at Hot Springs.--In the year 1883 the United States Government built a hospital known as the army and navy hospital at Hot Springs, Arkansas, on the Southwestern slope, near the base of Hot Springs mountain, since which time the soldiers and sailors of the army and navy have been sent there for treatment for such ailments as the waters may reasonably be expected to cure, or relieve. In his circular for the guidance of the officers of the army in sending the sick there, the surgeon-general of the United States enumerates the ailments for which the sick should be sent to the army and navy hospital at the Hot Springs. It says, "Relief may be reasonably expected at the Hot Springs in the following conditions: In the various forms of gout and rheumatism after the acute or inflammatory stage; neuralgia, especially when depending upon gout; rheumatism, metallic, or malarial poisonings, paralysis, not of organic origin; the earlier stages of locomotor ataxia; chronic Bright's disease (early stages only), and other diseases of the urinary organs; functional diseases of the liver; gastric dyspepsia, not of the organic origin; chronic diarrhea; catarrhal affections of the digestive and respiratory tracts; chronic skin diseases, especially the squamous varieties, and chronic conditions due to malarial infection." .

Approved, GEO. H. TORNEY, Surgeon-General U. S. Army.

J.M. DICKERSON, Secretary of War.

Privileges of Ex-Soldiers of the Civil and Spanish-American Wars.--Honorably discharged soldiers of thc Civil war, and the Spanish-American war, can obtain admission to the army and navy hospital at Hot Springs in the following manner, and under certain conditions:

First.--Write to the Surgeon-General, United States Army, Washington, D. c., for blank applications and instructions.

Second.--Upon receiving the blank application, fill it out properly, and return it to the Surgeon-General, when, if there is room in the hospital, he will forward to the applicant papers entitling him to admission to the hospital. The conditions are that such ex-soldier shall pay forty cents per day during the period he remains at the hospital. Such payment entitles him to board, lodging, baths, medical treatment and medicine.

Free Baths for the Indigent People of the United States.--By act of congress approved December 16th, 1878, the government maintains a free bath house for the indigent people of the United States of both sexes. No baths will be supplied except on written applications made on blanks furnished at the office of the bath house, making full answer to the questions therein propounded: then if the applicant is found to be indigent, in accordance with the common acceptations of the word, the manager will issue a ticket good for twenty-one baths, which may be reissued on the same application if necessary. The daily average of baths given at the free bath house for the year 1909 was more than six hundred.

The government is very broad and liberal in construing the meaning of the word indigent; and the fact that the applicant for free baths has some property, seems not to act as a bar to the privilege of free baths. Ninety per cent of the patients admitted to the Army and Navy Hospital are either cured or relieved. Taking into consideration the large number of old civil war veterans treated at the hospital, whose ailments have become chronic, this is a very remarkable showing.

Physicians' and Medical Regulations.--The United States Government, through the interior department, regulates and controls the practice of medicine in connection with the hot waters. A local federal medical board passes on the applications of physicians who wish to prescribe the hot waters. All who meet the requirements of the board are placed on the accredited list. Copies of this list are hung in all the bath houses and only those whose names appear thereon are permitted to prescribe the hot waters. For the benefit of visitors these lists are also kept at the office of the superintendent of the reservation near the Army and Navy Hospital. These regulations apply only to those who take medical treatment. Others get the baths without formalities of any kind. In addition to the Army and Navy hospital and the government free bath house, there are twenty-five bath houses operated by private parties, eleven of which are situated along the western base of Hot Springs mountains on the government reservation, and fourteen are on private property at various other points throughout the city. The relations of all the bath houses to the government are the same. They each pay the water rental to the Interior Department of the United States. The government's interests are looked after by a superintendent of the reservation, who is appointed by the President of the United States. He has charge of all improvements going on, on the reservation and enforces all government rules and regulations concerning the bath houses.

Cost of Living at Hot Springs.--Hot Springs is not located in a good agricultural section, and it is not a manufacturing city; therefore, the boarding and lodging of visitors is their only source of income. Upon nearly every house in the city is displayed the notice that board is furnished, or furnished rooms are for rent, with or without light housekeeping. A few places furnish board and lodging for $4.50 per week; the most general charge, however, is from $5.00 to $6.00 per week. Renting rooms, arranged for light housekeeping, is the cheapest method of living at Hot Springs. The above prices are intended to show the minimum cost of living.

Where to obtain additional reliable information relating to baths, board, etc., at Hot Springs, Arkansas.--First. Apply to the superintendent of the United States reservation, corner of Central and

Reserve Avenues, Hot Springs.

Second. The business men of the city have an organization known as the "Business Men's League," which is intended and prepared to furnish reliable information by letter or personal application to the secretary and managers of the Business Men's League. Persons visiting Hot Springs should not rely upon advice, information, or propositions from strangers either on the train or in the city.

MEDICAL USES OF SOME COMMON HOUSEHOLD ARTICLES.

SALT (Sodium Chloride).--This common household article is used in a great many different ways. In cooking it is used to season foods. The absence of salt gives rise to a bad state of the system, with the formation of intestinal worms. If used too freely, it produces in some persons excess of blood and corpulency. Salt renders the food more palatable in many instances and thus increases the flow of the gastric juice. Salt increases the flow of saliva also. For pin-worms, solution of salt injected is often effective.

Constipation.--One teaspoonful to a glass of water taken on arising is very good for some people troubled with constipation. For dyspepsia it tones the stomach and aids in digestion in some cases. Salt alone in teaspoonful doses will produce vomiting and is good after a spree or to empty the stomach in convulsions and poisoning. Mustard given with it makes it more effective. A salt solution is frequently injected into the rectum to keep up the strength after operating and it is also frequently put into the breast for same purpose.

A gargle and astringent in sore throat. For this purpose it is often of use and successful. Taken dry in teaspoonful doses it is often given in bleeding from the lungs. It is often used as an antiseptic to cleanse sores and wounds. Teaspoonful to a half pint of water. On bites of insects strong salt water or applied dry is often very good. In bites of snakes and animals dry salt applied freely upon the wound is often of value. It draws away some of the poison and also helps to burn out and cleanse the wound.

Fomentations.--Used in this way it is good for sprains and bruises.

Baths.--One pound of salt to four gallons of water forms a suitable salt water bath acting as a tonic and excitant to the skin.

Ague.--Homeopathic doctors claim that salt in the attenuations will cure some cases of ague.

Abuse of Salt.--Too much use of salt will cause a great many troubles. It produces a peculiar eruption on the skin, sore eyes, etc.

Want of Salt.--Domestic animals need it and may die for the want of it. Some animals may become sterile if deprived of it.

LEMON.--Lemons, owing to their pleasant flavor and agreeable acidity, are very useful in a sick room. The rind yields an oil of great fragrancy. Each lemon yields two to eight drams of acidulous juice and contains seven to nine per cent of citric acid, besides phosphoric and malic acids, in combination with potassa and other bases. Half an ounce of lemon juice should neutralize twenty-five grains of bicarbonate of potassium, twenty grains of bicarbonate of soda or fourteen grains of carbonate of ammonia. The rind of lemon when fresh, besides the oil above mentioned, contains a bitter crystalline glucoside.

Hesperidin.--Uses. Lemon juice applied to the surface of the skin removes freckles, moth spots, sunburn, pruritus, and ink-stains.

Internally.--This is a very good remedy to cure scurvy. It is a constant companion of sea-goers and scurvy is seldom seen when the regulation ration of lemon-juice is used regularly. It also cures the scurvy skin trouble or the form of muscular pains felt in scurvy.

Chronic Rheumatism.--In some cases several ounces of lemon-juice administered daily affords marked relief, and it is also sometimes useful in acute rheumatism. Lemonade is a useful drink during convalescence, as it increases the urine and reduces its acidity.

Hot lemonade is useful as a sweating agent to break up colds in their beginning. It satisfies the thirst and is very grateful to a stomach that is not normal. It makes a very pleasant drink in many cases of sickness.

ONION (Allium Cepa).--It is supposed that the onion is a native of Hungary. It is now found over the whole civilized world. It contains a white, acrid, volatile oil holding sulphur in solution, albumen, much uncrystallizable sugar and mucilage, phosphoric acid both free and combined with lime, citrate of lime. The Spanish onion contains a large proportion of sulphur and thus may be satisfactorily used in those cases where sulphur is needed. The action of the volatile oil enhances that of sulphur. Spanish onion boiled and eaten freely at bed-time is an excellent laxative. Moderately used the onion increases the appetite, promotes digestion, but in large quantities it causes flatulence, uneasiness in the stomach and bowels. The juice mixed with sugar is useful in cough, colds, and croup where there is little inflammation. Roasted or split it is excellent as a local application in croup, tonsilitis and earache. Boiling deprives the onion of its essential oil.

SODA (Bicarbonate of Soda).--Uses. It is used in stomach fermentation and in sick headaches arising from this condition. Useful in acidity of the stomach. Good for gas in the stomach. It is good as a local application to enlarged acute tonsils applied in powder. It is also used in preparing different articles of food. The best to get is the bicarbonate of soda at a drug store.

SULPHUR.--This is an important constituent in certain native mineral waters. On the bowels it acts as a mild laxative. It is very good in certain skin diseases and for itch in the form of an ointment it is often used. It is useful in chronic acne, and for lice, itch, barber's itch, etc. It is frequently used as a disinfectant after infectious diseases. Burning sulphur in a room destroys bed-bugs, chicken lice, etc.

TURPENTINE (Terebinthina).--Uses. It is a valuable counter-irritant in peritonitis, bronchitis, pneumonia, lumbago, pleurodynia, etc. Turpentine stupes are frequently used in abdominal inflammation, for flatulence and for bloating in typhoid fever. It is a valuable constituent of a great many liniments. Used in excess it produces bloody urine, painful urination and inflammation of the kidneys. The free use of barley water, hot bath and purgative relieve its bad effects.

VASELIN.--Under the name of Petrolatum is sold a semi-solid substance derived from certain kinds of petroleum called cosmoline or vaselin. It has very soothing powers and does not become rancid and is used as a soothing dressing in sores, boils, and skin affections. It is frequently used as a base for ointments. Fluid or liquid petrolatum is much used now in the form of a spray in the treatment of acute and chronic catarrh and after irritant applications to the nasal cavities. It is put up now in tubes and is much cleaner and purer. It is very soothing and healing when used in this pure form.

ALCOHOL (Spirit of Wine).--Alcohol is a liquid composed of ninety-one per cent by weight of ethylic alcohol and of nine per cent by weight of water. Alcohol dissolves alkaloids, fatty and resinous substances, and is largely used as a menstruum in obtaining the active principles of drugs in an available form for administration. It is the basis for spirits, tinctures and elixirs; spirits being solutions of volatile substances in alcohol; tinctures, solutions of active principles of plants, generally obtained by maceration and percolation. An elixir is a cordial flavored with orange and syrup, used as a vehicle for other remedies and as a stomachic.

Its action is very extensive. It is used extensively in medical preparations. It is a good application to prevent bed-sores. The addition of one dram of alum to a pint makes it more effective. Hot applications relieve pain in face neuralgia, cold in the face or toothache. It is often used after bathing in full strength or diluted to rub on the body to prevent taking cold. It stimulates the digestive organs, nervous system and the circulation. It is much used in snake-bite. Its constant use is a menace, as all know. It should never be taken for disease unless prescribed by a reputable physician.

ALUM (Alumen).--Dried alum is an astringent and mild "burner" for growths such as "proud flesh." The glycerite of alum is useful in tonsilitis or pharyngitis when it is not acute. In solution it condenses tissue by coagulating their albumin and acts as an astringent.

Uses of the Strength.--One dram to a pint of whisky and water aids in checking sweating in consumption when applied with a sponge. It is a good injection for the whites. A cotton plug soaked in alum often stops nosebleed by inserting it in the nostrils, or a solution may be thrown or snuffed into the nostrils. It is also good as a gargle for tonsilitis and sore throat.

Emetic for Croup.--Put a heaping teaspoonful in thirty-two teaspoonfuls of water or syrup and give a teaspoonful every fifteen minutes until vomiting is produced. It is often used stronger when quick action is desired. It is a mild astringent and thus used to check mucous discharges from the bowels, etc. Burnt powdered alum is often used to destroy "proud flesh."

BORAX (Sodium Borate).--This drug as it appears in commerce of America is derived entirely from natural deposits found on the shores of lakes of California and Nevada. This is purified.

Action.--It is antiseptic in its action. It renders the urine alkaline.

Gargle.--It is used as a gargle in sore mouth and throat in dose of a dram to a pint of water. It is very good used as a wash for fetid sweating, especially of the feet. It is often used in combination in catarrh of the nose. It can be combined with soda for this purpose in dose of one dram of each to two pints of pure water and used in an atomizer.

CAMPHOR.--This is distilled from the wood and bark of the camphor tree, cinnamomum camphora, which grows chiefly in China and Japan. It should be kept in closed bottles.

Uses.--It is good for cold in the head in the early stages. It may be snuffed up the nostrils in fine powder, or put in boiling water and the fumes inhaled. It is good used as a liniment in neuralgia, stiff neck, rheumatism and for boils and sores. Used in the form of camphor ice it is very good for sores, cuts, boils, etc. It is often of use to smell when one feels faint. It is one of the ingredients in many liniments. Its external use as spirits of camphor is extensive.

CASTOR OIL (Oleum Ricini).--This is derived from the beans of Ricinis Communis, a plant in the United States.

Action.-- It is bland and unirritating in its action as a purge and generally acts in four to five hours.

Uses.--It is used whenever irritant materials such as bad food, putrid flesh, decaying vegetables have been eaten, to move the bowels. It is good in diarrhea produced by above causes and others, such as corn, peanuts, cherry stones, berries. It is apt to produce piles and constipation if used constantly. It is often given in the form of capsules containing from one-fourth to one teaspoonful. Dip the capsules in water, as this renders them slippery and are easily swallowed. Dose is from one to six teaspoonfuls.

OLIVE OIL. Sweet Oil (Oleum Olivae).--This is expressed from the ripe fruit.

Action and Uses.--It is a lubricant. It is added to poultices as an emollient in pneumonia and skin diseases. Internally, olive oil is nutritious and laxative, and a purgative in infants in doses of one teaspoonful. In adults it is a useful remedy in many irritant poisons, excepting phosphorus. It is given in large doses for gall stones, three to six ounces at a dose.

GINGER (Zingiber).--Ginger is the rhizome of Zingiber Officinale, a plant of Hindostan, Jamaica and other tropical countries.

Action: It is an agreeable carminative and stimulant, in easing the secretions and stimulating the wavelike movement of the bowels. It acts as an irritant to the bladder and urethra.

Uses.--It is put in laxative pills to prevent griping and to disguise the taste of the salines. It is useful in dyspepsia of aged persons and also good in flatulence and diarrhea. For menstrual cramps, due to suppression from exposure to cold it is useful as a warm tea and also for colds. It is also used in the spice plasters.

HONEY (Mel).--This is a saccharine fluid deposited in combs by the honey bee (Apis Mellifica).

Action: It is slightly laxative and a pleasant article of food. Honey and water is used as a gargle and to relieve cough, dryness of the mouth and fauces. When used as a gargle it increases the secretion of the mucous membrane and so relieves the congestion. It is apt to disorder the stomach when used too freely. Honey mixed with lemon juice and water is very good for a cough, especially the tickling kind.

LARD (Adeps).--This is a common household article known to all. It is frequently used as the basis for ointments and cerates and in domestic practice as a lubricant. Tincture benzoin added to it prevents it from becoming rancid. It can be used in corrosive poisoning as an antidote except where phosporus and carbolic acid have been swallowed. It is also used in preparing articles of food. It has more penetrating power than petrolatum or vaselin. Washed lard, beaten up with an equal quantity of lime-water, and a few drops of oil of bitter almond, thymol, or carbolic acid added, is splendid for burns; stiffened with yellow wax it forms the simple ointment often used. It softens the hard skin and reduces its heat, when the natural secretion is suppressed. It also softens and removes scabs and lessens and prevents the effect of irritant discharges. The simple lard ointment relieves the intense heat and itching of the skin in scarlet fever. Dissolved and given in large doses it causes nausea and vomiting.

MUSTARD (Sinapis).--Mustard flour, two tablespoonfuls to a glass of water, acts as an emetic. If given largely it produces violent gastritis, and chronic gastritis is often set up by its constant use in excess. It should not be used in acute dyspepsia and bowel irritation.

External: It is applied for colic due to flatulence and for acute inflammation of different organs and is also good when applied to the nape of the neck in headache, neuralgia, etc. Lint soaked in limewater and olive oil relieves the excessive burning from the plaster. Mustard foot baths made by using one handful of ground mustard to half pail of hot water is useful in colds, sleeplessness, headache, convulsions, dysmenorrhea.

CREAM OF TARTAR (Potassii bitartras).--Uses: It is useful in kidney diseases to remove dropsy. In large doses of four teaspoonfuls it acts as a watery purge. It is useful where the urine is thick and alkaline to make it clear and normal. It is sometimes combined in equal parts with epsom salts to move the bowels, especially when an action on the kidneys is also necessary. It is given in teaspoonful doses before breakfast for prickly heat; it is cooling to the blood and is one of the old home remedies.

VINEGAR (Acetic Acid).--Vinegar contains from six to seven per cent acetic acid. Dilute acetic acid contains six per cent pure acetic acid. The pure or glacial acetic acid is a crystalline solid at 59 degrees F., takes up moisture readily so should be kept in well stoppered bottles. Acetic acid is a strong corrosive poison; if taken internally, causes vomiting, with intense pain, followed by convulsions and fatal coma. If the acid remains in the stomach for some time it may eat its way through the stomach wall. In cases of poisoning by acetic acid, milk or flour and water should be freely given and vomiting produced. Weak alkalies should also be given as antidotes. Glacial acetic acid is used as an application to cancer of the skin, ulcers, warts, growths in the nose, ringworm, lupus (Jacob's Ulcer) and other ulcerous growths. Vinegar or dilute acetic acid is given to check night sweats and to relieve diarrhea. It is also used in treating painter's colic after the constipation has been relieved, as an antidote to poisoning by caustic alkalies; externally to prevent bed sores, relieves headaches, checks moderate bleeding from leech bites, superficial wounds, nosebleed and in post-partum hemorrhage. It inhibits the growth of micro-organisms. Cases of catarrhal, membranous and diphtheric croup are benefited by the vapor of vinegar diffused through the sick room. A compress saturated in vinegar and placed over the nose until consciousness returns is recommended to prevent or relieve vomiting, nausea and headache following the inhalation of chloroform.

UNCLASSIFIED MOTHERS' REMEDIES

Received Too Late to Place in Proper Departments

Burns, Lime Water and Sweet Oil for.--"Put unslaked lime about the size of a hen's egg in three pints of water and strain; add one cup of sweet oil, shake and keep burn moist. Will heal without scar or scab." This is highly recommended by physicians.

Burns, Charcoal for.--"Powered charcoal put on thick. This gives quick relief," It is an antiseptic poultice and keeps air from burned surface.

Burns or Scalds, Grated Onions for.--"Grate onions and mix two parts pulp with one part salt; apply twice or three times a day, changing as soon as onions are wilted." The onions are very soothing and keep the air from the affected parts.

Burns, an Easily Prepared Remedy for.--"Spread pure lard, or any unsalted grease over burned surface: cover thickly with flour and wrap with soft cloth after pain has ceased. Remove the flour and spread again with lard or vaselin. Sprinkle over with boracic acid powder and wrap up." This is an old tried remedy and one we all know to be good. The grease helps to lessen the smarting, while the boracic acid is a good antiseptic and keeps the air out.

Bunions, Pulverized Salt Petre for.--"Five cents worth of pulverized saltpeter put into a bottle with sufficient olive oil to nearly dissolve it. Shake well and apply to parts night and morning."

Blisters from Burns or Scalds, White of Egg for.--"Apply immediately the white of an egg. Keep the part from being exposed as much as possible to the air." White of egg is soothing and forms a coating while blistered part is healing, also protects it from air.

Bites from Insects, Simple Remedies for.--"Tolerably strong solution carbolic acid and water. An onion cut in two and rubbed on will also do." Carbolic acid is an antiseptic; onion is soothing and helps to draw out poison by acting as a poultice.

Catarrh, Burnt Alum for.--"Burn alum and power finely or buy prepared burnt alum at the drug store and use as a snuff eight or ten times daily. Ten cents' worth will last a long time. My mother used this remedy and believes that she has cured her catarrh entirely with it." Alum is an antiseptic, is cleansing, as well as an astringent remedy.

Catarrh, Bad Case Cured by the following: "Inhale fumes of iodine crystals. This was given me by a friend, who claimed it cured a bad case of catarrh." Use moderately.

Catarrh, Borax and Camphor for.--"Inhale three times daily equal parts of borax, camphor and salt." These ingredients should be powdered very finely and a pinch of the powder snuffed carefully several times a day. This is a very simple but effective remedy.

Catarrh, Pure Lard for.--"Take a bit of pure lard size of a pea and draw it up each nostril every evening. It will require about a year of constant use." The grease helps to keep the affected parts moist and relieves any congestion present. Anyone suffering with this disease should make it a point to use grease in some form every night. It gives great relief.

Cancer, Yellow Dock Root for.--Scrape narrow leaf yellow dock roots and steep in cream to make a salve and apply externally. Add a little alcohol if you wish to keep it for sometime."

Colds.--

"Dover's Powders	20 grains
Capsicum	15 grains
Camphor	10 grains
Quinine	25 grains"

Mix. Make up into about 20 capsules or powders. Take one every 2 or 3 hours. This is recommended as a sure cure for colds. Keep bowels open with small doses of salts or oil.

Coughs and Colds, Mullein Remedy.--"Steep Mullein leaves in fresh milk. Drink of it just before going to bed. This makes a soothing drink."

Cough Syrup, an Easily Prepared Remedy for.--

"Fluid Wild Cherry Bark	1/2 ounce
Compound Essence Cordial	1 ounce
White Pine Compound	3 ounces"

Dose: Take twenty drops every half hour for four hours and then from one-half to one teaspoonful three or four times a day, children less according to age.

Constipation, Bran as a Cure for.--"Take each night two dessertspoonfuls of bran. Take a spoonful at a time and chew it slowly and thoroughly and swallow." This simple remedy has been known to cure cases of long standing if kept up faithfully for a while.

Constipation, an Old Tried Remedy for.--"One ounce of cream of tartar and two ounces of salts; pour quart of boiling water over mixture and stir till dissolved; drain off and take a wineglassful every morning." The cream of tartar is a good blood purifier and the salts carry off all impurities in the system and in that way relieve the constipation.

Constipation, an Effective Remedy for.--"Chop fine a half-pound seeded raisins and one ounce of senna leaves together; mix with a half ounce powdered sulphur in air-tight jar. Chew a piece the size of a walnut every night."

Constipation, Baby, Juice from Prunes for.--"Give baby a teaspoonful of juice from cooked dried prunes whenever a laxative is needed." This remedy will be found useful, not only for infants, but older children as well. When old enough let them eat the pulp as well as the juice.

Cramps, Turpentine for.--"A cloth dipped in turpentine and applied will relieve cramps in the limbs," Any one suffering with this difficulty will find the above treatment very beneficial.

Croup, Quick Cure for.--"A quantity of raw linseed oil should always be at hand in a family where the children are subject to croup. It is an unfailing remedy, and for quick results it beats anything else which can be given for that dread disease. Half a teaspoonful is a dose, unless the child is choking very badly; then give a teaspoonful. It acts two ways. In the first stage of croup, where there is not much mucus, it is loosened and carried off through the bowels. In the second stage it causes vomiting, but, unlike ipecac, it leaves no soreness of the throat as an after difficulty. It is rarely necessary to give more than one dose, when the child will get relief and go to sleep again. This simple remedy is one that is within the reach of every mother, and one that can be kept on hand at all times; and, while it is in the house the dreaded croup need cause no terrors."

Croup, Salt Water for.--"A handful of salt in a basin of cold water. Wring towel out of this solution and apply over the throat. Cover with warm flannel, keep patient warm." This simple but effective remedy has been known to give relief many times and has been thoroughly tried by a great many mothers.

Chapped Hands, an Inexpensive Remedy for.--"One-fourth ounce gum tragacanth, one-fourth ounce boracic acid, one ounce glycerin, one and one-half ounce alcohol, five cents' worth best white rose perfume. Soak gum in pint of rain water for thirty-six hours; let warm slowly until heated. Remove from the stove, strain through a cheese cloth, add the other ingredients, stir well and bottle."

Cholera Infantum, Chickweed For.--"Chickweed boiled and sweetened in milk. This cured my daughter when an infant. This recipe has been used by me and my mother and proved effectual." The above remedy is an inexpensive one and easily prepared. It will be found excellent for this trouble.

Dog Bite, Home Treatment for.--"Apply common salt." Salt eats and draws poison out. Use it freely.

Drunkenness, Chocolate for.--"Give patient all the chocolate he can or will eat. This cured one man I know."

Diphtheria, a Marine City Mother Gives the Following Cure For.--"One-fourth pound loaf sugar, one-fourth pound gum kino, one-fourth ounce alum; put in a covered porcelain dish on stove in a quart of soft water. Simmer down to one pint, gargle the throat every fifteen minutes, or for small children use a swab. Bandage the throat with onion poultices; this recipe has relieved when used as directed; was used by my mother and proved effectual."

Dropsy, Chestnut Leaves for.--"A tea made of chestnut leaves taken freely instead of water." These leaves can be purchased at any drug store in five-cent packages. Prepare the same as ordinary tea, only stronger.

Eczema, Lard and Sulphur for.--"Melt lard and sulphur. When cool add a little alcohol to keep sweet." This combination is very soothing to the parts affected.

Eczema, Gasoline for.--"Bathe the affected parts in gasoline; be careful not to use the liquid where there is fire or lamps."

Erysipelas, Antiseptic Wash for.--

"Hyposulphite of Soda	8 ounces
Carbolic Acid	(200 drops) 3-1/3 drams
Soft Water	1 pint"

The above wash has very strong recommendations as a local application. It was secured from a family that had used it at different times for twenty years. The family seemed to be susceptible to erysipelas and this medicine had been used for three generations, grandfather, son and grandson. In fact, it was the only remedy that helped their case, although many others had been tried. The entire prescription would cost about fifteen cents.

Fishbone, Choking from.--"Raw egg, taken soon as possible." It helps to carry bone out of throat and is a remedy ready at hand.

Goitre, a Good Remedy for.--

"Iodine	1 dram
Iodide of Potassium	4 drams
Soft Water	4 ounces

Apply night and morning. Rub on with feather or soft brush all around, as well as immediately on the lump." This is a counterirritant and often used for goitre.

Goitre, Iodine for.--"Blister with iodine. Heal with sweet cream, paint and blister again. This wore my sister's goitre away. It took time but was worth it." It should produce redness instead of a blister.

Headache, Lemon Juice and Coffee for.--"A teaspoonful of lemon juice in a small cup of black coffee will relieve." This is an old tried remedy and one that will be found beneficial.

Inflammatory Rheumatism, Salt Petre and Sweet Oil for.-- "One ounce salt petre pulverized, one pint sweet oil. Rub parts affected."

Ingrowing Toenail, Home Treatment for.--"Cut a notch in the top of the nail with a penknife, scrape the nail from base to top."

Ingrowing Toenail, a Good Canadian Remedy for.--"Paint part under flesh with four parts caustic potash, six parts warm water. Paint part and scrape with piece of glass or sharp knife. Repeat till thin enough to break off." The caustic potash makes parts soft.

Ingrowing Toenail, Camphor for.--"Cut part growing in with sharp knife and put camphor on intruding part. This eases the pain and prevents second growth."

Indigestion, Egg Shells for.--"Brown egg shells in oven and crush till very fine with a rolling pin, then take a teaspoonful at meal times three times a day."

Inflammation of the Bowels, a Grandmother's Remedy for.-- "Raw linseed oil and bean poultice. Use as hot as can be borne; keep repeating until relieved. This recipe has been used by my mother."

Kidney Trouble, an Easily Prepared Remedy for.--"Steep plantain leaves into strong tea. Take half cup every night. This has been found good for kidney trouble." Also good for ivy poisoning, burns, scalds, bruises, and to check bleeding; pound leaves to a paste and apply to parts.

La Grippe, Red Pepper Treatment from a Canadian Mother for.--"Take a bottle of alcohol, put enough red pepper in it so that when four drops are put in a half cup of water it is strong. This is what I always break up my grippe with." Peppers thus prepared stimulate and warm up the stomach and bowels and increase the circulation.

Rheumatism, Liniment Sent Us from Gentleman in Canada (says he paid $7.00 for it).--

"Capsicum Powdered	1 ounce
Camphor	1/2 ounce
Oil Hemlock	1/2 ounce
Spirits Ammonia	1/2 ounce
Chloroform	1/2 ounce
Oil Turpentine	1/2 ounce
Oil Wormwood	1 dram
Potassium Nitrate	1 dram
Add Alcohol to make	12 ounces

Good Liniment.--"Sweet oil, turpentine, hartshorn, equal parts. Keep corked."

Liniment, Sprains, Etc.--English Black Oil.

"Tanner's Oil	1 pint
Oil Vitriol	1 ounce
Spirits of Turpentine	1 ounce
Beef 's Gall, contents of	1 gall

Put oil vitriol in tanner's oil, let stand twelve hours and not cork tightly, then add balance."

Lumbago, Ointment for.--

Vaselin	1 ounce
Belladonna	15 grains
Salicylic Acid	1 dram
Sodium Salicylate	1 dram

Apply. Also good to rub on bunions."

Neuralgia, Soothing Ointment for.--"One ounce of laudanum, baking soda to make paste." Apply to parts and cover with flannel." Its virtue is in its soothing and quieting action.

Pain or Rheumatism, Tansy and Smartweed for.--"Boil handful each of tansy and smartweed together till strong tea is made. Dip cloths in the hot tea and apply." Good local and quieting application.

Pain, Horseradish Poultice for.--"Grate and make poultice. Apply to part where pain is." Makes a good drawing poultice and a counterirritant.

Pains, Liniment to Relieve.--

"Peppermint	1 ounce
Oil of Mustard	1/2 ounce
Vinegar	1 pint
White of one egg.	

Beat egg and stir all together."

Pain, Vinegar and Pepper for.--"Hot flannel cloths wrung from vinegar, to which a pinch of cayenne pepper has been added, applied hot to any part of the body, will relieve pain." This is very good. This remedy is always at hand and can be prepared quickly. It will most always give relief.

Palpitation of the Heart, Salt Baths for.--"Stop drinking tea and coffee. Add sea salt to water when bathing. This cured me and I have not been bothered for four or five years." Good when palpitation is due to nervousness.

Piles.-

"Extract Belladonna	15 grain
Acetate Lead	1/2 dram
Gum Camphor	1 dram
Gallic Acid	15 grains
Acetanilid	20 grains
Vaselin	1 ounce
Mix.	

In protruding, itching and blind piles this ointment will give almost instant relief; if kept up several days it will promote a cure."

Poison Ivy, Buttermilk and Salt Heals.--"Add considerable salt to buttermilk and bathe poisoned parts in it frequently."

Poison Ivy, Lead Water and Laudanum Relieves.-- "Application of cold lead water, made in proportions of two drams of sugar of lead, half an ounce of landanum to half a pint of water and applied by means of cloths. The patient should eat a cooling, light diet and use a good saline cathartic, such as rochelle salts, etc."

Poison Ivy, Excellent Cure for.--"Copperas mixed with sour milk; put in all the copperas the milk will dissolve. I knew of a very bad case to be cured by this after a few applications. Care should be taken not to let it get on the clothing, as it burns badly."

Poisonous Wounds, Ammonia Application for.--"Strong spirits of ammonia applied to the wounds of snake bite or rabid animals is better than caustic. It neutralizes the poison and is an excellent remedy."

Oak Poison, Gunpowder and Lard for.--"Mix small quantity of gunpowder and lard and apply. One application cured me." This is an old, tried, standard remedy.

Milk Poison, Popular Remedy for.--

Yellow Poplar Bark	4 ounces
Wild Gooseberry Roots	4 ounces
Slippery Elm Bark	4 ounces

Put in an earthern vessel with two quarts of water; put over a slow fire and simmer to one pint, then strain and add it to one gallon of the best rye whisky and give one wineglassful for the first dose, and thereafter give two tablespoonfuls every two hours. Move the bowels by pink and senna tea. Poultice the bottom of the feet with blue flag swamp root mashed fine to the consistency of a poultice. For the vomiting associated with the disease give one teaspoonful wild deer horn in a little water obtained by filing or grinding the horn of a wild deer. As this is not always to be obtained, a tablespoonful of pulverized chalk is good, or a little cold tea may be given. This recipe has been known to save many persons' lives, when the doctors had given up in despair. When the patient becomes sufficiently improved to warrant it, the dose may be decreased, but it should be taken quite a long time to kill the poison or counteract the poison in the system."

Poor Circulation, Alcohol Rub for.--"Rub vigorously night and morning with good whisky. Don't stop for a week or so after patient looks and feels well." Rubbing with alcohol would probably be preferred.

Ruptures, Herb Remedy for.--"Make a poultice of lobelia and stramonium leaves, equal parts, and apply to part, renewing as often as necessary." This poultice acts by relaxing the muscles, but in severe cases no application will do any good and the doctor should be consulted.

Rheumatism, Mountain Leaf Tea for.--"Tea made of mountain leaf taken frequently cures rheumatism."

Rheumatism, Beef Gall for.--"Two beef galls in pint bottle, fill bottle with whisky. Apply often."

Salt Rheum, a Well-Tried Remedy for.--"Teaspoonful of red precipitate to two tablespoonfuls of lard. Anoint the parts affected." This recipe has been used by my mother and myself and proved effectual.

Snake Bites, Simple Poultice for.--"Poultice of hops or salt and grease; grease is to keep salt together. Hops are always kept to be used in berry season." As a poultice it draws the poison out.

Snake Bites, Onions and Salt for.--"Good drawing poultice for snake bites is an onion and a handful of salt pounded together. We also use this for a common poultice."

Stings, an Old, Tried Canadian Remedy for.--"For the bee sting I put soda on and dampen it with honey." An old-time remedy and seems to do the work. Soda is an antiseptic and cleansing remedy. If no honey at hand, dampen soda with water.

Stings from Nettles, an Inexpensive Remedy for.--"Rub the affected parts, if of nettles, with berry juice and let dry. This is what I always do during the berry season." Berry juice is quieting and soothing; it contains tannin. It would be handy to use and is recommended.

Stye, Common Tea Leaves for.--" After steeping tea gather out a small handful of the steeped leaves, lay them in a cloth as you would any poultice, and apply warm over the stye." It is the tannin in the tea that cures the stye, although clear tannin bought at the drug store does not seem to do the work as well. Black tea may be preferable.

Splendid General Salve.—

"Resin	4 ounces
Beeswax	4 ounces
Lard	8 ounces
Honey	2 ounces

Boil slowly until melted, then remove and stir until cold."

Scrofulous Difficulties, a Good Remedy for.--"A tea made of ripe dried whortleberries and drank in place of water is an excellent remedy."

Sore Eyes, Camphor and Breast Milk for.--"When a tiny baby has sore eyes, add one-half drop of camphor to a teaspoonful of breast milk; bathe the eyes several times a day." Breast milk alone applied to the eyes of an infant is very healing, but the addition of camphor improves it.

Sore Throat, Mustard Plaster for.--"Mustard plaster applied on outside of the throat. I know it is good--have tried it." Care should be taken not to allow the plaster to remain on too long as it will blister.

Stammering, a Canadian Mother's Treatment for.--"I always stop my boy when I hear him stammering and make him say the words by syllables. I find he is getting much better." The above is one of the best plans and should be tried.

Sweating, to Cause.--"Wet flannel cloth in vinegar, lay it on a hot soapstone and wrap in cloth. Take it to bed and you will sweat." This creates a steam and of course will produce sweating very quickly.

Sweating, to Cause.--"Hot cornmeal mush applied as a poultice to parts, will cause sweating."

Splinter, to Extract.--"When a splinter has been driven deep into the hand, it can be extracted without pain by steam. Nearly fill a wide-mouthed bottle with hot water, place mouth of the bottle over splinter and press tightly. The suction will draw the flesh down, and in a minute or two the steam will extricate the splinter and the inflammation will disappear."

Toothache, Benzoin for.--"Compound tincture of benzoin applied on batting to tooth,"

Toothache, Oil of Cinnamon for.--"Oil of cinnamon rubbed on gum and on cotton batting and put in hollow tooth."

Weak Back, Turpentine and Sweet Oil for.--"Take one part of turpentine to two parts of sweet oil, mix together and apply to back several times a day. It is well to massage the back at night with this mixture just before retiring. Always apply warm."

Weak Back, Liniment for.--

"Tincture of Cayenne Pepper	1/2 ounce
Spirits of Camphor	2 ounces

Tincture of Arnica	1-1/2 ounce

No better liniment; is an excellent remedy to bathe the back with; will not blister."

MANNERS AND SOCIAL CUSTOMS

FOR

OUR GREAT MIDDLE CLASS

AS WELL AS

OUR BEST SOCIETY

Correspondence, Cards and Introductions, Dress for Different Occasions, Weddings, Christenings, Funerals, Etc.,

Social Functions, Dinners, Luncheons.

Gifts, "Showers," Calls, and

Hundreds of Other Essential

Subjects so Vital to Culture and Refinement of Men,

Women, School-Girls and Boys at Home and in Public.

By MRS. ELIZABETH JOHNSTONE

"The small courtesies sweeten life, the greater ennoble it."

The social code which we call etiquette is no senseless formula. It has a meaning and a purpose. It is the expression of good manners, and good manners have been rightly called the minor morals. This is true in the sense that they are the expression of the innate kindness and good will that sum up what we call good breeding. As to its importance, Sir Walter Scott once said that a man might with more impunity be guilty of an actual breach of good morals than appear ignorant of the points of etiquette.

Every social custom has a foundation established by usage as a recognition of social needs, and intended to prevent rudeness and confusion; intended also to make polite society polite. We must conform, according to our circle, to social conventions as thus established, since they are the ripened results of long and varied experience in what is most suitable and becoming. Not to observe them is to advertise our ignorance and expose ourselves to criticism.

Importance of Knowledge.--That the importance of a knowledge of social customs is widely felt is proved by the pathetic letters addressed to the editors of women's magazines and departments, asking for information to enlighten ignorance. Such letters range from the naive inquiry of the unsophisticated girl as to whether it is "proper" to allow her "gentleman friend" to kiss her good night, up to the plaint of the novice who doesn't know how to make her spoons and forks come out even at a dinner-party. Here in America, where circumstances may lift a family from poverty and obscurity to wealth, with a position to win in a few brief years, the first great anxiety of those not "to the manor born" is to learn how to comport themselves in their new situation, and educate their children in correct behavior.

Good manners are a necessary equipment of both men and women. In many circles, success is impossible without such equipment. An agreeable manner, a knowledge of what to do and when to do it, is indispensable to the woman in society, and any man who meets other men in a business way will willingly bear testimony to the reluctance with which he approaches the gruff, brusque man, whose manners are patterned after those of Ursa Major. The man whose manners are agreeable may be as ugly as Caliban, yet please everybody.

Moreover, there is no weapon so effective against the rude and ill-mannered as a calm politeness--a courtesy which marks the person who can practise it as superior to the one who cannot. For one's own peace of mind, one should learn the art of good manners.

A Matter of Habit.--Manners, like everything else in life, must be learned by rule, the only possible exception being in the case of those who have been brought up in what we call our best society, where what to do and how to dress and behave have been matters of habit from earliest childhood. When once the rules of etiquette are firmly fixed, they become instinctive and are obeyed unconsciously. The individual then has "good manners." No one can be easy and graceful who must stop to think how to do things. Familiarity with form breeds ease and grace of manner. Therefore those who would be letter perfect must practise the rules of good form at all times and places. Manners cannot be put on and off like a garment. Moreover, as has just been said, the politeness that comes of such observance is the best possible armor against the rudeness or boorishness of the ignorant and untrained.

Many books on etiquette are written, most of which are intended for those in fashionable society who have a number of servants and entertain both extensively and expensively. Other writers take too much for granted; they presuppose a knowledge of the subject which the novice who needs instruction does not possess. This department is intended for those who desire to add to their knowledge of social forms, who do not wish to appear ignorant and awkward, and who, in a more limited social sphere, still wish to entertain properly and pleasantly, and comport themselves in correct form.

CONCERNING INTRODUCTIONS.

The first and most positive rule in regard to introductions is that a man is introduced to a woman; never the reverse, no matter how distinguished the man may be.

The best form is the simplest. "Mrs. A., allow me to introduce Mr. B." If the introduction has been solicited, the hostess may say "Mrs. A., Mr. B. desires the honor of knowing you." If either party resides in another city, she may mention the fact, or any other little circumstance that may aid the two to enter into conversation. The woman does not rise when a man is introduced, but if she is standing may offer her hand. To say "How do you do" is much better form than "Glad to know you" or "Pleased to meet you,"

The person who performs an introduction should be careful to choose an opportune moment. Do not interrupt a conversation to introduce another party, unless, as hostess, you feel it has continued so long that it is time the talk became more general. It is not courteous to simply acknowledge an introduction, and not exchange a few words.

Women and Introductions.--In introducing women, the younger is introduced to the older; if nearly of the same age a distinction is immaterial. Young girls are introduced to matrons, and the younger matrons to those older.

If a woman is seated when another woman is introduced she should rise and offer her hand, and then invite the new acquaintance to a seat near her where they may converse. If a man has been talking with the lady who rises, he should rise also and remain standing until they are seated, when he may bow and take himself away unless requested to remain. Generally, this is the proper moment to leave.

When Calling.--If making a call, and another visitor enters, the lady of the house rises to greet her and introduces any other guests who may be present. A man must rise and find a scat for the newcomer, but the women bow without rising. If only one guest is present, she should rise if the hostess and latest caller remain standing, or if a change of seats seems desirable. Introductions of this kind are semi-formal; they do not establish a later acquaintance unless both are agreeable; the social intent is to bridge over a situation that might seem awkward. However, many pleasant friendships have been made by such casual encounters at the house of a mutual friend.

On the other hand, if two women who are not on friendly terms happen thus to meet and are introduced, it would be a most grievous breach of etiquette not to acknowledge the introduction courteously and exchange a remark or two. Neither has a right to embarrass a hostess by airing a private animosity under the roof of a friend--or in society generally.

General Introductions.--The only "collective" introduction possible is that of a speaker or essayist to an audience. At a club meeting or other assemblage where a stranger is present as guest of honor, the members should request the hostess or the president of the club to present them severally.

Men and Introductions.--Men seldom ask introductions. They have the privilege of speaking without them. A man's title should always be given him in an introduction. A man must request permission before bringing another man to be introduced to a woman or to a friend's house. In the latter case he will present his companions to the lady of the house and any of the family who are present; if others arrive, the hostess should introduce him to them.

After an introduction, the man waits for the woman to recognize him at their next meeting. She should bow, even if she does not care to establish an acquaintance. A casual introduction between women may not be recognized afterwards, though a slight bow is more courteous.

A Few Things Not To Do.--Do not introduce a person as your "'friend." It is not supposed you will introduce anyone who is not a friend. Moreover, in certain circles the term friend is employed in naming a companion, secretary, governess or managing housekeeper to one's guests. In this connection it may be mentioned that one should not speak of "visiting a friend" or "staying at a friend's house." Name the person referred to; or if you do not wish to do so, do not allude to the circumstance. Naturally, one visits only friends.

The indistinctness with which people who introduce often pronounce a name is not infrequently the cause of awkwardness. The failure to hear is no fault on the part of those introduced, but rather a mishap chargeable to the person who brings them together. In this case, try to think of something besides "I didn't catch the name;" that is so cut and dried. Say rather, "I'm sorry, but I didn't understand Mrs. A. when she presented me." Forgetting a name in the act of introducing someone is a much more grievous failure; it speaks for your own social unaccustomedness, and is a poor compliment to the person you introduce. Do not attempt an introduction unless you are sure of your names.

One of the society woman's most necessary accomplishments is the ability to remember names and fit them to the individual to whom they belong. It is an art she should sedulously cultivate.

It is not etiquette, but misplaced politeness, to perform what may be termed casual introductions--as in accidental encounters. Never introduce on the street, unless your acquaintance is to join you. Don't introduce in a street car or any public conveyance. In "our best society"--so-called--it is not considered good form to introduce people in church. People do not go to church for social purposes. In village neighborhoods and the less fashionable city churches, this rule is often violated in the vestibule, where acquaintances linger to greet each other and introductions are not infrequent. But in the body of the church--the space set apart for purposes of worship--an introduction is wholly out of place.

Try to remember family relationships and feuds, that you may not attempt to introduce those at enmity with each other. A woman once introduced, at a crowded function, two sisters who had not recognized each other for years, and afterwards exulted in having "made them speak." Their manners were far superior to hers.

In Company.--At a reception or dinner-party it is perfectly proper for those who have never been introduced to converse with each other without such formality. The roof under which they meet confers the privilege. Indeed, it is often the greatest kindness to speak to a shy person or one who evidently has few acquaintances present, relieving his embarrassment and putting him at ease. Not to reply courteously to such overtures is great rudeness. The story is told of a prominent society woman who addressed a stranger at such a function and actually received no reply. Later, the hostess brought up the strange person and introduced her. Then she explained that, not having been properly introduced, she felt she could not respond. The society woman quietly remarked, "Oh, was that the trouble? I thought you were deaf and dumb."

The late H. C. Bunner and the more recently deceased T. B. Aldrich cherished an aversion for each other. They were not acquainted, but disliked each other on general principles, both being engaged in literary work. They happened to meet at an entertainment where Bunner was in the house of his friends and Aldrich an outsider. Bunner's native kindliness and courtesy made it impossible for him to see anyone uncomfortable in a friend's house. He introduced himself, carried Aldrich to his host's "den," and over a cigar and a glass of "Scotch" began a friendship that was ended only by death.

School Girls' Etiquette.--Etiquette is not so formal among school girls, though its form remains the same. Propinquity in classes, and the being thrown together by mutual aims and interests, excuses informal friendliness. In some women's colleges there are what may be termed "unwritten laws"--school traditions--never set down in books but handed on from class to class. Thus a member of a lower class would not take precedence of a Senior, either on entering or leaving a room, or at table. She would introduce her friends, even her parents, to the Senior and to any member of the Faculty instead of the Senior to them. These little matters of punctilio have to be learned by observation, or by the grace of some friendly classmate who happens to be conversant with them.

CARD AND CALLING ETIQUETTE.

For Women.--Card etiquette has been jocosely termed "going into society in a pasteboard way." Yet cards have a very essential part in the social regime. They are the expedient resorted to by the woman with a large circle of acquaintances and many engagements, for keeping herself in mind.

A card represents a visit, or acknowledges a courtesy in the way of an invitation, There are well-defined rules which regulate the use of cards, familiarity with which is necessary to all who have social aspirations. And the questions most frequently asked by the novice relate to whom and when they should be sent or left.

A General Rule.--Though calling has, in a degree, "gone out of fashion," the general rule is that a woman should call on her friends and acquaintances once a year. This signifies the desire to continue the relationship. If she finds her friend at home she gives her name to the maid and at the conclusion of the visit leaves her card on a table or some convenient place. If her friend is out, the maid receives her card on a tray. In each case a visit has been paid and the card is a reminder that the obligation has been discharged. At this call, if it is the first, or expected to be the only one of the year, a married woman leaves one of her cards for each lady in the family, and one of her husband's for each lady and one for the man of the house. One card, of her husband's may include several grown daughters. If she calls again during the season, she may leave her own cards only, though she should acknowledge an invitation received by her husband by leaving his cards. Cards are never to be handed to the lady of the house or any member of the family.

After Social Functions.--Now here is the law as regards leaving cards after social functions: After receiving invitations to receptions, dinners, luncheons, card parties or evening entertainments, calls are to be made within a week after the event, whether one has accepted or not. However, in some localities, it is thought correct to leave cards at the time if one attends the function, or send them if not attending. It is safest to ascertain the local custom in advance. The correct etiquette is to call afterwards.

An invitation to a church wedding necessitates sending cards to those in whose name the invitation was issued and to the newly wedded pair. The same is true of announcement cards. Cards for an afternoon tea do not require reply; those present leave their own cards and those of any member of the family who was invited but did not attend.

After Absence.--Another use of cards is when one returns home after a long absence. Cards with one's address are sent to previous acquaintances, as a notification that the sender wishes to resume her social relations. In case of a friend's illness, one should call to make personal inquiries, leaving a card on which is written "To inquire."

After a death, cards may be left or sent, on which it is correct to write "With sincere sympathy." After the funeral, cards are sent by those bereaved to those who have thus manifested regard, with the words

"With thanks for kind inquiries" or remembrances.

Thus we see cards are not meaningless, but indicate courtesy, kindly interest and regard.

For Men.--Whereas the married man may discharge some of his social obligations through his wife, the bachelor has no such resource. In response to every invitation, accepted or otherwise, he must pay a visit, leaving cards. Unless he does this, his invitations will soon cease.

A man may pay Sunday afternoon visits, as he is not supposed to be at leisure during the week. An evening call indicates greater intimacy. If he calls upon a young lady he must leave two cards, one for her and one for her mother.

Letters of Introduction--Letters of introduction are never presented in person. The man must call and leave the letter, with his card, but on no account enter the house. The next step is to be taken by the recipient of the letter.

At a Hotel.--If a man calls on a lady at a hotel he sends up his card and waits in a reception room. It is not permissible to write on his card the name of the member of the family whom he wishes to see. That is to be the subject of later inquiry.

Styles in Cards.--Styles in cards vary, both for men and women. Usually the stationer will be a reliable guide as to size and style of engraving. A printed or written card should never be used, nor, according to strict etiquette, should acceptances, regrets or informal invitations be written on cards. Use note paper.

A woman's card should be of medium size and nearly square. Plain script, Old English or Roman are the only letterings used. Engraved plates, once obtained, may be used a long time. The street address, if used, is at the lower right-hand corner. This can be changed on one's plate, if necessary, by ways known to the maker. Men's cards are much smaller than women's, and must be engraved. The name is always prefaced by "Mr."

Use of Names.--A married woman uses her husband's full name on her cards. A widow who happens to be the oldest representative of the family may have her cards engraved without her own or her husband's name, as "Mrs. Astor;" this signifies her place as social head of the family. A clergyman's card may have Rev. as a prefix; a physician's Dr., never M. D. A young girl is always Miss, and pet names are without social recognition. For a year after she enters society a girl has her name engraved beneath her mother's; where there are several daughters "out," "The Misses Smith" may be engraved under the mother's name. A widow may act her pleasure as to using her Christian name or her late husband's on her card; the latter is customary. It would be a social convenience to use the Christian name, as with the prefix "Mrs." widowhood would be indicated.

THE ETIQUETTE OF CALLS.

As has been said, a woman is expected to call on her friends once a year at least. The "Day at Home" has rather gone out of fashion. It imposed an obligation on the hostess which often proved irksome, interfering with engagements she might wish to make. If, however, one has "a day," her friends should so far as possible observe it.

Time and Manner.--The time limit of a call is fifteen or twenty minutes, not to exceed the latter. This is the protection society affords us from bores. We can endure even the most tiresome of visitors for fifteen minutes.

If one does not wish to see callers, the maid or whoever answers the door should be so informed; the conventional "Not at home" being perfectly proper; it is merely a polite way of saying it is not convenient to receive anyone. But for the maid to say "I will see, if Mrs. A is at home," and return to say she is not at home or not receiving, is a grave discourtesy. Nor should one keep a visitor waiting while she makes an elaborate toilette; better say "Not at home." The call counts as a visit whether the lady is at home or not, and must he returned. It is not customary to invite a visitor to be seated, to come again, or urge a longer stay. It is supposed she will take the initiative in these particulars; and too, that the fact that the two exchange visits warrants a certain wontedness of habit. Still, among intimates it is by no means unusual for the hostess to say "Do come again soon; I always enjoy you so much I should be glad to see more of you," or for the departing visitor to say: "I shall hope to have the pleasure of seeing you at my home soon."

Men's Demeanor.--A man calling upon a lady either takes his hat and stick into the reception room with him, or deposits them in the hall; she does not instruct him what disposition to make of them. He removes his overcoat of his own volition, or retains it, as he pleases; the lady does not suggest its removal. This is the strict letter of etiquette. As a matter of fact, many a man would feel snubbed, and the hostess that she failed in cordiality, if she failed to invite him to lay aside his coat. One must be governed by the customs of one's circle. It is safe to say that unless it is a first call, which is the most formal, in our middle social stratum a man expects, if he is welcome, to be asked to remove his overcoat.

A man waits for the woman to invite him to call, since it is her privilege to choose her acquaintances. Such an invitation should not be given too hastily, nor too soon after a first introduction. It is well not to show too much eagerness to cultivate the acquaintance, and the woman should be reasonably sure that the man is desirous of having the pleasure. If invited, he should avail himself of the permission within a short time, by way of showing his appreciation of the compliment. Young girls do not invite young men to call on them; this is their mother's prerogative.

It is more correct in these days when everyone has a telephone, to call up and inquire whether it will be convenient for the lady to receive callers, unless, of course, one is paying duty calls, in which case a card discharges the obligation.

"Pour Prendre Conge."--In taking leave, it is well not to wait until one has exhausted the conversational gamut, and "that awful pause" in which neither seems to have anything to say, occurs. And having risen, do not "stand upon the order of your going;" do not linger for last words, or begin a fresh topic at the door, keeping your hostess standing and perhaps detaining her from other guests. "Parting is such sweet sorrow" in some cases that it becomes awkward and embarrassing because so prolonged. Especially does it seem difficult for the youth who has not yet attained the aplomb which makes him at ease in society, to "tear himself away." Remember that a too abrupt departure, though regrettable, is better than one too prolonged.

Girls' Manners.--When the young girl accompanies her mother on a calling expedition, she waits for the latter to take the initiative in regard to departure. She must allow the older person to precede her in entering and leaving, and she must be careful not to monopolize the conversation. Good manners give precedence to age.

"P. p. c."--The social novice is sometimes puzzled by "P. p. c." written in the lower corner of a card. The letters stand for the French phrase, "Pour prendre conge"--to take leave. Such cards are sent when one is to be absent from home for a considerable period. They are left to be mailed after departure. Thus the intending traveler is not incommoded by well-meant but ill-timed calls at an hour when she is most busy. "P. p. c." cards intimate the acquaintance is to be resumed on the sender's return.

The custom of turning down the corner to signify the call was made in person is now entirely obsolete.

First Calls.--It is desirable, when making a first call, to meet the lady called upon, and it is best to have been properly introduced. In the case of a stranger, the oldest or most prominent member of the social circle of the town should call first. A polite expedient by which a newcomer makes entree into the society of a new place of residence is by sending her cards to those whom she wishes to know. These are, if possible, to be accompanied by the card of some well-known friend, who thus becomes her social sponsor.

A first call must be returned, and within two weeks at the outside. Not to return such a call is a gross breach of etiquette. Even if one does not wish or intend to keep up the acquaintance the return call must be made. After this call she may act her pleasure. If a newcomer extends an invitation to an older resident, she should at once leave cards and send a regret or an acceptance. If the invitation comes through a friend, and she is unacquainted with the hostess, she must call soon; but if the call is not returned, or another invitation extended, she must understand the acquaintance is ended. The newcomer may invite her late hostess to some affair at her own house, and if the invitation is accepted, may understand the acquaintance is established.

A stranger often finds her social progress slow unless she has acquaintances in her new location who can help place her where she wishes to be. The easiest way is to identify herself with some church, attend regularly, and the pastor calling on the new member of his congregation and finding her acceptable, will ask some of the ladies of the church to call. These calls should be returned within two weeks; it would be a discourtesy to the pastor not to acknowledge them.

INVITATIONS.

The Formal Invitation.--A dinner-party is the most formal and most important of all social functions. We may invite all our acquaintances to a ball or a reception. We may select more carefully for our teas and luncheons, but the dinner is reserved as the greatest compliment to be paid those we wish to honor. Therefore an immediate acceptance or regret must be sent, and nothing but illness, accident or death should prevent us from presenting ourselves. If such obstacles intervene, immediate notice should be given the hostess, that she may supply the place at her table thus made vacant.

Do not write you will "try to come;" that you will come but your husband will not be able to do so, or in any way make your acceptance conditional. Your hostess may wish to invite another couple; she must know who will be present that she may arrange her table accordingly. Nothing is so annoying to a hostess as to be obliged to rearrange her table because of some slight excuse on the part of a guest who has once accepted,

Do not forget that an invitation to dinner is the highest social compliment, and value it accordingly; also answer at once.

Formulas for Invitations.

The formula for a dinner invitation is this:

Mr. and Mrs. John Henry Smith
request the pleasure of
Mr. and Mrs. George Brown's company at dinner,
127 Blank Avenue.
on March fifteenth at seven o'clock.

This invitation may be written on note paper or engraved on a card.

The correct form of reply is this:

Mr. and Mrs. George Brown
accept with pleasure the polite invitation of
Mr. and Mrs. John Henry Smith for dinner
on March fifteenth, at seven o'clock.

If the dinner is in honor of guests, the formula may be:

To meet
Mr. and Mrs. William Dash,
Mr. and Mrs. John Henry Smith request the pleasure of
Miss Anderson's
company at dinner,
on Wednesday, January twenty-sixth,
at seven o'clock.
R. S. V. P. 91 East Ninety-fourth street.

If the invitation must be declined, this form may be observed:

Mr. and Mrs. Brown
regret that owing to a previous engagement
they are unable to accept
Mr. and Mrs. John Henry Smith's
very kind invitation
for Tuesday evening, March fifteenth.

Any other reason, as illness, proposed absence, or the like, may be substituted for a "previous engagement."

In acknowledging invitations it is better to err on the side of over-politeness than the reverse.

If a dance or theatre party is to follow the dinner, words indicating the fact are written across the lower part of the card or in the lower left-hand corner.

"R. s v. p." stands for the French phrase, "Respondez, sit vous plait,"--meaning that a reply is desired.

Replies.--The reply to an invitation should be in the same form as the invitation; thus if in the third person the reply should also be made in the third person. Such invitations are the most formal. The reply is to be addressed according to the wording of the invitation: thus if Mr. and Mrs. John Henry Smith issue it, address the reply to them; if Mrs. John Henry Smith's name alone appears, address it to her. The same rule applies to a wedding invitation. The acknowledgement is sent to the parties issuing the invitation, not to those to be married.

Must Not Ask Invitations.--It is not allowable to ask for an invitation to a dinner, a luncheon or a card party for a guest or friend. These are functions arranged for a definite number of guests; to include another person is not possible. If your hostess knows you have a guest, she will, if her arrangements make it practicable, include her; if not, there is no slight to you or your guest. The presence of a guest does not excuse one from a dinner, luncheon or card party, the invitation having been already accepted. Provide some pleasure for your friend, or leave her to a quiet evening at home.

In case a guest drops out at the last moment, as sometimes happens, one may ask a very intimate friend, a relative, or some member of the family to fill the vacant seat. Such a "last minute" invitation is no compliment: one knows she is simply a substitute, but good sense and kindliness should prompt the recipient to help out in the dilemma, which may happen to her next time.

Other Particulars.--Dinner invitations are issued in the name of the host and hostess, so also those for luncheons to which both men and women are invited. Invitations to teas, card and garden parties, "at homes," balls, and women's luncheons are in the name of the hostess alone.

Guests should present themselves punctually at the hour named in a dinner or luncheon invitation, allowing themselves just time to remove wraps, etc., before the meal is announced. It is almost unpardonable to be late.

Invitations are sent to people in mourning after the month following bereavement, not because acceptance is expected, but as a compliment, except that cards for dinners, luncheons and balls are not sent. Wedding cards and announcements, and cards for large general receptions are sent. During the year of mourning people thus remembered send cards with a narrow black border in acknowledgment.

Unless an entertainment is exclusively for women, an invitation to a married woman should include her husband. That he is personally unknown to the hostess does not matter.

INFORMAL INVITATIONS.

Invitations by telephone are permissible for informal affairs, but why a woman should spend hours at the telephone, calling up various parties and losing her temper over "Central's" dilatoriness when she could sit comfortably at her desk and write notes, is difficult to understand.

Whereas the formal luncheon invitation simply substitutes the word "luncheon" for "dinner," the informal invitation is written in the first person and requires a reply in the same form. It may be said again that the response should follow the form of the invitation; this is an invariable rule. This model is usually employed:

My dear Mrs. Henderson:

Will you and Mr. Henderson dine with us informally on Tuesday evening, January twenty-seventh, at half-past six o'clock? Trusting we may have the pleasure of seeing you, I am,

Yours sincerely,
Mary Bronson.

In reply the recipient will write:

My dear Mrs. Bronson:

Mr. Henderson and I accept, with much pleasure your very kind invitation to dine with you on Tuesday evening, January twenty-seventh, at half past six o'clock.

Yours sincerely,
Helen Henderson.

If the invitation is for luncheon, that word is substituted; afternoon written in the place of evening, and Mr. Henderson is left out. In an acceptance, one should repeat the date and hour, that no mistake may occur. If the invitation must be declined, it is not correct to explain the nature of the engagement or whatever reason occurs for refusal. We say we "are unable to accept," not that we "will not be able;" the refusal rests in the present.

An invitation sent by mail is enclosed in an envelope addressed to Mr. and Mrs. A., and then in an outer envelope bearing full name and address. Informal notes of invitation are written on one's best notepaper and no outer envelope used.

Afternoon Tea.--The afternoon tea is a favorite method of paying off social debts. Elaborate refreshments are not served. Tea is poured at the dining table, by some friends asked to do so--it is thought quite a compliment to be asked "to pour" For a very informal "at home" the hostess may have a small table at hand and herself offer a cup of tea to her visitors. For such a small affair she sends her visiting card with the date written in the lower left hand corner. If many guests are expected servants must be at hand to remove soiled dishes and replenish the tea and cakes.

In acknowledgment of invitations, it is highly improper to send your card with "regrets" written on it. An invitation is a courtesy offered; it must be received courteously. You regret you "must decline the pleasure" of accepting somebody's "kind--or polite--invitation."

The Verbal Invitation.--Verbal invitations do not count for much.

"Come and dine with us some day" has no standing among invitations. The day and hour must be named if it is to be reckoned with. And then--suppose the hostess forgets she has given the invitation, or she prepares for a guest who does not come! Except among very intimate friends the verbal invitation should be looked upon with great caution. A verbal invitation should be followed by a note repeating it.

WEDDING INVITATIONS AND ANNOUNCEMENTS.

The number of wedding invitations often must conform to the size of the church or the house, and to the character of the wedding. If it is to be a large one, cards are usually sent as liberally as possible. An invitation to the church may not invite to the reception at the house afterwards, which may necessarily be limited because of the size of the house or the means of the family. No guest receiving cards for the church should let herself feel aggrieved because of failure to receive the other. Answers to invitations should invariably be sent; many omit this, not thinking it necessary, but why not?

Announcement cards are sent to everyone you know, or, more properly, to all those whom you wish to recognize socially. It is quite correct to send them to people you know but slightly. They are mailed immediately after the wedding. They imply no obligation in the way of gift or reply. If an "at home" card is enclosed, calls are expected.

Correct Form.

Wedding invitations of course must be engraved. The following form is employed:

Mr. and Mrs. Lawrence Harmon
request the honor of your presence
at the marriage of their daughter
Harriet
to
Mr. Harrison Richard Ames
on Thursday, the sixth of January,
at twelve o'clock.
Church of the Messiah.

If the wedding is at home, the street and number are given in place of the church.

If the bride has no mother, the invitations are issued in the name of the father; if no father, the mother's name is used. If an orphan, invitations are issued in the name of the nearest of kin in the town where the wedding occurs. If a married sister and her husband issue, the words "their sister" are used. If a girl has a stepfather her own name is engraved in full. Announcement cards follow the same rules as to who issues them, and are couched in these words:

Mr. and Mrs. Hughson Smith
announce the marriage of their sister
Bettina
to
Mr. James Rhodes Grayson,
on Monday, the tenth of January,
Nineteen hundred and ten,
at the Church of the Messiah,
in the City of Cleveland.

For a home wedding, this formula is correct:

My dear Mrs. Jennings:

My daughter Julia is to be married to Mr. George Bronson Holmes on Monday, the tenth of January, at twelve o'clock, and it will give Mr. Brush and myself much pleasure if you and Mr. Jennings will come.

Yours sincerely,
Eleanor
Graves Brush.

For informal church weddings, with small reception to follow, or for a simple home wedding, most people prefer to use the engraved cards, but personal notes may with perfect propriety take their place. For a home wedding, the above formula is correct.

The Bridegroom's Family.

In inviting the bridegroom's parents by note, the mother may write: "Will you and Mr. Holmes come to the quiet informal wedding of my daughter Julia and your son on Monday," etc. Such invitations are written by the mother. Other members of the family are included by adding "you and Mr. Jennings and your daughter will come." Written invitations may follow the form of the engraved, but for a small wedding at home, which will be of course more or less informal, the personal form seems more in keeping.

Other Items.

Formal wedding invitations and announcements are addressed, one to the head of the family, Mr. and Mrs. Jones; one to Miss Jones, or to The Misses Jones, if there are several daughters, and one to each young man of the family.

Note that the year is given in an announcement, but not in an invitation. Announcements are engraved on note-paper, as in the case of invitations.

A double wedding, which requires two ceremonies, also requires two sets of invitations and announcements.

It is quite correct for a girl who has been employed in an office to send an announcement of her marriage to her former employer, but if he is married, it must be addressed to "Mr. and Mrs." So-and-So.

Do not abbreviate in writing notes of invitation, nor permit it on engraved invitations. Doctor, Judge, Reverend, are to be in full. Mr. before a man's name is the only abbreviation permitted. The names of the month, day, year, and of the street or avenue are written out in full.

DINNERS AND LUNCHEONS

FORMAL DINNERS.

"A fig for your bill of fare; show me your bill of company,"

As has already been remarked, we ask our "dear Five Hundred" to our balls and receptions, reserving our dinner invitations for those whom we particularly wish to compliment. The dinner we provide is by no means of the comfortable "pot-Iuck" kind. It is, in society, an elaborate and expensive form of entertainment. A dinner to eight people, not specially elaborate and without wines, rarely costs the giver less than $25 or $30, and may easily run much higher. It requires delicacies for the palate, flowers and bonbons and other decorations for the table, and ceremonious serving. The finest of linen, cut glass and silver adorn it, and the repast may easily be prolonged through two or more hours. Such a dinner is served in courses; begins with an appetizer, extends through soup, fish, joint, salad and dessert courses at the very least, and ends with coffee, served at the table or in some other apartment--the library or drawing room--where the guests converse over their cups.

Such a meal cannot be prepared or served without competent service in the kitchen and dining-room. The cook must know how to prepare every dish in the best manner, and have it ready at the right moment; the waiter must be experienced and noiseless. The hostess must have such perfect confidence that everything will progress in perfect and proper order that she can give her full attention to the guests,

Serving the Dinner.--Let us suppose a dinner for eight people is to be served. The ceremonious dinner, the world over, is served a la Russe, that is, according to the Russian fashion. By this fashion nothing but the covers--a term which includes the china, silver and glass at each plate--flowers, dishes of bonbons, salted nuts and olives, occasionally small cakes, are on the table when the guests are seated,

The hostess has inspected the table, after it is laid, seeing that everything is correct, Silver must have had a fresh polish, the cut glass must shine and sparkle, There must be plenty of light, yet no glare; to prevent this, ground glass globes on the electric lights are preferred. The hostess herself will arrange the place cards, separating married people, and in so far as possible so seating her guests that each may be pleased with his or her neighbor. The centerpiece is of flowers; for this never choose a strongly scented flower like hyacinths or narcissi. The heat, the odor of the food, combined with the scent of the flowers, may induce lethargy, so that the dinner may be "garnished with stupidity."

There must be a service plate at each place. These are to be as handsome as you can afford. At the side of this is laid the dinner napkin, within which a roll is folded. The guest removes the napkin, unfolding it for use. The waitress removes the service plate and puts down another on which is a grapefruit, vermouth, or other kind of cocktail. This plate and glass removed, there comes another plate, and little dishes of caviarre are passed. These plates also disappear, others are substituted, and soup is served. After the soup is eaten the soup plates are removed, leaving the other plates, and celery and radishes and salted nuts and olives are passed, not necessarily all, but at least two, say celery and olives; nuts and radishes. If the little individual almond dishes are used, of course the salted nuts will not be passed.

These plates are again changed when the fish is served, the rule being that at no time during the dinner must a guest be without a plate before him until the table is cleared for dessert. Moreover, the waitress, in placing plates that have a monogram or heraldic device for decoration, must so place the plate before each guest that the design faces him. In taking up the plates, one is taken up with the right hand while with the left the waitress replaces it with another; one plate is never placed upon another.

The fish, meat, and other courses are served from the pantry, the portions being arranged for convenience in helping, and garnished with parsley or lemon. The dish is passed first to the guest seated at the host's right hand, next to the one on the left, and afterwards in regular rotation, irrespective of sex. All service is at the left; this leaves the guest's right hand in position to help himself. The waitress holds the dish upon a folded napkin on the flat of her hand, and low down. Vegetables are passed in the same fashion.

You will see how much depends upon having well trained servants at such a dinner. The service must be without haste, yet without delay; there must be no clatter of china and silver, no awkwardness in removing plates, etc. The waitress must be quick to refill glasses or supply whatever is needed.

The Help Required.--A dinner to twelve or fourteen guests cannot be served properly without two or three waiters--usually men at such large dinners--and additional help in the kitchen. So much thought and anxiety are required for the success of a home dinner party that it is small wonder many prefer to add a little to the expense, in cities at least, and order a dinner for the requisite number at hotel or club, where the responsibility rests with the management after the details of the menu are settled. Such a dinner is less of a compliment to one's guests than the entertainment at one's own home, however; and why should one possess stores of beautiful and expensive furnishings without their use?

One dinner generally means another a short time afterwards, since in selecting the small number who can be entertained one must necessarily leave out others who have equal claims to hospitality and whose sense of being slighted must be appeased. And if the hostess is socially prominent she may find herself embarked on a course of entertainments that will tax her time and her funds to a considerable degree.

Invitations to a dinner must be sent at least two weeks in advance. As has already been stated, an immediate and unconditional acceptance or regret is demanded.

Precedence.--At these formal dinners, the question of precedence engages the hostess's attention, If all the guests are about on equal terms, the host takes out the oldest or most prominent lady, seating her at his right. The other, guests are paired off according to the hostess's ideas of social propriety or congeniality. No man ever takes his wife in to dinner. The place of honor for men is at the hostess's right hand. Dinner cards, legibly written, are placed on the napkins. The men draw out the chairs and seat the ladies, then seat themselves. Generally, at a small dinner, the hostess tells each man before leaving the drawing room, whom he is to take out: at large functions, he finds in the men's cloak room an envelope addressed to him containing the lady's name. He seeks out his partner and gives her his arm when dinner is announced.

Be Prompt.--It is almost unpardonable for a guest to be late at a dinner. The arrival should be within fifteen minutes of the time named on the invitation, never earlier. The hostess must be ready in ample time, and must appear calm and untroubled. Nervousness bespeaks the novice in entertaining. Generally, however, even if the affair passes off without any contretemps she is ready to say "Thank heaven it's over!"

Now this is not to say that one may not serve a good and very enjoyable dinner or luncheon to a few friends, without as much trouble and expense as are here indicated. This is simply to state how such meals are served, formally and informally. Knowing the proper procedure one may adopt as much or as little as her circumstances and style of living warrant.

THE INFORMAL DINNER

The informal dinner resembles the formal, save that fewer courses are served, the menu is simpler, and the decorations less elaborate. The serving is on the same order--a la Russe. If one is fortunate enough to have a maid who combines the experience of a waitress with the qualities of a good cook, by ingenious planning it is possible to serve six persons acceptably in the approved fashion.

But there are thousands of households in which but one maid is kept, and in this case what may be termed "the family dinner" will be found better, because there will be no endeavor to do more than one can accomplish with the means at her command. Better by far serve well and simply than attempt something more elaborate and fall short in it.

Family Dinners.--At the family dinner, the grape fruit or oyster cocktail, or the raw oysters which form the first course, is on the table when the guests are seated. The grape fruit may be served in glasses, like the cocktail. If oysters are served, the maid passes the condiments. She then removes these plates, replacing them with service plates as she does so, and brings in the soup. This the hostess serves and the maid carries about. While this is being eaten--celery or olives being passed after the guests are helped--the maid slips out in the kitchen to dish up the vegetables unless these are already in the warmer. Returning, she removes the soup-plates, never taking more than two at a time. She then brings on the joint or roast, placing it before the host, who proceeds to serve it. (If oysters are served first, a fish course is generally omitted; indeed, so many courses tax one's resources too severely.) The maid carries about the dinner plates, removing the service plate with the right hand and placing the other with the left. She then passes the vegetables. The serving begins with the lady at the host's right hand. If the *piece de resistance* is a turkey, white and dark meat and a portion of dressing are placed on each plate; gravy and the vegetables, then cranberry or currant jelly, are passed. Here the waitress should refill water glasses.

The plates are then removed for the salad course, and the table cleared. This should be ready on the plates, and kept where it will be perfectly cold. While this is being brought on, the hostess will start dishes of salted nuts and bonbons down the table, the guests passing them. After the salad the plates are removed and the dessert brought in. This may be a mould of ice cream or a pudding; pie is seldom or never served. This the host or hostess serves. The coffee service may be brought in, and the hostess pours it; little cakes or wafers, or mints, are usually passed with it; then the maid is excused from further service. The hostess always gives the signal for leaving the table by a slight nod toward the lady on her husband's right, and rising.

Requirements.--A dinner of this kind requires a serving-table or sideboard where china and silver may be in readiness. Such an aid is even more indispensable where the hostess serves the meal herself. Many very enjoyable "company dinners" are served where the hostess is also the cook, and she and her husband serve. If one has daughters they should be taught how to serve, and may rise from the table to change plates and bring in courses with perfect propriety. In such case, the soup is served at the table and, as it is awkward to pass without spilling, some one should carry it about if more than two or three guests are present. The roast or fowl is carved by the host; vegetables are on the table and are passed from hand to hand. After this course the hostess, or the daughter delegated to do this, clears the table and brings in the salad. The dessert follows. Coffee is occasionally served with the meat course, but it is better to bring it on with the dessert. Cups, etc., should be in readiness on the side table, to be transferred to the table. There should be an apparent absence of formality at such a meal, though everything should progress in regular order, systematically, quietly, without orders or clash. Above all things, see that everything likely to be wanted is at hand; nothing looks worse than someone jumping up to get some article that has been forgotten. If dishes, spoons or forks must be washed during the progress of the meal, have warm water ready in the kitchen, wash them quickly, and wipe them out of cold water; then their heat will not betray your limited resources.

Setting the Table.--The "best cloth" and napkins are brought out for the dinner party. The cloth must be laid with mathematical exactness, its center exactly on the center of the table. The centerpiece, almost invariably of flowers, only occasionally of fruit, is also exactly placed. This should be low; it is awkward not to be able to see one's vis-a-vis, and the hostess should be able to command an uninterrupted view of her table, so that if the waitress omits any service she may by a glance direct her to supply it. The arrangement should be graceful and pretty, and, in summer, garden flowers may be used with propriety. The flowers give the keynote of the color scheme; dinner cards, bonbons, ices and creams and the decorations of the small cakes usually served with the dessert, conform to it. Candelabra are less used than at one time, but are by no means "out." A handsome silver candelabra may be used as a centerpiece, its base banked in flowers. On a square or oblong table, candlesticks with shades give a touch of color that relieves the whiteness of napery and glass.

There is a plate--your handsomest--at each place; a napkin squarely folded and lying flat; a row of forks at the left, oyster fork outside, then fish fork, dinner and salad fork, four in all, laid in the order in which they will be used. Knives are at the right of the napkin, always two, a large and a small one. Fashion has re-introduced the steel-bladed knife for the meat course; it is surprising to notice how much more tender meat is than it used to be when we tried to cut it with the silver knives. The soup-spoon is laid at the top of the plate. The salad fork may be brought in with the salad if preferred, spoons with the dessert and coffee. Grape fruit is eaten with an orange spoon, laid at the right. No "fancy folding" of napkins is permissible. The glasses stand at the top of the plate, a little to the right. Small cut glass or fancy dishes containing the relishes are placed near the corners of the table within the circle of plates if the table is square; if it is round they are so arranged so as to balance each other in the form of a square. There may be two of nuts and two of stuffed olives or of bonbons. Individual salt cellars are at the top of the plate; a roll is folded in the napkin, sometimes laid on the bread-and-butter plate, which is placed at the left. Such rolls should be small and well-baked. At formal dinners no butter is served, and the plates are omitted. Finger bowls are brought in after the ices or the pudding. They are on a small plate on which is a doily, and the fruit knife, if to be used, is on the plate. The guest lays bowl and doily at his right, lifting the two together, the plate being for fruit, if any is served. If no fruit, the bowl is left on the plate.

LUNCHEONS.

The luncheon is a less elaborate function than the dinner, but ranks next it in point of compliment and display. The "stand-up" or buffet luncheon is much less popular than formerly, in fact even at the so-called buffet luncheons the guests are now seated at small tables accommodating four. Invitations are sent out ten days or two weeks in advance, and require prompt replies.

Formal Luncheons.--Save in a less elaborate menu, the formal luncheon differs very little from the dinner, except that the latter is at seven o'clock, and the luncheon almost invariably at one. The menu generally begins with grape fruit, served in glasses on small plates and doilies, and on the table when the guests are seated. An orange spoon is used. The table is set as for dinner, save that less silver is laid. Bouillon, served in bouillon cups, with a spoon on the saucer may follow. Then may come lobster a la Newburg; sweet-breads and peas; salad; ices and coffee. In place of the sweet-breads one may serve squab on toast, fillet of beef, or broiled chicken; peas, beets, and potatoes cut in balls and cooked in deep fat may accompany anyone of these. The meat, cut in portions, and surrounded by mounds of the vegetables, is often served from a large platter, from which the guests help themselves. The hostess is served first; this is, that, in case any unfamiliar dish is served, she may show how it is to be handled. The lady on her right is next in order of serving. The same etiquette in regard to serving, changing plates, etc., is observed as at the dinner, save that the rolls are on bread-and-butter plates instead of being folded in the napkin. The decorations, ornamental dishes, candies, and the like are used as at a dinner.

Minor Particulars.--The roast never figures at a luncheon; the courses consist largely of what are called entrees, the idea being that the repast is of a lighter character than a dinner. The salad is a special feature; it may be chicken, Waldorf, fruit, or any kind preferred, but must be carefully studied in its relation to the other dishes.

The guests keep on their hats during the luncheon, removing the gloves as they are seated; at an informal luncheon the gloves are removed in the dressing room.

Very often bridge or some other card game follows the luncheon. If not, guests are not expected to remain more than half an hour after leaving the table.

The luncheon--never say lunch--is a favorite form of entertainment for girls. In this case the dishes served are light and delicate. Mushrooms on toast, oyster patties or croquettes, a salad, and ices; the menu prefaced by grape fruit and bouillon, are often thought sufficient for a girl's luncheon. Sweets are served freely for them.

It is no longer thought correct to go to extremes in carrying out a "color scheme." Sandwiches are not tied up with ribbons, nor cakes colored to correspond with the preferred hue. Flowers, ices, and the decorations on the small cakes passed with the dessert are quite sufficient. Candles, if used, should have shades to correspond.

Large Luncheons.--The large luncheon has few friends these days; it is too heterogeneous an affair. Those invited feel it is an easy way of paying off social obligations; few find it entirely enjoyable. There is more or less of a crush; one experiences difficulty in finding a table and being served; it is not appetizing to note evidences that others have eaten at the same table and departed. And one is likely to be seated with the wrong people and thus miss much that belongs with and makes pleasant the smaller affair.

No woman need hesitate at inviting a few friends to have luncheon with her. She may prepare a simple meal, and if it is nicely served and she herself gives the cordiality and the conversational impetus that "keeps things going," her guests will find it enjoyable. She may adopt as much of the regular method of serving as befits her home and its resources, but she must make her table as beautiful as possible, and she must not serve "stewed hostess."

TABLE ETIQUETTE.

We have seen how a table should be laid and a meal served; now let us see how it should be eaten:

There is no situation in which one's good breeding is so much in evidence as at the table. For that reason, mothers should begin to train their children in infancy to correct usage. As soon as a child is able to hold a spoon and fork, he should be taught how to hold them properly, and the training should be continued until the right habit is established.

One should not be seated until the lady of the house is seated, unless especially requested to do so. Children should observe this rule as rigidly as that which requires the removal of the hat on entering the house.

At the Table.--On being seated, the napkin is unfolded and laid across the lap. It is more correct to only unfold one-half, that is, open it at the center fold. One is not supposed to require further protection than from the accidental crumb. On no account should it be used as a bib, or be tucked in the dress or waistcoat.

Grape fruit is eaten from an orange spoon. If oysters are served raw, they must not be cut but eaten whole.

Soup must be taken from the side of the spoon, quietly, with no hissing or other sound, nor should the spoon be so full that it drips over. The motion of the spoon in filling it, is away from instead of towards the person; and tilting the plate to secure the last spoonful is bad form. Crackers are never served with soup: croutons--small squares of bread toasted very hard and brown, or small H. & P. biscuits are passed. These are never put into the soup, but are eaten from the hand. Neither soup nor fish should be offered the second time.

Fish is generally eaten with a fork and a bit of bread, though silver fish knives are in occasional use. The entree which follows the fish should be eaten with the fork only. A mouthful of meat is cut as required; it is never buried in potato or any vegetable and then conveyed to the mouth. Vegetables are no longer served in "birds' bath-tubs," as some wit once called the individual vegetable dishes, but are cooked sufficiently dry to be served on the plate with the meat. All vegetables are eaten with the fork, so also jellies, chutney, etc., served with the meat course.

Using the Fork.--The fork laid farthest from the plate is to be used for the first course requiring such a utensil; the others are used in their order. The knife is held in the right hand; by the handle, not the blade. The fork should not be held like a spoon, or a shovel, but more as one would hold a pencil or pen; it is raised laterally to the mouth. The elbow is not to be projected, or crooked outward, in using either knife or fork; that is a very awkward performance. The fork should never be over-burdened. The knife is never lifted to the mouth; it is said that "only members of the legislature eat pie with a knife nowadays." The handle of neither knife or fork may rest on the table nor the former be laid across the edge of the plate.

Tender meat, like the breast of chickens, may be cut with the fork. A bone is never taken in the fingers, the historic anecdote about Queen

Victoria to the contrary notwithstanding. The table manners of the twentieth century are not Early Victorian. Olives and celery are correctly laid on the bread-and-butter plate. The former is never dipped in one's salt cellar; a small portion of salt is put on the edge of the plate; both are eaten from the fingers.

Vegetables, Fruits, etc.--Green corn is seldom served on the cob at ceremonious dinners. If it is served, it is to be broken in medium-sized pieces and eaten from the cob, a rather messy process, and one not

45

pretty to observe. The fastidious avoid it. If eaten, the piece is held between the fingers of one hand. To take an unbroken ear in both hands and gnaw the length of it suggests the manners of an animal never named in polite society.

It is correct to take up asparagus by the stalk, and eat it from the fingers, but the newer and more desirable custom is to cut off the edible portion with knife and fork. Lettuce is never cut with a knife; a fork is used, the piece rolled up and conveyed to the mouth.

Hard cheese may be eaten from the fingers; soft cheeses, like Neufchatel, Brie, and the like, are eaten with the fork, or a bit is spread on a morsel of bread and conveyed to the mouth with the fingers.

A soft cake is eaten with a fork. The rule is that whatever can be eaten with a fork shall be so eaten.

Roman punch and sherbets require a spoon. Berries, peaches and cream, custards, preserves, jellies, call for the spoon. Strawberries are often served as a first course in their season. They are then arranged with their hulls and a portion of stem left on, dipped in powdered sugar and eaten from the fingers. A little mound of the sugar is pressed into shape in the center of the small plate and the berries laid around it.

Peaches, pears, and apples are peeled with the fruit knife, cut in quarters or eighths, and eaten from the fingers. Bananas are stripped of the skin, cut in pieces with a fork and eaten from it. Oranges are cut in two across the sections and eaten with an orange spoon. Plums, like olives, are eaten by biting off the pulp without taking the stone in the mouth. Pineapple, unless shredded or cut up, requires both knife and fork; it is usually prepared for more convenient eating. Grapes, which should be washed by letting water from the faucet run over them and laid on a folded towel until the moisture drips off, are eaten from behind the half-closed hand, which receives the skins and seeds, then to be deposited on the plate.

If the small cup of coffee--the demi-tasse--is served, the small after-dinner coffee spoon is necessary. Cream is seldom served with the black coffee--cafe noir--with which a meal concludes, cut loaf sugar is passed.

The Spoon.--The spoon must never be left in the cup, no matter what beverage is served. Most of us have seen some absent-minded individual (we will charitably suppose him absent-minded instead of ignorant), stir his coffee round and round and round, creating a miniature whirlpool and very likely slopping it over into the saucer; then, prisoning the spoon with a finger, drink half the cup's contents at a gulp. To do this is positively vulgar. Stir the coffee or tea very slightly, just enough to stir the cream and sugar with it, then drink in sips. To take either from the teaspoon is bad form. Bread is broken, not cut, and only a small portion buttered at a time. Do not play with bread crumbs or spoon, etc., during the progress of a meal.

Leave knife and fork on the plate, handles side by side, when it is passed for a second helping, and at a conclusion of a course, or the meal, lay them in the same position, points of the fork upward.

Finger Bowls.--When finger bowls are brought, the tips of the fingers are dipped in the bowl and dried on the napkin. Men may lift the moistened fingers to the lips; women seldom do this, but wipe the lips with the napkin. At any function the napkin is not folded, but laid at the side of the plate at the conclusion of the repast. If a guest for a day or so, or for more than one meal, note what your hostess does with her napkin and follow her. If a guest at only one meal, never fold the napkin. Be careful not to throw it down so carelessly that it is stained with coffee, fruit, or fruit juices; your hostess will thank you for your consideration.

Be ready to rise when your hostess rises; you do not push your chair into place; simply rise and leave it. Rise on the side of your chair so you will not have to go around it in following your hostess to the drawing room.

RECEPTIONS.

When invitations are sent out for a reception, the recipient dons her handsomest afternoon gown for the occasion. This may be a dressy tailored suit; by this is meant one not severely simple; or she may wear some handsome trained gown under a long coat. Small cards for presentation at the door are sometimes enclosed with invitations to a large reception or buffet luncheon, since "the pushers" have been known to present themselves at such functions without having been invited. These cards are handed to the man who opens the carriage door. An awning extends from the door to the curb, and strips of carpet are laid under it, A maid opens the door and directs guests to the dressing room, where wraps are laid aside, hats and gloves being retained.

Receiving.--The hostess stands near the door of the drawing room, welcoming her guests with hand and smile. Next to her stand the ladies who receive with her. During the hour of arrival there is seldom opportunity for more than a word of greeting, and one should not linger but pass on down the line. A reception is often given to some visiting stranger, who is introduced by the hostess.

The guests then circulate through the rooms, greeting acquaintances, and drifting eventually to the dining room, where refreshments are served. They may stay as long as they find it agreeable, within the hours named on the card of invitation, but people seldom stay more than an hour.

The hostess remains near the door after the rush is over to greet the belated guest and bid adieu to those who are leaving.

Decorations.--It is usual to decorate the rooms with flowers, and the services of the florist as well as the caterer are required if it is a large affair. Cards are usually left, as a token that one has been present, but in this case a card is manifestly not a visit, since it would be absurd for a woman to invite fifty, a hundred, or even five hundred people, who would expect her to call on them afterwards. Cards are sent by those who do not attend, on the day.

A reception given for forty or fifty people is less formal, perhaps, but requires flowers--in less profusion--and refreshments. The awning may be dispensed with if the day is fine, but seldom is. The door must be promptly opened, and the maid remains at her post during the affair if there are many guests, to open it for those who leave as well as those who arrive.

HOSPITALITY IN THE HOME.

"There is an emanation from the heart in genuine hospitality which cannot be described, but is immediately felt, and puts the stranger at once at his ease."

--Washington Irving.

Were we to look up the meaning of the word hospitality in the dictionary, we would find it defined as the act of receiving and entertaining guests kindly, generously, and gratuitously, without expectation of reward.

According to such a definition, much that passes for hospitality in the social realm does not deserve the name. Society is a give-and-take arrangement, somewhat resembling the gift exchange we practise at Christmas. If you do not give you do not get; if you do not entertain you are not invited, unless it is understood that circumstances prevent your doing so. Then one is asked for what one can contribute in the way of good company, promotion of gayety, and the like. One "pays her way" by being agreeable, well gowned, popular. Thus, in a way, much social hospitality is merely social bargaining. The woman who feels indebted to her circle--or circles, for these impinge upon each other--gives a large reception or "at home." She can seldom do more than welcome the coming and speed the parting guest. Her greeting is "So delighted to see you here;" her farewell, "Good-bye; so glad you were able to come." Her guests have greeted each other in much the same casual fashion, have had some refreshments warranted to destroy their appetite for dinner; have shown a handsome gown and hat--and perhaps had the former injured in the crush. One is reminded of Bunthorne's "Hollow! Hollow! Hollow!!"

Real Hospitality.--Quite different is this from what we offer when we invite our friends to visit us. Here is genuine hospitality--the receiving and entertaining gratuitously those whose companionship we enjoy. One of the chief joys of having one's own home is the pleasure of being able to welcome one's friends and afford them the privilege of enjoying it also. An invitation of this kind means we are willing to incommode ourselves, incur expense, and give a measure of our time to the entertainment of those of our friends whose society we wish to enjoy familiarly. Thus it seems that an invitation to visit a friend in her home is a compliment of no mean order, although Nicole says: "'Visits are for the most part neither more nor less than inventions for discharging upon our neighbors somewhat of our own unendurable weight."

Short Visits.--Visits are of much shorter duration than in those "old times" people talk about so enthusiastically--and would find so tiresome were they to return again. Then visitors stayed week after week; were urged to remain longer when they proposed departure. The story goes of a Virginia planter who invited an old war-time friend to visit him. At the end of a month the major proposed departure. His host objected so strenuously that he agreed to stay another month. And so it went on, the guest regularly proposing to leave, the host hospitably insisting on his remaining, until in the end the old veteran died in and was buried from his friend's house. This, however, is an example not to be emulated in these less hospitable days.

There is a saying, "Short visits make long friends," that is worth consideration by those who visit. Probably the truth of the saying has been so often attested that it has given rise to the custom of specifying the date of arrival and departure of a guest when giving the invitation. It has become to be understood that the vague, indefinite invitation "Do come and see us sometime," means nothing. No one would think for a moment of taking it in good faith. If the giver wishes to entertain her friend she will ask if it will be convenient for her to visit her at a certain specified date. Nothing less counts. An understanding of this might save the unexperienced from the awkwardness of making an unwelcome visit.

The Unexpected Visit.--Nothing is worse form than "the surprise visit." Generally you do surprise your hostess and very often most disagreeably. A housekeeper does not enjoy an intrusion--for such it is---of that kind any more than you would be pleased to have a chance caller rush unannounced into your private rooms. Even among relatives and the most intimate friends, there is nothing to justify the unexpected arrival. Nothing so strikes terror to a woman's soul as the thud of trunks on the piazza and the crunch of wheels on the gravel, meaning someone has "come to stay."

Such an arrival is a piece of presumption on the part of the visitor. She assumes she will be welcome at any time she chooses to present herself. This may be true; but at the same time there is an obligation of courtesy which requires her to consult her friend's convenience. Instead, she consults her own and utterly ignores that of her hostess, who is thus forced into entertaining her.

The Inopportune Arrival.--Many awkward and sometimes amusing anecdotes are told in connection with the inopportune visit. Thus not long ago the newspapers chronicled the plight of a woman who undertook to surprise an acquaintance from whom she had not heard for several years. She was driven to their house and dismissed the carriage. A strange face met her at the door, and she learned that her friend had removed to another city nearly a twelvemonth before. "Served her right" will be everybody's verdict.

Suppose one arrives unexpectedly and finds the friend's house full of other and invited company. Then, if ever, she ought to feel herself "a rank outsider." If she is tactless enough not to give notice of her intended arrival, she probably has not the good sense to depart as quickly as possible. The man of the house may have to sleep on the parlor sofa, or the children on the floor, and ninety-nine times out of a hundred the whole family will wish her in Halifax.

Or she may arrive to find some member of the family ill, or house-cleaning or repairing in progress, or the house in the hands of the decorators. Indeed, so many unforeseen accidents may occur to make her visit an unpleasant memory, both to herself and her hostess, that only the most selfish and inconsiderate of women will so violate the social conventions as to make "surprise visits."

Visits That Save Expense.--Something equally reprehensible is the visit we pay to a friend in town where we have business or desire a pleasure trip, and do not propose to have it cost us much of anything. We force hospitality on our acquaintances in order to save hotel bills. They know it, and they feel about it just exactly as we would in their places--that is, that it is an imposition on good nature and a mean and selfish thing to do.

"We gave up our house and went to boarding simply because my health and my husband's salary were inadequate to the demands made upon them by our out-of-town relatives and acquaintances, who used us as a restaurant and hotel. There was seldom a week when we did not give ten or twelve meals and two or three nights lodging to people better able to pay for them than we were to furnish them. So we gave up housekeeping." This is an actual experience.

WEEK-END VISITS.

The "house-party," as the week-end visit is now often styled, is a comparatively recent addition to social entertainments. It is a fashion imported from England, and a very good one. It is the "from Saturday to Monday" visit, and so universally recognized that during the summer extra trolley cars and railroad trains are in use to convey resorters and their guests to summer homes in the country.

Invitations to a house-party are given several weeks in advance, and great care should be taken to invite those who are congenial and will "mix well," since where a few are thrown together congeniality is absolutely essential to success. The invitations are informal; the length of the visit definitely fixed; even the train by which the visitor is expected to arrive and leave is mentioned, that there may be no misunderstanding.

The Invitation.--One may write to her friend: "Won't you give us the pleasure of entertaining you from Friday afternoon to Monday?

The 3:45 train will bring you here in time for tea. There is to be a musical in the evening; an automobile ride is planned for Saturday afternoon, to show you the beauties of our vicinity, and there is to be the usual Saturday evening dance at the hotel. A train leaves here at 10:30 Monday morning, which will take you back to the city in ample time for lunch. Hoping to have the happiness of seeing you on Friday, I am," etc., etc.

This not only suggests to your friend at what time she is expected to arrive and depart, but gives her an idea of what she should bring with her in the way of clothes. One should always take her prettiest gowns that will be suitable to the entertainments proposed for her pleasure--for a hostess naturally wishes to have her guests make a good appearance. From four to six is the number generally asked to a small house-party, since the usual summer cottage has few guest rooms. The guests are, if possible, evenly divided as to sex, and a hostess may, with perfect propriety, arrange that the men of the party shall be lodged at a hotel, coming over to breakfast with their entertainer.

Amusements.--Some amusements are always provided for the visitors at a house-party. Often a dinner-party is planned for Sunday, in which several other guests are included. Men who cannot leave business for even a week-end often come out Sunday for a dinner and a breath of country air. Now that automobiles are as plenty as blackberries the railroad train can be ignored. Young people living in the country should take advantage of this method of entertaining their city friends, who will find the change delightful in summer, and will gladly reciprocate by inviting them to the city during the social season. Remember that a hearty hospitality, a sincere joy in seeing your friends, and the fresh milk, eggs and fruits you can offer will do much toward counterbalancing your lack of "city conveniences."

The Hostess's Arrangements.--The hostess should arrange to have the guests met at the station. She will naturally try to have them arrive by the same train, is possible; but she must see that their baggage arrives at the house nearly as soon as they do, that they may at once remove the soil of travel and dress for the evening meal. She may or she may not meet them at the station, according to her own convenience, but she must be ready to receive them when they arrive at the home. If the journey has been long, a cup of tea may be offered; otherwise they are at once shown to their rooms. The hostess does this for her women guests, the host or a servant for the men.

If a visitor is so unfortunate as to miss her train she should immediately telegraph or telephone her hostess, explaining the accident, and saying she will arrange to have herself conveyed from the station to the house on her arrival by a later train. Of course, the hostess will not permit this, but will send some vehicle to meet the next train.

The matter of guest rooms and their conveniences, proper furnishings, etc., will be taken up in a later section.

What Is Expected of Guests.--One does not invite guests to make them uncomfortable, therefore it is best not to expect them to rise for an early breakfast. If they are expected to present themselves, as late an hour as possible should be named. But they may be served with coffee, rolls, fruit and any other easily prepared breakfast dish whenever they please to arise, being given to understand that a substantial breakfast is the price of the extra "forty winks." Guests at a house-party are expected to entertain themselves, among themselves, to a considerable extent. They may walk, or row, or play croquet or tennis, or read or gossip or play cards, while the hostess attends to her domestic duties. If the party is large, or if but one or no servants are kept, the women should quietly attend to their own rooms, making up the bed and picking up their own belongings. Whether they may do this or not depends upon circumstances of which they must judge.

The most enjoyable house-parties are given in these roomy old houses with broad verandas, surrounded with lawn and garden. But this need not deter those having less delightful surroundings from offering their best to their friends. It is not so much the elegance of what we offer as the manner in which it is offered that makes our friends remember their visit with pleasure.

Dress at Week-End Visits.--Women wear a simple tailored suit while traveling, with white waist or silk skirt to match. If the weather is warm, white duck, pique or linen skirts with white shirts are worn mornings; afternoons, foulard, or some of the fine and dainty fabrics suited to the season. For evening, nothing is prettier than white for the young--and, indeed, "everybody wears white." By change of accessories, the same white gown may be made to do for the two evenings. If an automobile trip is part of the entertainment, one should take an ulster or long loose coat and veil.

The woman's greatest trouble is to carry a second hat--something she may need under some circumstances, though the fashion of going bareheaded helps considerably. But if the entertainment includes a garden party, a tea or reception, she must have a hat. The trunk is uncalled for, and the suitcase is disobliging. What shall she do?

Her best plan will be to have a becoming shape covered with black tulle or malines, and a made bow attached to it to travel in. On arrival, she will detach the bow and pin on a couple of plumes, an aigrette, or flowers, converting it into a dress hat.

Men's Wear.--The man wears the ordinary business suit for travelling, sack or cutaway. He wears in the country in the morning a suit of flannel, tweed or cheviot, a straw hat and tan shoes. His shirt may be of striped madras or linen, with a white collar. The cutaway coat is correct for ordinary afternoon wear, with a white waistcoat, white shirt and four-in-hand tie. This takes the place in summer of the frock coat, which is the formal day wear. He will seldom, if ever, have occasion for a dress suit at a week-end visit in summer. Of course, the size of the party and the gayeties in which one will participate have a bearing on the dress question, but the tendency is for men's dress to be more comfortable and less formal in summer, especially in the country.

THE DUTIES OF A HOSTESS.

The woman who is entertaining guests must remember two things: that she must not neglect them, and that she must not tire them out with too much attention. There is a "happy mean" to be attained, which is the climax of pleasure and comfort to both.

One woman makes her visitor feel that "the domestic veal" has been slaughtered in her behalf. The usual manner of living and habits of life have been put aside that she may be "entertained." Elaborate meals are planned; there is a straining after hospitality which defeats its own purpose and makes the visitor uncomfortable, because the hostess has so manifestly incommoded herself. The fussy hostess puts too much endeavor into her entertainment.

On the other hand, there is the hostess who announces her intention of regarding her visitor as "one of the family," "making no fuss" on account of her being in the house. This sounds much better than it works out in actual practice. Unless we are prepared to modify our routine in accordance with our friend's pleasure and convenience, at least to some extent, we should not invite her. We do not ask people to our houses to make them more uncomfortable than they would be at home. A visit is in the nature of a holiday, or vacation, to the visitor; we are to see to it that she is deferred to and efforts made to please her.

The Visitor's Comfort.--It is hospitable to consult her tastes in the matter of food. It is uncomfortable for both hostess and guest if the principal dish at dinner is something the latter dislikes. Nor should we ask her to conform to the family breakfast hour if we know she is unaccustomed to early hours, or is very much fatigued. In that case it is best to say that the early breakfast is a family necessity and that she will not be expected to appear at it, but may have her coffee and toast in her own room or down stairs at the hour at which she wishes to rise. This, though it may necessitate the preparation of a tray to be sent up, is really a convenience to the hostess, who is then left free to attend to her domestic duties. As some one has said, "It is not hospitality to ask a guest to your rooftree and expect her to find sufficient delight in being there and doing as you do." Very often she would be far more comfortable at home, physically at least. Remember your object in inviting people is to make them happy. Unless you are willing to make some sacrifices to do this, do not invite them.

Preparing for Company.--An expected guest should always be met at the station by some member of the family. The guest room should be in readiness, closet and bureau drawers vacated for her use. The bed should be freshly made up, the bedding having been properly aired. It would seem that no one would offer a visitor a bed that has not been changed and aired after having been slept in, yet guests, exchanging experiences, acknowledge it has been done--let us hope through inadvertence, though it is really inexcusable.

There should be plenty of fresh towels and water; a fresh cake of soap, a candlestick and matches, and a waste paper basket. On the dressing-bureau there should be a spotless spread, a pincushion well stocked with pins, hand mirror, comb and brush. The guest will bring her own, but may need to use these before her luggage arrives. The brush and comb should have been washed after a previous using.

A lounge, preferably placed at the foot of the bed if there is room; a light quilt or blanket for use upon it; an easy chair, and a clock in good working order are desirable furnishings. Writing materials should be provided. Some careful and painstaking hostesses include a small writing desk, well stocked with paper, pens and ink, postage stamps, even picture postal cards already stamped and ready to be addressed. A new magazine and a few books, and a little basket containing thimble, needles, scissors and several spools of cotton complete the conveniences arranged for the guest. A potted plant, or a few flowers in a vase, give a personal touch that bespeaks the hostess's solicitude for the pleasure of her friend.

There is no more delicious flattery than that of having one's personal tastes remembered and recognized.

The Visitor's Entertainment.--The entertainment of a guest is, of course, dependent on the hostess's means, mode of life, social standing, the season of the year, and whether one lives in town or in the country.

She will ask some of her friends to call on her guest; she will give a little entertainment for her, at cards, or a tea, or a reception, according to circumstances. No doubt her friends will include her visitor in their invitations during her stay. She will take her friend to see the sights of her home city if she is a stranger; she may give a theatre party, or at least take her friend several times. She will pay her guest's carfare, unless the other anticipates her, and pay for the theatre tickets. It will be perfectly correct for the guest to "stand treat" by inviting her host and hostess to accompany her to concert or play, paying for the seats herself.

The Hostess's Invitations.--It often happens that a hostess has invitations not extended to her visitor. She may have accepted; before her guest's arrival, an invitation to dinner, card party or luncheon. In neither of these may she ask to have her guests included. They are formal functions for which arrangements are made long in advance. She may say to an intimate friend who is giving a musical or an "At home" or any informal affair, that she has a visitor staying with her, and the friend will no doubt extend an invitation to the latter. It is proper for host and hostess to accept invitations in which a guest is not included if they make some provision for her pleasure during their absence.

She may be asked to invite some friend to dine with her, or someone provided to take her to the theatre. Nor has she a right to feel affronted at being left at home.

One thing must be carefully avoided, the hostess must not let her guest feel, for one moment, that she is the cause of inconvenience or trouble. Even if she is, the fact must be sedulously concealed. Bear with the annoyance until the visit ceases; then do not invite her again. It is the hostess's privilege to invite; having invited she must not allow her equanimity to be disturbed.

THE OBLIGATIONS OF A GUEST.

If it is the duty of the hostess to be attentive to the comfort of her guest, there is quite as much obligation resting on the guest to show a disposition to be pleased and to make herself agreeable. Some women--young girls more particularly--seem to think too much cannot be done for their entertainment. They make themselves burdensome by their wish to have "something doing" all the time. The visitor who conveys the impression that she is neglected unless some festivity is in the immediate future easily becomes tiresome.

The guest should accommodate herself to the ways of the family. Especially should she be punctual at meals and ready on time when going out with her friends. Her host may acquire a dislike to her if she keeps him waiting. She should always be neatly dressed, never appearing at the breakfast table in kimona or dressing-jacket if men will be present. She should respect the privileges of the host, not occupying his easy chair, appropriating the newspaper or the best position round the lamp. She should give as little trouble as possible and be especially careful about scattering her belongings about the house. This particularly applies to young girls, who are apt to be careless in this respect. It annoys a hostess to find Missy's rubbers kicked off in the hall, her hat on the piano, and a half eaten box of candy on the parlor sofa.

About Being Thoughtful.--She should be careful to avoid injury to any of her hostess' pretty things or her furnishings. The story is told of a girl who, conducted to her hostess's beautiful guest room, furnished with the utmost daintiness in white, threw her umbrella and dusty coat on the spotless counterpane, exclaiming: "What a lovely room!" It was not lovely when she left it. The wall was defaced by marks made by scratching matches; the bureau scarf was blackened by the curling-iron; there were ink spots on the hemstitched sheets where she had written letters in bed, and something that would not come out was spilled on the table cover. It does not show that you are accustomed to nice things to be so negligent and careless; it shows you are not accustomed to them and do not know how to treat them; and it makes you a visitor the hostess is glad to get rid of, and never invites again.

The guest, young or old, should take herself out of the way part of the time; she shouldn't be always in evidence. Let her go to her own room and write letters, read, or take her work out of doors; in other words, show an ability to entertain herself which releases her hostess from that responsibility for the time being. This is much better than having one's friend in one's constant presence.

Outside Acquaintance.--If one is staying with a friend and has other acquaintances in the same place she will naturally expect them to call on her. If her callers are strangers to her hostess, they should ask for her. The hostess may see them or ask to be excused with equal propriety. The guest is at liberty to accept outside invitations which do not include her hostess, but should always consult her in reference to them. She has no right to invite any of her friends to a meal without first mentioning her wish to her hostess and securing a cordial acquiescence. She must not make a convenience of her friend's house, and if a girl or young woman, she must not receive there any man or woman of whom her parents disapprove. This is disloyal to them, and an imposition upon her hostess.

Other Points to Observe.--If a visitor can play, sing, recite, tell stories, or in any way contribute to the pleasure of her friends or other guests, she should comply cheerfully with requests that she do so. On the other hand, she should not monopolize the piano. She should enter readily into any plans proposed for her entertainment; even though they may not be especially agreeable, she should subscribe to the kindly intent.

The question as to how much assistance the visitor should volunteer in case her hostess keeps but one servant, or does her own work, is dependent upon circumstances. She certainly shouldn't follow her hostess all over the house with offers of help: "Can't I do this?" "Shan't I do that?" Let her quickly and unostentatiously render such small services as are helpful without being obtrusive. She may care for her own room; she may fill the vases with flowers; she may tell stories to the children or take them for a walk, but she must carefully respect the hostess's privacy and not intrude in the rear regions where the domestic rites are performed, without her hostess's permission. And whatever aid she renders she should give according to her hostess's method, not her own.

A visitor should carefully avoid any comment on the cook's failures, should such occur; she must not criticise the children's manners: nor reprove them; nor should she criticise the chance caller or visitor, who is a friend of her hostess, but not of her acquaintance. Above all she must avoid comparisons. If she has been visiting more wealthy people it is not good form to wax eloquent over the elegance of their establishment or their more expensive mode of entertaining.

Concerning Departure.--If there has been no time named as the length of her visit, she should take an early opportunity to mention now long she will remain "if perfectly convenient." And it is almost invariably a mistake to remain beyond the date named. Better go, and have your departure regretted, than linger to find the later days give a flat ending and you and your hostess alike relieved at parting.

It is customary, on leaving, to give a small fee to the maid who has cared for one's room, and to the waitress, if one is employed. Anyone who has rendered personal service is generally remembered. A dollar is usually given at the close of a week's visit: something depends upon the style of the household. Men generally tip the chauffeur.

After having been received as a guest in a family it is the height of incivility and bad manners to criticise their mode of living, discuss the peculiarities of any member, or make unkind remarks in reference to a slight, real or fancied, or any negligence or oversight. Having eaten your hostess's salt, there is an obligation of silence imposed, unless one can speak in terms of praise.

At Home Again.--Immediately after one's return home it is obligatory to write what is sometimes called "the bread-and-butter letter"--that in which one expresses her pleasure in the visit and her appreciation of the hospitality received. A serviceable form for this follows:

My Dear Mrs. Blank:

I wish to tell you at once how much I enjoyed my visit to your charming home and how truly I appreciate all you did to make my stay so pleasant. I shall always remember my good times with you, and especially that most delightful picnic to Ferndale.

With kind remembrances to Mr. Blank and to Lois, who helped so much to make me happy, believe me,

Yours most sincerely,

Mary Annesley.

This recognition of hospitality enjoyed must on no account be omitted.

VISITING ETIQUETTE FOR GIRLS.

The best personal asset a girl can have is "nice manners;" they will contribute more to her lasting popularity than beauty or wealth. Girls sometimes wonder how it happens that a girl they have regarded as "too homely" to be accounted dangerous, still carries off the matrimonial prize of "her set." Ten chances to one it is because she has that charm of manner that makes a man overlook her physical deficiencies. Her manners, in such case, are the spontaneous expression of a kind and generous disposition, aided, of course, by a familiarity with the social code that prevents awkwardness. She has ease, and that puts others at their ease; she is companionable; and not being engrossed by her own good looks, she has had time to cultivate the intellectual graces.

Nothing is more becoming to a young girl than respect and deference to her elders. If for no other reason than that it gives observers an unfavorable opinion of her manners, she should avoid any disrespect or rudeness toward her parents or older sisters. The young girl is often negligent in this respect. Her own ego is exaggerated, owing to her youth and inexperience; she thinks

"What there is to know, I know it;
What I don't know isn't knowledge;"

and is much inclined to dub her own mother "old-fashioned." So she contradicts her, precedes her in entering a room, takes the easiest chair, monopolizes the conversation, and in other disrespectful ways endeavors to assert her own importance. Instead of crediting her with more social experience, bystanders consider her a very crude and untrained young person.

Deference to Age.--One reason why convent training is so highly esteemed in our best circles is because girls are taught such beautiful manners. No convent-bred girl would think of showing the slightest disrespect to an older person. They are taught all the little matters of etiquette that contribute to gentle and refined manners. A lady staying at a large summer hotel noted the charming manners of a young Southern girl, especially in regard to the unfailing deference paid to her mother and aunt. She rose when they addressed her and remained standing during the conversation. When the aunt came to the breakfast table the girl rose, standing until the elder lady was seated; if her mother entered one of the reception rooms she excused herself if conversing and advanced to meet her, finding a seat for her and perhaps asking permission to introduce an acquaintance. And it was all done so easily, so naturally, that it was plainly seen there was no affectation, but the unstudied courtesy due to good-breeding.

On the other hand, girls who undertake to show their respect for their seniors sometimes overdo the matter. No elderly person likes to be "fussed over." She doesn't want someone continually thrusting a cushion behind her shoulders or insisting on providing a foot-stool. The unwelcome service provokes a little resentment. One must have an intuitive sense of what to do and when to do it, and tact enough to perform a trifling service without the appearance of saying "See me! how polite I am!" As young men should rise when an elderly woman enters the room, so a young girl may pay the same pretty deference to her mother or an acquaintance. She should be careful not to take precedence of older women, not to interrupt them when speaking, and to render any small service unobtrusively.

THE YOUNG GIRL'S SOCIAL AFFAIRS.

There is no special code of etiquette for girls. Why should they be trained in one code, only to discard it for another when they enter society? Their etiquette is simply more informal. Until they are "out," they do not give formal invitations. Their functions are chiefly luncheons, invitations being given by telephone or personal notes, and the menu more simple. They may give theatre parties, but never without a chaperon. They do not invite young men to call on them; that is their mother's duty. They do not send written invitations to young men; these are in the mother's name. Thus:

> *My Dear Mr. Smith:*
>
> *My mother wishes me to say that it will give her much pleasure if you will spend Friday evening, March tenth, with us, quite informally. We hope to see you at eight o' clock.*
>
> *Yours sincerely,*
>
> *Mary Gray.*

Such an invitation presupposes the presence of other guests. If for cards, or music or games, mention may be made of the proposed entertainment.

A girl should not receive calls from young men without the presence of some member of the family, her mother by preference, at some time during the evening. A young man should not feel that the girl he calls upon is not properly looked after by her parents.

The Girl and the Chaperon.--Youth scorns the chaperon, regarding her as superfluous. "I can look out for myself," is the young girl's motto. Yet scandal has dimmed the fair name of many a girl through her disinclination to submit to proper chaperonage. The chaperon is much more of a social necessity in the East than she is in the South and West. If a girl proposes to "look ant for herself," there are some things she must carefully abstain from doing. She must not go to a restaurant with a young man alone; she must not travel about with him alone, even if she is engaged to him; she must not go "on excursions" unattended, nor go for a ride with a man and stop anywhere for refreshments; indeed, she should not accept such an invitation unless another couple or another girl are included in the party. This is not prudery; it is protection; and any young man's acquaintance is not desirable if he objects to such arrangements. He would not permit his sister to do what he asks some other man's sister to do. A young man loses in respect for a girl if she holds herself cheap.

If a girl receives invitations of the character just mentioned, it is far better to say frankly "My father (or mother) does not allow me to accept," than to make excuses or plead previous engagements time after time.

The Girl and the Young Man.--Do not ask a young man to call on the occasion of your first meeting. Young people often meet and make each other's acquaintance when the girl's mother, whose place it is to give the invitation to call, is not present. After several meetings the girl, having ascertained the young man's antecedents, may say, if he seems desirous of the invitation, "'My mother will be glad to know you," or "Mother and I will be pleased to have you call some evening."

The young man should acknowledge the compliment by calling at an early date, and should meet the girl's mother, The girl does not suggest when he shall call, though she may mention that she receives calls on a certain evening. She must not give him her card; if he is not sufficiently interested to remember her address he probably does not intend to call.

It is not correct for girls to suggest a walk, ride, hint a wish to dance or row, or tacitly invite a tete-a-tete. Let those who wish such favors ask for them. The girl who shows herself most anxious for young men's attentions generally receives fewest. Despite "the woman's movement," man still insists on his privilege of taking the initiative.

About Gifts.--It is not correct form for a girl to receive presents from young men, aside from flowers, candy and an occasional book or piece of music. In some circles, to offer a girl a piece of jewelry would be considered insulting. Not until he is engaged to her may a man offer expensive presents. This rule, it is lamentably true, is often violated by a certain order of young persons, who rather boast of the gifts of their gallants, and are thus the object of rather unkind criticism.

As a rule, a girl makes a mistake when she sends a gift to a young man. It is generally something that is as superfluous to him as a fifth wheel to a wagon, and it entails an irksome sense of obligation. It is presumed, if he has been very courteous and shown her many attentions, that it has been his pleasure to do so, and her gracious acceptance and pleasure in them is sufficient reward. A girl may give Christmas and birthday gifts to her fiance, but he should not give her any article of wearing apparel except gloves.

The Telephone.--A girl should be chary of calling up her young men acquaintances by telephone. If forced to do so, she should make her communication as brief as possible. It is annoying to a young man to be called from his business to answer social or "nonsense" calls--the latter when some idle, ennuied or "smitten" girl takes a notion she would like to chatter to somebody awhile. It exasperates an employer to have his men called from their duties to answer such calls, and fellow employees are likely to "guy" the man about his "mash." The "note habit" is just about as bad, though not quite as annoying, as the telephone habit, because a man can carry such missives in his pocket unopened.

A wise girl will not give her photograph to any young man until she is engaged to him. What nice girl would care to see her picture neighbored by ballet dancers and footlight favorites in a young man's rooms! She will be equally careful about corresponding with men, writing to but a few intimate and long-known friends, making her letters bright and gay, but carefully avoiding any warmer expressions of regard than those warranted by the friendship. Many a girl has bitterly regretted the affectionate missives sent to some young man who made "werry fierce love" to her for a time, and whose regard afterward cooled. When the man she truly loves comes along, she would give her most precious jewel to get those letters into her hands again. It is a great deal safer not to write them.

A young woman, receiving back her letters at the close of a mistaken engagement, once said:

"I sat down on the floor and read them over, and I tell you I was proud of myself. There wasn't one I wouldn't have been willing to have my father read--and you know what I think of my father!"

THE DEBUTANTE.

A large number of young girls enter society without formal introductions. After leaving school, they assume their social responsibilities with no formality. It is seldom that a girl enters the social world under eighteen, or over twenty-two. The early appearance implies no college career; the later, that, she has spent several years at college or finishing school.

Increasingly, however, it is becoming the custom to introduce the young aspirant for social recognition at some function given in her honor. This may be a ball, a reception, a "coming-out party," a dinner, a tea, at which the debutante is introduced to the older members of the circle in which she will move. Whereas her associates heretofore have been young folk of her own age, she now meets the people of all ages who constitute what we call society. Her circle of acquaintances will be much enlarged, and her breeding will be judged by the manner in which she accepts her new obligations.

A Grave Mistake.--The greatest mistake the debutante can make is to treat with carelessness and lack of respect the matrons, young or old, to whom she is introduced. In the arrogance of her youth and ignorance she may think them "old frumps" and devote herself to her mates in age and inexperience. But the "old frumps" hold the trump cards; she will be dependent on them for invitations to many pleasant little functions, especially those exclusive affairs to which it is an honor to be invited, and if she is not personally agreeable, there will always be some one else to take the place that might have been hers, for a chaperon often influences a young man's invitations. Moreover, by her disrespect for age and position she advertises her lack of good breeding and social training.

Her Dress.--The debutante dresses in white at her "coming-out party," as a rule; white being supposed to typify her virginal attitude in the social realm. The mother receives her guests with her daughter standing at her side. It is not uncommon for two girls of about the same age who are close friends to be introduced at the same function. The celebrant's friends send flowers; sometimes the number of bouquets is so great that a screen is arranged behind her on which they are displayed. Girls pique themselves on the number of such tributes.

46

If Not a Belle.--But suppose a girl is not pretty enough, nor rich enough, nor attractive enough to become a social success. She will suffer countless mortifications. In society, as in business, "Nothing succeeds like success." If she is popular, she will have a very happy time as debutante. If she is not "a success," her chaperon will despair of her. She will be partnerless when other girls have too many; she will have to retire to the dressing-room, deeply humiliated because unescorted to the supper-room. She will be a wall-flower while others dance. Young men are very selfish; unless a girl has some claim to consideration, personally, or they expect invitations through her parents, they often will selfishly neglect her.

What shall she do in such a case? She will be happier and more contented to give up the losing fight, find some sphere that is congenial, and determine to adorn it. There are many kinds of belles; she may make herself a belle of the home, a belle in out-door sports, a queen of the chafing-dish. Far better these humbler triumphs than neglect and unhappiness in the social world.

A girl looks forward to her debut with many joyous anticipations, but often finds her second social season a happier one than her first. She is more sure of herself, less shy and reserved; little things--the small mistakes made through ignorance--do not worry her so much; she has gained ease and grace of manner, having shed her self-consciousness.

THE ETIQUETTE OF BALLS.

"Dinner dances" have largely taken the place of balls, the latter having seemingly passed into the hands of clubs and assemblies or being known as "subscription dances." One must have a very large house, with ball-room, to give a ball successfully, so it is customary to engage private apartments at some fashionable restaurant or hotel, where there are accommodations for such an affair.

Invitations are formal, and of course engraved. If a debutante is to be presented her card may or may not be, but usually is, enclosed with the invitation. The patronesses of a subscription dance are entitled to invitations which they send to their friends, enclosing their card. The word "ball" never appears on an invitation; its nature is indicated by "Cotillion," the fashionable name for what was called "the German." The hostess or hostesses stand near the entrance to the ball-room, and should see that the guests receive a fair amount of attention. The supper is provided by a caterer, of course. Two orchestras, playing alternately, provide music; they are screened behind palms and other plants. Balls generally begin about eleven o'clock, the hour named on the cards being half after ten, and everybody waiting in the hope that someone else may arrive earlier. General dancing is in order until supper is served; afterwards the cotillion is danced.

At the dinner dance, the cotillion is preceded by a dinner, given by the hostess at her own house, or by several hostesses at some restaurant, where each presides over a table. Dinner and subscription dances are much favored by the younger set, as the hostesses act in the capacity of chaperons, and the company is gayer.

To bid one's hostess good night--or good morning--and express one's pleasure in her entertainment is obligatory.

GARDEN PARTIES.

Jupiter Pluvius apparently has a grouch against garden-parties, so often does he shake his sieve with deliberate intent to spoil the affair, which is after all, merely afternoon tea out of doors. The hostess anxiously consults "the probabilities" as to weather, and if storm threatens must hastily convert her garden fete into an in-door function. If blessed with a bright day, a garden party is a pretty affair. The women wear beautiful light gowns, en train by preference, and their flower-laden hats and gay parasols contribute to the charm of the scene.

The garden-party is the special prerogative of the out-of-town hostess. She has the lawn and the trees without which a party of this character cannot be undertaken. Invitations may be formal, or the hostess may use her card with the hour and the date and "Garden Party" written in the lower left hand corner. If guests from a distance are expected to arrive by train or trolley they must be notified of the train or car which will be met by carriages or automobiles she provides.

The hostess receives on the lawn, and hats are retained. Games, like lawn tennis, archery, croquet, should be provided. Guests wander about and entertain each other, and seek the refreshment tables when so inclined. The supper may be served under a tent or in the house. Seats are provided, and rugs spread on the grass. No matter if the weather is unfavorable the guests are expected to present themselves, as the hostess will quickly transform her out-door fete into an in-door affair in case of rain.

Refreshments.--A hostess is not expected to use her best china and linen at a garden party. She should have an ample supply of napkins, plates, cups and silver, but the expense of hiring them from a caterer is offset by the danger of breakage and loss.

She may serve salads, sandwiches, cakes, ices and ice creams, fruit, and claret cup; or sandwiches, cakes, ice cream and lemonade and fruit punch. Hot tea should be provided for those who prefer it, especially if rain drives the guests in-doors. The young matrons are invited to pour it. The maids should remove soiled dishes and napkins promptly, and keep the tables looking fresh. Music is usually provided.

AT SMALL ENTERTAINMENTS.

Many small, informal entertainments are more enjoyable than those larger affairs given for the purpose of paying off social debts. Good will and jollity prevail, and people "go in for a good time."

Card Parties.--The most stringent rule of etiquette at a card-party is to be punctual, that the tables may be filled up in good season. The second rule is to keep good-natured, even if your partner fails to return your lead or trumps your ace. Some people make themselves very disagreeable over cards, and are avoided as partners. If unfortunate enough to be paired off with such a person, at least control your own annoyance.

Never descend to the meanness of telegraphing information, hinting at your preferences in the way of trumps, overlooking a neighbor's hand, or taking any unfair advantage. A prize thus won is no honor. Nor do such violations of good breeding pass unnoticed.

At the Party.--If one accepts an invitation to a card party she is supposed to have sufficient proficiency to play the game proposed with some degree of credit; otherwise she should promptly send regrets. Invitations may be formal or informal, or the hostess may send her card with "Bridge, at half after two o'clock," or "Euchre," or "Five Hundred," written upon it. Replies are to be sent at once. Many such invitations are given by telephone. The guests are assigned to tables by the hostess, the names being written at the top of the scorecards. Two packs of cards are on each table, and small pencils attached to the score-cards. Playing begins when all are present. Or the hostess may fill the tables as the guests arrive, begin playing at the stated time, and assign late comers to places as they come in. Hats are kept on at an afternoon card-party. The usual limit for playing is two hours. The "progressive" fashion requires the providing of two prizes, the first prize and a consolation prize for the person having the lowest score. If prizes are given at each table they should be duplicates. These prizes are wrapped up in tissue paper and tied with ribbons, and are to be opened at once, displayed, and the hostess cordially thanked. It is not good form to be ostentatiously generous in the matter of prizes, nor should guests show themselves too eager to win.

It is customary to engage card tables and chairs for such an entertainment. The refreshments are served on these tables. Punch is sometimes served while the game is in progress.

Very often the hostess invites some of her friends who do not play cards to come in for refreshments at half after four or five o'clock.

Refreshments should not be too elaborate for either afternoon or evening card-parties. Sandwiches, coffee, and small cakes, or ices and cake, for the afternoon; salad of some kind with coffee, olives, and some sweet or fancy wafer, for evening. Men enjoy an oyster stew served hot in the dining room.

YOUNG GIRLS' PARTIES.

Until a girl is formally launched in society, her parties are of the simplest and most informal kind. She will invite a few friends to tea, or to a card-party, giving informal invitations and confining them to her school friends and most intimate acquaintances. Games, music, and the like are the usual amusements. Properly chaperoned, she may give a small theater party.

Birthday Party.--The largest of her social functions will probably be her birthday party. For this, her birthday flower will be chosen for decorations. Her young friends may give her little presents. Once in a season she may be invited to a small dance given for some schoolmate. This she will attend, prettily and simply gowned, and properly chaperoned. On no account will she go alone in a carriage, or with a young man alone. If she is a well bred girl she will not pique herself in dancing every dance, nor "split the dances" into fragments to please those who wish to dance with her. She will be careful not to romp nor laugh too loud; nor to permit herself to be held too closely in dancing, nor be served too often with punch.

"STAG" DINNERS.

The woman who wishes to give her husband a birthday party or anniversary will not go amiss if she makes it a "stag dinner"--that is, a dinner for men only.

To this she invites as many of his men friends as she can accommodate, and provides a good, substantial meal, without any "frills." It need not be elaborate if everything is good of its kind, well cooked and served hot. The menu may include oysters, roast fowl, two vegetables, several relishes, and an entree, with some simple dessert and good coffee. She will also see to it that the cigars are of the proper excellence. It is optional whether she sits at the table till the coffee and cigars are served, or stays in the kitchen to superintend the serving. Red is the most appropriate color for decorations, since a man's ideas of color are usually rather crude. Men always enjoy a dinner of this kind. The evening may conclude with cards.

A stag card-party sometimes takes the place of a dinner; it is followed by a substantial supper.

THE MUSICAL AND INFORMAL TEA.

At a musical, guests are seated, the hostess remaining near the door to welcome late arrivals. If these arrive while a selection is in progress, they stand till it is finished, then find seats. Guests do not leave their seats during the intermission, but converse with those in the vicinity. Refreshments are always served. Hats are removed.

For a very informal tea the hostess sends her card with the date and hour written across the lower corner. If a friend is staying with her, she may write "to meet Mrs. A." at the top. She will offer a cup of tea and cakes or wafers to each comer, or may ask some friend to do so for her, leaving her free to mingle with her visitors. Simplicity and informality characterize this form of receiving friends.

ETIQUETTE FOR CHILDREN.

"The future destiny of the child is always the work of the mother." -- Bonaparte.

Children reflect the manners of their homes. As they learn to talk after the fashion of their parents' speech, so they learn to be polite by example, aided by training, and in both cases the habit of youth persists in greater or less degree all through life.

To train children properly requires patience and persistence, but to have polite children, and to feel that they know what to do and how to do it when they begin to go out, is certainly a great source of satisfaction to a mother, on whom the burden of training falls.

The secret of success is beginning early. Before the baby is three years old he should be in process of training. When he comes into the use of spoon, knife and fork, he should be taught how to hold these properly, and how to feed himself. He should never be permitted to play with his food; out of that baby habit comes the later playing with crumbs, holding the fork in the hand when not eating, drinking tea from a spoon, and other little gaucheries resorted to in embarrassment or preoccupation. It is not necessary to wait until a child is ten or twelve years old before teaching him not to interrupt a conversation, and to make his wants known quietly and without iteration, nor yet that your yea means yea, and your nay, nay.

First Lessons.--The mother's first lesson is usually in regard to taking off his hat or cap. Teach him to remove this as soon as he enters the house, as soon as he begins to go out of doors alone, and the habit will become life-long. It is very charming to see a child of either sex rise to open the door for a visitor, or stand while she talks to him. One often sees boys of seven, nine and eleven years of age occupying the seats in a car while the ladies stand. No mother should permit this.

Whether a child should say "father" and "mother," or use the more babyish form of "papa" and "mama" is a matter of parental choice, but the preference in some circles is for the former. A blunt "yes" or "no" is not thought polite from a child; he should say "yes, father," "no, mama," "yes, Mrs. Smith." "Ma'am" as a form of address is quite obsolete.

Most parents make the mistake of believing their children as absorbingly interesting to other people as they are to them, and bring them forward so prominently that they become tiresome. A good rule is for the mother to allow children to greet the visitor and then send them away to their play. The spectacle of a little child primly seated on a chair and "taking in" the conversation with eyes and ears is not wholly edifying; while to allow a child to hang on a visitor or monopolize the attention makes the youngster a nuisance.

CHILDREN'S PARTIES.

There is nothing children love better than a party. It takes so little to make them happy that the exertion is well repaid by their pleasure. A few games, a light supper, an inexpensive souvenir, and they have had "a perfectly splendid time."

For children from five to twelve, the best hours for a party are from three to half past five. This gives time for all to return home by six o'clock. Few mothers wish to have their children out evenings at that age. Where the children are old enough they should write their own invitations. They should receive their guests themselves, the mother standing in the background to see that they do it properly and to second their welcome. The little host or hostess should early learn the lesson that she must study the pleasure of her guests, not her own, and be taught the courtesies required of her.

Games.--The first thing is the games, which are suitable to the children's age. Little ones play romping games, like "Cat and Mouse," "London Bridge," etc.; those a little older enjoy a peanut hunt or a peanut race, or supplying the donkey with a caudal appendage. Many novel games are possible. Or the children may be asked to a doll's party, or an animal party. To the one they bring their favorite doll; to the other their teddy bears and cotton elephants.

Supper.--The supper should be simple. Sandwiches, cocoa, jellies, and fancy cookies not too rich. After the supper they may dance "Sir Roger de Coverley," or some simple form all know, and then little souvenirs may be distributed in a way that leads to a hunt. Notes are written and put in a bag; each child takes one; the note directs where to look. All rush pell mell to that spot. There they find directions to look somewhere else, and finally each gets a little card or a note directing a search at some particular place, say in a basket in the hall or in the dining room, where each finds and unwraps a little gift. Or a large paper sack filled with wrapped bonbons is hung between folding doors, each child blindfolded in turn, given a cane and instructed to hit the sack if he can. Presently the paper is broken and the youngsters scramble for the contents. Each little guest should thank the giver of the party and the mother for the pleasure enjoyed. The little host or hostess should stand where they can make their adieus, for it is no longer proper to "take French leave" on any occasion except "a crush."

Games for Older Children.--Older children enjoy a peanut hunt, or a spider party where they follow a twine through a labyrinth of loopings and find a small prize at the end, or a book party, where each guest represents the title of some book. Thus Ouida's "Under Two Flags" could be very easily represented. Young folks always enjoy "dressing up," and any hostess can either find directions for some form of fancy dress, or invent something new for herself. St. Valentine's Day, St. Patrick's Day, May Day, the Fourth of July, Hallowe'en, have their traditional decorations, and games, and suggest their own refreshments. Elaborate refreshments have rather gone out of style.

CONCERNING ENGAGEMENTS.

A marriage engagement is one of the most serious contracts into which young people can enter, second only to actual marriage. It is not to be lightly entered upon. It is no credit to a girl to have been several times affianced; indeed, it almost invariably occasions unfavorable comment. There may be reasons for breaking one engagement, but when it comes to the second, Mrs. Grundy makes remarks, and is inclined to blame the girl, either for too great haste to wed, or for being fickle and capricious,

A girl should be very sure of herself before she gives her promise. She must respect the man, and have faith and confidence in him, and not permit herself to be carried away by considerations of wealth and position. If there is anything about him she dislikes, she may be sure dislike will become aversion after marriage, unless she has a genuine affection for him.

Parental Wishes.--She should not engage herself without consulting her parents. Where can she find better advice than from those who have cared for her so long and faithfully? Where there is parental disapproval, a girl should show her respect for her parents' opinion by avoiding a hasty decision. Men know men much better than women can ever know them; and the opposition of a father or older brother should have due consideration.

In these days and in this country, young women take their matrimonial affairs into their own hands. "In the good old times" the young man asked the consent of the girl's parents before he was sure of her sentiments toward him; he asked permission to woo, and if in his eagerness he forestalled the etiquette of the occasion she modestly referred him to her parents, first indicating her consent would accompany theirs. In the twentieth century the young people too often settle the matter between themselves, and announce their intentions to wed quite regardless of their parents' sentiments on the subject. So many youthful attachments are really youthful follies that the girl who submits her wishes to her parents' counsel often has reason to consider herself fortunate. Girls, however, almost invariably regard parental opposition as unreasonable; actually it is often founded on a better understanding of their temperaments and the character of the young men in the case than they imagine--or in many cases can be made to see.

A manly man will approach the father of the girl he wishes to make his wife, state his prospects, and ask the father's consent. If withheld, he will not urge the girl into a hasty marriage, but will wait until the opposition has diminished. In case this does not happen, the girl has at least had an opportunity to learn her own mind. Many who have married against their parents' wishes have lived happily; it must be admitted that others have not. Delay, at least, gives time for reason to outweigh romance.

It is especially awkward for the girl if the parents of her fiance do not approve his choice. In such case she should give ample time for their disapproval to have whatever effect it may on the young man's feelings towards her. Some girls refuse to enter a man's family unless made welcome.

No girl should engage herself to a man she has known but a short time; certainly not without searching inquiry into his reputation in his former place of residence. No man can reasonably object to such inquiries; indeed, he should welcome them; invite them by furnishing credentials. No matter how violently in love a girl may be, she should not throw prudence and discretion to the winds.

ANNOUNCEMENT OF ENGAGEMENTS.

An engagement may be announced soon after it is entered upon, or not until several weeks before the marriage. Usually the engagement is known to the two families some time in advance of the later formal announcement. This is to save the girl embarrassment in case it is broken off. Should this happen, the young man takes the blame upon himself, declaring the young lady discarded him. Only an out-and-out cad would intimate to anyone that he "threw her over."

The announcement of the engagement comes through the girl's family; the man waits until it is their pleasure to make it known. The usual way is for the girl and her mother to write notes to relatives and close friends. The man, of course, will know when this is done, and may send notes to his relatives and friends, or acquaint them by word of mouth, at the same date. No special form is employed for such notes; they are always informal and familiar.

How Disclosed.--Sometimes a girl announces her engagement to her most intimate girl friends at a small tea or luncheon her mother or some relative gives for her. In this case the decorations are suggestive.

Heart-shaped place cards, decorated with the entwined initials of the two parties; pink flowers, banked in heart-shape and pierced with silver arrows, for a centerpiece, and sandwiches and cakes in heart shape, the latter decorated in pink, are often used. At each plate may be a small cluster of pink carnations, tied with narrow ribbons, one end connecting with an arrow in the centerpiece. When these are drawn out some appropriate sentiment is found attached, which is read aloud by the guest.

Any novel form may be employed in communicating the joyous intelligence. Midway the repast some friend previously selected for the honor may propose a health to the two who are betrothed; someone may ask a moment's indulgence while she reads an interesting paragraph from a letter, or a mock telegram may be delivered. Congratulations are in order; sometimes the fiance has been held in reserve, and is brought in to share with his fiancee the good wishes of her friends.

All who receive notes are expected to call in person or send letters of congratulation. Flowers are often sent, and dinners, theater parties, and other entertainments given for the young couple. Engagement gifts are often given; china being a favorite choice, though any gift is in order.

After the Announcement.--Immediately upon the announcement of the engagement the parents of the young man call upon his fiancee and her mother, whether previously acquainted or not. His family takes the initiative in the exchange of hospitality which follows. Calls are to be returned within a week. In case the man's family live at a distance, the members should at once write cordial, kindly letters to the girl, to which she must reply within a few days. She should not "gush" but should show her desire to know them, and a cordial and friendly feeling. The prospective mother-in-law may invite the girl to visit her. She should remember that no matter how welcome the alliance she is under inspection, as it were, and do her best, through courtesy and tact and friendliness to create a favorable impression.

The Girl's Behavior.--The engagement ring is not worn until the engagement is announced. If the young man's means permit, it is usually as handsome a diamond solitaire as he can afford. No womanly girl would wish her fiance to go in debt to purchase her ring. Should it be less handsome than she had hoped or expected, she should not give the slightest evidence of disappointment. That would seem mercenary and grasping. Nevertheless, a girl does doubtless get much more joy out of her engagement ring than she does out of her wedding ring.

Though a girl may receive from her affianced gifts of jewelry, silver, etc., as well as the bonbons, books and flowers she was privileged to accept before her engagement, it is not in good taste for him to offer any article of wearing apparel to her. He is not to buy clothes for her until after their marriage. Nothing that cannot be returned to him uninjured in case the engagement is broken is really correct for her to receive.

She will naturally receive many notes, letters, etc., from her fiance, especially if he is called out of town often, or resides in another city. The inexperienced, very-much-in-love girl is quite likely to write very ardent and affectionate letters. Leave that to the man. If she knows her Thackeray she will remember the rose-colored billet-doux poor Amelia used to write to her George, and which lay unopened day after day, and will model her missives upon the style of Lucy Snowe's to the Professor--"a morsel of ice, flavored with ever so slight a zest of sweetness." Let her make them bright, chatty, kindly, but not too tender.

Length of Engagement.--As for the length of an engagement, it is often argued that if one has made a mistake, it is much better to find it out before marriage than after. A prolonged engagement, however, is not advisable. It embarrasses a girl to be asked "When is it going to be?" and be obliged to make evasive answers. Thc old saying "Absence makes the heart grow fonder" often proves untrue. The long engagement is a strain, undoubtedly. A year is quite long enough for the two to demonstrate their fidelity and for all necessary preparations.

Breaking Off.--If the two develop incompatibility, after being convinced it is irreconcilable the only thing to do is to sever the tie. This is often heart-breaking if caused by the infidelity of one party, and always humiliating, especially to the girl. To spare her as much as possible, the man assumes the breaking-off was her act. He never allows himself to speak of her save in terms of the most perfect respect. The presents, letters, pictures, are returned, and Cupid retires discomfited. The girl's mother writes to her friends and tells them the engagement is broken; no reason is given and no person of tact or knowledge of social forms will inquire why or ever allude to the matter to either of the parties to the engagement or their parents.

"Being engaged" does not relax etiquette. It does not justify a journey or an excursion together, nor appearance in public places unchaperoned. Lovers refrain from caresses or evidence of their devotion in the presence of others; in short they should conduct themselves with decorum.

The Wedding Trousseau.--In case everything goes well when the wedding day is set it is the custom to announce the engagement in the society columns in the newspapers. The trousseau is nearly ready, the linen chest is filled, the details of the wedding settled. It is not customary now for the expectant bride to have dozens and dozens of undergarments, to be laid aside, turn yellow and go out of style. One dozen of each garment is an ample supply for the average bride; even half a dozen new garments of each kind have been known to answer every purpose. She should have a moderate supply of shoes, corsets, gloves, petticoats, both silk and cambric, and handkerchiefs. Fashions change so rapidly now that it is foolish to lay in a great stock of gowns. The supply of these must be in accordance with her social position and its requirements. After she is married, she will find her table-cloths and napkins, sheets, and pillow slips and towels a much greater source of satisfaction than a lot of passe gowns and wraps. Her silver and linen are marked with the initials of her maiden name. These initials are always embroidered on the latter.

The supply of table and bed-linen will depend upon the size of her house and the style in which she lives. Six sheets and six pillow and bolster slips are allowed to each bed, and twelve towels, half of them bath towels, to each bedroom. She should have dinner and lunch cloths, with napkins to match; it is usual to allow a dozen napkins to each cloth. It is good economy to purchase all these in a good quality. The dinner cloths and napkins should be of double damask, so called. The very large dinner napkins--seven-eighths of a yard square--are less in favor than the medium, three-quarter size. A fairly ample supply of comforts, down and silk quilts, and blankets, is often acquired by purchase before marriage.

WEDDING FESTIVITIES.

Very soon after the wedding invitations are out, the bride's friends bestir themselves and a number of entertainments are planned in her honor. These are dinners, luncheons, teas, and theatre parties, the latter often prefaced by a dinner at the house of the hostess. Often these include the bridal party--bridesmaids and "best man." To dinners and theatre parties the bridegroom-to-be is invited; luncheons and teas are given by the bride's friends to her. The bridegroom's bachelor friends frequently give a dinner for him--a farewell to the man so soon to rank as "Benedict, the married man."

These functions in honor of the bride are exclusive, rather than general, invitations being restricted to familiar friends. The bride's relatives are the entertainers. At such functions the bride expectant may wear one of the gowns of her trousseau. Because of these entertainments, which are really quite a tax on the girl's strength and vitality, the trousseau should be complete and the wedding preparations well under way before they begin. Most of them seem to be crowded into the week or ten days preceding the ceremony.

Engagement "Showers."--"The shower"--an entertainment that is somewhat on the order of an informal tea at which each guest brings some gift to the bride--has been called "provincial." It has a recognized place in middle class society, at least, and may be made an enjoyable function. No two "showers" are alike, hostesses vieing with each other in the endeavor to present something original and attractive. The linen shower is one of the most popular, each guest bringing some contribution to the bride's linen chest. These are the more valued if the handiwork of the giver, and some girls always have a bit of work in progress which may, when finished, be their offering at a linen shower.

Only intimate friends are asked to a linen shower and the occasion is entirely informal. The invitations may be couched in this form:

My Dear Miss Ames--

I am giving a linen shower for our mutual friend, Miss Gray, who is to be married next month, and would be very glad to have you with us. I am asking a few friends for luncheon on Thursday, January sixth, at one o'clock, and hope you will be able to come. As the "shower" is to be a surprise to Miss Gray, please do not mention it should you see her.

Very cordially,

Helen Brown.

The invitation should be promptly answered. Usually, the nature of the entertainment is not known to the guest of honor until she arrives; sometimes not until she is seated at the table.

How Presented.--The more unique the method of presentation the more amusing the surprise of the guest. The gifts are to be neatly wrapped up in white tissue paper, tied with ribbons, the card of the giver being enclosed. Often some sentiment is written on the card, or an original rhyme; this the recipient reads aloud when the gift is unwrapped.

At one long remembered shower, the centerpiece was a white linen parasol, beautifully embroidered and the gift of the hostess. This, open, was fastened upright, the block of wood which held it being hidden under asparagus plumosus interspersed with pink roses. Under this were arranged the several packages. Between each course the guest of honor was requested to draw and open a parcel, the remainder being opened before leaving the table. At another luncheon the gifts were brought in by a boy dressed as a messenger, one at a time, as if just delivered. The surprise of the guest at the first delivery greatly amused her friends. One guest contributed a handsome lunch cloth, another the napkins to match, each marked with embroidered initials. An embroidered white linen handbag, for use with a white gown, was enclosed in a box about a foot square; within this was another, neatly wrapped and tied, which, opened, contained another and still another, keeping expectancy at its height. The "Jack Horner pie" has been used, and the "showered" girl has been handed a white satin ribbon and been bidden to follow where it led her, discovering at the end the pile of presents.

Gifts for a linen shower may include towels of all kinds, the monogrammed damask and initialed guest towels, embroidered linen pillow slips; centerpieces, doilies, bureau scarfs and many other textile gifts suggest themselves. The "kitchen shower" suggests the useful; the handkerchief shower is dainty.

Refreshments.--The refreshments at such an entertainment may be as simple as one likes, unless the invitations are for a luncheon; in that case they should be more elaborate. Chocolate and sandwiches with cake and ices; sandwiches, cake and coffee, are allowable. The guests are seated at a table, which should be decorated with pink and white flowers. Pink carnations are beautiful for this use. The guest of honor is seated at the hostess's right hand and is served first. She must thank those who have presented the gifts individually, and express to her hostess her pleasure in the entertainment and her gratitude for the trouble she has taken for her.

WEDDING PREPARATIONS.

The Expense of a Wedding.--It may be said at the outset that no wedding should be more costly than the financial standing of the bride's family warrants. If the bridegroom's family is wealthy, and that of the bride in very moderate circumstances, there will be many to intimate that the bridegroom "put up for it." The intimation is a sneer, because the bride's family should pay all the expenses of a wedding. If the expense is manifestly beyond the resources of the bride's father, society lifts its eyebrows.

Of course her wedding is the one pageant in which the girl is the central figure--the admired of all beholders. It is quite natural for her to wish it to be beautiful, to look lovely herself, and not to go empty-handed to her husband. But no sensible girl will have a grand wedding if its cost will put her father in debt. If Mary's music lessons must be intermitted, or John's entrance into college postponed because of her trousseau and her wedding, she should assume some of the sacrifice herself and be content with a more modest outfit and a simple ceremony. Thousands of thoughtless girls leave their families to recover slowly from the financial strain of their wedding. It is selfish and inconsiderate for a girl to say, "You will never have to do it again for me," or "I shall be no further expense to you." That may be true, but it is no justification.

Nor is it permissible for the bridegroom to furnish any part of the bride's trousseau. If she is poor, and is to marry into wealth, good taste and public opinion counsel her to confine her wedding preparations to what she or her family can pay for. Let her make ready a simple wedding dress and going-away gown, or be married in the latter, and take with her to her new home only her under linen and the treasured keepsakes of her maiden days. As soon as she is wife, her husband may lavish silks and laces and furs upon her, but not before.

The Bride's Privileges.--It is the province of the bride to name the wedding day, subject of course to the insistence of her fiance, who will urge an early date. She decides whether her wedding shall be formal or informal, at church or at home. She chooses the clergyman who shall perform the ceremony, the bridegroom notifying him of her desire. Her family issues--and pays for--the wedding invitations and announcement cards. It is customary to ask the bridegroom to make out a list of those of his relatives and friends to whom he wishes these sent. The bride names her attendants, decides upon their number and if a bridal procession is contemplated, consults with them as to their gowns and the accessories. Here she is in duty bound to consider the expense to be incurred by those invited to take part in the affair, unless she is prepared to pay for their gowns herself; this however is seldom done. If she desires her attendants to wear some particular adornment which will be of no use to them afterwards, as a fancy muff or boa, she should pay for it herself. She may endeavor to arrange with her dressmaker to make their gowns if she can obtain a reduction on account of their being made alike, or the large order placed. To be invited to serve as bridesmaid is often an expensive compliment, as it usually involves a new gown and hat, the latter always being worn at a church wedding.

If the bride decides to have but one attendant, the latter is usually styled her maid-of-honor, and may be her sister or her most intimate friend. If she has more than one maid she should include the bridegroom's sister, if he has one. If a matron-of-honor is to participate, she should be a friend or sister of the bride who has been recently wedded. The bridesmaids are chosen from her unmarried friends.

Who Pays?--The question is often asked, "Who pays, for" this, that or the other item.

The bridegroom provides the marriage certificate, the wedding ring, pays the clergyman, and for the carriage in which he drives away with the bride. He sends a gift and the bouquet to the bride; usually gives gifts of jewelry to the bridesmaids and the best man, and often includes the ushers.

The bride's family pays for the wedding cards, pays the florist and the caterer, the expense of opening the church and the service of the sexton; the music, carriages for the bridal party, in short, the bills are for the family to pay. Where a wedding is very elaborate, the details are sometimes turned over to a "manager," who sees to everything, and receives a fat fee for his services.

The Wedding Gown.--Choice of a wedding gown depends upon the style of the wedding. At a church wedding it is as handsome as the bride can afford. Any girl is excusable for wishing her wedding to be "an occasion," and her bridal attire as beautiful as possible. White is suitable, and there are so many fabrics in that color that all purses can be accommodated. The gown may be of satin, crepe de chine, messaline, lace or chiffon, or of simple white organdie; all are appropriate for a church wedding. With any of these a veil should be worn. Two and a half yards of tulle will be sufficient; other accessories are white kid gloves, white slippers and white silk hose, if white is worn. White is suitable for the most elaborate church wedding and for the simplest ceremony at home. The gown is made en train, as a rule; always so for a church wedding, and always with high neck and long sleeves.

A bride may elect to be married in a traveling dress. For this some pretty light color, as light gray, champagne, tan or biscuit color is chosen. A hat must be worn with such a costume, and for a young bride is by preference trimmed with flowers. It is correct to carry flowers--not a shower bouquet, however--with such a gown, which is to be changed for a plainer one for actual travel. For this dark blue, brown, or gray are suitable colors; gloves match, and the hat is inconspicuously trimmed. It is the bride's greatest desire not to look "just married."

Later Wear of the Wedding Gown.--The wedding gown is worn at the more formal of the post-nuptial entertainments. The trousseau should include an evening dress and wrap. For the former, black lace, chiffon cloth or net will prove the most serviceable, and almost universally becoming. A traveling gown, a handsome suit for visiting, receptions, etc., a pretty gown for receiving at home, and several house gowns will be needed. Kimonas, bath-robes, dressing-jackets, are included in the less ornamental parts of the trousseau.

A girl often invites her intimate friends to inspect her wedding finery, rejoicing in their admiration. The privilege of such a view is highly valued.

Bridal Flowers.--Orange flowers are reserved for the bride, and she never wears any other in her hair, at least no other that are artificial. She may carry any flowers, she prefers; the florists make all seasons alike. Often an order is given months in advance for the bride's favorite flower to grace her wedding, and the florist forces it to bloom at the appointed time. White roses and carnations can be had at almost any season; sweet peas, white lilacs, lilies of the valley, are less easy to procure. The "shower bouquet" has many narrow white satin ribbons falling from it to the foot of the skirt, and knotted at intervals round flower sprays.

The rarest of bridal flowers are the orchids, so costly that only the rich may have them, though a few orchids, two or three, are sometimes put with lilies of the valley, or Roman hyacinths, intermixed with stephanotis or stevia, for the bridal bouquet. Bridesmaids may carry large clusters of flowers tied with ribbons, the flowers suiting their costumes. Or, if they all wear white, American Beauties may be chosen. The usual preference is for flowers in more delicate hues.

The Widow's Bridal Attire.--A widow does not wear white at her second wedding, nor a veil, nor does she have bridesmaids. Her usual choice is to be married in a handsome traveling gown of some light color, wearing hat and gloves to match. The material may be silk or broadcloth for a church wedding. She wears her wedding ring up to the day of her second marriage. Though she may have no bridesmaids she may have a matron-of-honor, some married friend, who wears a street or reception dress, with suitable hat and gloves.

A woman who has entered her fourth decade does not, as a rule, wear white when married.

It is no longer customary for a woman to go into semi-retirement preceding her marriage. She does not parade herself; no lady would do that, but she accepts invitations and appears at all the fetes planned for her up to the wedding day. As a result, she is often very tired and fagged before the event.

The Man's Wedding Garments.--One of the most frequent inquiries made of the editors of women's departments in magazines relates to the proper attire for the bridegroom. "When is it correct to wear a dress suit?" and "What should the bridegroom wear at a day wedding?"

"The dress suit," so called, is the man's evening clothes. Naturally, then, he will not don his evening attire until evening--after or for a six o'clock dinner,' This should dispose of the question of "the dress suit." For a man to wear evening clothes at a noon wedding would be as absurd as for a woman to appear in a ball dress at that hour.

For a day wedding a man wears a black frock coat and gray trousers; his waistcoat may match the coat or be of white duck or marseilles, white shirt with standing collar, and tie of the fashionable cut in pearl gray or soft white silk. Pearl-colored kid gloves are worn, and a silk hat. The overcoat is black. A boutonniere of white flowers is usually worn.

The above is the correct dress for best man and ushers at a day wedding, in church or at home.

For a formal evening wedding, full evening dress is worn by bridegroom, best man and ushers. The suit is of fine black worsted, silk faced as to the coat. The waistcoat may be of the same material, or white duck or marseilles may be worn. A fine white linen shirt with standing collar, and pearl or white enamel studs, white lawn tie, white or pearl-gray kid gloves stitched in the same color, and patent leather pumps complete the attire. A black overcoat, single breasted, and silk hat are the additions for out-of-door wear.

The Bride's Mother.--The bride's mother wears a handsome reception dress. Black with much jet and lace, pearl gray, mauve and lavender are favorite colors for her. White gloves are worn. Mourning attire should never be seen at a wedding. If the bride's mother, or any of the family, are in mourning, it must be laid aside for the occasion. Black may be worn, but it must be lightened with white lace, jet, or other accessories that will take it out of the conventional garb of grief. Guests of course gown themselves handsomely.

THE FORMAL CHURCH WEDDING.

Let us suppose that the church has been decorated with flower and palms, arranged by experienced hands to form a background for the bridal party. The seats for the respective families have been roped off with wide white satin ribbons; those on the right for the bridegroom's family, those of the left for the bride's. The bridegroom and the best man are with the clergyman in the vestry; the bridesmaids have assembled at the bride's house, and have entered their carriages; the relatives, including the bride's mother, and guests are in their seats. The carriages containing the bridesmaids precede that of the bride to the church; they alight and await her in the vestibule. The bride, accompanied by her father, arrives. The bridal procession is quickly formed, the vestibule doors having been closed by the ushers on the arrival of the wedding party. At the signal the organ breaks into the familiar strains of the wedding march; the clergyman, followed by the groom and best man, enter from the vestry, and stand on the chancel step facing the guests, awaiting the bride, the bridegroom being slightly, in advance.

The ushers, walking two and two, lead the way up the aisle; the bridesmaids follow at a distance of ten or twelve feet, also walking in pairs; then comes the maid-of-honor, walking alone. She is followed by the bride, leaning on the arm of her father or nearest male relative. At the chancel the ushers separate to right and left, remaining below the chancel step; the bridesmaids separate in the same manner, but ascend the chancel step. The maid-of-honor places herself at the left

47

of the place left for the bride, in readiness to hold her bouquet and remove her glove. The bridegroom descends the chancel step, meeting the bride. The two place themselves before the clergyman, the bride standing on the bridegroom's left; the best man stands at the right of the bridegroom a step or two in the rear.

The Bride's Father.--The place of the bride's father is at the left somewhat in the rear. As the clergyman asks: "Who giveth this woman to be married to this man?" he steps forward and places the bride's right hand in that of the clergyman, who in turn places it in that of the bridegroom. The father steps aside, and as the bridal procession forms to retire after the ceremony, he joins his wife and escorts her from the church.

At the proper moment the maid-of-honor removes the bride's glove and takes her bouquet. The best man gives the ring to the bride, who passes it to the clergyman; the latter gives it to the bridegroom, who places it on the bride's finger, holding it there while repeating the formula, "With this ring I thee wed," etc. The significance of this transfer is the forming of a circle, to indicate the endlessness of the contract.

Another Form.--A form sometimes introduced is for the bridal party to stand below the chancel while the clergyman reads the service up to and including the sentence, "If any man can show just cause," etc. After the customary moment's pause, there being no unseemly interruption, the party ascends the chancel step and the ceremony proceeds.

The order of the procession after the ceremony is this: The just married pair lead the way, the wife taking her husband's arm; the maid-of-honor follows; then the bridesmaids, after them the ushers. Such is the conduct of a church wedding, a thousand times repeated. The ceremony is often rehearsed a night or two previous to the event, to make sure each will be familiar with his or her part.

The Best Man's Duties.--The best man has charge of the ring. At the conclusion of the ceremony he disappears into the vestry, where he places the wedding fee, enclosed in an envelope, in the clergyman's hands. He then hastens to his carriage and is driven to the house, where he assists in the reception of the guests, and takes the maid-of-honor or the bridesmaid to luncheon. Or he may escort the maid-of-honor from the church.

The best man also sees to it that the agitated bridegroom's clothes are in order, packs his suitcase, orders the baggage to be called for, buys the tickets for the wedding journey and sees that they are in the bridegroom's possession, and orders the carriage in which the newly wedded pair drive to the station. He takes as many of the details of the affair as possible off his friend's mind and hands, and stands by manfully to the last. The best man should fully acquaint himself with the duties of his position before assuming it The sexton of the church takes the groom's hat from the vestry to the vestibule, and hands it to him at the door.

Duties of Ushers.--An usher escorts each lady to her seat, giving her his arm. The guests should stand during the ceremony, rising as the procession enters, and remaining in their seats until it has retired. The ushers often pass ribbons along their seats, not removing them until the bridal party and the relatives have left the church. Having seen the bridal party to their carriages, the ushers return to escort the relatives to theirs, and then hasten to the house, where they meet the guests on arrival and escort them, severally, to the receiving party. The bride's mother welcomes them first; they are then presented to the newly married pair. The bride offers her hand; the guest wishes her much happiness, congratulates the bridegroom, shaking hands the while, greets the maid-of-honor and the bridesmaids with a smile and bow, and passes on, making way for the next.

The Wedding Reception.--The wedding reception follows the ceremony, guests coming at once from church to the house. There should be no undue haste in presenting one's self; the party requires a little time to arrange itself in proper order for receiving. At a day wedding reception women lay aside wraps, retaining their hats. At an evening reception they remove both, and wear full dress.

After greeting the bride and groom, as indicated in the preceding paragraph, the refreshment room is sought. If the reception is a large one, a buffet or "stand-up" repast is often served, though it is more desirable to provide small tables seating four people. If these are not furnished the men may assist the ladies, though the service should be adequate. No tea, coffee, or chocolate is poured at the table.

Refreshments.--The refreshments may be simple or elaborate. The table is laid in the dining-room, and decorated with flowers. On it are the refreshments, and plenty of napkins, plates and silver, in piles. Bouillon, creamed oysters or oyster patties; salads, cold salmon or lobster with mayonnaise dressing, ices and cake are suitable. Usually one hot dish is passed. Or one may serve a salad, ice cream and cake, with punch. If wine is offered it is always champagne.

The wedding cake, neatly packed in white boxes bearing the monogram of the bride and groom and tied with white satin ribbon, is arranged on a table in the hall, and each departing guest takes a box. Wedding cake is no longer sent.

Going Away.--When the last guest has been greeted, the bridal party may be served with refreshments. Their supper is laid in a private room, and they are seated, a most welcome rest after the fatigue of the ceremony and the reception. The bride then retires to change to her traveling dress; the bridegroom, who has had his valise sent to the house in the morning, retires for the same purpose. The maid-of-honor accompanies the bride; the best man assists the groom, and packs his suit worn during the ceremony, either to be taken with him or to be sent to his home.

At the time agreed upon the bridegroom awaits the bride at the head of the stairs. Adieus to the family are said in the bride's room and should be brief. The bridesmaids and ushers are awaiting the departure in the hall. Half way down the stairs the bride throws her bouquet. The bridesmaid who catches it will be married next, according to the old superstition. The bride and groom enter their carriage amid a shower of rice or confetti, the carriage door bangs; the caterer has removed the debris of the feast; the maids have restored the house to its wonted order and the wedding is over--all except paying the bills.

Guests at a wedding do not remain until the departure of the bride. They congratulate, partake of refreshments, chat a few minutes with friends, and depart.

At a church wedding it is customary--and usually necessary to keep out the uninvited--to enclose small cards which are presented at the church door to ensure admittance. If the reception is large, the same thing is sometimes done as a measure of protection.

Calls after Wedding.--It is expected that the guests at a wedding breakfast or reception will call on the mother of the bride within three weeks after the marriage, and upon the bride on one of her "At Home" days, or soon after her return from the wedding journey, if no days are specified.

Cards bearing the date of the bride's "At Home" days, or "At Home after"--a certain date, are enclosed with the announcement cards, or the date named on the card. If sent they must be ready to mail immediately after the wedding.

THE HOME WEDDING.

While the home wedding is modeled in its essentials along the lines of the church wedding, much less formality is observed. The invitations to the church wedding are always in the third person and engraved. Those for the home wedding, though often following the same formula, may be informal notes in the first person, written by the bride's mother.

Correct Attire.--It is sometimes supposed that a bride married at home may not wear a veil nor be "given away." On the contrary, if she wears white she may with perfect propriety wear a veil, and the Episcopal marriage ceremony always, and nearly all other forms of the service include the giving away, as implying parental sanction and consent. The "giving away," then, is customary, even at the simplest home wedding.

If the bride wears a traveling dress she has a maid-of-honor, the one attendant being so-called. The groom is attended by his best man. There are usually two ushers, though these may be omitted, The maid-of-honor wears some pretty costume which is in keeping with that of the bride. If the latter wears white, the attendant also wears white with colored trimmings. If the bride wears a veil, the maid wears a hat; the veil being the head covering of the bride.

The bridegroom wears a black frock coat, gray trousers, white waistcoat and tie, silk--not lawn, gray or white gloves, and patent leather shoes at a day wedding, The ushers are similarly attired, save that they may wear black waistcoats. Silk hats are worn.

Minor Particulars.--The bridegroom and best man will require a room. The clergyman expects a room where he may don his surplice or gown. The ushers may also require a room.

The bride's mother receives the guests, her father remaining with his daughter to conduct her to the room where the ceremony is to be performed. A mother may perform this office if the father is not living. After placing his daughter's hand in that of the clergyman, the father steps back a pace or two, awaiting the end of the service. Wedding music is played when the party is ready to enter, and may be continued, very softly, through the ceremony; it must not overpower the voices of the participants.

Guests should arrive at the hour named, leave wraps in hall or dressing room, and descend to the parlors. It is not expected that all will be seated, though a few chairs are provided for the elderly. The ushers stretch two lengths of white ribbon from end to end of the room, making an aisle for the little procession.

The clergyman, groom, and best man enter and take their places at one end of the room, when the music begins. Then come the ushers, next the maid-of-honor, walking alone; then the bridesmaids, if any, followed by the bride on the arm of her father. The groom steps forward to receive her and the two face the clergyman. The best man stands on the bridegroom's right. The maid-of-honor will hold the bride's bouquet and her glove, if this is removed; the ring is in the custody of the best man.

Etiquette to be Observed.--At the close of the ceremony the clergyman congratulates the pair and steps aside. They face about and the bride's mother is the next to offer her good wishes, then the groom's parents. The guests then extend felicitations. It is thought in better taste to wish the bride happiness and congratulate the groom, it being supposed that he is the most fortunate in having been able to secure such a prize.

It is no longer customary for everyone to kiss the bride; she is not compelled to suffer to that extent.

The best man assists the ushers--whose first duty is to remove the white ribbons--in escorting guests to the bride and groom. His duties are the same as those of the best man at a church wedding.

The maid-of-honor stands at the bride's left as she receives.

The bride and bridegroom lead the way to the dining room, the best man offering his arm to the maid-of-honor.

The bride's father escorts the bridegroom's mother, the guests follow in such order as is convenient, and the bride's mother and the bridegroom's father are the last.

If only twenty-five or thirty guests are present the wedding breakfast is preferably served at small tables. The clergyman and his wife, who should always be invited, are seated at the bride's table. So also the maid-of-honor, the best man, the ushers, and the parents of the pair, with sisters and brothers if convenient. Or, the bride's table may be reserved strictly for the bridal party.

The bride may cut her own cake if she chooses, or the wedding cake may be dispensed in boxes as at the reception following a church wedding.

The departure of the newly wedded pair is on the order already indicated.

After the Wedding.--It may be said here that the "horse play"--for it is nothing else--sometimes indulged in as "an after clap" to a wedding, in which practical jokes are played on the pair, is not only unkind and ill-bred, but in most execrable taste. To placard the luggage "Just married;" to tie white ribbons on it and the carriage in which they are driven away; to substitute a suitcase packed with the things a man doesn't want on his journey for one containing what he does, is not at all "smart."

Why should some coarse, ill-bred persons, whether they have or have not been favored with invitations, strive to embarrass and make uncomfortable those to whom the situation is already sufficiently trying? Why, after so much pains and expense have been employed to make the occasion beautiful and impressive, should the "practical joker" take it upon himself to spoil it all by an ill-timed "pleasantry" which is the acme of rudeness and discourtesy? It is a curious character that can enjoy perpetrating what are really outrages upon other people's sensibilities.

Wedding Gifts.--Very soon after the wedding invitations are out the presents begin to pour in. The fashion of gift giving on such an occasion is not as prevalent as at one time; it was overdone, carried beyond the limits of good taste, and of course a reaction was inevitable. Some men profess to share the feeling of the Scandinavian immigrant who was so deeply affronted at the offerings made by his bride's friends--as if he were not able to furnish his home with the necessary articles--that in his Berserker rage he was with difficulty restrained from casting gifts and donors together into the street.

Generally speaking, only relatives and intimate friends send gifts, though there is no interdict as regards others who may wish to testify to their interest in the bride in this way. An ostentatious gift from a person not in the family is in bad taste. The words "No presents" on wedding invitations are in the worst possible form.

An invitation to a church wedding and not to the reception precludes the necessity of making a gift; indeed, it would be thought rather "pushing" to send one.

What to Give.--The flat silver is generally given by the bride's family. In order to avoid duplicates, it is best for the friends and relatives to consult together in regard to their gifts. It is not thought good form to offer articles of wearing apparel. Anything the bride's immediate family has to offer in this line is best included in the trousseau. Cut glass, silver, bric-a-brac, napery, books, pictures, fans, rugs, clocks, handsome chairs and tables, are things that may be chosen with propriety.

The question of the correct form of marking silver and napery often comes up. The rule is to have it engraved with the initials of the bride's maiden name--not the single initial of her family name, as is sometimes ignorantly done--because it is her own private property. If a wife dies, the silver bearing her name is packed away for the future use of her child, especially if it is a girl. The second wife would be forbidden by good taste and convention, from using the first wife's silver.

Acknowledgments.--Wedding gifts are usually packed where they are bought, and sent direct from the shops. The card of the donor is enclosed, within a tiny envelope. It is a rule that the wedding gift must be acknowledged immediately, before the marriage, and by a personal note from the bride. This is not always possible, but the note should be written at the earliest moment the bride's engagements will permit. Such notes are always in the first person, and should be pleasant and cordial. The writer must be careful to render thanks for the article sent. Amusing mistakes sometimes happen; thus a lady who had sent a pair of handsome candlesticks was mystified by expressions of gratitude for a silver berry spoon she had not sent.

A cordial form of acknowledging a gift is this:

1

2 Canton Avenue.

My Dear Mrs. Bruce:

The beautiful cut glass vase sent by you and Mr. Bruce has just arrived, and I hasten to thank you most sincerely for your kind thought of me. It will be a constant reminder of your goodness to Mr. Waters and myself, and a most lovely ornament to our new home.

Gratefully yours,

Marion Moore.

July tenth, nineteen hundred and nine.

The wedding gifts may or may not be displayed, according to the personal preference of the bride. They are commonly shown to intimate friends. A room is given up to their display. Cards are to be removed.

Wedding Decorations.--At a church wedding it is customary, and wisest, to put the matter of decorating the church and house into the hands of a florist, who can furnish the palms and others plants required for the chancel, and carry out any color scheme desired. He has the paraphernalia requisite to effective disposition of flowers. Usually large clusters of foliage and flowers, ribbon tied, are attached to the pews reserved for the relatives; often they are arranged the entire length of the aisle, The mantels in the house are banked with flowers, southern smilax is used in profusion, and flowers are arranged upon the tables at which the supper is served.

At a church wedding in the country the bride's friends must come to the rescue, and their gardens be robbed to beautify church and home. Flowers may be sought in the fields. Large jars of daisies, wild ferns, tall grasses, autumn tinted boughs, or in the blooming season, boughs of fruit trees, can be used most effectively. At one pretty home wedding the decorations were boughs of the wild crab-apple in bloom, pink and pretty, and kept so by having the stems inserted in bottles of water, suspended by wires and concealed by other foliage. A large screen sometimes forms a background for the bridal party. If covered with wire netting flowers can be very easily attached.

Walls are not festooned; "wedding bells" and canopies are out of date. The most approved setting is tall palms, ferns on standards concealed by a lower grouping, with a few potted plants in bloom to relieve the sombreness of the green. Large flowers like lilies, hydrangeas, chrysanthemums and peonies are most effective. Tulips are often employed at a spring wedding. One little country girl made good use of ordinary field clover in decorating her home for her marriage.

After a wedding, the flowers are often sent to the hospitals, or to those who are known to be ill, at the request of the bride.

THE SIMPLEST OF WEDDINGS.

Now, although we have told how the church wedding and the ordinary home wedding are conducted, it does not follow that one may not have a much simpler and yet a pretty wedding, with less "pomp and circumstance" and consequent expense.

Wherever a girl has a home, she should be married from it. This is her due, as "daughter of the house."

She may make the simplest possible preparations; may be married in her best dress, not new for the occasion. She may omit all attendants, and invite less than half a dozen of her friends; she may receive them herself and at the appointed hour simply stand up and be married to a blushing young man in a business suit, and afterwards cut her own cake, and then proceed to her new home, which may be a little flat or a cottage. But she should have the ceremony performed by a clergyman in her father's house.

If she has no parents, no home, merely a room in a boarding house, she and her affianced may go to a clergyman's house and be married there. The church and the law should sanction the rite; therefore she will not permit herself to be married by a magistrate or a justice of the peace.

As for "sneaking off" and being married without the knowledge of one's parents, this is both disrespectful and unkind--a poor return for their care of her.

WEDDING ANNIVERSARIES.

The fashion of celebrating a succession of wedding anniversaries has passed its high tide and is on the wane. Nevertheless, the custom is not out, by any means. The tenth, twenty-fifth and fiftieth anniversaries, known as the tin, silver, and golden, are those most frequently observed.

The first anniversary of the wedding day gives occasion for a paper wedding; the second is cotton; the third leather. The fourth is omitted; the fifth is the wooden wedding; next to be observed is the tin, celebrating the close of the first decade. The next skip is to the china, when twenty years have elapsed; and the quarter century of wedded happiness is recognized in the silver wedding.

The wooden and tin weddings are occasions of great hilarity, and mean a general frolic. The former began years ago with the gift of a rolling-pin and a step-ladder. The gifts are of those practical, useful articles that replenish the kitchen, though handsome gifts are of course easily selected. Carved wooden boxes, handsome picture frames, articles of furniture, are at the service of those who choose to pay their price.

Invitations to a wooden wedding are sometimes written or printed on birch bark or thin strips of wood, or are engraved on cards which imitate wood in appearance. The refreshments have been served on wooden plates procured from the grocer. So far as possible the wooden idea is carried out.

Tin Weddings.--Gifts for the tin wedding are of course in that material, and there is a wide range of choice. The tinsmith is often called upon to manufacture fantastic articles, anything to raise a laugh. Thus one couple were adorned, the wife with a set of tin curls, the man with a tin hat. A tin purse enclosing a check for "tin" was once presented to a tin bride on the occasion of her tin wedding. The freakish fancy of one's friends is generally much in evidence at a tin wedding. As at the wooden wedding, the bride cuts a wedding cake decorated with a monogram formed of the initials of her own and her husband's name, and the year of the wedding and of its anniversary. Refreshments may be served from tin dishes, and the guests provided with tin plates.

The Silver Wedding.--Cards for a silver wedding are printed in silver, or in black on silvered cards--the former being in better taste. The form--which may be used for all with the variation of but one word--that designating the nature of the anniversary, is as follows:

1885 Mr. and Mrs. Smith 1910
request the pleasure of your company on
Thursday, February the twenty-fourth,
at eight o'clock.
Silver Wedding.

George Smith Anna Hall As the couple who celebrate are generally in the prime of life, and their friends of about the same age, a silver wedding is usually a very enjoyable function. The many beautiful articles now made in silver afford a wide range of choice in the way of gifts, both valuable and in those inexpensive trifles that please everybody because so artistic. Silverware is marked with the initials of the married pair, often enclosed in a true lover's knot. Toilet articles, pomade jars, silver jewelry, spoons, silver parasol and umbrella handles, picture frames in silver, rings and bracelets, besides the manifold pieces for table use, offer a wide individual range in choice and price.

The supper at a silver wedding is quite elaborate. The bride that was cuts a wedding cake in which a silver piece is baked; the person who gets it being expected to live to celebrate his or her silver wedding. Speeches are made, often an original poem read, and not infrequently the health of the pair pledged in a glass of wine.

Golden Weddings--Occasions for the celebration of fifty years of union are much rarer than any other. Nor are they wholly joyful. The aged couple are looking from "life's west windows" at a fast declining sun. A few short years and it must set for them. The festivities are usually planned and carried out by their descendants, who so far as possible summon to the celebration the friends of "Auld lang syne," the clergyman who performed the ceremony and any of the bridal party yet alive, and the dearest friends of the present. Invitations in the conventional form are printed in gold letters; often a monogram formed of intertwined initials is placed between and a little above the years at the top of the invitation. The wedding cake has a yellow frosting, or if in white, the monogram and the years--1860-1910--are in yellow to represent gold.

Gifts in this precious metal are naturally circumscribed, but a gold coin is apropos, particularly if Fortune has been chary of her favors. In the seventh and eighth decade people have small use for bijouterie.

A golden wedding must be a sad anniversary to the participants. When they were wedded, they were looking forward, joyously; now they recall the past, its losses and trials and misfortunes. They remember the children who are dead, or far away; or the prosperity once theirs, but now fled. Few old folks would care to celebrate their golden wedding; it is usually some well-meaning grandchild who sees in it "an occasion." Often, too, the excitement, the fatigue, the unusual strain on mind and body, result in illness which sometimes proves fatal.

The Courtesies of the Occasion.--There is no formal etiquette for any of these anniversaries. Friends, as they arrive, are greeted by members of the family; then, in the case of the elderly celebrants, are conducted to them as they sit side by side, and presented. Failing eyesight and dulled ears demand this. The congratulations are offered, and good wishes for the future. If any speeches are made, they should be brief, that neither the old couple or their guests be over-fatigued. The stay should be brief.

Gifts.--Gifts for the anniversary wedding are sometimes sent the day previous, sometimes carried in person. Anything fantastic is generally presented at the gathering, to contribute to its hilarity. The silver wedding gifts are nearly always sent in advance, and are displayed on a table, the cards of the donor usually being left on them. The recipients are to tender their thanks in person or by note.

Every effort should be made to have these festivities joyous. Especially should the wife subdue her emotion if the review of the years since her bona fide wedding day have seen the loss of beloved children. She must stifle her sad recollections for the sake of her guests.

The members of the bridal party, the more honored guests at the first wedding, the clergyman who officiated, are sought as welcome guests at the anniversary. The bride that was wears something she wore on the first occasion. If the wedding dress and the bridegroom's suit have been preserved they are worn--and wonderfully quaint they often look, so great the change in fashion.

CHRISTENING CEREMONIES.

"Our birth is nothing but our death begun, as tapers waste the moment they take fire."--Young.

The arrival of the stork with the new baby is an event of vast family interest, especially if it is the first visit of the bird to the domicile. In America it is not customary to announce a birth in the newspapers, as is often done in England, especially among the nobility. The personal friends of the parents receive the visiting card of both, or of the mother only, to which is attached a small card bearing the baby's full name and the date of his arrival. These are enclosed in an envelope, this again in an outer one, and mailed.

It is proper for those thus notified to call at an early date to inquire as to the well-being of mother and babe. As it is not customary for the mother to receive any but a very few of her nearest relatives under at least three weeks, callers should not be expected to see her, but are to leave cards. A note of congratulation is often sent instead of calling, and offers to the ingenious and witty an excellent chance for the display of delicate pleasantry. Thus it is entirely proper to address the note to the baby, and congratulate him on having chosen such charming parents, and such a lovely home. Flowers are not infrequently sent to the mother, and little gifts--soft booties, little gold pins for sleeve and neck, little crocheted or knitted sacks, or dainty bibs--to the baby.

The Ceremony.--The baby is usually christened when it is six or eight weeks old. Clergymen prefer this should be done at the church, and generally arrange to perform several baptisms at the same time---Children's Day being a favorite time. Otherwise, the christening usually takes place after the congregation is dismissed at the conclusion of a service. Only those interested and a few specially invited friends remain for it. There is no objection, however, to having a child christened at home, when the affair is made one of more festivity.

Most young married people prefer to have the clergyman who married them christen their first baby, when practicable.

Sponsors.--The baby's sponsors are chosen, by the parents' agreement, from among their relatives and close friends, almost always those of their own communion. The request is preferred verbally or by personal notes. A boy has a godmother and two godfathers; a girl two godmothers and a godfather. Occasionally this rule is broken and a godmother alone chosen for a girl, and one godfather for a boy. Godparents are supposed to stand in a more intimate relation to their godchildren than to others, and to take a more personal interest in them, especially in case of the parents' death. It is a serious relation, involving a certain religious responsibility, and is not to be lightly entered into.

The godparents are expected to make christening gifts to the child on his baptismal day. They are usually in the form of silver cups, porringers, silver spoons, forks, etc.; these should be solid, never plated ware. If the babe is named for one of its godparents, the latter is expected to do something handsome in the way of a christening gift. Sometimes a bank account is opened in the child's name, the sum deposited being left at interest until he becomes of age.

Church Christenings.--At a church christening, the babe is dressed in its handsomest robe and cap. Formerly the robes were very long and miracles of lace and embroidery; at present the finest of linen lawn or batiste, with a little real lace at neck and sleeves, and a bit of fine French embroidery, is thought in better taste, even in the case of the very wealthy. And many a blessed baby is given his name in a simple little lawn robe with no embellishment beyond a little tucking--done by the mother's own hands, perhaps.

The nurse carries the child into the church. Sponsors and parents group themselves around the font, which is often decorated with white flowers. The godmother has the privilege of holding the babe until it is time to lay him in the clergyman's arms, the cap having been removed. The parents make the responses; after the naming the godmother takes the little one again, holding him until the close of the service. She should not wipe away any of the water placed on the child's head. A good baby is expected not to cry during the ceremony, and one advantage of an early christening is that the little fellow is less liable to be alarmed at strange surroundings.

The same forms are observed at a home christening, the hour being usually in the afternoon.

A luncheon to which the clergyman and the christening party, and a few friends if desired, are invited, customarily follows the church ceremony--unless several children of other families are baptized at the same time--and always follows the home christening. It is not unusual to make some recognition of a clergyman's services at a church christening, and always is in order at the home rite, though it is not expected as a clergyman counts on his wedding fee.

If church or house is decorated for a christening, white flowers only are employed, in conjunction with palms and ferns to relieve them. White lilies are particularly beautiful. The table is adorned with white flowers; the cakes and bonbons are white. Any desired refreshments may be served, those for afternoon tea being suitable. That old-fashioned beverage known as caudle is never served at any other time. It is dispensed in bouillon cups.

MOURNING ETIQUETTE.

Conduct of Funerals--

So brief the span between our birth and death that the etiquette of burial may fittingly follow that of the christening ceremony. It might be supposed that the funeral, especially the private, could be conducted without formality. But informality often means disorder, and simplicity without order is confusion. There is no time where lack of order and system so grate on one's nerves as at a funeral. The less "fuss" on such an occasion the better, and for that reason, the routine of meals should go on as usual, though no one seems to have the heart to eat them. Still, it is in a way a comfort to most people to feel the chain of accustomed habit; it brings a trifling sense of relief.

Save in the case of a person who has been prominent in the public eye, there is no excuse, or reason, for any but a private funeral. Time was when not to hasten to the house of death was thought unkind; not to attend the funeral of an acquaintance a mark of disrespect. We have changed all that. We do not expect the uninvited to attend our weddings and receptions, why should they come at times of much more intimate and personal emotion--those times when we can hardly endure the words and presence of those we love best? What the sensitive have endured at the hands--or tongues--of well-meaning but clumsy sympathizers--not infrequently curious as well as sympathetic--only those who have suffered can relate. In addition to the natural grief experienced, the members of the family are usually worn out with nights of watching and days of anxiety; it is a fresh strain to be obliged to see people, relate sick-room details and listen to stereotyped condolences.

The Undertaker.--Cases are rare where there is not some "next friend" who is competent to see the undertaker, and arrange details with him. In fact, the undertaker may well be put in charge. He should be competent and experienced. A clumsy, fussy undertaker is an affliction.

The undertaker will obtain the physician's certificate as to the cause of death, without which in many cities a burial permit cannot be issued. He will secure the necessary permit, see to the preparation of the grave, and the purchase of a lot if necessary, arrange the house for the funeral, furnish the bearers, and secure the requisite number of carriages; and, before the family returns from the cemetery, have the funeral paraphernalia out of the house, so that the maids or whoever is left in charge can restore the rooms to their wonted order. Everything possible is done to spare the grief-stricken.

The Duties of the Next Friend.--The actual duties devolving upon the person representing the family include ascertaining their wishes as regards the officiating clergyman and his notification of their desire and the hour of the funeral; for music, if any is desired; the selection of a casket, and determining the number of carriages to be ordered. A written list of relatives and friends who will go to the cemetery, arranged in order of their relationship, four in a carriage, is given the undertaker for his guidance in assigning those present to their places. The friend of the family will accompany the undertaker to the cemetery if a lot must be purchased, or he may go alone, the undertaker receiving his instructions from the cemetery authorities. If any special position is desired for the new grave, this will be definitely stated.

With this knowledge, an undertaker will conduct a burial so quietly and decorously that as a bereaved wife once remarked, it was "a real comfort to have John buried." She did not quite mean what she implied, however.

Where means suffice, a black cloth-covered casket with silver mountings is chosen. If the interment is in a vault, a metallic casket is obligatory. The child's casket is white; that for a young person is white or pearl-gray.

It is no longer necessary to call on friends and neighbors to bear the dead to their last resting-place, though it may be done. Honorary pall-bearers are chosen among the associates of the dead in case he is a prominent personage; the active may be relatives, or undertaker's assistants. A child is sometimes borne by his or her little school friends, though it seems a pity to call on children for such offices.

The House Funeral.--At the house funeral the family remains upstairs, or is seated in the room with the casket, the former more customary. The clergyman stands at the head of the casket, or in the doorway, that his voice may be heard. At the conclusion of the service, those not going to the cemetery quietly disperse; the carriages drive up; the undertaker in a low voice assigns the relatives to them in proper order, and the cortege moves off. At the grave, the remainder of the solemn service is read, the casket lowered, and all is over.

That dreadful custom known as "viewing the remains," by which those present file past the casket for a last look at the dead, is obsolete. The bereaved take their farewell before any arrivals; those who desire to behold the face of the dead do so as they enter, then are seated in another room. Sometimes the casket is closed before the funeral.

Church Funerals.--The church funeral is more dignified, perhaps, but much less common than a few years ago. Good taste counsels that our leaving, like our arrival in this world, be a purely family affair. Those who attend a church funeral are in their seats when the cortege arrives. The organ is softly played as the casket is borne up the aisle, the clergyman preceding it; its rests before the chancel, the clergyman reads the burial service from the step, the mourners, who have followed the casket, being seated in the front pews. The procession retires in the same order, the congregation dispersing afterwards.

Flowers.--Flowers are usually ordered the day before the funeral, to arrive in the morning, that they may be fresh. Cards are removed before they are taken to the cemetery. Colored flowers, preferably those of pale tints, are admissible, though American Beauties are not infrequently sent. Wreaths of galax leaves are often ordered for the funeral of an elderly person; sometimes half of the wreath is of the leaves and the remainder of flowers. Wreaths and sprays are almost invariably sent by private individuals, the stereotyped "emblems" like "the broken wheel," "gates ajar," etc., being the offerings of clubs, or other organizations to which the deceased may have belonged. Where there is a great quantity of flowers, the loose sprays are often sent to the sick in hospitals, only enough to cover the grave being reserved. The visitor to a cemetery could find it in his heart to wish that when the beauty of these floral offerings has departed, the sodden remnants might be speedily removed. They speak so forcibly of forgetfulness.

MOURNING GARMENTS.

The custom of wearing mourning after a bereavement is almost universal. Even the poorest endeavor to show their grief by donning a few shreds of black, while among the well-to-do an entire new wardrobe is felt to be obligatory. However our religion bids us look forward to a more perfect existence in the beyond, however truly death may be a relief from pain and suffering, custom, that makes cowards of us all, must be followed. Often too, mourning garb is but the visible evidence of the gloom that oppresses us spiritually. In spite of our faith, our sense of loss and loneliness is best expressed in sad raiment and abstinence from pleasures. Often it would be kindness to the living to go our way as usual, but that is not in harmony with our hearts.

Mourning is in a manner a protection to a woman. Strangers respect her sorrow and refrain from the jocular. Behind her crepe she may defy intrusion. But it often becomes a hardship to the young.

"I missed all my youth," complained a middle-aged woman. "We were a large family. A brother died when I was sixteen and we went into mourning and shut ourselves away from entertainments. Then my father died; next a sister, and another brother, so that, looking back, I can remember but one gown I had, between the age of sixteen and thirty-one, that was not black--and the one exception never had a chance to get worn out."

The Expense of Mourning.--Mourning, however, is sometimes a distraction. In deciding about trimmings and the width of crepe hems many a woman forgets her woe, for a time at least. Mourning wear is expensive, and to clothe a whole family in black totals no inconsiderable sum. Many families have been financially swamped through the expenses of an illness, a burial, and the conventional mourning. In this instance, as in the case of weddings, all these things should be regulated by common sense. A costly casket, a profusion of flowers and a long funeral procession merely gratify a foolish and ostentatious pride on the part of the survivors, and often entail a heavy burden on the father or husband.

It is quite customary to borrow the black garments worn at the funeral. These should be returned immediately after the funeral, with a message or note of thanks.

It is well to look over one's wardrobe to see what garments may be colored for use during the period of mourning. The art of the dyer has made such progress that very satisfactory results are obtained, and quite wealthy people do not hesitate to resort to this expedient.

Mourning Wear.--Crepe, ugly, expensive and easily ruined by dust and dampness, is no longer indispensable to a mourning outfit. If used at all, it is in the form of hems or narrow bands on face veils and as borders or facings, on gowns. Even widows, who wear the deepest mourning, no longer wear crepe veils.

All dress materials for mourning wear have a dull finish. Henrietta, imperial serges, tamese cloth and nun's veiling are the standard fabrics. A lusterless silk is sometimes employed, also crepe de chine.

Crepe is used as a trimming only during the first period of mourning. Hats have almost entirely replaced bonnets, except for elderly widows, who often adopt the close-fitting Marie Stuart bonnet, with the white ruche inside the brim. A long veil of fine silk nun's veiling is worn with this, with a tulle or net face veil with a narrow fold of crepe. Veils of crepe or nun's veiling are not worn over the face except at the funeral.

Hats with crepe folds and trimmings, with veils arranged to fall in folds in the back are usually selected; with them is worn a plain net face veil. Dotted veils are not mourning. Black furs, lynx, fox or Persian lamb are worn.

Many women wear narrow lawn turn-over collars and cuffs; they are hemstitched, with no other decoration. Black-bordered handkerchiefs are no longer carried; if, however, one's woeful trappings must extend to this detail, the narrower the edge the better.

Either black glace kid or suede gloves are worn. Shoes and slippers must be in a dull kid finish.

All white may be worn in summer during the later period of mourning, but combinations of black and white are not mourning; thus a white dress with black ribbons is not correct.

Jewelry (in gold), ostrich feathers, velvet, lace, satin, and jet trimmings, except in dull jet, are barred. One may wear a diamond or pearl ring or two, but no colored jewels set in rings. Some women have outer shells made in black enamel to enclose diamond ear-rings they are accustomed to wearing.

If one wears mourning, she should hold to the correct form. If, however, she elects to wear black, more license is permitted her. Whatever is done, should be consistent. Thus if she simply adopts black she may have a net or all-over lace yoke in a gown, may wear hats with wings and quills or fancy feathers in black, or black flowers--which are botanical monstrosities--whereas in correct mourning she could not.

The Period of Mourning.--The length of time during which mourning is to be worn has been considerably shortened of recent years. Widows formerly wore deep mourning-crepe, bombazine, etc., for two years, and "second mourning" for another year. Now, even among the most rigid sticklers for form, two years is the limit, and there is a tendency to diminish this period. Eighteen months of woe inconsolable; six months of grief assuaged. Nor are all recreations debarred the widow, as formerly; she may go to concerts, small entertainments, even to matinees, after some months have elapsed. This is as it should be. Many women have settled into gloom and despondency which have darkened their homes because there has been nothing to lift them out of their low frame of mind.

For a parent, a grown son or daughter, the conventional period is two years, one year of deep mourning. For a young child a mother wears black for a year. The same time suffices for a brother or sister. Six months answers for grandparents; three for an uncle or aunt. Often one does not wear mourning except for husband, child or parent.

Young girls need not wear mourning as long as an adult does, nor do they wear crepe, unless it be a hat with crepe trimmings, or one with ribbon bows and face veil with crepe border. It seems as unnecessary as it is unkind to put young children into black.

French Mourning.--The French, with characteristic cheerfulness, greatly abridge the mourning attire, dividing it into three grades, deep, ordinary and half-mourning. For the first only woolen materials in black are employed; the second, silk and woolen; the third gray and

violet. The wife laments her husband for a year and six weeks,--six months of deep mourning; six of ordinary, and six weeks of gray and violet melancholy. The bereaved husband, on the other hand, is let off with six months of sorrow, three in deep mourning, three in ordinary; he has not to pass through the gray-and-violet stage at all.

Six months is also the period for parents, evenly divided between deep and ordinary. One gets off with two months for brother, sister or grandparent, and three weeks suffices for a mere uncle or aunt. Good taste decrees mourning should be discarded gradually. From black one may go to quiet costumes in dark colors, gray being an approved hue.

Mourning for Men.--Custom sets more lightly upon men than upon women in the matter of mourning. Here, as elsewhere, the details of etiquette devolve upon women. A widow would incur censure if she married within two years after her husband's death; indeed, if her marriage followed soon after the expiration of that term, Mrs. Grundy would infer some surreptitious courting had been going on. A man, however, may marry again after a year has elapsed. A widower would abstain from society and the theater for six months. A parent is mourned for a year.

The correct attire for men is a black suit, black gloves and tie of grosgrain or taffeta silk, and a black band upon his hat. The tailor adjusts this hat band with scrupulous nicety to the depth of his affliction. It is deepest for a wife; it diminishes mathematically through the gamut of parents, children, brothers or sisters.

The widower is not expected to wear mourning for two years, unless he prefers to do so. If he goes into the niceties of the garb he will wear black enamel shirt studs and cuff buttons, and a plain black watch fob. After a year he may wear a gray suit, retaining the black accessories.

The custom, followed in some circles, of wearing a black band on the left coat sleeve, is to be emphatically condemned. The place for the band is on the hat. If not placed there, let it be nowhere. On a gray or tan coat the effect is startling. The custom of wearing such a band as emblem of mourning for a fellow member in a lodge, or any organization, whether worn by man or woman, is more honored in the breach than the observance. Better drape the departed member's seat in black, or hang crepe on the charter than follow this foolish fad.

The Duties of Friends.--Where there is sickness in a family, friends call to make inquiries or to proffer assistance. Kindness counsels that such calls should be brief; often duties press heavily upon the well, and the time spent in receiving visitors may be sadly needed for rest, or for other duties. To stay to a meal or to take children on such a visit is inconsiderate, to say the least. If help is needed, give it quietly, unobtrusively, and as efficiently as possible. A little service rendered by a thoughtful neighbor is always appreciated, whereas the person who goes "a-visiting" where there is sickness comes near being a nuisance.

In town, friends call at the door to make inquiries. Unless very intimate, they do not expect to see any member of the family. Cards are left, and it is correct to write "To inquire" on the card. If death follows, cards are properly left, either before the funeral or within a week after the event. Upon these may be written "with deepest sympathy." One does not ask to see one of the family. Cards of this character are often sent by mail, and are acknowledged within three weeks by sending one's visiting card with narrow black edge and envelope to match. Across the top of the card is written "With grateful appreciation of your sympathy," or "It is a comfort to feel that we have your sympathy in our loss." Cards are sometimes especially engraved for this purpose. Such cards have a mourning border and are enclosed in an envelope and mailed. One's visiting card, with narrow black edge and black-bordered envelope, is sent in acknowledgment of invitations to weddings, receptions, etc. If a note is necessary in reply to an invitation, it is written on note-paper having a narrow mourning border, and follows the customary formula, the border being an indication of the reason it is declined.

In case the request "Kindly omit flowers" is made in the obituary notice, the wish of the family should be observed.

Letters of condolence should be written as soon as possible. Friends should not be afraid to intrude. If they feel a sincere sympathy it should be allowed expression, for such tributes, coming from the heart, are always grateful to the stricken. Answers to such letters should not be expected; it is customary to acknowledge them by a card, as above mentioned.

Friends who send flowers should be thanked, either by note, or word of mouth.

THE ETIQUETTE OF CORRESPONDENCE.

"Letters should be easy and natural, and convey to the persons to whom we send just what we would say if we were with them."--Chesterfield.

They say nobody has time to write letters these days, and yet the post office department handles millions of them each year. True, they are not the formal, lengthy, somewhat stilted epistles of a century ago, when a lad began his home letters "Honoured Parents," and your correspondent announced, "I take my pen in hand to inform you," etc. The letter of today, however, is not less the messenger of good-will and remembrance than it was in those days. It remains largely the bulletin of business and of family affairs.

The postman's bag! What may it not contain? News of birth or tidings of death, of lover's vows made or broken, of achievements or misfortunes. Every letter is like a new day; we cannot tell what its message may be.

It is no mean accomplishment to be able to write a good letter.

The Essentials.--The first essential to letter-writing is to have something to say, and the ability to say it well. This is a talent that may be cultivated. The next requisite is good paper. Better curtail in some other item and allow yourself good, plain, heavy paper and envelopes. Avoid all fancy papers, whether in tint or design. Plain white or cream laid paper is always good form. Whatever the vagaries of the stationer, the plain white, fine quality paper is to be preferred. The intertwined initials of the writer are often placed at the top of the first page, either in the center or at the left-hand corner where the water-mark used to be. These are done in gold or silver, or some pale tint. Just now, the street address of the writer is often engraved across the flap of the envelope. The form of the latter, whether square or oblong, varies according to the passing fashion. Whichever is used, the letter sheet is folded once to fit it. Sealing-wax is little used at present; if at all, the "blob" of wax is small, only large enough to receive the impress of a single initial on the seal.

Use a good black ink. Violet and purple inks are as passe as colored stationery. There is a certain writing-fluid, bluish when first used, and turning black after a few hours' exposure, that is standard.

Write legibly. Handwriting may or may not be an index of character, but it certainly does indicate certain attributes. A cramped, slovenly, awkward handwriting is naturally associated with a careless and uneducated person; whereas a free, graceful and trained hand indicates culture and refinement in the writer. We say again, write legibly. Nothing is more exasperating than certain examples of modern fad-writing, where one might as well attempt to translate a page of Chinese script. Despite the typewriter, one should endeavor to be a good penman, because the typed letter or note is inadmissible in polite society, being reserved for the world of business. Avoid also the microscopic calligraphy with a fine pen; it is very trying to your correspondent's eyes, unless she happens to have a reading-glass conveniently near.

Take pains to make your signature easily decipherable. Remember that while a word may be puzzled out by the context, or by the analogy of its letters to others, the signature has no context, and is often so carelessly written that the letters composing it are indistinguishable. One should be particularly careful in this respect where writing business letters or letters to strangers.

Letter Forms--Ceremonious letters, and notes in the first person are addressed to My dear Mrs. Smith. If Mrs. Smith is a friend or an acquaintance, she is addressed as "Dear Mrs. Smith." This is the American custom, and is an exact reversal of the English. which is, by the way, being more generally adopted in our society. "My dear" certainly seems to the uninitiated, at least, more intimate and familiar than "Dear." A business communication to a stranger begins--

Mrs. Joseph Smith,

Dear Madam:--

There are shades of courtesy to be observed in signing letters. "Sincerely yours" is a little more formal than "Yours sincerely;" "Yours with much regard" is more familiar than "Yours sincerely." "Yours truly" is for the business letter; "Yours affectionately" for the family or those to whom we are much attached. The rule has been to capitalize all the words of the address, but only the first word of the conclusion, as "My Dear Friend Mary" and "Yours sincerely," but of late this rule seems to be broken in regard to the address, which is now often written "My dear Mrs. Smith."

Abbreviations.--Abbreviations are always incorrect. The month, day and date must be spelled out; the street number and the year are correctly indicated in numerals. The year is sometimes spelled out on formal invitations, but is regarded as an affectation in private correspondence. To indicate a date in numerals, as 3: 18: '12, is bad form. "Street" is not shortened to "St." and "Avenue" is to be spelled out. The city and state should be written in full. "Cal." and "Col." are often wrongly read by busy railway clerks, and your Colorado letter goes to California.

The character and (&) is never to be employed. "Hon.," "Dr." and "Rev." are permissible on an envelope; "Rev. Father" is incorrect; write "Rev." We do not use "Esq." in America as much as it is used in England, where it is always employed in addressing a letter to an equal, "Mr." being reserved for tradesmen. Here we use "Mr." almost entirely. Christian names are not abbreviated in an address; one should write "George" or "Charles" rather than "Geo." or "Chas."

What Not to Do.--A woman is never to be addressed by her husband's title, either verbally or in writing. "Mrs. Dr. Smith" is "Mrs. Lewis Smith"; "Mrs. Judge Morris" is "Mrs. Henry Pond Morris." Of course she would not think of signing herself "Mrs. Dr. Smith." She should sign herself by her own name, "Marion Morris." If necessary to convey the information, she may, in a business note, place Mrs. in brackets, before her name, or after signing her own name, write below it, "Mrs. Henry Pond Morris." This is never done in a social note. Often, upon her marriage a woman includes her maiden name in her signature, thus, "Marion Ames Morris." A hyphen is not used. The four-storied name, as "Marion Helen Ames Morris," is too cumbersome for common use.

A woman uses her husband's full name on her cards. The man, in signing himself, writes his full name "Henry Pond Morris" or "R. P. Morris," rather than "Henry P. Morris."

The postscript has been laughed out of existence. If a few words must be added the "P. S." is omitted. Dodging about on the pages, from first to third, then to second and fourth, is to be avoided. Don't write across your written pages; a plaided letter is so difficult to decipher that one is justified in destroying it unread. One is supposed to have sufficient letter paper on hand. A half sheet should never be used as a means of eking out an epistle. Don't send a blotted, smeared letter.

Placing the Stamp.--Several years ago silly girls occasionally inquired through the newspapers as to "the significance" of the postage stamp when placed in certain positions on the envelope. One paper made reply that to place it anywhere but on the upper right hand corner of the envelope indicated that the sender was a first-class idiot. The answer was widely copied and the inquiries ceased. The stamp is placed there for convenience in canceling, that being done by a machine in all but the smaller offices.

The last item to be remembered is, spell correctly, though it is one of much importance. A mis-spelled word is a grievous error in a letter--worse than a blot. Keep a dictionary on the desk; when in doubt look up the word, and then take pains to fix it in mind so as to have no further trouble with it.

When to Write.--Notes of invitation should be promptly answered. So should business letters. As for friendly letters, were they answered at once, by both parties, the exchange would be so brisk that too much time would be thus occupied. One may let a reasonable time elapse before replying; this depending upon the intimacy. Friends whose time is much taken up with other cares, but who do not wish to lose touch with each other, not infrequently agree to exchange letters at certain dates or anniversaries. Both may write simultaneously, or one write and the other reply.

Make it a point to re-read the letter you are about to answer, and take pains to reply to any questions your correspondent may have asked. Nothing is more maddening than to make several important inquiries and find them wholly ignored while your friend tells you how busy she is, how many engagements she has in the future, how tired she is, and prefaces these uninteresting details with a long apology for her silence. Who was it said "An apology is a mistaken explanation"?

Postal cards are not considered in correspondence. They are to be used only for business, or where one is traveling and wishes to inform her friends of her whereabouts. The picture or souvenir postals are largely used for this purpose. But the postal card, in correspondence, is like a call when the lady is out and you do not leave your card--it doesn't count.

In regard to love-letters, bear in mind what Rousseau says:

"To write a good love-letter you ought to begin without knowing what you mean to say, and finish without knowing what you have written." Then, having unbosomed yourself, don't send it.

Care in Writing.--It is well to remember, that once you have dropped a letter into the box, it is no longer yours. It belongs to the person to whom it is addressed. If you have been indiscreet, the matter is out of your hands. Therefore, he careful what you write. You cannot tell what use your correspondent may make of it. Your friend may be trustworthy, but careless; some one may be dishonest enough to read it; it may be lost. It is a good plan to write nothing you would not be willing to have read before a roomful of people who know that you wrote it.

Avoid personalities. Don't commit your unflattering opinions of other people to paper. The letter is a witness whose veracity is unquestioned.

Don't read your letters to others, unless they are family letters in which all may rightly have a share. A letter is a private communication.

Keeping Letters.--It is a bad plan to keep old letters, especially if they are of a personal nature, or if they contain confidences or secrets. When the owner dies, there is no knowing to what use they may be put. One regrets the publication of the private letters of great men and women, showing, as they so often do, the foolish, silly, conceited side of a character we have admired. Private letters are often disillusioning, or betray the presence of the skeleton of the family, unhappiness or disgrace.

The safest way is to keep a letter till it is answered, then destroy it, This does away with a lot of useless lumber.

Letters of Congratulation and Condolence.--It is not possible to give forms for letters of this character. They are meaningless unless they come from the heart, and should be characterized by sincerity. Nevertheless, they should be written, and promptly, as also letters of acknowledgment of gifts, favors offered, and the "bread-and-butter letter"--the missive you write to your hostess after a few days' visit.

Letters of condolence are especially difficult to write. One so fears to wound instead of comforting. If one can offer some quotation that has been a personal help in time of sorrow, it is often gratefully appreciated. But because we "don't know what to say" we must not omit writing. The letter is often a greater kindness than the call, which is a tax upon the strength of the mourner.

"The path of sorrow, and that path alone, leads to the land where sorrow is unknown; no traveler ever reached that blessed abode who found not sorrows in his road."

"Wherever souls are being tried and ripened in whatever commonplace and homely way, there God is hewing out the pillars for His temple."

Do not think you must write a long letter. A few well chosen phrases, sincere expressions of feeling, are more grateful to one who grieves. One may say:

My dearest Friend:--

It is with sincerest sorrow I have just heard of your great bereavement. I cannot hope to comfort you; God only can do that, but I want to say how deeply and tenderly I feel for you in your sad affliction.

Believe me, most faithfully yours, On the other hand, if we must congratulate, we may write:

> *I have just heard of your engagement to Mr. Blank, and wish to be among the first of your friends to express my sympathy with you in your happiness. I have known Mr. Blank for some time, and greatly admire his many good qualities. I am sure you are very happy with him, and will be more so as you grow together in marriage. Hoping good fortune and joy may always be your portion in life, and present bliss an earnest of more in store for you, I* am, *Most sincerely yours,*

MANNERS FOR MEN.

"Politeness and good breeding are absolutely necessary to adorn any or all other good qualities or talents."--Chesterfield.

Though what we call society is largely vested in women, and women's customs regulate etiquette, men are by no means exempt from the necessity of knowing and practising what we call good manners. A man can have no greater charm than that easy, unstudied, unconscious compliance with social forms which marks what we call "a man of the world"--the man who knows what a good manner requires of him in any situation, and does it quietly and with the grace of habit.

There has been no time in the history of the world when good manners counted for more than at the present. This is true of both men and women. It is so true that in certain fields it is practically impossible to succeed without their aid. The value of a pleasing manner can hardly be overestimated. Such a manner is as far from the self-assurance and presumptuous familiarity which some men assume under the idea that these are impressive, as night is from day.

Value of Courtesy.--Courtesy has a commercial value, and exerts no little influence upon a man's success in business. Polite attention and readiness to oblige bring customers again and again, where their lack would send people to rival houses.

We can forgive, in the intellectually great, or in the man of affairs who has done things worth doing, a lack of social training that would not be endured in a man with no such claim. Yet this is not saying that the great man would not command more unqualified admiration were he to practise the social graces instead of ignoring them. The truth is, the fact that we have to overlook the absence of these graces induces a more critical attitude toward his achievements. Great though he be in spite of his lack of courtesy, we feel he would have been greater had he known and practised the art of gentle manners.

The Manners of the Gentleman.--These "gentle-manners," that make the "gentle man" are an indispensable requisite to success in society. They testify to a man's good breeding, to his social affiliations; they "place him." They often bring a man many things that wealth could not.

The rich boor is despised in spite of his money. The poor man may be popular because of his pleasing personality and his fine manner.

Men sometimes profess to despise those refinements that are associated with good manners, saying they detest affectations. But these things are not to be affectations. They should be the outward expression of inward kindness and good-will and unselfishness. The cultivation of good manners is a duty; somebody has said that "the true spirit of good manners is so nearly allied to that of good morals that they seem almost inseparable." John G. Holland says somewhere: "Young men would be thoroughly astonished if they could comprehend at a glance how greatly their personal happiness, popularity, prosperity, and usefulness depend on their manners." Emerson remarked that,--"Manners should bespeak the man, independent of fine clothes. The general does not need a fine coat."

A Matter of Training.--It may be that politeness is instinctive with some, but with most men (women also), it is a matter of training and habit, and careful discipline. In process of time courtesy becomes perfectly natural, so gracefully spontaneous it seems to be.

Here is where the mother's work in the early training of her sons comes in. Taught from childhood, by example and precept, the observances that make for good manners, the young man wears them as easily and as unconsciously as he does his clothes.

Politeness an Armor.--There is no better armor against rudeness and discourtesy than politeness. The individual is impervious to slights and snubs who can meet them with the courtesy which at once puts the common person in his proper place as the inferior.

A woman is shocked and repelled by disagreeable manners in a man, manifested in discourtesy toward her, by an awkward manner, coarse speech, incivility, neglect of the little attentions she expects of a man and which men of breeding render as a matter of course. A woman is more likely to fall in love with a homely man of pleasing address than with an Adonis so clad in self-complacency that he thinks politeness unnecessary, or one who does not know its forms.

THE ETIQUETTE OF THE HAT.

The first rule a man should observe in regard to his hat is never to wear it in the presence of women, save in the open. If mothers would take the trouble to train their small sons to rigid observance of the rule of removing their head covering the moment they enter the house there would, be fewer adults guilty of this particular discourtesy, which is at once the greatest and the most common. One occasionally sees a man wearing his hat and preceding a woman down the aisle of a theatre.

The expression, "tipping the hat," is a vulgarism. A man doesn't "tip" his hat, he raises it quite off his head.

The Coachman's Salute.--The semi-military salute--raising the hand to the hat as if to lift it, but merely approaching the forefinger to the brim--is a discourtesy to a woman. Such a salute would bring a reproof in military circles; it is objectionable among men. Actually it is the manner in which a man-servant acknowledges an order from his master or mistress, and is not inaptly called "the coachman's salute."

A man wears his hat on the street, on the deck of the steamboat, in a picture-gallery or promenade concert-room. He removes it in a theatre, the opera-house, and the parlors of a hotel.

When to Raise the Hat.--Men raise their hats to each other on the street. They extend the same courtesy to all members of their family, of both sexes. A well-bred man raises his hat to his little daughter, as he would to his wife.

On the street, a man must wait for a lady to recognize him, but should be ready to remove his hat simultaneously with her greeting, raising and replacing it quickly. The fashion of removing the hat after meeting a lady is absurd. How does she know the courtesy has been extended?

When a man is with a lady who recognizes an acquaintance, he must raise his hat, whether he knows the individual or not. He should, however, keep his eyes straight ahead, not looking at the person.

If he meets a man walking with a lady whom he does not know, he waits the man's recognition.

A man removes his hat in an elevator if women enter or are already inside. This rule is often ignored in large public buildings.

If a woman bows to a man in any place where it is his privilege to wear his hat, he removes his hat and does not replace it while she is talking with him. This rule applies everywhere except on the street. "A gentleman of the old school" will stand bareheaded on the street if exchanging a word or two with a lady; in such case she may request him to replace his hat.

A man when driving or motoring cannot remove his hat. He bends forward slightly and touches his hat brim with his whip, held upright, in the first case, and raises his hand to the visor of his cap in the latter.

At Other Times.--When he is able to render some slight service to a woman whom he does not know, she will thank him with a slight inclination of the head and a smile, and he should raise his hat. When he relinquishes his seat in the street car, he should give the lady a chance to acknowledge his courtesy, and then raise his hat.

Men raise their hats and stand uncovered as a funeral cortege passes into the church or from a house, and at the grave.

They also stand uncovered when the United States flag is borne past, or the national hymn--the "Star Spangled Banner"--is played in public, at a military review, etc.

When a man passes a lady in the corridor of a hotel, or on the stairway, he should raise his hat.

When he takes leave of a lady, the same act of deference is expected.

Hat and Coat When Calling.--When calling, the man looks after his own hat, overcoat and stick. His hostess does not offer to relieve him of them, nor suggest the removal of his coat. He deposits his hat and stick on table or seat in the hall before entering the drawing-room, and takes off his overcoat if his call is to be prolonged. Or, he may take them all with him into the drawing room if his call is to be brief. In any event, it is his business to dispose of them according to his own pleasure.

RULES FOR PRECEDENCE.

A man precedes a woman in going down-stairs and follows her in going up. This is that he may be in readiness to catch her should she fall.

He allows a woman to precede him on entering or leaving a room, and should open the door for her.

On entering a hotel dining-room the man may precede the lady to the table assigned them, on the occasion of their first meal, standing until she is seated. Afterwards, he may follow her as the head-waiter leads the way. Sometimes he permits her to precede him in the first case.

The question is sometimes asked who should follow the usher on entering church or theatre. The rule above stated obtains. The woman follows the usher; the man follows her.

The man allows the lady to enter the carriage first, but descends before her that he may assist her to alight. The same rule prevails in regard to entering and leaving a street car, etc.

ABOUT SMOKING.

The old rule of good manners: "A gentleman does not smoke in the presence of ladies," is many times violated in these modern times. There is a story of an elderly woman who, being asked if smoke was offensive to her, replied: "I do not know. No gentleman has ever smoked in my presence." The woman of today is more likely to answer "Oh, dear no! I love the odor of a good cigar." The truth is the cigar has become such a constant and apparently necessary adjunct to a man that to banish it is in effect to banish the man. And women prefer to endure the smoke rather than have the man absent himself. There are very few cafes and restaurants where men do not conclude their repast with a good cigar, even when entertaining ladies.

Where Not to Smoke.--Nevertheless, there are times and places when and where a man should not smoke. When he is about to meet a lady he knows he removes his cigar before removing his hat and bowing. If he wishes to join the lady, walking a short distance with her, he throws away his cigar before doing so. He does not smoke, when driving with a lady, unless possibly in the country. He should not smoke when walking with her--but he often does, with her full consent and permission. In fact, women, as has been said, are responsible for men's lapses in the way of smoking.

A guest does not smoke in his host's house unless especially invited to do so, by his host, not some younger member of the family or another visitor.

At a dinner party at which ladies are present, men do not smoke until the ladies have left the dining-room.

It is a bad form to smoke when anyone is singing, unless in those free-and-easy places of amusement where "everything goes."

About Expectoration.--No man should smoke, anywhere or at any time, who cannot smoke without using a cuspidor. It is a practice so much worse than smoking, so thoroughly abominable in itself, that no man with any claim to good breeding or good manners permits himself to indulge in it.

In most homes, nowadays, men are permitted to smoke "all over the house." It is better, wherever possible, to let the man have a "den" where he may smoke with his friends. The practice of smoking in bedrooms is reprehensible; the air one will breathe through the night should not be vitiated.

BACHELOR HOSPITALITY.

"A bachelor's life is a splendid breakfast; a tolerably flat dinner; and a most miserable supper."

Being a bachelor does not excuse a man from certain forms of hospitality. Many "society men" live in apartments, at the present time, and may entertain the ladies who have favored them with invitations; in fact, it is expected that a man who has often been entertained will reciprocate in some fashion.

If a bachelor's quarters are too restricted for any other form of entertaining, he may give a theatre party, followed by a supper at some cafe. Or he may do this without the theatre party. Of course, such an entertainment is expensive, but he must remember that the ladies who have entertained him have spent a good deal of money on their fetes.

The Bachelor and the Chaperon.--The first thing the bachelor must do is to secure a chaperon. She must be a married woman of unimpeachable reputation. Having done this, he invites the other members of the party, first submitting his list to her approval. The usual number is six, three men and three women, or two men and four ladies. Two men may join forces to entertain a quartet of ladies, or more, and thus halve the expense. The carriage or taxicab is sent first to the residence of the chaperon; the host accompanies it or may meet it there. The other ladies are called for, the other men generally meet the carriages at the theatre. The host sits next the chaperon at the theatre and at the supper, placing her on his right.

If a supper is to follow, and it almost always does, the host has reserved a table at the hotel or cafe and has perhaps ordered flowers and a special menu in advance. He has also settled the account, so that he has only to cross the waiter's palm with silver at the conclusion of the repast, in acknowledgment of faultless service.

Cheaper Ways of Entertaining.--In summer there are cheaper ways in which a bachelor may payoff his social obligations. Most bachelors belong to clubs, where they may give luncheons or suppers. There are roof-gardens and outdoor vaudeville, open-air concerts, etc., that may be made pleasurable occasions. He may charter a yacht, in company with several friends, and entertain a dozen or half score ladies with a sailing party. At all these, however, he must provide a chaperon.

A very pleasant and informal way for a bachelor to entertain is to invite some of his more intimate women acquaintances to afternoon tea at his apartments. For this he writes personal notes or gives verbal invitations. He asks some married, lady to assist him, placing it in the light of a favor to himself. She must arrive early, and remain until the last guest has left. The host pays the chaperon special deference, asking her to pour the tea, and either escorting her home or ordering a carriage for her.

Elaborate refreshments are not necessary at such an affair. Sandwiches, cakes, tea, served in the American fashion or a la' Russe, are sufficient. The chaperon presides at the refreshment table. All things needed for the refreshment of the guests may be ordered from a caterer. If the affair is in the evening, chocolate and coffee may be served instead of tea, or cakes, coffee and ices.

The Bachelor's Chafing Dish.--If the circumstances of the bachelor permit, he may give a chafing-dish supper, presiding over the manufacture of a Welsh rarebit or lobster a la Newburg, making the coffee himself in a machine. This might take the place of the supper at a restaurant after the play. After such a supper, or a dinner in his rooms, the host escorts the ladies to their carriages, and accompanies the chaperon to her home.

If none of these methods of entertaining chance to be within the man's means--for many poor men of pleasing address are social favorites--he may fall back on the pretty compliment implied in sending flowers or bonbons, remembering that matrons as well as "buds" appreciate such attentions.

In Village Society.--In small towns and in the country, the young man would ridicule the idea of having a chaperon along. He seldom considers the question of repaying social invitations, or paying calls after an entertainment. He should be careful to show courtesy to the host and hostess, to dance with the latter and her daughter at a dancing party, and may escort mother and daughter or the mother and some one of her friends, to a lecture or concert. Generally he ignores all claims of this character. But he should not.

Should He Offer His Arm?--A man seldom offers a woman his arm nowadays, unless she is so elderly or infirm that she needs the support. For a couple to walk arm in arm in daylight is decidedly provincial. For a man to take a woman's arm is a liberty not permissible unless she is a member of his family. He should offer his arm if holding an umbrella over her at night, on a poorly lighted street or a country road at night. A woman, unless very infirm or ill, should not walk arm-in-arm with a man in daylight.

The Outside of the Walk.--A man usually walks on a woman's right, in order to protect her if necessary, It looks absurd, however, for him to be dodging around her to keep on the outside of the walk unless some danger is to be encountered.

Minor Matters of Men's Etiquette.--A man should not carry a girl's parasol; he should however assume any parcel she may be carrying.

When a man escorts a woman to her home it is not correct for him to linger at the door. He should accompany her up the steps, ring the bell and wait until she is admitted. If the hour is at all late he should not enter, even though invited.

It is extremely bad form for a man to speak of a woman by her Christian name while talking to casual acquaintances. Though long acquaintance may sanction the familiarity at home, or among intimate friends, to all outsiders she should be Miss.

The custom of leaving the theatre between acts is inexcusable. If a man is escorting a lady, he is guilty of great rudeness if he leaves her,

Cards and Calls.--If calling on a lady who is visiting a person who is a stranger to him, he must ask for her hostess, sending up a card for her as well as for his friend. If calling with a lady, he should wait for her to give the signal for departure.

The man who attends an afternoon tea should leave a card for each lady mentioned in the invitation, and for the host, whether the latter was present or not. He must send the same number of cards if unable to be present, enclosing them all in an envelope which fits the cards, addressing it to the hostess, and mailing it so that it will be received on the day of the function. He must call upon his hostess within two weeks after an invitation to a dinner or ball.

In attending a tea or afternoon reception, the right-hand glove must be removed before entering the drawing room, as it is bad form to offer a gloved hand to one's hostess on such occasions.

If, when calling on a lady, another visitor arrives, the first comer must not attempt to "sit him out." He should make his adieux within a reasonable time after the second arrival, even though a friend in more intimate standing.

Bad Habits.--A man should carefully avoid mannerisms, such as twisting his mustache, fussing with his tie, fidgeting with some little article taken from a table, as a paper knife, etc. These awkwardnesses are the outcome of nervousness. He should strive at all times to be simple, at ease, and unconscious of himself. If he tries to "show off" he makes himself obnoxious.

Picking the teeth, chewing a toothpick, cleaning the finger nails in company, are gross violations of propriety.

The Car Fare Question.--A girl occasionally appeals to writers on social forms to find out when she should permit a man to pay her car fare. It is expected that he will pay for her if he is escorting her, and she should allow him to do so without comment. If they happen on the same car by chance she should pay her own fare. If the man anticipates her, handing the change to the conductor and saying "For two," she should thank him simply and let the matter pass. Really, it is not entirely good form for a man to pay a woman's fare under such circumstances, unless she has difficulty in finding her purse, or her change. Then he may say "Allow me" and pay for her. If she finds her money she may return the amount, and he should take it without protest.

THE ETIQUETTE OF DRESS.

"The best possible impression that you can make with your dress is to make no impression at all; but so to harmonize its material and shape with your personality that it becomes tributary in the general effect, and so exclusively tributary that people cannot tell after seeing you what kind of clothes you wear."--Holland.

MEN'S DRESS.

A man--lucky creature--is not expected to change his clothes as frequently as a woman must. He wears morning dress until dinner, unless he is to attend some afternoon function, like a wedding or a reception. Dinner is now almost universally at six or half after six o'clock. Before that hour, save in the exception noted above, he wears a business suit, a derby or "soft" hat, tan shoes if he prefers them, or laced calf-skin shoes with heavy soles. The coat may be sack or cutaway. Such an outfit is correct for traveling wear. A white shirt, or one of striped madras, is worn, with a white linen collar. The tie is usually a four-in-hand in some dark shade.

The cutaway coat is correct for church wear. In summer it largely takes the place of the frock coat, which, with the silk hat, is usually "out of season," so to speak, from about the middle of May until about the same time in September. Straw or felt hats are worn.

Tweed flannel and cheviot suits are favorite summer wear for men, Flannel trousers, white with flannel shirt and leather belt, constitute the usual wear for tennis, golf, etc., and blue cheviot or serge for yachting.

Afternoon Wear.--For formal afternoon wear the double-breasted frock coat of black worsted, with waistcoat of the same or of white duck, is reserved, dark gray pin-stripe trousers are worn with it, patent leather shoes, gray gloves, silk hat and standing linen collar. The standing collar is for formal wear. This attire is suitable for all social affairs between noon and evening.

After dinner evening clothes--the "dress suit"--are worn. This has been fully described in the chapter on wedding etiquette, under the head of correct dress.

Incongruity in Dress.--A man must avoid incongruities in dress. Tan shoes are inadmissible with formal afternoon dress. They do not accompany a silk hat. A lawn tie is never worn save with evening clothes, nor a turn-down collar with them. Gloves should be inconspicuous. A man's hands encased in bright tan gloves make one think of sugar-cured hams.

The Tuxedo is a dinner coat, hence never seen before six o'clock; it must not be worn at a theatre party, or if a man escorts ladies. It may be worn in summer at informal dinners, and at summer hotels. Silk hat, white waistcoat, or white lawn tie are not correct wear with a Tuxedo.

APPROPRIATE DRESS FOR WOMEN.

The real beauty of dress resides in being suitably gowned. Suit the attire to the time and place. Fashion prescribes and regulates styles; etiquette settles the appropriate garb for the occasion. Every detail, from shoes to hat, should be harmonious and suited to the occasion and consequently to the hour of the day. But how many, many violations of this rule we see! Ostrich feathers worn with shirtwaists; low shoes on the street; dressy hats in the morning; jewels at breakfast--all inappropriate and unrelated!

The correct street wear in the morning in the winter is a tailored suit with medium sized hat in felt or beaver, walking shoes, and rather heavy gloves in glace kid. More elaborate suits or gowns in fine smooth cloth or velvet are worn at afternoon functions, for calling and receptions. One does not choose light or showy colors for these if she must walk or take a street car. Ostrich feathers can be worn on the velvet or satin hat that accompanies this costume, which is completed by patent leather shoes and white or pearl-gray gloves.

When Decollete Gowns are Worn.--High-necked and long-sleeved gowns are worn at every daytime function.

At balls, cotillions, formal dinners, evening parties, and in the large cities in opera boxes, decollete gowns may be worn.

No "nice" woman wears a low gown when dining at restaurant or hotel. The neck may be cut low, under a lace yoke, unlined, and the sleeves finished from the elbow with lace. Hats are worn.

One chooses a handsome velvet or other dressy material for a dinner dress, and wears with it her rarest jewels. Good taste and modesty forbid too lavish a display of shoulders. As a rule, in our average social life, the unlined lace yoke and collar and lace sleeves are preferred for dinner wear, the decollete gown being reserved for balls and cotillions.

Young girls' dancing gowns are never cut very low; the "Dutch" neck and the slightly low round cut being preferred. A string of pearls, a fine gold chain and locket, or gold beads, which have been restored to favor, are the usual ornament.

For theatre wear, where one is not to occupy a box, one may wear a handsome reception gown, or a handsome bodice and skirt. Shirt and lingerie waists are not appropriate theatre wear, unless one patronizes some second-class house of amusement.

Wearing the Hat.--The rule to bear in mind as to the wearing of hats is this: At all daytime affairs, hats are kept on. At all evening affairs--musicales, concerts, receptions, the play, they are removed.

Tea-gowns and negligees are for the boudoir; the kimona is for the bedroom.

Gloves are removed at a luncheon or dinner. Of course they would not be kept on at a card-party or a tea. One may retain them at a stand-up supper.

Ornaments.--An abundance of ornament is in bad taste. Don't be one of the See-me-with-'em-all-on type. A cheap ornament spoils a handsome costume, better none at all; too many ornaments, even if good, look tawdry.

At a certain fashionable summer hotel a young woman was seen dancing in high shoes and wearing a demi-trained lingerie gown over a petticoat of ordinary walking length. She was certainly "the observed of all observers," but hardly the object of admiration.

The Debutante's Dress.--The debutante usually wears white on the occasion of her introduction to society. The material should be light and youthful--crepe de chine, some soft white silk like messaline, chiffon or organdie being the usual choice, made with high neck and long sleeves if the affair takes the form of an afternoon reception. Only a ball or cotillion permits a low gown, and then the gown is not "low" in the usual sense: it is merely cut out modestly in the neck

49

and the sleeves are short. In the afternoon her mother, who presents her, wears a handsome reception gown; her young friends, who "assist," wear light colored, dressy gowns of chiffon, net, etc. At such an affair guests remove wraps but retain hat and gloves.

Dressing on a Modest Allowance.--The woman who wishes to be well dressed but must produce that effect on a moderate allowance, must be particularly careful in her purchases. She should confine herself to two colors, of which black will be one. She must choose conservative styles as well as colors, and above all, she must study very closely the relationship of her purchases in order to avoid incongruities. A hat may be beautiful and becoming and within her means, yet a very unwise purchase because it will not harmonize with or be suited to the costume with which it is to be worn.

Neat gloves and good shoes are items of dress not to be disregarded by the woman who wishes to look well dressed. Shabby gloves are ruinous to a well-dressed appearance.

DRESS FOR ELDERLY WOMEN.

The woman who has been "dressy" in her youth must curb her fancy as she grows older, and carefully avoid things that are "too young" for her. She may "love pink" or pale blue, and because she could wear it when a girl, unwisely clings to it in her fifth and sixth decades. A bedizened old woman dressed in a fashion suitable for one twenty years younger, is a sight more pitable than admirable. She must not permit the milliner or costumer to convince her that she is still young enough to "wear anything" but must try to have sense enough to distinguish what is suitable from what appeals to her because she would have looked well in it in her youth.

Ermine furs, for instance, are absurd on a woman of forty-five or fifty. The dead white brings out the yellow in her complexion and the faded color of eyes and hair. A very light "dressy" hat makes the wrinkles more obvious.

The Suitable.--Dark, unobtrusive colors, relieved by white lace at throat and wrists, hats modest in size and coloring, set off gray hair and matronly figure far better than showy and more youthful garb. No elderly woman should attempt to wear brown; somehow it kills her complexion if she is sallow. Black, very dark blue, the softer shades of gray, are generally becoming if relieved with white. Lavender and mauve can be becomingly worn by those dear old white-haired ladies who have pretty complexions. The lemon-colored lady must avoid them. We must remember Joubert's saying: "In clothes fresh and clean there is a kind of youth with which age should surround itself."

Materials must be as handsome as can be afforded; soft wool materials may be chosen, cashmere, henrietta, voile, make up suitably. In summer most old ladies can wear white to advantage.

Simplicity should be the guide as to styles. Leave the fussy and elaborate to younger women, and adopt a dignified simplicity.

DUTIES OF A CHAPERON.

"The art of not hearing should be learned by all." Young America flouts the chaperon. The young girl of the middle class guesses she can "look out for herself," and knows "how to behave." Very often she doesn't know, and sadly demonstrates her lack of the knowledge of life and good sense that would enable her to avoid situations that create gossip. In European society the chaperon is indispensable and has an acknowledged and honored position. In America, young women ridicule the idea and young men are decidedly impatient of her presence. And yet in our more conventional circles it is understood that she is a protection to the girls in her charge, and an oft-needed restraint on young men who are inclined to be too free and familiar.

Mothers as Chaperons.--A mother is her daughter's best chaperon. Very often her health, her home duties and her own lack of social experience unfit her for such a duty. In that case, she should be glad to put her girls in charge of some more experienced woman. If all young men were honest and honorable and temperate, the unchaperoned girl would meet with fewer embarrassments. Think of the awkward plight of a girl should the carriage or the taxicab break down as she is returning home, or the miserable state of the girl whose escort at play or party has taken too much wine! These things don't often happen, some one says. They do happen--far more frequently than the world at large is aware.

Chaperon's Lot Not Easy.--The duties of a chaperon are so onerous that she deserves much gratitude, rather than revilement, for undertaking them. She must stay at balls and parties when she would infinitely prefer her bed; she must frequent places of amusement that are tiresome to her but agreeable to her young charges; she must remain in the parlor, or in the adjacent room separated only by draperies from it, while the girt entertains men callers, and no woman enjoys being "gooseberry;" she must check too high spirits and prevent "loud" behavior. And she will many times know that her presence is resented, and sad to say, endure slights in the discharge of her duties.

Chaperons a Social Help.--Nevertheless, if girls only knew it, the chaperon may be very helpful and aid them materially in having a good time. She should be a woman of wide acquaintance, accustomed to good society. Then she will introduce the girls under her charge to nice men whom they should know, and to partners for the dance; see that they are invited to nice places, and that they are correctly dressed. She must have tact combined with dignity, and be able to reprove little lapses in decorum so tactfully that youth will not take umbrage. She must make her charges like her, and win and hold their respect. And it is very important that she should know what not to see--"the art of not hearing"--yet she should never overlook anything vital, It will be seen that she should be a person of infinite tact, good nature and courage.

The Chaperon of the Motherless Girl.--Nowdays, the wealthy widower, instead of putting his young daughter at the head of the household, secures some woman of good reputation and social standing as his daughter's chaperon. She is, practically, the feminine head of the house, and in so far as possible, takes a mother's place with the girl. She sees to it that the girl has proper companionship and does not make undesirable acquaintances. She accompanies her on shopping expeditions, travels with her, attends theatres and parties with her, takes the head of the table if the girl gives a luncheon, and everywhere strives to make life pleasant for her young charge, giving up her own pleasure and convenience for that purpose.

Even the young woman of twenty-five or twenty-seven, at the head of her father's household, or living in a hotel, should have a companion.

Avoid Espionage.--And yet, with all this responsibility, the chaperon must avoid anything like espionage. She must not open letters; she must not be prying and inquisitive; she must not give reasons for the girl she chaperons to regard her as "a dragon."

A giddy, flirtatious chaperon is a disadvantage to a girl. She is so desirous of securing attention and having a good time herself that she neglects her charge. Often she undertakes chaperonage chiefly or entirely in order to go about herself. Such a chaperon is worse than none at all.

The Girl and the Chaperon.--A girl should remember that her chaperon stands in the relation of a mother to her for the time being, therefore any disregard of her chaperon's suggestions or wishes is the same as disregarding her mother's. No well-bred girl ever does this---well, at least not publicly. If her chaperon gently intimates that it is time to go home, that she is dancing too many times with the same man, or "sitting out" too long, she should cheerfully comply with the hint. She should not vanish with an escort, leaving her chaperon and others--to wonder at her absence, but at the close of every few dances, before the beginning of another, ask to be taken to her chaperon. There her next partner will naturally look for her.

She must at all times treat her chaperon with the utmost respect and deference, remembering the lady is bestowing a favor by taking charge of her, and that it is often at her parents' request.

At a theatre party, bachelor's tea, sailing party, excursion, etc., one married woman is sufficient chaperon.

The girl who works, the art and music student, may look after herself, but the society girl must submit to the thralldom of the chaperon.

The Chaperon in Middle Class Society.--While the rules of etiquette are intended to be of general application, there are certain relaxations in middle class society not permissible in more fashionable circles. This is the case as regard the chaperon. Many young men on moderate salary would not feel they could afford to buy a ticket to the theatre or concert for a chaperon, or order a carriage. But is a girl then to be denied permission to accept the invitation? Under such circumstances middle class etiquette requires that the young man shall be well known to the family as a person of good habits and reputation. The girl, however, is not supposed to accept an invitation to a supper afterwards. She may go to a dancing party at a private house or a club in case proper chaperons are provided for the affair and they almost invariably are. But it is better taste for a party of young people to go together under the care of a chaperon.

When a girl receives a young man visitor, her mother should always meet him. She should enter the parlor, be introduced if he is a stranger, converse for fifteen or twenty minutes, and excuse herself, leaving the young people to their tete-a-tete. No girl ever loses a young man's estimation through being properly looked after.

Under no circumstances should the young girl be allowed to accompany a young man on an excursion without a chaperon. She should not motor with him alone; another pair of young people should go with them unless a chaperon is included.

GOOD FORM IN SPEECH.

"It isn't so much what you do; it is how you do it. Not so much what you think as how you clothe your thoughts that enables you to make a pleasant impression."

Good breeding is shown in the use of words, quite as much as in manners. Correct use is evidence of culture and personal refinement.

Use of Slang and Colloquialisms.--Slang, we are often reminded, is common--meaning vulgar. And yet, there are some slang phrases that are so expressive, and convey so much meaning in few words that the temptation to use them is irresistible. Much use of slang, however, is very undesirable, indicating lack of refinement. We may be colloquial, but must eschew the vulgar.

Among the words that are bad form we find "folks," used instead of "family" or "relatives." "Ain't" is one of the most common improprieties of speech and one that has no standing whatever in good language. "Gentlemen friend." "lady friend," are vulgarisms. We should not speak of young men as "fellows."

We should say "shops" instead of "stores," and "station" instead of "depot." A depot is a place where provisions and stores are accumulated. Just how it came to be applied to a railway station is an etymological puzzle. The use of "learn" for "teach" is incorrect. "Pupil," "student" and "scholar" are often used interchangeably, but incorrectly so. "Pupil" refers to the younger classes in a school.

Those in the most advanced grade of a high school, and those in college are students; while scholar signifies those who are learned and out of school. "Dresser," "bureau" and "dressing case" are incorrectly applied to a chest of drawers. "Vest" for "waistcoat," and "dress suit" for "evening clothes" are incorrect. "Visitors" is in better taste than "guests." "Got" is a word often used superfluously and always inelegantly. "I have it" sounds much better than "I have got it"; leave out "got" wherever you can. As for "gotten"--it ought to be unspeakable.

"Don't" for "doesn't" is, perhaps the most common grammatical error. "I don't," "you don't," "they don't,' are correct. "Don't" is a contraction of "do not." You wouldn't say "he do not," "she do not," would you? Then don't say "he don't," or "she don't."

As a rule the simpler the speech the better. "Residence" for "house," "peruse" for "read," "retire" for "going to bed"--all these and their like sound stilted.

The use of French words and phrases is to be avoided, both in writing and speaking. Generally they are mispronounced--as in the case of the very affected lady who spoke of "Mrs. Brown, nee Smith," pronouncing "nee" as if spelled "knee."

Form of Address.--To acquaintances, a woman speaks of "my husband"; to friends, she calls him by his Christian name. To servants, he is "Mr. Smith." This is a rule often violated, so often in fact, that few are aware of the impropriety of saying "Mr. Smith" to friends and acquaintances. The man employs the converse of the rule; it is "my wife" to acquaintances, etc. To speak of a daughter as "Miss Mary" or "Miss Jane" to anyone but a servant is insulting, placing the person thus spoken to on a par with an inferior. If formality is desirable one should say "my daughter Mary." The same rule applies to a son.

It has already been said that we do not address a wife by her husband's title. He is Dr. Brown; she is Mrs. Brown. Mrs. General, Mrs. Judge, are not current in polite circles.

We do not use "Sir" in addressing equals. Children no longer say "sir" or "ma'am" to their parents, but "Yes, father," or "No mother." Ma'am is seldom heard now except from old-fashioned servants. Maids and men-servants say "yes, Mrs. Smith," or sometimes, "No, madam."

Courtesy in Conversation.--"Things said for conversation are chalk eggs," said Emerson. There are many chalk eggs on the market. Most of us feel that to "be sociable" we must talk incessantly. True, there are sometimes dreadful pauses in conversation when no one seems able to think of anything to say, and the longer the pause the more vacuous one's mind.

What passes for conversation at receptions, dinners, ordinary social affairs, is merely chatter made up, of persiflage and repartee. One must be able to furnish it, however, for small talk is conversational "small change," without which it is not easy to "do business." Lacking it, one is like Mark Twain's man with the million dollar check and not change enough to buy a postage stamp.

SUBJECTS OF CONVERSATION.

No one can tell another person what to talk about. Advice on that subject is valueless. There are some things we may do, however, to make ourselves agreeable in conversation. We may study the art of expressing ourselves clearly,--saying what we wish to say without circumlocution. Some people seem to begin in the middle of a subject and talk both ways.

Avoid personalities in your conversation. Don't talk about yourself; nobody is interested in your personal perplexities and troubles. Don't recite your "symptoms" nor tell what the doctor says, nor what diet he has prescribed. Nothing, positively nothing, is so tiresome. Don't indulge in animadversions upon the absent, nor make sarcastic remarks about them.

Try to discover some subject in which your companion is interested, and get him to talking. Then show yourself a good listener. A woman may get the reputation of being bright and clever if she will simply show herself a good listener. To do this, she must give her attention to the person who is talking. She must seem interested. Her eyes must not wander around the room; she must not take up picture or book and glance over it; her questions must be intelligent and to the point. Then, unless the speaker is a well-known bore, she need never suffer under the imputation of being neglected in society, and she will be thought courteous and intelligent.

Discourtesies.--To interrupt a speaker, to take the words out of his mouth and finish the sentence for him, to broach a new topic, irrelevant to that in hand, unless the latter is in danger of leading to thin conversational ice,--all these are discourtesies.

To yawn while listening to anyone; to show lack of interest in a story or anecdote that is being told, or let the attention wander, is marked impoliteness. We are not to remind a speaker that his story is an old one, or that he has told it before.

Some Things to Avoid.--A man should avoid raving over the perfections, the beauty or chic of one woman to another. He shouldn't talk golf to one who doesn't know the language of the game, nor discourse on music to the unmusical. Above all, he shouldn't undertake to entertain the whole company, nor introduce a topic in which he only is interested or informed. The more serious questions of life are barred in society; people wish to be amused, not instructed. An inveterate talker, especially one of a didactic turn, is a bore. So is the man who puts a hobby through its paces. Avoid exaggerations in conversation, also extravagances, such as "beastly this" or "awfully that," also avoid over emphasis. Don't talk in italics.

The Speaking Voice.--A clear, distinct enunciation should be cultivated. The voice need not--should not--be raised above the ordinary conversational level to make one perfectly understood, if only one speaks clearly. This is something that can be cultivated. So also a discrimination in the use of words, so that which most nearly expresses the meaning of the speaker comes to him readily.

A pleasant voice is a charm, either in man or woman. A noted teacher of singing once remarked that the cultivation of the speaking voice is a positive duty, and possible to almost everyone. Certainly a harsh, squeaky, shrill or affected tone of voice may be improved by care and endeavor.

CHURCH ETIQUETTE.

Surely the church is the place where one day's truce ought to be allowed to the vanities, the dissensions and animosities of mankind."--Burke.

The church is sometimes sarcastically referred to as "the social stepping-stone." It is a fact that the newly made rich and the vulgar often choose a church attended by the people of fashion whose acquaintance they most desire, rent a high-priced pew, and become prominent through their benefactions and their services in church work. They are "taken up," after a time, in a fashion, and unless too socially impossible through lack of good breeding, may, from "fringers," become "climbers." "I might go to that church for a hundred years and no one would notice me," bitterly complained a woman who had undertaken the social uplift via the church. The woman in question defeated her own object. She dressed in the extreme of style; she always came in late, with much rustle of silk and rattle of bangles; her hair was "touched up" and her face rouged. The well-bred and refined members condemned her on these grounds. Nevertheless, where a stranger comes who bears the hall-mark of culture and refinement, the church connection is often an aid to social habilitation, though it should never be sought as such.

Friendly Advances.--Friendly advances generally come from pew neighbors. Respond to them courteously but without undue eagerness. Do not expect your pastor to become your social sponsor with his congregation, and remember that though he will probably call after letters of church membership are presented, you have no claim upon his family, nor the families of any of the church officers through acquaintance in business life. This is often a grievance to people from smaller towns who, moving to a city, expect the families of their business associates to assist them socially. Two men may be partners for ten years without their wives knowing each other by sight, if they chance to move in different social circles.

Demeanor.--One should dress quietly at church, give attention to the service and the clergyman, and not linger unduly in the vestibule to gossip or greet friends. To notify the usher if one's pew will not be occupied is a courtesy if the preacher is popular and the church crowded. To be disagreeable in case strangers are shown to one's pew, or mistakenly seated there, is unkind and unchristian. Giggling, smiles, exchange of smiles or bows in the church proper are regarded as bad form.

NEIGHBORHOOD ETIQUETTE.

Neighborliness is a quality little exercised in cities, where one may live next door to people for years and merely know their names. Some people prefer not to know their neighbors, fearing undue familiarity on their part. The relationship may be a very pleasant one if both parties observe certain restraints. It is not well to become too intimate. Nobody wants a neighbor running in at all hours, with or without an errand. Sometimes to sit on the back porch with a book or paper seems to invite a neighbor to "run over" and the hour's rest or mental recreation is given over to small talk.

A neighbor has no more right to enter without knocking than any other caller, whether by kitchen or front door. It is an intrusion, a disregard of the reserve that should characterize neighborly intercourse.

No matter how friendly, friendship will last longer where the forms of decorum are observed.

Borrowing.--The exchange of "kitchen-kindnesses" should be ventured upon rarely. By these is meant the plate of cookies or biscuit or doughnuts we send our neighbor on baking-day. Some families prefer their own cooking. A woman who had been annoyed by many unsolicited donations of this kind, persisted in though unreciprocated, finally piled the sent-in biscuit rather ostentatiously on the garbage can in full sight of her neighbor's window. Other hints had failed, this was effective--a rather violent remedy, but after all not undeserved. In case of illness, where one has no maid, or the family must care for the sick, a fresh cake or a tasty dessert may be offered, and will seldom fail of appreciation. Knowing the circumstances, one need not hesitate over the proffer of a neighborly kindness.

There is little excuse in the city for the borrowing of kitchen staples which is the bane of some country neighborhoods. A borrowing neighbor is an affliction--a nuisance which unfortunately doesn't come under the jurisdiction of the Board of Health.

CARRIAGE ETIQUETTE.

A story is told of a certain great lady who visited at the court of a reigning monarch on a secret matrimonial mission. The monarch had three daughters; the emperor of her own country had a marriageable son. Before overtures were made for an alliance, the lady was to see the three princesses and decide which one should be honored by the proposal. It was her whim to rely upon "the carriage test." She watched the young princesses as they alighted from the royal carriage. The oldest one descended clumsily, displaying too much of the royal lingerie. The second skipped out, disdaining the step. The third descended gracefully and with dignity, and Cupid's ambassador decided she would make the most fitting empress.

At certain finishing schools, lessons in deportment include training in how to enter and leave a vehicle gracefully. Stepping out on the right-hand side, the right foot is placed on the step, the left naturally falls on the ground. Entering, the left foot is first advanced. In this way the other foot clears the body of the carriage without awkwardness.

Minor Items.--The rule that the owner of the carriage occupies the right-hand seat even when accompanied by a guest, is almost universally observed. The only exception seems to be when the guest is a person of unusual distinction.

To place one's carriage at the disposal of a friend is a great courtesy, and should never be abused by the recipient. In case of accident the occupant should pay the bills for repairs, or at least urge that she be allowed to do so.

If a lady invites a friend to pay calls with her, dropping her companion to call on some acquaintance while she goes on to see a friend of her own, the lady thus favored must not keep her waiting on her return, more than the few moments necessary to make her adieux.

CIVILITY IN PUBLIC.

One is shocked, often, at the prevalence of rudeness in human intercourse. People who are courteous in the drawing-room are sometimes horribly uncivil in public. They crowd and jostle and elbow in thc endeavor to secure better places for themselves, violating every canon of politeness. Women have fainted, gowns have been ruined and valuable articles lost in "crushes" incident to gatherings in "our best society."

Many people carry an umbrella with utter disregard of the eyes and headgear of the passing crowd. Closed, it is tucked under the arm, the ferrule projecting behind on a level with the face of a pedestrian. They go through a heavy door, pushing it open for themselves and letting it swing back against the next comer. They step in advance of those who have prior claim to be shown to seats, and accept civilities and service without so much as a "Thank you." They endeavor to obtain "something for nothing" by piling their luggage into seats they have not paid for on the train; on the boat they fortify themselves in a circle of chairs that are "engaged"--generally to hold their wraps and lunch-boxes, while others look in vain for seats.

Rude Tourists.--Tourists have a reputation for a disregard of the rights of others, which makes them obnoxiously uncivil. They enter a church where worshipers are kneeling and audibly criticise the architecture and decorations, or the faith to which it is consecrated. They comment flippantly on great pictures in art galleries, and snicker over undraped statues, evincing the commonness of their minds and their lack of knowledge of art. But one of the worst lapses of decorum is to sit in a theatre and anticipate the action of the play, or the development of a musical number, by explanations to a companion. To do so may show familiarity with the play or the score, but it also shows a painful lack of good breeding, and a disregard of others' rights to peaceful enjoyment. On a par with this is the incivility of a person who undertakes to accompany a soloist with his (or her) own little pipe, to the annoyance of those who prefer to listen to professional rather than amateur efforts.

Of course all these rude people excuse themselves by saying they "get left" if they don't "rush," and that they "paid for their seats," as if this atoned for their disregard of those who, equally with themselves, have paid for a pleasure spoiled for them by the greed or impertinence of their fellow men--and women.

Telephone Etiquette.--"Central" could disclose how discourteous many women who pique themselves on their good manners can be when they are "calling down" the tradesman who has made a mistake in filling their order. And how often a party line is held for a lengthy "telephone visit" while others wait their really important affairs because the "line's busy!"

The manners of the public need reforming. Civility is a public good. Without it, we would be barbarians. It is the practical application of the Golden Rule to everyday life. To lay aside our own courtesy because we are in a crowd, or among people who do not know us, reduces us below the level of those who are not versed in the social requirements, because we know them and should practise them, whereas they do not know.

DUTIES AND DRESS OF SERVANTS.

In many large and well-to-do households in this country only one maid, the "girl for general housework" is engaged, the mistress and her daughters assisting with the lighter parts of the work. In such case each must have a certain definite portion of the daily duties and be responsible for its performance. Very few maids are capable enough to do all the work of a good sized family without assistance, even though the linen be sent to the laundry.

The One Maid.--Where but one maid is kept she must rise early and put in a couple of hours' work before breakfast, airing the house and perhaps putting in order and dusting the living rooms, then preparing breakfast. She will probably serve it unless everything is put on the table, in which case she may busy herself in the kitchen, washing the rougher dishes used in preparing the meal. The mistress of each household must make out her own schedule for the week, according to the convenience of the family.

The maid is supposed to have her dress changed by three o'clock. She will wear a simple but neat cotton gown about her work, mornings;

in the afternoon she will put on a black dress with white apron, collar and cuffs. She is expected to keep a clean apron in the kitchen to slip on if summoned to the door before luncheon. She should never answer the bell with her sleeves rolled up. The mistress provides the white apron with shoulder pieces, the linen cuffs and collar worn by the maid of all work in the afternoon and evening. These are the mistress's property, remaining in the family through the changes of servants. So many girls object to the cap that it is seldom seen save in very formal establishments. If worn, the mistress furnishes it.

Instructing the Maid.--If the mistress finds her maid's education in her duties is deficient, she should teach her to open the door wide, as if the visitor were welcome; to have her tray ready to receive cards;

to be informed as to whether the mistress is at home or not that she may answer the visitor's inquiry at once. She is to usher the visitor into the drawing room or parlor, take the card to her mistress and return to say that "Mrs. Blank will be down in a few minutes," never alluding to her mistress as "she," as some ill-trained girls do.

If a lady who keeps but one maid entertains at all she must instruct the girl in the proper serving of meals. In the first place, everything that is necessary for the service must be ready; there must be no getting out of extra silver or china at the last moment, with its upsetting confusion. The menu must be so carefully planned that most of the food to be served can be prepared beforehand. For a six o'clock company dinner, the soup may be hot in the kettle; the fowl or joint in the oven; the entree waiting the finishing touches on the back of the range, the vegetables in the warmer, and the dessert in the ice-box. All the china and silver being in readiness and the table properly laid, the maid slips into her black dress and apron, and presents herself at the drawing-room door, announcing "Dinner' is served."

The Maid's Serving.--The guests being seated, she brings in the soup tureen, uncovers it, taking the cover to the pantry as she goes for the hot soup plates. She then stands at the left of the mistress with a tray, covered with a doily, in her left hand, a folded napkin under the tray; takes the soup plates as they are filled, passing them to the left of each guest, taking the plate from the tray with the right hand. She then removes the tureen. Removing the plates she takes them from the left side of the guest. The roast is brought in and served in the same manner as the soup; the vegetables are passed, each guest helping himself from the dish. The salad is usually served on the plates upon which it has been arranged. After the salad the table is cleared and the crumbs brushed with a napkin upon a plate or tray, and the dessert brought on for the hostess to serve, The latter starts the little dishes of bonbons or salted nuts on their travels, guests passing them along.

Chocolate is a good beverage to serve on such occasions; it can be made in the morning, or even the day before, and heated without in the least impairing its quality.

Given a capable, willing girl, one anxious to learn and not too self-conscious, a woman may entertain two or three or four guests very adequately if she will plan her menu carefully and see, personally, that everything is in readiness. She should, however, avoid any over-elaboration. Better a simple meal well prepared and served than a more pretentious one that fails in these particulars.

Duties of Waitress and Cook.--Where two maids are kept they are waitress--"second girl" or "housemaid," sometimes so-called--and cook. The housemaid--we will so style her--opens and airs the house and dusts and arranges the rooms before breakfast. She serves the breakfast, clears the table and washes the dishes taken from it. She then proceeds to the bedrooms, putting them in order, dusting, making beds, etc. She will probably have fine lingerie waists, etc., to wash and iron on certain mornings. She does the sweeping, unless there is a man to take out and beat the rugs, and wipes up hardwood floors. She must clean the silver once a week and rub up brass; keep the pantries in order, clean the bathrooms, wait on table, answer the bell, both the door bell and her mistress's bell, and usually assist the latter in dressing. She is expected to do part of the family mending, keeping table linen and bed linen in good condition, and in some households is expected to wash and iron the napkins and dish-towels, unless a laundress is employed.

The Cook's Work.--The cook must prepare the meals, and put the food into the proper dishes and these in the pantry, ready for the waitress, who is not expected to enter the kitchen during the service of a meal. She washes the dishes used in the kitchen and the meat dishes from the table; she must keep the kitchen and its adjuncts, including back stairs, refrigerator, back porch and closet in order. Her mistress plans the meals with her, and she is expected to make good and economical use of left-overs. She often does the ordering by telephone, and sees to the milk, ice, etc., as they are delivered.

Should Understand Duties.--Most of the difficulties between servants arise from misunderstanding of and friction about their respective duties. It is best to have a definite and thorough understanding as to the work expected of each before engaging her. Both cook and housemaid have one afternoon and one evening each week and every other Sunday afternoon. When one is off duty the other must necessarily assume part of her work. Some mistresses allow a girl the afternoon and evening of one day; others give one afternoon, and the evening of another day, requiring the cook to return to prepare dinner on her "day" and the maid to come back to serve it on hers. If afternoon and evening go together the cook is expected to leave everything in readiness for the evening meal; the cook, on the housemaid's day out, must wait upon the table.

Servants always respect a mistress who knows her rights, exacts them, and respects her servant's rights. She should permit no familiarities;

at the same time she must not regard her household assistants as mere machines, beyond her sympathy, Good mistresses make good servants.

The Nurse.--The nurse must wash and dress the children; keep their clothes in order, washing and ironing the finer articles; eat with them, keep the nursery in order; sleep in the room, or in a room adjoining them with the door open, and take care of them when they are ill. A nursery governess teaches them, and is excused from the laundry work and from keeping the nursery in order.

The mistress who can conduct her domestic menage with two servants only is usually better served and with less friction than where more are employed. Rarely can three servants get on harmoniously. The more servants there are, unless there is a housekeeper, the more shirking there is, and the more waste and extravagance.

SUMMARY.

Remember--

That, in introducing people the man must always be introduced to the woman.

That the younger woman, the unmarried, the less socially prominent, are introduced to the older, the married and the more renowned..

That to pronounce names distinctly avoids much awkwardness to those introduced.

A casual meeting on the street does not necessitate an introduction.

Never present yourself with a letter of introduction. Leave it at the door.

That a card represents a visit, and that leaving your name in this way makes your friend your debtor.

That after dinners, luncheons, theatre and card parties a call is required, whether the invitation is accepted or not.

An invitation to a wedding must be acknowledged by sending cards to those in whose name the invitation was issued, and may, if she so pleases, call on the bride on her return from her wedding journey.

One should send announcement cards rather than invitations to those with whom acquaintance is slight.

An invitation to afternoon tea does not require reply. Leave cards if present.

The etiquette of calling on an "at home" day does not differ from that of an ordinary call, save that some light refreshment is offered, as a rule.

That the bachelor and the widower should respond to every invitation whether accepted or declined, by calling and leaving cards, whereas the married man's wife may leave his cards with her own. Men ignore this rule a great deal, however.

Cards must be engraved, never written or printed.

That a married woman uses her husband's full name on her cards; that a man's name always has the prefix Mr., and an unmarried woman's or young girl's that of Miss, and that "pet" names are not "good form" on cards.

The extreme limit of a call is twenty minutes, and the first caller to arrive should be the first to depart.

That you should not prolong your leave-taking.

That the lady invites the man to call, and being thus complimented he should soon avail himself of the permission.

It is the mother's place to invite young men to call, not the daughter's, though she may say "My mother would be pleased to have you call on us," The mother must then meet and assist, for a time at least, in entertaining him.

A first call must always be returned. Afterwards the acquaintance need not be continued.

"Not at home" is no discourtesy to a caller if she is so informed when the maid opens the door. The maid should know whether her mistress wishes to see callers or not.

P. p. c. on a card means "To take leave," and intimates your friend is leaving town for a season.

It is customary for mother and daughter to use a card on which hath names appear when calling together. A debutante, in our most conventional society, has no separate card of her own. If she calls without her mother, she uses this double card, running a pencil mark lightly through her mother's name.

Sisters may use a card in common; it should be engraved "The Misses Jones," and used when calling together or sending gifts.

The divorced woman, if she drops her husband's name by permission of the court, uses her maiden name on her cards, with the prefix Mrs. If she retains her husband's name, she usually combines her family name with it, as Mrs. Jones Brown.

A card should never be handed to a hostess or any member of the family. Lay it on the table. If a member of the family opens the door, a card need not be used, though one is often left as above.

At afternoon teas, receptions and "At Homes" the visitor leaves a card for the hostess on the tray in the hall, and one for the guest of honor, or the debutante if one is being introduced.

A card to an "At Home" or an afternoon reception does not require either acceptance or regret. If the person invited attends she leaves her card; if not, she sends it by mail to reach the home on the day of the reception.

An invitation to a dinner must be answered immediately, and unconditionally accepted or declined.

If, having accepted, it becomes absolutely impossible to keep the engagement, the earliest possible notice must be given to the hostess.

It is unpardonable to be late at a dinner party. Arrivals are expected within ten minutes of the hour named.

One wears the best she has that is suitable for a dinner party.

The reply to an invitation must follow the style of the invitation. If formal, that is, in the third person, the reply must also be in the third person. If informal, the personal form being employed, the reply is also informal.

Do not send your card with "Regrets" written upon it, in response to any invitation, formal or informal.

Telephone invitations are admissible only for informal affairs. General invitations, given verbally, have no social footing. "Do come and dine with us some day," unless followed by a definite date or note of invitation, means nothing.

An invitation given by a man to dine or visit, or to a home entertainment, is not to be accepted unless seconded by his wife.

A girl, sending invitations to commencement exercises, encloses her card.

It is bad form to show that one feels slighted or affronted at not having been invited to any function, or not given the precedence one feels herself entitles to. The hostess, in her own home, obeys such rules as she believes correct.

A visitor is expected to contribute her share to the pleasure of the occasion by being conversationally agreeable.

If hostess, one must overlook every awkwardness on the part of the guest or servant, and any accident to one's belongings, but be deeply solicitous and apologetic if an accident happens to a guest,

The guest of honor at a dinner party should take leave first. Other departures follow speedily.

Remember--

That an invitation to spend a few days with a friend requires a speedy reply. It is not allowable to say one will come either earlier or later than the time specified.

A visitor should adapt herself to the ways of the household, be punctual at meals, and make no plans or arrangements without consulting her hostess.

She may not invite a friend of her own to a meal without requesting permission of her hostess.

She should be careful not to infringe upon the privileges and prerogatives of the man of the house.

She may accept invitations in which the hostess is not included, but never without due consultation with her hostess.

She should show herself pleased with the efforts made to entertain her and enter into them readily.

She should leave promptly at the expiration of the time set for her visit. It is almost invariably a mistake to outstay the limit. If no limit was named in the invitation, she should, within a day or two of her arrival, state the date on which she will leave.

On her return home, her first duty is to write her hostess, announcing her arrival and expressing her pleasure in the visit. To omit this is a grave discourtesy. A hostess once said of a woman who failed in this particular: "We don't know whether she reached home or not; we never heard from her after she left."

On departure, maids or servants who have attended one should receive a gratuity, proportioned to the means of the visitor and the style of the establishment.

The hostess should arrange to have the visitor met, either meeting her in person at the station or being first to greet her on her arrival at the house.

Guest rooms should be in perfect order and equipped with every possible convenience for the comfort of visitors.

The hostess arranges whatever pleasures are possible for her guest's enjoyment, invites her friends to call on her, and probably gives a tea or reception in her honor.

Do not forget that it is ill-bred as well as unkind to discuss the family affairs of one's hostess with others; to criticise or complain of her arrangements; or gossip about her or her family.

Remember--

The announcement of an engagement comes from the family of the girl.

The parents and relatives of the bridegroom-elect should call on the girl and her mother, or if living in another city write cordial letters without delay.

The bride-elect should respond to these advances with cordiality.

She should try to make her future husband's family like her.

Etiquette is not relaxed in the case of an engaged couple. They do not make calls together except on relatives or very close friends. They may not make journeys together unchaperoned.

The cost of a wedding, whether at church or at home, is borne by the bride's family, the bridegroom paying for the wedding ring, the clergyman's fee, and the carriage in which the pair leave the church after the ceremony.

Though it may be necessary to limit the number of invitations to a wedding, announcement cards should be sent to all the friends and acquaintances of the two families.

50

The "giving away" of a bride by her father is no mere form; it is a recognition of family authority, the claim of a father upon his daughter. It should therefore be a part of the ceremony.

Invitations to the church ceremony do not necessitate a wedding gift. Those invited to the reception may send gifts if they so desire.

Cards are usually removed from gifts, but in some cases are left on.

All gifts should be acknowledged before the ceremony if possible, by the bride herself.

If the bridegroom's parents live out of town, it is customary for the parents of the bride to invite them to their home as guests of the occasion. If this is not practicable, they may engage rooms for them at a hotel, paying the bill in advance.

It is thought unlucky to postpone a wedding. Better withdraw the invitations in case of severe illness or death, and have a quiet home ceremony with few present.

A bridal procession always moves up the central aisle of the church. In case there is no center aisle, it moves up one aisle and retires down the other. The relatives of the bridegroom are seated in the body of the church on the right; those of the bride are similarly placed on the left.

The hats of the father and ushers are left with the sexton in the vestibule and handed to them as they leave.

At a church wedding a bride almost invariably wears a veil. Her attendants wear hats. The maid-of-honor may wear a short veil.

The dress of the bridal party has already been fully described in a preceding chapter.

It is the custom for the bridegroom to give a gift, almost invariably a piece of jewelry, to his bride; and a small gift of silver or jewelry to each of the ushers and to the best man. The bride generally gives some souvenir of the same character to each of her attendants.

The bridegroom sends the bride her bouquet, and often one of violets or her favorite flower to the bride's mother.

The bride's father seems a rather subordinate figure at the fashionable wedding. After he has given away the bride, he retires into the background, escorting his wife to her carriage at the conclusion of the ceremony. He does not assist her in receiving the guests at the house, but circulates among them after congratulations have been tendered the newly wedded pair.

Formal afternoon dress is necessary for men who attend a day wedding, at church or at home. At an evening wedding they wear evening clothes.

After a wedding, the members of the bridal party are expected to call on the bride's mother within ten days or two weeks.

A bridal party always stand with their backs to the audience, the clergyman facing it.

Remember--

That men's evening clothes are not worn before six o'clock.

That women wear their hats at afternoon functions, teas, luncheons, bridge parties, etc., and remove them at evening affairs.

That in society, personal affairs, servants, dress, household difficulties, "symptoms," illnesses and bereavements, are not to be made a subject of conversation.

It is not good form to talk of the cost of articles or mention money affairs in company.

The social aspirant should cultivate the art of saying polite nothings acceptably. Small talk is the small change of social life.

One should be prompt at dinner, a card-party or a musicale.

At a dancing-party the hostess does not dance, as a rule, during the first part of the evening. She receives her guests and sees that the women are provided with partners.

A man who dances should pay his hostess the courtesy of inviting her to dance. He should certainly dance with her daughter.

Engaged couples should be careful to avoid demonstrations of affection or preoccupation in each other while in company.

Remember--

That the salt-shaker is out of favor; the open salt cellar and the salt-spoon are much preferred.

Never cut bread; break it with the fingers. Never butter a large piece, or spread it in the palm of your hand.

The finger-bowl will be brought on a plate with a doily under it.

Lift both from the plate to the table. The plate is then ready for the fruit course.

Black coffee--cafe noir--is usually served without cream. Cut loaf sugar is passed with it.

If a visitor for one meal only, the napkin is not folded at the conclusion of a meal. If staying a day or two follow the practice of the hostess.

Creme de menthe is served before the coffee, in small liquor glasses.

Do not break bread or crackers into the soup nor tip the plate to obtain the last of it. Do not play with crumbs, or finger knife or spoon.

Never touch a knife to fish or salad.

Remember--

Do not move glass, spoon, etc., when the maid brushes the crumbs from the cloth.

Knife and fork are laid upon the plate, tines of the latter upward, when the plate is passed for a second helping. This "second help" is permitted only at family or informal dinners.

A host must not urge food upon a guest after it has once been declined.

Lift the cup or glass to the lips, instead of bending toward it. Do not throw the head back and raise the cup to get the last of its contents.

Remember--

To prepare a list of the members of the family who will go to the cemetery at a funeral, for the undertaker's guidance, arranging them in the order of the relationship.

Flowers should be sent early in the morning of the day of interment, or on the previous afternoon. Acknowledgment by note or verbally is expected.

A letter expressive of sympathy in a friend's bereavement should be sent immediately upon learning of a death.

During an illness, make inquiries at the door, leaving a card with "To inquire" written upon it. This apprises a friend of your interest in her troubles, yet makes no claim upon her time.

Men wear mourning bands on their hats, not on the coat sleeve. Borders on mourning stationery and cards should be narrow.

Invitations to receptions, weddings, and general entertainments, excepting dancing parties, balls and cotillions, are sent to people in mourning. A response on black bordered stationery sufficiently indicates the reason for non-acceptance.

Remember--

That the typewriter does not figure in social correspondence.

A neat, well written letter or note is a credit to the writer, and a compliment to her correspondent.

Avoid "fancy" or bizarre stationery. A good quality of white or cream paper, in several sizes, is indicative of refined taste.

The forms of address, under the head of "Letter forms" may be profitably studied.

Abbreviations are incorrect. Write out the name of the state on your envelope; otherwise it may go astray.

To keep a dictionary on one's desk is a wise precaution unless one is sure of herself in regard to spelling.

Answer all notes of invitation promptly, and unconditionally; and all friendly letters within a reasonable time.

If you never say an unkind or hateful thing in a letter, you will never fear you may be some day condemned by your written evidence.

Don't keep old letters; it is unwise.

Avoid discussions on any subject on which people feel strongly, like politics and religion. Do not hold an argument in society.

Remember that good manners are made up of petty sacrifices, gracefully made.

A kind "no" is often more agreeable than a rough "yes." An assent, given grudgingly, is always ungracious.

Take note of this quotation: "Life is like a mirror. It reflects the face you bring to it. Look out lovingly upon the world and the world will look lovingly in upon you."

T. J. Ritter

BEAUTY AND THE TOILET

INCLUDING MANICURING, CARE OF THE COMPLEXION, TEETH, EYES, FEET, Etc.

"The one thing that woman prizes most is her beauty. Though she have none, she yet persuadeth herself that she possesses some charm upon which men's eyes rest admiringly."--Johnson.

"There is no wound a woman will not more willingly forget than a blow to her vanity."

Although woman's chief desire is to be beautiful, it is a historical fact that nearly every woman whose beauty has been renowned has either led an unhappy life or met a tragic fate. Strangely, too, the most famous attachments of which we have record have been inspired by women who were not only not beautiful, but who had some noticeable defect. So to be attractive, and to charm, it is not necessary to be beautiful. Beauty gives a woman a start in the race; her other qualities must enable her to keep her advantage.

THE FACE-HEALTH AS AN AID TO BEAUTY.

The first essential to good looks is good health. The clear complexion, the bright eyes, the lustrous hair that are such helps are born of good health rather than of creams and hair tonics. Health depends a good deal on wholesome diet and out-door exercise, which make pure blood. Pure air is invaluable. Country girls often have exquisite complexions because of the pure air they breathe--unless they eat too much heavy, greasy food.

Study hygiene, then, instead of relying upon "Bloom of Youth" and "Cream of Roses" as aids to a good complexion. Such things deceive no one, and by use ruin the skin, wrinkling and withering it. It is a good thing to drink plenty of water. A glass on retiring, another on rising, and a third an hour before the noon meal is little enough. Keep the stomach and bowels in good order.

BLACKHEADS.--The most frequent inquiry in the "beauty pages" of the papers is what to do for blackheads. In the first place, don't allow yourself to get them. Keep your face clean. A blackhead is simply a pore that is filled with oil and dirt. Sometimes they are as large as the head of a pin. When taken out they leave an enlargement known as a coarse pore. Do not steam the face to remove them. Wash the face well with soap and hot water; wring cloths out of hot water and hold to the face then massage with cold cream. Several treatments will soften them so they may be pinched out between the thumbs. Never attempt this treatment before going out; do it at night, before retiring.

Blackheads are a reflection upon one's personal cleanliness, therefore bathe the whole body often.

PIMPLES.--Pimples are due to an impure condition of the blood, for which sulphur is a good remedy, taken internally and applied externally. One dram each of camphor and flowers of sulphur in four ounces of rose-water is a good lotion for external use. Do not pick or squeeze pimples, unless pus has formed in them. Nothing is more disgusting than a face broken out in pus-filled pimples. See a physician if thus afflicted.

FRECKLES.--These have been poetically called "the kisses of the sun," but no girl cares for evidences of that sort of affection. Prevention is easier than cure. Simple home remedies are lemon juice and glycerin, sour buttermilk, and elderflower soap used in bathing.

A well-known application is six grains of bichloride of mercury in one ounce each of glycerin and alcohol, and a few drops, say ten or twelve, of oil of lavender. The trouble is that after using these remedies the skin is delicate and freckles more easily.

The fad for going bareheaded has ruined many a girl's complexion.

SUNBURN.--Avoid it when possible. If going on the water, apply magnesia to the face rather thickly. If sunburned, rub the skin with cold cream, leaving it on as long as you can before using water on it. A wash that is good for tan and sunburn requires half an ounce of borax and an ounce of lemon juice in a pint of rose water.

CHAPPED HANDS AND FACE.--Many cases of "chaps" may be avoided by the simple precaution of wiping the face and hands *perfectly dry.* If the skin chaps easily keep at hand a bottle of glycerin and lemon juice mixed in about equal proportions, and after wiping rub a little on the hands. Before going out in the cold, rub a little cold cream or oil of sweet almonds over the face; leave it on a few minutes, rub off lightly with a dry towel and dust with rice powder. Camphor ice is good for chapped lips.

A PURE FACE CREAM.--Set a bowl in a basin of hot water over the fire. In it put a quarter of an ounce of white wax and two and a half ounces of spermaceti, and the same quantity of oil of sweet almonds. When melted and hot, add a pinch of borax and an ounce and a half of rose-water. Beat these ingredients with a silver fork, briskly, till the cream is cold. Warm the jar before filling it and keep in a cool place.

ANOTHER GOOD CREAM.--One ounce each of white wax and spermaceti; two ounces each of lanolin and cocoanut oil and four ounces of sweet almond oil. Melt in a double-boiler or a bowl set in hot water, and stir in two ounces of orange flower water and thirty drops of tincture of benzoin. Stir briskly till cold, and of the consistency of a thick paste. This is to be used at night, after thoroughly washing the face. It is a good cleansing cream also.

WRINKLES.--It is a great deal easier to prevent wrinkles than it is to get rid of them after one has acquired them. A little study of women's faces will show how wrinkles, that no amount of massage will obliterate, are being made. They make perpendicular wrinkles between the eyes by drawing the brows together when sewing or reading, sometimes through habit and sometimes because of insufficient light. Some wrinkles are born of in-temper, of fretfulness, or sorrow. As the skin loses its elasticity, through age or ill-health, wrinkles come more and more easily. The best remedy for wrinkles is a light heart and a contented mind. Assist these with good, wholesome food that makes pure blood to feed the body, and render external aid through gentle massage and some good face cream and you have done the best you can. It is a good plan to some day take your hand-mirror with you as you go about your daily duties and watch the process of wrinkle-making. Say you are sewing and note the glass. Without changing your expression, take a look at yourself. The chance is it will be a revelation. You will realize why wrinkles come.

MASSAGE.--Unless properly done, massage may do more harm than good. If one can afford a few treatments by a scientific masseur and study her methods, it is a great help. The thing is not to rub in more than you rub out, by improper manipulation.

Rub the face up, not down. This is because of the tendency of the muscles to sag. Rub across, not with, the lines. Rub the "parentheses" around the month up and out, and give a rotary motion to the rubs given the checks, gently pinching and pulling them out.

But after all, there's nothing like good temper and steady nerves to prevent the tell-tale lines.

WRINKLED HANDS.--Wrinkled hands belong to age, and are due to loss of oil in the skin. After washing and wiping them, rub with a little cold cream or olive oil. Rub well into the skin. At night, use the cream or oil freely and put on a pair of old gloves.

Camphor is a good whitening agent for the hands, and a teaspoonful of spirits of camphor beaten into any greasy, cold cream will be beneficial. A piece of the gum camphor melted with the ointment blends more readily. A piece of camphor size of a walnut to two tablespoonfuls of the cream is about right proportions.

RED HANDS AND NOSE.--Sometimes a too tight corset, impeding the circulation of the blood, is responsible for the blemishes; sometimes poor circulation due to poor health. Cold feet may send the blood to the nose. Find out what is the cause and remove it. Local applications are ineffective.

COLD OR FEVER SORES.--These unpleasant afflictions may be cured if taken at the first indication of what is coming--a smarting or burning sensation--by frequent applications of dilute spirits of camphor.

FACE POWDERS.--There are few women who do not at times have occasion to use face powder. A woman once remarked: "It isn't decent not to in summer--one looks so greasy without." There are many face powders on the market, some of which are comparatively harmless, while others are deleterious. The injury done by powder is that it fills the pores, stopping them up and thus clogging the skin. Many powders contain lead or bismuth, both of which are very injurious. Magnesia is drying. Rice powder is most harmless, but does not adhere. The most innocent powder is probably a preparation of French chalk. Weigh a box of powder in your hand before purchasing. If heavy, it doubtless contains lead, and should be refused. Find some powder that agrees with your skin and then buy that brand. Suit the color of the powder to your complexion. Don't use flesh tint if you are sallow, the "outlying regions" of neck and ears betray you.

TO USE POWDER.--Wash the face; rub a little cold cream over it, rubbing it in well, wipe with a dry towel, gently, then apply the powder with a chamois--a clean one. Do not keep it on unnecessarily. Remove by rubbing with the cleansing cream, then wash the face. Never go to bed with powder on your face.

LIQUID WHITENERS.--Avoid these. They are "whitewashes" that wither and wrinkle the skin and make it prematurely old. Almost without exception they contain lead in some form. Constant use may produce a facial paralysis due to lead poisoning. Moreover they deceive no one, and give an unpleasing impression as regards one's good sense.

ROUGE.--Well, don't do it. There may be a few who can have a rouge especially prepared that is the exact tint that harmonizes with the skin, the hair, the eyes, and can apply it so carefully as to look "natural." But ordinarily the deception is evident, and rouge in conjunction with liquid washes and penciled eyes and brows, suggest the aids employed by women of the demi-monde.

If any rouge is used, let it be the "Spanish lady's rouge" or crepons--bits of white woolen crepe dyed with an ammoniacal solution of carmine. These are gently rubbed on the skin to produce the required glow.

THE HAIR.--Beautiful hair is woman's crown of glory. Thousands of the sex wear it unbecomingly. They follow the latest fashion in arrangement without reference to whether it suits the lines of the face and head or otherwise. One should never be satisfied with a front view alone. Study the back, the sides, the lines produced, just as you study the becomingness of a hat from all angles. If a new fashion is unbecoming, either avoid it, or modify it into becomingness if you can. So many women make guys of themselves by a slavish devotion to the freaks of fashion.

CARE OF THE HAIR.--The hair is kept in order by frequent brushings, which excite the natural oil by which it is fed, and by washing it. Dr. Leonard, an authority on the hair, says once a month is as often as the hair needs washing. As a shampoo, he advises yolk of egg, well rubbed into the scalp and roots of the hair, then washed out with tepid water and castile soap. A brisk rubbing with dry towels excites the blood-vessels of the scalp. There is no doubt that this simple shampoo is more beneficial than many new-fangled ones.

The hair should be taken down and well brushed every night, This removes dirt and makes it glossy. Use a brush with bristles as stiff as you can use without irritating the scalp too much, and *keep it clean.* Don't drag a fine comb through the hair. The proper comb has regular and even teeth, rounded, not sharp. If a tooth becomes split, remove it; it will break the hair. Wire brushes are nothing more or less than combs, and are not as good for the hair as good bristle brushes. Keep combs and brushes clean.

USE OF POMADES.--Hair that is dry and brittle really requires some oleaginous preparation, used in moderation. Yellow vaselin is good. Part the hair and rub it into the scalp with the tips of the fingers. A sufficient amount will find its way to the hair itself to relieve the dryness. Cocoanut oil is also good. Never apply anything of this kind to the hair itself, which is simply made greasy. The benefit should be to the roots. The application of vaselin may be made a couple of days before the monthly washing, or if the hair is very dry, may follow it. Remember not to overdo the matter. It does not follow that because a little is good, more is better.

A specialist on the hair who makes biennial trips abroad to advise himself as to the most recent methods and treatment, in a moment of confidence admitted to a customer that after all pure cold water was as good a hair tonic as he knew of. "Do not wet the hair." he said. "Dip the tips of your fingers in cold water and rub the scalp, wetting it and at the same time massaging it. Do this as faithfully as you would apply a tonic, and in all but certain exceptional cases it will be as beneficial."

CLIPPING THE HAIR.--It is a good plan to clip the ends of the hair once a month to keep the growth even. If the hair splits, trim to a point above it, as the tendency is for the split to extend further up the hair-shaft.

DANDRUFF.--Dandruff is the scaling off of dead cuticle. In excess, it becomes a disease, forming so thick a scale as to kill the roots of the hair and cause it to fall out. It is rightly called "itch dirt." Cleanliness therefore helps a cure.

An old-fashioned recipe for dandruff calls for five ounces of bay rum, one ounce of olive oil, one ounce tincture of cantharides. Dr. Leonard advises free applications of sweet oil for the purpose of softening the scales, then a washing with warm water and castile soap, or the "green soap" of the pharmacy. If the disease is bad, or obstinate, apply a little oxide of zinc ointment.

WASHING THE HAIR.--One suspects that those who advise washing the hair once a week have more of all eye to the increase of their business than to the welfare of their customers' hair. The egg shampoo has been advised. Use a soap made of vegetable oil if possible. Never rub soap in the hair, and be very careful to rinse thoroughly, to get all the soap out using hot water for washing, then graduating the temperature till the final douche of cold. Do not use ammonia, soda or borax on the hair.

COLOR OF THE HAIR.--Nature has suited the hair to the complexion in every case, and we cannot improve upon her idea of harmony. That is why any attempt to change the color is so unsatisfactory. The "bleached blonde" is always recognizable; so is the woman who dyes her faded locks in vain effort to retain her "youth." As the hair changes by natural processes the complexion changes to match it, so that we never get a chance to improve upon nature's handiwork.

In Elizabethan days, wigs were worn to harmonize or match with the costume. Queen Elizabeth had over eighty. Think of purple hair? Yet some dyes give a purple tinge to the locks.

DYED HAIR.--Dyed hair is a sorry makeshift at best. Far better let nature have her way. There is but one hair-dye that is not positively harmful, this is henna, and its use entails no end of trouble because it must be frequently renewed,--some use it every day.

To prepare the dye, get a quarter pound of henna leaves; to this add two quarts of cold water. Let stand on the back of the range where it will steep slowly for four or five hours. Add three ounces of alcohol and bottle. Apply with a tooth-brush. It gives a sort of reddish-brown color. Women whose hair is prematurely gray often use this, declaring their white hair prevents them from obtaining or holding business positions. But where hair has whitened prematurely there is always a freshness and vitality about eyes and complexion that bespeaks youth.

Physicians strongly deprecate the use of hair dyes. No matter how strenuously the label insists on "absolute harmlessness," the dye relies for its effectiveness upon the presence of lead in some chemical combination. The frequent application of lead to the scalp induces a certain dangerous form of poisoning, which results in paralysis. If "dye you must," pin your faith to henna.

GRAY HAIR.--"The only thing to do with gray hair is to admire it." This is true. Nothing so sets off an aged face like the crown of silver. To color it is a great mistake. There is absolutely no cure for it; the one thing we can do is to make it a beauty. Gray hair is due to the exhaustion of the pigment or coloring cells of the hair, supposed to be occasioned by the lack of a regular supply of blood.

For the progressive whitening of the hair due to the advance of age, curative agents are rarely of any avail, especially if the trouble is hereditary. Not that gray hair and baldness are handed down from father to son, but that the peculiarities of constitution which produce them are inherent in both. Nervousness, neuralgia, a low physical condition, aid the falling and blanching of the hair, and the victim should build up the general system. Preparations of iron and sulphur, taken internally, are supposed to supply certain elements of growth and pigment-forming power to the hair.

A solution of iron for external application to the hair, calls for two drams each of citrate of iron and tincture of nux vomica, and one and one-half ounces each of cocoanut oil and bay rum. It may be mentioned here, that faithfulness in treatment means even more than the tonic applied. To gain any real benefit, one must be persistent in application.

Hair often turns gray "in streaks" to the chagrin of the victim. Or it whitens above the forehead and temples and remains dark at the back. Nothing can be done for this.

Gray hair should be kept scrupulously clean, and requires more frequent washing than hair that holds its color. A very little blueing in the rinsing water gives a purer, clearer white. For this use indigo, not the usual washing fluid which is made of Prussian blue. Five cents worth of indigo will last a lifetime.

A HAIR TONIC.--A lotion Dr. Leonard recommends for the hair, especially where it is coming out calls for two drams tincture cantharides, half an ounce nux vomica, one dram tincture capsicum, one and a half ounces castor oil, and two ounces of cologne. Apply with a bit of sponge twice a day.

A preparation which is tonic in its properties and is also said to darken gray hair, and which certainly contains nothing injurious, calls for one ounce of sage and a pint of boiling water, allowed to stand twenty-four hours in an iron pot, and then filtered through filtering papers.

Digest half an ounce of pine tar in a pint of water for forty-eight hours, stirring occasionally; filter, and put with the other fluid, then add one pint of bay rum, one ounce each of cologne and tincture of cantharides, two ounces of glycerin and ten ounces of distilled water. Apply daily, using a tonic brush.

THE HAIR AND HEALTH.--The condition of the hair is largely predicated on the condition of the general health. In health, it should be abundant, glossy and bright--"live"--in color. A low physical condition may make it look dry and dead, and induce falling out. Take care of the general health for the sake of the hair as well as for the sake of the complexion.

THE HANDS.--One of the woman's continuous tasks is trying to keep her hands clean, and one thing that militates against their good looks is careless washing. They are washed indiscriminately in hot or cold water, the soap not properly rinsed off, nor the drying complete. To keep them soft and white, wash in soft, tepid water, dry thoroughly, then rub in a little cold cream or compound of glycerin, or fine cornmeal. Use rubber gloves in dish washing, and if you must have your hands in soapy water for a long time, after washing them in pure water rub over with a few drops of lemon juice or cider vinegar. This kills the potash in the soap that has been used.

CARE OF THE NAILS.--It is a luxury to have one's nails done by a manicure, and if one can not afford this, always, it is profitable to have it done a few times and carefully observe the process, because the nails are a very important part of the care of the hands.

Finger Nail Powder, Old Tried Remedy for--

"Violet Talcum Powder	1/2 ounce
Pulverized Boric Acid	1/2 ounce
Powdered Starch	1/2 ounce
Tincture of Carmine	15 drops

If the nails become hard or brittle, immerse them in warm olive oil every night or rub vaselin into them."

IMPLEMENTS.--The tools required are a pair of manicure scissors, which have small curved blades; get a good pair of steel scissors, the silver are not so good; a package of emery boards, an orange-wood stick, a flexible nail file, a small bottle of peroxide of hydrogen for bleaching, a bit of pumice stone, a cake of polishing powder, a chamois covered "buffer" and a box of rosaline or other paste.

THE PROCESS.--The nails are to be shortened by filing, as cutting thickens them. The orange-wood stick is then dipped in peroxide and run under the nail to bleach, then the pumice stone, powdered, is used in the same way to cleanse. During this the left hand is soaking in tepid, soapy water. Of course, if you do your own manicuring you will go on with the right hand, waiting while the cuticle at the base of the nail softens. This is then anointed with a little cold cream or vaselin; the cuticle is loosened and trimmed if necessary,--do not trim if you can avoid it, as cutting thickens it. When both hands have been thus treated, they are again soaked a few minutes, then a little of the rosaline paste--a very little--is put on each nail, the buffer dipped in the polishing powder and the nails polished. The hands are then washed, rubbed dry, and the fingers gone over a second time in search of roughness of nail or cuticle; they are then polished again with a clean buffer, and may be sprayed with perfume from an atomizer.

MOUTH AND TEETH.--Many young people owe their homely mouths to infantile habits. Sucking the thumb, and these horrible "pacificators" or "baby comforters" are responsible for some ill-shaped mouths. A large mouth, if not malformed, is not ugly unless filled with bad teeth or set in a disagreeable expression. Thus, in a way, we mould this feature ourselves, to a considerable degree.

CLEANSING THE TEETH.--A good brushing twice a day, using cold water and some pleasant antiseptic wash, like listerine, does much to keep the mouth and teeth clean. Particles of food lodged between the teeth should be removed with a bit of dental floss.

VISITS TO THE DENTIST.--Pain and expense are saved by consulting the dentist in good season. The smallest cavity should be filled as soon as discovered. At least once a year the teeth should be carefully examined by one's dentist; it would be better to go every six months. Let the dentist clean them and remove the tartar, if any, as commercial preparations often injure. Most dentists will save a tooth wherever possible. There is little excuse for bad teeth these days, since modern dentistry can work marvels.

CHILDREN'S TEETH.--On no account let a child's second teeth come in crowded, irregular or projecting. A good dentist can remedy all these malformations and though it may be troublesome at the time, the child, when grown, will blame you for not having relieved him of them. From babyhood, the child should be taught that cleansing the teeth is as important a part of the toilet as washing the hands.

THE EYES.--No gift is more precious than sight. Therefore take care of your eyes. Don't overstrain them, don't put anything in them, don't follow any casual prescription, nor use belladonna to brighten them. Consult an oculist, not an optician, if there is anything the matter with them. Bathe them in hot water when they feel tired and drawn. Eyesight is too precious to be tampered with. If a child is cross-eyed, a simple operation will straighten them, and it is a crime not to have it done.

EYELASHES AND EYEBROWS.--The best application for

these is the simplest. Just a little yellow vaselin, which encourages growth. Don't clip, either. Frequent brushing will generally train the brows into a shapely line. A heavy, coarse hair may be pulled out with the fingers.

THE FEET.--The three most frequent evils to which the feet are heir are corns, bunions or enlarged joints, and chilblains. Ingrowing nails are much less common, but make up in painfulness.

CORNS.--Corns are of three kinds: callous spots, soft corns, and corns. Callous spots may be rubbed or pared down and rubbed with cocoa butter. Soft corns come between the toes and are very painful. Soak absorbent cotton in a little turpentine and put between the toes; or sprinkle the cotton with powdered alum. These corns are supposed to be due to moisture between the toes and are sometimes cured and often prevented by keeping absorbent cotton between the toes. Prevention saves a lot of suffering. "Just corns" are calloused spots with hard center; pressure on this causes pain. Soaking in hot water, and shaving off as much of the hardened skin as can be removed with safety, affords relief. The little hard core should be taken out.

Precautions.--Be sure that your knife, razor, or whatever implement is used is perfectly clean (sterilized) and avoid drawing blood. If this happens, use some antiseptic. Cases of blood-poisoning that have resulted fatally have been caused by such wounds. If you wear colored hose, have them washed before wearing, as the dye may be injurious.

BUNIONS.--These painful enlargements are due to a too short shoe, or one that does not fit well. Better discard such footwear; it will be cheaper in the end. Paint the sore joint with a mixture of equal parts of glycerin, tincture of iodine and carbolic acid; using a camel's hair brush. Stockings that are too short may produce the same affliction.

CHILBLAINS.--People who have, or do not want chilblains should avoid woolen stockings. Neither should they "toast their toes" at the fire, wear bed-socks, or take a hot water-bottle to bed with them. Warm the feet by exercise, or vigorous rubbing. If very painful, try ice-cold applications, tincture of iodine, camphor, and tincture of chloride of iron are healing.

INGROWING NAILS.--A bad case should be taken to the chiropodist. Shaving the nail thin on the top, or cutting a V-shaped piece out of it, tend to relieve. Raise up the nail and put a bit of absorbent cotton under it. The best way is to avoid foot troubles by wearing well fitting shoes which are sufficiently large.

NURSERY HINTS AND FIRESIDE GEMS

For Mother and Her Little Family

TEN COMMANDMENTS FOR RAISING CHILDREN.

1. Thou shalt not frighten thy child by threats of punishment.

2. Thou shalt not visit thine own disappointments upon thy child, nor speak to him sharply without just cause.

3. Thou shalt not administer any rebuke while feeling anger toward thy child.

4. Thou shalt not require more of thy child than of thyself.

5. Thou shalt not speak discourteously to thy child.

6. Thou shalt not lie to thy child, neither break thy promise, nor deceive.

7. Thou shalt not waste thyself upon the effort to destroy evil tendencies and wrong activities in thy child, but shall remove temptation from him and cultivate his virtues and his righteous activities.

8. Thou shalt not curtail thy child's liberty but shall insist he respect the liberty of all others, even as his is respected.

9. Many hours shalt thou labor with thy child and do all thy work, dressing him, feeding him, teaching him, amusing him, but for one hour out of every seven waking hours shalt thou let him alone, and bother him not, neither thou, nor thy husband, nor thy nursemaid, nor thy friends, nor thy relatives nor any that are in thy house. For in that hour shall the Lord come unto him.

10. Thou shalt not force thy child in any respect, neither physically, mentally or morally. Thou shalt not force obedience, for forced obedience is not righteous; but thou shalt gently lead thy child along the way that he should go, having first passed over the road thyself.

THE PRAYING OF A CHILD.

Pray, little child for me tonight,
That from thy lips like petals white,
Thy words may fall and at His feet
Bloom for His path with fragrance sweet!
Pray, little child, that I may be
Childlike in innocence like thee,
And simple in my faith and trust
Through all the battle's heat and dust!
Pray, little child, in thy white gown,
Beside thy wee bed kneeling down;

Pray, pray for me, for I do know
Thy white words on soft wings will go
Unto His heart, and on His breast
Light as blown doves that seek for rest
Up the pale twilight path that gleams
Under the spell of starry dreams!
Pray, little child, for me, and say:
"Please, Father, keep him firm today
Against the shadow and the care,
For Christ's sake!" Ask it in thy prayer,
For well I know that thy pure word
'Gainst louder tongues will have been heard,
When the great moment comes that He
Shall listen through His love for me!
Oh, little child, if I could feel
One atom of thy faith so real,
Then might I bow and be as one
In whose heart many currents run
Of joyful confidence and cheer,
Making each earthly moment dear
With sunshine and the sound of bells
On the green hills and in the dells!
Pray, little child, for me tonight,
That from thy lips in sunward flight,
One word may fall with all its sweet
Upon the velvet at His feet,
That He may lift it to His ear
Its tender plea of love to hear,
And lay it, granted, on the pile
Signed with the signet of His smile!

Motherhood.--Motherhood is a profession that is overworked. The hours are long and holidays and vacations are few and far between. Mother gets a great deal of maudlin sympathy and not enough tangible aid, says a writer in the *Housekeeper.* Our poetic conception of the true mother is that her whole life is bound up in the welfare of her children and her family. At what age are her children not, for her, a matter of serious concern? She has ever had plenty of material which she can manufacture into worry and heartaches. Many mothers consume too much of their own nervous energy and jeopardize their health in what they think their bounden maternal duties. There is a judicious limit of all things even though they are virtues.

Mother.--The babe at first feeds upon the mother's bosom, but is always on her heart.--*H. W. Beecher.*

Baby's Layette.--The principal thing to be borne in mind regarding the baby's layette is that all the clothing should be light, soft, in both surface and texture, and porous also in order that the evaporation of perspiration and a certain ventilation of the skin may take place.

Perfect simplicity, not only in material and trimming, but in the whole plan of the little garments will testify to good taste and common sense, and at the same time tend to eliminate much fretfulness and wailing.

Baby.--A sweet new blossom of humanity, fresh fallen from God's own home, to flower on earth.--*Massey.*

51

Boy's Garments.--Don't burden the boy with a whole array of separate garments, but give him a few good, heavy things. The lessened number will allow him freedom, and his comfort, too, is to be considered. Boy's trousers are now fully lined, and these with the right sort of underwear will give him the requisite warmth with very little unnecessary weight.

Boys.--A torn jacket is soon mended, but hard words bruise the heart of a child.--*Longfellow.*

Pretty Things for Baby.--Among pretty articles for baby there are tiny ribbon garters to hold up the little sleeves, in colors to match the blue of the eyes or the pink of the cheeks, and there are huge soft rosettes of ribbon and hand embroidered strings for the cap, and gold baby pins and fleecy robes and bow-decked quilts.

Baby.--A rose with all its sweetest leaves yet folded.--*Byron.*

Baby's Outing.--It is always better for a baby, no matter how young, to go out in a carriage than to be carried. Young babies are much more comfortable lying full length on a pillow placed in the carriage and properly covered than when carried in the arms.

Baby.--A lovely bud, so soft, so fair, called hence by early doom; just sent to show how sweet a flower in paradise would bloom.--*Leigh Richmond.*

Wild Flowers.--Children who gather wild flowers should be taught that they must not put them in their mouths. The buttercup, which is harmless enough to handle, contains an acid poison that will produce sore mouth, and taken into the stomach worse effects might result. It also contains a narcotic principle, anemonin, which has the property of diminishing the respiration and heart action.

Flowers.--It is with flowers as with moral qualities, the bright are sometimes poisonous, but I believe never the sweet.--*Hare.*

Reasoning versus Punishment.--There is one great point that all mothers should observe and that is not to punish children when reasoning would bring the same results. For needless correction blunts a child's sensitiveness. To state that it brutalizes him is putting it too positively, but it tends to develop indifference and hardness that one does not want a child to possess,

Discipline.--Be ever gentle with the children God has given you.--Watch over them constantly; reprove them earnestly, but not in anger.--In the forcible language of Scripture, "Be not bitter against them." "Yes, they are good boys," said a kind father. "I talk to them much, but I do not beat my children: the world will beat them." It was a beautiful thought, though not elegantly expressed.--*Burritt.*

Baby's Kimono.--The little flannel kimonos or wrappers, so convenient to slip on the baby before the morning bath, or if the room is at all chilly, may be made up in pretty styles, in delicate colors, bound with silk, and tied with tiny bows to match.

Early Schooling.--Of ten infants destined for different vocations, I should prefer that the one who is to study through life should be the least learned at the age of twelve.

--*Tissot.*

Baby's Fine Dresses.--If the baby's dress is not made of the finest of handkerchief linen, French nainsook or a very fine batiste is usually chosen. These are the soft materials, soft as well as sheer. They are the materials on which embroidery is done most successfully and the baby dress de luxe is always hand embroidered. It may have on it the merest touch of hand work--scarcely more than a few eyelets and a tiny blossom and stem and yet follow the prescribed lines. The little round yokes are attached to the fulled on skirt portion with the tiniest of beading or else the yoke scallops are lapped down over the fullness. The neck is edged with the little hand-made scallops.

Nicknames.--A good name will wear out; a bad one may be turned; a nickname lasts forever.--*Zimmermann.*

Undergarments.--In buying the little wool shirts (wool being considered the most satisfactory for infants' undergarments) never get the heaviest weights; there are four usually offered, even for winter wear. The next to the heaviest is quite warm enough for winter, and for summer the lightest weight obtainable, preferably of a mixture of silk and wool; cotton and wool should not be used. In hot weather shirts of cotton gauze or a soft porous cotton stockinet are satisfactory.

Training.--The education of our children is never out of my mind. Train them to virtue, habituate them to industry, activity, and spirit. Make them consider every vice as shameful and unmanly. Fire them with ambition to be useful. Make them disdain to be destitute of any useful knowledge.--*John Adams to his wife.*

Baby's Nerves.--Never try to entertain a baby too vigorously. Little babies especially, but also children somewhat older, should never be subjected to unnecessary excitement. Older people seldom realize how exceedingly undeveloped the nervous system of a little child is, and any undue shock to it is apt to cause the direst consequence. Do not take very small children to the theatre or the circus. They don't understand it, and they can't enjoy it.

Intemperance.--Violent excitement exhausts the mind, and leaves it withered and sterile.--*Fenelon.*

Second Teeth.--When the baby's second teeth are cut there are often injurious influences to be combated. There is more or less chance for the formation of caries or tartar; care must be taken and counsel sought, and every effort made to prevent the aggravation of the evil.

Tears.--Tears are the safety-valves of the heart when too much pressure is laid on it.--*Albert Smith.*

Going Barefoot.--The careful mother does not let her child run barefoot, no matter how they clamor to do it. If they wish to go shoeless, let them wear bathing sandals without stockings, is the advice of the writer, who adds, the germ of tetanus, better known as lockjaw, is frequently found in the soil and a child with even a small scratch or cut takes big risks. For girls, especially, running barefoot should be a forbidden pleasure as it makes the feet broad and flat.

FROM JOHN GREENLEAF WHITTIER'S "BAREFOOT BOY."

Blessings on thee, little man,
Barefoot boy, with cheek of tan!
With thy turned-up pantaloons,
And thy merry whistled tunes;
With thy red lip, redder still
Kissed by strawberries on the hill;
With the sunshine on thy face,
Through thy torn brim's jaunty grace;
From my heart I give thee joy,
I was once a barefoot boy.

The Children's Sunday.--What can we do with the children on Sundays? Do not attempt to do anything unusual or make yourself miserable over their natural antics. Send them to the Sabbath School, never deny a child this privilege or be too negligent to give him the privilege, says the *Woman's National Daily.* A walk during the day to the park, woods or some place where the recreation is pleasant, is advisable. But do not get so modern in your views that you will permit them the riotous amusements in which they must usually indulge through the week. One cannot do wrong in impressing the sacredness of the day upon the children, for it is one of the deplorable features of modern life that the sacredness is sadly abused, and mostly by the young folk.

Idleness.--Idleness among children, as among men, is the root of all evil, and leads to no other evil more certain than ill-temper.---*Hannah More.*

Learning to Sew.--Every reasonable mother knows that it is wise to teach her little daughter to sew. Let her begin on the tiny garment of her doll. She will easily form the habit of mending torn places in dolly's clothes and replace absent buttons. With this experience, it will not be long before she will begin to take an interest in her own clothes, and so will not need to be warned that a button is coming off or that the hem of her skirt is coming out. But, of course, she could not begin by sewing or patching her own clothes, nor by mending intricate tears. First see that she sews on buttons correctly and then let her do some basting.

A Good Rule.--St. Edmund of Canterbury was right when he said to somebody. "Work as though you would live forever; but live as though you would die today."--*Henry Giles.*

Double Duties.--Children should never be required to do housework to the extent a housekeeper must do it, for the strength of a growing child should be applied almost wholly to duties at school. A growing child cannot do mental and hard physical labor at the same time. Wiping dishes and assisting in the dusting do not interfere with school work, and are really good exercises. But the young girl who is compelled to rise early in the morning, prepare breakfast, assist with the family washing or ironing and prepare herself for school will lose out somewhere.

THE BABY-CLASS TREE.

We little folks planted a wee, wee, tree,
    The tiniest tree of all;
Right here by the school-house door it stands
With two little leaves like baby's hands,
    So crumpled and soft and small.
And I really believe it is ever so glad
    That we planted it there to grow,
And knows us and loves us and understands,
For it claps them just like two little hands,
    Whenever the west winds blow.

The Flannel Binder.--The flannel binders for baby should be cut from the softest kind of flannel and on the bias to increase their elasticity. They should be about five inches wide and twenty inches long, with the edges raw, or pinked, perhaps, but not hemmed. After the first six or eight weeks the knitted, circular band which can be bought ready made or may be crocheted at home, is substituted for the flannel binder.

LOVE.

Over and over and over
These truths I will say and sing--
That Love is mightier far than Hate;
That a man's own Thought is a man's own Fate,
And that life is a goodly thing.
--*Ella Wheeler Wilcox.*

Wholesome Pleasures.--Pleasures for the little ones should be wholesome and sensible, and the dangers of excitement cannot be overestimated. Their minds so ready to receive impressions should receive only the best and most beneficial, the wholesome air play in the park, or the country, not too much company, nor too much noise, nor too many toys.

FROM "THE CHILDREN'S HOUR"

Between the dark and the daylight.
When the night is beginning to lower,
Comes a pause in the day's occupations,
That is known as the Children's Hour.
I hear in the chamber above me,
The patter of little feet,
The sound of a door that is opened,
And voices soft and sweet. --*Longfellow.*

Scrubbing Tender Faces.--Children have tender skins as a rule, and yet mothers are very apt to scrub the little faces with soap and water and send them out to play. Think of such treatment in connection with your own skin. If the children are going out at once after the washing, use warm water with plain unscented soap, then rub a little good cold cream into the skin.

FROM LONGFELLOW'S "VILLAGE BLACKSMITH"

Toiling.--rejoicing,--sorrowing,
Onward through life he goes;
Each morning sees some task begun,
Each evening sees it close;
Something attempted, something done,
He has earned a night's repose.

Saving the Coverlet.--It is discouraging to the mother to find the eiderdown coverlets becoming soiled where the children rub their hands over them. This can be avoided by making a tiny sham of swiss or other similar material and basting it across the top of the coverlet. It can be pinned into place at the corners with tiny baby pins or caught with a few stitches. These shams edged with narrow lace add a really attractive touch to the coverlet, and they can be quickly removed and easily laundered.

The Greatness of Love.--There are no little events with the heart; it magnifies everything. It places in the same scale the falling of an empire and the dropping of a woman's glove; and the glove generally weighs more than the empire.

--Honore De Balzac.

Oranges as Medicine.--One of the most valuable adjuncts in acquiring a generally good complexion in youth is that of eating oranges in quantities. Let the mother give her children two or three oranges every day, as they possess many virtues, especially upon the action of the liver. The mother who buys plenty of oranges for the children will note the reduction in her medicine bill.

THE HUMAN FACE.

When I meet a human face,
Lit for me with light divine,
I recall all loving eyes,
That have ever answered mine.--
Phoebe Cary.

The Art of Entertaining Children.--Entertaining convalescent children is quite an art in itself. Nurses who expect to make a specialty of caring for children sometimes take a brief course in kindergarten work, and certainly such knowledge is a valuable asset. Quiet games that do not call for too much exertion, paper-doll plays, the ever-delightful "cutting out" of pictures or fashion book people, making scrap books for children's hospitals and simple knitting or crocheting all help to amuse the little folk. Almost all children enjoy being read to, but care must be taken not to select stories that will depress the child or so excite him as to keep him awake at night or cause unpleasant dreams.

Tireless Talkers.--A sick man that gets talking about himself, a woman that gets talking about her baby, and an author that begins reading out of his own book, never know when to stop.--O. *W. Holmes.*

Unselfishness.--Unselfishness is the key of a happy and beautiful life, and this is one of the first things that should be taught to the little one, says a writer in *The Woman Beautiful.* Insist upon her sharing her pleasures, even at a great sacrifice with other children. One mother whom I know has trained her baby to extend an entire box of bon-bons to her little friends with the words "Hop yourself," and she does this with a charm and spontaneity which makes her irresistible.

A Cheerful Giver.--We should give as we would receive, cheerfully, quickly, and without hesitation; for there is no grace in a benefit that sticks to the fingers.--*Seneca.*

Indulgence.--It takes far more than the mere mother love to bring up children. It takes training, study, knowledge, says the *New York Tribune.* It takes self-control in the parents themselves. The mother who spoils a child through weak indulgence does not truly love her child. She loves her own pleasures in going along the line of least resistance.

Selfishness.--When parents spoil their children, it is less to please them than to please themselves. It is the egotism of parental love.--*Carlyle.*

Method.--Now that school days are here, mark umbrellas by writing name on muslin with ink and sewing to inside of top with black thread; overshoes and rubbers by writing name on the lining, and handkerchiefs by writing name across the center with ink.

System.--Marshal thy notions into a handsome method. One will carry twice more weight packed up in bundles, than when it lies flapping and hanging about his shoulders.--*Fuller.*

Baby's Meals.--To make a healthy baby of eighteen or twenty months wait for the meal times of adults before feeding, is putting too great a strain on the little system. Its diet should be adapted to its needs, says a careful mother. Five light feedings are much more scientific, the first at about six-thirty in the morning since baby keeps early hours. Milk and toast should be given at this time. At ten-thirty a. m., well cooked and well strained cereal might be served with rich milk. Cream is for older children. Stewed prunes, baked apples, and oranges are also good. Dinner at one-thirty might include meat broth, or soft boiled eggs, and bread and toast. Soups must be free from grease. Crackers or toast with a cup of milk should be served for the five o'clock supper, and another cup of milk at bedtime.

Forbearance.--There is a limit at which forbearance ceases to be a virtue.--*Burke.*

The Romper.--The romper has become an essential part of the young child's wardrobe. They are developed mostly in linen, galatea, and less expensively still in chambray. The best colors are dark blue, brown, green, tan and natural colored linen; green perhaps is best for summer. It is cool looking and it does not show grass stains. Short flowing sleeves are most satisfactory.

BABY'S PURPOSE.

With mighty purpose in his mind,
He clambers up. And then,
With purpose quite as well defined,
He scrambles down again.

From *"Seven Ages of Childhood."*

Picnic Supplies.--Women taking small children to picnics should carry along a heavy quilt or blanket to place on the ground for the babies to sit on. There is always more dampness in the woods than out in the open, and summer colds are not pleasant for grown folk, much less wee tots. A few safety pins, needle and thread will not take up space in the big basket, and how often such articles are needed.

THE MYSTERIOUS FUTURE.

I've been a little girl so long,
That, somehow, it seems almost wrong
To think how grown-up I shall be
In days that have to come to me.

--*Carolyn Wells.*

Zweiback Noodles.--When making soup for children zweiback or Jew's bread is excellent for making noodles. Pound the bread to a powder, roll it with the rolling pin, sift and use the same as flour. It can also be used in milk as a baby food, and is often given to children with very delicate stomachs.

AFFECTION.

In the soft soil of little lives
Affection quickly springs and thrives
And grows like anything;
Its tiny tendrils Love puts out,
Not knowing what it's all about
But glad to smile and sing. --*Carolyn Wells.*

Playgrounds for Boys.--In a certain Ohio city there is a large placard "Boys, you can play here," It is a large corner lot thronged the whole day through during the good weather with boys playing ball and other games. This lot which could be sold for thousands of dollars, has been donated to the boys for a playground near their homes, The owner realized that the streets are not suitable playgrounds for the children and that accidents occur there almost daily. The streets of our cities are poor places in which to play, bad for the boys, and still worse for the community, If you have vacant lots turn them over to the boys this summer. A boy never forgets a favor, and American boys are not going to abuse good privileges. The loneliest boys are those who are not allowed to play on the beautiful lawn at home, are not allowed on the streets, and wander about from place to place to be told "Move on," every place they go.

ALL GIRLS AND BOYS.

Fourscore, like twenty, has its tasks and toys;
In earth's wide school-house all are girls and boys.

--*O. W. Holmes.*

Disinfection of Toys and Books.--All toys that have been used by a child suffering from an infectious disease should be either burned or thoroughly disinfected before they are used again. Books read by the little patient should be especially guarded against.

FROM LOWELL'S "AFTER THE BURIAL."

In the breaking gulfs of sorrow,
When the helpless feet stretch out
And find in the deeps of darkness
No footing so solid as doubt,
Then better one spar of Memory,
One broken plank of the Past,
That our human heart may cling to,
Though hopeless of shore at last!

Keep Dainties Away from the Beginning.--The well-trained child does not crave unaccustomed dainties. It is natural that he should feel a curiosity with regard to a dish with which he is not familiar, and ask some questions about it. But that does not mean that any of it is to be given to him. A boy whose digestive organs were very delicate was taught from babyhood to sit in his high chair at the table and eat what was on his tray and was perfectly content with what he had, as he knew no other diet. Once in awhile he would ask: "Is that good for little boys?" and when his mother would answer gently, "No. darling, that would make little boys sick," he was perfectly satisfied. Never having tasted things not suited to his age he did not crave them. One cannot miss that which he has never had. As he grew older he reaped the benefit of the strict regime and his digestion was perfect.

PROGRESS.

New occasions teach new duties; Time makes ancient good uncouth;
They must upward still, and onward, who would keep abreast of Truth;
Lo, before us gleam her camp-fires! we ourselves must Pilgrims be,
Launch our Mayflower, and steer boldly through the desperate winter sea,
Nor attempt the Future's portal with the Past's blood-rusted key.

--James Russell Lowell.

Temperature of Nursery.--Sixty degrees Fahrenheit is the proper temperature for the nursery, either in summer or in winter. This is not sufficiently warm to be weakening nor sufficiently cool to cause chills. Of course, when the natural heat of the atmosphere is higher than sixty degrees the temperature of the nursery cannot be kept that low, but with darkened windows during the heated portion of the day and good ventilation the room can be kept at a reasonably comfortable temperature.

ROCK ME TO SLEEP.

Backward, turn backward, O Time in your flight,
Make me a child again just for to-night!
Mother, come back from the echoless shore,
Take me again to your heart as of yore;
Kiss from my forehead the furrows of care,
Smooth the few silver threads out of my hair;
Over my slumbers your loving watch keep;
Rock me to sleep, mother,--rock me to sleep!

--Florence Percy.

The Pinafore.--The ideal dress for children is, of course, the pinafore style. It is so easy to renew the overdress and under bodice as required and it is, moreover, invaluable to suit the weather changes from day to day. The serge overdress can have a little cotton or flannel blouse, just as thermometers demand.

WEDDING CELEBRATIONS.

Three days--Sugar.

Sixty days--Vinegar.

1st anniversary--Iron.

5th anniversary--Wooden.

10th anniversary--Tin.

15th anniversary--Crystal.

20th anniversary--China.

25th anniversary--Silver.

30th anniversary--Cotton.

35th anniversary--Linen.

40th anniversary--Woolen.

45th anniversary--Silk.

50th anniversary--Gold.

75th anniversary--Diamond.

Afternoon Gowns.--Short afternoon gowns are proper for formal wear; especially for those who can wear the full skirts attached to narrow hem-bands. The dresses escape the floor by several inches and reveal the slippers and an inch of the colored hosiery.

A SONG OF LONG AGO.

A Song of Long Ago:
Sing it lightly--sing it low--
Sing it softly--like the lisping of the lips we used to know
When our baby-laughter spilled
From the glad hearts ever filled
With music blithe as robin ever thrilled! --*Riley.*

Rather Hard on the Baby.--Here is some advice that appeared in a paper for mothers the other day: "The bottle must be kept perfectly clean. When the babe has finished drinking it should be unscrewed and laid in a cool place under the tap." One feels rather sorry for any babies thus treated.

Learning Wisdom.--We learn wisdom from failure much more than from success; we often discover what will do, by finding out what will not do; and probably he who never made a mistake never made a discovery.--*S. Smiles.*

Nursery.--Today the nursery is looked upon as an essential apartment in a house where children abide, and from a hygienic standpoint, it may justly be called a sensible room, for children after they walk should not sleep in the mother's room. Whether the room is large or moderately small it should, by an means, have plenty of ventilation, the more windows the better. The room should be papered in light colors, also painted in light tones, though the blinds should be the darkest shade, to darken the room when necessary.

Cares of Matrimony.--Husbands and wives talk of the cares of matrimony, and bachelors and spinsters bear them.--*W. Collins.*

Awkwardness Due to Eyes.--A school teacher has remarked that many children are awkward, not through being ungainly in walking, but wholly because of impaired vision. It has been her experience with children in her department who were usually awkward and who had their eyes examined that there was something wrong with the vision, which was quickly overcome when glasses were purchased.

Medicine.--The disease and its medicine are like two factions in a besieged town; they tear one another to pieces, but both unite against their common enemy, Nature.--*Jeffrey.*

Baby's Petticoats.--Fine white flannel is the best material for baby's petticoats. They may be made in one piece, in princess style, or may consist of a flannel skirt attached to a loose cambric waist. These are decidedly preferable for summer and are really quite warm enough for any season.

Charity.--Prayer carries us half way to God, fasting brings us to the door of His palace, and alms-giving procures us admission.--*Koran.*

Tub for the Playroom.--Every playroom should be provided with a galvanized tub to hold water for sail boats. What boy does not like to play with water, boats and artificial fish? Do not expect him to be contented with toys or plays that amuse the little girl. The boy prefers splashing in water or making a noise with a hammer. Aquatic toys are numerous and reasonably cheap.

NOW OR NEVER.

Gather the rosebuds while ye may,
Old Time is still a-flying;
And this same flower that smiles today
To-morrow will be dying.

--*R. Herrick.*

Cleaning the Rug at Home.--Baby's fur rug may be cleaned at home by giving it a thorough bath in dry cornmeal. Rub the meal in as though it were soap, shake it out and rub in more meal, letting it remain in the rug for a day or two. Then shake out and the appearance of the rug will be much improved.

The Value of Wise Conversation.--A single conversation across the table with a wise man is better than ten years' mere study of books.--*Chinese Proverb.*

Tooth Powder.--Look well at the teeth of the little ones. Charcoal and tincture of myrrh are very beneficial to the teeth of the young, and both are easily procured at any drug store.

Silence.--Silence is one of the hardest arguments to refuse.--*Show.*

A Dish for Children.--An old-fashioned dish which never fails to delight the children may be prepared as follows: One quart of cornmeal, one pint of ripe chopped apples, three tablespoonfuls of butter, pinch of salt, one and one-half cups of water. Sweeten the apples to taste and bake as ordinary corn bread.

THE NOON OF LIFE.

What! grieve that time has brought so soon
The sober age of manhood on?
As idly might I weep, at noon,

To see the blush of morning gone. --*Bryant.*

Mouth Breathing.--Little ones who habitually breathe loud or snore in their sleep may be troubled with an adenoid growth.

Family.--A happy family is but an earlier heaven.--*Bowering.*

Obedience.--Prompt, unquestionable obedience in children seems to be a thing of the past, is the criticism of a recent writer, who adds: The up-to-date mother no longer tells her offspring that they must do or leave undone certain things because it is right. She enters into elaborate explanations and they need no longer blindly obey. This is not the wise preparation for the adult life. Unless we have taught our children the necessity for life's discipline, which they cannot at the time understand, it will make them rebellious and fail to work out the peaceable fruits of righteousness.

The Value of a Laugh.--A laugh is worth a hundred groans in any market.--*Lamb.*

Sanitary Drinking Cups.--Supply the youngsters on going to school with folded paper cornucopias which come in sealed packages for a small sum. These are used for drinking cups instead of those found in public places. Teach the children to make these useful little drinking cups from clean white paper, and there will be no danger of contracting disease from a drinking cup used by everyone who passes.

Easy to Misjudge Men.--Every heart has its secret sorrow which the world knows not, and oftimes we call a man cold when he is only sad.--*Anon.*

Night Petticoats.--Night petticoats for baby have sleeves. If no petticoat is worn, then an extra short jacket is provided in the coldest weather, for most babes sleep best with hands and arms uncovered.

A Bathrobe.--A large Turkish bath towel makes a nice bathrobe for a baby or small child. Use white cotton curtain cords for the girdle and make the hood of the Turkish face cloth. This little robe is very serviceable and convenient, and is easily laundered.

An Easy Task.--It is easy finding reasons why other people should be patient.--*George Eliot.*

Money to Children.--Instead of paying children for doing work let them understand that they have little duties that they must perform, but give them money at intervals. Teach them the value of money and the principles of saving.

Be Discreet.--Thy friend has a friend; thy friend's friend has a friend, therefore, be discreet.--*Anon.*

Methods of Cooking Eggs.--If you find that your baby, who is just beginning to eat solid food will not eat soft cooked eggs, and there are many who do not like them, try scrambling them until they are well done. If not found palatable in that form make an egg custard. A baby usually enjoys this and receives the same amount of nourishment that he would if the egg were cooked in any other way.

Politics and Veracity.--Politics and veracity have the same number of letters, but there the resemblance ends.--*Anon.*

Songs and Story Telling.--It is an unusual child indeed who does not delight in listening to story telling or bright little songs at bedtime and the nurse who is much with children will do well to treasure up all such material that comes in her way. Being used to children and having a sincere love for them makes one's work much easier, as even very little children seem to know instinctively who their real friends are and to be more easily controlled by them.

Friendship.--Two persons cannot long be friends if they cannot forgive each other's little failings.--*Bruyere*

Harsh Commands.--Can a parent who habitually speaks to his children in tones of harsh authority, and gives his commands to them in a manner of an officer addressing refractory troops, expect that they will feel for him the affection that they would give to one who took the trouble to draw out their better natures by loving treatment? The above is a question to be considered by parents who govern wholly by "authority."

Maidenhood.--No padlock, bolts, or bars can secure a maiden so well as her own reserve.--*Cerantes.*

Baby's Sleeves.--When baby's arms grow too large for the shirt sleeves, while the body of the shirt is still large enough, purchase a pair of infant's white cashmere hose. Cut the feet off and overcast neatly into the armholes; putting in a little gusset under the arms is necessary to enlarge armhole. The leg of the stocking makes the sleeves and the top fits nicely around the little wrist,

Reading.--To read without reflecting, is like eating without digesting.--*Burkc.*

Princess Skirt.--For long skirts, both flannel and white ones, the princess skirt adds to comfort of the body; no bands or fullness around the body or neck. Cut the material same as for princess slip, coming narrow on the shoulder and low neck back and front, and to flare at the bottom, which may be finished as desired. The flannel ones add to warmth, having flannel to neck baby needs no little jackets,

The Two Symptoms of Love.--The first symptom of love in a young man, is timidity; in a girl, it is boldness. The two sexes have a tendency to approach, and each assumes the qualities of the other.---*Victor Hugo* **Securing Covering at Night.**--If a delicate child has a habit of kicking the clothes off at night and so contracting chills, it is a good plan to sew a large button to each corner of the coverlet and attach a long tape loop to each corner of the bed. When fastened this will keep the bedclothes securely in place, however much the child may toss in its sleep.

Honesty.--Socrates being asked the way to honest fame, said, "Study to be what you wish to seem."

Amusing Baby.--A simple device for keeping the baby amused and happy is to fasten at intervals upon a broad, bright ribbon the toys of which he is most fond, suspending the ribbon above the bed upon which he lies, within reach of his little hands, by securing one end to the head of the bed and the other to the foot. He will then entertain himself by the hour pushing the toys back and forth, and watching them swing above him.

Prominent Ears.--Prominent ears should always be corrected in childhood by putting a thin cap on the child at night.

Disappointing a Child.--A day in a child's life is equal to a week in ours; so think twice before you condemn a child to a whole day's disappointment or unhappiness.

Baby's Veil.--Baby's veil, which should only be used in cold or windy weather, may be either a Shetland veil or made of bobbinet.

Sweaters.--There are cunning little sweaters exactly like those made up for older children, which come in sizes to fit an eight-months old baby.

Wild Flowers.--Every garden should contain a few wild flowers. The busy mother will find that they grow without care if proper soil is provided and will bloom where there is too much shade for other flowers. March brings forth the lovely hepatica, and wild phlox or sweet william soon follows. Next comes the wild geranium cranes bill, but as its petals fall rapidly, it is not as effective as sweet william, which will be a mass of delicate bloom for five weeks or more. The trillium or wake robin is another desirable flower, and wild violets thrive where the cultivated kind will not grow. The Indian turnip or Jack-in-the-Pulpit is an interesting plant and a curiosity to many who never ramble in the woods to see it in its native abode. All of these bear transplanting and are satisfactory as garden plants, but choose sweet william if you wish the most desirable for color, fragrance and duration of bloom.

Making Friends.--Blessed is the man who has the gift of making friends, for it is one of God's best gifts.--*Thomas Hughes.*

Baby's Nose.--But the most pliable of baby's features is the nose. By gently massaging this feature every day with the thumb and forefinger a tendency to broadness may be promptly subdued. The bridge should be gently pressed between the fingers in the course of an upward massage movement.

Flowers.--They are wreathed around the cradle, the marriage altar, and the tomb.--*Mrs. L. M. Child.*

Bed Time.--One little chap was constantly being deceived as to his bed hour, which was 7:30 o'clock. He could not tell the time, and his mother or nurse would tell him that it was bedtime when in reality it was only seven o'clock. He would look puzzled and only half convinced as his reason told him it could not be that late; but he had no choice but to obey. It would have been far wiser to set seven o'clock as his bed hour and to have stuck to it.

Little Minds.--Minds of moderate calibre ordinarily condemn everything that is beyond their range.--*La Rachefoucauld.*

Tea and Coffee.--Don't give your two-year-old child tea and coffee to drink. What if she does cry for them? The crying will harm her far less than the drink.

FOUR THINGS.

Each man has more of four thing than he knows.

What four are these? Sins, debts, fears and woes.

--From the French.

Sanitary Care of Baby's Bottles.--To wash and cleanse baby's bottles satisfactorily, have a good stout bottle brush; make a strong suds of hot water and soap or soap powder; wash the bottles thoroughly, using the brush, then rinse several times, using the hot water and borax, and drain. Before using bottles, always rinse again with hot water. With this care there should be no trouble with sour or cloudy bottles.

Moulded by Circumstances.--In all our reasonings concerning men we must lay it down as a maxim that the greater part are moulded by circumstances.--*Robert Hall.*

Forming Habits.--The trouble with most bad habits is that they are so quickly formed in small children. The mother relaxes her care for a day or two, and a new trick appears, or the work of weeks on an old one is undone. What is true of physical habits is equally so of the moral habits. A tiny baby of a few months old knows very well if the habit of loud crying will procure for it what it wants, and if not cheeked will develop into the irritable whining adult we are all acquainted with. Habits of disrespect, of indifference to the rights of others, of cruelty, may all be irresistibly formed or dispelled in the first few years of life.

Chains of Habit.--The diminutive chains of habit are seldom heavy enough to be felt, till they are too strong to be broken.--*Samuel Johnson.*

Unique Table Protector.--Many mothers prefer to bring their young children to the family table on ordinary occasions when there are no guests. At the same time they dislike to mar the appearance of their table with the tin waiter which is usually set before the children to protect the cloth against the depredations of dropped bread and milk.

A clever device for this purpose is made of two oblong pieces of butcher's linen sewed together in the form of a case, with an oilcloth interlining. The linen is hemmed neatly so that it looks like an oblong napkin, and while it protects the cloth and the table it protects the table underneath; being white, like the cloth itself, it does not spoil the looks of the table. When soiled the oilcloth is slipped out and wiped off with a damp cloth, and the linen case goes with the tablecloth and napkin. Several of these cases will be needed, for the ordinary enterprising baby, but one piece of oilcloth will be sufficient for a long time.

Banish Tears.--Banish the tears of children; continual rains upon the blossoms are hurtful.--*Jean Paul Richter.*

Folding Bathtub.--The thing most desired by a young mother in these days is a bathtub for the baby made of sheet rubber that is attached to a campstool foundation. It can be folded up and put out of the way when not in use, and it telescopes into a small bundle when one wants to travel.

Flowers.--Flowers are the sweetest things God ever made and forgot to put a soul into.--*Henry Ward Beecher.*

Correct Length of Clothes.--In making long clothes for the baby it is well to remember that the correct length for long dresses is one yard from the shoulder to the hem. The petticoats should be made the same lengths as the dresses, or perhaps a half inch shorter.

Life.--A pendulum betwixt a smile and tear.--*Byron.*

DOMESTIC SCIENCE DEPARTMENT.

The Theory and Practical Methods of Preserving Foods.

MARMALADES AND BUTTERS. CANNING. JAM JELLIES. PICKLES. CHAFING DISHES.

By EDNA GERTRUDE THOMPSON,

Director of Domestic Science Department, Thomas Normal Training School,

Detroit, Michigan.

Theory and Practice of Domestic Science.--Domestic Science has come to be considered one of the most important factors in our public school education of today. We have just awakened to the fact that our daughters should receive training in those things which will best fit them for housewives and mothers. While many of our girls are earning their own livelihood, the majority ultimately settle into homes of their own. Many girls have an excellent opportunity to get the training they need as homemakers from their mothers, but many of the children in this country lack this home training. There are two reasons for this neglect on the part of the mothers: first, the mother may not know how to do these things herself; and, second, she may be a wage-earner and of necessity cannot train her daughter.

Its Moral Influence.--In the early life of the child it is susceptible to influences which may be brought to bear upon it, and if the home-making instinct is instilled early much is done toward moral growth of the child. The public school is expected to develop the child along these lines and consequently the cookery class, together with the class in housekeeping, has a mighty influence toward developing noble women. All the home duties are developed and made a pleasure and not a duty to the child, so that the home is looked upon with favorable eyes.

There is an old saying that "the way to a man's heart is through his stomach." This contains much more truth than it would seem on the surface. Investigators who have made careful research into the divorce question, which has assumed such large proportions, state that if women knew more of the science of home making there would be fewer homes broken up. What man or woman either would not be utterly discouraged to come home day after day to poor meals and untidiness everywhere, conditions which in time bring poor health and disease. The public school aims through domestic science to teach the importance and dignity of being a good housewife.

Economy of Domestic Science.--Then again, domestic science makes a plea for recognition on the ground of economy. Many times debt and trouble come to homes, not through lack of sufficient funds, but through lack of knowledge on the part of the dispenser of the funds. One of the principles which domestic science emphasizes in its teaching is to show how some of our cheaper foods furnish more nutriment to our systems than do some of our more expensive articles of diet. With this fact thoroughly established and understood domestic science tries to develop new and simple methods of cooking such foods and of making them attractive and appetizing. It is a well-known fact that it is not the amount of food we eat but the amount that we digest that gives nourishment to our bodies, and it has been proven that food that is not attractive and palatable to us gives only one-half the value to our bodies as when it is made attractive and palatable.

Greatest Food Value from Proper Cooking.--Then also students along this line of study have discovered that some of our common foods lose much of their value to us through improper cooking and preparation.

If we are going to prepare food and use it as part of our diet, why should we not obtain the most of its value? Is that not true economy? For an example of this fact let us take eggs, one of our most common articles of diet. We commonly cook eggs to harden the white, or albumen, so as to make them more palatable. One common method of doing this has been to boil them. Through experiments it has been proven that boiling makes this albumen so hard to digest that our bodies get practically no value from it. The newer method advanced proves that the same results can be obtained by cooking eggs in water which is kept just below the boiling point, and eggs cooked this way are easily and readily assimilated by our bodies. Why should we not endeavor then to give to our bodies food so prepared that it gives the most nourishment. To take another example,--when salt is added to vegetables it draws out from them into the water their mineral salts and any proteid which will build tissue for us. In most vegetables the cooking water is thrown away so that much of the value of the vegetable is lost. Why should we not try to devise a method of cooking which will save for us this food value? Salt is added for flavor only, so why cannot the salt be added a short time before the cooking is finished so that it will not have time to draw out the food value?

How to Save in Cooking Meats.--Again we cook different kinds of meats in different ways. Perhaps you think these different kinds of methods have simply come down to us through the ages. It is, however, interesting to know that our mothers probably developed these methods through thought. Tough meats, we know, require long cooking, but do we know why? The fibers and tissues have become strong through constant use on the part of the animal, and to be of use to us must be softened, so we cook tough meats long and usually with moisture to accomplish the softening. Tough meats are our cheap meats, but have you stopped to consider that they contain more nourishment than our tender meats. As has been stated, the tough meats are the parts of the body of the animal most used and consequently have been developed and nourished. Why not learn how to cook these pieces which give us more nourishment, and which are cheaper, in such a way as to be attractive and palatable? This is what the Domestic Science Course in our public school aims to teach our girls so that as housewives they can get the most value for the least money and be economical and intelligent buyers.

Our Winter Supply.--From an instinct, which ought to be common to all of us, in time of plenty we lay something aside for the time of need. As housewives this truth comes home to us, especially in the summer when we have an abundance of fruit which, without care, would soon become worthless. By reason of which fact we have developed methods of canning, preserving, etc., which at the present time have become so advanced that we can retain a very large share of the original color, flavor and shape of the fruit.

Preserving Foods.--All food products, on exposure to air, undergo certain changes which unfit them for use as food. It was once thought that these changes were due to oxidation, but they are now known to be caused by minute living organisms present in the air, in the water, in the ground and in the food itself. To preserve food two things are necessary; first, to either kill or render harmless those organisms already present; and second, to exclude others from entering. The first we usually accomplish by cooking, and the second by sealing. In order to live these organisms require three conditions; first, a particular temperature; second, a certain amount of moisture; third, the right kind of food. By taking away all or anyone of these requirements we may stop the growth or, in other words, we may preserve the food. For example: with the familiar method of cold storage the factor of temperature is removed; in the drying of the fruits and vegetables the factor of moisture is removed; by salting the factor of food is taken away.

The fruits and vegetables, commonly preserved in the home, are divided into five classes:

1.--Canning.

2.--Jellies.

3.--Jams.

4.--Marmalades and Butters.

5.--Pickles.

CANNING.--Under this head there are four common methods:

1. Steaming.--By this method the fruit is put into the sterilized jars, the jars filled with boiling water and the covers loosely set on. Then the jars are set on small blocks of wood in a pan of cold water. Cover this pan and let the water come to a boil and boil for 15 minutes. Remove the jars and fill them with boiling water, if necessary. Seal tightly. Small berries, such as strawberries and raspberries, retain their color and are especially good done in this manner. Whole tomatoes done in this way are especially attractive for winter salads, and corn will keep indefinitely.

2. Boiling in Syrup.--This is the common household method of preserving fruits, such as peaches and pears. A syrup is prepared of sugar and water, into this the fruit is dropped and cooked until soft; it is then put into sterile jars, sufficient syrup added to fill jar and the jar then sealed.

3. Preserving.--This is the same as boiling in syrup, except that equal quantities of sugar and fruit are used. Small fruits such as berries are usually done in this way.

4. Cold Water Process.--This is a simple and easy method to use, and is especially desirable for vegetables such as rhubarb. Great care must be taken to use only perfect fruit, because in this method of canning bacteria are merely excluded, not destroyed, and if any are present in the food there is nothing to prevent it from spoiling. If fruit is over-ripe, or not perfectly fresh one of the other methods, such as boiling or steaming, is preferable.

To Can by the Cold Water Process.--Pack the fruit in a sterilized jar; pour over it water which has been boiled and cooled, seal your jar and keep in a cool place. Sometimes a solution of salt and water is used in place of pure water. When salt water is used food will need to be freshened by being allowed to stand in cold water for some time before using. Vegetables, such as beans, put up in this way are very similar to the fresh product.

Utensils.--Among the utensils most necessary for use in preserving foods in the home are scales, measuring cups, porcelain or agate ware sauce pans; earthen or agate ware bowls; silver, agate or wooden spoons; an agate colander; small dipper and funnel; new rubbers and perfect covers for the jars.

To Sterilize Jars.--Wash the jars, fill with cold water, place them on rests, such as small blocks of wood on the bottom of the kettle or boiler and surround them with cold water. If blocks of wood are not obtainable the jars may be wrapped in brown paper to prevent them knocking against each other. Be sure the mouths of the jars are uncovered. Heat gradually until the water boils, boil 15 minutes or until ready to fill them. Sterilize the covers of the jars also, and dip the rubber bands in boiling water just before using.

Directions for Filling Jars.--Remove the jars from the boiling water--the handle of a wooden spoon is good to use in removing them. Wring a cloth out of hot water and place it on a plate, put the jar to be filled on the hot cloth, put a silver spoon in it,--silver being a good conductor of heat absorbs the heat from the fruit and lessens the danger of breakage. Fill the jar with fruit and then add enough syrup or boiling water, as the case may be, to fill the jar to overflowing. Run a silver knife or spoon down the sides of the jar to allow any enclosed air to escape; add more syrup or water, if necessary. Put on the sterilized rubber and seal tightly.

Tomatoes Canned Whole by Steaming.--Select medium sized, firm, ripe tomatoes. Wash and peel. Pour boiling water over the tomatoes and they will peel easily. Pack in sterilized jars, fill with boiling water and put on the lid lightly. Set in cold water on rests and let boil about fifteen minutes. If necessary, fill the jar with boiling water to overflowing. Put on the sterilized rubbers and seal tightly. These tomatoes are especially good for winter salads.

Canned Corn.--Cut the corn from the cob while fresh, pack in sterilized jars, and fill with boiling water. Put the cover on lightly and set on a rest, such as small blocks of wood, pieces of thick paper or the corn husks, in a pan of cold water. Let boil from two to three hours. Remove the can, fill to overflowing with boiling water and seal tightly.

Canned String Beans.--Select medium sized beans and string. Pack in a sterilized jar, fill to overflowing with a brine and seal tightly. This brine may be made in two ways: First, by mixing cold water and salt; second, by mixing salt and boiling water and then letting it cool before pouring over the beans. This method is best as the salt dissolves more readily in boiling water than in cold water. One part salt to two parts water makes a strong brine. Keep in a cold place and freshen before using by letting the beans stand in cold water for an hour. In winter these beans make an acceptable substitute for fresh ones.

Canned Rhubarb.--Select medium stalks, skin and cut either into one-inch pieces, or eight-inch lengths. Pack in sterilized jars, fill to overflowing with cold water and seal. Rhubarb put up in this way has been known to keep for over a year, and is especially good for pies and sauce.

Steamed Strawberries.--Wash and hull the strawberries, and for every quart of strawberries use one cup of sugar. Pack the berries in a sterilized jar, cover with sugar and fill with boiling water. Cover the jar lightly, put in a pan of cold water, on a rest and let the water boil for about fifteen minutes. Remove, seal tightly, and keep in a cool place.

Canned Strawberries.--Wash and hull the berries. Make a syrup of sugar and water, using one cup of sugar to every three of water. Boil 10 minutes. Drop the berries in the boiling syrup and cook until soft. This will require only several minutes. Fill the jars to overflowing with fruit and syrup, then seal.

Canned Cherries.--Follow the method for strawberries. Cherries can be pitted or not, as desired. If pitted, add a few stones for flavor.

Canning Raspberries.--Use the same method as for strawberries. The large number of seeds in raspberries are objectionable, and the berries are more often made into jam than canned.

Canned Pears.--The pears should be ripe and of fine flavor. Wipe and pare the fruit. If the pears are large they may be cut in halves. Make a syrup of sugar and water, using one cup of sugar to one cup of water. Boil 10 minutes. Put in the pears, cook until soft. Fill sterilized jars and seal.

Canned Peaches.--Follow the directions for pears. Peaches may be canned by the steaming method by cutting them in two and removing the stones.

Strawberry Preserves.--Wash and hull the berries, then weigh. Make a syrup by boiling three-quarters of their weight in sugar with water, allowing one cup of water to each pound of sugar. Cook syrup 15 minutes, fill glass jars with the berries, add the syrup to overflow the jars. Let stand 15 minutes. By this time the fruit will have shrunk; add enough more fruit to fill the jar. Put on a cover; set on a rest in a pan of cold water, heat to the boiling point, and keep just below boiling for one hour. Raspberries may be done in the same way.

Raspberry and Currant Preserves.--

3 lbs. Currants. 3 lbs. Sugar. 4 qts. Raspberries.

Pick over, wash and drain the currants. Put into a preserving kettle and mash. Cook one hour and strain through cheesecloth. Return to the kettle, add the sugar, heat to the boiling point, cook 20 minutes. Add the raspberries and cook until soft. Fill jars to overflowing and seal. If the seeds of the currants are not objectionable the mixture need not be strained.

JELLIES.--Fruits to be used in making jelly should be underripe, rather than over-ripe. Green fruit contains two substances, called "pectase" and "pectose" and, by the action of the sun in ripening, these substances change into pectin which makes fruit jelly. If the fruit is over-ripe the pectin breaks down into pectosic acid which has not the power of jellying; and as a result the fruit does not jell. If the fruit is a little under-ripe pectin is formed through cooking, and it is often advisable to add some green fruit to the ripe fruit in making jelly. Nearly all failures in jelly making are due either to over-ripe fruit or to the use of too much heat, because in both cases the pectin is lost.

To Prepare Glasses for Jelly.--Wash the glasses, put in a kettle of cold water, heat the water gradually to the boiling point, and boil for fifteen minutes. Remove the glasses and drain; place, while filling, on a cloth wrung out of hot water. If the glasses are wrapped in brown paper with the mouths uncovered they will not break.

To Cover Jelly Glasses.--First: with paraffin. Melt the paraffin over hot water and pour over the jelly when cold about one-fourth inch thick. Be sure to use hot water in melting the paraffin, as it is apt to explode if heated to too high a degree.

Second.--Cut two pieces of white paper, one just the size of the glass and the other larger; dip the first cover in brandy or alcohol and press down tightly over the jelly. White of egg or water may be used, but it is not so good. Then cover with the second paper, sealing edges with white of egg. A tin cover could be used in place of the last paper.

To Make a Jelly Bag.--Take a piece of flannel about three quarters of a yard long, fold the opposite corners together and sew in the shape of a cornucopia, rounding at the end; if the seam is felled it will be more secure. Bind the top with tape and finish with two or three heavy loops by which it may be hung.

Good Fruits for Making Jelly.--Crab apples, snow apples, early summer apples, grapes, currants, blackberries, raspberries, quinces, barberries are the fruits most commonly used for making jellies.

General Directions for Making Jelly.--Wash the fruit, remove the stems and imperfections. Cut large fruit into pieces. With fruit such as apples or quinces add enough water to cover them, but with watery fruits, such as grapes and currants, omit any water. Cook the fruit, until the juice flows, keeping it just below the boiling point. Remove from the fire and strain through a pointed bag, hung at some height. Allow all the juice possible to drip through before squeezing the bag and keep this juice by itself. Then squeeze the bag and use the juice thus obtained for second grade jelly, which, while it is not as clear as the first lot, can be used for jelly cakes, etc. Measure the juice, bring to the boiling point, boil slowly two or three minutes, then add an equal quantity of heated sugar. Boil until the jelly thickens when dropped upon a cold plate. Pour slowly into sterilized jelly glasses and set away to harden. The jelly bags should be sterilized before using.

Apple Jelly.--Wipe the apples, remove the stem and blossom ends and cut into quarters. Put into granite or, porcelain lined preserving kettle and add enough cold water to come nearly to the top of the apples. Cook slowly until the apples are soft. Mash and strain through a coarse sieve. Allow the juice to drip through a jelly bag. Boil slowly for about 20 minutes, add an equal quantity of heated sugar, cook for about five minutes or until the jelly will harden when dropped on a cold saucer. Pour into sterilized jelly glasses and seal when cold. If the apples are pared a very light colored jelly is obtained.

Crab Apple Jelly.--Follow the recipe for apple jelly and use red cheeked crab apples, if possible.

Quince Jelly.--Follow the recipe for apple jelly, substituting quinces for apples. Remove the seeds from the fruit. Sometimes apples and quinces are used in combination and make an excellent jelly.

Grape Jelly.--Pick over the grapes, wash and remove stems. Heat to the boiling point, mash and boil 30 minutes. Strain through a jelly bag, return the juice to the kettle and boil *slowly* for about five minutes. Add an equal quantity of heated sugar. Boil three minutes or until it hardens on a cold plate. Skim if necessary. Pour into sterilized jelly glasses; seal when cold. Be very sure the grapes are not over-ripe. It is very desirable to add a few green grapes. Wild grapes make excellent jelly to serve with game.

Barberry Jelly.--This is considered quite a delicacy, and is made the same as grape jelly, except that a very little water,--about one cup to one peck of berries--is sometimes added.

Currant Jelly.--Pick over the currants but do not remove the stems, wash and drain. Put into a preserving kettle and mash. Cook slowly for about 20 to 30 minutes. Strain through a coarse strainer and then through a jelly bag. Follow directions for grape jelly.

A combination of currants and raspberries makes a good jelly.

Raspberry Jelly.--Follow the directions for grape jelly. Raspberry jelly is hard to make and should not be tried if the fruit is not perfectly fresh or if it is at all over-ripe.

JAMS.--The pulp, seeds and skins are all retained in jams; often material that is left from jellies, and so on, can be used in this way by adding spices and nuts to give flavor. Sterilization and the exclusion of air are not quite so important in this class of preserving on account of the large amount of sugar used which takes away food from the bacteria. Equal amounts of sugar and fruits are used in making jams.

Raspberry Jam.--Pick over the raspberries, mash in a preserving kettle with a wooden masher. Heat slowly to the boiling point, and add an equal quantity of heated sugar. Cook slowly for about 45 minutes. Put into sterilized jars.

Strawberry Jam.--Wash and hull the berries. Add the sugar gradually so that the juice of the berries will dissolve it. Boil about 20 minutes, or until it will harden when dropped on a cold plate. Pour into sterilized glasses.

Grape Jam.--

8 Cups of Grapes. 4 Cups of Sugar.

Wash the grapes, remove the stems and squeeze the pulp from the skins into a preserving kettle. Put the skins on a granite plate and save them. Boil the pulp until the seeds separate easily, stirring constantly. Strain through a sieve, add the skins to the strained mixture, measure, return to the kettle, and add an equal amount of sugar. Boil gently for 15 minutes or until the jam is very thick. Pour into sterilized glasses and seal when cold. The mixture needs careful watching and stirring, as it will burn easily, especially after the sugar is added.

Rhubarb Conserve.--

2 lbs. rhubarb. 2 oranges.
3 lbs. sugar. 1 lb. shelled nuts.
Juice of 3 Lemons.

Remove the leaves and pieces of root from the rhubarb and wash the stalks in cold water. Cut into one-inch pieces. Do not remove the skin unless it is fibrous. If the skin is removed do this before cutting in pieces. Wash the oranges and either grate the rind or cut the yellow into strips thin enough to be seen through. Wash the lemons and use only the juice. A little rind may be used, if desired, but it will take away from the orange flavor. The nuts need not be blanched, but should be broken into pieces of medium size. Any nut may be used, but walnuts are especially good. Mix all the materials, except the nuts, with the sugar. Cook slowly, stirring constantly, until the mixture is thick,--about three-quarters of an hour. After the first half hour's cooking, add the nuts. Pour into sterilized jelly glasses and seal when cold.

MARMALADES AND BUTTERS.--Marmalades and butters are really strained jams and the same rules hold true as for jams.

Apple Marmalade.--Pare and core the apples. Cook until tender with just enough water to keep from burning. Force through a fine sieve, return to the fire with a scant pound of sugar and the juice and rind of one lemon for each pound of pulp. Cook, stirring with a wooden spoon until the marmalade is thick when dropped on a cold saucer. Pour into sterilized glasses.

Peach Marmalade.--Follow the recipe for apple marmalade, adding spices, such as cinnamon, nutmeg and cloves.

Crab Apple Marmalade.--When making crab apple jelly, core the apples and after straining, use the pulp that is left to make marmalade. Various seasonings can he added. Among the best are cinnamon, cloves, nutmeg, grated rind and juice of oranges and lemons. When seasoned according to taste, add sugar to the pulp, and cook until of the desired consistency. Seal in sterilized jars.

Rhubarb Marmalade.--

2 lbs. rhubarb. 3 lbs. sugar. Rind and pulp of 6 oranges.

Boil the ingredients together until thick. The rind of the orange may be grated and cooked by itself until tender before adding to the rest of the materials. Pour into sterilized glasses and seal.

Pineapple.--Pare and remove the eyes from pineapple, then grate. Weigh the pulp and heat two-thirds of its weight in sugar. Cook the pineapple in an uncovered dish for some time. Then add the juice of one lemon for each pound of fruit. Then add the sugar and boil until thick,--about five minutes. Pour into sterilized jelly glasses.

PICKLES.--Under this heading are classified pickles and relishes, such as chili sauce, chow chows and catsups. Pickling is preserving in salt or acid liquor. Pickles do not contain much nutritive value, but add much to a meal in making it attractive. Cucumber pickles should never look as green when pickled as the fruit on the vine; if they do it is almost certain that some preservative has been used.

Sweet Pickled Pears or Peaches.--

1 peck peaches. 4 lbs. brown sugar.
1 quart vinegar. 2 ozs. stick cinnamon.
Cloves.

Boil sugar, vinegar and cinnamon for 20 minutes. Dip peaches quickly in hot water and rub off fur with a towel. Stick each peach with three or four cloves, put into syrup and cook until soft. Cook only enough fruit at a time to fill one jar. Seal in sterilized jars. Pears may be prepared in the same way.

Chili Sauce.--

25 ripe tomatoes (medium sized). 1/2 cup brown sugar.
4 large white onions. 6 peppers. (chopped fine)
4 teaspoons of ginger. 4 teaspoons of allspice
1 teaspoons of cloves. 2 tablespoons of salt.
1 qt. vinegar.

Mix these materials and cook for one hour, stirring occasionally. The consistency should be quite thick and more than an hour's cooking *may* be necessary. Strain or not as desired, but if strained put back in the kettle and bring to the boiling point before scaling. Use tall wide necked bottles and fill to overflowing, using the same precautions as you would in canning fruit. The chili sauce is quite "hot," but this can be remedied by altering the number of peppers and onions. In preparing, the tomatoes should be washed; scalded and peeled. The peppers should be washed in cold water, the stems removed and the peppers chopped finely. Chop the onions finely in the same bowl as the peppers.

Olive Oil Pickles.--

8 qts. sliced cucumbers.
1 cup olive oil.
1 cup sugar.
1 teaspoon mustard seed.
One dozen onions.
1 teaspoon cloves.
1 teaspoon allspice.
1 teaspoon celery seed.
4 teaspoons cinnamon.

Slice the cucumbers thin and let stand over night in a weak brine. In the morning drain, add the onions sliced thin. Mix the ingredients given. Put the cucumbers and onions in a crock, pour over the mixture and add enough vinegar to cover. Mix well.

Sweet Cucumber Pickles.--Select small cucumbers. Wash well but do not peel. Put into a crock one cup of salt and 4 quarts of cucumbers. Cover with boiling water and let stand over night. In the morning remove from the brine, put in a granite kettle, cover with vinegar to which has been added mustard seeds, whole cloves, stick cinnamon, two cups of sugar and other desired seasonings. Let it come to the boiling point, but not boil. Seal while hot.

Green Tomato Pickles.--Remove a thin slice from each end of the green tomatoes. Slice and sprinkle one peck of tomatoes with one cup of salt and let stand over night. Drain, boil 15 minutes in two quarts of boiling water and one quart of vinegar. Drain again. Cook for 10 minutes the following: one gallon of vinegar, 2 pounds or less of sugar, 1 red pepper, 10 teaspoon mustard seed, 3/4 cup cinnamon bark, and any other seasonings desired. Add the tomatoes and simmer for about one hour, stirring occasionally. The spices should be removed; this is easily accomplished if they are tied in a muslin bag. Pack in sterilized jars.

SOME HINTS ON CHAFING DISH COOKERY.

The Use of the Chafing Dish and Some Favorite Recipes.

Within recent years the chafing dish has become very familiar to us. It is, however, not a recent invention, for in the time of Louis XIV it was very commonly used. To the housekeeper who wishes to save herself and to serve her guests with food at its best, the chafing dish comes as an acceptable friend for use at the breakfast table in the preparation of eggs and dishes which should be served immediately. Toast can be served fresh and hot by using a toaster over the burner of a chafing dish. At luncheon a hot dish can easily take the place of the cold meat course if the chafing dish is at hand. However, the chief use of the chafing dish is in the preparation of late suppers, and is largely in use by those who have limited facilities for housekeeping, such as college girls. By those who entertain the chafing dish is looked upon as a true friend of hospitality.

Chafing dishes vary in price from the common ones made of tin which can be bought for about a dollar, to the more expensive ones made of silver. Various wares are utilized for the chafing dish. Among those most satisfactory are graniteware, earthenware, nickel, copper and aluminum.

To get satisfactory results with the chafing dish you must have certain parts. There should be a pan to use for hot water, and it should be furnished with a handle. The cooking pan or blazer, as it is called, should have a handle also. Until one becomes an expert the hot water pan should be in constant use but later one need only use the hot water pan for keeping food warm. The burner should be carefully looked after and be in readiness. Alcohol, electricity and gas are all used as fuel, but denatured or wood alcohol is probably the most common of all. If care is taken in the use of alcohol there need be no danger. Fill the lamp with sufficient alcohol to cook the dish desired, and if necessary to refill during cooking shut off the flame and let the burner cool somewhat before replenishing with the alcohol. A large tray upon which to set the chafing dish prevents danger of fire and protects the table. Large forks and spoons, made especially for the chafing dish, can be obtained at a small price, but any table spoon and fork can he used. It is well to have a napkin and extra spoon and fork at hand if it is necessary to taste the preparation.

That a chafing dish supper may be a success, care should be taken on the part of the hostess to have everything in readiness. The table should be set with the required dishes, silver, etc., and all ingredients should be at hand for the preparation that is to be made on the chafing dish. Most chafing dishes will not supply portions for more than eight, so that a larger number should not be included at a chafing dish supper. Unless skilled in the use of a chafing dish, it is best not to prepare new dishes for guests. If one will observe some care and have everything in readiness, a chafing dish supper can be a very enjoyable source of entertainment for informal affairs.

To use the following recipes with success level measurements of all ingredients must be made--level teaspoon, level cup, etc.

SOME FAVORITE CHAFING DISH CONCOCTIONS.

Cream Sauce.--

2 tablespoons flour.
2 tablespoons butter.
1 cup milk.
1/2 teaspoon salt.
1/4 teaspoon pepper.

Melt the butter and stir in the flour and seasonings until smooth; add the scalded milk slowly, stirring constantly. Cook until of the right consistency. This makes a medium thick sauce, the thickness of which can be varied by increasing or diminishing the amount of flour. This is the foundation for a great number of chafing dish recipes, such as creamed dishes. A richer sauce may he made by substituting cream for milk and omitting most of the butter.

Creamed Chicken.--

1 cup cold flaked chicken.	1/2 teaspoon celery salt.
1 cup thin cream sauce.	1/4 teaspoon curry powder.

Prepare one cup of thin cream sauce and season with the celery salt and curry powder. Add the chicken and when heated through pour over slices of toast or into timbal cases. Garnish with parsley. Any desired seasonings can be used in place of the celery and curry.

Chicken a la Goldenrod.--

1 cup cold flaked chicken.	2 cups thin cream sauce.
6 hard cooked eggs.	1/2 cup mushrooms.
Seasonings.	

Cut the eggs in slices, putting two yolks through a potato ricer. Make a thin cream sauce, season as desired with celery seed or curry. Add the chicken and mushrooms, drained from their liquor. When hot, and just before serving, add the eggs. Pour the mixture over rounds of toast and over the top of each portion sprinkle some of the yolk which was forced through the potato ricer as a garnish. A bit of parsley improves the appearance.

Creamed Beef.--

1 cup shredded dried beef.	1 cup medium cream sauce.
4 hard cooked eggs,	Seasonings as desired.

Prepare the cream sauce, add the beef and hard cooked eggs, cut into slices. When heated through pour over toast diamonds. Garnish with parsley and serve hot.

Cheese Fondue.--

2 cups grated cheese.	2 tablespoons butter.
1 cup soft bread crumbs.	1/2 teaspoon salt.
1 cup cream or milk.	1 teaspoon dry mustard.
3 eggs.	1/2 teaspoon paprika.
6 slices buttered toast.	

Melt the butter and add the seasonings. When hot add the cheese and the bread crumbs which have been soaked in the milk. When very hot add the egg yolks which have been well beaten. Mix thoroughly, then fold in the whites of eggs beaten stiff. Let cook several minutes over the hot water, then pour over the buttered toast.

Curried Toast.--

1 cup cream sauce.	1 teaspoon curry powder.
4 hard cooked eggs.	6 slices buttered toast.

Make a cream sauce using the curry as seasoning. Chop the eggs fine, add to the cream sauce and when hot pour over the toast. Garnish with parsley.

Eggs and Cream.--

6 eggs. 1 cup cream.
1/4 teaspoon salt. 1/8 teaspoon cayenne.
2 teaspoons Worcestershire Sauce. 1 tablespoon butter.
6 slices toast.

Put the cream and seasonings in a dish. When almost boiling drop in the eggs and put in the butter cut in bits. When the eggs are poached serve on the toast which has been dipped in melted butter. Garnish with parsley.

Creamed Oysters.--

1 qt. oysters. 4 tablespoons butter.
1 cup cream. 1/4 teaspoon salt.
1 teaspoon parsley, minced. 6 slices toast.

Remove the hard muscles from the oysters, scald and drain. Melt the butter, add the cream and seasonings. Cayenne, celery salt, Worcestershire sauce and onion juice are good seasonings. When this is hot add the oysters, cook two minutes and serve on the toast. The bread should be toasted on one side only. Sprinkle with the minced parsley.

Welsh Rarebit.--

1 tablespoon butter. 1/4 teaspoon mustard.
1 cup soft mild cheese. 1/4 teaspoon salt.
1 egg. Few grains cayenne.
1/2 cup ale or beer.

Cut the cheese into small pieces and beat the eggs slightly. Put the butter in the chafing dish, and when it is melted add the cheese and seasonings, stirring constantly. Add the ale slowly and when smooth the slightly beaten egg. Much of the success of a rarebit depends upon the cheese. It should be smooth and creamy, and never stringy. Cook over hot water. The rarebit may be served on toast or wafers.

Cream Welsh Rarebit.--

1 tablespoon butter. 1 cup soft mild cheese.
1/4 teaspoon salt. 1/4 teaspoon mustard.
Few grains cayenne. 1/2 cup milk.
1 egg. 1/8 teaspoon soda.

Follow directions for welsh rarebit (above) adding the soda with the cheese and the milk in place of the ale. Curry powder and celery salt make good additions as seasoning.

Curry of Tomato.--

4 tomatoes. 1 tablespoon butter.
1 tablespoon flour. 2 teaspoons curry.
1/2 teaspoon onion juice. 1/2 teaspoon salt.

Select large, firm, fresh tomatoes. Peel and cut in slices. Melt the butter in the blazer. Add the tomatoes and cook for several minutes. Add the cream, flour and curry and seasonings. When hot serve on toast. Care must be taken or the acid in the tomato will curdle the cream.

Salted Almonds.--

1 cup almond meats. 1/2 cup olive oil.

Cover the almonds with boiling water. Remove the skins, then soak for several hours in strong salted water. Drain and dry. Put in enough olive oil to cover the bottom of the blazer. Put in the nuts and cook until brown. Drain on paper. A shorter method is to remove skins and dry the nuts, then cook in olive oil until brown, and while draining to sprinkle them with salt. Peanuts, pecans and walnuts can be prepared in the same way. Butter may be substituted for olive oil, if desired.

T. J. Ritter

ONE HUNDRED CHOICE RECIPES

on

CANNING, PICKLING, PRESERVING, JELLIES, JAMS, MARMALADES, RELISHES, CATSUPS, SPICES.

FOREIGN WORDS IN THE MENU.

In this list are many of the foreign words used on menu cards in hotels, with their translation:

Cafe--Coffee.

Demitasse--After-dinner cup of coffee.

Frappe--Semi or half-frozen.

Fricasse--Stew.

Fromage--Cheese.

Glace--Frozen.

Cafe au lait--Coffee with hot milk.

Neufchatel--A soft Swiss cheese.

Timbale--Pie crust baked in a mould.

Croutons--Bread toasted in squares, used for soup and in garnishing.

Bouillon--A clear broth, usually of beef.

Au Gratin--Dishes baked, prepared with cheese.

Menu--Bill of fare.

Puree--Ingredients rubbed through a sieve; usually the term given a thick strained soup.

Tutti Frutti--Various kinds of fruits (chopped fine).

Consomme--Clear soup.

Jus--Gravy or juice of meats.

CANNING.

1. Apples and Quinces.--Pare and cut the apples and quinces, the same amount of each. Cook the quinces in enough water to cover them until tender. Remove these from the water and cook the apples in the same liquid. When these are done put in a jar or kettle a layer of quinces, then of apples until all are used. Pour over them a syrup made of a half pound of sugar to pound of quinces, dissolved in a little water and let it stand over night. The next day heat them thoroughly and seal in cans.

2. Apple Sauce.--Take as many apples as desired, pare them and cut in quarters. Put in a stew pan filled about two-thirds with water and cook until tender. Remove from the fire and beat up thoroughly, adding a teaspoonful of butter to a quart of apple sauce, half cup sugar and grate in a quarter of nutmeg. Serve with or without cream.

3. Apples to Can.--Cook the same as for apple sauce, leaving out all seasoning and sugar. Put in glass jars and seal. When these are opened in the winter, just add such seasoning as may be desired.

4. Apple Butter.--Five pounds of brown sugar, three gallons of cooked apples, one quart of cider vinegar. Boil this down to about two gallons and season with cinnamon.

5. Canned Pears.--Prepare a syrup of one pint of water and one cup sugar to one quart of fruit. Before doing this, have your pears all pared and ready for the syrup when done. As you pare each piece of fruit drop it into a dish of cold water. This will prevent the fruit from turning dark. When the syrup has come to a fast boil, put in the pears carefully and boil until they look clear and can be easily pierced with a fork, which will probably be about twenty minute. Then done place in glass jars.

6. Canned Pineapple.--Pare the pineapple and cut in slices about one-half inch thick. Be sure that all the eyes are cut out, as the fruit will spoil quickly if these remain in. Make a syrup of one pound of sugar to quart of water. When this syrup becomes thick enough, add the fruit and let boil about fifteen minutes. When done place in glass jars and seal while hot.

7. Canned Peaches.--Pare the peaches and cut in halves and lay in a dish of cold water until ready to put in the syrup. Make a syrup of one quart of hot water to a pound of sugar. Let this cook to a syrup, then add the fruit. Cook about eight minutes. Put in glass jars and seal while hot.

8. Brandy Peaches.--Drop the fruit into hot water. Let it remain there until the skin can be taken off easily. Make a very thin syrup and cover the peaches, after skin has been removed. Boil in this thin syrup until the fruit can be pierced with a straw. While these are cooking make another syrup, very rich, into which put the fruit after it is done. Remove this from the fire and add an equal quantity of brandy while the syrup is still hot.

9. Canned Plums.--Wash the fruit well in cold water, then add one pound of sugar to a pound of fruit and let boil ten minutes. When done put in glass jars and seal while hot.

10. Canned Strawberries.--Wash the berries thoroughly before removing the stems. Then weigh them, and to each pound of berries allow a half pound of sugar. Let these boil about ten minutes, and they are ready for the cans.

11. Canned Rhubarb.--Take rhubarb when it is young and tender, or even the later plant will do, cut into pieces about an inch long. Wash well and put in glass jars, into which has been poured a cupful of cold water. Fill the jar full of the rhubarb and then cover completely with water. Seal and put in a cool place. When opened in the winter time a few minutes' boiling with sugar added will make a delightful sauce.

12. Canning Corn.--The following is one of the safest and surest ways of canning sweet corn, without the use of acids or the necessity of putting up the corn with tomatoes, etc. Cut the corn from the cob and put in glass jars, pack down tightly and screw covers on loosely to allow the air to escape. Set the jars in a boiler and fill the boiler with cold water until it reaches the rim of the jars and let boil for four hours. Remove the cans and when sufficiently cool tighten the lids and set them away. A good plan is to place a board or some corn husks in the bottom of the boiler on which to set the jars to prevent them from cracking. Corn will keep as long as you want it if canned in this way.

13. Canned Grapes.--Take the grapes and wash them thoroughly. Have two dishes on the table. Put the seeds in one dish and the skins in the other. Boil the pulp until all the seeds come out easily, then put through a sieve. Add the skins, allowing one-half pound sugar to one pound of fruit. When done put either in glass jars or crocks, taking precaution to see that they are sealed tightly in either case.

TABLE FOR CANNING FRUIT.

	Quantity of sugar per quart.	Time for boiling fruit.
Apricots	2 teacupfuls	10 minutes
Sour Apples	1-1/2 "	10 "
Crab Apples	2 "	25 "
Black Berries	1-1/2 "	6 "
Gooseberries	2 "	8 "
Raspberries	1 "	6 "
Huckleberries	1 "	5 "
Strawberries	2 "	8 "
Cherries	1-1/2 "	5 "
Currants	2 "	6 "
Wild Grapes	2 "	10 "
Sour Pears (whole)	2 "	30 "
Bartlett Pears	1-1/2 "	20 "
Peaches (in halves)	2 "	8 "
Plums	2 "	10 "
Peaches (whole)	1 "	15 "
Pineapple (sliced)	1-1/2 "	15 "
Quinces	3 "	30 "
Rhubarb	3 "	10 "
Tomatoes	0 "	20 "

PICKLING.

1. Tip-Top Pickles.--Take one peck green tomatoes, one dozen large onions. Slice both of these in separate kettles, sprinkling salt between the tomatoes, then letting them stand two hours. Pour scalding water over the onions and let stand until wanted. After the tomatoes have stood the desired length of time squeeze the liquid off from them, also the onions and arrange in a crock in alternate layers, sprinkling celery seed between them (white and black mustard seed). Pour over this a quart of vinegar and a pint of sugar brought to a boil. This is ready for use when cold.

2. Chow-Chow.--Two quarts tomatoes, half dozen green peppers, one dozen cucumbers, two white onions, two heads cabbage. Chop these all fine and let stand over night, sprinkling a cup of salt on it. In the morning drain off the brine and season with one ounce tumeric, one tablespoon celery seed, half teaspoonful cayenne pepper, one ounce of the following spices, cinnamon, allspice, one ounce black pepper, one quarter ounce cloves, one cup brown sugar, vinegar enough to cover, then boil two hours.

3. Sweet Apple Pickle.--Pare the apples, leaving them whole, then take three pounds of sugar, two quarts of vinegar, one-half ounce each of cloves and cinnamon. Boil them in part of the vinegar and sugar until tender; then take them out, heat the remainder of the fluid and pour over them. Care should be taken not to boil the apples too long, as they will fall to pieces.

4. Sweet Tomato Pickles.--Peel and slice eight pounds of tomatoes, four and a half pounds of sugar, one pound of mace and cinnamon mixed, one quart of vinegar and one ounce cloves. Mix all together and boil one hour.

5. Standby Pickles.--Chop fine one gallon green tomatoes, twelve onions, slice fine two gallons of cabbage, one gallon vinegar, one pound brown sugar, half an ounce turmeric powder, one tablespoon black pepper, one ounce celery seed, one tablespoonful ground allspice, also ground cloves, white mustard, one quarter pound, and one gill salt. Boil all these together for two hours except spices, stirring well. When taken from the fire add the spices, put in air-tight jars. If this pickle is kept in a cool, dry place, you will find them in perfect condition at the end of the winter.

6. Pickled Peppers.--Select nice large peppers, cut off the stems and rind. Then put into strong hot brine, repeating this for three mornings, and then drain off and cover with hot vinegar. When wanted to use, take out of brine and stuff with creamed sweetbreads and mushrooms and serve on a lettuce leaf. This makes a very attractive and appetizing dish.

7. Piccalili.--One-half peck green onions, sliced, one peck green tomatoes, one cauliflower, one peck small cucumbers. Leave in salt water twenty-four hours; then put in a kettle with a handful of scraped horse-radish, one ounce tumeric, one ounce cloves (whole), one-quarter pound whole pepper, one ounce cinnamon, one pound white mustard seed, one pound English mustard. Place in kettle in layers and cover with cold vinegar, boil fifteen minutes, stirring constantly.

8. Sweet Pickled Peaches.--Make a liquid of three pounds brown sugar, one pint strong cider vinegar, and small handful each of cinnamon and cloves and bring to a boil. Wash clean, but do not peel, several pounds of peaches. Put in as many peaches as the liquor will cover; cook until moderately soft and put into jars. Cook all alike, and pour liquid over them. These are delicious.

9. Chopped Pickles.--Chop and mix together one peck green tomatoes, two large heads of cabbage, three green peppers, one small cup salt, let stand over night and drain. Then cover with cider vinegar and boil until soft; drain again and mix with one tablespoon cloves, same amount of mustard, two pounds each of raisins and sugar, one-half cup grated horse-radish, three chopped onions, celery and salt to taste. Hot vinegar enough to make moist, can rather dry.

10. Pickled Onions.--Select small white onions, peel and boil them in equal portions of sweet milk and water for ten minutes, or until tender, drain and pour scalding spiced vinegar on them immediately. Never use allspice, as it darkens the onions.

11. Pickled Red Cabbage.--Choose purple red cabbage, slice into a colander, sprinkle each layer with salt, let it drain two days, then put into a jar, pour boiling vinegar enough to cover, put in a few slices of red beet-root. A few spices in bunches and thrown in after being salted, will look red and pretty.

12. Pickled Grapes.--Select grapes that are not quite ripe, but dark colored, pick from the stem and wash, put in glass jars; in a separate kettle make a syrup of sugar and vinegar and boil a few minutes, add spices to suit the taste; pour over grapes and seal jars.

13. Spiced Cherries.--Take nine pounds of fruit, one pint cider vinegar, four pounds sugar, one-half ounce cinnamon bark, one-half ounce whole cloves, let the syrup come to a boil before putting in the fruit; cook the fruit until the skin breaks, then take out the fruit and boil the syrup down until thick, pour over the fruit hot.

14. Beet Pickles.--Cook beets in hot water until tender. Then remove the skin and if the beets are large slice them, as you would for table use. Place these in a glass jar. Take a quart of cider vinegar, one cup granulated sugar, teaspoonful of salt, let this come to a boil, then pour over beets. If vinegar is very strong dilute about half. When these are opened in the winter, you will think you are eating fresh beets from the garden.

15. Pickled Cauliflower.--Choose good firm cauliflower, and full size. Cut away all the leaves and pare the stalks. Pull away the flowers in bunches. Steep in brine two days, then drain them, wipe dry and put in hot pickle.

16. Pickled Cabbage.--The cabbage should be sliced and salted for two or three days, then placed before the fire for twenty-four hours, spread upon a dry cloth, after which they are put into a jar, and covered with spiced vinegar.

17. Cantelope Sweet Pickle.--Select melons not quite ripe, weighing about seven pounds in all, put them in a weak brine over night. Then boil in weak alum water until transparent. Take them out and place in a jar. Then take 1 quart cider vinegar, 2 ounces stick cinnamon, 1 ounce cloves, 3 pounds granulated sugar; let this boil, then add the cantelope, cooking it twenty minutes longer. Pour in a jar and close tight. Scald it over for two mornings.

18. Mother's Pickled Blackberries.--Take three quarts of blackberries, one quart of sugar, one quart vinegar. Put all together at the same time into your kettle and boil ten or fifteen minutes. No spices are required. After standing a few weeks they are very nice.

19. Pickled Brocoli.--Choose the whitest, closest and finest vegetables before they are quite ripe, pare off all green leaves and the outside of the stalks. Parboil them about five minutes in well-salted water. Then drain well and pull the branches in convenient sized pieces and put into a jar of pickle, prepared as follows: Heat vinegar to boiling point, add a little mace and whole red peppers, and pour hot over the brocoli.

20. Mixed Pickles.--One quart boiled beets, chopped fine, one quart raw cabbage chopped fine, two cups sugar, tablespoon of salt, one teaspoonful red pepper, one cup grated horse-radish. Cover with cold vinegar and keep from the air.

21. Mustard Pickles.--One quart small cucumbers, one quart large cucumbers, cut in pieces, one quart large tomatoes, two quarts small onions, three heads cauliflower, six red and six green peppers cut in strips. Put these in separate dishes and let stand over night. In the morning drain off and cook in separate dishes of clear water until nearly tender. Then put together and boil a short time in the following paste: One ounce pulverized tumeric seed, half pound ground mustard, two cups flour, seven cups sugar, one gallon vinegar. This is an excellent recipe.

22. Sweet Pickled Peaches.--Boil together four pounds sugar and one pint vinegar to twelve pounds of fruit. Add the fruit and let it come to a boil; the next day drain off the liquor and boil again; do this three times and your pickles are delicious; add cinnamon to the liquor and stick two or three cloves in each peach.

23. Sweet Pickled Prunes.--Soak four pounds prunes for two or three hours, then steam them ten or fifteen minutes. While the prunes are soaking, boil together for ten minutes two pounds sugar, one pint vinegar, one ounce each of cloves and cinnamon and one-fourth of an ounce of ginger. After the prunes have been strained, pour the hot vinegar over them and boil all together until the prunes are soft. These are delicious.

24. Celery Sauce that Mother Used to Make.--Take fifteen large ripe tomatoes, two red peppers, two onions, two and one-half cups vinegar, two stalks (arrowroot) celery, eight tablespoons sugar, two spoons salt; chop all fine and boil one and one-half hours.

25. Spiced Tomatoes.--Take red and yellow pear-shaped tomatoes; prick two or three times with a fork, sprinkle with salt, let stand over night, pack in a glass jar and cover with vinegar, prepared as follows, for a half-gallon jar: 1 pint vinegar, 1 teaspoon ground cloves, 1 teaspoonful ground cinnamon, 1 teaspoonful ground allspice, 1 teaspoonful pepper, 1 tablespoon sugar. Let this come to a boil and pour over the tomatoes; after they get cold tie strong paper over them.

26. Ripe Cucumber Pickles.--Take twelve large cucumbers and remove the pulp. Cut them in strips about two inches wide and four inches long. Let these stand while you boil for a few minutes the following: 2 pounds sugar, 1 ounce cinnamon, 1/2 ounce cloves, 1 pint vinegar. Be sure and skim this while it is boiling, then put in the cucumbers, letting them cook until tender. Take the cucumbers out and let the liquor boil for fifteen minutes. Pour this over the cucumbers and cover tight.

27. Green Tomato Pickles.--Chop a peck of green tomatoes and stir in half a cupful of salt. Let these drain over night. Then add 3 green peppers, chopped, 1 teacup of grated horseradish, 2 quarts of vinegar, 1 teacupful of sugar. Let this all boil, stirring occasionally, gently, until the tomatoes are tender, then add a large spoonful of cinnamon and cloves. These are very good and easily kept.

28. Pickled Tomatoes.--Select tomatoes that are thoroughly ripe, and let them lie in strong salt and water for four days; then put them down in layers in jars, mixing with them small onions and pieces of horseradish; then pour on vinegar, cold, after having spiced it. Be sure and use plenty of spices, cover carefully and let stand for a month before using.

29. Green Tomato Sauce, for Meats or Fish.--Slice two gallons of green tomatoes without peeling; slice one dozen good sized onions; one quart of sugar, two quarts vinegar, two tablespoons each of salt, ground mustard, and ground black pepper, one tablespoonful of cloves and allspice. Mix all together and stew until tender, stirring frequently to prevent scorching. Put up in small glass jars.

30. Chili Sauce.--One peck ripe tomatoes, one pint vinegar, one cup sugar, two red peppers, three sweet peppers, six large onions, one tablespoon each of cinnamon, pepper and salt. Chop the onions and peppers fine. Boil for two hours.

31. Tomato Relish.--One peck good ripe tomatoes, chop and drain, 3 large onions, a peppers, red or green, 3 heads celery, chopped fine, 3/4 cup salt, 2 pounds brown sugar, 2 oz. white mustard seed, 1 oz. cinnamon, a pints vinegar. After the tomatoes have drained thoroughly, mix in the balance of the recipe. Do not cook; keep in a jar. This relish cannot be beaten. Everyone will like it.

32. Tomato Catsup No. 1.--Take one gallon ripe tomatoes, peel them, one teaspoon allspice, one tablespoon mustard, one red pepper; let all boil, then strain and to this add one tablespoon salt, one teaspoon ground pepper, one teacup vinegar, two pounds granulated sugar. Let all of this boil until reasonably thick, or as thick as desired.

33. Aunt Mary's Catsup.--One cup onions, one peck ripe tomatoes (chopped), one and one-half cups celery, one cup horseradish (grated), one cup sugar, half cup salt, one cup white mustard seed, two red peppers, one teaspoon each of black pepper, ground cloves, mace, cinnamon and celery seed, one quart vinegar. Drain tomatoes thoroughly, before adding spices. Keep this in stone jars and tie closely and it will keep nicely for a year or more.

34. Gooseberry Catsup.--To one pound of gooseberries, use three-fourths pound sugar and spices to taste. One pint of vinegar to ten pounds of the fruit. Boil two hours. This is delicious.

35. Spiced Vinegar for Pickles.--(This can be used generally for pickles.) 1 gallon of vinegar, 1 pound of sugar, 2 tablespoonfuls of allspice, 2 tablespoonfuls mustard seed, 2 tablespoonfuls celery seed, 2 tablespoonfuls salt, 1 tablespoonful of tumeric powder, 1 tablespoonful of black pepper, 1 tablespoonful mace, 2 nutmegs, grated, 3 onions, 1 handful grated horseradish. This can always be relied upon as good.

36. Tomato Catsup No. 2.--1 gallon tomatoes (strained), 6 tablespoons salt, three tablespoons black pepper, 1 tablespoon cloves, 2 tablespoons cinnamon, 2 tablespoons allspice, 10 pints vinegar, boil down to half. One peck tomatoes will make one gallon strained.

37. Bottled Pickles.--Wash the pickles and pour boiling water over them, letting them stand for four hours; to every gallon of vinegar take 1 teacup of sugar, 1 teacup of salt, 1 teaspoonful of pulverized alum, one ounce of cinnamon bark, 1/4 of an ounce of whole cloves. Boil spice and vinegar and pour over the pickles. Seal while hot.

38. Sliced Cucumbers.--Peel and slice one gallon of cucumbers and soak them over night in weak salt water. Drain and put them in weak vinegar on the stove and let them get hot; drain and pack in glass jars. Then bring to a boil, one quart vinegar, a few slices of onions, sugar and spices to taste. Then pour this over the cucumbers, while hot, and seal.

39. Grandmother's Dill Pickles.--Fill a stone jar with alternate layers of grape leaves, fresh cucumbers, dill and salt. Cover with water and an inverted plate; place a brick on the plate to keep all under water. The cucumbers will be ready for use in about two weeks.

40. Mustard Pickles.--Wash the pickles and put in fruit jars, then cover with the following dressing, do not cook the pickles or dressing: 1 cup salt, 2 cups dark brown sugar, 1 cup Colman's mustard, 1 gallon vinegar, mix together and put over pickles.

41. Green Tomato Pickles.--One bushel tomatoes, slice and put in salt water over night. The next morning put tomatoes in kettle after draining them, with five pounds of brown sugar, 1/4 cup cloves, ten cents worth cinnamon stick, two quarts vinegar. Boil until the tomatoes are tender.

42. Oyster Catsup.--Squeeze through a sieve 1 pint of oysters with the juice, then add 1 pint of sherry or white wine and salt to taste. Flavor with garlic, celery, etc., if desired. Add two or three ounces of mixed spices. Simmer fifteen or twenty minutes, strain and bottle when cold.

43. Pepper Catsup.--Select about twenty-five red bell peppers without removing the seeds. Add 1 pint of vinegar and boil until tender, stirring constantly. Rub it all through a sieve. Set aside the juice. Pour over the pulp another pint of vinegar with two tablespoonfuls brown sugar, 2 or 3 ounces mixed spices. Stir altogether and boil down one-half. Strain through cheese-cloth and bottle when cold.

44. Grape Catsup.--Select grapes that are ripe, but not soft. Pick them over carefully and add to five pounds of grapes, half as much sugar (by weight), 1 pint vinegar, two or three ounces of mixed spices, and salt to taste. Boil until it thickens. Bottle when cold.

45. Pickled Cherries.--Select firm and medium ripe cherries. Fill a wide-mouthed glass bottle or jar with them, then add two tablespoons of salt, and fill the jars with cold vinegar. Seal and let stand six or eight weeks before using. These are very good.

46. Sweet Mixed Pickles.--For sweet mixed pickles, scrape and wash half a dozen young carrots, and parboil in salted water for three or four minutes, then drain and set aside to cool; meanwhile cut into strips. Then take six green tomatoes, three large white onions, one large red pepper, (taking out the seeds) three sour apples, one small cupful of tender string beans, and finally the carrots treated in the same manner; place all these ingredients together in the preserving kettle in which they are to be cooked, adding salt and a very little paprika and allow them to stand for twelve hours. When ready to cook drain off the water that will have formed, adding sufficient vinegar to well moisten, one cupful of sugar, a tablespoon olive oil and two teaspoonfuls of celery seed tied in a piece of muslin, for about five minutes. Remove from the fire and mix in quickly half a teaspoonful ground English mustard blended with a little vinegar; seal immediately in small well-closed jars.

47. Corn Relish.--One dozen ears of corn, one large cabbage, one large red pepper, chop all these up fine together, mix thoroughly and add one pound of brown sugar and one quart of vinegar, salt to suit taste. Let this all come to a boil.

48. Mustard Pickles.--One hundred small cucumbers (if you get the larger ones cut them in two), one-half peck of the tiny white onions, large head of cauliflower, one pound brown sugar, 1-1/2 cups flour, 1/2 pound mustard, five cents worth of tumeric powder, one cup salt. The cucumbers are to be soaked in salt and water over night and drained in the morning, put in the vinegar and let come to a boil, then add your onions and cauliflower. Take the flour, mustard and tumeric powder, work to a cream with a little vinegar, then gradually stir into the boiling vinegar to thicken it. Boil this all about fifteen minutes. Watch every minute as this scorches very easily.

49. Spiced Currants.--Steam and wash the fruit carefully, and for every four pounds of currants take two pounds of brown sugar, one pint cider vinegar, one tablespoon each of ground cinnamon, cloves, mace, nutmeg and allspice. Put in the fruit and boil all together for a half hour. Fill into wide mouthed bottles, lay a paper wet with vinegar over the currants and tie up the mouth of the bottle with paper.

50. Spiced Grapes.--Five pounds of grapes, three pounds of granulated sugar, half pint of vinegar, two teaspoonfuls each of cinnamon, allspice and cloves. Pulp the grapes, boil skins until tender. Cook the pulp soft and strain through a sieve, add to skins. Put in spices, sugar and vinegar and boil thoroughly. Seal.

51. Ginger Pears.--Peel a dozen large pears which are not quite ripe and cut into long, thin strips. Add two-thirds as much sugar as you have fruit, the juice of a lemon, two-thirds cupful of water and a desertspoonful of ginger. Boil all together until the fruit is transparent, and serve as a relish.

52. Tomato Soye.--One peck of ripe tomatoes, one dozen large onions, three large red peppers, one gallon best vinegar, twenty-four tablespoonfuls brown sugar, twelve teaspoonfuls ground cinnamon, twelve teaspoonfuls of salt, six teaspoonfuls of ground ginger and six teaspoonfuls of ground cloves. Chop the tomatoes, onions and peppers fine and add the other ingredients. Let simmer for three hours.

53. Spanish Pickles.--One peck of green tomatoes, one dozen onions, sprinkle with salt and let stand over night and strain off the juice. Allow one pound of sugar, one-fourth pound whole white mustard seed, one ounce ground black pepper, one teaspoonful ginger and one of cinnamon. Mix dry. Put a layer of tomatoes and onions in a kettle and sprinkle with spices, then tomatoes and so on until all are used. Cover with vinegar and let boil two hours, after which pack in jars and set in cool place.

54. Chili Sauce.--Take five large onions, eight green peppers, and chop fine with thirty ripe tomatoes. Add five tablespoonfuls of brown sugar, three tablespoonfuls of salt and eight cupfuls of vinegar. Boil all together two and a half hours and bottle for use.

55. Green Tomato Pickles.--Half bushel green tomatoes, six large onions, six large peppers, one-fourth pound white mustard seed, and three tablespoonfuls celery seed. Chop all fine together, put in layers, one of tomatoes and onions and one of salt, using in all a half cupful of salt. Let stand over night. In the morning squeeze dry and put on to boil in two quarts of vinegar. Cook until tender, when nearly done, add one pound of sugar, put in cans and seal.

Green Beans Pickles.--"Green beans with the strings taken off and placed in a kettle, salted and cooked until tender, then place in jars, fill with good cider vinegar and seal tightly."

PRESERVES.

1. Rhubarb Preserve.--1/4 lb. almond or walnut meats, chopped, 3 lbs. rhubarb, 3 lbs. sugar, rind and juice of 2 lemons, boil until thick. Serve with meats.

2. Preserved Pears.--Pare the fruit and drop into a bowl of cold water to preserve the color. When all are pared, put into a pan of clear, cold water, and boil until almost tender. Make a syrup of the water in which the pears were boiled, allowing one pound of sugar to each half pint of water. Drop the pears into the syrup and cook them slowly until they can be pierced with a silver fork. Put the fruit into hot jars and cover with boiling syrup. Seal.

3. Fig and Rhubarb Preserve.--Wash dry and cut up three pounds of figs and seven pounds of rhubarb, put them into a basin, add six pounds of sugar, one cupful of water, two heaping teaspoonfuls of ground ginger and the juice of two large lemons. Cover and leave for twelve hours. Boil for half an hour. Divide into jars and cover. This is an excellent preserve and keeps well.

4. Preserved Cherries.--Select large, rich, red cherries; stone and weigh them, adding three-fourths of a pound of sugar for each pound of fruit. After the stones have been taken out, allow them to stand in a stone jar over night; in the morning put them in a preserving kettle and cook until clear. Put in glass tumblers and cover the tops when cool with melted paraffin, before putting on covers.

5. Strawberry Preserves.--The fruit for this must be solid, and must be used as soon as they are gotten ready, and not sugared down. To one pound of sugar add one pound of fruit. Use just enough water to keep them from sticking, and put fruit, sugar and water all on at the same time, and let them cook twenty minutes. Then spread on flat dishes and set in sun for three or four days, and then put in glass jars. They will need no more heating or cooking. These are considered fine.

6. Lemon Butter.--Take two nice large lemons, grate the rind and use the juice, two eggs, two cups of sugar, small lump of butter. Boil ten minutes in double boiler.

7. Apple Preserves.--Make a syrup of three-fourths pound of sugar to each pound of apples. Add a little lemon juice or sliced lemon; keep skimming this as it boils, and put in only a few apples at a time into the syrup, and boil until they are transparent; skim out and put in a jar. When the apples are done, boil the syrup down thick, then pour boiling hot over the apples and cover closely. Well flavored fruit, not easily broken, should be selected.

8. Apricot Preserves.--Pare the fruit very thin and stone it. Place the fruit in a porcelain or granite kettle, first a layer of fruit, then a layer of sugar, using pound for pound of sugar. Let this stand in the kettle for a day. The next day boil very gently until they are clear. Then place the fruit in a large pan or bowl and pour the liquor over them. The following day pour the liquor into a quart of codlin liquor, this being made by boiling and straining a pound of fine sugar with just enough water to make a syrup. Let the whole boil quickly until it will jelly. Put the fruit into it and bring to a boil, being careful to remove all the scum. Then put up in small jars.

9. Citron Preserves.--Select sound fruit, pare it and divide into quarters, (carefully take out the seeds) and cut in very small pieces, any shape you desire, and weigh it. To every pound of fruit allow a half pound of loaf sugar; put the citron on to cook until it is quite clear, then remove it from the kettle where it can drain, and pour out the water it was cooked in. Then put on the sugar you have weighed, with water enough to wet it through; let it boil until very clear, and before putting in the citron again add to the syrup two large lemons sliced, and a small piece of ginger root, to give it a fine flavor; then add the citron and let all cook together about fifteen minutes; fill the jars with citron and pour over the hot syrup, then seal up.

10. Citron and Quince Preserves.--Pare and cut the citron into inch pieces; boil hard in a medium strong alum water thirty minutes; drain and boil in fresh water till the color is changed and they are tender; wash the quinces carefully, pare, quarter, core and halve the quarters; boil the cores and parings in water to cover them, an hour and a half; remove them and add the prepared juice to the liquid; boil, and when they begin to be tender, add the citron and three-fourths of a pound of white sugar to every pound of the fruit. These are delicious.

11. Preserved Pears.--Have a pan of cold water ready to drop pears into after they are pared, halved and the cores removed. This will prevent them from turning black. Select smooth, sweet pears of a kind which will not break when cooked. Put a little over one quart of granulated sugar into your preserving kettle; add just water enough to moisten the sugar; when warm put into this two quarts of pears; let them cook very slowly several hours; when the syrup is thick put your fruit in jars.

12. Pineapple Preserves.--Pare and slice the pineapple. Then weigh the fruit and allow a pound of sugar to a pound of fruit; then put a layer of the slices in a jar and cover them with a layer of sugar; do this until the apples and sugar are used up; let them stand over night. The next morning take the apples out of the syrup, cook the syrup until it thickens, replace the apples and boil fifteen minutes; remove the pineapple from the syrup and let them cool, then put in jars and pour the syrup over them. A few pieces of ginger root boiled in the syrup will improve it.

13. Tomato Preserves.--Select small, pear-shaped tomatoes, not too ripe. Prick with a needle to prevent bursting, and put their weight in sugar over them. Let this stand over night, then pour off the juice into a preserving kettle and boil until it is a thick syrup, clarifying it with the white of an egg; add the tomatoes and boil until they look transparent. One lemon to a pound of fruit, sliced thin and cooked with the fruit, together with a piece of ginger root, will improve it.

14. Preserved Strawberries. No. 1.--Take a couple of quarts of berries at a time, remove the stems, and place in a colander. Pour water over them to cleanse them. Make a syrup of two pounds of white sugar and a half cup of water. Drop the berries into this and allow them to boil rapidly for twenty minutes, removing all scum that rises, but do not stir the fruit. Pour into tumblers, and when you are done cook your syrup and juice to a jelly and fill up your jelly glasses. Keep in a dry place.

15. Preserved Strawberries. No. 2.--To one pound of berries use three-fourths of a pound of sugar,--in layers (no water). Place in a kettle on the back of the stove until the sugar is dissolved into syrup; then let it come to a boil, stirring from the bottom. Spread on platters, not too thickly and set out in the hot sun till the syrup thickens--it may take two or three days. Keep in tumblers or bowls like jelly. Strawberries done in this way retain their color and flavor.

16. Spiced Currants.--Three pounds white sugar, five pounds ripe currants, one tablespoonful each of cinnamon, nutmeg, cloves and allspice. Boil currants one hour, then add sugar, spices and a half pint vinegar, boil a half hour longer.

17. Spiced Gooseberries.--Six quarts gooseberries, nine pounds sugar, cook one and a half hours, then add one pint vinegar, one tablespoonful each cloves, cinnamon and allspice. Boil a few minutes. When cold they should be like jam. Boil longer if not thick enough.

18. Tomato Preserves.--Peel the tomatoes and to each pound add a pound of sugar and let stand over night. Take the tomatoes out of the sugar and boil the syrup, removing the scum. Put the tomatoes in and boil gently twenty minutes; remove fruit again and boil until the syrup thickens. On cooling put the fruit into jars and pour the syrup over. The round yellow variety of tomato should be used and as soon as ripe.

19. Preserved Pears.--Peel the fruit which should not be overripe, cut into halves, extract cores and throw at once into a dish of cold water.

From the water put into jars, arranging the pieces as compactly as possible, cover with cold water and then drain off. Make a syrup of sugar and water, allowing a teacupful of sugar to a jar and fill the jars to the brim; put on the covers, without rubbers and place in a kettle of cold water over the fire. The water in the kettle should come to the neck of the jars. Note carefully when the water comes to a boil, and let it boil twenty minutes or more, according to ripeness of the fruit. Take the jars from the water, adjust the rubbers and screw on the tops tighter and tighter as the jars cool. A plated knife should be used in peeling the fruit as a steel one discolors the fruit.

20. Preserved Peaches.--Plunge the fruit into boiling water to make the skins come off easily, then throw into cold water. For three pounds of fruit use one pound of sugar and half a teacup of water. When the syrup boils put in the peaches, a few at a time, and cook until tender. Fill jars as for pears. The stones will add to the flavor.

21. Brandied Peaches.--Put the peaches in boiling water for a few minutes, when the skin will peel off easily. Make a syrup of half a pound of sugar and half a teacupful of water for each pound of peaches. Skim as the scum rises in boiling, then put in the peaches and boil them gently until tender, no longer. Take them out carefully and fill your cans or jars. Remove the syrup from the fire, and add to it half a pint of best brandy to every pound of peaches.

22. Preserved Quinces.--Pare and quarter, taking out cores and all hard parts. Boil in clear water until tender; spread out to dry. Allow a half pound of sugar and one-third cup water to a pound of fruit. When the syrup boils, put in the fruit, set back on stove and cook very slowly for an hour or more if not too tender, as the longer it cooks the brighter will be the color. Put in jars, the same as other fruit.

23. Preserved Grapes.--A delicious preserve can be made of California grapes. Cut each grape with a knife and extract the seeds; add sugar to the fruit, pound for pound; cook slowly for half an hour or longer until the syrup and pulp of the grape are perfectly clear and transparent.

24. Purple Plums Preserved.--A very fine preserve can be made from these plums, if you take equal weight of fruit and sugar. Take a clear stone jar and fill it with the fruit and sugar. First a layer of fine granulated sugar, then the plums and so on until the jar is filled. Cover them and set the jar in a kettle of water over the fire. Let them stand in the boiling water all day, filling up the kettle as the water boils away. If at any time they seem likely to ferment, repeat this process. Any housewife trying this recipe will be greatly pleased with the results.

25. Spiced Grapes.--Select five pounds of nice grapes, pulp them, and boil until tender. After the pulps are thoroughly cooked, strain through a sieve, then add to it three pounds of sugar, two teaspoonfuls of cinnamon and allspice, and half teaspoonful of cloves. Add enough vinegar and spices to suit the taste. Boil thoroughly and cool. This is very nice.

26. Spiced Peaches.--Take five pounds of peaches, wipe them thoroughly and boil until tender in one quart of vinegar and two pounds of brown sugar. When done remove them from the liquid, and add one ounce each of cinnamon, cloves and mace. Boil the liquid for some time after the spices have been added, then place the fruit in jars and pour this over them.

27. Pear Chips.--Ten pounds of pears sliced thin, seven pounds of sugar, four lemons boiled soft; press out the juice and pulp; chop the peel very fine. Boil the fruit and sugar together until soft, then add the lemon, a half pound green ginger root scraped and cut into small pieces. Let the above mixture boil until quite thick. This can be placed in jelly glasses, and will keep nicely. This is an excellent recipe.

JAMS AND JELLIES.

1. Crab Apple Jelly.--Select nice ripe apples, wash and cut out any imperfections; place on the stove and cover with water, cook slowly until soft enough to strain, then take them off and drain through a jelly bag. To every four pints of juice use three pints of sugar; heat the sugar very warm in the oven. Boil the juice fourteen minutes, stir in warm sugar, and boil altogether three to five minutes, then turn into moulds or jelly glasses.

2. Apple Jelly.--After you have selected nice tart, juicy apples of good flavor, pare them, core and quarter, then put them with the skins and cores, in a jar in a slow oven. When they are quite soft, strain all through a coarse muslin bag, pressing hard to extract all the flavor of the fruit. Put a pound of loaf sugar to every pint of juice and the juice of one lemon, and put the liquor over the fire in a preserving kettle. Boil steadily for twenty minutes or so, skimming occasionally. Boil the jelly glasses in hot water and fill them with the jelly while hot. This jelly will keep for an unlimited time if kept in a cool, dry place.

3. Currant Jelly.--The currants should be washed very thoroughly, but do not stem; put in a kettle, scald them but do not cook. Cool and strain; boil the juice alone for twenty minutes. Weigh the sugar, and to a pint of juice use a pound of sugar. Have the sugar in the oven browning lightly and heating thoroughly. When the juice has boiled twenty minutes stir in the sugar until it dissolves; then put into glasses and keep in a cool place.

4. Blackberry Jelly.--Cook the berries until tender, then strain the juice from them. Add an equal quantity of sugar. Boil hard for twenty minutes, then pour into moulds or jelly glasses.

5. Cranberry Jelly.--Take two pounds of sugar, granulated, one quart of water and three quarts of cranberries. Cook thoroughly, mashing all the berries fine, then put all through a fine sieve. Return the juice to the stove and cook fifteen minutes more; pour into glasses and seal when cool.

6. Grape Jelly.--Select grapes that are partially ripe, as they make the prettiest jelly, and to every eight pounds of fruit take a large cupful of water; put them into a porcelain-lined kettle and boil until quite soft; strain through a cloth. Measure the juice, then measure and put away the same quantity of sugar. Let the juice boil half an hour, then add the sugar and let it boil five or ten minutes longer. All jellies to be good, should have nearly all the boiling done before the sugar is added.

7. Rhubarb and Apple Jelly.--Cut up your rhubarb and wash it; put on the fire without any water at all. Take good sour apples, pare and quarter and cook in a very little water. Strain the juice from both and put them on the stove to cook for fifteen minutes. Then add the heated sugar, using three-fourths as much sugar as juice. Boil hard for twenty minutes, turn into glasses and set in the sun, if possible, for half a day. Seal the next day.

8. Spiced Grape Jelly.--Take grapes half ripe, crush all the juice out well and strain. Take equal quantities of juice and sugar; to each quart of juice add one-half teaspoonful of cloves and one tablespoonful cinnamon. Cook very hard for twenty minutes, then remove from the stove and pour into glasses.

9. Rhubarb Jelly.--After the rhubarb has been thoroughly washed and cut up in small pieces, stew until tender in a preserving kettle. Strain through a jelly rag and flavor with extract of lemon. Put in enough to suit the taste. To each pint of juice add a pound of sugar; boil until it jellies on the skimmer, then remove and place in glasses. Keep in a cool place.

10. Orange Marmalade.--Cut the oranges in half; remove the pulp with a spoon, take one lemon to five oranges, preparing the same way. Then cut the shells of the oranges in two, scrape out the white lining and put the skins on to boil; weigh the pulp, take half as much sugar, and simmer together fifteen minutes. When the skins are transparent and tender, take up, putting several pieces together, cut it quickly into the narrowest possible strips. Mix these with pulp and sugar; cook until very thick. Put in glasses and then when cold, seal.

11. Blackberry Jam.--Take two quarts of blackberries, one quart fine cooked apples, two quarts of sugar, boil these all together for twenty minutes. This is very easily made and is very good.

12. Plum and Apple Jam.--After canning plums, there is often some left, not enough to fill a can; a very nice jam can be made of this by putting it through a sieve; and adding the same quantity of good apples, cooked. Sweeten to taste and put in a very little cinnamon and cloves. Cook an hour, then tie up in jars when cold.

13. Tomato Marmalade.--Pare and slice without wetting four pounds of unripe tomatoes, Give them a slow boil for several hours until a large portion of the water has evaporated; add for each pound of tomatoes three-quarters of a pound of sugar and two sliced lemons. Boil for one hour longer.

14. Raspberry Jams.--To three or four pounds of ripe red raspberries add an equal quantity of white sugar. Crush the whole well in a preserving kettle; add one pint of currant juice and boil gently until it jellies upon a cold plate; put into a small jar and cover with brandied paper. Tie over them a thick paper and keep in a dark, cool, dry place.

15. Strawberry Jam, with Red Currants.--Take four pounds of strawberries, one pint of red currant juice, and two pounds of sugar. Place in a porcelain kettle and boil the berries and currant juice first, then add the sugar and boil up again, skimming well. Put in jars, cover with paraffin and keep in a cool place.

16. Peach Jelly.--Cook peaches and add a few kernels; when done strain. To one pint of peach liquor add one lemon and one pound of sugar. Dry and heat the sugar in a separate pan and let the peach liquor boil twenty minutes. Then add the sugar and boil a few minutes longer. This is very nice.

17. Gooseberry Jam.--To one pound of pulped fruit, add three-fourths pound of sugar. Stew the berries in a little water, press through a coarse sieve or colander. Then place on the stove again and add sugar. Boil three-quarters of an hour, stirring constantly. Pour in jars or jelly glasses.

CANDY MAKING

CONFECTIONERS' AND COMMON CANDY.

From the Following Recipes and Formulae, Hundreds and Even Thousands of Candies Can Be Made.

Candy Making at Home.--The proverbial "sweet-tooth" is a characteristic of the American people. Hundreds of tons of candy are annually consumed, and fortunes have been made in the business. The range of price is from ten cents to a dollar a pound, with some specially wrapped and boxed bon-bons exceeding the latter price, not because of intrinsic excellence, but because of the ornamental form in which they are presented. Cheap candies are adulterated and hence more or less detrimental to health. Good candies are not harmful, unless eaten to excess. Delicious candy may be made at home at much less cost, and some famous candies, like the "Mary Elizabeth" and others, had their beginnings in a home kitchen and grew into popular favor because of their known purity and uniform excellence. The cost of ten one-pound boxes of candies is estimated at $1.50 when materials are bought in small quantities; such candies, placed on sale at church fairs, bazars, etc., are sold at forty and fifty cents per box. Even at twenty-five cents a box there is a profit of ten cents on each box. Any girl can prepare bon-bons for a luncheon or a party at home, if she is willing to take the trouble,--which is, after all, a pleasure to many. She may save her own candy boxes and by getting a supply of paraffin paper, fill them again with candies quite as good as those they originally contained; or buy new boxes of the paper box manufacturers at two or three cents apiece. A box of home-made candy makes a nice Christmas or birthday gift.

Boiling the Sugar.--Confectioners recognize seven degrees in boiling sugar for candy, only four of which, however, are practically important. The first of these is the "thread" at about 215 degrees, by the sugar thermometer, when a short thin thread forms when thumb and forefinger are separated with a drop of syrup between them. This passes very quickly into a second stage, known as the large or long thread, when it can be drawn out to a considerably greater length without breaking. In a moment more it can be extended as far as the thumb and forefinger can be separated. The next stage is the "pearl," shown when the surface of the syrup is covered with bubbles, and is the stage at which much candy is made. The "blow" and "feather" come next; then the "ball" or fondant stage at 235 to 245 degrees; this is the third important stage. To discover when the boiling has progressed to this stage, drop a little of the syrup on to ice water, or dip the tips of the thumb and forefinger into ice water and then into the syrup and instantly into the ice water again with the syrup between. One can use a small stick in the same way. If the syrup can be rolled into a soft, but not sticky ball, it is in the soft ball stage; half a minute more of boiling will convert it into the "hard ball," if tested in the same manner. For fondant, the "soft ball" is chosen. The next is the "crack" or brittle stage, at about 300 degrees; when testing as above the syrup remains dry and hard on the fingers. This is the stage for candy that is to be pulled. At the caramel stage the syrup begins to brown, and must be quickly taken from the fire or it becomes "burnt sugar;" dropped in water it crackles and snaps.

Making the Fondant.--Fondant ("foundation") is the basis of all French bon-bons, so-called. An endless number of varieties may be made from it in combination with other material. There are two ways of preparing it. The easiest and simplest way is to add to the white of an egg an equal bulk of cold water and a teaspoonful of vanilla; beat until it froths, then add, gradually, one pound or more, of confectioners' XXX sugar; if the egg is large, one and one-half pounds may be required. Ordinary sugar will not do. Add sugar until the mixture forms a stiff paste; work this with a spoon until it is very smooth, then put away in a cool place for at least twenty-four hours, letting it stand in an earthen dish, and cover with a doubled napkin wrung out of cold water.

French, or Boiled Fondant.--Put into a porcelain lined kettle a pint of the best granulated cane sugar, half a pint of cold water and a salt spoon of cream of tartar dissolved in warm water. Stir it till the sugar is dissolved and boil rapidly without stirring or moving the kettle. Without a sugar thermometer it is impossible to tell exactly how many minutes it should boil, but usually in about ten minutes a little of the syrup dropped into cold water will form a soft waxy ball between the moistened fingers. It should then be removed from the fire and put in a cool place until the hand can rest with comfort on the bottom of the kettle. If too hot, it will turn back to sugar; if too cold, it will not thicken properly. In either case it is not spoiled, try again; add boiling water, stir until dissolved, and repeat the boiling. A little experience makes one to seize "the psychological moment" when the syrup is in the right condition. When the syrup has cooled to the degree indicated above, begin to stir it, using a long-handled wooden spoon. It will turn milky at first, then thick and white, finally dry on the edge of the dish and get so stiff it is difficult to stir. Then take the mass out on a marble slab and knead as you would bread dough; if you have no marble slab you may work it in the hands.

Flavor and Color.--At this point add the flavoring. Make little holes in the fondant with the fingers and put in each a little of the flavoring, working it through the mass. The essential oils are better than extracts. Three or four drops of any of the oils will flavor a pound of fondant. Three cents worth would be sufficient for a number of pounds. The flavor should not be strong. About a teaspoonful of any extract will be sufficient. If it is desirable to have two or more flavors, divide the fondant into the required number of portions, and have an assistant take up the kneading of each. Work the fondant until it is creamy. The pure food laws discourage the use of colorings, and it is difficult for the amateur to procure them in economical quantities. Cochineal can always be had and provides any number of shades of pink. Spinach heated over steam, and the juice expressed, gives a pretty green which is perfectly harmless. Work into the fondant as you used the flavoring oil or extract. The above ingredients will make one pound of fondant, all the beginners should undertake at one time. It may be kept for some time by packing it in glass cans and sealing tightly. The fondant should "mellow" for at least twenty-four hours before being used, especially as centers for chocolate creams, etc.; and these in turn should stand as long before being dipped. It is also advisable to let the bon-bons stand a day at least before being wrapped and packed. Choose a dry, clear, quiet day to make fondant, and do not attempt to work with it in wet weather; it is very sensitive to atmospheric conditions.

Making the Bon-bons.--After the fondant has stood the required interval it is ready to make up. Here comes in play the ingenuity of the candy maker in the employment of various accessories. Candied cherries, candied violets and rose petals, angelica, dates, figs, hard jellies, raisins, white grapes, crystallized ginger, cocoanuts, marshmallows, nuts, all are employed, while chocolate is used in so many forms that it gives rise to an entire class of candies. When ready to make up the bon-bons, roll the fondant out evenly and cut in squares of equal size; shape these with the fingers. The hands must be frequently dipped into ice water and wiped dry, but never greased. Roll the fondant into a ball; while still in the hand, press into the top an English walnut meat, or whatever decoration is desired, and lay on paraffin paper to harden. Another class is made by using a nut meat, say a blanched almond or pecan meat, a raisin, etc., as center, and rolling the fondant round it. The ball may be rolled in beaten white of egg and then in coarse white sugar. By using various centers, and ornamenting the tops differently a great variety of bon-bons may be made; in fact, hundreds or even thousands can be worked out by changing the flavor, nuts, coloring, etc.

Chocolate Candies.--If the American girl had to be restricted to one class of candies, there would be little doubt she would profess a preference for those prepared with chocolate.

Chocolate Creams.--To make chocolate creams, roll the fondant into balls of uniform size; let them stand on paraffin paper twenty-four hours or more. Also coat nut meats, raisins, candied cherries, etc., with fondant. In making a small quantity of chocolate dipped candies, get a small bowl that will fit into the top of the teakettle; into this cut half a pound of unsweetened chocolate and a lump of paraffin as large as a black walnut, and let them melt; when smooth and well mixed let cool a little, and then set on a hot soapstone. Have ready a colander and a long darning needle. Cover the bottom of the colander with paraffin paper, stick the point of the needle into the piece to be dipped, immerse in the melted chocolate, let it drip a moment, then push the eye of the needle through one of the holes in the colander, reach the other hand under and pull out the needle. There then remains no disfiguring hole in the bottom of the cream. When the colander is filled, lift the paper very, very carefully, and put in a cool place to harden. Unless the colander must be used again it is best to let the creams stand in it to harden. Nut meats, white grapes, candied cherries and the like, may be dipped in the melted chocolates and coated like the creams. If the chocolate gets too thick, thin it with a little olive oil or unsalted butter;

not with water which will make it grain.

Chocolate Creams. No. 2.--Put two cups of granulated sugar into half a cup of sweet cream. Boil five minutes from the time it begins to boil hard. Set the pan into cold water and stir in the flavoring, a teaspoonful of vanilla, usually. Stir until the candy is so stiff that stirring is difficult; drop from a spoon on waxed paper; as it hardens, mould into balls, and dip in chocolate as above.

Chocolate Candy, Plain.--Melt a square of unsweetened chocolate and stir into plain fondant, flavoring generously with vanilla.

Chocolate Caramels.--Put together over the fire one cup of molasses and two teacupfuls of sugar. Add a quarter of a pound of grated chocolate and a piece of butter the size of an egg. Boil, without stirring, fifteen to twenty minutes; pour into flat buttered dishes to a depth of one-third of an inch, and when nearly cold cut into squares. Wrap each in a square of paraffin paper.

Chocolate Nut Caramels.--Boil together a cup of molasses, a cup of sugar and half a cup of sweet milk until a little hardens in cold water. Cut into it a piece of butter the size of an egg and add a cup of chopped nuts. Proceed as above.

Chocolate Fudge.--Put into a porcelain lined pan two cups of granulated sugar, four sections of unsweetened chocolate, grated, one cup of milk and two rounded tablespoonfuls of butter. Cook, stirring constantly, for twenty minutes. Dip out a little of the mixture, put on a cold plate, and if it is done it will form a soft pliable paste. Flavor generously with vanilla, beat hard for a few minutes, then turn into buttered pans and cut into squares while warm.

CHOCOLATE CANDIES. Cocoanut Cream Bars.--Boil three pounds of granulated sugar, one cup of cold water and half a teaspoonful of cream of tartar until thick--or in the "ball" stage. Let cool slightly, then beat until creamy. Have ready a large cocoanut, grated; mix and stir well, then pour into shallow tins covered with buttered paper. When cold, cut into bars. Let stand a day or two before using.

Cocoanut Caramels.--Three pounds of granulated sugar, one cup of milk, a tablespoonful of butter and two teaspoonfuls of lemon extract. Put into a kettle, stir till dissolved; add one grated cocoanut and boil to the "pearl" stage. Pour into buttered pans, after it has cooled a little mark off into squares, and when cold break apart. Use when quite fresh.

Cocoanut Snow Balls.--Knead dessicated cocoanut into fondant; make into balls, and roll in grated cocoanut. Dessicated cocoanut may be used but is not as good as grated cocoanut.

MAPLE CANDIES. Maple Creams.--Beat thoroughly one cup of the best maple syrup and the while of one egg. With XXX confectioners' sugar, make it into a stiff fondant or paste. Use as the centers for bon-bons, or make into balls to be dipped into chocolate.

Maple Creams No. 2.--To two pounds of maple sugar add a cup of water and a quarter teaspoonful cream of tartar. Shave the sugar, and stir till dissolved. Boil without stirring to the soft ball stage; let stand in the kettle until cool, not cold; beat until creamy and pour into a shallow buttered pan.

Maple Balls.--Boil without stirring, two cups of shaved maple sugar and a cup of water. At the hard ball stage add a heaping tablespoonful of good butter. Beat till creamy. As soon as it can be handled form into balls and press the half of an English walnut or pecan on one side.

WAFERS.--To make wafers, boil without stirring two cups of granulated sugar, a half cup of water. When it will "spin a thread" set the kettle in cold water and beat till creamy. Flavor with peppermint, wintergreen, cinnamon, or any flavor you choose. Squeeze through a pastry tube upon paraffin paper in quantities that will spread to the size of a quarter dollar.

Chocolate Peppermint Wafers.--Take some of the fondant prepared as above, flavor rather strongly with peppermint and dip in sweet chocolate.

MOLASSES CANDIES.--Nothing pleases children more than a "candy pull." Turn them loose in the kitchen and let them make molasses taffy.

Molasses Taffy.--Boil a cup of good Porto Rico molasses, a cup of brown sugar and a piece of butter the size of an egg until a little will harden, in cold water. Cool on buttered plates, and as soon as it can be handled grease the fingers and pull till hard and light colored. To prevent boiling over, grease the edge of the pan or kettle in which it is boiled.

Molasses Taffy No. 2.--Four cups of sugar, two of molasses, half a cup of vinegar. Boil till it hardens in cold water, then add a tablespoonful of soda dissolved in a little water. Pour into buttered dishes and pull when sufficiently cool to handle.

Butter Scotch.--One cup of each of sugar and molasses, half a cup of vinegar, one tablespoonful of butter and a quarter teaspoonful of soda.

Nougat.--Nuts intended for nougat should be blanched, skinned and dried. Melt in a porcelain lined vessel, one pound of fine white sugar with two tablespoonfuls of water, stirring continually with a wooden spoon. Heat the nuts in the oven, after chopping them, add to the syrup, and stir for five minutes. Remove from the fire and add a little grated lemon rind. Oil a flat pan; place it in a warm place on the range and pour the candy into it. When brown, turn out of the mould, cut in cubes and wrap in oiled paper.

Nut Bars.--Chop any kind of nutmeats you prefer, or a mixture of nuts, moderately fine. Butter a shallow pan and spread the nuts evenly over the bottom. Boil one pound of granulated sugar with half a cup of water and a pinch of cream of tartar till thick, but not too brittle. Pour over the nuts and set aside to cool. When it begins to harden mark into bars with a sharp knife. Let stand several days, when it becomes soft and delicious.

Nut Loaf.--Chop nutmeats into small pieces and work into fondant. Make into a roll, and after standing a day or two, cut into slices. Chopped dates, figs and raisins may be used in the same way.

Peanut Candy.--Carefully remove the shells and brown skins from roasted peanuts. Put them an inch thick in a buttered pan. Boil a pound of crushed loaf sugar with three gills of water and a salt spoon of cream of tartar (to prevent graining) dissolved in water, to the caramel stage. The instant the sugar reaches that point, shown by its beginning to brown, it must be removed from the fire and the pan set in cold water to check the boiling; then pour over the nuts.

Pop Corn Candy.--Boil two cups of sugar, two tablespoonfuls of butter and a cup of water until it threads. Stir in four quarts of nice popped corn, rejecting all hard kernels, take from the fire and stir till cool. Make into balls.

Popcorn Baskets.--Prepare the corn as above, instead of making into balls, butter the bottoms of tumblers and press the candy around them to form little baskets, in which ice cream may be served or which may be filled with candies.

Sour Drops.--Strain the juice of three or four large lemons into a bowl, and stir in powdered loaf sugar till it is quite thick. Put into a pan and let boil five minutes, stirring constantly. Drop from the end of a spoon upon writing paper, and when dry keep in tin cannisters. Tartaric acid is generally used by commercial candy makers, but is much more injurious to health.

Crystallized Fruits.--Other Candies.--Boil two cups of granulated sugar with two-thirds of a cup of water until it hardens in cold water, do not stir. When it is brittle without being sticky, it is ready to use. Dip the fruit to be candied, sections of oranges, white grapes, cherries, squares of pineapple, etc., into this, and lay on paraffin paper. Dip a second time after the first has hardened, to ensure a good coat. Use the same rule for the syrup to glace nuts.

Cream Dates.--Remove the stones from nice dates. Replace them with the roll of flavored fondant. Or roll a blanched almond in fondant and stuff the date with it.

Hoarhound Candy.--Boil the hoarhound in a little water till the strength is extracted. Make a sugar syrup, adding the hoarhound to it; let it boil up and stir against the sides of the pan until it thickens. Pour out on paraffin paper dusted with fine sugar, and cut into squares.

Marshmallows.--Dissolve over a slow fire eight ounces of best gum arabic in three gills of water. Boil one ounce of marshmallow roots in a little water for half an hour. Strain, and boil down. Put this and the gum arabic solution with half a pound of loaf sugar, let it cook slowly till it makes a paste that can be rolled between the fingers to the "soft ball" stage. Then add the beaten whites of two eggs; when well mixed pour in a pan which should be lined with white paper, with enough projecting over the sides so that as the mixture cools it can he lifted out and cut in cups with a sharp knife, then rolled in powdered sugar.

Marrons Glaces.--Remove the shells from a quart of large Italian or French chestnuts. Let stand fifteen minutes in boiling water. Drain; rub off the skin; cover again with boiling water and simmer gently half an hour or till tender, but not soft. Drain in a sieve. Boil together one cup of granulated sugar and one cup of water; add the nuts and simmer until they begin to look clear. Make another syrup of one pound of granulated sugar and one cup of water; boil till it will spin a thread, add a teaspoonful of lemon juice and set aside till it cools a little; then beat till it begins to turn white. Set in a basin of hot water, flavor with vanilla, and when melted to a syrup, dip each nut. When coated, lay on paraffin paper to dry. These sugared chestnuts are highly esteemed as a sweetmeat and are expensive to buy.

Stick Candy.--Three pounds of granulated sugar, two cups of water, one teaspoonful of cream of tartar dissolved in a little warm water. Stir over the fire till the sugar is dissolved; cover the kettle while the syrup is boiling and skim carefully a few drops. When it will harden in cold water, take from the fire and add the flavoring and coloring, then pour on well buttered plates. When cool, pull, and make into sticks or mark off into squares.

School Girl's Delight.--Two cups of white sugar, three-fourths cup of golden color corn syrup and a quarter cup of water. Put into a granite sauce pan and boil till a little will crisp in cold water. Beat the whites of two eggs very stiff in a large bowl; pour the syrup very slowly into the bowl, beating the while, and beat and stir until it begins to harden. Then add one teaspoonful of vanilla, half a cup of chopped nutmeats, and five cents worth of dates, cut up with the scissors. Pour upon oiled paper in a flat pan and cut in squares. Those who eat this candy will ask to have it made again.

A Few Hints.--Many candy makers consider coffee A sugar, better than the granulated, as being purer. Choose a sugar that is dry, uniform in quality and with hard, sparkling crystals. Cane sugar is greatly to be preferred over beet sugar. When you can, let the sugar and water stand together for some time. The syrup may be stirred until it reaches the boiling point, but not afterward. Unless otherwise specified, cook over a hot fire. The syrup passes quickly from one degree to another and must be tested often and carefully. Cream of tartar must be dissolved in a little warm water before being put into the syrup. So also must soda. If you use nuts, be careful to remove every particle of shell and skin before putting them into the syrup. Almonds are blanched by letting them stand in boiling water for a few minutes and then nipping off the skins between the fingers. They should be warmed in the oven before being put into the syrup. Dessicated cocoanut should be steamed a few minutes before being used; put in a dish in a colander over boiling water. Use the fresh cocoanut if you can get it. Bonbons made of fondant are probably the easiest form of candy making for the amateur to attempt, and the most interesting on account of the variety possible through the use of other materials in combination.

OVER THREE HUNDRED MISCELLANEOUS RECIPES

A GOLD MINE OF INFORMATION FOR PROGRESSIVE HOUSEWIVES

HOUSEKEEPERS' ALPHABET.

Apples.--Keep in a dry place, as cool as possible, without freezing.

Brooms.--Hang in the cellarway to keep soft and pliant.

Cranberries.--Keep under water in cellar; change water monthly.

Dish of hot water set in oven prevents cake from scorching.

Economize health, time, and means and you will never beg.

Flour.--Keep cool, dry and securely covered.

Glass.--Clean with a quart of water mixed with a tablespoonful of ammonia.

Herbs.--Gather when beginning to blossom; keep in paper sacks.

Ink Stains.--Wet with spirits of turpentine; after three hours, rub well.

Jars.--To prevent, coax husband to your will rather than order him.

Keep an account of all supplies with cost and date when purchased.

Love lightens labor.

Money.--Count carefully when you receive change.

Nutmegs.--Prick with a pin and if good oil will run out.

Orange and Lemon Peel.--Dry, pound and keep in corked bottles.

Parsnips.--Keep in ground until spring.

Quicksilver and white of an egg destroys bedbugs.

Rice.--Select the large, with a clear fresh look; old rice may have insects.

Sugar.--For family use, the granulated is the best.

Tea.--Equal parts Japan and green are as good as English breakfast.

Use a cement made of ashes, salt and water for cracks in stove.

Variety is the best culinary spice.

Watch your back yard for dirt and bones.

Xantippe was a scold. Don't imitate her.

Youth is best preserved by a cheerful temper.

Zinc lined sinks are better than wooden ones.

Regulate the clock by your husbands watch, and in all apportionment of time remember the Giver.

1. Charcoal to Prevent Rust.--Charcoal absorbs all dampness, for which reason it should be kept in boxes with silverware to prevent rust.

2. A Needle Holder.--A guest of ours kept all her needles in a bottle in which was a pinch or two of emery. She said that it keeps them always bright and free from rust, and she finds it much easier to pick out the needle she wants from the bottle than from a tray.

3. Care of a Scrubbing Brush.--Scrubbing brushes should never be put away with their bristles upward, for thus the water would soak into the wooden part and the bristles would soon become loose.

4. In Case of Sickness.--In our home, when hot cloths are needed wet ones are put in a steamer, and water kept boiling underneath. In this way the cloths are more easily handled and can be applied as hot as needed.

5. To Tighten Cane-Seated Chair Bottoms.--Cane-seated chair bottoms that have sagged may be made as tight as ever by washing them with hot water and leaving them to dry in the open air.

6. For Chilblains.--To relieve the chilblains bathe the feet in warm water at night, then rub them with castor oil. This method will cure very bad cases.

7. Paint, Smoked by Kerosene Lamps.--Paint that has been smoked by kerosene lamps may be cleaned with kerosene, which can afterward be rubbed off with a clean brush.

8. A Use for Sacks.--Save all salt and sugar sacks; wash and boil them and they can be put to various uses. Salt sacks are nice to strain jellies through; are also nice to bake veal or beef loaf in. Sugar sacks make nice dish-towels.

9. Soap With Stove Blacking.--Use a half bar of laundry soap, and one cake of blacking. Put in an old kettle with three quarts of water. Boil down until thick. This will last a year.

10. To Remove White Spots from Tables.--Wring cloths out of very hot water, lay them over spot and remove quickly. Repeat if necessary. When dry, rub the furniture with some of the good polish.

11. To Clean Mirrors.--To clean a French mirror which has grown dull, rub with a cloth soaked in alcohol; follow this by rubbing with a dry cloth. The dullness will vanish, and the mirror will look like new. This method is used for cut glass with excellent result.

12. To Whiten Linen.--If you want your table linen to last do not use bleaching preparations. Use only clean soap and soft water. If the water is not soft, add a little ammonia.

13. Velveteen for Polishing Cloths.--Old pieces of velveteen that have served their original purpose should be saved for polishing cloths. They will answer perfectly the purpose of chamois and save buying anything fresh. When soiled the cloths may be washed in soapy water and dried in the open air.

14. For Clearing Vinegar.--Should your home-made vinegar refuse to settle, try this: To each gallon stir in a half pint of fresh milk and let stand undisturbed for twenty-four hours. The milk will form a curd at the bottom and all the dregs will settle with it, leaving the vinegar clear. Pour off very carefully.

15. Uses for Old Velvet.--A bit of velvet is a fine polisher for brass. It quickly removes the dust from woodwork, or shoes soiled from walking which do not need reblacking. For dusting a felt hat there is nothing better than a piece of chiffon velvet. It is also good to keep the bottom of a silk skirt free from the dirt. One housekeeper even uses a big piece of old velvet to rub her stove to a high polish after it has been blackened.

16. Removing Warts.--Warts can be removed permanently and safely by an application of a salve made by mixing common table salt into a yolk of an egg. Change the application daily, and within the week they will all drop out.

17. To Save Time by Sewing.--When sewing on plain garments, cut out several garments at a time, and save time by stitching all the straight seams, then doing all the basting, etc.

18. To Remove Stains from Blankets.--Stains on blankets and other woolen materials may be removed by using a mixture of equal parts of glycerin and a yolk of an egg. Spread it on the stain, let it stay for half an hour or more, then wash out.

19. Burn from Acid or Lye.--In case of a burn with carbolic acid or lye, the speedy application of sweet oil or olive oil will give almost instant relief.

20. To Wash Laces.--To wash delicate or tender laces put the lace in a fruit jar with shavings of some good soap, cover with warm water, let soak for awhile then shake, using if necessary several waters, then rinse in same manner, spread between pieces of muslin and roll up on a bottle or jar, and leave to dry. They will not be torn in this way and will look like new.

21. For Cut or Bruise.--Bind sugar and turpentine on the wound or bruise at once. The healing properties of this simple remedy cannot be surpassed.

22. Lemons; How to Obtain More Juice.--Lemons placed in a moderately hot oven, for a few minutes will yield a greater quantity of juice than if used in the ordinary way.

23. Whipping Cream.--If cream does not whip well, add to it the white of an egg, and the result will be very satisfactory.

24. To Clean Lamp Burners.--To remove the black gummy coating which sometimes comes on the brass parts of lamp burners, moisten the cloth with common household ammonia, rub it on sapolio, and apply it to the coated surface with the aid of a little elbow grease. A bright brassy surface will soon appear.

25. To Preserve Hot Water Bottle.--Fill with air, cork tightly, and hang in a cool dry place. This keeps the walls of the bottle from coming in contact with each other and prevents deterioration and decay.

26. Sweep Stairs with Paint Brush.--My mother uses a paint brush with long bristles for sweeping her stairs. With its use the work is more quickly and thoroughly done than by the old way, because the bristles reach every corner and crack as a cloth cannot do.

27. Washing Hair Brushes.--To wash hair brushes take a piece of washing soda, dissolve it in warm water, and stand the brush in it, taking care that the water covers only the bristles. It will almost instantly become clean and white. Place it in the air to dry, bristles downward, and it will be as firm as a new brush.

28. Loops on Towels.--Always have a loop on each end of the kitchen towel, where a roller is not used. Otherwise all the soil and the wear come on the lower end.

29. Changing Pillow Slips.--To change pillow slips without scattering the feathers all over the house, sew up the clean tick, all except a space of about twelve inches. Take the full pillow unopened and baste one side of the empty one to the full one. Then with a knife slit open the seam of the pillow, the twelve-inch space. Quickly baste the other sides together so they will not come apart easily. Then slowly push the feathers into the clean and empty tick, and when finished undo the basting and sew tightly. Soak the soiled ticks in cold water immediately to remove remaining feathers.

30. Use of Old Linen Collars.--Cut them up into narrow strips and use them for gas-lighting instead of using wax tapers. They make a steady flame and do not drip grease.

31. Discarded Toys.--My baby came in the other day hugging to his breast a toy tin goat. It was evidently one of the discarded playthings of a neighbor's child. On inquiry I found that the toy had been given to my boy, and he has taken so much pleasure in this castoff plaything that I have been saving his old toys and passing them on to other children of the neighborhood. I have discovered that in their baby hearts these are as good as new, because they have never played with them. It is nothing to them that they are not just out of the store.

32. To Clean Silver.--Try curdled milk for cleaning your silverware. Let the silver stand for several hours in the milk, and you will be surprised at the result.

33. Removing Stains.--Damp salt will remove egg stains from silver and tea stains from cups.

34. To Keep Free from Mould.--Jelly and jam can be kept entirely free from mould by pouring a thin layer of melted paraffin on top. This paraffin can be saved when the jelly is taken from the glass and used the next season so the cost is very small.

35. Hanging Out Clothes.--The other day I came across a peculiar clothes bar. It was the same as any other, except that the crossbars had been removed, and for them ropes had been substituted. The owner told me she had had her husband fix it for her the previous winter when she was bothered with salt rheum. "I hang up all the baby's little things, fastening them with clothespins, right here in the house where it is warm," she explained. "Then it is but the work of a moment to take the whole thing out of doors, and there is no fishing around for the tiny things when my hands are so cold they feel as though they would drop off."

36. A Fine Cutting Board.--I measured the top of my kitchen cabinet, and had a piece of zinc cut to fit it, allowing an inch for turning over the edges. My husband tacked it on, and I can cut meat and bread or anything on it, without harming it in the least, besides using it as a moulding board.

37. Convenient Place for Stiletto.--It will he found a great convenience to have the stiletto tied to the embroidery hoop by a ribbon about a foot long, when that little instrument is necessary for the work in hand.

38. Cleaning Paint and Varnish.--Many housekeepers have been annoyed by finding their paint and varnish brushes dry and hard. To soften them, heat to the boiling water point some good cider vinegar, immerse your brushes and allow them to simmer in it for a few minutes, then wash out in strong soapsuds and your brushes will be soft and pliable.

39. How to Keep Cookies from Burning.--To keep cookies from burning on the bottom, turn the baking pan upside down and bake on the bottom of the pan.

40. Non-Sticking Cake Tins.--Cake layers will not stick in cooking if a little meal is scorched on the cake tins and rubbed off with paper.

41. To Clean Sieve.--Hold a sieve which has been used for straining oatmeal, tomatoes, fruit, etc., at once under the faucet, or shake it in enough water to cover it, then slap it, and it is easily cleaned; if it dries first it is almost impossible to get it clean even by more time and effort.

42. Washing Clothes.--After the clothes have been soaked a while to loosen the dirt, spread on washboard, soap, and then rub with a common scrub brush. The dirt comes out easier and with much less wear on the clothes. Even when the washing machine is used, this is a help for the wrist bands that are not quite clean.

43. Discoveries.--When old clothes, like worn-out aprons or waists or linings come to hand, and are absolutely good for nothing else, cut them into small pieces, say eight or twelve inches square, some larger, and put them into a bag or box easily accessible. Then when something is spilled over on stove or floor, or mess of any kind is made, use these bits for cleaning up and drop them into the fire.

44. To Stretch Curtains.--Take curtains while wet and put on a curtain rod; also put a heavy rod as a weight on the lower hem. Hang one on curtain at a time at an open window and stretch the desired width.

45. Cleaning Windows in the Winter.--It is a hard task in the winter time to wash windows in the old way, but if it is very cold, windows can be cleaned by using "Bon Ami," The same is useful for cleaning bright pieces on stoves.

46. How to Kill Black Ants.--A request for information as to how to rid plants and trees of black ants, which was received at the Pennsylvania department of agriculture's division of zoology, elicited the following from Prof. H. A. Surface, State Zoologist. You can do this by finding the nesting places of the pests and making holes into the interior of them with a sharpened stick like a broom handle and pouring into each hole a half tea cup of carbon bisulphide. Fill the hole with earth and cover with a wet cloth or blanket to keep down the fumes and the ants will be destroyed at once. This is the best possible method for destroying ants of any kind.

47. Washing Windows.--It is better to wash windows on a cloudy day or when the sun is not shining directly on them. Before washing, dust them thoroughly inside and out, then wash the woodwork without touching the glass. For the glass use warm water, to which add a table-spoonful of kerosene to each pailful of water used. Dry with a cloth or chamois skin, wrung very dry; then polish with a soft cloth or soft old newspapers.

48. Home-made Soap Shaker.--A baking powder can with holes punctured in both cover and bottom, makes a fine soap shaker. Put all the small scraps of soap in this, and when you wash dishes, just put box and all in your dishpan and shake about. You will have a nice suds and no soap rubbing off on the dishes.

49. Cleaning Rugs.--When cleaning rugs first lay them out straight and brush with a stiff dry scrubbing brush. You will be surprised at the amount of dirt that is loosened and comes out in this way.

50. Clean Leather Furniture.--A good way to clean leather furniture is to add a little vinegar to some warm water and wash the leather, using a clean soft cloth. Wipe with a dry cloth. To restore the polish, mix two teaspoonfuls of turpentine with the whites of two eggs; beat a little and apply with a soft flannel cloth. Dry with another cloth and rub well.

51. Ironing Board, Conveniences for.--Try tacking a pocket on the under side of your ironing board to keep your holder, stand and sheet of sand paper in.

52. Clean Gilt Furniture.--Gilt furniture can be cleaned with sifted whiting made into a cream with alcohol. Cover a small space at a time and rub off before it hardens. To clean brass fixtures rub them with cut lemon and then wash off in hot water.

53. For Tufted Furniture.--For tufted furniture use a bicycle pump to remove dust. Garments to be stored for the summer months should first be aired well on a bright breezy day. Brush thoroughly and shake free of dust. Do not leave clothing out in the air after three o'clock in the afternoon, as from that time until dark all sorts of insects are seeking their beds. A trunk or box that has been thoroughly cleaned and sunned and then lined with fresh newspapers will prove an ideal place in which to store winter clothing. Sprinkle each layer with cloves and tuck newspapers well around them, moths detest printer's ink.

54. Clean Linoleum.--To clean linoleum add one cupful of bees-wax, shaved fine, to two cupfuls of turpentine and set on the back of the stove to melt. When cool it will be thick and ready for use. First thoroughly clean the linoleum and then apply the paste with a soft cloth. Rub in well, then polish with a dry cloth, preferably flannel. Linoleum treated in this manner will look like new.

55. For Broken Needles.--A receptacle for broken needles in her work basket would be a boon to any woman, and this one which I am about to describe is very easily made, takes up little space and is really very convenient, when one is busy sewing and dislikes to get up to take care of the dangerous bits of steel. Take a little two dram bottle (homeopathic style), crochet for it a snug covering made of embroidery silk or silkaline, crocheting it tightly and covering the bottle completely, using some bright color if desired. When you break a needle just slip the pieces right through the meshes of silk into the bottle; they will go in easily, but the holes will close up after them, retaining them in safety till the receptacle is full.

56. How to Carry House Key.--The pocketless woman often finds it troublesome to carry a key, especially the house key, when she goes out. If an old-fashioned split metal ring can be found, use it to connect the key to be carried to the circular end of a strong, sure acting safety pin, not necessarily of the largest size. If such a ring cannot be found, fasten pin and key together with a bit of fine wire, string or thread will be sure to break just at the wrong time. Then the pin may be fastened to the inside of the jacket or slipped inside of the shirtwaist band pinned to the undergarment, or attached to the skirtband and allowed to hang down outside.

57. A Sewing Room Hint.--Thread will not become knotted so often if the newly-cut end is put into the needle instead of the other end, which is already broken.

58. Convenient Addition to Kitchen.--One of the most highly-prized helps in our kitchen is a bird cage hook, one which can be hung on a nail, and thus easily changed from place to place. On this when placed over the sink, I hang macaroni, greens, etc., to drain; and when placed over the kitchen table, it is an ideal arrangement for holding the jelly bag.

59. To Remove Candle Grease.--A simple way to remove candle grease is to scrape off all that will come off in that way, lay over the spot a piece of heavy brown wrapping paper (butcher's paper) and press with a very hot iron.

60. Using Silk on the Machine.--When sewing on the machine with silk, it often unwinds and twists around the spool spindle in a very trying manner. To avoid this make a hole in a small piece of felt and slip it on the spindle before the silk is put on.

61. A Shoe Cover.--When packing my trunk for a journey, I have found it to be a good scheme to use my stockings for shoe covers, this saves the added bulk of paper, and the shoes will be found less liable to muss up other things if protected by this clean and handy stocking covering. A stocking occupies practically no room when drawn over a shoe, and the two together will be found quite handy to tuck into chinks into which they alone can fall.

62. To Press Skirts.--An easy way to press skirts is to use a sheet of paper in place of a cloth; lay the folds, or plaits and in place of ironing over a wet cloth take a sheet of common magazine paper lay it on the goods and iron. This presses the skirt very well and keeps the shine off and will, I think, give more satisfaction than if pressed with a damp cloth or ironed on the wrong side.

63. How to Attach Holders to Kitchen Apron.--Pin two holders with long tape at each side of the apron when cooking. They are convenient for handling hot kettles or dishes.

64. To Pack Music.--An excellent place in which to pack away sheets of music that are not in constant use is a large box fitted with a hinged cover and upholstered in cretonne, after the manner of shirtwaist boxes so much in vogue. Such a box is kept in the hallway of a small flat, where room is at a premium. The music cabinet was full to overflowing and there was no closet shelf that could be utilized, as so often happens in an ordinary house. An unused shirtwaist box was suggested and has been found to answer every purpose, besides providing an extra seat when such a seat was desirable. The box seems to fit in as an article of furnishing and the reason for its being there would never be asked.

65. Pie Crust, How to Bake.--Bake empty pie crusts on the outside of the tin, instead of the inside, and they won't shrink.

66. Let the Poison Bottle Tinkle.--A wise house mother with half a dozen little folk needing all sorts of medicines and medical applications, has purchased in a toy shop a handful of little bells, and when a bottle containing poison is added to the medicine closet it is adorned with a bell tied around its neck with a narrow ribbon. No danger with the bottle thus equipped of taking by mistake, in the dark, the dangerous medicine. The moment the poison bottle is touched the little bell tinkles its warning.

67. A New Night Lamp.--Mothers who have timid little ones will appreciate the new night lamp, the apparatus of which may be carried to the country in a trunk or handbag. This apparatus consists of a small wooden float through which passes a tiny wick. An ordinary china teacup is half filled with cottonseed oil, the little floating wick placed in this, and a match touched to the upright wick. While the sides of the cup prevent thc direct light of the flame being visible to the person in bed, a pleasant dim light is cast over the room.

68. Time Saved in Sewing.--In a family of small children there are a great many buttonholes to be made. A quick way to make them in the everyday underwear, is on the sewing machine. Sew back and forth, leaving a small space in the center, three or four times where the buttonhole is wanted, and cut in the space left, being careful not to cut the stitching. In making little dresses, or slips after the skirts are sewed up, attach the gatherer to the machine and gather the top and bottom of sleeves and skirt. In this way work is quickly done.

69. Stews and Hash, How to Make.--Stews and hash made of fresh meat or round steak instead of scraps, are delicious. When the steak is to be used without being ground, select only tender, young, pinkish pieces; otherwise it will be tough in spite of prolonged cooking.

70. Dusters.--Another good idea about dusters. Do not use anything that comes handy, but get squares of five-cent cheese cloth or silkoline, fold a neat hem, and whip it nicely around, then turn and go back the other way. These materials are the best one can use, as they do not leave lint behind. Always wash the dusters after the sweeping day. No one can do clean work with soiled tools; besides dusters ruin the hands.

71. Broom Bags.--Good material for a broom bag or cover is old gauze underwear. The goods takes up dust very readily, and is easily rinsed out; or a piece can be thrown away without waste.

72. To Settle Coffee.--An economical and satisfactory way to settle coffee is as follows: Beat one egg well with an egg beater and pour over one pound of freshly-ground coffee, mix very thoroughly and no trace of dampness then remains. The coffee may then be put away as usual, and when used it will be found as clear as amber.

73. Stocking Tops for Convenient Holders.--For soft, convenient holders use old stocking tops. Take two thicknesses, cut in squares, bind all around with some bias pieces left from calico dresses and sew a brass ring on one corner.

74. Hat Hangers.--It is often convenient to hang up hats, even "Sunday-go-to-meeting ones." To make sure that everyone will stay hung up, and not fall to the floor to be soiled or crushed under foot, sew a loop of narrow ribbon or elastic braid or even shoestring, to the middle of the lining, making the loop long enough so that it will reach to the edge of the hat crown when the loop is pulled out. This can be done and passed over hook or nail or peg, and the hat hung over it, and even if the hat gets a hard knock, it's a case of "sure on" every time.

75. To Freshen Bread.--To freshen bread pour cold water all over the loaf, drain quickly, and place in the oven. When the outside is dry and hot remove the loaf and it can scarcely be detected from a new one.

76. Renewing Wringer Rollers.--A neighbor rejuvenated a worn-out wringer the other day by covering the rolls with white felt. She cut the felt so that it would just come together, not overlap anywhere, and caught the edges together with close stitches. It bids fair to last her as long again, and it is certain that just now the wringer does as good work as any new one.

77. To Prevent Cake Tins Sticking.--Flour the baking tins after greasing them. If the flour is shaken all over the grease, and the tins rapped, you will have no difficulty with sticky cakes which break when you try to get them out. Lard is just as good as butter, for it will not taste through the flour.

78. Substitute for Chopping Bowl.--When chopping mincemeat, tomatoes, or large quantities of other fruit, you will probably find that your chopping bowl is a good deal too small. Get a clean wooden box with a thick bottom, from your grocer and use it instead of your bowl. You will notice a great saving of time is effected.

79. Save the Gas.--Cut strips of asbestos paper an inch and a half wide and long enough to go around the burners of the gas range. Pin together to form a ring, slip over the burner, and all the heat will be concentrated where wanted. In this way the gas can be half turned off and the same results obtained.

80. To Prevent Pitchers Dripping.--Syrup or other liquids will not drip from a pitcher if a little butter or grease is rubbed on the edge and under the side of the lip.

81. Medicine Cupboard.--An array of ordinary medicine bottles is always unsightly, and a nuisance, too, on cleaning days. Have a tiny cupboard with tight closing door, or a well-fitted curtain, and there is gain in looks and convenience.

82. To Prevent Tablecloths from Blowing Off.--We had some pieces of brass chain, and found them splendid to run through the hems of the tablecovers when in use on the porch in summer. Such "loaded" covers do not blow off easily, consequently they save quite a bit of annoyance and laundering.

83. To Mark Poison Bottle.--When you purchase a bottle of poison run a brass-headed tack into the top of the cork. It serves as a marker, and children will be more cautious of the marked bottle. If the label comes off or is discolored, the marker remains as a warning that the bottle contains poison.

56

84. To Remove White Spots Caused by Hot Dishes.--For polishing tables after hot dishes leave a white spot, take a cloth wet in alcohol, then have one wet in sweet oil. Do it quickly and spots will disappear at once.

85. Stains from Fly Paper, to Remove.--Almost anything that has come in contact with sticky fly paper can be thoroughly cleansed by sponging with kerosene. The odor will soon evaporate if the article is exposed to the air for a short time.

86. A Use for Ravelings.--In trimming a tablecloth to be hemmed or stitched, one very frequently has to cut off quite a piece of the linen. Ravelings from these pieces are invaluable for mending old cloths, and ought to be saved for that purpose,

87. How to Remove a Glass Stopper.--The obstinate glass stopper in a glass bottle will yield to a string of seaweed around the neck of the bottle. Friction, heat, slight outside expansion solve the problem.

88. To Prevent Starch from Boiling Over.--Add a small piece of butter the size of a walnut when the starch comes to a good boil. This not only gives a nice, smooth finish and makes the ironing easier, but it prevents the starch from boiling over.

89. To Hold Sheets in Place.--I worked out a little scheme which has saved me a lot of trouble and inconvenience, so I thought I would pass it on. The sheets and bed clothes are constantly pulling out at the foot, so one day I sewed three buttons on to my mattress with strong thread, and worked buttonholes in the hems of the sheets to correspond, and since then have not had trouble with their pulling up in the middle of the night.

90. Hints for Bathing the Baby.--It is a great advantage when bathing the baby to have all the towels heated before using, as they absorb the moisture much more readily and are very pleasant and soothing to the delicate skin. This is also excellent for bathing an invalid as it greatly hastens the work and lessens the danger of catching cold. It acts like a charm for the child who dreads a bath, this is usually a nervous child who does not like the feeling of the towel, on the wet surface of its skin; complains of feeling damp; and refuses to don its clothing when a less sensitive child would be perfectly comfortable.

91. A Satisfactory Shoe Polisher.--Not long since I ripped up a velvet covered hat, only to find the velvet impossible for further use in the millinery line. A threw it into the big waste basket that stands near my husband's shoe cleaning apparatus. He caught up the velvet in a hurry one day to take a spot off a shoe, and now has it laid away as a treasure in his shoe kit. He says it is the best polisher he ever had, and uses it on my fine shoes to his own entire satisfaction.

92. Tasty Way of Preparing Beef-tea.--Beef-tea will not prove so monotonous to an invalid if a different flavoring is used each day, as dove, bay leaf, or celery.

93. To Preserve Silk Gloves.--If white or delicately tinted silk gloves are wrapped in blue paper, then in brown they will not discolor. The chloride of lime in white paper is injurious.

94. Red Ants to Destroy.--Dry sulphur, sprinkled about in cupboards or flour chests where small red ants frequent, will rid the place of the pests.

95. Kitchen Account Book.--I have found a kitchen account book is a very useful record. I have a small vestpocket note book hanging by a string and pencil near my kitchen range. A page or two is devoted to each month's use. The month and year are entered at the top of page. When groceries are purchased, the date, article and price are noted, and summed up at the end of each month. It makes a handy, permanent record, showing how long supplies last, the expense of one month compared with another, and the monthly average of each year.

96. A Brick Pincushion.--A brick pincushion was a dressmaker's ingenious way of making easy work of basting and sewing long seams. She took a common red brick, topped it with a flat oblong cushion size and shape of the brick, covering the whole neatly with a bright chintz cover. This standing on the edge of her cutting table was in constant use, and proved a great convenience.

97. Fruit Stains, to Remove from Hands.--When your hands become stained from paring fruit or vegetables, dip them in soap suds then rub thoroughly with coarse salt, and they will become smooth and white.

98. Eyelet Embroidery, Suggestions for.--For some time after I began doing "eyelet work" I wondered if there was not some way to fasten the thread after completing an eyelet. A friend of mine showed me a solution of my problem. It was to leave the last three loops loose enough so that I could pass the thread back through them after completing the eyelet. Then I carefully pulled each of these loops down and cut off the thread. This obviates the necessity of any knots that are so unsightly, and at the same time, the thread is firmly secured.

99. To Prevent Stockings from Wearing Out.--Paste pieces of velvet soft side up, into the heels of your shoes, bottom and back, and you will find your stockings darning reduced by a big per cent.

100. Needle Sharpener.--I know a woman who always keeps a small piece of whetstone in her machine drawer for sharpening needles when they become blunted. It is a great scheme, and saves a lot of needles, as I have proved to my own satisfaction.

101. Burned Kettles.--If you have had the misfortune to burn your kettle it may be made smooth and clean by filling it with ashes and water, leaving it for an hour or so, then washing with clear water.

102. Children's Petticoats.--When making washable petticoats for her small daughters, a mother whom I know attaches two skirts to one belt, which in turn is sewed to a little lace trimmed waist.

The lower skirt is made of white cambric, and the top skirt is of swiss embroidery. This arrangement saves time in dressing the little ones and their upper and lower petticoats are always of the same length and set evenly.

103. Systematic Housekeeping.--A friend of mine who has a six-room apartment delights in taking care of it in sections, one room a day. On each of the six days in the week one room is thoroughly cleaned and put in order. She plans, if possible, to add some little touch of adornment, a new rocker, or vase, or table cover, or pin-cushion. In this way there is always something new to notice and admire, and yet no new and startling changes and never any accumulation of hard work.

104. To Keep Grape Fruit After Cutting.--When half a grape-fruit or melon is left from a meal, place it cut side down on a china or agate plate, so that no air can reach it, and the fruit will keep as though it had not been cut.

105. How to Freshen Nuts.--We had a lot of nuts that became too dry to be good, and were about to throw them away, when a friend told us of a very easy and practical way to freshen them. It was this: to let them stand over night in a solution of equal parts of milk and water, then dry them slowly in a moderate oven. They tasted so fresh and proved to be such an economy, that we thought the idea well worth passing along.

106. Measure the Eggs.--Try measuring the whites of eggs for angel food instead of counting them, for best results.

107. Kerosene Lamps.--A neighbor who has to use kerosene for lighting purposes told me the secret of her bright lights. After cleansing the lamps well and trimming the wick she fills the oil chamber, and drops into it a piece of camphor gum about as large as a marble. It is a very simple method of securing a splendid light.

108. Baking Help.--When creaming butter and sugar for cake or cookies, add two tablespoonfuls of boiling water, then deduct this amount from the other liquid used. Beat hard with a spoon, and the mixture will become a light creamy mass in one-third of the time it otherwise would take.

109. To Destroy Disagreeable Odors.--The cooking of onions, cabbage, or frying articles always leaves a disagreeable odor in our house. To get rid of this I place an old tin over a lighted burner and sprinkle some ground cinnamon on it. When the tin is very hot I carry it through the house on the dustpan, leaving behind me the pleasant pungent odor of the spice.

110. The Last Step.--A great many times last winter I had to go into the cellar to tend to the furnace when it was too light to light a lamp, and too dark to enable one to see easily. Almost every time I had to feel around to be sure that I was on the bottom step. One day my husband was doing some painting in the cellar and happened to think that a little white paint on that step would help. Now we wonder why we did not think of it before.

111. Truth spoken with malicious intent is greater error than keeping of silence where wrong is meant.

112. Boiled Potatoes.--Boiled potatoes should be served as soon as they are cooled. To make them dryer, drain off the water quickly, shake them in a strong draught of air and do not put back the lid of the kettle.

113. To Prevent Ripping.--When hemming table cloths, sheets, etc., on the machine, try the following plan: Sew the hem as you always do, but when you come to the end, instead of leaving a long thread to tie it, to keep from ripping, simply lift the presser-foot, turn the goods around, place the presser-foot down again and sew back over the same seam again, and sew about half an inch more. It makes a neat finish and no danger of the hem ever fraying out.

114. To Mix Corn Bread.--To mix corn bread more easily warm the bowl that it is to be mixed in.

115. Mending Table Linen.--To mend table cloths and napkins, take the sewing machine, loosen the tension, lengthen the stitch, place embroidery rings over the place to be mended, and stitch back and forth closely. You have a neat darn, easily done. When laundered you can scarcely see it. Do the same with stockings.

116. Children's Toy.--Save all the empty spools, and when any dyeing is done in the household, drop the spools into the fluid for a few minutes, and they will make fine playthings for the children on a rainy day.

117. To Keep Coffee From Boiling Over.--To keep coffee from boiling over add a lump of butter about the size of a small marble.

118. Sour Milk Pancakes.--We are very fond of sour milk pancakes, and have often had to go without any in the winter when the weather was cold, just because the milk would not sour. I have learned to put a teaspoonful of vinegar in a pan of milk, that I wanted to use for the cakes the next morning, and find that it never fails me in making the milk sour. Placing the pan over the register for the night helps matters along.

119. When the Wooden Scrub Bucket Leaks.--When the wooden scrub bucket leaks pour sealing wax into the crevice and paint on the outside. This will make it last for a longer period.

120. Rust Spots on Clothes.--Many rust spots on clothes are caused by bits of soap adhering to the latter when they come in contact with the bluing water. The discovery has been of great help to me because I can now easily avoid having these unsightly marks. I merely cut the soap into small pieces, and tie them in a salt bag I keep for the purpose. With this treatment the soap dissolves just as quickly but does not come into direct contact with the clothes.

121. Cleaning Stoves.--Before blacking my stove I rub soap on my hands, as if washing them, letting the soap dry on. When washing my hands after the work is done, the blacking and the soap come off together easily, leaving no stain on the hands.

122. Left-Over Peaches.--If there are not peaches enough left from an opened can to go around, mix them with orange pulp and a little sliced banana and the family will find them improved.

123. Substitute for Cream in Coffee.--For a substitute for cream in coffee put a pint of fresh milk into a double boiler and let it come to a boil, stirring often. Beat the yolk of one egg very light and pour it into the boiling milk and mix well.

124. Cooking cauliflower.--Soak cauliflower an hour before cooking. Put into boiling water to which a tablespoonful of salt is added. Boil from twenty to thirty minutes according to size of the head.

125. Uses for Child's Broom.--A child's broom should find place in the bath room. It can be kept in the clothes hamper, and will be useful in sweeping under the bath-tub.

126. Dish Cloths.--Dish cloths are often neglected. They should be kept scrupulously clean, and in order that they may be so they should be washed out carefully with soap, and well rinsed each time they have been used. After this has been done they may be hung in the air to dry. Some people, however, like to have a stone jar containing a solution of soda by the sink and to keep the dish cloths in it when not in use.

127. Watch for the wishes of the customers and not the hands of the clock, and some day you will have your boss's job.

128. We judge our neighbor as queer and eccentric, but with the same measure comes back his judgment of us.

129. Uses for Men's Worn Out Collars.--Men's collars when worn out, can be opened and bound together as a memorandum book which can be laundered each Monday.

130. Broiling Meat.--A little salt thrown on the coal flame will clear it for broiling meat.

131. Combinations of Cherries and Pineapple.--A combination of cherries and pineapple makes a most-delicious pie.

132. Crepe Paper for Dish Closet.--A pretty effect for the dish closet may be found in crepe paper. Some prefer white, but a tint harmonizing well with the china is pretty too. Have it to fall about three inches below the edge of the shelves and ruffle the edge of the paper by stretching it lightly between forefinger and thumb.

133. Boiling Rice.--One cook always puts a very little lemon juice in the water in which she boils the rice. She claims that it keeps the rice white and the grams whole and separate. It may be worth trying.

134. To Remove Grease from Silk.--Grease may be removed from silk and woolen clothes by the use of magnesia. Scrape a quantity upon the spot, cover with a brown paper and place a hot flat-iron over it. The heat of the iron acts upon the magnesia and when the iron and the paper are removed and the magnesia brushed off the spot will have disappeared.

135. Hemstitching.--When hemstitching wears out, take serpentine braid and stitch it across twice on the sewing machine. This makes the hem look neat and last a long time.

136. Moths.--When moths get into dresser drawers, sweep them clean, expose the wood to the sunlight and with an atomizer spray turpentine where the pests are liable to be. A lighted match or sulphur candle will kill them.

137. To Remove Putty.--To remove putty, rub a red hot poker over it, and cut off the putty with a steel knife.

138. New Method for Sprinkling Clothes.--Turn the nozzle of the hose to a fine spray and sprinkle the clothes while they are on the line; a very quick and good method. All plain pieces may then be rolled up and laid in the basket as they are taken down, while starched articles need but a little further hand sprinkling on portions not exposed.

139. To Open Packages of Breakfast Food.--To open packages of breakfast food and keep boxes in a dust proof condition until empty, make an opening in the side of box close to top by forcing a tablespoon through cardboard and turn flap downwards. The flap will fit back snugly in place each time package is used.

140. Preparing Oranges for the Table.--In preparing oranges for the table take a sharp knife, cut the skin straight around, insert the handle of a spoon turned over flat to fit the orange and loosen shell by forcing spoon to within one-half inch of the end, around one side, then the other, after which cut the orange through the center, making two parts. Then turn the skin back in cup form, making a pretty decoration for the table and serving as handles. Always serve in halves.

141. To Make a Muddy Skirt Wash Easily.--To make a muddy skirt wash easily and look white, take sour milk and dilute with water;

soak the skirt in it over night, then wash in the usual way; the skirt washes easier and looks white.

142. To Make Stained Water Bottles Clean.--To make stained water bottles clean and bright, put in salt and pour on vinegar, let stand a few minutes then shake. Rinse in clear water.

143. Sanitary Window Screen.--Try tacking cheese cloth on the pantry window screen frame. This admits air that is sifted free from smoke and soot, before it comes into the pantry.

144. Cheerfulness at Meals.--Cheer during the meals will do away with the need of digestive tablets. Make it a rule to come to the table smiling, and continue to smile, though the food does not suit you and everyone else is down on their luck. Your smile will prove contagious.

145. Uses for Stale Bread.--Take stale biscuits and grind them with a food chopper; toast in oven to a delicate brown. Serve with plenty of sugar and cream. Makes fine breakfast food and saves the stale bread.

146. Washing Lemons.--Always wash lemons before grating them, not only to remove any foreign matter sticking to them, but in order to remove the tiny insect eggs so often seen on them in the disguise of black specks. They may be kept fresh indefinitely, if wiped perfectly dry and placed in a sealed top glass jar.

147. To Give Vinegar a Nice Flavor.--A small button of garlic in a quart of vinegar will give it a mysterious delicious flavor, and it will immensely improve salads or anything in which it is used.

148. If Mice are Gnawing Holes.--If mice are gnawing holes in the house, rub common laundry soap around the gnawed places, and you may depend on it they will cease labor in that district.

149. To Teach Darning.--If young girls are taught to darn on canvas, the method of weaving the stitches is easily explained and put into practise.

150. Bed Sheeting.--Sheeting should never be cut, but should be torn into lengths, usually two and a half yards for medium beds.

151. Browning Potatoes.--For some kinds of frying the griddle is better and has a less tendency to grease than the frying pan. Among the other things potato cakes browned on a hot greased griddle are especially crisp and delicious.

152. To Keep Bread from Souring.--You will find that light bread will not sour so quickly in summer if it is not covered when taken from the oven. This steam is unnatural and should be allowed to escape or it soaks into the bread, making it clammy and more liable to sour. Let the bread cool gradually then put a clean cloth in a large stone jar, place the bread in and cover with the cloth, before covering with the stone, or wooden lid. This keeps bread fresh and moist from one bake day to another.

153. Never Pour Scalding Water into Milk Vessels.--Never pour scalding water into milk vessels; it cooks the milk on the sides and bottom of the vessels making it more difficult to clean such articles. Rinse them first with cold water. This same rule applies to cleansing of catsup bottles.

154. The Water Pipes in the Kitchen.--The water pipes in the kitchen will not be so unattractive, if painted the color of the kitchen woodwork.

155. To Brush Fringe of a Doilie.--Do not use a comb for the fringe of doilies as it pulls out the fringe, but brush it with a nail brush.

156. Wash Suits.--Large buttons should be removed from wash suits before they are sent to the laundry.

157. Sewing Machine Conveniences.--Always leave a piece of cloth under the presser foot of the sewing machine. This will save wear on the machine. Also it will absorb any drop of oil which might gather and spoil the first piece of fabric stitched, and will keep the needle from becoming blunted.

158. To Make a Ruffle Easily.--To make a ruffle easily, just above depth of the ruffle make a quarter inch tuck. Insert edge of ruffle under tuck, flatten down tuck over the ruffle edge and stitch on edge of tuck. If the ruffle is desired on very bottom of garment, make a quarter of an inch of tuck, leaving about half of an inch of goods underneath. Baste and stitch wrong side of ruffle to wrong side of half-inch piece, about quarter of an inch from edge. Turn back, making edge come under tuck. Flatten tuck and stitch on the edge. This will save all the trouble of bias bands, so dreaded by the dressmaker.

159. Greasing Cake Tins.--In making a cake, grease the tin with sweet lard rather than butter and sift a little dry flour over it.

160. Making Children's Petticoats.--When making children's petticoats gather the skirt to waistband before hemming the backs and then turn in with the hem, and when band gets too small and narrow across the back, all you have to do is rip out the hem and face back, and the gathers are already there properly placed; and no ripping skirt from band to adjust fullness is necessary.

161. After Cake is Removed from Oven.--A cake which has been removed from the oven should be placed on a wire stand on the stove and the steam allowed to thoroughly escape from it so as to obviate any chances of it becoming heavy.

162. When the Top Cannot be Removed from Fruit Cans.--When the top cannot be removed from a fruit can, if the lid is carefully pried at one point, so the gum can be caught, the rubber can easily be removed. It is not difficult to pull the band from beneath the metal cap.

163. Darning.--When darning must be done in the evening it is more easily done if a light colored darning ball be used.

164. In Pressing a Plaited Skirt.--In pressing a plaited skirt one will gain time and have more satisfactory results if the plaits are basted before the pressing is done. Clean the skirt and brush it on the inside. Next baste the seams, cover with a damp cloth and press on the right side with a medium warm iron. Dampen the cloth, when necessary and press until the cloth is dry.

165. Stitching Down a Seam.--After stitching down a seam, press with a hot iron, and if no seamboard is at hand, it is useful to know that a rolling pin, wrapped in a clean cloth, will answer this purpose equally as well.

166. The Color Meat Should be.--Meat should be red with the fat a clear white. The fat besides being white should be firm, and suety, and never moist. Good meat has very little smell. Bad meat shrinks considerably in boiling. Meat which is fresh and good does not loose an ounce of weight, but swells rather, when it is being boiled.

167. Buying a New Oil Cloth.--When you are ready to buy a new oil cloth for your kitchen table, take your old one and cut it up for aprons. Have it cover the whole front of your skirt, and make a large bib on it, and you will find, when you are through doing a washing, that you will be as dry as you were before you began.

168. Galvanized Tub.--The popularity of the galvanized tub due to its weight and durability, is the cause of a great many people discarding the wringer on account of their inability to fasten it to the tub securely. If a piece of heavy cloth is hung across the tub where the wringer fastens to it, you will find that it will fasten and hold as securely as to the old-fashioned wooden tub.

169. To Remove Mildew.--Mildew, if not of too long standing, can be removed by the use of raw tomato and salt. Rub the stains with raw tomato, sprinkle thickly with salt and lay in the sun. It may be necessary to repeat the process two or three times.

170. Closed Cupboards in the Pantry.--If there are closed cupboards in the pantry use them for storing provisions kept in screw top jars. There should be brass hooks for hanging up all the articles that can be suspended from the walls.

171. Keeping a House Account.--There are fewer reckoning days if housekeepers pay cash. If they persist in running accounts for groceries and other staples they should have a book and see to it that the right price is put down the minute anything is bought.

172. Chestnuts as a Vegetable.--Chestnuts have considerable food value. The boiled and mashed pulp may be used as one would use meat or vegetable, even croquettes being made of it.

173. To Give Starch a Gloss.--A little sugar added to boiled starch will give a desirable gloss to the clothes when ironed.

174. Apples Cored for Baking.--Apples cored for baking are delicious filled with orange marmalade and a little butter and sugar.

175. Beating Eggs.--When heating eggs observe that there is no grease on the beater, as it will prevent the eggs from frothing.

176. If you judge as evil the actions of another, through the judging comes evil to you.

177. A Toy Saw.--A toy saw may be utilized many times in the kitchen for sawing meat bones which are too large.

178. If a White Dress Has Turned Yellow.--If last summer's white dress has turned yellow, put it in a stone jar, cover with buttermilk and let it stand a day and night. Then wash well and starch with blued starch. This is better to whiten goods than freezing, sunshine, or the use of borax.

179. Scorched Food.--A practical cook says: When food has been scorched remove the pan from the fire and set into a pan of cold water. Lay a dish towel over the pan. The towel will absorb all the scorch taste sent up by the steam and the family need never know it was burned.

180. Mutton Chops to Make Tender.--Mutton chops can be made tender quite as much as lamb, if before they are boiled or fried they are allowed to simmer in just a little water on the back of the stove. This also makes the flavor more delicate.

181. Hollowing Out a Tomato.--For hollowing out a tomato, previous to stuffing, a pair of scissors enables a person to remove all the pulp without breaking the skin. They are equally useful for fruit salads as the fine skin which separates the sections of the grape fruit and oranges is easily clipped off.

182. The Easiest Way to Blacken a Stove.--The easiest way to blacken a stove is to use a flat paint brush about one and a half inches wide, and a tin or jar, large enough to receive the brush, to mix the blacking in. Apply the blacking to the stove as you would paint, and use a newspaper to polish with, which can be burned. In this way the hands do not come in contact with the blacking during the whole operation, and unsightly cloths and brushes, which soil the hands, are done away with.

183. Making Gravies.--For making gravies, thickening of roast gravies, it will be found useful to have browned flour on hand at all times, which can readily be kept in a mason jar or any covered vessel.

184. Kitchen Mittens.--Kitchen mittens can be bought in several thicknesses and sizes for various branches of housework. There are thick ones, with straps across the wrist to wear when polishing the ranges, then there are others to put on when scrubbing the sink or floors, and still thinner ones with chamois cloth inside to use for polishing silverware. These mittens are a great protection to the hands and finger-nails, and they really simplify the work to a great extent.

185. To Improve Baked Potatoes.--To improve baked potatoes let them stand in a pan of cold water for about an hour, then put them in the oven while wet. This seems to steam them and cook them much quicker.

186. Meat Shortcake.--Give your household a meat shortcake sometimes. Make the shortcake as you would for a fruit filling, a rather short biscuit dough, and put between the layers creamed chicken or creamed veal, and have it served with plenty of gravy.

187. Put a handful of coarse oatmeal in the water bottle and half fill with water. Let stand half an hour, then shake well and rinse. The bottle will look like new.

188. Making a Kitchen Apron.--In making a kitchen apron, provide it with an immense pocket in which can be carried a large dustcloth. Often one notices dusty places, on the furniture, windows or banisters while doing the morning work, and the dust-cloth is at hand.

Again one has to pick up numerous little articles to throw into the waste basket and the pocket holds such articles until the waste basket is reached. It is equally handy for holding a few clothes pins, while hanging out the clothes; in fact the large pocket is recognized as something decidedly useful in the kitchen apron.

189. To Make a Neat Buttonhole.--To make a neat buttonhole in thin white material that is likely to ravel when cut, take a piece of white soap and apply it to the back of the goods using enough to make a generous coat. Cut the buttonhole and work; you will find that the work is easily done and the buttonhole will not ravel.

190. To Mark Scallops.--To mark scallops place your thimble or spool just outside the circle line and mark around it with a pencil. In this way, any sized scallop can be made.

191. Delicate Fabrics to Clean.--Delicate fabrics can be cleaned perfectly by using gasoline with a teacupful of corn meal. The meal scours out all the spots. Place the meal in a dish, pour gasoline over it, then press and rub through the hands. Apply to soiled spots, rubbing carefully. Brush out with stiff brush.

192. When Using a Lap-Board.--While sewing a garment with the material lying on the lap-board, use glass top push pins to hold the goods on the board. One pin will oftentimes be sufficient. The pin is very sharp, and is easily thrust through the material into the board, and leaves a hole about the size of that made with a needle.

193. To Shape Cookies.--Cookies can be shaped with the bottom of a "star" tumbler. Flour the bottom of the glass and press it into the unbaked cookie until the indentions are imprinted upon the cake.

194. Have You Been Hoarding an Old Foulard Dress--One of that kind of dresses which you liked and hated to part with, but it went out of style. Get it out, clean it, rip it, and if there is not enough in it to make a scant shirt-waisted one-piece empire dress, make it into a pretty shirt-waist, with knife plaiting down the front.

195. To Wash Tarnished Brass.--Save the water in which the potatoes have been boiled, and use it to wash tarnished brass. It will come out as bright as new.

196. Sewing Lace.--When sewing two raw edges of fine lace together, like the tiny lace ruffles on lingerie blouses or dresses, do not fell it in the old-fashioned way, but place the two right sides together and bind the edge with the finest thread, making a buttonhole stitch along the edges. Put a stitch in each mesh, and you will have a neat lace seam which, when pressed, can scarcely be observed, and it will not fray.

197. Roasted Chestnuts.--Roasted chestnuts are said to be very delicious when salted the same as peanuts.

198. Mud Stains, to Remove.--Mud stains will disappear from cloth by the following method of cleansing: After brushing the dry mud away sponge the remaining stain with a weak solution of ammonia and water. This is absolutely safe to apply to black cloth. Colored goods, however, should be sponged with a solution of bicarbonate of soda as the latter does not affect coloring matter.

199. Drop Table for Kitchen.--A woman can have a kitchen made in a very cramped quarter if she provides it with a small work table, and a drop leaf table attached to the wall. If the stationary table is covered on all sides with a curtain and furnished with an undershelf, it will hold as much as a cupboard. Two large shelves will be found very convenient, even though it will be necessary to mount a chair or stool to reach the kitchen articles. Usually extremely small kitchens are more convenient than large ones, in which many steps must be taken.

200. A Convenience for Ironing Day.--The laundress who knows how to take care of herself has a high stool with rungs for her feet, on which she may sit when she is ironing the light pieces. It will help reserve her strength for the next day's work.

201. Quickest Way to Core Apples.--One of the simplest and quickest ways to core apples for baking is to use an ordinary clothes pin.

202. To Remove Iron Rust.--Tartaric acid will remove almost any iron rust blemish from material and is excellent for removing yellow marks.

203. The Kitchen Apron.--The kitchen apron should cover the skirt and the front of the waist, though not necessarily the sleeves, as most house dresses are made with short sleeves.

204. Cookies, to Keep.--Cookies put in an earthen jar lined with clean cloth, while they are still hot, and kept covered closely, will be much more melting and crumbling than if they were allowed to cool in the air.

205. Discolored China Baking Dishes.--Discolored china baking dishes can be made as clean as when new by rubbing them with whiting.

206. Care of Drippings.--The care of drippings in the kitchen, with the price of food so high, should receive more attention. In cooking all meats, poultry, and in making soup the grease should be carefully skimmed off and saved. Render it out once a week and after a good boiling, strain through cheesecloth. When cool skim the fat off and use in place of lard,--except for pie and biscuit.

207. To Mend Rubber.--To mend rubber, use soft kid from an old glove and paste to the patch the gum of automobile paste. The leather adheres better to the gum than a gum patch.

208. Cleaning Black Woolen Clothing.--The following is a good recipe for cleaning black woolen clothing: Dissolve borax in water and saturate a sponge or cloth in the solution. Wash the greasy spots by rubbing vigorously, then rinse in clear water the same way and dry in the sun. This is especially good for cleaning men's coat collars.

209. To Prevent Tinware Rusting.--To prevent tinware from rusting rub over with fresh lard and put in a hot oven for a few minutes before using it. If treated in this way it will never rust.

210. To Remove Machine Grease.--Cold water and a teaspoonful of ammonia and soap will remove machine grease when other means would not answer on account of the colors running.

211. To Keep Cheese From Drying.--Wring a cloth from vinegar and wrap several thicknesses around the cheese to keep it from moulding and drying.

212. Small Hand Churn.--A small hand churn makes home-made butter and cheese possible. It is no trouble whatever to make a pot of yellow butter, fresh and sweet, by the aid of one of these convenient little churns. After it is made it may be rolled into a delicate little pat and kept in an earthen jar made purposely for butter.

213. Larding a Piece of Meat.--Larding a piece of meat is a simple operation, and it is one which will greatly add to the juiciness of the dish. Cut a piece of salt pork into strips quarter of an inch thick and two or three inches long. Slip these into a larding needle and draw the needle through the meat, so either end of the pork will protrude beyond the meat.

214. To Make Vegetables Tender.--Cutting onions, turnips, and carrots across the fiber makes them more tender when cooked.

215. Clear black coffee diluted with water containing a little ammonia, will clean and restore black clothes.

216. To Make Linen Easier to Write on.--To make linen easier to write on when marking, dip the pieces you wish to mark into cold starch, rub over with hot iron and you will be able to write without the pen scratching.

217. To Air Pillows.--To air pillows, rip the corner of the ticking an inch or more. Insert a piece of rubber hose pipe a few inches long, first covering the exposed end of the tube with strong netting. Sew the ticking firmly to it and then hang all day on the line, in the air punching and shaking many times during the day. They will be light and fluffy besides being thoroughly aired and sweet and clean.

218. Uses for Pea-Pods.--Never throw away pea-pods; they give a delicious flavor to the puree for the next day.

219. To Remove the Skins of Tomatoes Quickly.--To remove the skins of tomatoes quickly, put them into a wire basket and sink it quickly into a kettle of hot water. Do not let the tomatoes stand in the water long enough to heat through, and plunge into cold water immediately from the hot. Another way is to rub the skins backward with the blunt edge of a knife. In this way the tomato does not need scalding, and according to epicures is more tasty.

220. Dyeing at Home.--In dyeing at home amateurs often make the mistake of putting the dyed article through the wringer, possibly to avoid staining the hands for one reason, or perhaps hoping to dry the garment more quickly. This however, should never be done, for the creases so formed are most obstinate and in fact, often only disappear with wear, despite all pressing. Dyed articles should be squeezed and hung out of doors to dry.

221.--To Save Children's Shoes.--To save children's shoes wash them occasionally to remove the dirt and old polish, and soften them with oil. When any part of the sole becomes badly worn, it should be mended at once, for usually a shoe will wear out at one point more quickly than elsewhere, and by paying ten or fifteen cents to have that part mended it saves dollars in time. Gunmetal shoes are preferable for everyday wear, for such shoes are lusterless and can be cleaned with oils instead of polish, which is destructive to the best leather, even when sparingly used.

222. A Systematic Housewife.--It is a handy plan for the business woman or the housewife who has much domestic accounting to do to keep two calendars, one to tear off day by day, the other to refer back to past dates when necessary. The reference calendar which can be very small and inconspicuous should have its special hook on the desk or table.

223. To Keep Candles in Warm Weather.--Keep your candles in the ice box this warm weather. They will remain beautifully upright through a whole evening's use, if they are hardened first in this way.

224. Tea Towels.--Keep the tea towels in sight, then have them fresh, clean, and whole, and hang them on a long metal curtain pole, in a convenient place, say back of the sink. This is better than placing the towels on a nail against the wall as is usually done, and it permits them to dry out quickly.

225. A Spotless House.--A house that is spotless at the price of the family's peace or of the housekeeper's best self, is the worst sort of an investment. You, the woman, are of vastly more importance than your surroundings. If you feel yourself becoming a mere drudge, if your family is growing away from you mentally, if your nerves are weakening under a fetish of cleanliness, get time to read.

226. To Keep Flooring in Place.--Strips of moulding may be tacked around the edges of a room at the baseboard, so as to cover the edge of oilcloth or linoleum. This holds the floor covering in place and prevents dust from getting beneath it.

227. Light Colored Wall Paper.--Light colored wall paper may be cleaned by a careful rubbing with a very clean rubber of the kind which artists use. If the spot cleaned seems lighter than the surrounding color it may be toned down by a gentle rubbing with a clean chamois skin.

228. To Keep Canary Seed Away from Mice.--If there are any mice in the house, the best way to keep the canary from being robbed of its food is to empty the contents of a cardboard box of bird seed into a quart preserve jar and cover with a screw top.

229. Convenient Scrub Bucket.--The most convenient scrub bucket is light, and is made of galvanized iron with a wide flaring top. The bucket is to be fitted with a wire soap tray on the outside, for often the soap is wasted while floating in the water if there is no convenient place to put it, while scrubbing. Holes can be punctured in the bucket and the wire tray fastened on with a heavy cord or a pliable wire,

230. Fruit Stains on Table Linen.--Fruit stains on table linen should be taken out before the cloth is put in the wash tub. Soap and water will set the stains.

231. Wicker Furniture.--Do not scrub your unpainted wicker furniture with soap and water, as it will turn it yellow and ruin its looks. Instead, try scrubbing it with a strong solution of salt water. If you have pieces that are so shabby that they must either be painted or thrown away, try the salt water treatment first. Scrub well and put in the sun and air and dry quickly.

232. Removing Dirt from Carpet.--Of all the ways to remove dirt from a carpet, the worst is by the use of the ordinary short brush which involves the housemaid's kneeling down in the dust.

233. How to Preserve the Household Broom.--The ordinary household broom will last twice as long, if care is taken of it, as it will if it is just used anyhow. When it is new, before using it, put it in a pail of hot water and let it remain there until the water is quite cold. Then thoroughly dry--in the sun if possible. Always clean it after sweeping, by dipping in water and shaking well before putting it away and occasionally give it a thorough washing in hot soda water.

234. A Good Furniture Polish.--A good furniture polish may be made of paraffin oil and turpentine. Kerosene too is very good, while crude oil may be used to darken wood that has not been varnished.

235. Delicious Salad.--Seeded raisins cut in pieces, broken nut meats, and a small part of celery in thin bits make up a delicious salad.

236. To Clean Light Rugs.--Rugs with white or very light ground may be cleaned by sprinkling with cornstarch, mixed with one-sixth its bulk of prepared chalk. Let the starch remain several hours and brush it out with a fine whiskbroom, then hang in the sun and heat well before putting down. This method is recommended for fine, silky rugs, as it injures neither tint nor texture and makes a beautifully clean surface.

237. To Light a Closet of Any Kind.--To light a closet of any kind, but especially a linen closet, the safest thing--next to electricity is a light clear glass lantern with wire guards outside the glass. Swing it by a light chain pulley, some little way in front of the shelves. Thus a touch sends it up or down, throwing the light wherever it may be needed.

238. To Remove White Marks on Furniture.--A mixture composed of equal parts of turpentine and linseed oil will remove the white marks on furniture caused by water. Rub it on with a soft rag and wipe off with a perfectly clean duster.

239. If Your Paint Has Been Marred.--If your paint has been marred by careless scratching of matches, try rubbing it with the finest sand paper. Use a half lemon for removing match marks from paint.

240. To Remove Inkstains from Cotton.--To remove ink-stains from cotton material, place the stain over the steam and apply salt and lemon juice which will soon remove the ink.

241. To Clean Plaster-of-Paris.--To clean plaster-of-paris figures, cover with a thick coating of starch and water, let it dry on the surface and the dirt will brush off with the dry powder.

242. To Clean Piano Keys.--A cloth moistened with alcohol will clean piano keys.

243. Washing Veils.--When veils are washed at home they usually come out quite limber and flimsy. To give them the stiffness add a pinch of sugar to the rinse water.

244. To Take Candle Grease Out of Linen.--To take candle grease out of linen, place the linen between two sheets of thick white blotting paper, and set a hot iron on it, leaving it there long enough for the iron to become perceptibly cooler. If necessary repeat this until the grease is removed.

245. Cleaning the Sweeping Brush.--Try cleaning the sweeping brush with an old comb. It is a good plan, for it preserves the brush and keeps it clean, and at the same time saves your hands.

246. Bright Wood Berries May be Preserved.--Almost any kind of bright wood berries may be preserved for decorative use in the winter, by dipping in melted paraffin and putting away in a cool place until needed. Treated in this way berries will remain firm and bright for a long time, and may be used in many ways.

247. Old Wood Work to Keep Clean.--Old woodwork, that is so hard to keep clean, can be made to look like new grained wood, by first painting it with cream colored paint to give a body alike, and when dry go over it with a dark oak varnish stain; with a little practice it can be made to look like grained wood. The varnish dries quickly and leaves it darker in some places. Any old furniture can be treated in the same way.

248. To Prevent Chairs Marring the Floor.--One should have all rockers covered with half rounds of rubber to prevent the scratching of the porch floor. These rocker tires are procurable at any furniture establishment and are easily adjusted.

249. Summer Homes.--Some of the wealthiest women are furnishing their summer homes with rag rugs, instead of the handsome oriental floor coverings, that are a mark of luxury; and what seems odd to those who cannot afford to please each whim, the rooms are being

56

repapered with simple sprigged effects and all evidences of up-to-dateness are being eliminated, to be in keeping with these copies of the colonial rag carpets.

250. To Destroy Flies.--Flies will get into the house during the summer in spite of the greatest care. One method of catching and killing them, without having disagreeable looking fly paper lying around is to prepare a mixture of cream, sugar and pepper. Put this on a plate and they will eat greedily of it and die. They will instantly seek the open air and it is easy to brush them from the screen doors. This is an old method and a good one.

251. Successful Fern Growing.--A woman who has had her refrigerator placed on the porch has a long drain pipe to carry off the melted ice, and this is made to flow right into a large bed of ferns. The cold water in no way destroys the plants, in fact, they can endure the coldest water, and last year her ferns grew to an enormous size all due to the daily supply of water from the refrigerator.

252. Faded Crepe.--Faded crepe can be dipped into a solution of water and indigo, the water made very dark with blueing for the purpose. Dissolve in one quart of water, a teaspoonful of sugar. Lift the crepe out, and shake it and pin it to the bed to dry. As it can not be ironed pin it carefully over soft muslin with needles.

253. Sweeping as a Beautifier.--The average woman who does her own housework gets exercise enough, only it is not under the best conditions, for the air, as a rule, is not sufficiently fresh. If she wants to be benefited physically, while putting her house in order, let her make it like outdoors, with the windows wide open so the fresh air can sweep through the rooms. If necessary she can wear a jacket while making beds and sweeping, and by the time her work is done she is bound to be in a healthy glow. If she does not do housework she must go outdoors, and walk, and indeed, a little walking is desirable even for the housekeeper.

254. Putting Screens Away.--If screens were carefully put away last fall there should be little difficulty in getting them in place on the first hot fly-breeding day. The wise housekeeper writes on the top of her screen, where it is hidden from view by the upper sash, the room and window where it belongs. She also covers the wires with a coating of vaselin and stores them in a dry place with a cover thrown over them. Should the wire have become shabby and rusty looking it can be freshened up with a coat of paint. If the wires have gone into holes and are badly bulged, replace with copper wire netting. It costs more than the ordinary kind, but does not wear out nearly so soon.

255. Attractive Living Room.--The living room is sure to have a cheery atmosphere if provided with a wooden seat at either side. The wooden shelf is a good place for the clock, candlesticks, and a few simple flower vases.

256. Finger Bowl.--A finger bowel should always have a few flowers or a leaf floating around on the surface.

257. Raw Oysters.--Raw oysters are further improved by sections of lemon or sprigs of mint among the cracked ice.

258. Cheerfulness at Meals.--Meals should be something more than the consumption of food. All work stops at those times and people meet together. Nothing that can be done should be omitted to make it an occasion of agreeable interchange of thought and conversation, and when this is done, not only the body, but the mind and nerves are refreshed.

259. To Keep a Rug from Curling.--The edge of the heavy rug will not curl if treated to a coat of shellac on the under side.

260. Grease Stains on Silk.--For grease stains on silk, rub the silk with French chalk or magnesia, and then hold it to the fire. Thus the grease will be absorbed by the powder, which may then be brushed off.

261. Ironing Centerpieces.--When ironing centerpieces of tablecloths, see that the iron moves with the straight grain of the cloth. If this method is followed the circular edge will take its true line.

262. Tucking Children's Dresses.--When hand tucks are to be used on children's dresses, they should be very carefully made, and the first one kept perfectly straight to use as a guide for the others. A good way to do this is to loosen one thread, not to pull out but sufficiently draw it to show the straight line, and crease the tuck in this line. After the width of the tuck and space between each is decided use a notched card as a measure for all the other tucks.

263. A Neat Way to Mend Table Linen.--A neat way to mend table linen is to darn it with linen threads off an older tablecloth. It will look much neater than a patch sewed on. It is advisable to keep a piece of a discarded tablecloth in the mending basket for that purpose.

264. A Good Substitute for a Toaster.--If the toaster is suddenly lost, you can find a very good substitute in the popcorn popper. It can be held over the gas or before the coal fire, and the bread will toast in a few minutes.

265. To Prepare Cauliflower.--To prepare cauliflower remove all the large green leaves and greater part of stalk. Soak in cold water, to which has been added one teaspoonful of vinegar and a half teaspoonful of salt to each quart.

266. Preserving Dress Patterns.--Some women, after they have used a pattern, just roll it up and tuck it away wherever it happens, and when they want to use it the next time, it curls up and acts so that there is no doing anything with it. If they would just lay the patterns out flat and put them where they might stay that way, all this trouble would be avoided.

267. Lace on Centerpieces.--Lace that is used on centerpieces is not fulled, but is just held in enough to lie flat. The best way to get this flatness is to draw the thread of the lace and fasten one end to the linen, leaving enough to make a neat seam, and then to adjust fullness so that it lies evenly. When right side is up one cannot see that any fullness exists.

268. Uses of Mop Handles.--Most women have found the mop handle with the handy clasp, a general utility tool. There is a great deal of unnecessary bending of the knees to the household gods. It is a painful attitude, and work that can be done just as well in a standing position, should never be done in a kneeling one.

269. Iron Holders Made from Asbestos.--Iron holders made from a piece of asbestos the desired size, and covered with drilling or heavy unbleached muslin are light and keep out the heat. There should be a ring or loop sewed to one corner to hang up the holder.

270. Washing Quilts.--To wash quilts a housekeeper gives the following directions: Dissolve a bar of white soap in a cupful of water. Run into your bath-tub sufficient water to cover one quilt; make a good suds, and put in the quilt, and let it soak for a few minutes. Do not rub, but use the washboard, top end down, to press or pound out the water and dirt. Never wring but with the wash-board press out the water. Rinse several times. When you have pressed out as dry as you can pin the quilt closely on the line to drain. When thoroughly dry, whip with a carpet beater until fluffy, before removing from the line. This method is especially fine for tied quilts. The bath tub is preferred, because of shape and water conveniences.

271. Shrinking Dress Goods.--Before making the white linen dress skirt, or any material that is liable to shrink, fold the goods carefully and place it in a tub and cover with water. Let it get thoroughly wet, stretch the clothes line as tightly as possible, hang the goods through the center, and pin perfectly straight on the line. When dry, let two persons stretch the goods as curtains are stretched, fold it with the wrong side of the material out and iron double with the seam running through the center of the goods on the length of the material. In shrinking colored prints add turpentine to the water, and it will set the color. A teaspoonful is used to a gallon of water.

272. Fixing Worn Corsets.--For stitching over worn corset stays, a wide white tape is unequaled.

273. Cooking Breakfast Food.--Don't leave the tin lid on the saucepan if you start the cereal in the evening for breakfast. It will rust and the moisture drip into the food.

274. Tough Meat to Make Tender.--Tough meat can be made

tender by adding a teacupful of lemon juice to the water in which it is boiled.

275. To Preserve Pineapple.--To preserve pineapple allow only three-quarters of a pound of sugar to each pound of pineapple.

276. Hemstitching Underclothing.--Hemstitching forms a dainty finish for the household linen and underclothing, but the busy woman often will not undertake it because of the difficulty of drawing the threads. If a piece of white soap be rubbed on the underside of the cloth, where the hemstitching is to be done, the threads may be drawn with ease, in half the time that is usually required.

277. To Boil Eggs Without Cracking Them.--To boil eggs without the risk of cracking, hold them in a spoonful of boiling water before immersing them.

278. Save the Basting Thread.--Basting threads, when saved, should be wound on a spool, otherwise they get hopelessly tangled and are not used again.

279. Threading Needles.--Thread will knot less easily, if the end that is broken from the spool is run through the eye of the needle.

280. Measuring Dress Goods.--Do not measure dress goods and laces with a tape line, as it stretches the material. Use a yardstick.

281. Do Not Use Coarse Thread.--An expert needlewoman says that the reason why so much embroidery does not look attractive is that too coarse a thread is used for the work. It is not a bad rule to use a cotton a number or two finer than is recommended, unless the advice comes from one who understands embroidery perfectly.

282. Putting in a Temporary Hem.--The hem of a dress that must be lengthened after it is laundered should be turned perfectly straight and stitched with number one hundred thread. It can be easily ripped and the fine threads will not leave the usual stitched lines that one often sees when a hem is lowered.

283. Serviceable Child's Dress.--A quaint little frock that will be serviceable, can be made from a remnant of demi flouncing hemstitched on the embroidered edge. This placed at the hem, of course, and the top is gathered in Mother Hubbard style into a neck band edged with a little frill. The sleeves are in bishop style confined with bands trimmed to match the neck.

284. Convenience for the Sewing Room.--A good sized waste basket should be continually close to every sewing machine. Then it is easy to form the habit of dropping all scraps into it just as the scissors make them, instead of leaving them to litter about the floor.

285. Buttons for Future Use.--When buttons are removed from a dress for future use they should be loosely strung on a thread before being put in the button box. This is a time-saver as well as keeps the buttons from getting lost or several of a set from being used.

286. Basting Long Seams.--When basting long seams, if the edge of the material is slipped under the machine needle and the needle is lowered it firmly holds the two pieces, and one can more quickly do the work.

287.--Mending Table Linen.--A woman who is expert in mending table linen does it in this manner: A piece of linen is coated with white soap, to make it stiff and the patch is evenly trimmed. This is placed under the hole in the damask after the edges around the hole in the tablecloth are soaped and trimmed to remove the rough edge.

288. Washing Cooking Utensils.--All the cooking utensils should be washed with soda immediately after they have been used, which will remove every trace of grease.

289. To Make Soft Soap.--Soft soap made from half a pound of shaved hard soap and two quarts of water will save the soap bill at - cleaning time.

290. Separate Night and Day Pillows.--If separate night and day pillows are not used, as is now generally done, the bed will look neater if special pillow slips are kept to put on over the wrinkled pillow cases by day.

291. To Keep An Iron Sink in Good Condition.--To keep an iron sink in good condition, scrub once or twice a week with hand soap and kerosene. Every night put a little chloride of lime in the strainer and pour through it a kettleful of boiling water.

292. Steaming or Boiling Pudding.--In steaming or boiling puddings, as the water boils away add more boiling water. If cold water is added, for a short time at least, the foodstuff will not be boiling, and this state of affairs may prove disastrous to the pudding.

293. Cooking Peas.--When cooking peas do not shell them. Wash the pods and put them on to boil. When they are done the pods will break and rise to the top of the kettle leaving the peas at the bottom. They have a better flavor cooked this way.

294. Troubled With Ants.--When troubled with ants in your pantry and kitchen pour kerosene around on the edge of your shelves and on your doorstep. They will soon disappear.

295. To Exterminate Roaches.--A housewife says that a few drops of turpentine sprinkled around where roaches gather will exterminate them at once.

296. How to Economize on Gas.--More gas is wasted in the oven than elsewhere. Often one burner will suffice after the oven has been well heated. It is better to run one burner than to burn two low, as they frequently go out.

297. Less Noise in Washing Dishes.--If your cook insists in washing the dishes in the pantry while the family is still at dessert, insist upon her placing the dishes to drain upon a heavy turkish towel. It will lessen much of the clatter.

298. A Useful Article in the Kitchen.--A useful article in the kitchen is a small microscope. Show the cook how to use one. She will be so horrified if shown dates, prunes, or figs that are germ infested that she will take special pains in washing them. The microscope is also useful to examine cereals, cornmeal, buckwheat and other things which unless kept tight may be unpleasantly infected.

299. To Restore Freshness to Vegetables.--For the housewife who must practise strict economy, as well as for her who lives at a distance from the market, it is well to know that cabbage, celery or lettuce and their like which have lost the first freshness, may be restored by putting first into warm water, just comfortably warm to the hand, and after fifteen or twenty minutes, you will be surprised to note that it will have the original snappy crispness so much desired. Often the grocer will sell the second day celery and lettuce at half price. The above method will freshen same, and may make quite a saving of bills.

300. Worn Brooms or Whisks.--Worn brooms or whisks may be dipped into hot water and uneven edges trimmed off with shears. This will make the straw harder, and the trimming makes the broom almost as good as new.

301. Making Over a Heatherbloom Petticoat.--When you make over a heatherbloom petticoat, do not cut it off at the top and place the drawing string in again, and do not plait it to fit the band. Instead, place a band around the waist of the person being fitted, pin the petticoat to the band, then make large darts at each seam and cut off that superfluous material that otherwise would need to be put into gathers. It does not destroy the shape and permits the petticoat to lie smoothly over the hips.

302. The Gingham Apron for the Housewife.--The gingham apron for the housewife at her daily tasks, especially if the maid is out and she has any kitchen work to do, is imperative, and she will find the long apron that buttons over the shoulders the most acceptable.

303. After Cleaning the Sewing Machine.--After cleaning the sewing machine, several yards of stitching must be accomplished before the machine runs smoothly and without leaving marks. If you have any long seams on dark material to sew up, sew them now before attempting any light work.

304. To Remove Tangled Threads.--No doubt you often have stopped sewing and patiently picked the threads out of the bobbin under the machine plate, or around the wheels, for this often occurs, says the *Woman's National Daily.* Save time in the future by lighting a match and burning out the threads, then brush the ashes off and oil the parts.

305. Clothes Rack for Children.--In one home, in the rear hall, is a low rack on which children can hang their coats, hats and mittens when they come in from school. The hanger was made with two stout steel brackets and a curtain pole fitted up with hooks on which the articles were held. On one end of the pole was hung a whiskbroom, and each tot was taught its use.

306. To Remove Dust from Any White Fabric.--To remove dust from any white fabric lay the spot over a tea-kettle of boiling water.

Place a cut lemon over the spot, pressing firmly. Remove occasionally, in order to allow the juice to evaporate, and the stain will disappear before one's eyes, no matter how stubborn or how deep set.

307. Amateur Dressmakers.--Amateur dressmakers will probably find it difficult to decide just how to finish the necks of the collarless frocks and waists that will be worn this summer. If the material is net, there is no prettier decoration than a band of the net piped with silk or satin and braided in a simple design. Necks of tub dresses while there is to be no contrasting yoke, may be trimmed with a threaded beading.

308. To Prevent Marks on the Dining Table.--If you have a highly polished dining table which you are afraid of spoiling, lay a piece of oilcloth on the table under the pad and you will have no trouble.

309. For Cupboard Shelves.--Put a white oilcloth on kitchen shelves instead of paper. The cloth will not turn yellow as the paper does, and can be kept clean while washing dishes.

310. Cleaning Gilt Frames.--When gilt frames or mouldings of the rooms have specks of dirt on them they can be cleaned with white of an egg, rubbed on with a camel's hair brush.

311. To Clean Kid Gloves.--Take a fine soft cloth, dip it into a little sweet milk, then rub it on a cake of soap, and rub the gloves with it. They will look like new.

312. Washing Fine Woolens.--To keep baby's sacques and socks and your own shawls and scarfs as fluffy as when new, dry and put in oven of range, shaking often between the palms while drying.

313. To Wash Grained Woodwork.--To wash grained woodwork take a half pail of hot water, add half a pound of soap chips, and boil until dissolved. Take from fire, add one pint kerosene, then boil for five minutes longer. Add one quarter of this to a half pailful of warm water. Wash woodwork thoroughly, wipe and dry, and lastly use a flannel to polish with.

314. Sewing on Buttons.--How often the mother hears the complaint: "I do wish you wouldn't sew these buttons on so tightly that I can't button them." When you start to sew on a button, before you take a stitch, lay a pin across the face of the button, and sew over the pin. Fasten your thread before you remove the pin, else you will draw the last stitch and spoil it. You will find there is a good shank to the button and yet it is perfectly secure.

315. Airing House After Meals.--After each meal, there should be another thorough airing of the lower floor in the home. No matter how perfectly the system of ventilation, it is impossible to prevent cooking odors. This airing is doubly necessary should there be smokers in the family.

316. House Cleaning Hints.--For the last few days before house cleaning, ornaments and pictures can be washed at one's convenience.

They need only be removed or covered when a room is cleaned. With these preparations, the actual cleaning can be done quickly and with much less disturbance of the family routine.

317. Uses for Men's Old Silk Handkerchiefs.--Men's old silk handkerchiefs should never be thrown away when worn thin. They are just the thing for dusting the polished surface of the piano, ornaments and fine china and glass and bric-a-brac.

318.--Cleaning Fine Fabrics.--In cleaning fabrics great care should be taken not to rub them roughly between the hands. The gentle rubbing on of the solvent with a fresh cloth is sufficient.

319. To Wash White Woolen Blankets.--To wash white woolen blankets, dissolve four tablespoonfuls of good washing powder in a dipperful of boiling water and pour into a tub of warm water. Open the blanket out wide and put it in the tub and let it soak all over for a half an hour. Then rub it all over between the hands, and if there are any stains left, rub them with soap. Rinse in clear water of the same temperature as the wash water. If you do this your blankets will be soft and will not shrink. Do not rub blankets on a washboard, as it makes them hard, and blueing added makes them a dull gray color.

320. To Take Out Wagon Grease.--To take out wagon grease, which is of two kinds, that made from coal tar may be removed from cloth by an application of petroleum; the other, made from animal fat, responds to a sponging of ether.

321. Old Perspiration Stains.--Old perspiration stains may be removed by applying oxalic acid and water in solution, one part of the former to twenty parts of the latter.

322. Eyelet Embroidery.--Eyelet embroidery is one of the daintiest as well as the simplest of embroideries, and, best of all, with a little practice the work can be accomplished quite rapidly. Eyelet embroidery is equally effective done on sheer or heavy material; and neat sewing is all that is required to gain good results.

323. A Convenience for the Household.--A convenience for the household, that will be appreciated by men as well as women, is a wire rack to hang in the closet. It has a series of projecting arms upon which coat hangers may be placed without interfering with each other. This greatly augments the closet room. This rack may be slipped over an ordinary closet hook, and will accommodate five coat hangers.

324. To Turn the Hems of the Table Linen Easily and Accurately.--To turn the hems of the table linen easily and accurately, remove the needle from your sewing machine, adjust the hemmer to the desired width and pass the goods through. They are then ready for hemming by hand. You will find this saves a great deal of time, and gives you a straight, even hem.

325. Soft Wood Floors to Paint.--If a soft wood floor is glue sized, before painting, it will take less paint.

326. Hanging Out Quilts.--When hanging out quilts and pillows, pound and brush them the first thing, and let the fresh air get into them all day. Most people do this just before taking them in. Consequently the beds did not get the proper airings.

327. Paint that Sticks to Glass.--Paint that sticks to glass can be removed with hot vinegar.

328. Books with Delicate Bindings.--Books with delicate bindings which have become soiled through much handling, can be satisfactorily cleaned by rubbing with chamois skin dipped in powdered pumice stone.

329. Cleaning Silverware.--Old tooth brushes and nail brushes, and old knitted underwear should always be reserved for cleaning silver. Nothing is better than a tooth brush for brushing the dried whiting out of the heavily chased silver or repousse work. The chamois skin is best for the final polishing. If table silver be steeped in hot soap suds immediately after being used, and dried with a soft clean cloth, a regular cleaning will not be needed so often.

330. Cleaning Crockery and Enamel.--By immersing, for a day or two in sour milk, glass, crockery or enamel ware articles may be perfectly cleaned of stains or limey accumulations from hard water. This is much better than a scouring, as the surface is not injured in any way, and every part can be reached.

331. Going to Market.--The housekeeper who goes to market rather than order by telephone will find she gets better things for less money.

332. Moths in Carpets.--If moths have attacked the carpet try putting gasoline on the edges, soaking the nap of the carpet. Also work powdered borax into the carpet wherever there is a sign of moths or under heavy pieces of furniture, which cannot easily be moved in the weekly sweeping.

333. A Serviceable Furniture Brush.--A serviceable furniture brush is made of turkey tail feathers. Take a stout twine and needle, sew the quills tightly together and cover the handle with a piece of oilcloth, smoothly stitched into place, or wrap the handle with cloth and stitch. A brush of this kind is very soft and may be used to dust any highly polished piece of furniture.

334. Uses of a Wooden Spoon.--Never use any but a wooden or silver spoon to stir anything with in cooking. Many a dish is spoiled by the cook stirring it with an iron or metal spoon. Wood is the best when any acid, such as vinegar, is used in the ingredients to be stirred.

335. Boiling Vegetables.--Boil parsnips and such vegetables with thin skins; then peel when cold. The flavor is preserved and your hands are not stained.

336. To Wash Furniture.--Furniture washed with castile soap and tepid water and rubbed with a piece of old silk will look like new.

337. Old Suitcases and Purses.--When suitcases and purses begin to show wear, coat all the spots with tan water color paint, and when perfectly dry rub over with a little sweet oil. Let stand for an hour, then rub with woolen cloth. Tan and brown shoes which have become scuffed may be treated in the same way.

338. Putting up Lunches.--Those who find the putting up of lunches a part of the daily routine may take comfort in the suggestion of one resourceful woman. When using eggs she sees to it that only a small piece of the shell is broken off from the end of one egg. The egg shell from which the piece has been cut is then washed and kept as a receptacle for jelly or jam for the noon lunch basket. The open end being protected by a piece of paper dipped in paraffin.

339. Paint Wicker Furniture.--If you must paint wicker furniture see that you buy paint that is well mixed and thinned to the proper consistency. If too thick it gets lumpy and the paint is apt to rub off on the clothes. Porch chairs which are exposed to weather should be finished with a coat of enamel to make them last longer. The coat of enamel is also more easily dusted.

340. Bureau Drawers that Stick.--Wax is better to use on the bureau drawers that stick than soap. It works better and will not catch dirt so much.

341.--Uses for Old Envelopes.--Cut out the corners from all heavy envelopes, for they are excellent for holding coins sent by mail. They always make good corner protection.

342. To Prevent Fruit from Moulding.--A layer of absorbent cotton laid over the fruit in the mouth of the fruit cans is an excellent preventive against the mould. If mould should form, it will cling to the cotton and leave the fruit clean.

343. Linoleum or Oilcloth That is Cracked.--Linoleum that is badly cracked may be improved by a filler made of ochre and boiled flour paste. After the filling is dry the linoleum may be painted.

344. Borax as a Purifier for Ice Box.--Borax is an invaluable aid to the woman who wishes to keep her ice box immaculate. It is especially desirable for use in small refrigerators where little food is kept, and where ice is kept more for the purpose of preserving butter and milk and keeping bottled water cool. Cold water with plenty of pure borax, is preferable to hot water to use in wiping off the walls of the refrigerator. It does not heat the box and, being a germ killer, it purifies everything it touches. It may also he put in the corners of the refrigerator. Its best use of all is perhaps in keeping the receptacle for the ice itself and the outside tube in pure and sanitary condition. It may be sprinkled freely over the bottom of the ice box proper and on the rack holding the ice.

345. To Clean Gilded Surfaces.--To clean gilded surfaces, dip a soft brush in alcohol to which a few drops of ammonia water have been added, and with it go over the surface. Do not rub roughly or harshly. In about five minutes the dirt will have become soft and easy of removal. Then go over the surface again gently with the same or similar brush dipped in rain water. Now lay the damp article in the sunlight to dry. If there is no sunlight place it near a warm (but not hot) stove, and let dry completely in order to avoid streaks, taking care that the position of the article, during the drying is not exactly vertical.

346. Hints for the Housewife.--Every housewife should have plenty of waxed paper or paraffin paper about the house. It is of the greatest value in preserving eatables from the air and keeping them properly moist. In the sandwich basket it is indispensable. Cake wrapped in it will keep moist and fresh for a much longer time than if put directly into the box. When the paper has become sticky run cold water on it, and it may he used again. Cheese wrapped up in it and put in the refrigerator will keep fresh for a week.

347. Excessive Gas Light Weakens the Eyes.--When the excessive light of the gas light or the electric bulb tires weak eyes, resort to the tallow candle. For the sick room wax candles are preferred, as they never produce smoke or smell. They seem to soothe the nerves of the invalid and in this way help to produce a restful night.

348. Handy Disinfectant for the Household.--Chlorate of lime moistened with vinegar and water, equal parts, is a handy disinfectant for the household. It can be kept in the cellar, and in case of sickness a few drops scattered around the house will purify the air.

349. For Closing Windows.--A piece of bamboo, an old blind roller, or any strong smoothly rounded stick about three feet long, with a small flat piece of wood about the same thickness, twelve inches long and covered with flannel, nailed across the ends, makes an admirable and useful article for closing top windows without either going outside or standing on a stool or a chair to reach, or straining one's self with the weight to be raised upward.

MEDICAL DICTIONARY

SIMPLE and PLAIN DEFINITIONS of MEDICAL TERMS

For Reference in your Newspaper and General Reading and Throughout this Work.

Abdomen (ab-do'men). That portion of the body, lying between the thorax and the pelvis, or "belly."

Ablution (ab-lu'shun). The act of washing or cleansing.

Abnormal (ab-nor'mal). Contrary to the usual structure or condition. Not normal.

Abortion (ab-or'shun). The expulsion of the fetus before the sixteenth week.

Abrasion (ab-ra-zhun). A spot rubbed bare of the skin or mucous membrane.

Abscess (ab'ses). A localized collection of pus in a cavity formed by the disintegration of tissues.

Absorbent (ab-sor'bent). Taking up by suction. A medicine or dressing that promotes absorption.

Acid (as'id). Sour, having properties opposed to those of the alkalies.

Acidity (as-id'it-e). The quality of being acid or sour.

Acrid (ak'rid). Pungent; producing an irritation.

Acetabulum (as-et-ab'u-lum). The rounded cavity in the innominate (hip) bone which receives the head of the femur.

Accoucheur (ah-kosh'er). An obstetrician. One who attends a woman in confinement.

Actual Cautery (kaw'tere). Fire, a red hot iron, or the moxa, used as a cauterizing agent.

Acholia (ah-ko'leah). Lack or absence of the secretion of bile.

Acupuncture (ak-u-punk-tur). The insertion of needles into a part for the production of counter-irritation.

Adhesive (ad-he'siv). Sticking or adhering closely.

Adipose (ad'ip-os). Of a fatty nature; fat.

Adjuvant (ad'ju-vant). An auxiliary remedy.

Adult (a-dult'). A person grown to full size and strength or to the years of manhood.

Affection (af-ek'shun). A morbid condition or diseased state.

Affusion (af-u'shun). The pouring of water upon a part or upon the body for reducing fever or correcting nervous symptoms.

Ailment (al'ment). Any disease or affection of the body.

Albuminose (al-bumin-os). A primary production of the digestion of a proteid, not coagulable by heat.

Aliment (al'im-ent). Food, or nutritive material.

Alimentary Canal (al-imen'ta-re). The portion of the digestive apparatus through which the food passes after mastication. The canal from the mouth to the anus; gullet, stomach, bowel, anus.

Alkali (al'kal-i). A compound which forms salts with acids and soaps with fats. Potash, soda, lithia, ammonia.

Alterative (awl-ter-at-iv). A medicine that produces a favorable change in the processes of nutrition and repair.

Alveolar (al-ve'o-lar). Pertaining to an alveolus.

Alveolus (al-ve-olus). Bone socket of a tooth; air sac of the lungs, etc.

Amaurosis (am-aw-ro'sis). Blindness without any visible defect in the eye, from disease of the optic nerve, retina, brain.

Amenorrhea (am-en-or-re'ah). Absence or abnormal stoppage of the monthly sickness.

Amniotic Liquid (am-ne-ot'ik). A fluid enclosed within the amnion which nourishes and protects the foetus (unborn child).

Amputation (am-pu-ta'shun). The surgical cutting off of a limb or other part.

Amylaceous (am-il-a'she-us). Starchy.

Analysis (an-al'is-is). Separation. into compound parts or elements.

Anchylosis (Ankylosis) (ang-kil-o'sis). Abnormal immobility and consolidation of a joint (stiff joint).

Anemia (an-e'me-ah). A condition in which the blood is deficient either in quantity or quality.

Anastomose (an-as'to-moz). Communicating with one another, as arteries and veins.

Anastomosis (an-as-to-mo'sis). The surgical or pathological formation of a passage between any two normally distinct spaces or organs.

Anasarca (an-ah-sar'kah). An accumulation of serum in the cellular tissues of the body. General dropsy.

Anesthesia (an-is-the-zhe-ah). Loss of feeling or sensation of a part or whole body.

Anesthetic (an-es-thet-ic). A drug that produces anesthesia, without the sense of touch or pain.

Aneurism (an'u-rizm). A pulsating tumor consisting of a sac or pouch into which blood flows through an opening in an artery.

Animalcule (anim-al'kul). Any minute animal organism.

Anodyne (an'o-din). A medicine that relieves pain.

Antacid (an-tas'id). A substance that counteracts or neutralizes acidity.

Antiphrodisiac (ant'af-ro-diz-e-ak). An agent that allays sexual impulses.

Anthelmintic (an-thel-min'tik). Destruction to worms.

Anthrax (an'thrax). A carbuncle.

Antibilious (an-te-bil'yus). Good against bilious conditions.

Antidote (an'te-dot). A remedy for counteracting a poison.

Antidysenteric (an'te-dis-en-ter'ik). Relieving, curing or preventing dysentery.

Antiemetic (an'te-e-met'ik). Arresting or preventing emesis or vomiting.

Antilithic (an-te-lith'ik). Preventing the formation of stone or calculus.

Antimorbific (anti-mor-bif 'ic). Preventing disease.

Antiperiodic (an'te-pe-re-od'ik). Serviceable against malarial or periodic recurrence.

Antiscorbutic (an'te-skor-bu'tik). Correcting or curing scurvy.
Antiseptic (an-te-sep'tik). A substance destructive to poisonous germs.
Antispasmodic (an'te-spaz-mod'ik). An agent that relieves spasms.
Antisyphilitic (an'te-sif-il-it'ik). Useful in cases of syphilis.
Anus (a'nus). The distal end and outlet of the rectum.
Apathy (ap'ath-e). Lack of feeling or emotion; indifference.
Apparatus (ap-ar-a'tus). A number of parts acting together in the performance of some special function.
Aphasia (ah-fa'ze-ah). Defect or loss of the power of expression by speech, writing, or signs.
Aphthous (af'thus). Pertaining to, characterized by, affected with aphthae (thrush).
Apex (a'pex). The top or pointed extremity of any conical part.
Apnea (ap-ne'ah). The transient cessation of breathing that follows a forced respiration.
Aperient (ap-e're-nt). A gentle purgative or laxative.
Appetite (ap'et-it). A natural longing or desire, especially that for food.
Areola (ar-e'o-lah). The colored circle round the nipple or round a pustule. A minute space or interstice in a tissue.
Aromatic (ar-o-mat'ik). A medicinal substance with a spicy fragrance and stimulating qualities.
Aroma (ah-ro'mah). The fragrance or odor, especially that of spice or medicine, or of articles of food or drink.
Arthrodia (ar-thro'de-ah). An articulation or joint which allows a gliding motion of the surfaces.
Articulation (ar-tik'u-la'shun). A connection between two or more bones whether allowing motion between them or not.
Articulated (ar-tik'u-la-ted). Connected by joints.
Arthritic (ar-thrit'ik). Pertaining to or affected with gout or arthritis. Relating to inflammation of a joint.
Ascaris (as'kar-is). A worm found in the intestines.
Ascites (as-si'tez). Dropsy of the abdominal cavity.
Aspirate (as'pi-rat). To treat by aspiration. To pronounce with full emission of breath.
Assimilation (as-sim-il-a'shun). The transformation of food into living tissue.
Asthenic (as-then'ik). Characterized by weakness or feebleness.
Asthmatic (az-mat'ik). Affected with asthma.
Astringent (as-trin'gent). An agent that arrests discharges by causing contraction, such as tannic acid, alum, zinc, etc.
Attenuant (at-ten'u-ant). Causing thinness, as of the blood.
Atony (at'on-e). Lack of normal tone or strength.
Atrophy (at'ro-fe). A wasting or diminution in the size of a part.
Auricle (au'rik-l). The pinna or flap of the ear. The chambers of the heart on either side above the ventricles.
Auscultation (aus-kul-ta'shun). Listening with the ear or an instrument to organs, such as the lungs, heart, etc.
Autopsy (au-top-se). The post-mortem examination of a body.
Axilla (ak-sil'lah). The arm-pit.
Axillary Glands. Lymphatic glands situated in the arm-pit.

Balsamic (bawl-sam'ik). Of the nature of balsam.
Biennial (bi-en'ni-al). Happening Once in two years.
Bifurcation (bi-fur-ka'shun). Division into two branches.
Bile or Gall (Bil). The golden brown or greenish yellow substance secreted by the liver.
Bilious (bil'yus). Characterized by bile. Full of bile.
Blister (blis'ter). A collection of serous, bloddy or watery fluid beneath the epidermis (outer skin).
Bonchioles. A minute bronchial tube.
Bronchia (brong'ke-ah). Bronchial tubes smaller than the bronchi, and larger than the bronchioles.
Bougie (boo-zhe'). A slender instrument for introduction into the urethra or a large one for the rectum or other opening.
Bronchial (brong'ke-al). Pertaining to the bronchi.
Bronchitis (brong-ki'tis). Inflammation of the bronchial tubes.
Bright's Disease (britz). Inflammation of the kidneys. Any disease of the kidneys associated with albumen in the urine.
Bulbous (bul'bus). A bulb.
Cachexia (kak-ek'seah). A profound and marked state of constitutional disorder. A depraved condition of general nutrition due to some serious disease such as cancer, tuberculosis (cancerous cachexia).
Cacumen (kak-u'men). The top or apex of an organ.
Callous (kal'us). Hard.
Calcareous (kal-ka'reus). Chalky. Pertaining to or having the nature of limestone.
Callus (kal'lus). The new growth of bony matter between the extremities of broken bone serving to unite them.
Capillary (kap'il-la-ri). Pertaining to or resembling a hair. A minute blood vessel connecting the arterioles with the venules; very minute blood vessels.
Capsicum (kap'si-kum). Cayenne pepper.
Capsule (kap'sul). A soluble case for enclosing a dose of medicine. A fibrous or membraneous covering as of the spleen or kidneys.
Carbon (kar'bon). Charcoal.
Carbonic Acid Gas (kar-bon'ik). An acidulous liquid made by dissolving carbon dioxide in water.
Cardiac (kar'de-ak). Pertaining to the heart.
Carminative (kar-min'-a-tiv). A medicine to relieve flatulence, such as anise, cinnamon, cloves, peppermint, soda.
Caries (ka're-ez). Rottenness. The molecular decay or death of a bone. It becomes soft, porous and discolored.
Carotid Artery (kah-ro-tid'). The large artery in the neck.
Carpus (kar'pus). The wrist.
Cartilage (kar'til-ej). Gristle. The gristle attached to joint surfaces and forming certain parts of the skeleton.
Catamenia (kat-ah-me'ne-ah). Monthly sickness.
Cataplasm (kat'ap-lazm). A poultice.
Catarrh (kat-ahr'). Inflammation of a mucous membrane with a free discharge.
Cathartic (kath-ar'tik). A medicine that produces free movements of the bow-

els.
Catheter (kath'it-er). A hollow tube for introduction into a cavity through a narrow canal or channel.
Caustic (kaws'tik). Burning; destructive to living tissues.
Cautery (kaw'ter-e). Application of a caustic substance or hot iron.
Cauterize (kaw'ter-iz). To scar or burn with a caustic or cautery.
Cell (sel). A small hollow cavity in any one of the minute protoplasmic masses which form organized tissues.
Cellular (sel'u-lar). Relating to or composed of cells.
Cerebellum (ser-e-bel'um). The inferior part of the brain lying below the cerebrum and above the pons and medulla.
Cerebro Spinal (ser'e-bro-spi'nal). Pertaining to the brain and spinal cord.
Cerebral (ser'e-bral). Relating to the cerebrum.
Cerebrum (ser'-e-brum). The main portion of the brain occupying the upper part of the cranium, and consisting of two equal portions, called hemispheres.
Cerumen (se-ru'men). Ear-wax.
Chalybeate (kal-ib'e-at). Containing or charged with iron.
Chancre (shang'ker). The primary lesion (or sore) of syphilis.
Cholagogues (ko'ia-gog). A medicine causing an increased flow of bile.
Choleraic (kol-er-a'ik). Of the nature of cholera.
Chorea (ko-re'ah). St. Vitus' dance.
Chordee (kor-dee'). Painful deflection of the penis in gonorrhea.
Chronic (kron'ik). Long continued; not acute.
Chyle (kile). The milky juice taken up by the lacteals from the food in the intestines after digestion.
Chyme (kim). The thick grayish liquid mass into which the food is converted by stomach (gastric) digestion.
Circulation (sir-ku-la'shun). Passing in a circle, as the circulation of the blood.
Cicatrix (sik-a'trix). A scar; the mark left by a sore or a wound.
Clavicle (klav'ik-l). Collar-bone.
Climacteric (kli-mak-ter'ik). A period of the lifetime at which the system was believed to undergo marked changes. Now generally applied to the "change of life."
Clinical (klin'ic-al). Pertaining to bedside treatment or to a clinic.
Clonic (klon'ik). Applied to spasms where the parts are rigid and relaxed in succession.
Clyster (kli'ster). An injection into the rectum; an enema.
Coagulation (ko-ag-u-la-shun). The process of changing into a clot.
Coagulum (ko-ag'u-lum). A clot or curd.
Coagulate (ko-ag'u-Iat). To cause a clot.
Coalesce (ko-al-es'). The union of two or more parts or things.
Collapse (kol-laps'). A state of extreme prostration and depression with failure of circulation.
Colon (ko'lon). That part of the large intestine which extends from the caecum to the rectum.

Colostrum (ko-los'trum). The first fluid secreted by the "breast" (mammary gland) after confinement.
Colliquative (kol-liq'wah-tuv). Characterized bv an excessive fluid discharge.
Collyrium (kol-lir'e-um). An eye-wash.
Coma (ko'mah). Profound stupor occurring during a disease or after a severe injury.
Comatose (ko'mat-os). Pertaining to or affected with coma.
Combustion (kom-bust'yun). Burning; rapid oxidation with emission of heat.
Concussion (kon-kush'un). A violent jar or shock, or a condition resulting from it.
Concretion (kon-kre'shun). A calculus or inorganic mass in a natural cavity or in the tissues of an organism.
Condiment (kon'di-ment). A seasoner.
Condyle (kon'dil). The rounded eminence at the joint (articular) end of a bone.
Confluent (kon-flu'ent). Becoming merged together.
Congenital (kon-jen'it-al). Existing at or before birth.
Congestion (kon-gest'jun). Excessive or abnormal accumulation of blood in a part.
Conjunctiva (kon-junk-ti'vah). The delicate membrane that lines the eyelids and covers the eyeball.
Constipation (kon-stip-a'shun). Infrequent or difficult evacuation of feces (bowel material).
Constriction (kon-strik'shun). A constricted part or place. Tight feeling.
Contagious (kon-ta'jus). Propagated by contagion or by immediate contact or effluvia.
Contusion (kon-tu-zhun). A bruise.
Contamination (kon-tam-in-a'shun.) Infection of the person or of matter by contact.
Convalescence (kon-val-es'ens). Getting well after an illness.
Convoluted (kon'va-lut-cd). Rolled together or coiled.
Convulsion (kon-vul'shun). A violent involuntary contraction or series of contractions of the voluntary muscles.
Cordial (kord'yel). Stimulating the heart; invigorating.
Cornea (kor'neah). The transparent anterior portion of the eyeball.
Corpse (korps). The dead body of a human being.
Corrective (kor-ek'tiv). Modifying or changing favorably.
Corroborants (kor-ob'er-ants). Aiding in proving.
Corrosive (kor-ro'siv). Eating away. A substance that destroys organic tissue either by direct chemical means or by causing inflammation and suppuration.
Counter Irritation (kown'ter-ir-rit-a'shun). A superficial irritation.
Cosmetics (koz-met'ik). Beautifying substances.
Costiveness (kos'tiv-nes). Constipated bowels.
Cranium (kra'neum). The skull or brain-pan.
Crassamentum (kras-sam-en'tum). A clot, as of blood.
Crepitus (krep'it-us). The grating of broken bones.
Crisis (kri'sis). Turning point of a disease for better or worse.
Cutaneous (ku-ta'ne-us). Pertaining to the skin.
Cuticle (ku'tik-l). The epidermis, outer or scarf skin.
Cyst (sist). A cavity containing fluid and surrounded by a capsule (covering).

Debility (de-bil-i-ti). Lack or loss of strength.

Decoction (de-kok'shun). A medicine, etc., made by boiling.

Decomposition (de-kom-po-zish'-un). Putrefying. The separation of the component parts of the body.

Deglutition (deg-lu-tish'un). The act of swallowing.

Dejection (de-jek'shun). Discharge of excrementitious material; mental depression.

Deleterious (del-e-te're-us). Hurtful; injurious.

Deliquium (de-lik'we-um). A fainting or syncope.

Delirium (de-lir'e-um). A condition of mental excitement with confusion and usually hallucinations and illusions.

Demulcents (de-mul'sents). Soothing; allays irritation, especially of mucous surfaces.

Dentition (den-tish'in). Teething; cutting of teeth.

Dentrifice (den'trif-is). A substance for cleansing teeth.

Duodenum (du-o-de'num). The first part of the small intestine.

Deobstruent (de-ob'stru-ent). A medicine to remove obstruction.

Depletion (de-ple'shun). Diminished quantity of fluid in the body or in a part, especially by bleeding, conditions due to excessive loss of blood or other fluids.

Depuration (dep'u-ra-shun). Purify or cleanse.

Derm (derm). The skin.

Desiccate (des-ik-at). To dry thoroughly.

Detergent (de-ter'gent). A cleansing, purifying medicine.

Desquamation (des-kwam-a'shun). Scaling; shedding of the epithelial elements, chiefly of the skin.

Determination (de-term-in-a'shun). Tendency of the blood to collect in a part.

Diagnosis (di-ag-no'sis). The art of distinguishing one disease from another.

Diaphragm (di'af-ram). The membrane that separates the abdomen from the chest cavity.

Diaphoretics (di-af-o-ret'ik). Sweating remedies.

57

Diathesis (di-ath'es-is). Natural or congenital predisposition to a special disease.

Dietetics (di-ct-et'iks). The science or study and regulation of food.

Dilatation (di-la-ta'shun). Stretched beyond the normal dimension.

Diluent (dil'u-ent). Makes less irritant; an agent that makes less irritant.

Discutients (dis-ku'te-ent). Remedies that scatter.

Disinfectant (dis-in-fek'tant). Agent that destroys disease germs or renders ferments inactive.

Dislocation (dis-lo-ka'shun). The displacement of any part, especially a bone.

Diuretic (diu-ret'ik). Agent to increase secretion of the urine.

Dorsal (dor'sal). Pertaining to the back or back of any part.

Drastic (dras'tic). Powerful acting remedy or agent.

Dyspepsia (dis-pep'se-ah). Difficult digestion. Impairment of the power or function of digestion.

Dysuria (dis-ur'e-ah). Painful or difficult passing of urine.

Dyspnoea (disp-ne'ah). Difficult or labored breathing.

Dyspragia (dys-pra'je-ah). Difficulty in swallowing.

Dyscrasia (dis-kra'ze-ah). A depraved state of the humors; abnormal composition of the blood and humors.

Ebullition (eb-ul-ish'un). The process of boiling.

Ecstacy (ek'stas-i). A kind of trance or state of fixed contemplation, with mental exaltation, partial abeyance of most of the functions and rapt expression of the countenance.

Edema (e-de'mah). Swelling due to the accumulation of serous fluid in the tissues.

Effervesce (ef-fer-ves'). To bubble; sparkle.

Efflorescence (ef-flo-res'sens). A rash or eruption.

Effluvium (ef-flu've-um). An ill-smelling exhalation, especially of a noxious character.

Effusion (ef-fu-zhun). The escape of fluid into a part or tissue.

Electrization (e-lek-tri-za'shun). The act of charging with, or treatment by, electricity.

Electuary (e-lek'tu-a-re). A medicinal preparation consisting of a powdered drug made into a paste with honey, syrup, etc.

Elimination (e-lim-in-a'shun). The act of expulsion from the body.

Emaciation (e-ma-se-a'shun). Leanness, or a wasted condition of the body.

Embryo (em'bre-o). The foetus (unborn child) in its earlier stages of development, especially before the end of the third month.

Emesis (em'e-sis). Vomiting.

Emetic (e-met-ik). Any substance that causes vomiting.

Emmenogogue (em-men'ogog). Any agent stimulating or favoring the monthly flow.

Emollient (e-mo'le-ent). Soothing or softening.

Emphysema (em-fis-e'mah). A swelling or inflation due to the presence of air in the interstices of the connective tissues.

Emulsion (e-mul'shun). An oily or resinous substance divided and held in suspension through the agency of an adhesive, mucilaginous, or other substance.

Enamel (en-am'el). The white substance that covers and protects the dentine of the crown of the teeth.

Empirical (em-pir-ic-al). Based on experience.

Encephalon (en-sef'al-on). That portion of the central nervous system which is contained within the skull or cranium.

Encysted (en-sis'ted). Enclosed in a sac, or cyst.

Endermically (en-der-mik'ally). Absorption through the skin.

Enema (en'em-ah). An injection thrown into the rectum.

Enervation (en-er-va'shun). Languor; lack of nervous energy.

Enteritis (en-ter-i'tis). Inflammation of the intestine, usually the small intestine.

Enteric (en-ter'ik). Pertaining to the intestines or bowels.

Epidemic (ep-id-em'ik). A disease which attacks many people in any district at the same time.

Epidermis (ep-id-er'mis). Outer skin; scarf skin; cuticle.

Ephemeral (ef-em'er-al). Transient; for one day or less.

Epigastrium (cp-a-gas'tre-um). The upper middle portion of the abdomen (belly); over or in front of the stomach.

Epigastric (ep-e-gas'trik). Pertaining to the epigastrium.
Epileptic (ep-e-lep-tik). A person troubled with epilepsy.
Epiglottis (ep-e-glot'tis). The lid-like structure covering the entrance into the larynx (upper windpipe),
Epiphora (e-pif-o-rah). An abnormal overflow of tears down the cheek, usually due to lachrymeal stricture.
Epispastic (ep-e-spas-tik). A congenital defect in which the urethra opens on the dorsum (back) of the penis. On the female, a fissure of the upper wall of the female urethra.
Epistaxis (ep-e-stax'is). Nose-bleed.
Epithelium (ep-ith-ele'um). The covering of the skin and mucous membrane consisting wholly of cells of varying form and arrangement.
Erethism (er'e-thizm). Excessive irritability or sensibility.
Erosion (er'o-zhun). An eating or gnawing away; a kind of ulceration.
Eructation (e-ruk-ta'shun). The act of casting up wind from the stomach; belching.
Eruption (erup'shun). A visible lesion on the skin due to disease and marked by redness, etc.
Errhine (er'rin). A medicine that promotes a nasal discharge.
Erysipelations (er-is-ip'el-a-shuns). Pertaining to or of the nature of erysipelas.
Eschar (e's-kar). A slough produced by burning or by a corrosive application.
Escharotic (es-kar-ot'ik). A caustic substance capable of producing a slough.
Esophagus (e-sof 'a-gus). Gullet, extends from pharynx to stomach.
Eustachian Tube (u-sta'ke-an). The bony cartilaginous canal that extends from the middle ear to the throat.
Evacuation (e-vak-u-a'shun). The act of emptying, especially of the bowels.
Evacuant (e-vak'u-ant). A medicine that causes the evacuation.
Exacerbation (eks-as-er-ba'shun). An increase in the symptoms of a disease.
Exanthema (ex-an-the'mah). An eruption upon the skin; An eruptive disease.
Excision (ex-sizh'on). The cutting out of a part.
Excitant (ek-si-tent). Stimulating.
Excoriated (ex-ko-re-ated). Any superficial loss of substance, such as that produced on the skin by scratching.
Excrement (eks-kre-ment). Fecal matter; matter cast out as waste from the body.
Excretion (eks-kre'shun). The discharge of waste products.
Excrescence (ex-kres'ens). An abnormal outgrowth upon the body.
Exfoliate (ex-fo-le-ate). A falling off in scales or layers.
Exhalation (cx-ha-la'shun). The giving off of matters in a vapor form.
Expectorate (ex-pec'to-rat). The act of coughing up and spitting out materials from the lungs and wind-pipe.
Expectorant (ex-pec-to'rant). A remedy that promotes or modifies expectoration.
Exostosis (cks-os'to-sis). A bony outgrowth from the surface of a bone or tooth.
Expiration (eks-pi-ra'shun). The act of breathing out or expelling air from the lungs.
Extravasation (eks-trav-as-a'shun). The passing of fluid (blood, etc.) outside of the cavity or part normally containing it.
Extremities (eks-trem'it-ies). Pertaining to an extremity or end.
Exudation (eks-u-da'shun). The passing out of serum or pus in or upon the tissues.
Facial (fa'shal). Pertaining to the face.

Facet (fa'set). A small plain surface on a bone or hard body.
Fauces (faw'sez). The passage from the mouth to the pharynx (throat).
Faeces. Same as feces.
Fecal (fa'kal). Pertaining to, or consisting of feces.
Fascia (fa'she-ah). A sheet or band of tissue which invests and connects the muscles, or the areolar tissue, forming layers beneath the skin or between muscles.
Farinaceous (far-in-a'se-us). Of the nature of flour or meal.
Febrifuge (feb'rif-ug). A remedy that allays fever.
Febrile (feb'ril). Feverish; pertaining to fever.
Femur (fe'mur). The thigh-bone. The bone from the hip to the knee.
Ferruginous (fer-ru'gin-us). Containing iron or iron-rust.
Fetid (fe'tid). Having a rank or foul smell.
Fetor (fe'tor). Stench or offensive odor.
Fibrin (fib'rin). A whitish proteid from the blood and serous fluids of the body.
Filtration (fil-tra'shun). The passage of a liquid through a filter.
Fistula (fis'tu-lah). A narrow canal or tube left by the incomplete healing of abscesses or wounds and usually transmitting some fluid, either pus or the secretions or contents of some organ or body cavity.
Flaccid (flak'sid). Weak, lax and soft.
Flatulence (flat'u-lense). Distended with gas in stomach or bowels.
Flatus (fla'tus). Gas, especially in the stomach and bowels.
Flexible (flex'ib-l). That which may be bent without breaking.
Flocculent (flok'u-lent). Flaky, downy, or wooly.
Flooding (flud'ding). A copious bleeding from the womb.
Flush (flush). A redness of the face or neck.
Flux (flux). An excessive flow of any of the excretions of the body, especially feces.
Foetus (fe'tus). Same as fetus, The child in the womb after the end of third month, called embryo before that time.
Fomentations (fo-men-ta'shun). Treatment by warm and moist applications to a part to relieve pain or inflammation.
Formula (for'mu-lah). A prescribed method of preparing a medicine.
Fracture (frak'tur). The breaking of a part, especially of a bone.
Friction (frik'shun). The act of rubbing.
Fumigation (fu-mig-a'shun). Disinfection by exposure to the fumes of a vaporized disinfectant.
Fungus (fung'gus). Anyone of a class of vegetable organisms of a low order of development, including mushrooms, toadstools, moulds, etc.
Function (funk'shun). The normal, special or proper action or office of any part or organ.
Fundament (fun'da-ment). The foundation or base of a thing.
Fungous (fung'us). Of the nature or resembling a fungus.
Galvanization (gal-van-iz-a'shun). Treatment by galvanic electricity.
Ganglion (gang'le-on). Any mass of gray nervous substance that serves as a center of nervous influence.
Gangrene (gang'gren). The mortification or non-molecular death of a part.
Gargle (gar'gle). A solution used for rinsing the mouth and throat.

Gastric (gas'tric). Pertaining to the stomach.
Gestation (ges-ta-shun). Pregnancy.
Gelatinous (gel-at'in-us). Like jelly or softened gelatine.
Genital (gen'it-al). Pertaining to the organs of generation or reproduction.
Gland. An organ that separates any fluid from the blood; or an organ which secretes something essential to the system or excretes waste materials the retention of which would be injurious to the body.
Glottis (glot'is). The space between the vocal cords, together with the larynx, which is concerned in voice production.
Gluteus (glu-te'us). One of the large muscles of the buttock.
Glandular (glan'du-lar). Pertaining to the nature of a gland.
Granular (gran'u-lar). Made up of, or containing granules or grains.
Granulation (gran-u-la'shun). The formation in wounds of small rounded fleshy masses.
Grumous (gru'mus). Clotted. Lumpy.
Guttural (gut'tur-al). Pertaining to the throat.
Habit (hab'it). The tendency to repeat an action or condition.
Hallucination (hal-lu-sin-a'shun). Perception of an object, etc., which has no external existence, as by sight, sound, smell, taste, or touch.
Hectic (hek'tik). Associated with consumption and with septic poisoning. Due to absorption of toxic substances.
Hematemesis (hem-at-em'es-is). The vomiting of blood.
Hemorrhage (hem'-or-rej). Bleeding. An escape of blood from the vessels.
Hepatic (hep-at-ik). Pertaining to the liver.
Hereditary (her-ed'-it-a-re). Derived from ancestry or obtained by inheritance.
Heredity (he-red'-it-e). The inheritance of qualities or of diseases from ancestry.
Hematuria (hem-at-u'-reah). The discharge of urine containing blood.
Hematosis (hem-at-o'sis). The process of the formation of blood; also its arterialization in the lungs.
Hemiplegia (hem-e-ple'jeah). Paralysis of one side of the body.
Hernia (her'neah). Rupture. Breach.
Hydragogue (hi'drag-og). A purgative that causes copious liquid discharges.
Hydrargyrum (hi-drar'gir-um). Mercury or quicksilver.
Hydrogen (hi'-dro-gcn). A light inflammable gaseous element, odorless and tasteless.
Hydrothorax (hi-dro-tho'rax). The presence of a serous fluid in the pleural cavity.
Hydrophobia (hi-dro-pho'bia). Acute infectious disease communicated to man by the bites of an animal suffering from rabies.
Hygiene (hi'-gen). The science of health and its preservation.
Hyperesthesia (hi-per-es-the'zeah). Excessive sensibility of the skin or of a special sense.
Hypochondrical (hi-po-kon'-dri-kal). Affected with hypochondriasis, morbid anxiety about the health.
Hymen (hi'men). The fold of mucous membrane that partially occludes the vaginal orifice.
Hypnotic (hip-not'-ik). Inducing sleep.

Hypertrophy (hi-per'tro-fe). An increase in the size of a tissue or organ independent of the general growth of the body.
Hypodermic (hi-po-der'mik). Applied or administered beneath the skin.
Hypogastrium (hi-po-gas'treum). The lower median anterior region of the abdomen.
Hysterical (his-ter'ikal). Pertaining to or affected by hysteria.
Ichor (ikor). An acrid thin puriform discharge. [transcriber's note: pus]
Idiopathic (id-eo-path'ik). Not dependent upon another disease or upon a known or recognized cause.
Idiosyncrasy (id-eo-sin'kras-e). A habit or quality of body or mind peculiar to any individual.
Ileum (il'-e-um). The tower portion of the small intestine terminating in the cecum.
Ileus (il'-e-us). Severe colic due to intestinal obstruction.
Iliac (il'-e-ak). Pertaining to the ilium or to the flanks.
Iliac Region. One of the regions into which the abdomen is divided. Flank region.
Illuminant (il-lu'min-ant). That which aids in lighting up a part, cavity or organ for inspection.
Impotence (im'-po-tens). Lack of power. Especially of sexual power in the man.
Imbecility (im-bes-il'-it-e). Feebleness of mind, congenital or acquired.
Immersion (im-mer'shun). The plunging of the body into a liquid.
Inanition (in-an-ish'un). Emptiness; wasting of the body from starvation.
Incontinence (in-kon'tin-ens). Inability to restrain natural discharges like the urine, feces, etc.
Incubation (in-ku-ba'shun). The period between the implanting of an infectious disease and its manifestation.
Incisor (in-sis'-or). Any one of the four front teeth of either jaw.
Incubus (in'-ku-bus). A heavy mental burden.
Indigenous (in-dij'-en-us). Native; originating or belonging to a certain locality or country.
Indigestible (in-dij-es'tibl). Not susceptible of digestion.
Indisposition (in'-dis-po-zish'-un). Slight illness.
Induration (in-du-ra'shun). Hardening. The process of hardening.
Infection (in-fek'-shun). The communication of disease from one person to another, whether by effluvia or by contact, mediate or immediate.
Infiltration (in-fil-tra'-shun). The accumulation in a tissue of substances not normal to it.
Inflammation (in-flam-ma'shun). A morbid condition characterized by pain, heat, redness and swelling, etc.
Infusion (in-fu'shun). Steeping; to extract the active principles of substance by means of water, but without boiling.
Ingestion (in-gcs'-shun). The act of taking food, etc., into the body.
Inguinal (in'gwin-al). Pertaining to the groin.
Injection (in-jek'-shun). The act of throwing a liquid into a part, such as the rectum or a blood vessel.

Inoculation (in-ok-u-la'shun). The insertion of a virus into a wound or abrasion in the skin in order to communicate the disease.
Inspiration (in-spi-ra'shun). The act of drawing air into the lungs.
Inspissation (in-spis-sa'shun). To make thick by evaporation or absorption of fluid.
Integument (in-teg'um-ent). The covering of the body; the skin.
Intercostal (in-ter-kas'tal). Situated between the ribs.
Intermittent (in-ter-mit'-ent). Occurring at intervals.
Intestines (in-tes'-tins). The bowels.
Ischuria (is-ku're-ah). Suppression or retention of the urine.
Joint. An articulation between two bones; more especially one which admits of more or less motion in one or both bones.
Jugular (ju'gu-lar). Pertaining to the neck.
Labia (la'beah). Two folds of skin, etc., of the female genital organs; lips.
Labium (la'-bi-um). A lip or lip-shaped.
Lacerated (las'er-a-ted). Torn; of the nature of a rent.
Laceration (las-er-a'shun). The act of tearing; a wound made by tearing.
Lactation (lak-ta'shun). Suckling. The period of the secretion of milk.
Lachyrmal (lak'ri-mal). Pertaining to the tears or to the organs secreting and conveying tears.
Lacinating (la'sin-a-ting). Tearing; darting or sharply cutting.
Lacteal (lak'-te-al). Pertaining to milk
Larynx (lar'inx). The organ of the voice, situated between the base of the tongue and the trachea.
Larva (lar'-vah). The first stage of the insect development after leaving the egg and in which the organism resembles a worm.
Laxative (lak'-sat-iv). Mildly cathartic. Loosening.
Laryngoscope (lar-in'-go-skop). A mirror attached to a long handle for examining the interior of the larynx.
Laryngotomy (lar-in-got'ome). The operation of cutting into the larynx (incising the larynx).
Lesion (le'zhun). An injury, wound or morbid structural change.
Lethargy (lith-ar-gi). A condition of drowsiness or stupor that cannot be overcome by the will; also a hypnotic trance.
Leucorrhea (lu-kor-re'-ah). A white, muco-purulent discharge from the vagina and womb, popularly called "the whites."
Ligature (lig'-at-ur). A thread or wire for tying a vessel, etc.
Ligament (lig'-am-ent). Any tough fibrous band which connects bones or supports viscera (internal organs).
Linctus (link'-tus). A thick syrupy medicament to be taken by licking.
Liniment (lin'-im-ent). Any oily preparation to be rubbed upon the skin.
Lithontriptic (lith-on-trip'-tik). An agent that dissolves renal stones.
Lithotomy (lith-ot'o-me). The removal of a stone by cutting into the bladder (cystotomy).
Lithotrity (lith-ot'ri-te). The crushing of a calculus (stone) within the bladder by a lithotrite (instrument).
Livid (li'vid.) Discolored from the effects of congestion or contusion.
Lochia (lo'keah). The discharge from the vagina that takes place during the first week after child-birth.
Lumbago (lum-ba'go). Neuralgia of the loins.

Lumbar (lum'bar). Pertaining to the loins.
Lymph (limf). A transparent slightly yellow liquid of alkaline reaction which fills the lymphatic vessels.
Lymphatic (limfat'-ic). Pertaining to or containing lymph.
Maceration (mas-er-a'shun). The softening of a solid by soaking.
Macula (mak'-u-lah). A stain or spot; especially one upon the skin not elevated above the surface.
Malaria (mah-la'riah). A fever disease, now known to be caused by a blood parasite.
Malarial (mal-a'real). Pertaining or due to malaria.
Malformation (mal-for-ma'shun). Deformity. An abnormal development or formation of a part of the body.
Malignant (mal-ig'nant). Bad. Threatening life.
Malleolus (mal-le'o-lus). A hammer-headed process of bone.
Mania (ma'ne-ah). A variety of insanity characterized by wild excitement, hallucinations, delusions and violent tendencies.
Mamma (mam-mah). The breast. Mammary gland.
Marrow (mar'o). The fatty substance contained in the medullary canal of long bones and in the interstices of the cancellous bone.
Mastication (mas-tik-a'shun). The chewing of food.
Maturation (mat-u-ra'shun). The formation of pus.
Matrix (ma'trix). The womb. The groundwork in which anything is cast.
Meatus (me-a'tus). A passage or opening.
Medulla Oblongata (med-ul-lah oblong-at'-a). An organ or ganglion of the brain which connects the spinal cord with the pons.
Menses (men'sez). Monthly flow from the womb.
Menstrual (men'stru-al). Pertaining to menstruation.
Menstruum (men'stru-urn). A solvent.
Metastasis (met-as'tas-is). The transfer of a diseased process from a primary focus to a distance by the conveyance of the causal agents through the blood vessels or lymph channels, like mumps from face to the scrotum.
Metatarsus (met-ah-tar'-sus). The bones of the foot--situated between the (instep) tarsus and toes.
Miasm (mi'asm). Anything harmful contaminating the air.
Micturition (mik-tu-rish'-un). The act of passing urine.
Midwife (mid'wif). A female nurse who attends women in childbirth.
Minim (min'-im). About a drop.
Mitral valves (mit'ral). The valves that control the opening from the left auricle to the left ventricle.
Morbid (mor'bid). Pertaining to disease or diseased parts.
Morbific (mor-bif 'ik). Producing disease.
Morbus (mor'bus). Disease.
Mucous Membrane (mu'kus). A membrane that secretes mucus.
Mortification (mor-tif-ik-a'shun). See gangrene.
Mucilage (mu-cil'ij). A solution of gum in water.
Mucus (mu'kus). A viscid liquid.
Narcotic (nar-kot'-ik). A drug that produces stupor.
Nausea (naw'sheah). Sickness at the stomach with an inclination to vomit.
Navel (n-a'vet). The umbilicus.
Nauseant. (naw'she-ant). Nauseating; producing nausea.

Necrosis (nek-ro'sis). The death of cells surrounded by living tissue.
Nephritic (nef-rit'-ik). Pertaining to nephritis (inflammation of the kidneys).
Nervine (nur'-vin). Acting upon the nerves.
Neuralgia (nu-ral'-jeah). Severe pain along a nerve without any demonstrable structural changes in the nerve.
Neurasthenia (nu-ras-then-iah). A group of symptoms resulting from debility or exhaustion of the nerve centers.
Nocturnal (nok'-tur-nal). Pertaining to the night.
Node (nod). A knob. Protuberance.
Normal (nor'-mal). Conforming to natural law or order.
Nostalgia (nos-tal'-je-ah). Homesickness.
Nostrum (nos'trum). A quack; secret medicine.
Nutritious (nu'trish'us). Nourishing.
Obtuse (ob-tus'). Dull.
Obesity (obes'it-e). An excessive development of fat.
Oedema (e-de'mah). An infiltration of serum in a part; watery swelling.
Obstetrics (ob-stet'-riks). Care of women during pregnancy, confinement and after.
Occipital (ok-sip'it-al). Pertaining to the back part of the head (occiput).
Olfactory Nerves (ol-fak'-to-re). Nerves of smell.
Omentum (o-men'tum). An apron. A fold of the peritoneum connecting the abdominal organs with the stomach.
Ophthalmia (off-thal'-meah). Inflammation of the eye.
Opiates (o'-pe-ats). A preparation of opium.
Optic (op'tik). Pertaining to vision or to the science of optics.
Optic nerve. Nerve of sight.
Orthopnea (or-thop-ne'ah). A condition marked by quick and labored breathing and relief is only had by remaining in an upright position.
Ossific (os-if '-ik). Producing bone.
Ossification (os'if-ik-a'shun). The formation of bone.
Ovary (o'var-e). One of a pair of glandular organs giving rise to ova (eggs).
Ovariotomy (o-va-re-ot'-o-me). Removal of an ovary.
Ovum (o'vum). An egg; the reproductive cell of an animal or vegetable.
Oxygen (oks'e-gen). A colorless, tasteless, odorless gas.
Palate (pal'-at). The roof of the mouth.
Palpitation (pal-pit-a'shun). A fluttering or throbbing, especially of the heart, of which a person is conscious.
Palliative (pal'-e-a-tiv). An agent that relieves or soothes the symptom of a disease without curing it.
Panacea (pan-a-se'ah). A cure-all.
Papilla (pap-il'-ah). A small nipple-like eminence.
Paracentesis (par'-ah-sen-te'-sis). Puncture of the wall of a cavity of the body, such as the chest, drum membrane, etc.
Paralytic (par-ah-lit'ik), Affected with paralysis.
Paralysis (par-al'-is-is). "Palsy." A loss of motion or of sensation in a part.
Paraplegia (par-ah-ple'jeah). Paralysis of the lower half of the body or of the lower extremities.
Parasite (par'ah-sit). An animal or vegetable living upon or within another organism, termed the host.

Paroxysm (par'oks-izm). The periodic increase or crisis in the progress of a disease.
Patella (pat-el'-ah). The knee cap.
Pathology (path-ol'-oje). The branch of medical science that treats of the modifications of functions and changes of structures caused by disease.
Pathognomonic (path-og-no-mon'ik). Characterized by a disease distinguishing it from other diseases.
Parturient (par-tu're-ent). Giving birth; being in labor.
Parturition (par-tu-rish'-un). The act of giving birth to young.
Pediculus (pe-dik'-u-lus). The louse.
Pelvis (pel'-vis). A basin or basin-shaped cavity. The bony ring formed by sacrum and coccyx and innominate bones.
Pepsin (pep'-sin). A ferment found in the gastric juice, and capable of digesting proteids in the presence of an acid.
Percussion (per-kush'-in). Striking upon a part to ascertain the condition of the underlying organs.
Pericardium (per-e-kar'de-um). The closed membranous sac enveloping the heart.
Pericarditis (per-e-kar'-di-tis). Inflammation of the pericardium.
Perineum (per-e-ne'um). That portion of the body included in the outlet of the pelvis, bounded in front by the pubic arch, behind by the coccyx, and ligaments and on the sides by the projections of the ichium.
Periodicity (pcr-e-o-dis'ite). Recurrence at regular intervals.
Periosteum (per-e-os'teum). Covering of parts of the bone except where the tendons and ligaments are attached to the joint surfaces.
Peristaltic (per-e-stal'tik). Pertaining to peristalsis, an wave-like motion seen in the tubes, like bowels, etc.
Perflation (per-fla-shun). To blow through.
Petechia (pet-e-keah). A small spot beneath the epidermis due to an effusion of blood.
Permeate (per'me-at). Passing throughout.
Permeable (per'me-able). Capable of affording passage.
Phagedenic (fag-ed-en'ick). Relating to phagedena, a rapidly spreading destructive ulceration of soft tissues.
Phalanges (fa-lan'ges). Plural of phalanx. Bones of the fingers or toes.
Pharynx (far'-inx), The throat.
Phlegmatic (fleg-mat'-ik). Indifferent, apathetic.
Phlebotomy (fleb-ot'o-me). Opening of a vein for blood letting.
Phlegmon (fleg'mun). An inflammation characterized by the spreading of a purulent or fibro-purulent exudate within the tissues.
Phthysical (tiz'ik-al). Pertaining to consumption (phthisis).
Physiognomy (fiz-e-og'no-me). The countenance.
Plethoric (pleth'o-rik). A state characterized by an excess of blood in the vessels and marked by a reddish color of the face, full pulse, etc.
Pleura (plu'rah). The serous membrane enveloping the lung and lining the inner surface of the chest cavity.
Pleurisy (plu'rise-e). Inflammation of the pleura (pleuritis).
Plexus (plex-us). A network, especially an aggregation of vessels or nerves

forming an intricate network.
Polypus (pol'e-pus). A tumor having a pedicle, found especially on mucous membranes, as in the nose, etc.
Pregnancy (preg'nan-se). Woman with child; state of being pregnant.
Prescription (pre-skrip-shun). A formula written by a doctor to the druggist, designating substances to be administered.
Post-mortem (post-mor'tem). An examination of a body after death.
Potable (po'ta-bl). Drinkable.
Prognosis (prag-no'sis). A judgment in advance concerning the duration, course and termination of a disease.
Prophylactic (pro-fil-ak'tik). An agent that prevents the development of disease.
Prolapsus (pro-lap'sus). Falling downward.
Pruritus (pru-ri'tus). Intense itching.
Pseudo (sudo). A prefix meaning false.
Ptyalism (ti'-al-izm). Salivation.
Puberty (pu'ber-te). The period at which generative organs become capable of exercising the function of reproduction.
Purperal (pu-ur'per-al). Pertaining to, caused by, or following childbirth.
Pulmonary (pul'mon-are). Pertaining to the lungs.
Pulmonitis (pul-mon'itis). Inflammation of the lungs. Better term is pneumonia.
Pulp. The soft part of fruit.
Pungent (pun'jent). Acrid, penetrating, producing a painful of prickling sensation.
Purgative (pur'ga-tiv). A drug producing copious discharges from the bowels.
Purulent (pu'rul-ent). Having the character of or containing pus.
Pus (pus). A liquid inflammation product made up of cells (leukocytes) and a thin fluid called liquor pures.
Pustules (pus'tuls). Small circumscribed elevations of the skin containing pus.
Putrid (pu'trid). Rotten.
Putrefaction (putre-fak'shun). The decomposition of animal or vegetable matters effected largely by the agency of nucro-production of various solid, liquid and gaseous matters.
Pylorus (pi-lo'rus). The circular opening of the stomach into the duodenum.
Pyrosis (pir'os-is). Heartburn; a burning sensation in the gullet and stomach with sour eructation, due to acid dyspepsia.
Rectum (rek'tum). The lower part of the bowel (of the large intestine).
Recurrent (re'kur'ent). Returning.
Refrigerant (re-frig'er-ant). Coating, lessening fever.
Regimen (rej'im-en). The systematic regulation of the diet and habits for some special purpose.
Regurgitate (re-gur-je'-tat). Flowing back or against a normal direction.
Resolution (rez-o-lu'shun). The return of a part to a normal state after a pathologic (disease) process.
Resolvents (rez-ol'vent). An agent that causes resolution.
Respiration (res-pir-a'shun). The act or function of breathing; the act by which air is drawn in and expelled from the lungs, including inspiration and expiration.

Restorative (res-tor'a-tiv). Prompting a return to health or consciousness.
Resuscitation (re-sus-sit-a'shun). The bringing back to life of one apparently dead.
Retina (ret'in-ah). The delicate innermost tunic and perceptive structure of the eye, formed by the expansion of the optic nerve and covering the back part of the eye as far as the "ora serrata."
Revulsion (re-vul'shun). The diverting of disease from one part to another by the sudden withdrawal of the blood from the part.
Rheum (rum). Any watery or catarrhal discharge.
Rubefacient (ru-be-fa'shent). An agent that reddens the skin.
Rigor (rigor). The rigidity or stiffening which follows after death, due to congestion of the "muscle plasm."
Saccharine (sak'kar-in). Sugary; of a sweet taste.
Salvia (sal've-ah). Sage.
Salutary (sal'u-ta-re). Favorable to the preservation and restoration of health.
Sanative (san'at-iv). Promoting health; health.
Sanies (sa'ne-ez). A fetid, ichorous discharge from a wound or ulcer, containing serum, pus and blood.
Scab (scab). The crust of a superficial sore.
Sanitary (san'it-are). Promoting or pertaining to health.
Sanitation (san-it-a'shun). The establishment of conditions favorable to health.
Sanguine (sang-gwine). Abounding in blood. Ardent; hopeful.
Scarf-skin (scarf-skin). The epidermis.
Scirrhus (skir'rus). A hard cancer.
Sciatic (si-at'ik). Pertaining to the ischium (bone).
Scorbutic (skor-bu'tik). Pertaining to or affected by scurvy.
Scrotum (skro'tum). The pouch which contains the testicles and their accessory organs.
Scrofulous (skrof 'u-lous). Affected with or of the nature of scrofula.
Sebaceous (se-ba'shus). Pertaining to sebum or suet.
Sedative (sed'at-iv). A remedy that allays excitement.
Sedentary (sed'en-ta-re). Sitting habitually; of inactive habits.
Seminal (sem'in-al). Pertaining to seed or semen.
Serum (se'rum). The clear portion of any animal liquid separated from its more solid elements; especially the clear liquid which separates in the clotting of blood from the clot and the corpuscles.
Serous (si'rus). Pertaining to or resembling serum.
Semiflexion (sem-e-flek'shun). The position of a limb midway between bending and extension.
Senile (se'nil). Of or pertaining to old age.
Septic (sep'tik). Produced by or due to putrefaction.
Sialagogues (si-al'-ag-og). An agent that produces a flow of saliva.
Sinapism (sin'ap-izm). A mustard plaster.
Sinew (sin'yu). The tendon of a muscle.
Slough (sluf). A mass of dead tissue in or cast out from living tissue.
Sewerage (su'er-ej). Drainage.
Solution (so'lu'shun). A liquid containing dissolved matter.
Solvent (sol'vent). Capable of dissolving.
Sordes (sor'dez). The dark brown foul matter which collects on the lips and teeth

in low fevers (typhoid, etc.).
Spasm (spazm). A sudden, violent, involuntary rigid contraction due to muscular contraction.
Speculum (spek'u-Ium). An instrument for dilating the opening of a passage or cavity of the body to view the interior.
Specific (spe-sif 'ik). A remedy especially indicated for any particular disease.
Sphincter (sfingk'ter). A ring-like muscle which closes a natural orifice.
Spinal Cord (spi'nal). The cord-like structure contained in the spinal canal.
Spleen (spleen). One of the so-called ductless glands.
Sporadic (spo-rad'ik). Occurring here and there, scattered.
Squamous (skwa'-mus). Scaly or plate-like.
Stertorous (ster'torus). Snoring. breathing.
Sternum (ster'num). Breast bone.
Stertor (ster'tor). Snoring or sonorous breathing, especially that of sleep or of coma.
Stethoscope (steth'o-skop). An instrument for ascertaining the condition of the organs of circulation and respiration.
Stimulant (stim'u-lant). Producing stimulation. Increasing the heart's action.
Stool (stool). The fecal discharge from the bowel.
Stomachic (stom'ak-ik). Pertaining to the stomach.
Strangury (stran-ju-re). Slow and painful discharge of the urine.
Stricture (strik-tur). Abnormal narrowing of a canal, duct or passage.
Strumous (stru'mus). Scrofulous.
Struma (stru'mah). Scrofula.
Stupor (stu-por). Partial or nearly complete unconsciousness.
Styptic (stip-tik). Astringent. To arrest hemorrhage by means of astringent quality.
Subcutaneous (sub-ku-ta'neus). Beneath the skin.
Submaxillary (sub-max'il-la-ri). Situated beneath the jaw.
Sudor (su'dor). Sweat or perspiration.
Sudorifics (sudor-if-iks). Sweaters.
Suppurate (sup'pu-rat). To produce pus.
Suture (su'tur). A surgical stitch or seam; an unmovable joint.
Symptom (simp'tom). Any evidence of disease or of a patient's condition.
Synocha (sin'-o-kah). A continued fever.
Syncope (sin'-co-pe). A swoon, fainting, or a faint. Sudden failure more or less of the heart's action.
Syphilis (sif'i1-is). A venereal disease (pox).
Syringe (sir'inj). All instrument for injecting liquids into any vessel or cavity.
Tepid (tep'id). Luke warm.
Tetanic (tet'an-ik). Pertaining to or of the nature of tetanus.
Tertian (tur'shan). Recurring every third day.
Tetanus (tet'an-us). An acute disease due to the bacillus tetani, in which there is a state of more or less persistent tonic spasm of some of the voluntary muscles.
Tibia (tib'eah). The inner bone of the leg (below the knee).
Therapeutics (ther-ap-u'tiks). The science and art of healing.
Thorax (tho'raks). The chest.
Testicles (tes'tik-kl). The two glands which produce semen.
Tendon (ten'don). A band of dense fibrous tissue forming the termination of a

muscle and attaching the latter to a bone.
Tense (tens). Stretched.
Tension (ten'shun). The act of stretching.
Tincture (tink'tur). A solution of the medicine principle of a substance in a fluid other than water or glycerol.
Tonsils (ton'sils). Small almond-shaped masses between the pillars of the fauces on either side.
Torpid (tor'pid). Not acting with normal vigor and facility.
Torpor (tor'por). Sluggishness.
Tormina (tor'minah). Griping pains in the bowels.
Trachea (tra-ke-ah). The wind-pipe.
Tracheotomy (trake-ot'o-me.) The formation of an artificial opening into the trachea, cutting into the trachea.
Transpiration (tran-spi-ra'shun). The discharge of air, sweat or vapor through the skin.
Tubercles (tu'ber-kl). Any mass of small, rounded nodules produced by the bacillus of tuberculosis.
Transudation (trans'-u-da'tion). The passing of liquid through a membrane.
Tumefaction (tu-me-fak'-shun). A swelling. Puffiness.
Tumor (tu'mor). Morbid enlargement.
Tympanum (tim'pa-num). The middle ear.
Typhoid (ti'foid). Resembling typhus.
Typhus (ti'-fus). A contagious fever characterized by a petechial (spotted) eruption, high fever and great prostration.
Ulcer (ul'-ser). An open sore other than a wound.
Ulna (ul'nah). A bone of the forearm on the side opposite that of the thumb.
Urea (u-re'ah). A white, crystallizable substance from the urine, blood and lymph.
Ureter (u-re'-ter). The tube that conveys the urine from the kidney to the bladder.
Urethra (u-re'thra). A membranous canal extending from the bladder to the surface.
Urine (u'rin). The fluid secreted by the kidneys, stored in the bladder and discharged through the urethra.
Uric Acid (u'rik a'sid). One of the nitrogenous end products of metabolism, found in the urine and spleen.
Uterus (u'ter-us). The womb.
Uvula (u'vu-lah). The pendulum (tip) of the soft palate.
Vaccine (vak'sin). The virus used in vaccinating.
Variolus (va-ri'o-lus). Pertaining to or of the nature of smallpox.
Varicose (var'ik-os). Swollen, knotted and tortuous blood vessels.
Vagina (vaj-i'-nah). A sheath. The canal from the slit of the vulva.
Vaginismus (vaj-in-iz'-mus). Painful spasm of the vagina due to local oversensitiveness.
Valetudinarian (val'e-tu-din-a-re-an). A person of infirm or feeble habit of body.
Vascular (vas'ku-lar). Pertaining to or full of vessels.
Venery (ven'er-e). Sexual intercourse.

Venous (ve'nus). Of or pertaining to the veins.
Venesection (ven-a-sek'shun). The opening of a vein for the purpose of bleeding.
Ventilation (ven-til'a-shun). The act or process of supplying fresh air.
Vermifuge (ver'mif-uj). Having the power to expel worms.
Ventral (ven'-tral). Pertaining to the belly side.
Ventricle (ven'trik-l). Any small cavity.
Vertebra (ver'te-brah). Anyone of the thirty-three bones of the spinal column.
Vertigo (ver'tig-o). Giddiness; dizziness.
Virulent (vir'u-lent). Exceedingly noxious or deleterious.

Virus (vi'rus). Any animal poison; especially one produced by and capable of transmitting a disease.

Viscus (vis'-kus). Pl.-Viscera (vis'-er-a). Any large interior organ in either of two great cavities of the body, especially the abdomen.

Vesiccant (vis'ik-ant). Causing blisters.

Vesication (ves-ik-a'shun). The process of blistering.

Vesicle (ves'ik-al). A small sac containing fluid.

Veterinary (vet'-er-in-a-re). Pertaining to domestic animals and their diseases.

Vitreous Humor (vit'-re-us yu'-mor). The transparent jelly-like substance filling the posterior chamber of the eye.

Volatile (vol'-at-il). Tending to evaporate rapidly.

Vulnery (vul-ne-ra-re). Pertaining to or healing wounds.

Vulva (vul'-vah). The external fleshy part of the female organs of generation.

Whites (whitz). Leucorrhea or leukorrhea.

Zymotic (zi'mot'ik). Caused by or pertaining to zymosis.

Zymosis (zi-mo'sis). Fermentation. The propagation and development of an infectious disease known by the growth of bacteria and their products. Any infectious or contagious disease.

MEDICAL INDEX

INCLUDING PAGES 1 TO 728

INDEX TO MANNERS AND SOCIAL CUSTOMS

INCLUDING PAGES 730, TO 841

MISCELLANEOUS INDEX

PAGES 841 TO 970

Including Chapters on "Beauty and the Toilet," "Nursery Hints and Fireside Gems," "Domestic Science," "Canning and Pickling," "Candy" "General Miscellaneous" and "Glossary"

Black Beauty, Young Folks' Edition - abridged with original Illustrations
Anna Sewell
Benediction Classics, 2011
112 pages
ISBN: 978-1-84902-394-8

Available from www.amazon.com, www.amazon.co.uk

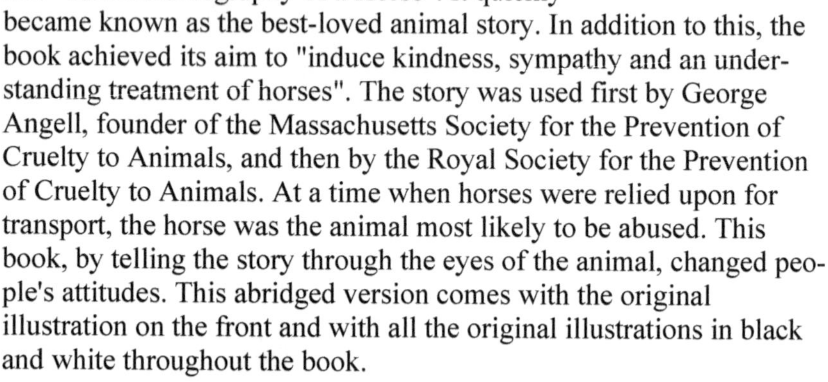

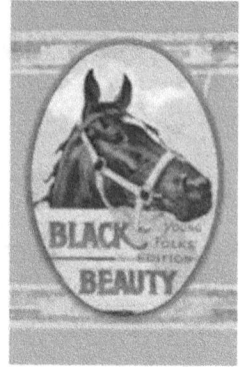

Black Beauty was written in 1877 and was subtitled "The Autobiography of a Horse". It quickly became known as the best-loved animal story. In addition to this, the book achieved its aim to "induce kindness, sympathy and an understanding treatment of horses". The story was used first by George Angell, founder of the Massachusetts Society for the Prevention of Cruelty to Animals, and then by the Royal Society for the Prevention of Cruelty to Animals. At a time when horses were relied upon for transport, the horse was the animal most likely to be abused. This book, by telling the story through the eyes of the animal, changed people's attitudes. This abridged version comes with the original illustration on the front and with all the original illustrations in black and white throughout the book.

Hurlbut's Story of the Bible
Unabridged and fully illustrated in BW
Jesse Lyman Hurlbut
Benediction Classics, 2011
976 pages
Size 11 x 8.5 inches
ISBN: 978-1849024556

Available from www.amazon.com, www.amazon.co.uk

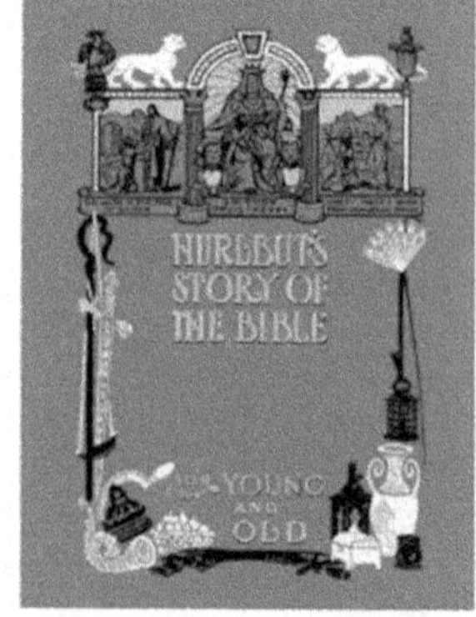

In the tradition of parents telling their children stories from the Bible, this new edition of a delightful book presents a continuous narrative of the Scriptures that brings the great heroes and events from the Bible to life. It is unabridged and features 168 stories from the Old and New Testaments, copious BW illustrations, a presentation page and a retouched version of the 1904 cover. Since it was written in 1904 by an American Methodist Episcopal Clergyman, Jesse Lyman Hurlbut, over 4 million copies have been distributed.

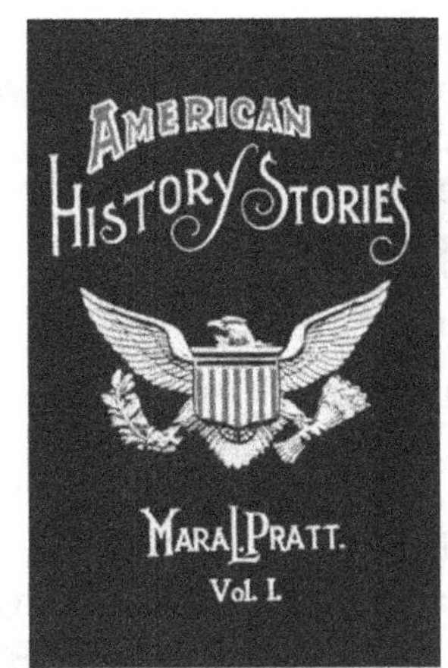

American History Stories Volumes I-IV

Mara L. Pratt

Benediction Classics,2011

Each c200 pages

ISBN:

Vol I 978-1-84902-412-9

Vol II 978-1-84902-410-5

Vol III 978-1-84902-409-9

Vol IV 978-1-84902-407-5

Available from www.amazon.com, www.amazon.co.uk

History is brought to life in these four volumes of Mara L. Pratt's retelling of the history of America, first published in 1891. The recommended reading age is 8-12, and the chapters are short with black and white illustrations, providing a wonderful introduction for children to American history. They are so compelling that adults will enjoy them as much as the children.

The first volume begins with the story from Long Ago and ends with how the colonies great together.

The second volume tells tales of the Revolutionary times, including the reasons for the American Revolution, the courage of those defending liberty, the early battles and the heroes who led the colonists to victory.

The third volume covers the period from the end or the Revolutionary War to the middle of the 19th Century. The chapters cover the Washington and Jefferson administrations, the War of 1812 and some Indian Wars, as well as a series of fascinating well-known characters of the period.

The final volume covers the period of great conflict from Lincoln becoming president and the southern states seceding until the end of the civil war.

Also from Benediction Books ...

Wandering Between Two Worlds: Essays on Faith and Art
Anita Mathias
Benediction Books, 2007
152 pages
ISBN: 0955373700

Available from www.amazon.com, www.amazon.co.uk

In these wide-ranging lyrical essays, Anita Mathias writes, in lush, lovely prose, of her naughty Catholic childhood in Jamshedpur, India; her large, eccentric family in Mangalore, a sea-coast town converted by the Portuguese in the sixteenth century; her rebellion and atheism as a teenager in her Himalayan boarding school, run by German missionary nuns, St. Mary's Convent, Nainital; and her abrupt religious conversion after which she entered Mother Teresa's convent in Calcutta as a novice. Later rich, elegant essays explore the dualities of her life as a writer, mother, and Christian in the United States-- Domesticity and Art, Writing and Prayer, and the experience of being "an alien and stranger" as an immigrant in America, sensing the need for roots.

About the Author

Anita Mathias is the author of *Wandering Between Two Worlds: Essays on Faith and Art*. She has a B.A. and M.A. in English from Somerville College, Oxford University, and an M.A. in Creative Writing from the Ohio State University, USA. Anita won a National Endowment of the Arts fellowship in Creative Nonfiction in 1997. She lives in Oxford, England with her husband, Roy, and her daughters, Zoe and Irene.

Anita's website:
http://www.anitamathias.com, and
Anita's blog Dreaming Beneath the Spires:
http://dreamingbeneaththespires.blogspot.com

The Church That Had Too Much
Anita Mathias
Benediction Books, 2010
52 pages
ISBN: 9781849026567

Available from www.amazon.com, www.amazon.co.uk

The Church That Had Too Much was very well-intentioned. She wanted to love God, she wanted to love people, but she was both hampered by her muchness and the abundance of her possessions, and beset by ambition, power struggles and snobbery. Read about the surprising way The Church That Had Too Much began to resolve her problems in this deceptively simple and enchanting fable.

About the Author

Anita Mathias is the author of *Wandering Between Two Worlds: Essays on Faith and Art*. She has a B.A. and M.A. in English from Somerville College, Oxford University, and an M.A. in Creative Writing from the Ohio State University, USA. Anita won a National Endowment of the Arts fellowship in Creative Nonfiction in 1997. She lives in Oxford, England with her husband, Roy, and her daughters, Zoe and Irene.

Anita's website:
    http://www.anitamathias.com, and
Anita's blog Dreaming Beneath the Spires:
    http://dreamingbeneaththespires.blogspot.com

www.ingramcontent.com/pod-product-compliance
Lightning Source LLC
Chambersburg PA
CBHW071350290326
41932CB00045B/1269

* 9 7 8 1 8 4 9 0 2 2 8 0 4 *